T0192560

Nutrition and Cardiometabolic Health

Nutrition and Cardiometabolic Health

Edited by
Nathalie Bergeron, Patty W. Siri-Tarino, George A. Bray,
and Ronald M. Krauss

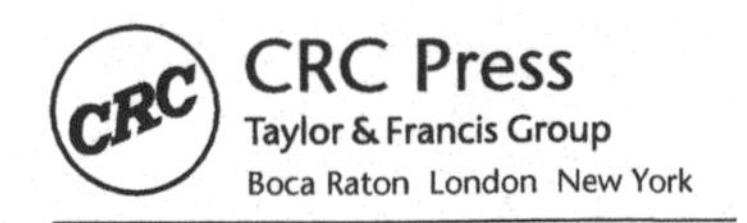

CRC Press is an imprint of the
Taylor & Francis Group, an **informa** business

CRC Press
Taylor & Francis Group
6000 Broken Sound Parkway NW, Suite 300
Boca Raton, FL 33487-2742

First issued in paperback 2021

ISBN 13: 978-1-03-209613-1 (pbk)
ISBN 13: 978-1-4987-0426-7 (hbk)

Publisher's Note
The publisher has gone to great lengths to ensure the quality of this reprint but points out that some imperfections in the original copies may be apparent.

Library of Congress Cataloging-in-Publication Data

Names: Bergeron, Nathalie, editor. | Siri-Tarino, Patty W., editor. | Bray, George A., editor. | Krauss, Ronald M., editor.
Title: Nutrition and cardiometabolic health / [edited by] Nathalie Bergeron, Patty W. Siri-Tarino, George A. Bray, and Ronald M. Krauss.
Description: Boca Raton : Taylor & Francis, 2017. | Includes bibliographical references.
Identifiers: LCCN 2017020806 | ISBN 9781498704267 (hardback : alk. paper)
Subjects: | MESH: Obesity, Metabolically Benign--diet therapy | Cardiovascular Diseases--prevention & control | Risk Factors | Nutrition Therapy—methods
Classification: LCC RC628 | NLM WD 210 | DDC 616.3/980654--dc23
LC record available at https://lccn.loc.gov/2017020806

Visit the Taylor & Francis Web site at
http://www.taylorandfrancis.com

and the CRC Press Web site at
http://www.crcpress.com

Contents

SECTION II Dietary Fats and Cardiometabolic Health

SECTION III Dietary Carbohydrates and Cardiometabolic Health

SECTION IV Dietary Protein and Cardiometabolic Health

SECTION V Dietary Food Groups, Patterns, and Cardiometabolic Health

SECTION VI Other Nutritional Influences of Cardiometabolic Health

Preface

Nutrition is the major environmental influence on metabolic systems that impact cardiovascular health and disease. Past decades have seen major advances in the identification of specific dietary effects on these systems. However, as this knowledge has grown, and the tools for studying these effects have become more diverse and powerful, there has been growing appreciation of the complexities and challenges facing those seeking to gain an in-depth yet comprehensive understanding of dietary effects on cardiometabolic health. Intensifying this concern is the imperative of addressing the global increase in the incidence of cardiovascular disease, coupled with the diet-related metabolic conditions—dyslipidemia, diabetes, and obesity—that play key roles in its pathogenesis. In preparing this textbook, we have called on the expertise of scientists across a broad range of topics and disciplines to assemble information aimed at researchers, clinicians, and other health professionals who have interests in this important field.

The chapters in the first section of the textbook are clustered around the theme of energy balance and adiposity as they relate to cardiometabolic health. An overview of the regulatory mechanisms that determine energy balance is provided in Chapter 1 followed by a chapter on the critical role of behavior in regulating eating (Chapter 2). The debate of whether "a calorie is a calorie" regardless of food source is addressed in the next two chapters (Chapters 3 and 4), along with methods for weight loss. Caloric restriction is addressed in Chapter 4 and bariatric surgery in Chapter 5. The benefits of physical activity on cardiometabolic health, with or without weight loss, are addressed in Chapter 6. The effects of diet on body fat distribution and the significance of the more metabolically active central versus peripheral adiposity are the topics for Chapter 7. This section concludes with Chapters 8 and 9 on nutritional considerations at different stages of the lifespan—in childhood and adolescence, and in the elderly.

Sections II through IV of the book are devoted to evaluating macronutrient effects on cardiometabolic health. In Section II on dietary fats, the effects of polyunsaturated fatty acids, specifically omega-3 and omega-6 fatty acids, are discussed in Chapter 10. The role of dietary saturated fats, along with the need to evaluate them in the context in which they are consumed, is reviewed in Chapter 11. The effects of *trans* fatty acids on blood lipids and cardiovascular disease risk, with consideration for industrially produced vs. ruminant *trans* fats, are discussed in Chapter 12, the third and final chapter of this section.

In Section III, Chapters 13 and 14 on dietary carbohydrates and cardiometabolic health pay particular attention to the role of sugar—consumed in quantities 40 times what was consumed at the time of the American Revolution in 1776. The quantity and quality of carbohydrates and the role of carbohydrate restriction in improving metabolic health are reviewed in Chapters 15 and 16.

Section IV's focus, dietary protein in relation to cardiometabolic health is covered in Chapters 17 through 19, with a focus on its role in energy balance, skeletal muscle function, and cardiovascular and diabetes risk.

A renewed interest and focus on whole foods and overall dietary patterns as a means toward cardiovascular health has led to the development of unique and validated methods of analysis as presented in Section V, Chapters 20 and 21. The two dietary patterns with the strongest evidence base for cardioprotective effects, namely, the Mediterranean and DASH diets, are reviewed in Chapters 22 and 23. Food groups that have been heavily touted and consumed include tree nuts and dairy foods, and the evidence for effects of these food groups on cardiometabolic health are reviewed in Chapters 24 and 25. The Section V concludes with Chapters 26 and 27 that present more debated approaches toward cardiometabolic health, including Paleolithic diets and intermittent fasting regimens.

In the last section of the textbook, Section VI, other nutritional factors impacting cardiometabolic health are considered. Chapter 28 focuses on the role of nutrition in modulating gene expression and epigenetics. Chapter 29 reviews gene–diet interactions that may contribute to interindividual differences in dietary needs and responses. An assessment of the role of the intestinal microbiome in modulating metabolic traits is provided in Chapter 30. Chapters 31 and 32, the final two chapters discuss alcohol and endocrine disruptors as diet-related influences on cardiometabolic health.

We are grateful to the individuals who contributed well-researched and incisive chapters to this textbook. It is our hope that the information assembled here will have value to those who share our goal of applying nutritional science to reducing the burden of cardiovascular disease.

Editors

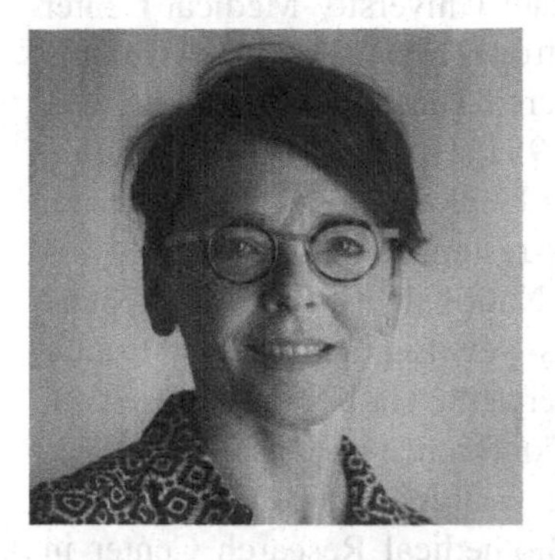

Nathalie Bergeron, PhD, is professor of biological sciences at Touro University California College of Pharmacy and associate staff scientist in the Atherosclerosis Research Program at Children's Hospital Oakland Research Institute. She was trained in dietetics and nutritional biochemistry and graduated from Laval University, Canada, with a PhD in nutrition. She pursued her postdoctoral training at the Cardiovascular Research Institute of the University of California, San Francisco, where she specialized in postprandial lipoprotein metabolism. Dr. Bergeron began her academic career as a research professor at Laval University in 1996. She was a visiting professor in the Department of Nutritional Sciences and Toxicology at the University of California, Berkeley, from 2000 to 2002 and joined the Touro University, California College of Pharmacy, at its inception in 2005. At Touro, Dr. Bergeron teaches in the areas of pathophysiology of metabolic diseases, as well as nutrition. She also holds a staff scientist position at the Children's Hospital Oakland Research Institute. Her research is clinical in nature and focuses on dietary composition, with a special emphasis on carbohydrate quantity and quality, and its relationship to features of atherogenic dyslipidemia. Her more recent research activities include looking at variations of the DASH and Mediterranean dietary patterns and their relationship to cardiometabolic health. Over the course of her academic career, she has received research grants from the Medical Research Council of Canada, the Heart and Stroke Foundation of Canada, the American Diabetes Association, and the National Institutes of Health, along with investigator-initiated funding from the Dairy Farmers of Canada, the Dairy Research Institute, and the Almond Board of California.

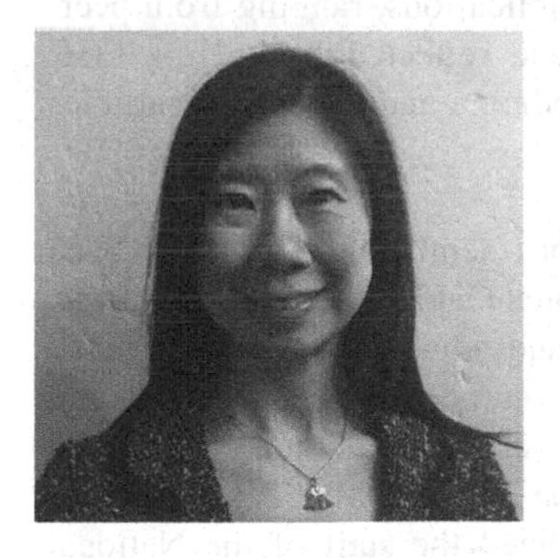

Patty W. Siri-Tarino, PhD, is an associate staff scientist in the Atherosclerosis Research Program and program director of the Family Heart & Nutrition Center at the Children's Hospital Oakland Research Institute. She earned her undergraduate degree in biology at Tufts University, a Master of Science in epidemiology at the Netherlands Institute of Health Sciences, and a PhD in nutrition and metabolic biology at Columbia University, where she developed a transgenic mouse model of insulin resistance, obesity, and dyslipidemia. Dr. Siri-Tarino began her postdoctoral work by developing and conducting studies in humans aimed at understanding variability in the postprandial response to high-fat meals and the role of cholesterol absorption inhibitors in its modulation. She subsequently worked on dietary intervention studies evaluating macronutrient effects on CVD risk profiles in the context of weight loss and stability as well as studies evaluating genetic effects on energy metabolism at rest and during exercise. Dr. Siri-Tarino has spoken nationally and internationally on the role of diet on lipoprotein profiles as biomarkers of cardiovascular disease and published peer-reviewed journal articles, reviews, book chapters, and popular media articles on diet, lifestyle, and genetic determinants of heart health. She is interested in community engagement and education.

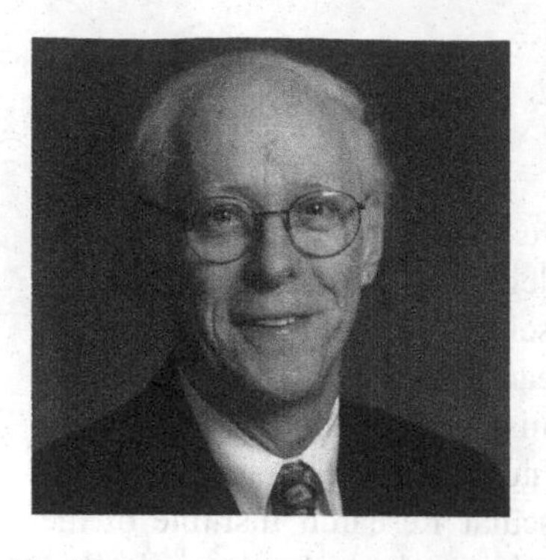

George A. Bray, MD, MACP, MACE, is a Boyd professor emeritus at the Pennington Biomedical Research Center of Louisiana State University in Baton Rouge, Louisiana, and professor of medicine emeritus at the Louisiana State University Medical Center in New Orleans. After graduating from Brown University summa cum laude in 1953, Dr. Bray entered Harvard Medical School, graduating magna cum laude in 1957. His postdoctoral training included an internship at the Johns Hopkins Hospital, Baltimore, Maryland, a fellowship at the NIH, residence at the University of Rochester, and fellowships at the National Institute for Medical Research in London and at the Tufts-New England Medical Center in Boston. In 1970, he became director of the Clinical Research Center at the Harbor UCLA Medical Center and the organizer of the First Fogarty International Center Conference on Obesity in 1973. Dr. Bray chaired the Second International Congress on Obesity in Washington, DC, in 1977. In 1989, he became the first executive director of the Pennington Biomedical Research Center in Baton Rouge, a post he held until 1999. He is a Master of the American College of Physicians, Master of the American College of Endocrinology, and Master of the American Board of Obesity Medicine. Dr. Bray founded the North American Association for the Study of Obesity in 1982 (now The Obesity Society), and he was the founding editor of its journal, *Obesity Research*, as well as cofounder of the *International Journal of Obesity* and the first editor of *Endocrine Practice*, the official journal of the American College of Endocrinologists. He has received many awards during his medical career, including the Johns Hopkins Society of Scholars Award, Honorary Fellow of the American Dietetic Association, the Bristol-Myers Squibb Mead-Johnson Award in Nutrition, the Joseph Goldberger Award from the American Medical Association, the McCollum Award from the American Society of Clinical Nutrition, the Osborne-Mendel Award from the American Society of Nutrition, the TOPS Award, the Weight Watchers Award, the Stunkard Lifetime Achievement Award, and the Presidential Medal from The Obesity Society. During his 50 academic years, he authored or coauthored more than 1900 publications, ranging from peer-reviewed articles and reviews to books, book chapters, and abstracts reflected in his Hirsch (H) Index of 89. Dr. Bray has had a long interest in the history of medicine and has written articles and a book on the history of obesity.

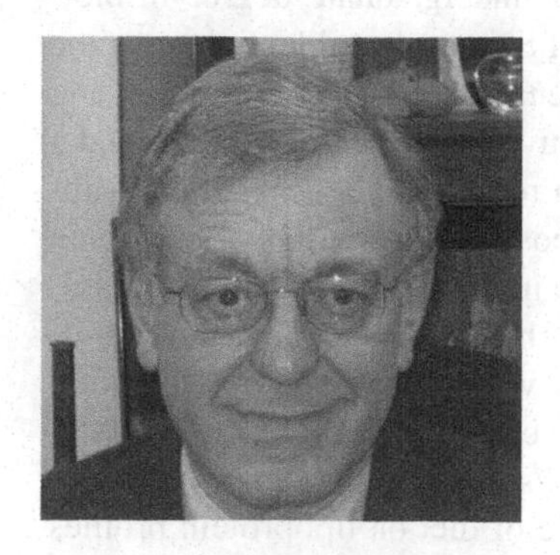

Ronald M. Krauss, MD, is senior scientist and Dorothy Jordan Endowed Chair at Children's Hospital Oakland Research Institute, professor of medicine at UCSF, and adjunct professor of nutritional sciences at UC Berkeley. He earned his undergraduate and medical degrees from Harvard University with honors and served his internship and residency in the Harvard Medical Service of Boston City Hospital. He then joined the staff of the National Heart, Lung, and Blood Institute in Bethesda, Maryland, first as clinical associate and then as senior investigator in the Molecular Disease Branch. Dr. Krauss is board certified in internal medicine, endocrinology, and metabolism, and is a member of the American Society for Clinical Investigation, a fellow of the American Society of Nutrition and the American Heart Association (AHA), and a distinguished fellow of the International Atherosclerosis Society. He has served on the U.S. National Cholesterol Education Program Expert Panel on Detection, Evaluation, and Treatment of High Blood Cholesterol in Adults; was the founding chair of the AHA Council on Nutrition, Physical Activity, and Metabolism; and is a national spokesperson for the AHA. He has also served on both the Committee on Dietary Recommended Intakes for Macronutrients and the Committee on Biomarkers of Chronic Disease of the Institute of Medicine of the National Academy of Sciences. He has received numerous awards, including the AHA Scientific

Councils Distinguished Achievement Award, the Centrum Center for Nutrition Science Award of the American Society for Nutrition, the Distinguished Leader in Insulin Resistance from the International Committee for Insulin Resistance, and the AHA Award of Meritorious Achievement. In addition, he has been the Robert I. Levy Lecturer of the AHA, the Edwin Bierman Lecturer for the American Diabetes Association, and the Margaret Albrink Lecturer at West Virginia University School of Medicine. Dr. Krauss is on the editorial boards of a number of journals and has been associate editor of *Obesity*, the *Journal of Lipid Research*, and the *Journal of Clinical Lipidology*. He has published nearly 500 research articles and reviews on genetic, dietary, and drug effects on plasma lipoproteins and coronary artery disease. Among his accomplishments is the identification of atherogenic dyslipidemia, a prevalent lipoprotein trait (high triglyceride, low HDL, and increase in small, dense LDL particles) that is associated with risk of cardiovascular disease and type 2 diabetes. In recent years, his work has focused on interactions of genes with dietary and drug treatments that affect metabolic phenotypes and cardiovascular disease risk.

Contributors

Brian J. Bennett
Western Human Nutrition Research Center
Agricultural Research Service
United States Department of Agriculture
Davis, California

Silvia Berciano
Faculty of Pharmacy
Universidad Autonoma de Madrid, Spain
Madrid, Spain

and

Jean Mayer USDA Human Nutrition Research Center on Aging
Tufts University
Boston, Massachusetts

Nathalie Bergeron
College of Pharmacy
Touro University California
Vallejo, California

and

Children's Hospital Oakland Research Institute
Oakland, California

Bruce Blumberg
Department of Developmental and Cell Biology
and
Department of Pharmaceutical Sciences
University of California, Irvine
Irvine, California

George A. Bray
Pennington Biomedical Research Center
Baton Rouge, Louisiana

and

Children's Hospital Oakland Research Institute
Oakland, California

Andrea M. Brennan
School of Kinesiology and Health Studies
Queen's University
Kingston, Ontario, Canada

Julie Brothers
Division of Cardiology
The Children's Hospital of Philadelphia
Philadelphia, Pennsylvania

Pedro Carrera-Bastos
Center for Primary Health Care Research
Lund University
Lund, Sweden

Elizabeth M. Cespedes Feliciano
Kaiser Permanente Northern California
Oakland, California

Raquel Chamorro-Garcia
Department of Developmental and Cell Biology
University of California, Irvine
Irvine, California

Catherine M. Champagne
Pennington Biomedical Research Center
Baton Rouge, Louisiana

Peter Clifton
Alliance for Research in Exercise, Nutrition and Activity (ARENA)
Sansom Institute for Health Science
School of Pharmacy and Medical Sciences
University of South Australia
Adelaide, South Australia, Australia

Stephen R. Daniels
Department of Pediatrics
University of Colorado School of Medicine
Aurora, Colorado

Michel de Lorgeril
Laboratoire Cœur et Nutrition
Faculté de Médecine
Grenoble, France

Lynda Frassetto
School of Medicine
University of California, San Francisco
San Francisco, California

Clint Gray
Liggins Institute and Gravida: National Centre for Growth and Development
University of Auckland
Auckland, New Zealand

Kevin D. Hall
National Institute of Diabetes and Digestive and Kidney Diseases
National Institutes of Health
Bethesda, Maryland

William S. Harris
Department of Internal Medicine
Sanford School of Medicine
University of South Dakota
and
OmegaQuant Analytics, LLC
Sioux Falls, South Dakota

Peter J. Havel
Department of Molecular Biosciences
School of Veterinary Medicine
and
Department of Nutrition
University of California, Davis
Davis, California

Frederick M. Hecht
Department of Medicine
University of California, San Francisco
San Francisco, California

Charlotte Holst
National Institute of Public Health
University of Southern Denmark
Copenhagen, Denmark

Frank B. Hu
Department of Nutrition
and
Department of Epidemiology
Harvard University School of Public Health
Boston, Massachusetts

Grace Marie Jones
College of Medicine
Touro University California
Vallejo, California

Sangeeta Kashyap
Department of Endocrinology, Diabetes and Metabolism
Cleveland Clinic
Cleveland, Ohio

Karim Kheniser
Department of Endocrinology, Diabetes and Metabolism
Cleveland Clinic
Cleveland, Ohio

Ronald M. Krauss
Children's Hospital Oakland Research Institute
Oakland, California

Penny Kris-Etherton
Department of Nutritional Sciences
The Pennsylvania State University
University Park, Pennsylvania

Sofia Laforest
School of Nutrition
Laval University
and
Quebec Heart and Lung Institute
Québec City, Québec, Canada

Benoît Lamarche
Institute of Nutrition and Functional Foods
School of Nutrition
Laval University
Québec City, Québec, Canada

Donald K. Layman
Department of Food Science and Human Nutrition
University of Illinois at Urbana-Champaign
Urbana, Illinois

Staffan Lindeberg
Center for Primary Health Care Research
Lund University
Lund, Sweden

Christina Link
Department of Nutritional Sciences
The Pennsylvania State University
University Park, Pennsylvania

Caitlin Lynch
Department of Nutritional Sciences
The Pennsylvania State University
State College, Pennsylvania

Geneviève B. Marchand
School of Nutrition
Laval University
and
Quebec Heart and Lung Institute
Québec City, Québec, Canada

Eveline A. Martens
Dutch Kidney Foundation
Bussum, the Netherlands

Ashley E. Mason
UCSF Department of Psychiatry
UCSF Osher Center for Integrative Medicine
San Francisco, California

Richard D. Mattes
Department of Nutrition Science
College of Health and Human Sciences
Purdue University
West Lafayette, Indiana

Ronald P. Mensink
Department of Human Biology
NUTRIM School of Nutrition and Translational Research in Metabolism
Maastricht University Medical Center
Maastricht, the Netherlands

Katie A. Meyer
Department of Nutrition
Nutrition Research Institute
University of North Carolina at Chapel Hill
Chapel Hill, North Carolina

Jasper Most
Division of Clinical Sciences
Pennington Biomedical Research Center
Baton Rouge, Louisiana

Kathleen Mulligan
College of Medicine
Touro University California
Vallejo, California

and

Department of Medicine
University of California, San Francisco
San Francisco, California

Jose M. Ordovas
IMDEA Alimentación
and
Centro Nacional de Investigaciones Cardiovasculares
Madrid, Spain

and

Jean Mayer USDA Human Nutrition Research Center on Aging
Tufts University
Boston, Massachusetts

Jennifer Panganiban
Division of Gastroenterology, Hepatology, and Nutrition
The Children's Hospital of Philadelphia
Philadelphia, Pennsylvania

Elizabeth Prout Parks
The Children's Hospital of Philadelphia
and
Perelman School of Medicine
The University of Pennsylvania
Philadelphia, Pennsylvania

Surya Panicker Rajeev
Institute of Ageing and Chronic Disease
University of Liverpool
and
Aintree University Hospital NHS Foundation Trust
Liverpool, United Kingdom

Leanne M. Redman
Division of Clinical Sciences
Pennington Biomedical Research Center
Baton Rouge, Louisiana

Clare M. Reynolds
Liggins Institute and Gravida: National Centre for Growth and Development
University of Auckland
Auckland, New Zealand

Robert Ross
School of Kinesiology and Health Studies
and
Division of Endocrinology and Metabolism
Department of Medicine
Queen's University
Kingston, Ontario, Canada

Jordi Salas-Salvadó
Hospital Universitari de Sant Joan de Reus
Universitat Rovira i Virgili
Reus, Spain

Jean-Marc Schwarz
College of Medicine
Touro University California
Vallejo, California

and

Department of Medicine
University of California, San Francisco
San Francisco, California

Ian W. Seetho
Institute of Ageing and Chronic Disease
University of Liverpool
and
Aintree University Hospital NHS Foundation Trust
Liverpool, United kingdom

Patty W. Siri-Tarino
Children's Hospital of Oakland Research Institute
Oakland, California

Kimber L. Stanhope
Department of Molecular Biosciences
School of Veterinary Medicine
and
Department of Nutrition
University of California, Davis
Davis, California

André Tchernof
School of Nutrition
Laval University
and
Quebec Heart and Lung Institute
Québec City, Québec, Canada

Alyssa Tindall
Department of Nutritional Sciences
The Pennsylvania State University
University Park, Pennsylvania

Janne Schurmann Tolstrup
National Institute of Public Health
University of Southern Denmark
Copenhagen, Denmark

John F. Trepanowski
Department of Kinesiology and Nutrition
University of Illinois, Chicago
Chicago, Illinois

Krista A. Varady
Department of Kinesiology and Nutrition
University of Illinois, Chicago
Chicago, Illinois

Mark H. Vickers
Liggins Institute and Gravida: National Centre for Growth and Development
University of Auckland
Auckland, New Zealand

Maelán Fontes Villalba
Center for Primary Health Care Research
Lund University
Lund, Sweden

Margriet S. Westerterp-Plantenga
Department of Human Biology
School of Nutrition and Translational Research in Metabolism
Maastricht University
Maastricht, the Netherlands

John P.H. Wilding
Institute of Ageing and Chronic Disease
University of Liverpool
and
Aintree University Hospital NHS Foundation Trust
Liverpool, United Kingdom

Edward Yu
Department of Nutrition
and
Department of Epidemiology
Harvard University School of Public Health
Boston, Massachusetts

Section I

Energy Balance, Adiposity, and Cardiometabolic Health

1 Regulation of Food Intake
The Gut–Brain Axis

Surya Panicker Rajeev, Ian W. Seetho, and John P.H. Wilding

CONTENTS

ABSTRACT

Regulation of food intake is a fundamental biological homeostatic process and is regulated at multiple levels. The process begins with sight, smell, and taste of food, the act of ingestion evoking either pleasurable or unpleasant sensations via these routes, which can themselves enhance, decrease, or even stop intake. Once food enters the gastrointestinal tract, it evokes a cascade of responses to its mechanical and chemical properties that have the function of coordinating orderly digestion, ensuring an appropriate metabolic fate for nutrients, and activating the process of satiation that ultimately leads to the end of the meal. This process of satiation involves signaling to the brain via neural, humoral, and hormonal signals from the gut. Brain signals are primarily detected in the brainstem and hypothalamus, which contain networks of neurons that are able to respond both to these messages and to important long-term signals of energy stores, most importantly the fat-derived hormone, leptin. These biological processes are also sensitive to and modulated by higher brain centers that are sensitive to hedonic signals, social context, and mood. Ultimately body weight is regulated by the net balance between intake and energy expenditure, the latter also being modifiable by many of the same neurotransmitter signals that influence food intake. The system seems biased toward weight gain, as a negative energy balance evokes a strong corrective response with a drive to increase intake and reduce expenditure; in contrast, the response to excess is weak and may be more easily overridden by hedonic and other higher centers. This may explain the difficulty many people have in maintaining a healthy weight.

INTRODUCTION

The mechanism of energy homeostasis is complex and influenced by various factors including nutrient availability and loss, hormone levels, genetic factors, and environmental stimuli. The system is also set in such a way to be more responsive to energy loss than gain [1], which poses a challenge in combating the obesity pandemic. The fundamental control of intake of energy/food starts with the sight, smell, and taste of food, the process of digestion in the gut, and finishes in the brain with physiological interactions at multiple levels.

The "gut–brain axis" describes the channels of communication between the gastrointestinal tract and the appetite control areas of the central nervous system (CNS). The gut responds to nutrients and mechanical stretch by generation of neural and hormonal signals to the brain with its homeostatic and hedonic regions. Apart from the gut and brain, adipose tissue and its hormones, notably leptin, play a major role in the regulation of appetite control and energy homeostasis.

The brain, through its hypothalamic nuclei as well as brainstem connections, plays an important part in regulating energy homeostatic mechanisms and hence is a potential target for drug therapy, although "off target" effects may limit this approach. The hypothalamus has orexigenic and anorexigenic neurons and can sense nutrient changes and alterations in the hormonal milieu including gut hormones. There are homeostatic and non-homeostatic systems involved in appetite control. While the former operate through the hypothalamus, brainstem, and gut, the non-homeostatic (environmental and hedonic) mechanisms influence food intake via the corticolimbic system.

The gastrointestinal (GI) system secretes various endocrine hormones and apart from exerting effects on several aspects of GI function, the gut sends neural and humoral signals to various brain regions, which are initially processed in the hypothalamus and brainstem. The gut–brain axis is the two-way interaction between the gut (through neural, nutrient, and hormonal factors) and the CNS (mainly in the hypothalamus and brainstem) and plays an important role in the maintenance of energy homeostasis by the human body. Short-term signals including gut hormones and neural pathways (vagal and spinal visceral afferents) moderate meal intake and satiation. Long-term humoral signals involved in the regulation of energy homeostasis include leptin, the adipose tissue hormone, and insulin, the pancreatic hormone.

CENTRAL NERVOUS SYSTEM REGULATION OF FOOD INTAKE

In this part of the chapter, we review the literature describing the role of the CNS in the control of food intake and show how this integrates peripheral signals from the gut and elsewhere to regulate energy homeostasis (Figure 1.1).

Brainstem Regulation

The CNS mediates energy balance in the body and is a key regulator of energy homeostasis. The brain receives signals from the gastrointestinal tract via both the nervous system and the circulation. Vagal afferents from the gut converge at the brainstem dorsal vagal complex (DVC), composed of the dorsal motor nucleus of the vagus, the area postrema, and nucleus of the tractus solitarius (NTS).

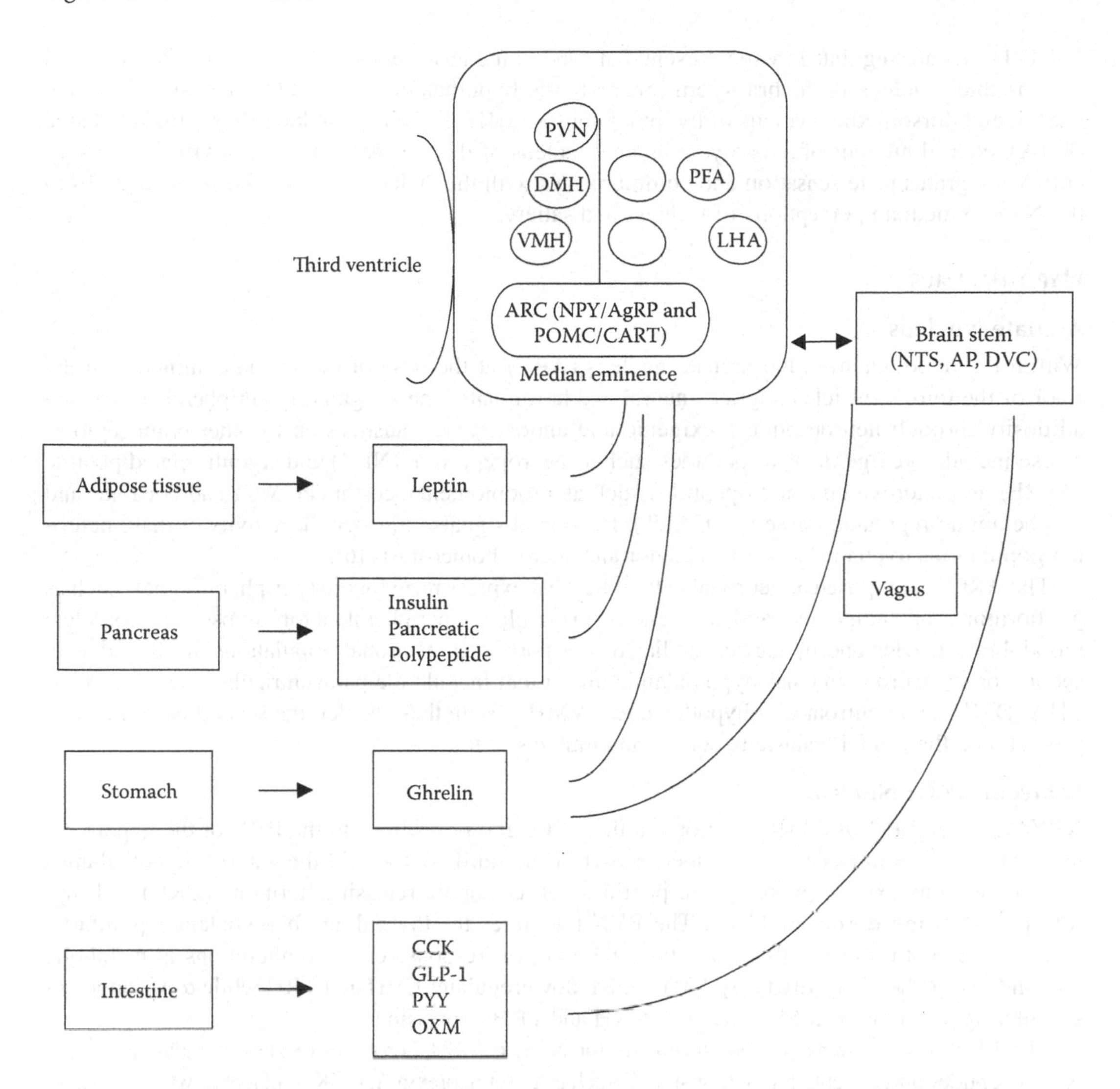

FIGURE 1.1 Links between the peripheral signals and central regulation of feeding. Numerous neural pathways transmit sensory information from the upper gastrointestinal viscera. Inputs are relayed to the NTS, AP, and DVC; signals from mechanical and chemical stimuli from the stomach and intestine initially via vagal afferents. Signals are relayed to the hypothalamus and appetite-regulating areas of the brain. ARC, arcuate nucleus; AgRP, agouti-related peptide; AP, area postrema; CART, cocaine- and amphetamine-regulated transcript; CCK, cholecystokinin; DMH, dorsomedial nucleus of hypothalamus; DVC, dorsal vagal complex; GLP-1, glucagon-like peptide 1; LHA, lateral hypothalamic area; NPY, neuropeptide Y; NTS, nucleus of tractus solitarius; OXM, oxyntomodulin; POMC, proopiomelanocortin; PP, pancreatic polypeptide; PVN, paraventricular nucleus; PYY, peptide YY; PFA, perifornical area; VMH, ventromedial hypothalamus.

The NTS is in close proximity to the area postrema with an incomplete blood–brain barrier and also responds to peripheral signals in the circulation as well as vagal afferents from the gastrointestinal tract [2]. The DVC subsequently projects to the hypothalamus and higher brain centers [3]. Leptin, insulin, and glucose-sensing receptors are expressed in the brainstem [3,4].

The NTS in the medulla receives afferent gustatory signals via vagal nerve stimulation (e.g., from mechanoreceptors detecting gastric distension and chemoreceptors detecting changes in nutrient composition and pH). The vagus also facilitates transmission of gut hormone signals such as cholecystokinin (CCK), ghrelin, pancreatic polypeptide (PP), and glucagon-like peptide-1

(GLP-1) that are regulated by the presence of food in the gastrointestinal tract [3,5]. The NTS and parabrachial nucleus in the brainstem innervate the hypothalamic paraventricular nuclei, arcuate nuclei, and dorsomedial nucleus of hypothalamus (DMH), as well as the lateral hypothalamic area (LHA), central nucleus of the amygdala, and nucleus of the stria terminalis. The visceral sensory cortex integrates taste sensation and communicates with the thalamus, which has projections from the NTS to mediate perceptions of fullness and satiety.

Hypothalamus

Arcuate Nucleus

Within the hypothalamus, the arcuate nucleus (ARC) at the base of the median eminence in the floor of the third ventricle integrates neural and hormonal signals regulating peripheral satiety and adiposity through neuropeptide orexigenic and anorexigenic transmission to other brain regions. These include orexigenic neuropeptides such as neuropeptide Y (NPY) and Agouti-related peptide (AgRP) and anorexigenic neuropeptides such as proopiomelanocortin (POMC) and cocaine- and amphetamine-regulated transcript (CART). Peripheral signals influence the activity of these neuronal populations to change feeding behavior and energy homeostasis [6].

The ARC is composed of neuronal cell bodies that express receptors for peripheral signals such as gut hormones and adipokines and is accessible to circulating peripheral factors across the incomplete blood–brain barrier and by carrier-mediated transport. ARC neuronal populations are linked with second-order neurons in other hypothalamic nuclei that include the paraventricular nucleus (PVN), LHA, DMH, and ventromedial hypothalamus (VMH). From these nuclei, the second-order neurons project onto the caudal brainstem, cortex, and limbic system.

Paraventricular Nucleus

NPY/AgRP and POMC/CART neurons in the ARC send projections to the PVN of the hypothalamus. The PVN is adjacent to the superior part of the third ventricle in the anterior hypothalamus and the neurons express anorexigenic peptides corticotrophin-releasing hormone (CRH) and thyrotropin-releasing hormone (TRH). The PVN integrates the thyroid and hypothalamic–pituitary–adrenal axes with nutritional signals, thus allowing for responsiveness to alterations in metabolic rate and sympathetic activity [7,8]. NPY/AgRP downregulates CRH and TRH while α-melanocyte-stimulating hormone (α-MSH) increases CRH and TRH expression.

The PVN also contains synaptic terminals for NPY, α-MSH, serotonin (5-HT), noradrenaline, and opioid peptides and appetite-regulating signals such as ghrelin, orexin A, CCK, and leptin, which can alter food intake and body weight [9]. The PVN may have an inhibitory role in food intake as hyperphagia is produced by central administration of NPY into the PVN and by destruction of the PVN [10]. The PVN has projections to the midbrain, prelocus coeruleus in dorsal pons, and NTS in the ventral medulla [3].

Lateral Hypothalamus

The LHA comprises populations of nuclei that receive projections from the ARC and express the orexigenic neuropeptides melanin-concentrating hormone (MCH) and orexin [3]. NPY neurons synapse with orexin and MCH nuclei in the LHA. MCH levels rise during fasting and stimulate appetite [11]. Excess MCH expression in transgenic mice leads to obesity [12], while mice with MCH deficiency are lean [13]. Orexins A and B stimulate appetite and are produced by neurons in the LHA that project to the olfactory bulb, cerebral cortex, thalamus, hypothalamus, brainstem, locus coeruleus, tuberomammillary nucleus, and raphe nucleus [2]. Glucose-sensing neurons have been found in the LHA, ARC, and ventromedial nucleus of hypothalamus that respond to fluctuations in local extracellular glucose concentration [3,4].

Dorsal Medial Nucleus and Ventromedial Nucleus of the Hypothalamus

The DMH is dorsal to the VMH and receives neuronal NPY/AgRP projections from the ARC and projects α-MSH to the PVN [3]. α-MSH activates catabolic pathways to reduce food intake and enhance energy expenditure.

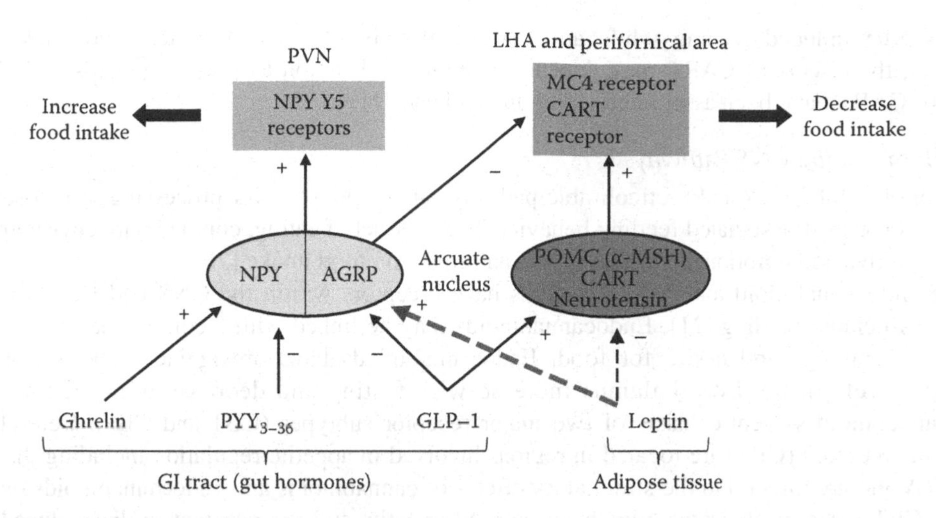

FIGURE 1.2 Schematic of the hypothalamic nuclei and interactions with peripheral signals. LHA, lateral hypothalamic area; PVN, paraventricular nucleus; NPY, neuropeptide Y; AGRP, agouti-related protein; POMC, pro-opiomelanocortin; CART, cocaine and amphetamine-related transcript; α-MSH, α-melanocyte-stimulating hormone; MC4, melanocortin 4.

The VMH has connections with the PVN, DMH, and the LHA. In the VMH, brain-derived neurotrophic factor is expressed and acts to suppress food intake through MC4 receptor activation. Hyperphagia and obesity have been found in mice with selective loss of brain-derived neurotrophic factor pathways in the VMH and DMH [3] (Figure 1.2).

Neurotransmitters and Homeostatic Control of Food Intake

Neuropeptide Y and Agouti-Related Peptide

The ARC contains NPY and AgRP neuronal populations that express receptors for circulating satiety signals. Neuronal activation leads to positive energy balance, lower energy expenditure, and increased food intake. NPY is a neuropeptide that has orexigenic effects mediated by G-protein coupled receptors (hypothalamic Y1 and Y5 receptors) and levels are associated with nutritional status, with levels being increased during fasting and reduced following food intake [14]. Studies have shown that the administration of NPY in the CNS of rats stimulates food intake and increases body weight [15]. The AgRP is expressed in the ARC and is secreted with NPY. AgRP is an antagonist of melanocortin receptors in the melanocortin system (MC3 and MC4 receptors) and stimulates appetite. Increased expression occurs in periods of fasting and acts to increase food intake [16].

Proopiomelanocortin and Cocaine- and Amphetamine-Regulated Transcript

The POMC and CART neuronal populations respond to satiety and their activation promotes negative energy balance, increased energy expenditure, and decreased food consumption. POMC is a precursor polypeptide of melanocortins such as the α-MSH that act at MC3 and MC4 receptors to control appetite. Nutritional status regulates mRNA POMC expression and this is decreased during fasting periods and conversely increased with feeding. Administration of agonists for MC3 and MC4 receptors reduces food intake and of antagonists at the receptors produces hyperphagia [10]. α-MSH acts as the agonist at the hypothalamic MC3 and MC4 receptors to suppress appetite [3]. In murine models of POMC deficiency, obesity and decreased metabolic rate occur and these effects are reversed by administration of melanocortins that suppress food intake. In humans, perturbations such as congenital POMC deficiency and MC3 and MC4 receptor mutations have been associated with obesity [17].

CART has anorexigenic properties and regulates energy homeostasis as neuronal expression responds to nutritional status. It modulates the actions of NPY and leptin. Administration of CART inhibits NPY-induced feeding while anti-CART antibody infusion promotes food intake [18]. However, the effects of CART may depend on signaling location as polymorphisms and altered levels of CART have been associated with human obesity [19].

Non-Homeostatic CNS Pathways

The orbitofrontal cortex and corticolimbic pathways are responsible for processing somatosensory stimuli and reward-associated feeding behavior. The very act of eating, coupled with environmental cues, cognitive and emotional state may have an impact on food intake [20].

The endocannabinoid and opioid systems have receptors within the CNS and have a role in reward-associated feeding [21]. Endocannabinoids may be linked with feeding behavior, possibly mediating cravings and desire for food. Endocannabinoids have orexigenic properties, and in rodents, levels in the hypothalamus increase with fasting and decrease with feeding [15]. The cannabinoid system consists of two major receptor subtypes (CB1 and CB2). Central cannabinoid receptors (CB1) are located in regions involved in appetite regulation including the ARC and LHA and are integral to the stimulatory effects of cannabinoids and endocannabinoids on food intake. CB1 receptor–deficient mice have reduced appetite and are resistant to diet-induced obesity. In humans, the RIO-Europe trial was a randomized double-blind trial that compared treatment of obese subjects with rimonabant and a calorie-restricted diet versus placebo over 2 years. Rimonabant was associated with a significant reduction in weight, waist circumference, and the presence of metabolic syndrome compared with placebo [22]. Rimonabant was approved for the treatment of obesity in Europe in 2008 but subsequently withdrawn due to concerns about increased risk of anxiety, depression, and suicide with its use.

Dopamine has central signaling pathways that are mediated by dopamine D1, D2, D3, and D5 receptors. It may have complex effects on feeding and may be associated with reward-associated behavior [2,23]. It is noteworthy that the D1/D5 receptor antagonist, ecopipam, was withdrawn from clinical trials for obesity due to depression [24], although the combination of the μ opioid antagonist drug naltrexone with the dopamine/noradrenaline reuptake inhibitor bupropion is approved for obesity treatment [25].

GASTROINTESTINAL SIGNALS THAT REGULATE FOOD INTAKE

The GI tract is the largest endocrine gland in the human body and secretes gut hormones that have a significant role in the maintenance of energy equilibrium. The main gut hormones that act on the central hypothalamic and brainstem pathways are ghrelin, CCK, PP, peptide YY (PYY), GLP-1, and oxyntomodulin (OXM).

A criterion for the physiological endocrine action of gut hormones on energy intake was proposed by Geary [26]. He suggested that

1. Hormone secretion should be associated with changes in eating—secretory effect.
2. Receptors should be expressed at the site of action of the relevant hormone—receptor-mediated effect.
3. Effects on appetite should be reproduced by the parenteral administration of a hormone, similar to its endogenous effects—physiological dose–related effect.
4. Removal of the hormone or receptor should prevent the effect on appetite, and replacement of the hormone should reinstitute the effect—removal and replacement effect.
5. Selective, potent antagonism of the hormone should prevent the effect of endogenous hormone as well as hormone treatment—antagonistic effect.

However, not all the gut hormones identified fit all these criteria.

Gut hormones were originally thought to have significant roles in regulating endocrine and paracrine aspects of gut function, such as motility, pancreatic exocrine secretion, and gall bladder contraction, as well as actions as incretins take on pancreatic endocrine activity. However, more recent work has demonstrated their fundamental role in the maintenance of energy equilibrium as peripheral signals of energy status (depletion or surge) through communication to the hypothalamus and brainstem. Local effects of gut hormones on motility such as delay in gastric emptying may also contribute to changes in energy intake. Mechanical effects include activation of stretch receptors through gastric distension contributing to decrease in food intake. Thus, neuroendocrine signaling through the gut–brain axis has a vital role in controlling food intake.

Enteroendocrine cells (EECs) are distributed throughout the gastrointestinal tract and are responsible for the secretion of these peptide hormones. There are open and closed types of EECs that are located throughout the GI tract. Open EECs are cone-shaped cells with microvilli at their open end while the closed end lies abutting the basal lamina. The microvilli at the open end sense the macronutrients in food via G-protein-coupled receptors (by stimulating the chemosensors on these receptors). This leads to release of gut hormones that act through endocrine, paracrine, and neural mechanisms to regulate food intake and energy homeostasis. Closed EECs do not have direct contact with luminal contents but utilize the neural mechanisms to exert their role. Sensory information from the gastrointestinal tract and abdominal viscera as well as taste information from the oral cavity are initially integrated by the NTS.

Due to their role in energy homeostasis, gut hormones (Table 1.1) are a major therapeutic target for the development of antiobesity drugs.

TABLE 1.1
Effects of Gut Peptides on Appetite and Other Physiological Effects

Gut Hormone	Site of Synthesis	Effect on Food Intake	Other Physiological Effects
Ghrelin	Gastric fundus	+	1. Stimulates GH release from pituitary 2. Increases gastric motility 3. Positive inotropic effect on heart 4. Reduction of glucose-stimulated insulin secretion
CCK	Small intestine	–	1. Contraction of gall bladder 2. Inhibition of exocrine pancreatic secretions 3. Delayed gastric emptying
PP	Endocrine pancreas	–	1. Relaxation of gall bladder 2. Inhibition of exocrine pancreatic secretions 3. Delayed gastric emptying
GLP-1	Ileum and proximal colon	–	1. Glucose-induced insulin secretion/incretin effect 2. Inhibits glucagon production 3. Delays gastric emptying 4. Trophic effects on pancreatic beta cell mass 5. Inhibition of gastric acid secretion 6. Cardiovascular effects—increases heart rate
PYY	Distal small and large intestine	–	1. Inhibits gall bladder contraction 2. Inhibits exocrine pancreatic secretion 3. Delays gastric emptying 4. Inhibits gastric acid secretion
Oxyntomodulin	Distal small and large intestine	–	1. Delays gastric emptying 2. Inhibits gastric acid secretion
GIP	K cells of duodenum and jejunum	Not known	1. Stimulates insulin secretion 2. Increase beta cell proliferation 3. Inhibits beta cell apoptosis 4. Increase lipogenesis 5. Increase bone formation

Gut Hormones

Ghrelin

Ghrelin is the only identified orexigenic hormone. Ghrelin, originally discovered as an endogenous ligand for the growth hormone secretagogue receptor (GHS-R) [27], is a 28-amino-acid peptide hormone secreted principally by the X/A like cells in the oxyntic glands of the gastric fundus [28]. Ghrelin is cleaved from preproghrelin by prohormone convertase. Though ghrelin is synthesized in many tissues, the stomach is the largest source of circulating ghrelin. The presence of an acyl side chain attached to the serine amino acid at position three of ghrelin is necessary for its orexigenic effects [27] through binding to GHS-R as well as enhancing its ability to cross the blood–brain barrier. Ghrelin O-acyltransferase (GOAT) is the enzyme responsible for the acylation of ghrelin. Des-acylated ghrelin (which lacks the serine-3 acylation) is not orexigenic and reduces food intake in rodent models with central or peripheral administration [29]. Though des-acyl ghrelin was originally thought to be the inactive form of ghrelin, recent data has demonstrated its physiological roles in the regulation of adiposity as well as glucose homeostasis through agonistic action at the growth hormone secretagogue receptor [30]. Obestatin was identified in 2005 from the ghrelin precursor [31]. Though initially thought to have opposing effects to ghrelin, the anorexigenic effects of obestatin were subsequently not proven from clinical studies.

Peripheral administration of acylated ghrelin in rodent models increases food intake [32], and chronic intracerebroventricular administration induces weight gain [33]. This was replicated in humans and intravenous administration of ghrelin increased food intake and appetite with no effect on gastric emptying, suggesting a central role as the possible explanation for its orexigenic effects [34]. This is through its effects on the hypothalamic ARC [33] via the bloodstream, and NTS via the vagal route. Vagotomy in rats as well as humans abolishes the effects of ghrelin [35–37]. GHS-R-knockout mice as well as ghrelin-deficient mice are resistant to diet-induced obesity further confirming the orexigenic effects of ghrelin. Ghrelin-deficient mice also selectively metabolize fat as a fuel, which provides evidence that ghrelin has other metabolic effects [38].

Circulating ghrelin levels are increased with fasting and fall in the postprandial period [39]. The macronutrient composition of the meal is important in ghrelin-induced postprandial suppression, with carbohydrate-rich meals causing more suppression of ghrelin than protein or fat [40].

In obesity, fasting ghrelin levels are low and the postprandial suppression of ghrelin is attenuated [41]. Moreover, peripheral administration of ghrelin stimulates appetite in obesity [42] and hence, unlike leptin resistance associated with obesity, the obese are not ghrelin resistant. Interestingly, patients with Prader–Willi syndrome (a genetic obesity syndrome associated with hyperphagia, short stature, mental retardation, and pituitary hormone deficiencies) have higher fasting as well as postprandial ghrelin levels [43–45]. However, the search for ghrelin antagonists for obesity treatment has so far been unsuccessful.

Fasting ghrelin levels are high in anorexia nervosa [46] and in patients who have lost weight through diet or gastric bypass surgery [47]. Though ghrelin antagonists may not be a successful therapeutic option in obesity, agonists might be of use in managing select patient groups with anorexia. Ghrelin agonists have also been shown to be of potential benefit in treating malnutrition associated with congestive cardiac failure, chronic obstructive pulmonary disease, renal failure [48], and cancer [49]. However, a concern regarding the use of ghrelin in patients with malignancy as an appetite stimulant is its potential to stimulate growth hormone and thus other growth factors.

Apart from its effect on energy homeostasis as a short-term signal, other physiological roles of ghrelin include stimulation of growth hormone release, increase in gastric motility, possible role in glucose homeostasis, and its positive inotropic effect on the heart [50]. The satiety effect of glucagon is also thought to be ghrelin-mediated [51]. Ghrelin along with insulin and leptin acts as a mechanism to combat energy deficit via its orexigenic signal as well as metabolic switch from carbohydrate to fat metabolism, thus facilitating the storage of carbohydrate. However, these metabolic effects of ghrelin are more pronounced during stages of energy deficit (i.e., fasting and starvation) than at the other end of the spectrum (fed and obese states) [52]. The effects of ghrelin on glucose homeostasis are more pronounced than on body weight [53]. Exogenous ghrelin administration resulted in reduction of glucose-stimulated insulin secretion [54]. Hence, ghrelin antagonism could be another untapped therapeutic approach for the management of type 2 diabetes.

In conclusion, ghrelin plays an important role in the regulation of energy homeostasis through its gut–brain interaction, acting on homeostatic as well as non-homeostatic centers. Manipulation of the ghrelin system could be a potential therapeutic approach for the management of obesity, other eating disorders, and type 2 diabetes but has not been successful so far. Ghrelin agonism, antagonism, anti-ghrelin vaccines, des-acyl ghrelin analogues, and GOAT enzyme inhibition are being investigated and could be potential pharmacotherapies in the future.

Cholecystokinin

CCK was the first gut hormone demonstrated to influence appetite control [55]. Secreted by the L cells of the duodenum and jejunum after meals, it is involved in contraction of the gall bladder, inhibition of exocrine pancreatic secretion, delays in gastric emptying, and increases in motility of the intestine, apart from its currently discussed role as a satiety signal. CCK exerts its gastrointestinal and other physiological effects through CCK_1 and CCK_2 receptors (previously named as CCK_A and CCK_B receptors), which are located in the gastrointestinal tract and select brain centers [56]. CCK_1 receptors are mainly located in the pancreas, pylorus, vagus, NTS, and hypothalamus and contribute to post meal satiety signaling. This is thought to be vagally mediated due to activation of vagal CCK_1 receptors [57]. CCK might also affect mechanoreception, augmenting the local stretch signals and conveying them to the hypothalamus. According to Geary's criteria, CCK was thought to be the gut hormone with the best-established physiological endocrine action [26].

CCK has a short half-life (1–2 minutes) and its levels increase 10–30 minutes after food intake, returning to basal levels after 3–5 hours [58]. With respect to the macronutrient composition of the meal, fat and protein are the major stimulants of CCK release, while carbohydrates are weak stimuli [58].

CCK levels in obesity have been shown to differ between studies with some studies showing increased levels while others had demonstrated opposite results [59,60]. There are data from animal studies that CCK might work synergistically with leptin [61] and insulin [62] in the maintenance of energy homeostasis.

CCK infusion (the C-terminal octapeptide of CCK) decreased food intake in lean individuals [63] suggesting its possible role as an appetite suppressant. The OLETF (Otsuka Long-Evans Tokushima Fatty rat) lacking the CCK_1 receptor was demonstrated to be obese and diabetic with defective control of meal sizes, and CCK receptor deficiency was thought to be the reason for obesity in these rodents (along with NPY overexpression) [64]. This suggested that CCK might have a physiological role in meal intake. However, chronic administration of CCK (2 weeks of intraperitoneal infusion) in rodent models was not associated with any changes in body weight or food consumption [65], and trials of CCK agonists in humans have not proceeded beyond phase 2 due to adverse effects. Thus, the therapeutic potential of CCK as an antiobesity agent may be limited.

Pancreatic Polypeptide

PP is a 36-amino-acid peptide secreted mainly from the endocrine pancreas (by the PP cells of the islets of Langerhans). It is a member of the PP family, all of which bind to the Y family of receptors. NPY and PYY are members of the same family. PP is released postprandially and has been demonstrated to reduce appetite in rodents [66] as well as humans [67]. This is receptor mediated, through its effect on the Y4 receptors (to which it has the highest affinity) in the brainstem and hypothalamus [68] as well as vagally [69]. The Y receptors are G-protein-coupled receptors of which there are five subtypes, Y1–Y5, that are all coupled to adenylate cyclase. Y4 receptors are expressed in abundance in area postrema in the DVC, and PP exerts its physiological effects by binding to these receptors. PP has a biphasic mode of release and its levels remain high up to 6 hours postprandially. PP also exhibits a diurnal rhythm with lowest levels at 02:00 and peaks at 21:00 hours [70]. The release of PP is stimulated by CCK, hypoglycemia, and exercise and inhibited by somatostatin.

The effect of PP on satiety is dependent on the route of administration with peripheral PP having anorexic effects while central administration causes orexigenic effects [71]. Transgenic mice overexpressing PP were lean with reduction in fat mass, reduction in food intake, delayed gastric emptying, and reduction in leptin levels [72]. Intraperitoneal administration of PP reduced adiposity in leptin-deficient *ob/ob* mice with a favorable metabolic profile for insulin resistance and hyperlipidemia [73].

PP also delays gastric emptying [74] that is thought to contribute to its anorectic effect. Other physiological effects of PP include inhibition of exocrine pancreatic secretions and inhibition of gall bladder contraction [75]. The concentration of PP post meal is markedly reduced in obese individuals [76] and is increased in patients with anorexia nervosa [77]. Prader–Willi syndrome patients have a blunted response to PP [78], and exogenous administration (PP infusion) reduces food intake in this condition restoring PP levels to normal [79].

PP is an anorexigenic peptide and transmits information related to food intake through vagus to the DVC as well as hypothalamic nuclei, thus playing a role in modulating energy homeostasis through the gut–brain axis. PP analogues have been investigated as antiobesity agents, but their therapeutic potential is still uncertain.

Glucagon-Like Peptide-1 and Peptide YY

The enteroendocrine L cells form an important part of the gut–brain axis. They express the preproglucagon gene, which undergoes tissue-specific posttranslational processing, that is, it generates different hormonal products when processed in different organs, such as the pancreas or intestine. The prohormone convertase 1 is responsible for the production of GLP-1, glucagon-like peptide-2 (GLP-2), and OXM from proglucagon in the intestine [80]. L cells in the intestine co-secrete different gut peptides depending on their location. The upper small intestinal cells secrete gastric inhibitory polypeptide (GIP). The lower small intestinal cells co-secrete GLP-1 and PYY, and these are important for energy homeostasis. Both GLP-1 and PYY are secreted in a biphasic manner with a first phase of release on arrival of food in the proximal small intestine, which is neurally mediated, and a second phase when food reaches the distal intestine through a nutrient receptor–mediated process [81].

Glucagon-Like Peptide-1

The peptide hormone GLP-1 is derived from the posttranslational processing of preproglucagon, which is also the source of glucagon, GLP-2, and OXM. GLP-1 is produced in the L cells of the distal small intestine (jejunum) and proximal colon and is secreted following a meal. GLP-1 secretion is proportional to caloric intake, especially the glucose content of the meal. Fat as well as protein also promotes GLP-1 responses [81]. GLP-1 is secreted 5–30 minutes following meal intake. It exists in two biologically active forms—GLP-1 (7-37) and GLP-1 (7-36) amide; the latter is the most abundant form in human circulation.

GLP-1 exerts its effects through the GLP-1 receptor, which is a G-protein-coupled receptor. GLP-1 receptors are widely distributed in the body, including pancreas, gastrointestinal tract, heart, lung, kidney, brain, as well as vascular endothelium and arteriolar smooth muscles. In the brain, these are mostly expressed in the supraoptic, paraventricular, and arcuate nuclei of the hypothalamus [82], brainstem, substantia nigra, and striatum. The demonstration of GLP-1 receptors in the brain indicates that the physiological effects of the GLP-1 system are at least partly, centrally mediated. GLP-1 is expressed in neurons in the NTS that project to the POMC and amphetamine-regulated transcript (CART) neurons in the arcuate nuclei of the hypothalamus, as well as to the paraventricular and dorsomedial nuclei.

The binding of GLP-1 to its receptors in the pancreas leads to a cascade of events.

There is an increase in cyclic AMP levels causing an increase in intracellular calcium levels leading to exocytosis of insulin-containing vesicles [83]. Similar to CCK, ghrelin, and PYY, the vagus nerve plays a significant role in the effects of GLP-1 on energy intake. Vagotomy in rodents has been demonstrated to abolish the effects of GLP-1 on food intake and its hypothalamic effects [84] demonstrating the significance of this gut–brain axis, that is, an intact vagal–brainstem–hypothalamic connection.

GLP-1 is an incretin hormone and its effect to stimulate insulin secretion in response to oral glucose is described as the "incretin effect." GLP-(7-36) and GIP are the incretin hormones and the circulating levels of both of these have been shown to rise following intake of carbohydrate or mixed meals. Incretin deficiency has been suggested as part of the pathophysiological process leading to the development of type 2 diabetes. Consequently, incretin-based therapies are now widely used in the management of type 2 diabetes.

Apart from its insulin stimulatory and glucagon inhibitory effect, GLP-1 also causes satiation [85], delays gastric emptying [86], and promotes weight loss in humans by decreasing energy intake [87]; all of these properties make it suitable as a treatment for obesity. It acts synergistically with PYY in the ileal brake phenomenon, which aids nutrient digestion. GLP-1 also has trophic effects on beta cells of the pancreas.

GLP-1 levels are low in obesity and increase after weight loss. GLP-1 secretion is low in anorexia nervosa [88].

Endogenous GLP-1, the most abundant incretin, has, however, a short half-life of 2–3 minutes and is susceptible to degradation by endopeptidases, notably dipeptidyl peptidase 4 (DPP-IV). Hence, pharmaceutical development has focused on the synthesis of GLP-1 analogues resistant to the action of DPP-IV, thus increasing its half-life. Available GLP-1 analogues include exenatide, lixisenatide (short-acting), liraglutide (intermediate-acting) and exenatide QR, dulaglutide (in development), and semaglutide (long-acting GLP-1 analogues, which are administered once weekly).

The therapeutic benefits of GLP-1 analogues include a glucose-lowering effect without increasing the risk of hypoglycemia (since its insulin secretory effect is only seen above blood glucose levels of 3.5–4 mmol/L), weight reduction, moderate reductions in systolic and diastolic blood pressure [89], and a favorable effect on the lipid profile (reduction in total cholesterol, low density lipoprotein-cholesterol, triglycerides, free fatty acid, and increase in high density lipoprotein cholesterol) [90].

Exendin-4 (4-39) is a purified derivative from the saliva of *Heloderma suspectum*, the Gila monster lizard, and was discovered in 1992. Exendin-4 shares only 53% homology with human GLP-1 but is a potent analogue and is resistant to the action of DPP-IV. Subsequently, exenatide, a synthetic form of exendin-4, became the first approved GLP-1 analogue for the treatment of type 2 diabetes in 2005. It has a short half-life of 2.4 hours and is administered subcutaneously, twice daily. In addition to improving glycemic control, exenatide treatment reduces body weight in patients with type 2 diabetes [91].

The GLP-1 system is the only successfully manipulated component of the gut–brain axis as a therapy for the treatment of obesity. Liraglutide, which shares 97% structural homology with endogenous GLP-1, is the first GLP-1 analogue to get the approval of regulatory authorities as a weight loss drug. Liraglutide 3 mg along with increased physical activity and reduced caloric intake resulted in significant weight loss in overweight and obese individuals without type 2 diabetes [92]. Liraglutide-induced weight loss was associated with improvement of overall cardiometabolic profile, including waist circumference, blood pressure, lipids, and inflammatory markers. Liraglutide was given FDA approval in December 2014 and EMEA approval in March 2015 and is currently marketed as a weight loss drug, Saxenda (liraglutide 3 mg). Low-dose liraglutide (0.6–1.8 mg) is marketed as Victoza and has been used for the treatment of type 2 diabetes since 2009. The cardiovascular safety of liraglutide was demonstrated in the LEADER (Liraglutide and Cardiovascular Outcomes in Type 2 Diabetes) trial, which randomized 9340 patients and followed up for 3.8 years [93].

Peptide YY

PYY is a 36-amino-acid peptide hormone co-secreted postprandially with GLP-1 from the enteroendocrine L cells of the GI tract. The name PYY is derived from its tyrosine residues at the C and N terminals. PYY exists in circulation in two forms, PYY_{1-36}, which has affinity to all the Y receptors, and PYY_{3-36}, the N-terminally truncated form which is the major circulating and biologically active form of PYY with the highest affinity to the Y2 receptors. Though PYY-expressing cells are distributed all along the intestine, they are most abundant in the distal part. Data from radioimmunoassay have demonstrated that PYY levels are low in the duodenum and jejunum, and high in the ileum and colon with the highest levels in the rectum [94].

PYY is another anorexigenic hormone with low levels in the fasting state and increasing in concentration postprandially. PYY levels rise after 30 minutes of food intake, plateau by 1–2 hours, and remain high for up to 6 hours. This rise in PYY is greatest with protein-rich meals. The satiety-enhancing effect of dietary protein is thought to be mediated by PYY. Dietary protein increased PYY levels in mice, resulting in decreased food intake and weight gain. PYY-deleted mice were resistant to this satiety effect of protein and developed obesity, which was in turn reversed by exogenous PYY administration [95]. Peripheral administration of PYY_{3-36} was shown to reduce food intake as well as weight gain in rodents [96], and these results have been replicated in humans [97]. PYY levels are low in obesity and there is a blunted postprandial rise in PYY levels. The circulating levels of PYY are increased in anorexia nervosa and this has been postulated to contribute to decreased food intake and increased bone turnover in such patients [98]. In women with anorexia nervosa, an increase in the PYY level is associated with diminished bone mineral density, especially at spine. Fasting PYY levels are high in inflammatory bowel disease, steatorrhea, tropical sprue, and cardiac cachexia, and high PYY levels could be a reason for the loss of appetite in such states.

The anorectic effects of PYY could be through the stimulation of the POMC neurons in the ARC of the hypothalamus or due to inhibition of the NPY neurons [99], which is likely to be Y2 receptor mediated. Vagotomy can dampen the anorectic action of PYY, thus demonstrating the role of vagus nerve in this gut–brain communication [84]. Direct administration of PYY into the third ventricle however has been shown to be orexigenic [100] likely due to the effects of PYY on the NPY neurons in the hypothalamic arcuate nuclei.

PYY along with GLP-1 mediates the "ileal brake" explained as follows.

Oxyntomodulin

OXM is a 37-amino-acid peptide that derives its name from its inhibitory effect on the oxyntic glands of stomach. It is secreted by the intestinal L cells along with GLP-1 and PYY by the post-translational processing of preproglucagon. Apart from the intestinal L cells, OXM is also expressed in the pancreas and the CNS. OXM exerts its physiological effects via the GLP-1 receptor though its affinity for GLP-1 receptors is low compared to GLP-1 [101]. The anorectic effect of OXM was blocked when it was coadministered in rats with exendin 9-39, a GLP-1 antagonist [102]. OXM signaling through the gut–brain axis is likely to be mediated through the vagus nerve as vagotomy abolished the effect of OXM on CCK-induced pancreatic secretion [103]. It is secreted postprandially with levels peaking in 30 minutes and remains elevated for several hours. Its secretion is stimulated by dietary fat [104].

Central (intracerebroventricular) [102] and peripheral (intraperitoneal) [105] administration of OXM in rats inhibited feeding. OXM also increases energy expenditure apart from its effects on energy intake, thus affecting long-term energy homeostasis. The anorexic effects of OXM have been replicated in human studies with OXM reducing both ad libitum energy intake at a buffet meal as well as 12-hour cumulative energy intake in healthy volunteers [106]. It was also noted that fasting ghrelin levels were suppressed by OXM, which might be responsible for its anorectic effects.

Similar to GLP-1, OXM is also inactivated by the DPP-IV enzyme and OXM analogues, which are resistant to the action of this endopeptidase, are under investigation [107].

GIP

GIP is a 42-amino-acid peptide secreted by the K cells in the duodenum and jejunum. GIP is mainly secreted after the ingestion of carbohydrates and fat [108] depending on the rate of absorption of nutrients rather than their presence. Fat is the major stimulator of GIP release in humans. Like GLP-1, GIP is an incretin hormone and is inactivated by the DPP-IV enzyme. GIP does not have a direct effect on energy intake. GIP-receptor-knockout mice on a high-fat diet have lower respiratory quotient (due to the use of fat as a metabolic fuel) and consequently are resistant to obesity and insulin resistance [109]. GIP has anabolic and lipolytic effects on adipose tissue.

Amylin

Amylin is co-secreted with insulin from the beta cells of the pancreas in response to food ingestion. In humans, amylin binds to AMY-receptor subtypes, which are calcitonin receptor complexes with receptor activity-modifying proteins [110]. In rats, amylin reduced the meal size and meal duration, thus demonstrating its anorectic effects [111]. Meal-induced amylin release activates area postrema neurons in the brain [112]. It enhances the anorectic effects of CCK, and this is likely to be via modulation in area postrema. Apart from reducing food intake, amylin delays gastric emptying, decreases gastric secretion, and reduces postprandial glucagon secretion. As such, pramlintide, a synthetic amylin analogue, is approved in the United States as an adjunct therapy in type 1 and type 2 diabetes [113,114].

Mechanical Mechanisms

The Ileal-Brake Reflex

The ileal-brake reflex is an inhibitory intestinal control mechanism whereby unabsorbed dietary constituents in ileum and colon inhibit proximal GI motility, thus increasing the digestion and absorption of nutrients [115]. Both GLP-1 and PYY may contribute to the ileal brake, which can reduce energy intake. Though fat was thought to be the most potent stimulator of the ileal brake, subsequent studies illustrated that all three macronutrients (carbohydrates, proteins, and lipids) influenced the ileal brake [116].

The Role of Mechanoreception in Appetite Control

Apart from communication through gut peptides, the hypothalamus also receives information from mechanical stimuli due to stretching of the stomach. The gastrointestinal tract is abundantly innervated with mechanoreceptors that can sense the mechanical stretch stimulus due to food intake and communicate information to the higher centers in the brain through vagal and splanchnic connections. Animal studies have demonstrated that gastric volume is an important factor for mechanoreception, which in turn regulates food intake. Male rats implanted with gastric catheters and pyloric cuffs were given specific volumes of saline or milk and decreased food intake was shown to be secondary to the volume or rate of infusion rather than related to a specific nutrient [117]. Because such techniques cannot be replicated in human studies, evidence for the contribution of mechanical factors to appetite control is scanty. Nevertheless, human data have demonstrated that energy density and portion size of food independently contribute to energy intake [118]. Energy-dense foods thus contribute to overconsumption, and reducing energy density of the diet is one possible dietary strategy to deal with the public health problem of obesity. Gastric antral area and antral distension are important in determining satiation as well as satiety [119] in humans.

Effect of Bariatric Surgery on Gut Hormones

Bariatric surgery is the most effective therapeutic intervention for obesity and results in significant, sustained weight loss as well as metabolic improvement in the majority of patients. The mechanisms of post-bariatric surgery weight reduction (reviewed in Chapter 7 of this textbook) are not completely unraveled but are thought to be mediated by more than caloric restriction and malabsorption. Alterations in circulating gut hormones may contribute; an increase in GLP-1, PYY, and OXM levels has been observed, and changes in ghrelin and GIP hormones could also play a role in weight reduction.

Bariatric surgical procedures involving the intestine (Roux-en-Y gastric bypass [RYGB] and biliopancreatic diversion [BPD]) and those that expedite nutrient delivery (sleeve gastrectomy) resulted in an increase in GLP-1 and PYY levels, whereas no increase was demonstrated after gastric banding [120]. Hence, rapid delivery of nutrients to the distal gut might be responsible for this phenomenon. Sleeve gastrectomy increases gastric emptying that in turn could result in fast passage of nutrients to the intestine, stimulating L cells to release these gut hormones. RYGB and BPD that are the surgical procedures associated with maximum weight loss had greater elevations in GLP-1 and PYY levels. Similar reductions in body weight via caloric restriction did not elicit these hormonal changes, thus demonstrating that these are solely related to bariatric surgery. Elevation in OXM levels was noticed after RYGB. However, changes in ghrelin levels were inconsistent from different studies and may be due to differences in surgical approaches.

Hormones from Adipose Tissue

Adipose tissue is an important source of hormones that regulate hypothalamic energy homeostasis. Though leptin is an adipose tissue hormone, it needs mentioning due to its significant role in the maintenance of energy homeostasis as well as carbohydrate, lipid, and bone metabolism. Leptin is predominantly expressed by white adipose tissue and acts as a circulating satiety factor, promoting negative energy balance. Circulating leptin levels correspond to fat mass, thereby reflecting the energy status of an individual. Leptin exerts its effects through the ARC by stimulation of POMC and CART neurons and inhibition of the NPY and AgRP neurons. The leptin-deficient *ob/ob* mouse model was found to be associated with hyperphagia and obesity, which was reversed with leptin administration. Recombinant leptin is used as a therapeutic strategy in congenital leptin deficiency (where it reduces body weight and fat mass) [121] and in congenital as well as acquired lipodystrophy, which is associated with leptin deficiency (where it improves insulin resistance and decreases triglyceride levels) [122]. However, obesity and type 2 diabetes are associated with leptin resistance, thus limiting the therapeutic potential of leptin in these conditions. It should be noted that although circulating leptin levels are associated with adiposity, leptin resistance may occur as obese individuals have high leptin levels (REF). In these individuals, the expected anorexigenic effects of leptin are diminished and may be due to leptin receptor overstimulation and activation of negative feedback loops that block leptin signaling contributing to leptin resistance [6].

Adiponectin is also secreted from white adipose tissue but in contrast to leptin, levels are decreased in obesity and inversely related to adiposity and are increased in fasting. Adiponectin receptors (AdipoR1 and R2) are expressed in the hypothalamus and induce AMP kinase phosphorylation and activity. Adiponectin promotes energy expenditure and fatty acid oxidation. Conversely, adiponectin deficiency induces insulin resistance and hyperlipidemia. Central administration of adiponectin increases expression of uncoupling protein 1 in brown adipose tissue, with increases in brown adipose tissue thermogenesis, thus promoting energy expenditure. Conversely, adiponectin administered peripherally resulted in increased food intake, reduced energy expenditure, and weight gain.

Circulating resistin levels are higher in obesity and its receptors are expressed in the hypothalamus. Resistin acts centrally to decrease food intake, an effect associated with suppression of the normal fasting-induced increase in NPY/AgRP expression and the normal fasting-induced decrease in CART expression [123].

Proinflammatory cytokines found in adipose tissue, such as TNF-α and IL-6, also inhibit feeding and induce thermogenesis by modulating expression of hypothalamic neurotransmitters; they may play a role in the anorexia associated with febrile illness, but their role in day-to-day appetite regulation is unproven.

Diet and the Gut–Brain Axis: Are All Macronutrients Equal?

The relative proportion of dietary macronutrients (protein, carbohydrate, and fat) as well as the glycemic index has a significant role in appetite and energy balance mechanisms. A high-protein, low-carbohydrate, low–glycemic index diet has been demonstrated from numerous clinical studies to be superior to a normal-protein, high-GI diet for the induction as well as maintenance of weight loss [124,125]. A high protein intake also promotes a negative energy balance due to the greater satiating effect of protein compared to other macronutrients. Dietary thermogenesis, which is a component of total energy expenditure, is also more for protein compared to carbohydrates and fat. The protein content of a meal produces a dose-dependent increase in GLP-1, PYY, and glucagon levels, which might contribute to the satiety-stimulating effects of this macronutrient [126].

CONCLUSION

The gut–brain axis is a vital link between the peripheral and central pathways facilitating the complex neuroendocrine regulation of energy homeostasis. Gut hormones have a crucial role in the maintenance of energy homeostasis. Modulation of one component of the system (GLP-1) has finally proven to be fruitful as an antiobesity therapy, and others, perhaps with multiple targets for action, seem likely to follow. As the obesity epidemic continues to be one of the major public health problems in all parts of the world, unraveling of this complex neuroendocrine network will help us in understanding appetite control mechanisms and, hopefully, more successful therapeutic strategies in the future.

REFERENCES

1. Schwartz MW, Woods SC, Seeley RJ, Barsh GS, Baskin DG, Leibel RL. Is the energy homeostasis system inherently biased toward weight gain? *Diabetes*. 2003;52(2):232–238.
2. Wynne K, Stanley S, McGowan B, Bloom SR. Appetite control. *Journal of Endocrinology*. 2005;184:291–318.
3. Suzuki K, Jayasena CN, Bloom SR. Obesity and appetite control. *Experimental Diabetes Research*. 2012;2012:824305.
4. Gonzalez JA, Reimann F, Burdakov D. Dissociation between sensing and metabolism of glucose in sugar sensing neurones. *The Journal of Physiology*. 2009;587(1):41–48.
5. Owyang C, Heldsinger A. Vagal control of satiety and hormonal regulation of appetite. *Journal of Neurogastroenterology and Motility*. 2011;17(4):338–348.
6. Perry B, Wang Y. Appetite regulation and weight control: The role of gut hormones. *Nutrition and Diabetes*. 2012;2:e26.
7. Cegla J, Tan TM, Bloom SR. Gut-brain cross-talk in appetite regulation. *Current Opinion in Clinical Nutrition and Metabolic Care*. 2010;13(5):588–593.
8. Neary NM, Goldstone AP, Bloom SR. Appetite regulation: From the gut to the hypothalamus. *Clinical Endocrinology*. 2004;60(2):153–160.
9. Stanley S, Wynne K, McGowan B, Bloom S. Hormonal regulation of food intake. *Physiological Reviews*. 2005;85(4):1131–1158.
10. Williams G, Harrold JA, Cutler DJ. The hypothalamus and the regulation of energy homeostasis: Lifting the lid on a black box. *The Proceedings of the Nutrition Society*. 2000;59(3):385–396.
11. Qu D, Ludwig DS, Gammeltoft S, Piper M, Pelleymounter MA, Cullen MJ et al. A role for melanin-concentrating hormone in the central regulation of feeding behaviour. *Nature*. 1996;380(6571):243–247.
12. Ludwig DS, Tritos NA, Mastaitis JW, Kulkarni R, Kokkotou E, Elmquist J et al. Melanin-concentrating hormone overexpression in transgenic mice leads to obesity and insulin resistance. *Journal of Clinical Investigation*. 2001;107(3):379–386.
13. Marsh DJ, Weingarth DT, Novi DE, Chen HY, Trumbauer ME, Chen AS et al. Melanin-concentrating hormone 1 receptor-deficient mice are lean, hyperactive, and hyperphagic and have altered metabolism. *Proceedings of the National Academy of Sciences of the United Stated of America*. 2002;99(5):3240–3245.
14. Swart I, Jahng JW, Overton JM, Houpt TA. Hypothalamic NPY, AGRP, and POMC mRNA responses to leptin and refeeding in mice. *American Journal of Physiology Regulatory, Integrative and Comparative Physiology*. 2002;283(5):R1020–R1026.
15. Lopaschuk GD, Ussher JR, Jaswal JS. Targeting intermediary metabolism in the hypothalamus as a mechanism to regulate appetite. *Pharmacological Reviews*. 2010;62(2):237–264.
16. Ollmann MM, Wilson BD, Yang YK, Kerns JA, Chen Y, Gantz I et al. Antagonism of central melanocortin receptors in vitro and in vivo by agouti-related protein. *Science*. 1997;278(5335):135–138.

17. Argyropoulos G, Rankinen T, Neufeld DR, Rice T, Province MA, Leon AS et al. A polymorphism in the human agouti-related protein is associated with late-onset obesity. *The Journal of Clinical Endocrinology and Metabolism*. 2002;87(9):4198–4202.
18. Kristensen P, Judge ME, Thim L, Ribel U, Christjansen KN, Wulff BS et al. Hypothalamic CART is a new anorectic peptide regulated by leptin. *Nature*. 1998;393(6680):72–76.
19. Kim GW, Lin JE, Valentino MA, Colon-Gonzalez F, Waldman SA. Regulation of appetite to treat obesity. *Expert Review of Clinical Pharmacology*. 2011;4(2):243–259.
20. Whitwell JL, Sampson EL, Loy CT, Warren JE, Rossor MN, Fox NC et al. VBM signatures of abnormal eating behaviours in frontotemporal lobar degeneration. *NeuroImage*. 2007;35(1):207–213.
21. Cota D, Tschop MH, Horvath TL, Levine AS. Cannabinoids, opioids and eating behavior: The molecular face of hedonism? *Brain Research Reviews*. 2006;51(1):85–107.
22. Van Gaal LF, Scheen AJ, Rissanen AM, Roessner S, Hanotin C, Ziegler O et al. Long-term effect of CB1 blockade with rimonabant on cardiometabolic risk factors: Two year results from the RIO-Europe Study. *European Heart Journal*. 2008;29(14):1761–1771.
23. Schwartz MW, Woods SC, Porte D, Jr., Seeley RJ, Baskin DG. Central nervous system control of food intake. *Nature*. 2000;404(6778):661–671.
24. Astrup A, Greenway FL, Ling W, Pedicone L, Lachowicz J, Strader CD et al. Randomized controlled trials of the D1/D5 antagonist ecopipam for weight loss in obese subjects. *Obesity*. 2007;15(7):1717–1731.
25. Yanovski SZ, Yanovski JA. Naltrexone extended-release plus bupropion extended-release for treatment of obesity. *JAMA—Journal of the American Medical Association*. 2015;313(12):1213–1214.
26. Geary N. Endocrine controls of eating: CCK, leptin, and ghrelin. *Physiology & Behavior*. 2004;81(5):719–733.
27. Kojima M, Hosoda H, Date Y, Nakazato M, Matsuo H, Kangawa K. Ghrelin is a growth-hormone-releasing acylated peptide from stomach. *Nature*. 1999;402(6762):656–660.
28. Date Y, Kojima M, Hosoda H, Sawaguchi A, Mondal MS, Suganuma T et al. Ghrelin, a novel growth hormone-releasing acylated peptide, is synthesized in a distinct endocrine cell type in the gastrointestinal tracts of rats and humans. *Endocrinology*. 2000;141(11):4255–4261.
29. Asakawa A, Inui A, Fujimiya M, Sakamaki R, Shinfuku N, Ueta Y et al. Stomach regulates energy balance via acylated ghrelin and desacyl ghrelin. *Gut*. 2005;54(1):18–24.
30. Heppner KM, Piechowski CL, Muller A, Ottaway N, Sisley S, Smiley DL et al. Both acyl and des-acyl ghrelin regulate adiposity and glucose metabolism via central nervous system ghrelin receptors. *Diabetes*. 2014;63(1):122–131.
31. Zhang JV, Ren PG, Avsian-Kretchmer O, Luo CW, Rauch R, Klein C et al. Obestatin, a peptide encoded by the ghrelin gene, opposes ghrelin's effects on food intake. *Science*. 2005;310(5750):996–999.
32. Wren AM, Small CJ, Ward HL, Murphy KG, Dakin CL, Taheri S et al. The novel hypothalamic peptide ghrelin stimulates food intake and growth hormone secretion. *Endocrinology*. 2000;141(11):4325–4328.
33. Wren AM, Small CJ, Abbott CR, Dhillo WS, Seal LJ, Cohen MA et al. Ghrelin causes hyperphagia and obesity in rats. *Diabetes*. 2001;50(11):2540–2547.
34. Wren AM, Seal LJ, Cohen MA, Brynes AE, Frost GS, Murphy KG et al. Ghrelin enhances appetite and increases food intake in humans. *The Journal of Clinical Endocrinology and Metabolism*. 2001;86(12):5992.
35. Date Y, Murakami N, Toshinai K, Matsukura S, Niijima A, Matsuo H et al. The role of the gastric afferent vagal nerve in ghrelin-induced feeding and growth hormone secretion in rats. *Gastroenterology*. 2002;123(4):1120–1128.
36. Williams DL, Grill HJ, Cummings DE, Kaplan JM. Vagotomy dissociates short- and long-term controls of circulating ghrelin. *Endocrinology*. 2003;144(12):5184–5187.
37. le Roux CW, Neary NM, Halsey TJ, Small CJ, Martinez-Isla AM, Ghatei MA et al. Ghrelin does not stimulate food intake in patients with surgical procedures involving vagotomy. *The Journal of Clinical Endocrinology and Metabolism*. 2005;90(8):4521–4524.
38. Cummings DE. Ghrelin and the short- and long-term regulation of appetite and body weight. *Physiology & Behavior*. 2006;89(1):71–84.
39. Cummings DE, Purnell JQ, Frayo RS, Schmidova K, Wisse BE, Weigle DS. A preprandial rise in plasma ghrelin levels suggests a role in meal initiation in humans. *Diabetes*. 2001;50(8):1714–1719.
40. Koliaki C, Kokkinos A, Tentolouris N, Katsilambros N. The effect of ingested macronutrients on postprandial ghrelin response: A critical review of existing literature data. *International Journal of Peptides*. 2010;2010:710852.
41. le Roux CW, Patterson M, Vincent RP, Hunt C, Ghatei MA, Bloom SR. Postprandial plasma ghrelin is suppressed proportional to meal calorie content in normal-weight but not obese subjects. *The Journal of Clinical Endocrinology and Metabolism*. 2005;90(2):1068–1071.

42. Druce MR, Wren AM, Park AJ, Milton JE, Patterson M, Frost G et al. Ghrelin increases food intake in obese as well as lean subjects. *International Journal of Obesity*. 2005;29(9):1130–1136.
43. Cummings DE, Clement K, Purnell JQ, Vaisse C, Foster KE, Frayo RS et al. Elevated plasma ghrelin levels in Prader–Willi syndrome. *Nature Medicine*. 2002;8(7):643–644.
44. Goldstone AP, Patterson M, Kalingag N, Ghatei MA, Brynes AE, Bloom SR et al. Fasting and postprandial hyperghrelinemia in Prader-Willi syndrome is partially explained by hypoinsulinemia, and is not due to peptide YY3-36 deficiency or seen in hypothalamic obesity due to craniopharyngioma. *The Journal of Clinical Endocrinology and Metabolism*. 2005;90(5):2681–2690.
45. Patterson M, Bloom SR, Gardiner JV. Ghrelin and appetite control in humans—Potential application in the treatment of obesity. *Peptides*. 2011;32(11):2290–2294.
46. Otto B, Cuntz U, Fruehauf E, Wawarta R, Folwaczny C, Riepl RL et al. Weight gain decreases elevated plasma ghrelin concentrations of patients with anorexia nervosa. *European Journal of Endocrinology/European Federation of Endocrine Societies*. 2001;145(5):669–673.
47. Cummings DE, Weigle DS, Frayo RS, Breen PA, Ma MK, Dellinger EP et al. Plasma ghrelin levels after diet-induced weight loss or gastric bypass surgery. *The New England Journal of Medicine*. 2002;346(21):1623–1630.
48. Wynne K, Giannitsopoulou K, Small CJ, Patterson M, Frost G, Ghatei MA et al. Subcutaneous ghrelin enhances acute food intake in malnourished patients who receive maintenance peritoneal dialysis: A randomized, placebo-controlled trial. *Journal of the American Society of Nephrology (JASN)*. 2005;16(7):2111–2118.
49. Neary NM, Small CJ, Wren AM, Lee JL, Druce MR, Palmieri C et al. Ghrelin increases energy intake in cancer patients with impaired appetite: Acute, randomized, placebo-controlled trial. *The Journal of Clinical Endocrinology and Metabolism*. 2004;89(6):2832–2836.
50. Korbonits M, Grossman AB. Ghrelin: Update on a novel hormonal system. *European Journal of Endocrinology/European Federation of Endocrine Societies*. 2004;151(Suppl 1):S67–S70.
51. Arafat AM, Weickert MO, Adamidou A, Otto B, Perschel FH, Spranger J et al. The impact of insulin-independent, glucagon-induced suppression of total ghrelin on satiety in obesity and type 1 diabetes mellitus. *The Journal of Clinical Endocrinology and Metabolism*. 2013;98(10):4133–4142.
52. Pinkney J. The role of ghrelin in metabolic regulation. *Current Opinion in Clinical Nutrition and Metabolic Care*. 2014;17(6):497–502.
53. Sun Y, Asnicar M, Saha PK, Chan L, Smith RG. Ablation of ghrelin improves the diabetic but not obese phenotype of ob/ob mice. *Cell Metabolism*. 2006;3(5):379–386.
54. Tong J, Prigeon RL, Davis HW, Bidlingmaier M, Kahn SE, Cummings DE et al. Ghrelin suppresses glucose-stimulated insulin secretion and deteriorates glucose tolerance in healthy humans. *Diabetes*. 2010;59(9):2145–2151.
55. Gibbs J, Young RC, Smith GP. Cholecystokinin decreases food intake in rats. 1973. *Obesity Research*. 1997;5(3):284–290.
56. Wank SA. Cholecystokinin receptors. *American Journal of Physiology*. 1995;269(5 Pt 1):G628–G646.
57. Moran TH, Baldessarini AR, Salorio CF, Lowery T, Schwartz GJ. Vagal afferent and efferent contributions to the inhibition of food intake by cholecystokinin. *The American Journal of Physiology*. 1997;272(4 Pt 2):R1245–R1251.
58. Gibbs J, Young RC, Smith GP. Cholecystokinin elicits satiety in rats with open gastric fistulas. *Nature*. 1973;245(5424):323–325.
59. Baranowska B, Radzikowska M, Wasilewska-Dziubinska E, Roguski K, Borowiec M. Disturbed release of gastrointestinal peptides in anorexia nervosa and in obesity. *Diabetes, Obesity & Metabolism*. 2000;2(2):99–103.
60. Milewicz A, Bidzinska B, Mikulski E, Demissie M, Tworowska U. Influence of obesity and menopausal status on serum leptin, cholecystokinin, galanin and neuropeptide Y levels. *Gynecological Endocrinology: The Official Journal of the International Society of Gynecological Endocrinology*. 2000;14(3):196–203.
61. Matson CA, Wiater MF, Kuijper JL, Weigle DS. Synergy between leptin and cholecystokinin (CCK) to control daily caloric intake. *Peptides*. 1997;18(8):1275–1278.
62. Riedy CA, Chavez M, Figlewicz DP, Woods SC. Central insulin enhances sensitivity to cholecystokinin. *Physiology & Behavior*. 1995;58(4):755–760.
63. Kissileff HR, Pi-Sunyer FX, Thornton J, Smith GP. C-terminal octapeptide of cholecystokinin decreases food intake in man. *The American Journal of Clinical Nutrition*. 1981;34(2):154–160.
64. Bi S, Moran TH. Actions of CCK in the controls of food intake and body weight: Lessons from the CCK-A receptor deficient OLETF rat. *Neuropeptides*. 2002;36(2–3):171–181.

65. Crawley JN, Beinfeld MC. Rapid development of tolerance to the behavioural actions of cholecystokinin. *Nature*. 1983;302(5910):703–706.
66. Malaisse-Lagae F, Carpentier JL, Patel YC, Malaisse WJ, Orci L. Pancreatic polypeptide: A possible role in the regulation of food intake in the mouse. Hypothesis. *Experientia*. 1977;33(7):915–917.
67. Batterham RL, Le Roux CW, Cohen MA, Park AJ, Ellis SM, Patterson M et al. Pancreatic polypeptide reduces appetite and food intake in humans. *The Journal of Clinical Endocrinology and Metabolism*. 2003;88(8):3989–3992.
68. Parker RM, Herzog H. Regional distribution of Y-receptor subtype mRNAs in rat brain. *The European Journal of Neuroscience*. 1999;11(4):1431–1448.
69. Taylor IL, Impicciatore M, Carter DC, Walsh JH. Effect of atropine and vagotomy on pancreatic polypeptide response to a meal in dogs. *The American Journal of Physiology*. 1978;235(4):E443–E447.
70. Track NS, McLeod RS, Mee AV. Human pancreatic polypeptide: Studies of fasting and postprandial plasma concentrations. *Canadian Journal of Physiology and Pharmacology*. 1980;58(12):1484–1489.
71. Clark JT, Kalra PS, Crowley WR, Kalra SP. Neuropeptide Y and human pancreatic polypeptide stimulate feeding behavior in rats. *Endocrinology*. 1984;115(1):427–429.
72. Ueno N, Inui A, Iwamoto M, Kaga T, Asakawa A, Okita M et al. Decreased food intake and body weight in pancreatic polypeptide-overexpressing mice. *Gastroenterology*. 1999;117(6):1427–1432.
73. Asakawa A, Inui A, Yuzuriha H, Ueno N, Katsuura G, Fujimiya M et al. Characterization of the effects of pancreatic polypeptide in the regulation of energy balance. *Gastroenterology*. 2003;124(5):1325–1336.
74. Schmidt PT, Naslund E, Gryback P, Jacobsson H, Holst JJ, Hilsted L et al. A role for pancreatic polypeptide in the regulation of gastric emptying and short-term metabolic control. *The Journal of Clinical Endocrinology and Metabolism*. 2005;90(9):5241–5246.
75. Hazelwood RL. The pancreatic polypeptide (PP-fold) family: Gastrointestinal, vascular, and feeding behavioral implications. *Proceedings of the Society for Experimental Biology and Medicine Society for Experimental Biology and Medicine*. 1993;202(1):44–63.
76. Lieverse RJ, Masclee AA, Jansen JB, Lamers CB. Plasma cholecystokinin and pancreatic polypeptide secretion in response to bombesin, meal ingestion and modified sham feeding in lean and obese persons. *International Journal of Obesity and Related Metabolic Disorders*. 1994;18(2):123–127.
77. Fujimoto S, Inui A, Kiyota N, Seki W, Koide K, Takamiya S et al. Increased cholecystokinin and pancreatic polypeptide responses to a fat-rich meal in patients with restrictive but not bulimic anorexia nervosa. *Biological Psychiatry*. 1997;41(10):1068–1070.
78. Zipf WB, O'Dorisio TM, Cataland S, Dixon K. Pancreatic polypeptide responses to protein meal challenges in obese but otherwise normal children and obese children with Prader-Willi syndrome. *The Journal of Clinical Endocrinology and Metabolism*. 1983;57(5):1074–1080.
79. Berntson GG, Zipf WB, O'Dorisio TM, Hoffman JA, Chance RE. Pancreatic polypeptide infusions reduce food intake in Prader-Willi syndrome. *Peptides*. 1993;14(3):497–503.
80. Dhanvantari S, Seidah NG, Brubaker PL. Role of prohormone convertases in the tissue-specific processing of proglucagon. *Molecular Endocrinology*. 1996;10(4):342–355.
81. Herrmann C, Goke R, Richter G, Fehmann HC, Arnold R, Goke B. Glucagon-like peptide-1 and glucose-dependent insulin-releasing polypeptide plasma levels in response to nutrients. *Digestion*. 1995;56(2):117–126.
82. Shughrue PJ, Lane MV, Merchenthaler I. Glucagon-like peptide-1 receptor (GLP1-R) mRNA in the rat hypothalamus. *Endocrinology*. 1996;137(11):5159–5162.
83. Ding WG, Renstrom E, Rorsman P, Buschard K, Gromada J. Glucagon-like peptide I and glucose-dependent insulinotropic polypeptide stimulate Ca^{2+}-induced secretion in rat alpha-cells by a protein kinase A-mediated mechanism. *Diabetes*. 1997;46(5):792–800.
84. Abbott CR, Monteiro M, Small CJ, Sajedi A, Smith KL, Parkinson JR et al. The inhibitory effects of peripheral administration of peptide YY(3-36) and glucagon-like peptide-1 on food intake are attenuated by ablation of the vagal-brainstem-hypothalamic pathway. *Brain Research*. 2005;1044(1):127–131.
85. Turton MD, O'Shea D, Gunn I, Beak SA, Edwards CM, Meeran K et al. A role for glucagon-like peptide-1 in the central regulation of feeding. *Nature*. 1996;379(6560):69–72.
86. Willms B, Werner J, Holst JJ, Orskov C, Creutzfeldt W, Nauck MA. Gastric emptying, glucose responses, and insulin secretion after a liquid test meal: Effects of exogenous glucagon-like peptide-1 (GLP-1)-(7-36) amide in type 2 (noninsulin-dependent) diabetic patients. *The Journal of Clinical Endocrinology and Metabolism*. 1996;81(1):327–332.
87. Jendle J, Nauck MA, Matthews DR, Frid A, Hermansen K, During M et al. Weight loss with liraglutide, a once-daily human glucagon-like peptide-1 analogue for type 2 diabetes treatment as monotherapy or added to metformin, is primarily as a result of a reduction in fat tissue. *Diabetes, Obesity & Metabolism*. 2009;11(12):1163–1172.

88. Tomasik PJ, Sztefko K, Starzyk J. Cholecystokinin, glucose dependent insulinotropic peptide and glucagon-like peptide 1 secretion in children with anorexia nervosa and simple obesity. *Journal of Pediatric Endocrinology & Metabolism (JPEM)*. 2004;17(12):1623–1631.
89. Fonseca VA, Devries JH, Henry RR, Donsmark M, Thomsen HF, Plutzky J. Reductions in systolic blood pressure with liraglutide in patients with type 2 diabetes: Insights from a patient-level pooled analysis of six randomized clinical trials. *Journal of Diabetes and Its Complications*. 2014;28(3):399–405.
90. Plutzky J, Garber A, Falahati A, Toft AD, Poulter NR. Reductions in lipids and CV risk markers in patients with type 2 diabetes treated with liraglutide: A meta-analysis. *Canadian Journal of Diabetes*. 2009;33(3):209–210.
91. DeFronzo RA, Ratner RE, Han J, Kim DD, Fineman MS, Baron AD. Effects of exenatide (exendin-4) on glycemic control and weight over 30 weeks in metformin-treated patients with type 2 diabetes. *Diabetes Care*. 2005;28(5):1092–1100.
92. Pi-Sunyer X, Astrup A, Fujioka K, Greenway F, Halpern A, Krempf M et al. A randomized, controlled trial of 3.0 mg of liraglutide in weight management. *New England Journal of Medicine*. 2015;373(1):11–22.
93. Marso SP, Daniels GH, Brown-Frandsen K, Kristensen P, Mann JF, Nauck MA et al. Liraglutide and cardiovascular outcomes in type 2 diabetes. *The New England Journal of Medicine*. 2016;375(4): 311–322.
94. Ekblad E, Sundler F. Distribution of pancreatic polypeptide and peptide YY. *Peptides*. 2002;23(2):251–261.
95. Batterham RL, Heffron H, Kapoor S, Chivers JE, Chandarana K, Herzog H et al. Critical role for peptide YY in protein-mediated satiation and body-weight regulation. *Cell Metabolism*. 2006;4(3):223–233.
96. Batterham RL, Cowley MA, Small CJ, Herzog H, Cohen MA, Dakin CL et al. Gut hormone PYY(3-36) physiologically inhibits food intake. *Nature*. 2002;418(6898):650–654.
97. Batterham RL, Cohen MA, Ellis SM, Le Roux CW, Withers DJ, Frost GS et al. Inhibition of food intake in obese subjects by peptide YY3-36. *The New England Journal of Medicine*. 2003;349(10):941–948.
98. Misra M, Miller KK, Tsai P, Gallagher K, Lin A, Lee N et al. Elevated peptide YY levels in adolescent girls with anorexia nervosa. *The Journal of Clinical Endocrinology and Metabolism*. 2006;91(3):1027–1033.
99. Acuna-Goycolea C, van den Pol AN. Peptide YY(3-36) inhibits both anorexigenic proopiomelanocortin and orexigenic neuropeptide Y neurons: Implications for hypothalamic regulation of energy homeostasis. *The Journal of Neuroscience: The Official Journal of the Society for Neuroscience*. 2005;25(45):10510–10519.
100. Morley JE, Levine AS, Grace M, Kneip J. Peptide YY (PYY), a potent orexigenic agent. *Brain Research*. 1985;341(1):200–203.
101. Schepp W, Dehne K, Riedel T, Schmidtler J, Schaffer K, Classen M. Oxyntomodulin: A cAMP-dependent stimulus of rat parietal cell function via the receptor for glucagon-like peptide-1 (7-36)NH2. *Digestion*. 1996;57(6):398–405.
102. Dakin CL, Gunn I, Small CJ, Edwards CM, Hay DL, Smith DM et al. Oxyntomodulin inhibits food intake in the rat. *Endocrinology*. 2001;142(10):4244–4250.
103. Anini Y, Jarrousse C, Chariot J, Nagain C, Yanaihara N, Sasaki K et al. Oxyntomodulin inhibits pancreatic secretion through the nervous system in rats. *Pancreas*. 2000;20(4):348–360.
104. Read NW, McFarlane A, Kinsman RI, Bates TE, Blackhall NW, Farrar GB et al. Effect of infusion of nutrient solutions into the ileum on gastrointestinal transit and plasma levels of neurotensin and enteroglucagon. *Gastroenterology*. 1984;86(2):274–280.
105. Dakin CL, Small CJ, Batterham RL, Neary NM, Cohen MA, Patterson M et al. Peripheral oxyntomodulin reduces food intake and body weight gain in rats. *Endocrinology*. 2004;145(6):2687–2695.
106. Cohen MA, Ellis SM, Le Roux CW, Batterham RL, Park A, Patterson M et al. Oxyntomodulin suppresses appetite and reduces food intake in humans. *The Journal of Clinical Endocrinology and Metabolism*. 2003;88(10):4696–4701.
107. Druce MR, Minnion JS, Field BC, Patel SR, Shillito JC, Tilby M et al. Investigation of structure-activity relationships of Oxyntomodulin (Oxm) using Oxm analogs. *Endocrinology*. 2009;150(4):1712–1722.
108. Creutzfeldt W, Ebert R, Willms B, Frerichs H, Brown JC. Gastric inhibitory polypeptide (GIP) and insulin in obesity: Increased response to stimulation and defective feedback control of serum levels. *Diabetologia*. 1978;14(1):15–24.
109. Miyawaki K, Yamada Y, Ban N, Ihara Y, Tsukiyama K, Zhou H et al. Inhibition of gastric inhibitory polypeptide signaling prevents obesity. *Nature Medicine*. 2002;8(7):738–742.
110. Bailey RJ, Walker CS, Ferner AH, Loomes KM, Prijic G, Halim A et al. Pharmacological characterization of rat amylin receptors: Implications for the identification of amylin receptor subtypes. *British Journal of Pharmacology*. 2012;166(1):151–167.
111. Lutz TA, Geary N, Szabady MM, Del Prete E, Scharrer E. Amylin decreases meal size in rats. *Physiology & Behavior*. 1995;58(6):1197–1202.

112. Riediger T, Zuend D, Becskei C, Lutz TA. The anorectic hormone amylin contributes to feeding-related changes of neuronal activity in key structures of the gut-brain axis. *American Journal of Physiology Regulatory, Integrative and Comparative Physiology*. 2004;286(1):R114–R122.
113. Edelman S, Garg S, Frias J, Maggs D, Wang Y, Zhang B et al. A double-blind, placebo-controlled trial assessing pramlintide treatment in the setting of intensive insulin therapy in type 1 diabetes. *Diabetes Care*. 2006;29(10):2189–2195.
114. Riddle M, Frias J, Zhang B, Maier H, Brown C, Lutz K et al. Pramlintide improved glycemic control and reduced weight in patients with type 2 diabetes using basal insulin. *Diabetes Care*. 2007;30(11):2794–2799.
115. Spiller RC, Trotman IF, Higgins BE, Ghatei MA, Grimble GK, Lee YC et al. The ileal brake—Inhibitions of jejunal motility after ileal fat perfusion in man. *Gut*. 1984;25(4):365–374.
116. van Avesaat M, Troost FJ, Ripken D, Hendriks HF, Masclee AA. Ileal brake activation: Macronutrient-specific effects on eating behavior? *International Journal of Obesity*. 2015;39(2):235–243.
117. Eisen S, Davis JD, Rauhofer E, Smith GP. Gastric negative feedback produced by volume and nutrient during a meal in rats. *American Journal of Physiology Regulatory, Integrative and Comparative Physiology*. 2001;281(4):R1201–R1214.
118. Kral TV, Roe LS, Rolls BJ. Combined effects of energy density and portion size on energy intake in women. *American Journal of Clinical Nutrition*. 2004;79(6):962–968.
119. Sturm K, Parker B, Wishart J, Feinle-Bisset C, Jones KL, Chapman I et al. Energy intake and appetite are related to antral area in healthy young and older subjects. *American Journal of Clinical Nutrition*. 2004;80(3):656–667.
120. Korner J, Bessler M, Inabnet W, Taveras C, Holst JJ. Exaggerated glucagon-like peptide-1 and blunted glucose-dependent insulinotropic peptide secretion are associated with Roux-en-Y gastric bypass but not adjustable gastric banding. *Surgery for Obesity and Related Diseases: Official Journal of the American Society for Bariatric Surgery*. 2007;3(6):597–601.
121. Farooqi IS, Matarese G, Lord GM, Keogh JM, Lawrence E, Agwu C et al. Beneficial effects of leptin on obesity, T cell hyporesponsiveness, and neuroendocrine/metabolic dysfunction of human congenital leptin deficiency. *The Journal of Clinical Investigation*. 2002;110(8):1093–1103.
122. Oral EA, Simha V, Ruiz E, Andewelt A, Premkumar A, Snell P et al. Leptin-replacement therapy for lipodystrophy. *New England Journal of Medicine*. 2002;346(8):570–578.
123. Vazquez MJ, Gonzalez CR, Varela L, Lage R, Tovar S, Sangiao-Alvarellos S et al. Central resistin regulates hypothalamic and peripheral lipid metabolism in a nutritional-dependent fashion. *Endocrinology*. 2008;149(9):4534–4543.
124. Larsen TM, Dalskov SM, van Baak M, Jebb SA, Papadaki A, Pfeiffer AF et al. Diets with high or low protein content and glycemic index for weight-loss maintenance. *New England Journal of Medicine*. 2010;363(22):2102–2113.
125. Clifton PM, Condo D, Keogh JB. Long term weight maintenance after advice to consume low carbohydrate, higher protein diets—A systematic review and meta analysis. *Nutrition, Metabolism, and Cardiovascular Diseases (NMCD)*. 2014;24(3):224–235.
126. Belza A, Ritz C, Sorensen MQ, Holst JJ, Rehfeld JF, Astrup A. Contribution of gastroenteropancreatic appetite hormones to protein-induced satiety. *American Journal of Clinical Nutrition*. 2013;97(5):980–989.

2 Overeating Behavior and Cardiometabolic Health

Mechanisms and Treatments

Ashley E. Mason and Frederick M. Hecht

CONTENTS

ABSTRACT

Environmental and genetic factors are important influences on diet and its cardiometabolic effects, but overeating and unhealthy eating are ultimately malleable behaviors. Environmental- and individual-level factors are therefore key targets for intervention. In this chapter, we review current behavioral models of three types of overeating: *mindless overeating*, *stress-induced overeating*, and *compulsive overeating*. We define *mindless overeating* as overeating that occurs outside of one's awareness and without attention. We define *stress-induced overeating* as overeating that can occur with or without awareness in response to stress. We define *compulsive overeating* as eating that occurs with awareness and that typically involves (1) overeating of highly palatable foods for their hedonic properties, and (2) experiencing a loss of control over such eating. These forms of overeating can increase risk of metabolic syndrome. We review evidence that environmental interventions at both the institutional and individual levels can decrease overeating and improve cardiometabolic health. These interventions target food environments in which people make most of their food purchasing and consumption decisions and include workplaces, supermarkets, restaurants, and schools. Cognitive-behavioral intervention approaches, such as cognitive restructuring and self-monitoring of weight and food consumption, have been demonstrated effective in weight loss in the context of lifestyle interventions, such as the Diabetes Prevention Program, which typically employ a combination of such cognitive-behavioral approaches. Mindfulness-based interventions that target overeating by enhancing nonjudgmental awareness of eating behaviors and eating related to distressing emotions also hold promise, although more data are needed to better assess the effectiveness of these interventions. We conclude that current data support referral of individuals who are overweight or obese to high-quality behavioral intervention programs that include evidence-based components to promote improvements in cardiometabolic risk factors. In settings without high-quality group interventions, referral to a nutritionist with expertise in behavioral weight loss strategies may be helpful.

ABBREVIATIONS

ACTH	Adrenocorticotropic hormone
ADHD	Attention-deficit/hyperactivity disorder
ANS	Autonomic nervous system
BED	Binge eating disorder
BES	Binge eating scale
CBT	Cognitive behavioral therapy
CRH	Corticotropin-releasing hormone
DBT	Dialectical behavioral therapy
DSM-IV-TR	*Diagnostic and Statistical Manual for Mental Disorders*, 4th edition, Text-Revision
DSM-5	*Diagnostic and Statistical Manual for Mental Disorders*, 5th edition
GC	Glucocorticoid
HbA1C	Hemoglobin A1C
HDL	High-density lipoprotein
f-MRI	Functional magnetic resonance imaging
L-HPA	Limbic hypothalamic-pituitary-adrenocortical
LEARN	Lifestyle, Exercise, Attitudes, Relationships, Nutrition
MIDUS	Midlife in the United States
NAC	Nucleus accumbens
NHLBI	National Heart, Lung, and Blood Institute
SAM	Sympathetic-adrenal-medullary
TSST	Trier Social Stress Test
VTA	Ventral tegmental area
YFAS	Yale Food Addiction Scale

INTRODUCTION

As described throughout this volume, the qualities and quantities of food that people eat impact cardiovascular health via several complex and interactive metabolic processes. This chapter focuses on behavioral factors that promote overeating and intervention techniques that target these factors. We first review three types of overeating: *mindless overeating*, *stress-induced overeating*, and *compulsive overeating*. The modern food environment is replete with cues to eat and easy access to highly palatable foods, which generally contain high levels of sugar, salt, fat, caffeine, and/or flavor enhancers, and are typically highly processed (Gearhardt et al. 2011). Cues to eat such foods can operate outside of our awareness and powerfully impact how much we eat, resulting in *mindless overeating* (Wansink 2007). In the past three decades, increases in both psychosocial stress and weight among U.S. adults (Block et al. 2009) may reflect a situation in which some people overeat highly palatable foods to reduce psychological stress. Habitual *stress-induced overeating* may carry particular risk for abdominal adiposity (Dallman 2010), a key risk factor for poor cardiovascular outcomes (Ashwell, Gunn, and Gibson 2012; Carmienke et al. 2013). Finally, more than one-third of U.S. adults with obesity who seek weight-loss treatment self-report *compulsive overeating*, which involves overeating for the hedonic properties of food and experiencing a loss of control over one's eating (Davis and Carter 2009).

We then review behavioral intervention techniques that directly address the processes underlying each type of overeating. We first review environmental interventions at both the institutional and the individual level. Such interventions target food environments in which people make most of their food purchasing and consumption decisions, including the workplace, supermarkets, restaurants, and schools (Wansink and Chandon 2014). Next, we review cognitive-behavioral techniques commonly combined into intervention packages ("lifestyle interventions") for obesity. These techniques include cognitive restructuring, self-monitoring, and other practices rooted in the theoretical foundation of cognitive and cognitive behavioral therapy (CBT) (Beck 2011). We also review the CBTs specifically developed for pathological overeating as observed in binge eating disorder (BED). Finally, we review mindfulness-based interventions that target overeating by cultivating an open, nonjudgmental orientation toward present-moment experiences. This serves to disrupt habitual patterns of thoughts, emotions, and behaviors that underpin overeating by promoting awareness of bodily experiences related to physical hunger, satiety, taste satisfaction, and emotional triggers of overeating (Kristeller and Wolever 2010). We close this review with suggestions for future intervention development.

TYPES OF OVEREATING

Eighty-three percent of Americans report having overeaten, defined as eating more than one intends to eat at a given occasion, within the past 10 days (Wansink 2014). Overeating takes many forms; here, we outline three major types of overeating. We define *mindless overeating* as overeating that occurs outside of one's awareness and without attention. We define *stress-induced overeating* as overeating that can occur with or without awareness in response to stress (Adam and Epel 2007; Tsenkova, Boylan, and Ryff 2013). We define *compulsive overeating* as eating that occurs (1) with awareness and that involves overeating of (typically) highly palatable foods for their hedonic properties, and (2) experiencing a loss of control over such eating (Davis and Carter 2009). Next, we review these three types of overeating.

Mindless Overeating

Mindless overeating occurs in a myriad of settings, such as at the movie theater, while watching a baseball game, or when walking past a candy dish in the office for the tenth time. Indeed, people are unable to detect when they have eaten 15%–20% more or less than they typically do, and the modern food environment powerfully biases this margin of error toward overeating (Brownell and Horgen 2004). Consequently, people routinely underreport how much they eat: Pooled results from five validation studies of dietary self-report instruments indicate that people underreport caloric intake by as much as 28% and that greater body mass index (BMI) is associated with greater levels of underreporting (Freedman et al. 2014). These severe misperceptions of how much one has eaten make sense in light of the tremendous impacts of portion sizes, food proximity and visibility, ambient environments, palatability, distracted eating, and social influences, among other factors, on eating behavior.

Portion Size

Perception of portion size plays an important role in estimating how much food one is about to eat and how much food one has eaten. "Portion distortion," or the tendency to consider a portion to be smaller or less calorically dense than it actually is, can contribute to overeating and weight gain (Schwartz and Byrd-Bredbenner 2006). Although people tend to be more accurate when estimating small portion sizes, they routinely underestimate larger portion sizes by as much as 38% (Wansink and Chandon 2006). Doubling the size of a fast food hamburger or a product package makes it appear only 50%–70% larger (Chandon and Ordabayeva 2009). Unfortunately, simple knowledge of this effect does not reduce this misperception: Estimates by nutritionists and other diet experts are also affected by portion size cues. In one study, nutrition experts given a larger bowl, relative to those given a smaller bowl, served themselves 31% more ice cream (Wansink, van Ittersum, and Painter 2006b). The effects of packaging size on consumption effects exist beyond the impact of palatability: One study provided moviegoers with medium or large popcorn containers with fresh or stale, 14-day-old popcorn. Moviegoers given fresh popcorn in large containers ate 45% more than those given fresh popcorn in medium containers. Similarly, moviegoers given stale popcorn in large containers ate 33% more than those given stale popcorn in medium containers (Wansink and Kim 2005). Thus, portion size powerfully impacts how much people eat, regardless of expert knowledge of these effects and the palatability of the food being eaten.

Proximity and Visibility

Food proximity and visibility highly impacts the amount and frequency with which we eat (Sobal and Wansink 2007). In one classic study, researchers placed dishes of chocolates either within reaching distance (proximately) or 6 ft away (standing required for access) from where secretaries sat in their offices. Additionally, researchers placed the chocolates in clear dishes (highly visible) or opaque dishes (less visible). On days when the dishes were within reaching distance and clear, the secretaries ate 7.7 chocolates; on days when the dishes were within reaching distance and opaque, they ate 4.6 chocolates; on days when dishes were further away and clear, they ate 5.6 chocolates; and on days when dishes were further away and opaque, they ate 3.1 chocolates (Wansink, Painter, and Lee 2006a). Additionally, when the chocolates were within reaching distance, participants underestimated the amount of chocolates they had actually eaten. These effects have been replicated in several experimental studies (Sobal and Wansink 2007; Privitera and Creary 2013; Privitera and Zuraikat 2014). Thus, proximity and visibility each impact not only how much people eat, but also how much they believe they have eaten.

Ambient Factors

Environmental factors such as lighting, music, temperature, and odor can each impact the types and quantities of foods we eat outside of awareness (Stroebele and de Castro 2004; Spence 2012). For example, people dining in the harsh, bright lighting of fast-food restaurants consume more calories than when they dine in the soft, low lighting of fine dining restaurants (Wansink and van Ittersum 2012). Music loudness is also associated with consumption patterns: People tend to drink more soda (McCarron and Tierney 1989) and alcohol (Guéguen et al. 2008) when in conditions of loud background music. Studies report mixed associations between music and rate of eating that vary by type of music and/or music preference (Caldwell and Hibbert 2002). For example, the slower the tempo of country western music played in a bar, the more quickly patrons consume their drinks (Bach and Schaefer 1979). In contrast, the faster the tempo of piano music, the more time patrons spent drinking soda (McElrea and Standing 1992). Warmer ambient temperatures are associated with selection of less calorically dense food and reduced food intake overall, which may follow from reduced metabolic rates observed in warmer environs (Stroebele and de Castro 2004). For example, participants in a cafeteria study chose less calorically dense foods in the late spring and summer months relative to the fall and winter months (Zifferblatt, Wilbur, and Pinsky 1980). Finally, pleasant ambient odors can increase consumption, whereas noxious odors can decrease consumption: In one study, participants consumed more Pepsi Cola while watching a movie if they were exposed to a pleasant scent (air freshener) than if they were exposed to a noxious scent (ammonia; Wadhwa, Shiv, and Nowlis 2008). In sum, ambient factors such as lighting, music, temperature, and odor—that is, factors over which consumers have little control when eating outside of the home—can impact eating behavior outside of awareness.

Palatability

The modern food environment is replete with highly processed, highly palatable foods, and consumption of these foods can promote overeating (Sørensen et al. 2003; Gearhardt et al. 2011). For example, participants who sampled a sweet Hawaiian punch beverage before being allowed to drink as much Pepsi Cola ad libitum while watching a movie drank significantly more Pepsi Cola than those who did not sample the Hawaiian punch beforehand (Wadhwa, Shiv, and Nowlis 2008). These findings suggest that sampling highly palatable food cues stimulates subsequent consumption of similar palatable foods. Importantly, the amount of palatable food or drink that people consume correlates with their ratings of the food's palatability, but not with ratings of self-reported hunger (Yeomans 1996; Yeomans and Symes 1999). One study demonstrated this effect by adding highly palatable condiments to already highly palatable foods: Perceived palatability of highly palatable foods (French fries and brownies) decreased over time spent eating them; however, the addition of highly palatable condiments (mayonnaise and vanilla ice cream, respectively) led to renewed increases in perceived palatability and intake that were independent of self-reported hunger (Brondel et al. 2009). Thus, the innate satiety system does not regulate eating of highly palatable foods in ways that adjust consumption after caloric needs have been met; therefore, such hyperpalatability may increase overeating.

Categorization Cues and Health Halo Effects

Perceptions of foods as "healthy" and "unhealthy" significantly impact how much of them people eat. People often misinterpret specific health claims about foods (Mariotti et al. 2010). This contributes to the "health halo effect" whereby people overgeneralize or magnify a given food's healthful properties. Such halo effects can highly distort beliefs about caloric impact of a proposed snack or meal. For example, in one study, participants reported that a small snack of an unhealthy food (Snickers miniature candy, 47 calories) would promote more weight gain than a large snack of healthful foods (cottage cheese, carrots, and pears, 569 calories; Oakes 2005). Similarly, in another study, participants perceived a 1000-calorie meal from Subway to have 213 fewer calories than a 1000-calorie meal from McDonald's (Chandon and Wansink 2007). Importantly, these misperceptions correlate with actual intake: Participants ate 35% more oatmeal cookies when they were labeled as a "healthy snack" relative to when they were labeled as an "unhealthy snack" (Provencher, Polivy, and Herman 2009). Misperceptions of foods as more or less healthful can strongly impact overeating by focusing people's attention on perceived quality rather than measurable quantity.

Distracted Eating

Engaging in activities while eating, such as watching TV or listening to music, impacts eating. For example, people eat 12%–14% more food when they eat lunch while watching TV, and this increase in eating is not associated with commensurately larger changes in post-meal hunger or satiety (Bellisle, Dalix, and Slama 2004; Hetherington et al. 2006). Auditory distractions exert a similar effect: Listening to music (Stroebele and de Castro 2006) or a recorded story, such as a detective novel (Bellisle, Dalix, and Slama 2004), relative to eating in silence, is associated with longer time spent eating and greater caloric intake. Distracted eating can also promote greater eating throughout the day. This may follow from the distraction of attention away from a meal, which compromises the encoding of the memory of that meal. In one study, participants' abilities to accurately estimate the amount of food that they had eaten were significantly worse if they had eaten while watching TV rather than without watching TV (Moray et al. 2007). Poorer memory of a recent meal due to distracted eating has been linked with greater subsequent snacking: For example, in one study, women ate lunch while watching TV on one day and ate lunch without distraction on another day. On both days, women were offered cookies upon returning to the laboratory later in the day. Women ate significantly more cookies on the day they had eaten lunch while watching TV relative to the day they ate lunch without distraction (Higgs and Woodward 2009). In contrast, enhancing memory of a recent meal before an opportunity for an afternoon snack decreases snack consumption (Higgs 2002). Thus, engaging in activities that distract one's attention away from his or her food can contribute to overeating both at that time, and at later times, suggesting that distracted eating may have a broader impact on overeating than is typically considered.

Social Influences

Social factors impact the amount of food that people eat (Herman 2015). Two types of social influences on eating behavior are referred to as *social facilitation* and *social matching*, which are theorized to impact eating behavior via different mechanisms. Social facilitation of eating refers to the observation that people tend to eat more and for a longer period of time when with other people than when alone. This effect is commensurate with the size of the group and the relationship with other diners: Dining with a larger group of people and/or dining with people with whom one is closer (e.g., friends and family) is associated with eating more. Such increases in intake, which range from approximately 30%–50% (Herman and Polivy 2005), may be due to increased arousal or emotionality, disinhibition, distraction from consumption monitoring, or longer meal times (Herman, Roth, and Polivy 2003; Hetherington et al. 2006; Pliner et al. 2006).

Social matching of eating refers to the tendency for people to eat more when their dining partners eat more, and less when their dining partners eat less. Researchers theorize that the desire for social acceptance, ingratiation concerns, appropriateness, perceived eating norms, and nonconscious mimicry can play important roles in this phenomenon (Herman et al. 2005; Robinson et al. 2011; Robinson, Blissett, and Higgs 2013). For example, eating behavior is one important avenue of impression management (Vartanian, Herman, and Polivy 2007), which involves regulating one's own behavior so as to create a specific image for an external audience (Schlenker 1980). Along these lines, people may undereat or overeat, or may mimic actual eating behavior, so as to gain favor with their dining partners (Salvy et al. 2007). One early study of this phenomenon examined eating of crackers among obese and normal-weight people when in the presence of a confederate who ate many crackers (20 crackers in 20 minutes), few crackers (1 cracker in 20 minutes), or no crackers. All participants ate significantly more crackers when with a confederate who ate many crackers relative to when with a confederate who ate few crackers (Conger et al. 1980), suggesting mimicry of quantity eaten. Many experimental studies have replicated these findings (Herman, Roth, and Polivy 2003; Robinson, Blissett, and Higgs 2013). Recent data have further dissected social matching behavior and found that people tend to mimic the timing of each other's bites of food (Hermans et al. 2012) and that desire for social acceptance predicts the degree of mimicry when consuming alcoholic beverages (Caudill and Kong 2001). In summary, social factors impact the amount of food people eat, suggesting that improving eating behavior among some individuals holds the potential to impact many.

Stress-Induced Overeating

There is considerable overlap among the neurobiological systems that regulate food intake and those that mediate stress responses (Dallman 2010; Sinha and Jastreboff 2013). Acute, isolated stressors and chronic, ongoing stressors impact eating behavior in both animals and humans (Macht 2008). Rodent studies report increased eating of highly palatable food, especially foods high in sugar, after standard laboratory stressors (e.g., restraining; Dallman, Pecoraro, and la Fleur 2005; Foster et al. 2009). Human studies also report increased eating of highly palatable "comfort foods" after standard laboratory stressors (e.g., social performance tasks; Oliver, Wardle, and Gibson 2000; Epel et al. 2001; Rutters et al. 2009; Lemmens et al. 2011). In the following text, we review neurobiological mechanisms of stress-induced overeating, studies of stress-induced overeating in humans, and the effects of stress-induced eating on cardiometabolic health. We refer the reader interested in animal models of stress-induced overeating to reviews on the topic (Corwin and Buda-Levin 2004; Corwin, Avena, and Boggiano 2011).

Neurobiological Mechanisms Linking Stress and Overeating

Stress responses involve a neural network comprised of neurons in the hypothalamus, brainstem, and afferent nerves, as well as several areas within the limbic system and frontal cortex (Kaltsas and Chrousos 2007). Stress responses operate along two interacting pathways. One pathway is the sympathetic-adrenal-medullary (SAM) axis, which is a part of the autonomic nervous system (ANS) that involves the catecholamines adrenaline and noradrenaline. A second pathway is the limbic hypothalamic-pituitary-adrenocortical (L-HPA) axis, which produces a cascade of hormone secretions that comprise an endocrine stress response. These hormones include corticotropin-releasing hormone, adrenocorticotropic hormone, and glucocorticoids (GCs; Herman and Cullinan 1997; McEwen 2007). Chronic arousal of the L-HPA axis leads to dysregulation in physiological satiety mechanisms, which can result in stress-induced overeating. Specifically, although GCs increase the hormones leptin and insulin, which signal satiety, these increases promote insulin and leptin resistance, which can blunt satiety signaling, thereby leading to overeating (Maniam and Morris 2012). Researchers have therefore widely examined L-HPA axis activity in the context of cardiometabolic health (e.g., visceral adiposity) and found the L-HPA axis to play critical roles in the neural regulation of eating and peripheral energy balance (Kyrou, Chrousos, and Tsigos 2006; Sinha and Jastreboff 2013).

In addition to disrupting the regulation of the physiological satiety mechanisms that regulate energy homeostasis, stress-induced L-HPA activity impacts the mesolimbic reward area, which is highly innervated by dopaminergic neurons. The effects of L-HPA activity in the mesolimbic reward area can render the experience of eating highly palatable foods especially rewarding, therefore encouraging overeating in times of stress. For example, functional magnetic resonance imaging data show that upon viewing images of highly palatable food, individuals who report greater chronic stress showed exaggerated activity in regions of the brain involving reward, motivation, and habitual decision-making, as well as reduced activity in areas linked to strategic planning and emotional control (Tryon et al. 2013). Furthermore, these chronically stressed individuals also ate significantly more highly palatable food from a buffet than their less-stressed counterparts after an acute laboratory stressor.

L-HPA axis activity also amplifies neural experiences of reward by stimulating the release of endogenous opioids, which increase eating of highly palatable food and instigate further opioid release. Specifically, stress-induced eating stimulates (1) increases in GCs and insulin that then drive intake of palatable food, (2) increases in opioid release, which reinforce and promote intake of these palatable foods, and (3) increases in dopamine secretion in the mesolimbic pathway, including the ventral tegmental area and nucleus accumbens, which amplify the neural experience of reward that follows from eating of highly palatable food (Adam and Epel 2007; Dallman and Bhatnagar 2010).

The neural stress-reward pathways promote the development of habitual behavior focused on obtaining relief. Repeated and strong opioid responses in the neural circuitry of reward promote the encoding of habits in the limbic system, specifically the basal ganglia, which regulates habit-based behavior. The limbic system is especially likely to encode memories involving strong emotions and the solutions that people use to effectively cope with them. Thus, stress-induced overeating of hyperpalatable food, which effectively reduces stress responses, is easily learned, remembered, and repeated (Dallman 2010; Ulrich-Lai et al. 2015).

Studies of Stress-Induced Overeating in Humans

Researchers have used experimental methods and naturalistic settings to study the biology and behavioral patterns of stress-induced eating in humans. One laboratory study examined the impact of repeated (daily) exogenous administration of GC or placebo on food intake over the course of several days. Participants ate ad libitum from an automated food selection system that tracked their intake both prior to and on the days of administration of GC or placebo. The GC participants' increase in caloric intake from Day 0 to Day 4 (total) was >1600 calories more than the placebo participants' increase in caloric intake. Another laboratory study used a standard acute psychological stressor task, the Trier Social Stress Test (TSST), to examine the extent to which acute psychological stress impacts immediate post-stress eating behavior through GC changes. Results indicated that women with larger increases in GC (salivary cortisol levels) following the TSST ate more total calories and more sweet foods (after the TSST) than women with smaller increases in GC (Epel et al. 2001). In another study, participants completed a TSST task in the laboratory, and researchers assessed their GC responses (assessed using saliva). Researchers then collected participants' self-reported daily hassles (real-life stressors) and snack intake for the following 2 weeks. Data showed that among participants with larger increases in GCs following the TSST (but not among participants with smaller increases in GCs), greater frequency of daily hassles was associated with more frequent snacking (Newman, O'Connor, and Conner 2007). Thus, data indicate that increases in a marker of physiological stress (GC), induced either via exogenous administration or psychological stressor techniques, are associated with increased eating.

Stress-Induced Overeating and Cardiometabolic Health

Researchers have found direct links between stress-induced overeating and cardiometabolic outcomes. For example, in an observational cohort study, 81 of 131 (62%) medical students self-reported on their eating behavior in times of stress. Forty-seven of these 81 students (58%) reported eating more than usual in times of stress ("more-eaters") and 34 students (42%) reported eating less than usual in times of stress ("less-eaters"). Researchers assessed traditional biomarkers of students' metabolic health (e.g., insulin, lipids, BMI, and waist-to-hip ratio [WHR]) and nocturnal cortisol levels (assessed using urine) during a low-stress period (summer vacation) and also during a high-stress period (final exams). Relative to those eating less, those eating more evidenced significantly greater increases in nocturnal cortisol, total/high-density lipoprotein (HDL) cholesterol ratio, weight (~5 lb), and WHR (but only among women) from low- to high-stress periods (Epel et al. 2004). Population-level data also highlight the impact of stress-induced eating on metabolic health: The Midlife in the United States (MIDUS II) study asked participants how they usually experience a stressful event and to indicate the extent to which they (1) tend to eat more of their favorite foods to make themselves feel better, and (2) tend to eat more than they usually do. Higher scores on these items (i.e., endorsing eating more of one's favorite foods and eating more than usual) were associated with significantly higher levels of glucose, insulin, insulin resistance, and HbA1C, as well as higher odds of developing prediabetes and diabetes. After adjusting for waist circumference, these associations were no longer statistically significant, suggesting that stress-induced overeating may be an important mediator of the association between visceral adiposity and cardiometabolic risk (Tsenkova, Boylan, and Ryff 2013). Taken together, these studies suggest that stress-induced eating is associated with elevated glucose levels and insulin resistance, with the effects occurring largely through weight gain and central adiposity.

Compulsive Overeating

At least 30% of treatment-seeking obese individuals identify times when they feel out of control over their eating and when they overeat highly palatable food in the absence of physical hunger, regardless of a desire to not do so (Spitzer et al. 1992; de Zwaan 2001). Such compulsive overeating has behavioral similarities to drug addiction (e.g., Volkow et al. 2012, 2013). Researchers have thus designed self-report measures to assess behaviors that are core features of substance misuse disorders, but in the context of overeating. One measure, the Yale Food Addiction Scale (YFAS; Gearhardt, Corbin, and Brownell 2016, 2009), conceptualizes problematic eating behavior similarly to traditional substance-related and addictive disorders as defined by criteria in the Diagnostic and Statistical Manuals for Mental Disorders (DSM-IV-TR, DSM-5; American Psychological Association 2000; American Psychological Association 2013). Another measure, the Binge Eating Scale (BES, Gormally et al. 1982), assesses compulsive overeating behavior, and scores on this measure correlate with a DSM diagnosis of BED (Celio et al. 2004; Grupski et al. 2012). Measures of addictive-like eating, such as the YFAS, are highly correlated with measures of binge eating, such as the BES (Flint et al. 2014). Compulsive overeating might best be considered along a continuum, with the most extreme end encompassing severe overeating indexed by high scores on measures of binge and addictive-like overeating (Davis 2013a,b). In the following text, we review neurobiological mechanisms of compulsive overeating, investigations of compulsive overeating in animals and humans, and associations between compulsive eating and cardiometabolic health.

Neurobiological Mechanisms Underlying Compulsive Overeating

Food and drug reward activate pathways in the same neural structures in the brain, and researchers have thus posited neurobiological models of binge eating that parallel those of addictive processes (Volkow et al. 2012, 2013; Smith and Robbins 2013). Similar to processes of addiction, the dopamine and opioid systems play key roles in compulsive behavior (e.g., overeating) by motivating reward-seeking behavior and mediating the neural perception of hedonic reward, respectively (Avena, Rada, and Hoebel 2008; Volkow et al. 2008; Davis et al. 2009). Compulsive overeating, both in animals and humans, generally involves overeating of highly palatable foods, which exert physiologic effects that suggest addictive potential (Gearhardt et al. 2011). For example, eating highly palatable foods activates dopaminergic neurons and increases μ-opioid receptor binding within the nucleus accumbens and other reward centers in the brain (Nathan and Bullmore 2009; Volkow, Wang, and Baler 2011). Repeated stimulation of the neural reward system can alter dopamine and opioid receptor binding in ways that promote addictive behavior (Colantuoni et al. 2001; Rada, Avena, and Hoebel 2005; Koob and Volkow 2009). The combination of genetic factors and environmental exposures that encourage consumption of highly palatable foods may thus converge to reinforce neural circuitry that drives compulsive overeating in susceptible individuals.

One method of studying neurobiological models of compulsive overeating is to administer intermittent feeding schedules to rodents to condition binge eating. These schedules involve intermittent access to highly palatable foods, such as sugar/fat and "cafeteria diets" generally comprised of processed snacks and desserts (Heyne et al. 2009; Corwin, Avena, and Boggiano 2011). Researchers then examine rodents' behavior in experimental paradigms traditionally used to test models of drug addiction (Avena 2010). Such paradigms induce behaviors and symptoms such as bingeing and tolerance (increases in amount and frequency of substance use over time), withdrawal (behavioral symptoms induced by removal of substance or pharmacologic blockade of neural effects of substance), and craving (enhanced responding to cues and increased motivation to work for substance after removal of substance), among others (Davis 2013a). Following binge eating of highly palatable food, rodents administered the opioidergic antagonist naloxone show symptoms similar to those observed during withdrawal from addictive drugs (e.g., heroin), such as aggression, anxiety, teeth-chattering, and head-shaking (Colantuoni et al. 2002). Notably, greater self-reported compulsive overeating among humans is associated with larger nausea and GC responses following administration of naloxone (Daubenmier et al. 2014; Mason et al. 2016). Conversely, administration of an opioid agonist (butorphanol) increases overeating of highly palatable food (Boggiano et al. 2005), and rodents prone to binge eating tolerate significant discomfort in the pursuit of highly palatable food, such as higher levels of foot shock in order to access Oreo cookies (Oswald et al. 2011). Similarly, rodents formerly administered an intermittent sugar-feeding schedule work harder to obtain sugar after a two-week period of abstinence than they ever did before, and the amount of work that they will do to obtain the sugar increases over time (Grimm, Fyall, and Osincup 2005).

Finally, there is evidence that sugar intake cross-sensitizes with addictive drugs, and vice versa (Avena and Hoebel 2003; Avena, Rada, and Hoebel 2008). Thus, animal models have shed light on behavioral and biological overlaps between compulsive overeating of highly palatable food and drug addiction; clarification of these overlaps can inform intervention development.

There is evidence that compulsive overeating is a specific phenotype within human obesity that is characterized by biological and behavioral characteristics (Davis et al. 2011; Burmeister et al. 2013). Obese individuals who meet the YFAS diagnostic criteria for food addiction (relative to their obese counterparts who do not) self-report and show behavioral and psychological profiles similar to those observed among individuals with drug addictions. For example, individuals meeting YFAS criteria for food addiction score more highly on measures of impulsivity and emotional reactivity. They are also significantly more likely to meet criteria for a diagnosis of BED, severe depression, and attention-deficit/hyperactivity disorder (ADHD); to have more addictive personality traits; to experience stronger food cravings; and to more frequently snack on sweet foods and eat in response to emotions (Davis et al. 2011). These individuals also endorse greater sensitivity to the rewarding properties of hyperpalatable food, which aligns with research linking greater sensitivity to reward with greater binge eating (Davis et al. 2007; Mathes et al. 2009). This enhanced sensitivity to reward has been associated with genetic polymorphisms that (1) influence dopamine receptor binding in ways that increase motivation to engage in appetitive behavior, and (2) affect opioid receptors in ways that increase reactivity to the hedonic properties of food (Davis et al. 2009, 2012). Importantly, greater food addiction severity, as indexed by continuous scoring of the YFAS, is associated with poorer adherence to, and effectiveness of, behavioral weight-loss interventions (Burmeister et al. 2013).

Compulsive Overeating and Cardiometabolic Health

Compulsive overeating, defined in terms of BED or food addiction, carries nontrivial cardiometabolic health risks (Hudson et al. 2010; Abraham et al. 2014; Klatzkin et al. 2015). For example, obese individuals who report compulsive overeating, relative to those who do not, experience more weight cycling (de Zwaan, Engeli, and Müller 2015) and are at greater risk for hypertension (Schulz et al. 2005; Hudson et al. 2010), dyslipidemia (Hudson et al. 2010), poor glycemic control, and type 2 diabetes (Hudson et al. 2010; Abraham et al. 2014; Raevuori et al. 2015), all of which increase risk for poor cardiovascular outcomes (DeFronzo and Ferrannini 1991).

BEHAVIORAL INTERVENTIONS FOR OVEREATING

Standard behavioral treatments that target reductions in overeating in the service of weight loss typically involve dietary changes and behavioral intervention techniques to support these changes (Bray and Bouchard 2014). Genetic predispositions, family and cultural backgrounds, and a host of other factors impact weight status; however, the primary targets of behavioral interventions are environmental factors and patterns of learned behavior that impact eating. In the following text, we review behavioral (nonpharmacologic) interventions that target overeating, including environmental approaches, approaches based on and incorporating CBT techniques (e.g., "lifestyle interventions"), and both independent and combination mindfulness approaches.

Environmental Approaches

The proliferation of environmental barriers to healthy eating highlights the relevance of interventions that directly address these barriers (Brownell and Horgen 2004; Wansink and Chandon 2014). Environmental interventions are rooted in behavioral principles (e.g., conditioning and stimulus control) and have been a centerpiece of interventions targeting overeating since the 1960s (e.g., Stuart 1967). Classical conditioning principles hold that repeatedly presenting a stimulus prior to (or simultaneously with) a given behavior will associate that stimulus with that behavior. For example, repeatedly purchasing chocolates from a convenience store may stoke cravings for chocolates whenever one walks by the convenience store on the way to work. In this context, stimulus control involves the management of cues that are associated with overeating, such as walking a different way to and from work to avoid a cue to purchase and eat chocolates (Wadden, Crerand, and Brock 2005). Thus, behavioral principles form the basis of environmental approaches targeting reductions in overeating.

Large-scale changes to the food environment, such as decreasing the availability and portion sizes of highly palatable foods, and increasing the attractiveness, availability, and affordability of healthier alternatives, will require considerable time and other resources. Researchers have therefore emphasized methods by which (1) institutions can implement changes in financially feasible ways (Wansink 2014) and (2) individuals can modify their personal food environments (Lowe 2003). The *food radius* (Wansink 2014), defined as the five areas where people purchase or consume their food approximately 80% of the time, includes the home, supermarkets, restaurants, work, and, if applicable, school. In the following text, we review environmental interventions in the five food radius areas within the institutional and individual levels.

Institutional-Level Environmental Interventions

One environmental approach to reducing overeating involves implementing policies or practices at the institutional level. Such interventions strive to increase consumption of healthy foods by increasing the availability, accessibility, and/or attractiveness of these foods. These interventions have been tested across several types of institutions, including the workplace (Pratt et al. 2007), retailers (e.g., Glanz, Bader, and Iyer 2012), schools (e.g., Hanks, Just, and Wansink 2013), and restaurants (e.g., Wansink, van Ittersum, and Painter 2005). In the following text, we describe applications of environmental interventions tested in these settings and data on the effects of such interventions on cardiometabolic outcomes.

When given the option to select smaller portions of food in workplace and supermarket settings, people do choose this option (Vermeer et al. 2011); thus, providing smaller-sized options can reduce consumption. Preference for smaller portions may be fueled by widespread dissemination of research findings (in the lay press) showing that people eat dramatically more food when eating from larger versus smaller plates or containers (e.g., Leonhardt 2007). Indeed, workers purchase price-adjusted smaller versions of standard dishes (approximately $^2/_3$ of the standard option available) when offered the opportunity (Vermeer et al. 2011). Retailers have capitalized on consumer preferences by developing single-serving packages of snack foods, such as the 100-calorie package, which can reduce consumption by as much as 25% (Wansink, Payne, and Shimizu 2011).

Product placement in supermarkets can also dramatically impact purchasing behavior and therefore eating behavior. Approximately 30% of all supermarket sales result from end-aisle displays (Cohen et al. 2014) and placing potato chips at eye level, rather than higher or lower, is associated with more purchases (Sigurdsson, Saevarsson, and Foxall 2009). Replacing unhealthy items typically found at checkout stations (e.g., candy) with healthier options (e.g., dried fruit and nuts) increases purchasing of the healthy options at checkout stations (Sigurdsson, Larsen, and Gunnarsson 2014). In response to these data and customer complaints (e.g., children asking for candy placed at their eye level in checkout stations), some food retailers, such as Lidl and Tesco (the United Kingdom's largest retailer), have removed candy from checkout stations (Smithers 2014). These broad types of structural changes can benefit customers by reducing the constant burden of coping with environmental cues to purchase hyperpalatable foods at checkout stations, without compromising retailers' sales of food items (e.g., healthier snack foods, such as nuts).

Similar environmental effects can dramatically impact children's and adolescents' eating behavior in schools and adults' eating behavior in restaurants. High school students given the option to use a "convenience line" in the cafeteria that included only healthier foods (e.g., salad bar, whole fruits and vegetables), in addition to a standard line that offered less healthy foods (e.g., tacos, hamburgers), choose and eat different types and quantities of foods compared to when only offered a standard line. In one study, inclusion of the option to use this type of convenience line led to a 27.3% reduction in actual eating of less healthy foods (Hanks et al. 2012). Similarly, middle school cafeterias selling apples presliced rather than in whole form increased apple purchases by 71%, and students offered sliced apples ate more than half of their purchase (73%), whereas students offered whole apples ate less (48%; Wansink et al. 2013). Increasing attractiveness of healthy options also impacts eating behavior. Elementary school cafeterias that assigned attractive, fun names to healthier food options (e.g., X-ray Vision Carrots) led elementary students to eat twice the percentage of their carrots relative to when cafeterias assigned these foods generic names (e.g., Food of the Day; Wansink et al. 2012). Additionally, people selecting food from a buffet line take more of the foods offered earlier in the line. Thus, placing healthier options at the beginning of the line can dramatically impact food selection (Wansink and Hanks 2013). Similarly, restaurants that use descriptive menu labeling can dramatically increase sales (Wansink, Painter, and Van Ittersum 2001) as well as patron satisfaction. Restaurant patrons who ordered and consumed meals from a menu with evocative, descriptive item descriptions (e.g., "Succulent Italian Seafood Filet"), relative to those who ordered from a generic menu (e.g., "Seafood Filet"), reported their food to be more attractive and tasty, and also estimated that they had eaten more calories and reported feeling more full and satisfied. Thus, restaurants and cafeterias can capitalize on these effects to help patrons make healthier choices while also enhancing patron satisfaction.

Individual-Level Environmental Interventions

Interventionists have begun to test environmental adaptations as standalone interventions for weight loss. In the literature, such interventions have been termed "small-change" interventions (e.g., Phillips-Caesar et al. 2015) and designed to foster small, minimally burdensome changes in one's environment or interaction with one's environment. Such interventions have been administered in-person, via telephone, and over the Internet (Carels et al. 2008; Wansink 2010; Kaipainen, Payne, and Wansink 2012). They have also been adapted into guided self-help formats published in widely available books, such as *Mindless Overeating: Why We Eat More Than We Think* (Wansink 2007) and *Slim by Design* (Wansink 2014). In addition to their standalone interventions, small-change environmental adaptations have been investigated as adjuvant techniques to promote weight-loss maintenance following traditional cognitive-behavioral (lifestyle) interventions. In the following text, we review investigations of environmental interventions each as standalone and adjuvant interventions and their effects on weight loss.

Trials comparing environmental interventions and traditional CBT lifestyle interventions for weight-loss suggest that environmental interventions may be effective ways for individuals seeking alternatives to traditional CBT-based lifestyle interventions. In one study, overweight and obese participants were randomized to receive an in-person, 14-week environmental intervention (Carels et al. 2009) or an in-person, 14-week course of the LEARN (*L*ifestyle, *E*xercise, *A*ttitudes, *R*elationships, *N*utrition) program (Brownell 2004). All participants self-monitored their dietary intake throughout the study period. The LEARN program is a traditional CBT-based lifestyle intervention that targets changes in the domains of eating behavior and physical activity, as well as building and strengthening psychological tools to work with one's attitudes, goals, and emotions. The environmental intervention in this study focused on adapting one's food environments, including convenience, serving sizes, and cue exposure, among others. Participants in both groups experienced significant weight loss (approximately 8.6 lb [3.9 kg]) from pre- to post-intervention; however, both groups also experienced weight regain (approximately 3.3 lb [1.5 kg]) from postintervention to 6-month follow-up (Carels et al. 2011). These data suggest that the environmental intervention was as effective as the lifestyle intervention. Further data is needed to help identify which approach may work best for different people.

The incorporation of environmental interventions as maintenance-oriented interventions that follow traditional CBT-based lifestyle interventions may bolster the benefits of existing behavioral weight-loss interventions. In one study, overweight or obese participants received a 16-week course of the LEARN program, and then were randomized to receive (or not) a 6-week intervention focused on changing their food environments, such as the home kitchen and how they eat in restaurants. Participants experienced similar weight loss during the LEARN program; however, participants randomized to receive the post-LEARN 6-week intervention (relative to control) evidenced significantly greater weight loss, percent of body weight loss, and body fat reduction from baseline through the 6-month follow-up period (Carels et al. 2008). Researchers have yet to investigate the effects of providing environmental interventions prior to other interventions, which may prove especially beneficial. Other investigations have found that teaching weight-loss maintenance skills (e.g., learning about energy balance principles and fine-tuning lifestyle habits by making quick, small, and easy adjustments that do not require effort and attention) prior to introducing a phase of acute weight loss is associated with better long-term weight-loss maintenance (Kiernan et al. 2013).

Studies of environmental interventions underscore that personalizing intervention components to fit individuals' cultural, lifestyle, and otherwise personal preferences is critical for promoting intervention acceptability (e.g., Phillips-Caesar et al. 2015). For example, environmental adaptations and techniques that participants rate as "easy" garner greater adherence, suggesting that personalizing such techniques is needed to maximize participant retention and long-term behavior change (Wansink 2010; Kaipainen, Payne, and Wansink 2012).

Environmental Interventions and Cardiometabolic Outcomes

Though selected trials have examined the impact of environmental interventions on weight loss as reviewed earlier, the majority of studies that have incorporated environmental intervention techniques have done so in the context of larger institution-wide initiatives to improve employee health. The National Heart, Lung, and Blood Institute developed the Obesity Prevention in the Worksite initiative in 2004, which took a population-based approach to promoting behavior change through environmental interventions targeting prevention and control of weight gain (for a review of funded trials, see Pratt et al. 2007). The trials completed under this initiative generally included a variety of environmental intervention techniques that targeted behavior related to both eating and physical activity. Hence, it is difficult to parse the extent to which weight loss outcomes are attributable to environmental intervention components directed at eating versus other intervention components targeting physical activity. Nevertheless, these interventions have begun to report promising results. For example, the Images of a Healthy Worksite group-randomized trial (Fernandez et al. 2015) reported on 3799 employees assessed at baseline and post-intervention (2 years) at 10 worksites. There were statistically significant differences between control (3.3% increase in percentage of overweight or obese workers) and intervention (4.5% decrease in percentage of overweight or obese workers) worksites. Thus, intervening on the food environments in places where individuals do not control options available to them (e.g., workplace and schools) is a promising way to impact eating behavior.

Cognitive-Behavioral Approaches

Behavioral approaches to reduce overeating are predicated on a core assumption of social learning theory (Bandura and McClelland 1977), which is that health behaviors such as healthy eating and exercise constitute learned behaviors that can be modified. In the following text, we review cognitive-behavioral techniques commonly packaged into "lifestyle interventions" that target weight loss through eating behavior change.

Cognitive Restructuring

The cognitive model holds that dysfunctional or distorted thoughts are key determinants of mood and behavior (Beck 2011). For example, the thought "I'm a failure because I ate a cookie today" can lead to feelings of guilt and sadness, which may precipitate relief-seeking in reactive, generally maladaptive ways (e.g., eating more cookies), thus reinstating the feedback loop. There are several types of dysfunctional or distorted thoughts that are problematic for individuals struggling with overeating, such as all-or-nothing and catastrophic thinking (e.g., "I've had one bite so I might as well eat the entire pint of ice cream"), labeling (e.g., "I'm a failure because I ate one cookie"), and "should" and "must" statements (e.g., "I should only eat steamed vegetables for all meals"; for a review of thought distortions, see Greenberger and Padesky 1995). Cognitive restructuring is a core cognitive-behavioral technique and first involves the identification of (1) a maladaptive thought, (2) the feelings that follow from the thought, and (3) evidence for and against the thought. Individuals then use this information to develop alternative, adaptive thoughts (Beck 2011). Cognitive restructuring can therefore be used to uncover cognitive drivers of overeating by targeting maladaptive thoughts that lead to a cascade of negative mood and maladaptive behaviors that serve to reinforce problematic eating behavior. Indeed, in the context of treatment for overeating, interventions that include cognitive restructuring can increase self-efficacy (e.g., Wolff and Clark 2001), which predicts greater weight loss (Warziski et al. 2007).

Self-Monitoring

Self-monitoring, or deliberately attending to some aspect of one's behavior and recording details of the behavior, has been examined as both a cornerstone of lifestyle interventions and a standalone lifestyle intervention for weight loss (Burke, Wang, and Sevick 2011). The theoretical basis for self-monitoring is rooted in self-regulation theory (Kanfer 1970; Kanfer and Gaelick-Buys 1991), which posits that self-monitoring must occur before it is possible to evaluate progress toward a goal (self-evaluation). Such self-evaluation is what provides the self-reinforcement needed to maintain progress toward a goal. Truthful, consistent, and accurate self-monitoring is therefore needed for effective self-regulation of a given behavior (e.g., weight loss; Burke et al. 2008, 2012).

Self-monitoring of diet (dietary self-monitoring) directly targets mindless eating by increasing awareness of what, when, how much, and potentially where individuals are eating. A recent review of 15 studies testing the effects of dietary self-monitoring on weight loss found that more frequent or complete dietary self-monitoring records were associated with greater weight loss (Burke, Wang, and Sevick 2011). Dietary self-monitoring practices are highly conducive to mobile platforms, which can dramatically reduce burden associated with paper-and-pencil methods (Khaylis et al. 2010; Raaijmakers et al. 2015). This reduced burden may promote sustained dietary self-monitoring, as evidenced by data showing that mobile self-monitoring tools can lead to more consistent and longer-term self-monitoring than paper-and-pencil methods (Burke et al. 2012; Wharton et al. 2014). Importantly, such longer-term dietary self-monitoring is associated with long-term weight-loss maintenance (Klem et al. 1997); hence, further investigation of how to optimize long-term adherence to mobile dietary self-monitoring interventions is warranted (Turner-McGrievy et al. 2013).

Goal Setting and Goal Striving

Setting and striving toward goals, which are mental representations of desired end states to which people are committed (Fishbach and Ferguson 2007), are common components of lifestyle interventions. After setting goals related to eating behavior (e.g., eating fewer desserts) or consequences that follow from eating behavior (e.g., weight change), individuals engage in goal striving strategies that reduce the intention–behavior gap (Sheeran 2002) and bring them closer to their goals.

Goal setting involves determining which goal to pursue and the criteria to evaluate whether one has achieved the goal. There are several characteristics of goals that are particularly relevant to health behavior, including motivational orientation (approach versus avoidance), difficulty (simple versus challenging), and type (performance versus mastery; Mann, de Ridder, and Fujita 2013). Data on goal motivational orientation show that approach-oriented goals (e.g., "eat fruit for a snack in the afternoon") are more effective than avoidance-oriented goals (e.g., "do not eat donuts for a snack in the afternoon"; e.g., Sullivan and Rothman 2008). Data on the goal difficulty suggest that people are more likely to achieve goals that are *s*pecific, *m*easurable, *a*ttainable, *r*ealistic, and *t*imely (as indicated by the SMART acronym; Latham 2003). Finally, data on goal type suggest that performance-based goals (e.g., "lose 10 lb" [4.5 kg]) and mastery-based goals (e.g., "learn to prepare and enjoy healthy meals") differ in how they impact what individuals attend to, and what they perceive as setbacks. Individuals with performance-based goals focus on documenting goal-related abilities and therefore perceive setbacks as evidence of lacking ability to meet the goal. In contrast, individuals with mastery-based goals focus on improving their skillfulness in the service of a goal and therefore perceive setbacks as opportunities to learn how to become more skillful. Mastery-based goals promote self-efficacy, which is associated with more effective self-regulation in the context of eating behavior (Anderson, Winett, and Wojcik 2007). In sum, setting goals that are approach-oriented, SMART, and mastery-based is more likely to lead to effective health behavior change.

Goal striving is the process of planning and enacting behavior that enables individuals to narrow and ultimately close the gap between their intentions and their actual behaviors (Sheeran 2002). Teaching and building skills of effective goal striving, as done in lifestyle interventions targeting weight loss, include instruction in several strategies that enable individuals to reduce overeating (Mann, de Ridder, and Fujita 2013). One strategy is *prospection and planning,* which allows individuals to predict times when they will struggle to maintain behavior that will move them closer to, rather than further from, their goals, and to plan accordingly. For example, if an individual knows that he will find it very tempting to purchase oversized packages of unhealthy foods from convenience stores while traveling, he may therefore prepare portions of healthy snacks to bring on his travels. Another strategy is *automating behavior*, which involves identifying triggers and cues for behaviors that promote progress toward (or away from) goals and developing strategies to automate (or disrupt) these behaviors. For example, an individual may routinely overeat potato chips if he/she eats them directly from the bag but may be able to avoid such overeating if she pours the chips into a small bowl before eating them. She can, for example, promote her use of a small bowl by storing the bag of potato chips in a cupboard next to a stack of small bowls. *Construal* is a strategy that involves framing health behaviors to be in line with individuals' abstract, long-term goals (e.g., weight-loss and increased fitness) rather than their more concrete, short-term desires (e.g., enjoying a tasty cupcake). In sum, the cognitive-behavioral techniques of goal setting and goal striving increase awareness of overeating, thereby facilitating informed decision-making about when, where, and how to implement changes, and providing strategies to implement changes.

Stimulus Control

Stimulus control techniques provided a foundation for early treatments targeting behavioral control of overeating in obesity (Stuart 1967) and have remained important components of more recent interventions (Brownell 2000; Wadden, Butryn, and Wilson 2007; Wadden et al. 2012). Stimulus control techniques are predicated on the assumption that environmental factors stimulate behavior, and therefore altering environmental factors can change behavior. It follows that weight-loss interventions that include this technique focus on *increasing* exposure to cues that reduce overeating and *reducing* exposure to cues that encourage overeating. For example, individuals can choose to keep a bowl of washed and ready-to-eat fruit (rather than a cookie jar) on the kitchen counter, which may promote eating of a fiber-filled fruit rather than a sugar-laden cookie for an afternoon snack. Similarly, individuals can choose to dine at menu-based restaurants rather than buffet restaurants to avoid a smorgasbord of cues to overeat a variety of foods. We further discuss applications, adaptations, and extrapolations of stimulus control techniques when we review environmental interventions, in the following.

Problem Solving

Problem solving techniques focus on developing adaptive solutions for difficult problems and generally comprise a five-stage process: (1) conceptualization of the experience of having problems as normative, (2) identification of the problem that is leading to an undesired behavior, (3) generation of potential solutions, (4) selection of a solution for initial testing, and (5) evaluation of the tested solution as a solution to the identified problem (Perri, Nezu, and Viegener 1992; D'Zurilla and Nezu 1999, 2009). In the context of lifestyle interventions for weight loss, problem-solving techniques are often taught in therapist-led group formats. Such formats allow for collaborative discussions about solutions to participant-introduced barriers to weight loss, such as difficulties with overeating in particular situations (e.g., social gatherings) or coping with food cravings. Increases in self-reported problem-solving skills following lifestyle interventions are associated with greater weight loss (Murawski et al. 2009).

Cognitive-Behavioral Protocols for Binge Eating

CBT is a first-line treatment for BED (National Institute for Clinical Excellence 2004), particularly in the form of CBT-based guided self-help for binge eating (Wilson et al. 2010). Individuals meeting criteria for BED benefit from a more intensive course of cognitive-behavioral techniques in these protocols than that traditionally included in lifestyle interventions. For example, individuals meeting criteria for BED report larger reductions in binge eating when administered a guided self-help CBT protocol (Overcoming Binge Eating; Fairburn 1995) relative to when administered a guided self-help behavioral weight-loss (lifestyle) protocol (LEARN Program for Weight Management; Brownell 2000; Grilo and Masheb 2005).

Clinician-administered CBT protocols for binge eating behavior include CBT for bulimia nervosa (CBT-BN), CBT for binge eating disorder (CBT-BED), and, more recently, enhanced cognitive behavioral therapy (CBT-E; Fairburn et al. 2008; Murphy et al. 2010). CBT-E is a transdiagnostic treatment for eating disorders, meaning that it is based on a theoretical framework that identifies common factors that affect the maintenance of several related eating disorders, such as binge eating, bulimia, and anorexia (and is therefore used to treat a wide spectrum of such disorders). CBT interventions are effective when delivered in both individual and group formats (Brownley et al. 2007; Hay 2013), except for CBT-E, which is only administered individually (Fairburn et al. 2008). CBT-BN, CBT-BED, and CBT-E protocols include a more intensive emphasis on cognitive-behavioral techniques common to lifestyle interventions for weight loss, including dietary self-monitoring, cognitive restructuring, and exposure-based practices. Such techniques directly target both stress-induced and binge eating through the identification of (1) thoughts and feelings that precipitate overeating, (2) alternatives to overeating, (3) barriers to change in eating behavior, and (4) effective problem-solving strategies (Fairburn 1995). These treatment protocols also include treatment components that specifically target core symptoms of eating disorder pathology, such as dietary restraint, meal skipping, emotional and bodily avoidance, and pathological preoccupation with body shape and weight. CBT-E also includes strategies and procedures targeting barriers to change often observed in individuals with depression, such as clinical perfectionism, low self-esteem, and interpersonal struggles (Fairburn et al. 2008). In sum, CBT interventions have demonstrated widespread effectiveness in reducing binge eating, and meta-analytic data suggest that CBT interventions should be recommended as first-line treatments for BED (Vocks et al. 2010).

Cognitive-Behavioral Interventions and Cardiometabolic Outcomes

Lifestyle interventions that use the cognitive-behavioral techniques reviewed earlier (in combination with diet and physical activity recommendations) can significantly improve cardiometabolic health. The Diabetes Prevention Program (DPP) is one of the most widely examined behavioral weight-loss interventions (Diabetes Prevention Program Research Group 2002b). In the landmark 27-center ($N = 3234$) randomized controlled trial of people with prediabetes, the DPP achieved significant reductions in diabetes risk (58%) compared with placebo and was significantly more effective than metformin therapy, which reduced diabetes risk by 31% compared with placebo (Diabetes Prevention Program Research Group 2002a). Secondary analyses reported significant reductions in triglycerides and significant increases in HDL-cholesterol in the DPP group relative to the metformin and placebo groups (Diabetes Prevention Program Research Group 2005). A subsequent 16-center

(*N* = 5145) randomized controlled trial in people with type 2 diabetes, Look AHEAD (*A*ction for *HEA*lth in *D*iabetes), reported that a behavioral weight-loss intervention similar to the DPP led to significant reductions in several cardiometabolic risk factors, including weight and glycemic control with a median of 9.6 years of follow-up. This trial did not, however, find significant reductions in cardiovascular events (Look AHEAD Research Group 2013). The effects of the DPP and other interventions on weight loss, as well as diabetes prevention and control, have been reviewed extensively (Norris et al. 2005; Franz 2007; Franz et al. 2007). We refer the interested reader to these and other reviews of large-scale randomized clinical trials, many of which have documented the effects of lifestyle interventions on a broad array of cardiometabolic outcomes, including lipids (Aucott et al. 2011), weight-loss maintenance (Barte et al. 2010), and glycemic control in type 2 diabetes (Ismail, Winkley, and Rabe-Hesketh 2004). A recent review and meta-analysis suggests that overweight and obese adults with type 2 diabetes may require a more potent suite of diet-specific intervention components, including nutritional therapies, to achieve cardiometabolic improvements and that focusing on weight as a primary outcome in this population (e.g., >5% weight loss) might not be the optimal strategy with which to improve glycemic control (Franz et al. 2015).

Independent and Combination Mindfulness Approaches

Mindfulness approaches involve noticing, becoming curious about, and accepting unpleasant thoughts, rather than labeling such thoughts as dysfunctional and attempting to change them. These techniques have been applied in the treatment of problematic overeating as independent interventions (e.g., mindful eating for binge eating; Kristeller and Wolever 2010) and as combination approaches (e.g., packaged with cognitive-behavioral approaches, as in dialectical behavioral therapy [DBT] for binge eating; Telch, Agras, and Linehan 2001). There are several recent reviews of interventions testing these approaches (Katterman et al. 2014; O'Reilly et al. 2014; Godfrey, Gallo, and Afari 2015). The extent to which mindfulness approaches are more effective than existing cognitive-behavioral approaches, or whether mindfulness approaches are most effective when administered in combination protocols, remains unclear. In the following text, we review findings from studies of independent mindfulness approaches and combination mindfulness approaches for problematic overeating, as well as their effects on cardiometabolic outcomes.

Independent Mindfulness Approaches

Mindfulness, broadly defined as paying attention on purpose, in the present moment, and non-judgmentally, is a core component of mindful eating and acceptance and commitment techniques targeting problematic overeating (Kristeller and Wolever 2010; Forman and Butryn 2015). Such approaches seek to strengthen abilities to become aware of and tolerate uncomfortable sensations (e.g., food cravings) without reacting (e.g., indulging food cravings). Mindfulness protocols have demonstrated some effectiveness in reducing binge eating. Katterman et al. (2014) systematically reviewed mindfulness interventions targeting reductions in overeating (excluding acceptance and commitment therapy and DBT, which do not include mindfulness training in all sessions). Seven of fourteen eligible trials collected data on changes in binge eating using traditional self-report measures (e.g., BES, Eating Disorder Examination Questionnaire; Gormally et al. 1982; Fairburn and Beglin 1994). All seven trials reported reductions in binge eating among participants receiving the mindfulness interventions. Of these seven trials, four trials included comparison groups. Two of these four trials reported significant between-group differences in reductions in binge eating, with the mindfulness groups showing greater improvements compared to waitlist control groups (Alberts, Thewissen, and Raes 2012; Kristeller, Wolever, and Sheets 2014), and one showing a statistical trend in this same direction (Daubenmier et al. 2011). In one of these trials, relative to active control groups (i.e., CBT groups), the mindfulness groups showed no significant differences (Kristeller, Wolever, and Sheets 2014). The last of these four trials reported a statistical trend toward greater reductions in binge eating in the mindfulness group relative to the CBT group (Smith et al. 2008).

These data collectively suggest that mindfulness approaches may contribute to reductions in binge eating; however, whether these approaches are more effective than CBT techniques remains uncertain. We want to highlight the importance of the type of mindfulness training on eating behavior.

Combination Mindfulness Approaches

Mindfulness approaches for the treatment of overeating may prove more effective when combined with additional intervention components (Forman and Butryn 2015), such as cognitive-behavioral techniques and environmental adaptations. O'Reilly et al. (2014) reviewed mindfulness-based interventions for overeating, including those co-administered with other intervention techniques (e.g., cognitive-behavioral techniques). Of 12 eligible studies that targeted binge eating using mindfulness and/or acceptance techniques, 11 reported reductions in binge eating frequency and/or severity. These 11 studies tested combinations of mindfulness with cognitive-behavioral techniques (Baer, Fischer, and Huss 2005; Leahey, Crowther, and Irwin 2008; Courbasson, Nishikawa, and Shapira 2010; Woolhouse, Knowles, and Crafti 2012), mindful eating protocols (Dalen et al. 2010; Kristeller, Wolever, and Sheets 2014), acceptance-based practices (Tapper et al. 2009), and combinations of mindfulness exercises (Kristeller and Hallett 1999; Alberts et al. 2010). The only study that did not report reduced binge eating used a general mindfulness-based stress reduction protocol (Smith et al. 2006). Godfrey et al. (2015) recently conducted a systematic review and meta-analysis of mindfulness-based interventions specifically for binge eating and included DBT, which is a CBT intervention that includes mindfulness-based emotion regulation practices (e.g., DBT). Analysis of the 19 included studies supported large or medium-large effects of interventions on binge eating (within-group random effects mean Hedge's g [a standardized measure of effect size] = −1.12, 95% CI [−1.67, −0.80], $k = 18$; between-group mean Hedge's $g = -0.70$, 95% CI [−1.16, −0.24], $k = 7$). These data indicate that combination mindfulness approaches for the treatment of binge eating are promising, and future research should clarify the optimal combination approach.

Mindfulness Approaches and Cardiometabolic Outcomes

In one of the largest trials to date testing the long-term effects of a mindfulness intervention on weight loss, Daubenmier et al. (2016) randomized 194 obese adults to receive a 17-session program of diet and exercise information with either (1) training in select cognitive-behavioral techniques (active control group), or (2) training in mindfulness-based eating and stress reduction (mindfulness group). Relative to the active control group, the mindfulness group lost more weight (though not a statistically significant difference) and evidenced statistically significant reductions in fasting glucose at 18 months post-baseline. Analyses also revealed that increases in self-reported mindful eating among participants assigned to the mindfulness group, but not among participants assigned to the active control CBT group, were associated with larger reductions in self-reported eating of sweet and dessert foods, as well as larger reductions in fasting glucose levels, at 12 months post-baseline (Mason et al. 2016). While this trial suggests that mindfulness training may impart some benefit in terms of cardiometabolic health, it may require optimization to surpass the effectiveness of traditional CBT-based interventions. Alternatively, the benefits of mindfulness training may be most potent when combined with other intervention techniques, such as specific dietary recommendations or goal-setting.

In their reviews of mindfulness interventions, Katterman et al. (2014) and O'Reilly et al. (2014) each reported on 10 studies that included weight outcomes. The Katterman and O'Reilly reviews included 5 common studies, meaning that taken together, these reviews reported on 15 analyses of weight change following mindfulness interventions targeting eating behavior. Excepting one study (Miller et al. 2012; Cohen's d [a standardized measure of effect size] = −3.29), Katterman and colleagues reported Cohen's d's ranging from −0.17 to +0.04, and the average intervention effect size was small (Cohen's $d = 0.10$, favoring greater weight loss in mindfulness groups). O'Reilly and colleagues reported a slightly larger average effect size (Cohen's $d = 0.19$, favoring greater weight loss in mindfulness groups). Notably, 3 of the 10 studies included in Katterman and colleagues' review (2014) included treatment components targeting weight loss as a specific goal of the intervention, and all three of these interventions reported significantly greater weight loss in the mindfulness group (Dalen et al. 2010; Miller et al. 2012; Timmerman and Brown 2012). In summary, data suggest that mindfulness approaches may be more effective in the treatment of binge eating when in combination with other intervention components (e.g., cognitive-behavioral techniques); however, more definitive trials are needed to test the effectiveness of such combination approaches on cardiometabolic outcomes.

CONCLUSION

We have reviewed three types of overeating and three broad categories of interventions for overeating. Here, we reviewed types and interventions for overeating separately, though these types may co-occur and interventions may be most effective in combination. Indeed, we hypothesize that the intervention components we reviewed in this chapter might be most effective in targeting several types of overeating (and cardiometabolic health) when administered in combinations. We believe that current data support referral of overweight and obese persons with increased cardiometabolic risk factors to behavioral intervention programs (including programs that incorporate training in mindful eating, where available), to promote weight loss and weight-loss maintenance, as well as improvements in cardiometabolic risk factors. In settings without ongoing, high-quality group interventions, referral to a nutritionist with expertise in behavioral weight-loss strategies may be helpful. Referral to the lay books mentioned in this chapter, which, in plain language, detail simple environmental intervention techniques that can be adapted in ways that fit a variety of individual needs, may also be helpful. Future research is needed to optimize behavioral interventions, including mindfulness interventions, and to ascertain the most effective combinations of behavioral and environmental interventions for improving weight loss and weight-loss maintenance.

REFERENCES

Abraham, T. M., J. M. Massaro, U. Hoffmann, J. A. Yanovski, and C. S. Fox. 2014. Metabolic characterization of adults with binge eating in the general population: The Framingham Heart Study. *Obesity* 22 (11): 2441–2449.

Adam, T. C. and E. S. Epel. 2007. Stress, eating and the reward system. *Physiology & Behavior* 91 (4): 449–458.

Alberts, H. J. E. M., S. Mulkens, M. Smeets, and R. Thewissen. 2010. Coping with food cravings. Investigating the potential of a mindfulness-based intervention. *Appetite* 55 (1): 160–163.

Alberts, H. J. E. M., R. Thewissen, and L. Raes. 2012. Dealing with problematic eating behaviour. The effects of a mindfulness-based intervention on eating behaviour, food cravings, dichotomous thinking and body image concern. *Appetite* 58 (3): 847–851.

American Psychological Association. 2013. *Diagnostic and Statistical Manual of Mental Disorders (DSM-5®)*. Arlington, VA: American Psychological Association.

American Psychological Association. 2000. *Diagnostic and Statistical Manual of Mental Disorders: DSM-IV-TR®*. Arlington, VA: American Psychological Association.

Anderson, E. S., R. A. Winett, and J. R. Wojcik. 2007. Self-regulation, self-efficacy, outcome expectations, and social support: Social cognitive theory and nutrition behavior. *Annals of Behavioral Medicine* 34 (3): 304–312.

Ashwell, M., P. Gunn, and S. Gibson. 2012. Waist-to-height ratio is a better screening tool than waist circumference and BMI for adult cardiometabolic risk factors: Systematic review and meta-analysis. *Obesity Reviews* 13 (3): 275–286.

Aucott, L., D. Gray, H. Rothnie, M. Thapa, and C. Waweru. 2011. Effects of lifestyle interventions and long-term weight loss on lipid outcomes—A systematic review. *Obesity Reviews* 12 (5): e412–e425.

Avena, N. M. 2010. The study of food addiction using animal models of binge eating. *Appetite* 55 (3): 734–737.

Avena, N. M. and B. G. Hoebel. 2003. A diet promoting sugar dependency causes behavioral cross-sensitization to a low dose of amphetamine. *Neuroscience* 122 (1): 17–20.

Avena, N. M., P. Rada, and B. G. Hoebel. 2008. Evidence for sugar addiction: Behavioral and neurochemical effects of intermittent, excessive sugar intake. *Neuroscience & Biobehavioral Reviews* 32 (1): 20–39.

Bach, P. J. and J. M. Schaefer. 1979. The tempo of country music and the rate of drinking in bars. *Journal of Studies on Alcohol* 40 (11): 1058–1059.

Baer, R. A., S. Fischer, and D. B. Huss. 2005. Mindfulness and acceptance in the treatment of disordered eating. *Journal of Rational-Emotive and Cognitive-Behavior Therapy* 23 (4): 281–300.

Bandura, A. and D. C. McClelland. 1977. *Social Learning Theory*. Englewood Cliffs, NJ: Prentice Hall.

Barte, J. C. M., N. C. W. Ter Bogt, R. P. Bogers, P. J. Teixeira, B. Blissmer, T. A. Mori, and W. J. E. Bemelmans. 2010. Maintenance of weight loss after lifestyle interventions for overweight and obesity: A systematic review. *Obesity Reviews* 11 (12): 899–906.

Beck, J. S. 2011. *Cognitive Behavior Therapy: Basics and Beyond*. New York: Guilford Press.

Bellisle, F., A. M. Dalix, and G. Slama. 2004. Non food-related environmental stimuli induce increased meal intake in healthy women: Comparison of television viewing versus listening to a recorded story in laboratory settings. *Appetite* 43 (2): 175–180.

Block, J. P., Y. He, A. M. Zaslavsky, L. Ding, and J. Z. Ayanian. 2009. Psychosocial stress and change in weight among US adults. *American Journal of Epidemiology* 170 (2): 181–192.

Boggiano, M. M., P. C. Chandler, J. B. Viana, K. D. Oswald, C. R. Maldonado, and P. K. Wauford. 2005. Combined dieting and stress evoke exaggerated responses to opioids in binge-eating rats. *Behavioral Neuroscience* 119 (5): 1207–1214.

Bray, G. A. and C. Bouchard (Eds.). 2014. *Handbook of Obesity: Clinical Applications*. Vol. 2, 4th edn. Boca Raton, FL: CRC Press, Taylor & Francis Group.

Brondel, L., M. Romer, V. Van Wymelbeke, N. Pineau, T. Jiang, C. Hanus, and D. Rigaud. 2009. Variety enhances food intake in humans: Role of sensory-specific satiety. *Physiology & Behavior* 97 (1): 44–51.

Brownell, K. D. 2000. *The LEARN Program for Weight Control*. Euless, TX: American Health Company.

Brownell, K. D. 2004. *The LEARN Program for Weight Management: Lifestyle, Exercise, Attitudes, Relationships, Nutrition*. Euless, TX: American Health Publishing Company.

Brownell, K. D. and K. B. Horgen. 2004. *Food Fight: The Inside Story of the Food Industry, America's Obesity Crisis, and What We Can Do about It*. Chicago, IL: Contemporary Books Chicago.

Brownley, K. A., N. D. Berkman, J. A. Sedway, K. N. Lohr, and C. M. Bulik. 2007. Binge eating disorder treatment: A systematic review of randomized controlled trials. *International Journal of Eating Disorders* 40 (4): 337–348.

Burke, L. E., S. M. Sereika, E. Music, M. Warziski, M. A. Styn, and A. Stone. 2008. Using instrumented paper diaries to document self-monitoring patterns in weight loss. *Contemporary Clinical Trials* 29 (2): 182–193.

Burke, L. E., M. A. Styn, S. M. Sereika, M. B. Conroy, L. Ye, K. Glanz, M. A. Sevick, and L. J. Ewing. 2012. Using mHealth technology to enhance self-monitoring for weight loss: A randomized trial. *American Journal of Preventive Medicine* 43 (1): 20–26.

Burke, L. E., J. Wang, and M. A. Sevick. 2011. Self-monitoring in weight loss: A systematic review of the literature. *Journal of the American Dietetic Association* 111 (1): 92–102.

Burmeister, J. M., N. Hinman, A. Koball, D. A. Hoffmann, and R. A. Carels. 2013. Food addiction in adults seeking weight loss treatment. Implications for psychosocial health and weight loss. *Appetite* 60: 103–110.

Caldwell, C. and S. A. Hibbert. 2002. The influence of music tempo and musical preference on restaurant patrons' behavior. *Psychology and Marketing* 19 (11): 895–917.

Carels, R. A., K. Konrad, K. M. Young, L. A. Darby, C. Coit, A. M. Clayton, and C. K. Oemig. 2008. Taking control of your personal eating and exercise environment: A weight maintenance program. *Eating Behaviors* 9 (2): 228–237.

Carels, R. A., C. B. Wott, K. M. Young, A. Gumble, L. A. Darby, M. W. Oehlhof, J. Harper, and A. Koball. 2009. Successful weight loss with self-help: A stepped-care approach. *Journal of Behavioral Medicine* 32 (6): 503–509.

Carels, R. A., K. M. Young, A. Koball, A. Gumble, L. A. Darby, M. W. Oehlhof, C. B. Wott, and N. Hinman. 2011. Transforming your life: An environmental modification approach to weight loss. *Journal of Health Psychology* 16 (3): 430–438.

Carmienke, S., M. H. Freitag, T. Pischon, P. Schlattmann, T. Fankhaenel, H. Goebel, and J. Gensichen. 2013. General and abdominal obesity parameters and their combination in relation to mortality: A systematic review and meta-regression analysis. *European Journal of Clinical Nutrition* 67 (6): 573–585.

Caudill, B. D. and F. H. Kong. 2001. Social approval and facilitation in predicting modeling effects in alcohol consumption. *Journal of Substance Abuse* 13 (4): 425–441.

Celio, A. A., D. E. Wilfley, S. J. Crow, J. Mitchell, and B. T. Walsh. 2004. A comparison of the binge eating scale, questionnaire for eating and weight patterns-revised, and eating disorder examination questionnaire with instructions with the eating disorder examination in the assessment of binge eating disorder and its symptoms. *International Journal of Eating Disorders* 36 (4): 434–444.

Chandon, P. and N. Ordabayeva. 2009. Supersize in one dimension, downsize in three dimensions: Effects of spatial dimensionality on size perceptions and preferences. *Journal of Marketing Research* 46 (6): 739–753.

Chandon, P. and B. Wansink. 2007. The biasing health halos of fast-food restaurant health claims: Lower calorie estimates and higher side-dish consumption intentions. *Journal of Consumer Research* 34 (3): 301–314.

Cohen, D. A., R. Collins, G. Hunter, B. Ghosh-Dastidar, and T. Dubowitz. 2014. Store impulse marketing strategies and body mass index. *American Journal of Public Health* 105 (7): 1446–1452.

Colantuoni, C., P. Rada, J. McCarthy, C. Patten, N. M. Avena, A. Chadeayne, and B. G. Hoebel. 2002. Evidence that intermittent, excessive sugar intake causes endogenous opioid dependence. *Obesity Research* 10 (6): 478–488.

Colantuoni, C., J. Schwenker, J. McCarthy, P. Rada, B. Ladenheim, J.-L. Cadet, G. J. Schwartz, T. H. Moran, and B. G. Hoebel. 2001. Excessive sugar intake alters binding to dopamine and mu-opioid receptors in the brain. *NeuroReport* 12 (16): 3549–3552.

Conger, J. C., A. J. Conger, P. R. Costanzo, K. Lynn Wright, and J. A. Matter. 1980. The effect of social cues on the eating behavior of obese and normal subjects. *Journal of Personality* 48 (2): 258–271.

Corwin, R. L., N. M. Avena, and M. M. Boggiano. 2011. Feeding and reward: Perspectives from three rat models of binge eating. *Physiology & Behavior*, The Neural Basis of Feeding and Reward: A Tribute to Bart Hoebel 104 (1): 87–97.

Corwin, R. L. and A. Buda-Levin. 2004. Behavioral models of binge-type eating. *Physiology & Behavior*, Festschrift in Honor of Gerard P. Smith 82 (1): 123–130.

Courbasson, C. M., Y. Nishikawa, and L. B. Shapira. 2010. Mindfulness-action based cognitive behavioral therapy for concurrent binge eating disorder and substance use disorders. *Eating Disorders* 19 (1): 17–33.

Dalen, J., B. W. Smith, B. M. Shelley, A. L. Sloan, L. Leahigh, and D. Begay. 2010. Pilot study: Mindful eating and living (meal): Weight, eating behavior, and psychological outcomes associated with a mindfulness-based intervention for people with obesity. *Complementary Therapies in Medicine* 18 (6): 260–264.

Dallman, M. F. 2010. Stress-induced obesity and the emotional nervous system. *Trends in Endocrinology & Metabolism* 21 (3): 159–165.

Dallman, M. F. and S. Bhatnagar. 2010. Chronic stress and energy balance: Role of the hypothalamo-pituitary-adrenal axis. *Comprehensive Physiology*. Somerset, NJ: John Wiley & Sons, Inc.

Dallman, M. F., N. C. Pecoraro, and S. E. la Fleur. 2005. Chronic stress and comfort foods: Self-medication and abdominal obesity. *Brain, Behavior, and Immunity* 19 (4): 275–280.

Daubenmier, J., J. L. Kristeller, F. M. Hecht, N. Maninger, M. Kuwata, K. Jhaveri, R. H. Lustig, M. Kemeny, L. Karan, and E. Epel. 2011. Mindfulness intervention for stress eating to reduce cortisol and abdominal fat among overweight and obese women: An exploratory randomized controlled study. *Journal of Obesity* 2011: 1–13.

Daubenmier, J., R. H. Lustig, F. M. Hecht, J. L. Kristeller, J. Woolley, T. Adam, M. Dallman, and E. Epel. 2014. A new biomarker of hedonic eating? A preliminary investigation of cortisol and nausea responses to acute opioid blockade. *Appetite* 74: 92–100.

Daubenmier, J., P. J. Moran, J. L. Kristeller, M. Acree, P. Bacchetti, M. Kemeny, et al. 2016. Effects of a mindfulness-based weight loss program in obese adults: A randomized clinical trial. *Obesity* 24(4): 794–804.

Davis, C. 2013a. Compulsive overeating as an addictive behavior: Overlap between food addiction and binge eating disorder. *Current Obesity Reports* 2 (2): 171–178.

Davis, C. 2013b. From passive overeating to 'food addiction': A spectrum of compulsion and severity. *ISRN Obesity* 2013: 1–20.

Davis, C. and J. C. Carter. 2009. Compulsive overeating as an addiction disorder. A review of theory and evidence. *Appetite* 53 (1): 1–8.

Davis, C., C. Curtis, R. D. Levitan, J. C. Carter, A. S. Kaplan, and J. L. Kennedy. 2011. Evidence that 'food addiction' is a valid phenotype of obesity. *Appetite* 57 (3): 711–717.

Davis, C., R. D. Levitan, C. Reid, J. C. Carter, A. S. Kaplan, K. A. Patte, N. King, C. Curtis, and J. L. Kennedy. 2009. Dopamine for 'wanting' and opioids for 'liking': A comparison of obese adults with and without binge eating. *Obesity* 17 (6): 1220–1225.

Davis, C., R. D. Levitan, Z. Yilmaz, A. S. Kaplan, J. C. Carter, and J. L. Kennedy. 2012. Binge eating disorder and the dopamine D2 receptor: Genotypes and sub-phenotypes. *Progress in Neuro-Psychopharmacology and Biological Psychiatry* 38 (2): 328–335.

Davis, C., K. Patte, R. Levitan, C. Reid, S. Tweed, and C. Curtis. 2007. From motivation to behaviour: A model of reward sensitivity, overeating, and food preferences in the risk profile for obesity. *Appetite* 48 (1): 12–19.

DeFronzo, R. A. and E. Ferrannini. 1991. Insulin resistance: A multifaceted syndrome responsible for NIDDM, obesity, hypertension, dyslipidemia, and atherosclerotic cardiovascular disease. *Diabetes Care* 14 (3): 173–194.

de Zwaan, M. 2001. Binge eating disorder and obesity. *International Journal of Obesity and Related Metabolic Disorders: Journal of the International Association for the Study of Obesity* 25: S51–S55.

de Zwaan, M., S. Engeli, and A. Müller. 2015. Temperamental factors in severe weight cycling. A cross-sectional study. *Appetite* 91: 336–342.

Diabetes Prevention Program Research Group. 2002a. Reduction in the incidence of type 2 diabetes with lifestyle intervention or metformin. *The New England Journal of Medicine* 346 (6): 393.

Diabetes Prevention Program Research Group. 2002b. The diabetes prevention program (DPP) description of lifestyle intervention. *Diabetes Care* 25 (12): 2165–2171.

Diabetes Prevention Program Research Group. 2005. Impact of intensive lifestyle and metformin therapy on cardiovascular disease risk factors in the diabetes prevention program. *Diabetes Care* 28 (4): 888–894.

D'Zurilla, T. J. and A. M. Nezu. 1999. *Problem-Solving Therapy: A Social Competence Approach to Clinical Intervention*. New York: Springer Publishing Company.

D'Zurilla, T. J. and A. M. Nezu. 2009. Problem-solving therapy. In *Handbook of Cognitive-Behavioral Therapies*, 3rd edn., K. S. Dobson (Ed.), pp. 197–225. Guilford Press.

Epel, E. S., S. Jimenez, K. Brownell, L. Stroud, C. Stoney, and R. Niaura. 2004. Are stress eaters at risk for the metabolic syndrome? *Annals of the New York Academy of Sciences* 1032 (1): 208–210.

Epel, E. S., R. Lapidus, B. McEwen, and K. Brownell. 2001. Stress may add bite to appetite in women: A laboratory study of stress-induced cortisol and eating behavior. *Psychoneuroendocrinology* 26 (1): 37–49.

Fairburn, C. G. 1995. *Overcoming Binge Eating*. New York: Guilford Press.

Fairburn, C. G. and S. J. Beglin. 1994. Assessment of eating disorders: Interview or self-report questionnaire? *International Journal of Eating Disorders* 16 (4): 363–370.

Fairburn, C. G., Z. Cooper, R. Shafran, and G. T. Wilson. 2008. Eating disorders: A transdiagnostic protocol. In *Clinical Handbook of Psychological Disorders*, D. H. Barlow (Ed.), pp. 578–614. New York: Guilford Press.

Fernandez, I. D., N. P. Chin, C. M. Devine, A. M. Dozier, C. A. Martina, S. McIntosh, K. Thevenet-Morrison, and H. Yang. 2015. Images of a healthy worksite: A group-randomized trial for worksite weight gain prevention with employee participation in intervention design. *American Journal of Public Health* 105 (10): 2167–2174.

Fishbach, A. and M. J. Ferguson. 2007. The goal construct in social psychology. In *Social Psychology: Handbook of Basic Principles*, A. W. Kruglanski and E. T. Higgins (Eds.), pp. 490–515. New York: Guilford Press.

Flint, A. J., A. N. Gearhardt, W. R. Corbin, K. D. Brownell, A. E. Field, and E. B. Rimm. 2014. Food-addiction scale measurement in 2 cohorts of middle-aged and older women. *The American Journal of Clinical Nutrition* 99 (3): 578–586.

Forman, E. M. and M. L. Butryn. 2015. A new look at the science of weight control: How acceptance and commitment strategies can address the challenge of self-regulation. *Appetite* 84 (January): 171–180.

Foster, M. T., J. P. Warne, A. B. Ginsberg, H. F. Horneman, N. C. Pecoraro, S. F. Akana, and M. F. Dallman. 2009. Palatable foods, stress, and energy stores sculpt corticotropin-releasing factor, adrenocorticotropin, and corticosterone concentrations after restraint. *Endocrinology* 150 (5): 2325–2333.

Franz, M. J. 2007. The evidence is in: Lifestyle interventions can prevent diabetes. *American Journal of Lifestyle Medicine* 1 (2): 113–121.

Franz, M. J., J. L. Boucher, S. Rutten-Ramos, and J. J. VanWormer. 2015. Lifestyle weight-loss intervention outcomes in overweight and obese adults with type 2 diabetes: A systematic review and meta-analysis of randomized clinical trials. *Journal of the Academy of Nutrition and Dietetics* 115 (9): 1447–1463.

Franz, M. J., J. J. VanWormer, A. Lauren Crain, J. L. Boucher, T. Histon, W. Caplan, J. D. Bowman, and N. P. Pronk. 2007. Weight-loss outcomes: A systematic review and meta-analysis of weight-loss clinical trials with a minimum 1-year follow-up. *Journal of the American Dietetic Association* 107 (10): 1755–1767.

Freedman, L. S., J. M. Commins, J. E. Moler, L. Arab, D. J. Baer, V. Kipnis, D. Midthune et al. 2014. Pooled results from 5 validation studies of dietary self-report instruments using recovery biomarkers for energy and protein intake. *American Journal of Epidemiology* 180(2): 172–188.

Gearhardt, A., W. R. Corbin, and K. D. Brownell. 2016. Development of the Yale Food Addiction Scale Version 2.0. *Psychology of Addictive Behaviors* 30(1): 113–121.

Gearhardt, A. N., W. R. Corbin, and K. D. Brownell. 2009. Preliminary validation of the yale food addiction scale. *Appetite* 52 (2): 430–436.

Gearhardt, A. N., C. Davis, R. Kuschner, and K. Brownell. 2011. The addiction potential of hyperpalatable foods. *Current Drug Abuse Reviews* 4 (3): 140–145.

Glanz, K., M. D. M. Bader, and S. Iyer. 2012. Retail grocery store marketing strategies and obesity: An integrative review. *American Journal of Preventive Medicine* 42 (5): 503–512.

Godfrey, K. M., L. C. Gallo, and N. Afari. 2015. Mindfulness-based interventions for binge eating: A systematic review and meta-analysis. *Journal of Behavioral Medicine* 38 (2): 348–362.

Gormally, J., S. Black, S. Daston, and D. Rardin. 1982. The assessment of binge eating severity among obese persons. *Addictive Behaviors* 7 (1): 47–55.

Greenberger, D. and C. A. Padesky. 1995. *Mind over Mood*. New York: Guilford.
Grilo, C. M. and R. M. Masheb. 2005. A randomized controlled comparison of guided self-help cognitive behavioral therapy and behavioral weight loss for binge eating disorder. *Behaviour Research and Therapy* 43 (11): 1509–1525.
Grimm, J. W., A. M. Fyall, and D. P. Osincup. 2005. Incubation of sucrose craving: Effects of reduced training and sucrose pre-loading. *Physiology & Behavior* 84 (1): 73–79.
Grupski, A. E., M. M. Hood, B. J. Hall, L. Azarbad, S. L. Fitzpatrick, and J. A. Corsica. 2012. Examining the binge eating scale in screening for binge eating disorder in bariatric surgery candidates. *Obesity Surgery* 23 (1): 1–6.
Guéguen, N., C. Jacob, H. Le Guellec, T. Morineau, and M. Lourel. 2008. Sound level of environmental music and drinking behavior: A field experiment with beer drinkers. *Alcoholism: Clinical and Experimental Research* 32 (10): 1795–1798.
Hanks, A. S., D. R. Just, L. E. Smith, and B. Wansink. 2012. Healthy convenience: Nudging students toward healthier choices in the lunchroom. *Journal of Public Health* 162(4): 867–869.
Hanks, A. S., D. R. Just, and B. Wansink. 2013. Smarter lunchrooms can address new school lunchroom guidelines and childhood obesity. *The Journal of Pediatrics* 162 (4): 867–869.
Hay, P. 2013. A systematic review of evidence for psychological treatments in eating disorders: 2005–2012. *International Journal of Eating Disorders* 46 (5): 462–469.
Herman, C. P. 2015. The social facilitation of eating. A review. *Appetite* 86: 61–73.
Herman, C. P., S. Koenig-Nobert, J. B. Peterson, and J. Polivy. 2005. Matching effects on eating: Do individual differences make a difference? *Appetite* 45 (2): 108–109.
Herman, C. P. and J. Polivy. 2005. Normative influences on food intake. *Physiology & Behavior* 86 (5): 762–772.
Herman, C. P., D. A. Roth, and J. Polivy. 2003. Effects of the presence of others on food intake: A normative interpretation. *Psychological Bulletin* 129 (6): 873.
Herman, J. P. and W. E. Cullinan. 1997. Neurocircuitry of stress: Central control of the hypothalamo–pituitary–adrenocortical axis. *Trends in Neurosciences* 20 (2): 78–84.
Hermans, R. C. J., A. Lichtwarck-Aschoff, K. E. Bevelander, C. Peter Herman, J. K. Larsen, and R. C. M. E. Engels. 2012. Mimicry of food intake: The dynamic interplay between eating companions. *PLoS ONE* 7 (2): e31027.
Hetherington, M. M., A. S. Anderson, G. N. M. Norton, and L. Newson. 2006. Situational effects on meal intake: A comparison of eating alone and eating with others. *Physiology & Behavior* 88 (4–5): 498–505.
Heyne, A., C. Kiesselbach, I. Sahún, J. McDonald, M. Gaiffi, M. Dierssen, and J. Wolffgramm. 2009. An animal model of compulsive food-taking behaviour. *Addiction Biology* 14 (4): 373–383.
Higgs, S. 2002. Memory for recent eating and its influence on subsequent food intake. *Appetite* 39 (2): 159–166.
Higgs, S. and M. Woodward. 2009. Television watching during lunch increases afternoon snack intake of young women. *Appetite* 52 (1): 39–43.
Hudson, J. I., J. K. Lalonde, C. E. Coit, M. T. Tsuang, S. L. McElroy, S. J. Crow, C. M. Bulik et al. 2010. Longitudinal study of the diagnosis of components of the metabolic syndrome in individuals with binge-eating disorder. *The American Journal of Clinical Nutrition* 91 (6): 1568–1573.
Ismail, K., K. Winkley, and S. Rabe-Hesketh. 2004. Systematic review and meta-analysis of randomised controlled trials of psychological interventions to improve glycaemic control in patients with type 2 diabetes. *The Lancet* 363 (9421): 1589–1597.
Kaipainen, K., C. R. Payne, and B. Wansink. 2012. Mindless eating challenge: Retention, weight outcomes, and barriers for changes in a public web-based healthy eating and weight loss program. *Journal of Medical Internet Research* 14 (6): e168.
Kaltsas, G. A. and G. P. Chrousos. 2007. The neuroendocrinology of stress. In *Handbook of Psychophysiology*, J. T. Cacioppo, L. G. Tassinary, and G. Berntson (Eds.). New York: Cambridge University Press.
Kanfer, F. H. 1970. Self-monitoring: Methodological limitations and clinical applications. *Journal of Consulting and Clinical Psychology* 2 (35): 148–152.
Kanfer, F. H. and L. Gaelick-Buys. 1991. Self-management methods. In Pergamon General Psychology Series, Vol. 52. *Helping People Change: A Textbook of Methods,* F. H. Kanfer & A. P. Goldstein (Eds.), pp. 305–360. Elmsford, NY: Pergamon Press.
Katterman, S. N., B. M. Kleinman, M. M. Hood, L. M. Nackers, and J. A. Corsica. 2014. Mindfulness meditation as an intervention for binge eating, emotional eating, and weight loss: A systematic review. *Eating Behaviors* 15 (2): 197–204.
Khaylis, A., T. Yiaslas, J. Bergstrom, and C. Gore-Felton. 2010. A review of efficacious technology-based weight-loss interventions: Five key components. *Telemedicine and E-Health* 16 (9): 931–938.
Kiernan, M., S. D. Brown, D. E. Schoffman, K. Lee, A. C. King, C. B. Taylor, N. C. Schleicher, and M. G. Perri. 2013. Promoting healthy weight with 'stability skills first': A randomized trial. *Journal of Consulting and Clinical Psychology* 81 (2): 336.

Klatzkin, R. R., S. Gaffney, K. Cyrus, E. Bigus, and K. A. Brownley. 2015. Binge eating disorder and obesity: Preliminary evidence for distinct cardiovascular and psychological phenotypes. *Physiology & Behavior* 142: 20–27.

Klem, M. L., R. R. Wing, M. T. McGuire, H. M. Seagle, and J. O. Hill. 1997. A descriptive study of individuals successful at long-term maintenance of substantial weight loss. *The American Journal of Clinical Nutrition* 66 (2): 239–246.

Koob, G. F. and N. D. Volkow. 2009. Neurocircuitry of addiction. *Neuropsychopharmacology* 35 (1): 217–238.

Kristeller, J. L. and C. B. Hallett. 1999. An exploratory study of a meditation-based intervention for binge eating disorder. *Journal of Health Psychology* 4 (3): 357–363.

Kristeller, J. L. and R. Q. Wolever. 2010. Mindfulness-based eating awareness training for treating binge eating disorder: The conceptual foundation. *Eating Disorders* 19 (1): 49–61.

Kristeller, J. L., R. Q. Wolever, and V. Sheets. 2014. Mindfulness-based eating awareness training (MB-EAT) for binge eating: A randomized clinical trial. *Mindfulness* 5 (3): 282–297.

Kyrou, I., G. P. Chrousos, and C. Tsigos. 2006. Stress, visceral obesity, and metabolic complications. *Annals of the New York Academy of Sciences* 1083 (1): 77–110.

Latham, G. P. 2003. Goal setting: A five-step approach to behavior change. *Organizational Dynamics* 32 (3): 309–318.

Leahey, T. M., J. H. Crowther, and S. R. Irwin. 2008. A cognitive-behavioral mindfulness group therapy intervention for the treatment of binge eating in bariatric surgery patients. *Cognitive and Behavioral Practice* 15 (4): 364–375.

Lemmens, S. G., F. Rutters, J. M. Born, and M. S. Westerterp-Plantenga. 2011. Stress augments food 'wanting' and energy intake in visceral overweight subjects in the absence of hunger. *Physiology & Behavior* 103 (2): 157–163.

Leonhardt, D. 2007. Your plate is bigger than your stomach. *The New York Times*, May 2, sec. Business.

Look AHEAD Research Group. 2013. Cardiovascular effects of intensive lifestyle intervention in type 2 diabetes. *The New England Journal of Medicine* 369 (2): 145.

Lowe, M. R. 2003. Self-regulation of energy intake in the prevention and treatment of obesity: Is it feasible? *Obesity Research* 11 (S10): 44S–59S.

Macht, M. 2008. How emotions affect eating: A five-way model. *Appetite* 50 (1): 1–11.

Maniam, J. and M. J. Morris. 2012. The link between stress and feeding behaviour. *Neuropharmacology*, 63 (1): 97–110.

Mann, T., D. de Ridder, and K. Fujita. 2013. Self-regulation of health behavior: Social psychological approaches to goal setting and goal striving. *Health Psychology* 32 (5): 487.

Mariotti, F., E. Kalonji, J. F. Huneau, and I. Margaritis. 2010. Potential pitfalls of health claims from a public health nutrition perspective. *Nutrition Reviews* 68 (10): 624–638.

Mason, A., E. S. Epel, J. Kristeller, P. J. Moran, M. Dallman, R. H. Lustig, M. Acree et al. 2016. Effects of a mindfulness-based intervention on mindful eating, sweets consumption, and fasting glucose levels in obese adults: Data from the SHINE randomized controlled trial. *Journal of Behavioral Medicine* 2 (39): 201–213.

Mathes, W. F., K. A. Brownley, X. Mo, and C. M. Bulik. 2009. The biology of binge eating. *Appetite* 52 (3): 545–553.

McCarron, A. and K. J. Tierney. 1989. The effect of auditory stimulation on the consumption of soft drinks. *Appetite* 13 (2): 155–159.

McElrea, H. and L. Standing. 1992. Fast music causes fast drinking. *Perceptual and Motor Skills* 75 (2): 362.

McEwen, B. S. 2007. Physiology and neurobiology of stress and adaptation: Central role of the brain. *Physiological Reviews* 87 (3): 873–904.

Miller, C. K., J. L. Kristeller, A. Headings, H. Nagaraja, and W. F. Miser. 2012. Comparative effectiveness of a mindful eating intervention to a diabetes self-management intervention among adults with type 2 diabetes: A pilot study. *Journal of the Academy of Nutrition and Dietetics* 112 (11): 1835–1842.

Moray, J., A. Fu, K. Brill, and M. S. Mayoral. 2007. Viewing television while eating impairs the ability to accurately estimate total amount of food consumed. *Bariatric Nursing and Surgical Patient Care* 2 (1): 71–76.

Murawski, M. E., V. A. Milsom, K. M. Ross, K. A. Rickel, N. DeBraganza, L. M. Gibbons, and M. G. Perri. 2009. Problem solving, treatment adherence, and weight-loss outcome among women participating in lifestyle treatment for obesity. *Eating Behaviors* 10 (3): 146–151.

Murphy, R., S. Straebler, Z. Cooper, and C. G. Fairburn. 2010. Cognitive behavioral therapy for eating disorders. *Cognitive Behavioral Therapy for Psychiatric Clinics of North America* 33 (3): 611–627.

Nathan, P. J. and E. T. Bullmore. 2009. From taste hedonics to motivational drive: Central μ-opioid receptors and binge-eating behaviour. *International Journal of Neuropsychopharmacology* 12 (7): 995–1008.

National Institute for Clinical Excellence. 2004. National Institute for Clinical Excellence (NICE). Eating disorders: Core interventions in the treatment and management of anorexia nervosa, bulimia nervosa and related eating disorders. *Clinical Guideline* 9. https://www.nice.org.uk/.

Newman, E., D. B. O'Connor, and M. Conner. 2007. Daily hassles and eating behaviour: The role of cortisol reactivity status. *Psychoneuroendocrinology* 32 (2): 125–132.

Norris, S. L., X. Zhang, A. Avenell, E. Gregg, B. Bowman, C. H. Schmid, and J. Lau. 2005. Long-term effectiveness of weight-loss interventions in adults with pre-diabetes: A review. *American Journal of Preventive Medicine* 28 (1): 126–139.

Oakes, M. E. 2005. Stereotypical thinking about foods and perceived capacity to promote weight gain. *Appetite* 44 (3): 317–324.

Oliver, G., J. Wardle, and E. L. Gibson. 2000. Stress and food choice: A laboratory study. *Psychosomatic Medicine* 62 (6): 853–865.

O'Reilly, G. A., L. Cook, D. Spruijt-Metz, and D. S. Black. 2014. Mindfulness-based interventions for obesity-related eating behaviours: A literature review. *Obesity Reviews* 15 (6): 453–461.

Oswald, K. D., D. L. Murdaugh, V. L. King, and M. M. Boggiano. 2011. Motivation for palatable food despite consequences in an animal model of binge eating. *International Journal of Eating Disorders* 44 (3): 203–211.

Perri, M. G., A. M. Nezu, and B. J. Viegener. 1992. *Improving the Long-Term Management of Obesity: Theory, Research, and Clinical Guidelines*. Vol. xvi. Wiley Series on Health Psychology/Behavioral Medicine. Oxford, England: John Wiley & Sons.

Phillips-Caesar, E. G., G. Winston, J. C. Peterson, B. Wansink, C. M. Devine, B. Kanna, W. Michelin et al. 2015. Small changes and lasting effects (SCALE) trial: The formation of a weight loss behavioral intervention using EVOLVE. *Contemporary Clinical Trials* 41 (March): 118–128.

Pliner, P., R. Bell, E. S. Hirsch, and M. Kinchla. 2006. Meal duration mediates the effect of 'social facilitation' on eating in humans. *Appetite* 46 (2): 189–198.

Pratt, C. A., S. C. Lemon, I. D. Fernandez, R. Goetzel, S. A. Beresford, S. A. French, V. J. Stevens, T. M. Vogt, and L. S. Webber. 2007. Design characteristics of worksite environmental interventions for obesity prevention. *Obesity* 15 (9): 2171–2180.

Privitera, G. J. and H. E. Creary. 2013. Proximity and visibility of fruits and vegetables influence intake in a kitchen setting among college students. *Environment and Behavior* 45 (7): 876–886.

Privitera, G. J. and F. M. Zuraikat. 2014. Proximity of foods in a competitive food environment influences consumption of a low calorie and a high calorie food. *Appetite* 76: 175–179.

Provencher, V., J. Polivy, and C. P. Herman. 2009. Perceived healthiness of food. If it's healthy, you can eat more! *Appetite* 52 (2): 340–344.

Raaijmakers, L. C. H., S. Pouwels, K. A. Berghuis, and S. W. Nienhuijs. 2015. Technology-based interventions in the treatment of overweight and obesity: A systematic review. *Appetite* 95 (December): 138–151.

Rada, P., N. M. Avena, and B. G. Hoebel. 2005. Daily bingeing on sugar repeatedly releases dopamine in the accumbens shell. *Neuroscience* 134 (3): 737–744.

Raevuori, A., J. Suokas, J. Haukka, M. Gissler, M. Linna, M. Grainger, and J. Suvisaari. 2015. Highly increased risk of type 2 diabetes in patients with binge eating disorder and bulimia nervosa. *International Journal of Eating Disorders* 48 (6): 555–562.

Robinson, E., J. Blissett, and S. Higgs. 2013. Social influences on eating: Implications for nutritional interventions. *Nutrition Research Reviews* 26 (02): 166–176.

Robinson, E., T. Tobias, L. Shaw, E. Freeman, and S. Higgs. 2011. Social matching of food intake and the need for social acceptance. *Appetite* 56 (3): 747–752.

Rutters, F., A. G. Nieuwenhuizen, S. G. T. Lemmens, J. M. Born, and M. S. Westerterp-Plantenga. 2009. Acute stress-related changes in eating in the absence of hunger. *Obesity* 17 (1): 72–77.

Salvy, S.-J., D. Jarrin, R. Paluch, N. Irfan, and P. Pliner. 2007. Effects of social influence on eating in couples, friends and strangers. *Appetite* 49 (1): 92–99.

Schlenker, B. R. 1980. *Impression Management: The Self-Concept, Social Identity, and Interpersonal Relations*. Monterey, CA: Brooks/Cole Publishing Company Monterey.

Schulz, M., A. D. Liese, H. Boeing, J. E. Cunningham, C. G. Moore, and A. Kroke. 2005. Associations of short-term weight changes and weight cycling with incidence of essential hypertension in the EPIC-potsdam study. *Journal of Human Hypertension* 19 (1): 61–67.

Schwartz, J. and C. Byrd-Bredbenner. 2006. Portion distortion: Typical portion sizes selected by young adults. *Journal of the American Dietetic Association* 106 (9): 1412–1418.

Sheeran, P. 2002. Intention–behavior relations: A conceptual and empirical review. *European Review of Social Psychology* 12 (1): 1–36.

Sigurdsson, V., N. M. Larsen, and D. Gunnarsson. 2014. Healthy food products at the point of purchase: An in-store experimental analysis. *Journal of Applied Behavior Analysis* 47 (1): 151–154.

Sigurdsson, V., H. Saevarsson, and G. Foxall. 2009. Brand placement and consumer choice: An in-store experiment. *Journal of Applied Behavior Analysis* 42 (3): 741–745.

Sinha, R. and A. M. Jastreboff. 2013. Stress as a common risk factor for obesity and addiction. *Biological Psychiatry* 73 (9): 827–835.

Smith, B. W., B. M. Shelley, J. Dalen, K. Wiggins, E. Tooley, and J. Bernard. 2008. A pilot study comparing the effects of mindfulness-based and cognitive-behavioral stress reduction. *The Journal of Alternative and Complementary Medicine* 14 (3): 251–258.

Smith, B. W., B. M. Shelley, L. Leahigh, and B. Vanleit. 2006. A preliminary study of the effects of a modified mindfulness intervention on binge eating. *Complementary Health Practice Review* 11 (3): 133–143.

Smith, D. G. and T. W. Robbins. 2013. The neurobiological underpinnings of obesity and binge eating: A rationale for adopting the food addiction model. *Biological Psychiatry* 73 (9): 804–810.

Smithers, R. 2014. Tesco bans sweets from checkouts in all stores. *The Guardian*, May 21, sec. Business. http://www.theguardian.com/business/2014/may/22/tesco-bans-sweets-from-checkouts-all-stores.

Sobal, J. and B. Wansink. 2007. Kitchenscapes, tablescapes, platescapes, and foodscapes influences of microscale built environments on food intake. *Environment and Behavior* 39 (1): 124–142.

Sørensen, L. B., P. Møller, A. Flint, M. Martens, and A. Raben. 2003. Effect of sensory perception of foods on appetite and food intake: A review of studies on humans. *International Journal of Obesity* 27 (10): 1152–1166.

Spence, C. 2012. Auditory contributions to flavour perception and feeding behaviour. *Physiology & Behavior* 107 (4): 505–515.

Spitzer, R. L., M. Devlin, B. T. Walsh, D. Hasin, R. Wing, M. Marcus, A. Stunkard et al. 1992. Binge eating disorder: A multisite field trial of the diagnostic criteria. *International Journal of Eating Disorders* 11 (3): 191–203.

Stroebele, N. and J. M. de Castro. 2004. Effect of ambience on food intake and food choice. *Nutrition* 20 (9): 821–838.

Stroebele, N. and J. M. de Castro. 2006. Listening to music while eating is related to increases in people's food intake and meal duration. *Appetite* 47 (3): 285–289.

Stuart, R. B. 1967. Behavioral control of overeating. *Behaviour Research and Therapy* 5 (4): 357–365.

Sullivan, H. W. and A. J. Rothman. 2008. When planning is needed: Implementation intentions and attainment of approach versus avoidance health goals. *Health Psychology* 27 (4): 438–444.

Tapper, K., C. Shaw, J. Ilsley, A. J. Hill, F. W. Bond, and L. Moore. 2009. Exploratory randomised controlled trial of a mindfulness-based weight loss intervention for women. *Appetite* 52 (2): 396–404.

Telch, C. F., W. S. Agras, and M. M. Linehan. 2001. Dialectical behavior therapy for binge eating disorder. *Journal of Consulting and Clinical Psychology* 69 (6): 1061.

Timmerman, G. M. and A. Brown. 2012. The effect of a mindful restaurant eating intervention on weight management in women. *Journal of Nutrition Education and Behavior* 44 (1): 22–28.

Tryon, M. S., C. S. Carter, R. DeCant, and K. D. Laugero. 2013. Chronic stress exposure may affect the brain's response to high calorie food cues and predispose to obesogenic eating habits. *Physiology & Behavior* 120: 233–242.

Tsenkova, V., J. M. Boylan, and C. Ryff. 2013. Stress eating and health. Findings from MIDUS, a national study of US adults. *Appetite* 69: 151–155.

Turner-McGrievy, G. M., M. W. Beets, J. B. Moore, A. T. Kaczynski, D. J. Barr-Anderson, and D. F. Tate. 2013. Comparison of traditional versus mobile app self-monitoring of physical activity and dietary intake among overweight adults participating in an mHealth weight loss program. *Journal of the American Medical Informatics Association* 20 (3): 513–518.

Ulrich-Lai, Y. M., S. Fulton, M. Wilson, G. Petrovich, and L. Rinaman. 2015. Stress exposure, food intake and emotional state. *Stress* 18 (4): 381–399.

Vartanian, L. R., C. P. Herman, and J. Polivy. 2007. Consumption stereotypes and impression management: How you are what you eat. *Appetite* 48 (3): 265–277.

Vermeer, W. M., I. H. M. Steenhuis, F. H. Leeuwis, M. W. Heymans, and J. C. Seidell. 2011. Small portion sizes in worksite cafeterias: Do they help consumers to reduce their food intake? *International Journal of Obesity* 35 (9): 1200–1207.

Vocks, S., B. Tuschen-Caffier, R. Pietrowsky, S. J. Rustenbach, A. Kersting, and S. Herpertz. 2010. Meta-analysis of the effectiveness of psychological and pharmacological treatments for binge eating disorder. *International Journal of Eating Disorders* 43 (3): 205–217.

Volkow, N. D., G.-J. Wang, and R. D. Baler. 2011. Reward, dopamine and the control of food intake: Implications for obesity. *Trends in Cognitive Sciences* 15 (1): 37–46.

Volkow, N. D., G.-J. Wang, J. S. Fowler, and F. Telang. 2008. Overlapping neuronal circuits in addiction and obesity: Evidence of systems pathology. *Philosophical Transactions of the Royal Society of London B: Biological Sciences* 363 (1507): 3191–3200.

Volkow, N. D., G. J. Wang, J. S. Fowler, D. Tomasi, and R. Baler. 2012. Food and drug reward: Overlapping circuits in human obesity and addiction. *Current Topics in Behavioral Neurosciences* 11: 1–24.

Volkow, N. D., G. J. Wang, D. Tomasi, and R. D. Baler. 2013. Obesity and addiction: Neurobiological overlaps. *Obesity Reviews* 14 (1): 2–18.

Wadden, T. A., M. L. Butryn, and C. Wilson. 2007. Lifestyle modification for the management of obesity. *Gastroenterology* 132 (6): 2226–2238.

Wadden, T. A., C. E. Crerand, and J. Brock. 2005. Behavioral treatment of obesity. *Psychiatric Clinics of North America* 28 (1): 151–170.

Wadden, T. A., V. L. Webb, C. H. Moran, and B. A. Bailer. 2012. Lifestyle modification for obesity new developments in diet, physical activity, and behavior therapy. *Circulation* 125 (9): 1157–1170.

Wadhwa, M., B. Shiv, and S. M. Nowlis. 2008. A bite to whet the reward appetite: The influence of sampling on reward-seeking behaviors. *Journal of Marketing Research* 45 (4): 403–413.

Wansink, B. 2007. *Mindless Eating: Why We Eat More Than We Think*. New York: Random House LLC.

Wansink, B. 2010. From mindless eating to mindlessly eating better. *Physiology & Behavior* 100 (5): 454–463.

Wansink, B. 2014. *Slim by Design*. New York: HarperCollins.

Wansink, B. and P. Chandon. 2006. Meal size, not body size, explains errors in estimating the calorie content of meals. *Annals of Internal Medicine* 145 (5): 326–332.

Wansink, B. and P. Chandon. 2014. Slim by design: Redirecting the accidental drivers of mindless overeating. *Journal of Consumer Psychology* 24: 413–431.

Wansink, B. and A. S. Hanks. 2013. Slim by design: Serving healthy foods first in buffet lines improves overall meal selection. *PLoS ONE* 8 (10): e77055.

Wansink, B., D. R. Just, A. S. Hanks, and L. E. Smith. 2013. Pre-sliced fruit in school cafeterias: Children's selection and intake. *American Journal of Preventive Medicine* 44 (5): 477–480.

Wansink, B., D. R. Just, C. R. Payne, and M. Z. Klinger. 2012. Attractive names sustain increased vegetable intake in schools. *Preventive Medicine* 55 (4): 330–332.

Wansink, B. and J. Kim. 2005. Bad popcorn in big buckets: Portion size can influence intake as much as taste. *Journal of Nutrition Education and Behavior* 37 (5): 242–245.

Wansink, B., J. E. Painter, and Y.-K. Lee. 2006a. The office candy dish: Proximity's influence on estimated and actual consumption. *International Journal of Obesity* 30 (5): 871–875.

Wansink, B., J. Painter, and K. Van Ittersum. 2001. Descriptive menu labels' effect on sales. *The Cornell Hotel and Restaurant Administration Quarterly* 42 (6): 68–72.

Wansink, B., C. R. Payne, and M. Shimizu. 2011. The 100-calorie semi-solution: Sub-packaging most reduces intake among the heaviest. *Obesity* 19 (5): 1098–1100.

Wansink, B. and K. van Ittersum. 2012. Fast food restaurant lighting and music can reduce calorie intake and increase satisfaction. *Psychological Reports* 111 (1): 228–232.

Wansink, B., K. van Ittersum, and J. E. Painter. 2005. How descriptive food names bias sensory perceptions in restaurants. *Food Quality and Preference* 16 (5): 393–400.

Wansink, B., K. van Ittersum, and J. E. Painter. 2006b. Ice cream illusions: Bowls, spoons, and self-served portion sizes. *American Journal of Preventive Medicine* 31 (3): 240–243.

Warziski, M. T., S. M. Sereika, M. A. Styn, E. Music, and L. E. Burke. 2007. Changes in self-efficacy and dietary adherence: The impact on weight loss in the PREFER Study. *Journal of Behavioral Medicine* 31 (1): 81–92.

Wharton, C. M., C. S. Johnston, B. K. Cunningham, and D. Sterner. 2014. Dietary self-monitoring, but not dietary quality, improves with use of smartphone app technology in an 8-week weight loss trial. *Journal of Nutrition Education and Behavior* 46 (5): 440–444.

Wilson, G. T., D. E. Wilfley, W. S. Agras, and S. W. Bryson. 2010. Psychological treatments of binge eating disorder. *Archives of General Psychiatry* 67 (1): 94–101.

Wolff, G. E. and M. M. Clark. 2001. Changes in eating self-efficacy and body image following cognitive–behavioral group therapy for binge eating disorder: A clinical study. *Eating Behaviors* 2 (2): 97–104.

Woolhouse, H., A. Knowles, and N. Crafti. 2012. Adding mindfulness to CBT programs for binge eating: A mixed-methods evaluation. *Eating Disorders* 20 (4): 321–339.

Yeomans, M. R. 1996. Palatability and the micro-structure of feeding in humans: The appetizer effect. *Appetite* 27 (2): 119–133.

Yeomans, M. R. and T. Symes. 1999. Individual differences in the use of pleasantness and palatability ratings. *Appetite* 32 (3): 383–394.

Zifferblatt, S. M., C. S. Wilbur, and J. L. Pinsky. 1980. Influence of ecologic events on cafeteria food selections: Understanding food habits. *Journal of the American Dietetic Association* 76 (1): 9–14.

3 Energy Balance and Regulation of Body Weight

Are All Calories Equal?

Kevin D. Hall

CONTENTS

ABSTRACT

While the human body obeys the law of energy conservation, this alone does not imply that dietary carbohydrate, fat, and protein have contributed equally to the rise in obesity prevalence over the past several decades. Indeed, three scientific models of obesity have implicated each macronutrient as being the prime culprit, but the evidence supporting these models is, at best, mixed and, at worst, demonstrably false. This chapter reviews the concepts of energy balance and macronutrient balance as applied to the human body and presents the evidence for and against three scientific models that alternately place the blame for obesity on each dietary macronutrient. Finally, the chapter discusses putative mechanisms for why obesity prevalence has been increasing despite the likelihood that human body weight is actively regulated by a biological feedback control system.

INTRODUCTION

We live in an age where the developed world is becoming increasingly overweight and obese with potentially dire consequences for population health and the economy (Swinburn et al. 2011). At least a dozen putative causes of obesity have been proposed (Keith et al. 2006, McAllister et al. 2009), and media coverage of obesity has soared (Hilton, Patterson, and Teyhan 2012). Every comments section following an Internet article about obesity includes opinions from people who have avoided excess weight gain or have successfully lost weight and are convinced of their personal superiority over those who have succumbed to obesity. They often make strong claims about what really underlies obesity and how to solve it.

If your town still has a book shop, visit its nutrition and health section. You will find row upon row of books suggesting that the reader forget everything they have been told about diet and nutrition. The truth was somehow buried or unknown until now when the author will finally reveal that there is a painless way to melt the pounds away without feeling hungry or deprived. The science is surprisingly simple (and adequately covered in a couple of cursory chapters) as is the eating plan. Unfortunately, the truth is more complicated.

This chapter will attempt to clarify some popular misconceptions about the relationships between energy balance and body weight regulation as well as provide a brief overview of several models of obesity that purport causal relationships between dietary macronutrients and the accumulation of excess body fat.

ENERGY BALANCE AS A CONCEPTUAL FRAMEWORK

Any imbalance between the energy derived from food eaten and the energy expended to maintain life and perform physical work will be accounted for by changes in the body's energy stores, primarily body fat. This concept of energy balance as applied to body weight regulation is a useful bookkeeping device and is a necessary consequence of the physical law of energy conservation. However, energy balance is not a statement about causality and does not explain why some people have obesity.

In particular, it does not follow from the energy balance principle that the obesity epidemic has resulted from widespread moral failings or lack of willpower leading to population-wide increases in gluttony and sloth. Prevention of obesity is often erroneously portrayed as a simple matter of balancing calories in with calories out and that people with obesity should simply eat less and exercise more. Conversely, the fact that these failed concepts are incorrect does not imply that energy balance is an erroneous or useless concept.

Rather, the energy balance principle provides important constraints that are useful for experimental investigation of body weight regulation. For example, the complex biochemistry that derives energy from oxidation of macronutrients obeys the law of energy conservation and when these processes take place at constant pressure, as they do inside cells, the corresponding heat released is quantified by the enthalpy of the reactions. Furthermore, Hess's law of path independence dictates that the same net enthalpy change occurs in both the bomb calorimeter and the human body (although the reactions inside the calorimeter occur at constant volume and thermodynamics provides the means of accounting for this difference). In other words, "a calorie is a calorie" when it comes to macronutrients being oxidized either in the calorimeter through combustion or via the intricate biochemical pathways of oxidative phosphorylation inside cells. (Protein is incompletely oxidized in the body and the measurements can be corrected via application of Hess's law to account for the enthalpy of formation of the nitrogenous end products.)

The fact that the energy derived from macronutrient oxidation in the body can be equated to the energy derived from their combustion in a bomb calorimeter is a keystone for the study of in vivo energy metabolism. However, this equivalence does not imply that altering dietary macronutrients will necessarily have no effect on the body's energy expenditure or composition. Rather, manipulation of dietary macronutrients may alter overall calorie intake and/or expenditure with a corresponding requisite change in the energy stores of the body, likely primarily body fat changes.

Alternatively, changing dietary macronutrient composition may alter endocrine factors that influence the propensity to accumulate body fat or direct the storage of fat to particular locations. These possibilities do not violate the principle of energy balance since any changes in the body's overall energy stores must therefore also be accompanied by changes in calorie intake and/or expenditure.

REGULATION OF MACRONUTRIENT METABOLISM: IS A CALORIE A CALORIE?

The human body has been analogized to an automobile that runs on arbitrary mixtures of three different fuels (Hall 2010, 2012). Such a flex-fuel vehicle would allow the driver to fill the fuel tank with whatever fuel was cheaper or more readily available, regardless of the mixture already in the tank. Imagine the additional complexity if the vehicle was not allowed to have a fuel tank. Rather, the vehicle itself is composed of its fuel and is continually breaking down and reconstructing its components. Furthermore, despite the daily fluctuations of fuel delivery, the composition of the vehicle remains relatively stable and maintains similar performance characteristics, at least over the short term.

Exactly this remarkable engineering feat is accomplished by the human body through its use of the three dietary macronutrients (carbohydrate, fat, and protein) to both fuel metabolism and provide substrates for body constituents. The ability to adapt to a wide variety of diets was an evolutionary necessity that has allowed humans to thrive across the globe in widely different environmental conditions.

In the United States, roughly 50% of dietary energy is derived from carbohydrate, 35% from fat, and 15% from protein (Austin, Ogden, and Hill 2011). However, these average diet proportions can vary widely from person to person and also from day to day. Complex physiological control mechanisms maintain normal functioning of the body despite marked fluctuations of diet quantity and composition. However, these physiological adaptations may be imperfect and it is theoretically possible that sustained long-term manipulations of diet composition might lead to substantial alterations in body composition independent of calorie intake.

For example, isocaloric diets differing in macronutrient composition may result in preferential partitioning of energy storage toward body fat and away from other pools such as body protein. Such energy partitioning differences over the long term will thereby alter fat-free mass and influence energy expenditure. Dietary protein in particular is known to both influence body composition (Leidy et al. 2015) and is thermogenic (Bray et al. 2012, Ebbeling et al. 2012, Thearle et al. 2013, Wycherley et al. 2012).

Even with clamped dietary protein, varying the ratio of carbohydrate to fat between isocaloric diets is predicted to have an effect on energy expenditure by altering metabolic flux patterns through energy-requiring pathways such as gluconeogenesis (Veldhorst, Westerterp-Plantenga, and Westerterp 2009) and the triglyceride fatty acid cycle (Elia et al. 1987). For example, computational model simulations have found that wide variations in the proportion of carbohydrate to fat are predicted to result in modest changes in total energy expenditure and body fat in a non-monotonic pattern over a relatively narrow range (Hall et al. 2015). Thus, the nutritional aphorism that "a calorie is a calorie" (Buchholz and Schoeller 2004) may be only approximately true and the body achieves this near equivalence only as a result of major changes in the underlying metabolic flux patterns that adapt to the diet variations.

MODELS OF OBESITY THAT IMPLICATE INDIVIDUAL MACRONUTRIENTS

Scientific models seek to integrate a variety of data and explain a set of observations about a system within an overarching theoretical and mechanistic framework. Importantly, scientific models go beyond providing putative explanations and make experimentally testable predictions that are capable of falsifying the models.

Experimental confirmation of a model's predictions thereby provides additional support and repeated confirmations may eventually lead to widespread acceptance of the model as the scientific standard. However, models cannot be proven to be true but are rather provisional representations of our understanding. Countering evidence may lead to model corrections or possibly outright rejection.

Putative explanations of obesity abound (Keith et al. 2006, McAllister et al. 2009), but these are typically derived from observed correlations and scientific models of obesity that are amenable to experimental investigation in humans are rare. A few models of obesity have been proposed that focus on the macronutrient composition of the diet as the cause of excess adiposity. Unfortunately, while these macronutrient models are more amenable to scientific scrutiny, none appear to adequately explain the observations.

The Carbohydrate–Insulin Model

An increased proportion of refined carbohydrates in the diet has been purported to be particularly fattening due to the propensity of such diets to elevate insulin secretion (Ludwig and Friedman 2014, Lustig 2006, Taubes 2013, Wells and Siervo 2011). According to this "carbohydrate–insulin model" of obesity, elevated insulin suppresses the release of fatty acids into the circulation and directs circulating fat toward storage and away from oxidation by metabolically active tissues such as heart, muscle, and liver. The altered fuel delivery to such tissues has been suggested to result in adaptive decrease in energy expenditure and increased food intake (Astwood 1962, Ludwig and Friedman 2014, Pennington 1952, 1953, Wells and Siervo 2011). Therefore, the positive energy balance associated with the development of obesity is hypothesized to be a consequence of the insulin-driven shift in fat partitioning toward storage and away from oxidation due to an increased proportion of dietary carbohydrates.

The carbohydrate–insulin model of obesity has gained a following in recent years due to various popular accounts (Ludwig 2016, Taubes 2007, 2011) and commentaries in influential medical journals (Ludwig and Friedman 2014, Taubes 2013). Some epidemiological evidence appears to support the carbohydrate–insulin model since added sugars and sweeteners have increased in parallel to the development of the obesity epidemic (Wells and Buzby 2008), and self-reported carbohydrate intake has also increased (Austin, Ogden, and Hill 2011). However, correlations do not necessarily imply causation and there is little evidence that the overall carbohydrate fraction of the available food supply has substantially changed during the development of the obesity epidemic (Hiza, Bente, and Fungwe 2008).

Experimentally testing the carbohydrate–insulin model requires devising a study that mechanistically evaluates the model's predictions. For example, the carbohydrate–insulin model predicts that reduction of dietary carbohydrates will result in decreased insulin secretion, increased fat oxidation, increased energy expenditure, and greater body fat loss compared to an isocaloric reduction of dietary fat. Many of these predictions were recently tested in a study that confined adults with obesity to a metabolic ward where all food intake and physical activities were strictly monitored and controlled (Hall et al. 2015). The subjects were fed a standard baseline diet representing a typical habitual diet that provided 35% fat, 15% protein, and 50% carbohydrate with about 20% of total calories coming from sugar, and where calories were matched to participants' energy expenditure. In a randomized crossover design, diet calories were then cut by 30%, either entirely through restricting carbohydrates, keeping protein and fat at baseline, or selectively restricting fat and keeping protein, carbohydrates, and sugar at baseline.

The reduced-carbohydrate diet led to decreased insulin secretion and increased net fat oxidation as predicted by the carbohydrate–insulin model. However, despite no significant change in insulin secretion, the reduced-fat diet resulted in a significantly greater rate of fat loss than the reduced-carbohydrate diet, which is contrary to the carbohydrate–insulin model predictions. The small observed difference in body fat loss between the diets was detected using the metabolic balance method that is more precise than direct body composition assessment methods that were unable to measure significant differences between the diets (Hall et al. 2015).

The reduced-carbohydrate diet also led to a significant decrease in energy expenditure, both during sleep and throughout the day, whereas the reduced-fat diet had no significant effect on energy expenditure (Hall et al. 2015). Again, these results are contrary to the carbohydrate–insulin model but are in line with previous inpatient isocaloric diet studies employing clamped protein and varying carbohydrates from 20% to 75% of total calories that have either found small decreases in energy expenditure with lower-carbohydrate diets (Astrup et al. 1994, Dirlewanger et al. 2000, Horton et al. 1995, Shepard et al. 2001) or no statistically significant difference (Davy et al. 2001, Eckel et al. 2006, Hill et al. 1991, Rumpler et al. 1991, Schrauwen et al. 1997, Smith et al. 2000, Thearle et al. 2013, Treuth et al. 2003, Yerboeket-van de Venne and Westerterp 1996). Dietary carbohydrate restriction has only ever been observed to result in significantly increased energy expenditure if accompanied by an increase in dietary protein (Ebbeling et al. 2012, Veldhorst, Westerterp-Plantenga, and Westerterp 2009), which is known to be thermogenic (Bray et al. 2012, Ebbeling et al. 2012, Thearle et al. 2013, Wycherley et al. 2012).

In sum, the predictions of the carbohydrate–insulin model have been experimentally demonstrated to be false. However, this does not imply that dietary carbohydrates or insulin are unimportant for the development of obesity or its treatment. Diets with high amounts of insulinogenic carbohydrates may result in greater overall energy intake and cause obesity by mechanisms quite different from that proposed by the previous carbohydrate–insulin model, such as by increasing palatability or decreasing satiety. Conversely, prescribing very-low-carbohydrate diets appears to offer some short-term benefit for weight loss (Bueno et al. 2013), but this is unlikely due to increased metabolic rate (Hall et al. 2015, Johnston et al. 2006). Rather, such diets likely reduce appetite by promoting an increase in circulating ketones (Gibson et al. 2015), although the mechanism for this effect is unclear (Paoli et al. 2015). Furthermore, low-carbohydrate diets often result in comparatively greater protein intake that may increase satiety, decrease overall energy intake, increase energy expenditure, and beneficially influence energy partitioning and body composition (Leidy et al. 2015).

The Protein Leverage Model

The "protein leverage model" of obesity that postulates that the body seeks to consume a target amount of dietary protein, and if the protein fraction of diet is lowered then overall energy intake increases in an attempt to achieve the protein target, thereby resulting in positive energy balance and obesity (Simpson and Raubenheimer 2005). The protein leverage model of obesity is consistent with the observation that self-reported protein intake has decreased as a percentage of total calories since the 1970s (Austin, Ogden, and Hill 2011), but there is little evidence that the protein fraction of the available food supply has decreased (Hiza, Bente, and Fungwe 2008). Protein leverage may explain why higher-protein diets are more satiating and why increased dietary protein results in improved maintenance of lost weight (Leidy et al. 2015). However, the central tenet of the protein leverage model has recently been tested in three randomized controlled studies (Gosby et al. 2011, Martens, Lemmens, and Westerterp-Plantenga 2013, Martens et al. 2014) with the data from two of the three studies countering the model predictions.

Using a randomized crossover design, a total of 137 adults with a wide range of ages and degrees of adiposity were provided with ad libitum diets that varied the protein proportion of energy: 5%, 15%, or 25% of calories with a constant 33% fat for three periods of 12 days each (Martens, Lemmens, and Westerterp-Plantenga 2013, Martens et al. 2014). Contrary to the protein leverage model of obesity, the low-protein diet did not result in increased energy intake compared to the moderate-protein diet, whereas the high-protein diet led to a significantly decreased energy intake.

Another study was conducted by the originators of the protein leverage model who investigated 22 lean subjects in a randomized crossover fashion for three periods of 4 days each where the diets had 10%, 15%, and 25% of their energy as protein (Gosby et al. 2011). That study provided confirmatory evidence for the protein leverage model by demonstrating that the low-protein diet resulted in a significant increase in energy intake amounting to ~260 kcal per day compared to the moderate-protein diet, but the higher-protein diet did not result in a significant decrease in energy intake. If sustained for decades, such an increase in energy intake with the low-protein diet could fully account for the mean weight gain corresponding to the U.S. obesity epidemic (Hall et al. 2011). But considering the lack of effect of decreased dietary protein in the longer-term studies (Martens, Lemmens, and Westerterp-Plantenga 2013, Martens et al. 2014), the overall weight of the evidence does not appear to support the protein leverage model of obesity. Nevertheless, higher-protein diets may play an important role in weight loss interventions, maintenance of lost weight, and prevention of obesity (Leidy et al. 2015).

The Dietary Fat Model

The dietary fat model of obesity postulates that an increased proportion of the diet coming from fat results in elevated energy intake along with efficient storage of the excess energy as body fat (Astrup et al. 2000, Bray and Popkin 1998). It has long been recognized that dietary fat contains more than twice the calories per gram compared to carbohydrate and protein. Furthermore, naturally low-fat foods contain dietary carbohydrate and protein that are associated with large amounts of water that further decreases their energy density. Dietary fat is also less satiating than protein or carbohydrate (Stubbs 1998) and results in a smaller increment in energy expenditure compared to isocaloric feeding of dietary carbohydrate or protein (Westerterp 2004). Covert experimental increases in dietary fat content have been demonstrated to result in increased energy intake, positive energy balance, and accumulation of body fat (Stubbs et al. 1995a,b). Dietary fat does not directly promote its own oxidation (Flatt et al. 1985, Schutz, Flatt, and Jequier 1989) and body fat accumulates efficiently with added dietary fat and is relatively unopposed until adipose tissue has sufficiently expanded such that daily lipolysis increases to an extent sufficient to elevate circulating fatty acids and balance fat oxidation with fat intake (Flatt 1988). Furthermore, decreasing the fat content of meals leads to lower ad libitum energy intake (Rolls 2009, Williams, Roe, and Rolls 2013) and experimental overfeeding of dietary fat results in greater increases in body fat compared to isocaloric carbohydrate overfeeding (Horton et al. 1995). Therefore, several aspects of the dietary fat model have been confirmed.

The dietary fat model of obesity, along with concerns about saturated fat being linked to increased cardiovascular mortality, helped lead to public health messages to decrease our intake of dietary fat (Walker and Parker 2014). Unfortunately, the food industry capitalized on this opportunity to increase the production and marketing of highly processed, inexpensive, and convenient low-fat foods with high sugar content that lacked the benefits of foods naturally low in fat (Moss 2013, Roberts 2008, Swinburn et al. 2011). As a result, while self-reported fat intake decreased as a proportion of calories, absolute fat intake was relatively unchanged (Austin, Ogden, and Hill 2011) and added sugars, fats, and oils in the food supply have increased (Wells and Buzby 2008) in parallel with the rise in obesity prevalence. Furthermore, prescriptions to reduce dietary fat have not resulted in improved weight loss over the long term (Tobias et al. 2015). Thus, while the dietary fat model of obesity appears to be supported by physiological studies, the epidemiological and weight loss studies provide contrary evidence.

BODY WEIGHT REGULATION

Over the long term, all weight loss diets appear to be similarly ineffective for obesity treatment regardless of the prescribed changes in macronutrient composition (Hu et al. 2012, Johnston et al. 2014, Tobias et al. 2015). This is likely because the body actively resists weight loss by increasing appetite due to the action of feedback circuits influencing energy intake in response to weight changes (Gautron, Elmquist, and Williams 2015, Woods and D'Alessio 2008). These adaptations make it extraordinarily difficult to adhere to a diet over the long term (Hall 2015). Furthermore, weight loss results in a suppression of energy expenditure beyond what would be expected based on the body weight or composition changes alone. This phenomenon, called "metabolic adaptation" or "adaptive thermogenesis," has been repeatedly demonstrated in humans and both resting energy expenditure and physical activity energy expenditure are altered in parallel (Westerterp 2013). Therefore, achieving large sustained weight losses is difficult and weight regain is typical in the absence of vigilant efforts to maintain behavior changes (Greenway 2015).

If both energy intake and expenditure are controlled by feedback systems that regulate body weight, why have these systems been unable to prevent the obesity epidemic? A likely explanation is that the feedback system is only one part of a complex neurobiological system including hedonic and cognitive factors that act in concert to determine overall human food intake behavior (Berthoud 2012, Hall,

Hammond, and Rahmandad 2014). The feedback circuits were effective for body weight regulation in the environments that were prevalent in the distant evolutionary past.

However, over the past several decades, the feedback system may have been overwhelmed by the increased availability and marketing of inexpensive, convenient, energy-dense, palatable food (Moss 2013, Roberts 2008, Swinburn et al. 2011). In addition, occupations have become more sedentary (Church et al. 2011), food has progressively become cheaper (Putnam 2000), fewer people prepare meals at home (Lin and Guthrie 2012, Smith, Ng, and Popkin 2013), and more food is consumed in restaurants (Lin and Guthrie 2012). Food availability has increased by approximately 750 kcal per day that is so much more than enough to explain the observed increase in body weight that per capita food waste has increased by 50% (Hall et al. 2009).

Consider the analogy to a thermostat that attempts to control the temperature of a home through operation of a heating and air-conditioning system (Hall, Hammond, and Rahmandad 2014). A system that is adequately powered for the year-round temperate climate of Northern California may be insufficient to maintain a comfortable indoor temperature of the same home in Minnesota during the winter or in Florida during the summer. Nothing is inherently "wrong" with the heating and air-conditioning system, it is merely underpowered for the new environment and the temperature will be maintained at a level that is different from the set point of the thermostat.

Similarly, the feedback circuits that evolved to regulate body weight eons ago may have been overwhelmed in recent decades by the obesogenic environment of today. Whether such changes or the elevation of body weight itself additionally resets the homeostatic set point of the body weight "thermostat" upward is an interesting question.

CONCLUSION

While a multitude of environmental changes offer a plausible explanation for the rise in obesity prevalence, causality has not been demonstrated. Indeed, it is difficult to imagine how one could devise practical experimental tests of these putative explanations since such complex changes in the environment are difficult to manipulate. In contrast, the simpler macronutrient models of obesity discussed earlier have all been found to be contrary to some observations and, at best, incomplete.

Therefore, there has yet to be a model of obesity that has been adequately experimentally tested, repeatedly confirmed, and commensurate with all of the observations. In other words, there is presently no scientifically accepted standard model of obesity. It is possible that the obesity epidemic resulted from a complex confluence of multiple causes, or that a simple comprehensive model has been too difficult to adequately experimentally investigate. What appears to be clear is that no single macronutrient is the culprit or the cure for obesity.

ACKNOWLEDGMENT

This research was supported by the Intramural Research Program of the NIH, National Institute of Diabetes and Digestive and Kidney Diseases.

REFERENCES

Astrup, A., B. Buemann, N. J. Christensen, and S. Toubro. Failure to increase lipid oxidation in response to increasing dietary fat content in formerly obese women. *Am J Physiol* 266(4 Pt 1) (April 1994): E592–E599.

Astrup, A., L. Ryan, G. K. Grunwald, M. Storgaard, W. Saris, E. Melanson, and J. O. Hill. The role of dietary fat in body fatness: Evidence from a preliminary meta-analysis of ad libitum low-fat dietary intervention studies. *Br J Nutr* 83(Suppl 1) (March 2000): S25–S32.

Astwood, E. B. The heritage of corpulence. *Endocrinology* 71 (August 1962): 337–341.

Austin, G. L., C. L. Ogden, and J. O. Hill. Trends in carbohydrate, fat, and protein intakes and association with energy intake in normal-weight, overweight, and obese individuals: 1971–2006. *Am J Clin Nutr* 93(4) (2011): 836–843.

Berthoud, H. R. The neurobiology of food intake in an obesogenic environment. *Proc Nutr Soc* 71(4) (November 2012): 478–487.

Bray, G. A. and B. M. Popkin. Dietary fat intake does affect obesity! *Am J Clin Nutr* 68(6) (December 1998): 1157–1173.

Bray, G. A., S. R. Smith, L. de Jonge, H. Xie, J. Rood, C. K. Martin, M. Most et al. Effect of dietary protein content on weight gain, energy expenditure, and body composition during overeating: A randomized controlled trial. *JAMA* 307(1) (January 4, 2012): 47–55.

Buchholz, A. C. and D. A. Schoeller. Is a calorie a calorie? *Am J Clin Nutr* 79(5) (May 2004): 899S–906S.

Bueno, N. B., I. S. de Melo, S. L. de Oliveira, and T. da Rocha Ataide. Very-low-carbohydrate ketogenic diet. V. Low-fat diet for long-term weight loss: A meta-analysis of randomised controlled trials. *Br J Nutr* 110(7) (October 2013): 1178–1187.

Church, T. S., D. M. Thomas, C. Tudor-Locke, P. T. Katzmarzyk, C. P. Earnest, R. Q. Rodarte, C. K. Martin, S. N. Blair, and C. Bouchard. Trends over 5 decades in U.S. occupation-related physical activity and their associations with obesity. *PLoS One* 6(5) (2011): e19657.

Davy, K. P., T. Horton, B. M. Davy, D. Bessessen, and J. O. Hill. Regulation of macronutrient balance in healthy young and older men. *Int J Obes Relat Metab Disord* 25(10) (October 2001): 1497–1502.

Dirlewanger, M., V. di Vetta, E. Guenat, P. Battilana, G. Seematter, P. Schneiter, E. Jequier, and L. Tappy. Effects of short-term carbohydrate or fat overfeeding on energy expenditure and plasma leptin concentrations in healthy female subjects. *Int J Obes Relat Metab Disord* 24(11) (November 2000): 1413–1418.

Ebbeling, C. B., J. F. Swain, H. A. Feldman, W. W. Wong, D. L. Hachey, E. Garcia-Lago, and D. S. Ludwig. Effects of dietary composition on energy expenditure during weight-loss maintenance. *JAMA* 307(24) (June 27, 2012): 2627–2634.

Eckel, R. H., T. L. Hernandez, M. L. Bell, K. M. Weil, T. Y. Shepard, G. K. Grunwald, T. A. Sharp, C. C. Francis, and J. O. Hill. Carbohydrate balance predicts weight and fat gain in adults. *Am J Clin Nutr* 83(4) (April 2006): 803–808.

Elia, M., C. Zed, G. Neale, and G. Livesey. The energy cost of triglyceride-fatty acid recycling in nonobese subjects after an overnight fast and four days of starvation. *Metabolism* 36(3) (March 1987): 251–255.

Flatt, J. P. Importance of nutrient balance in body weight regulation. *Diab Metab Rev* 4(6) (September 1988): 571–581.

Flatt, J. P., E. Ravussin, K. J. Acheson, and E. Jequier. Effects of dietary fat on postprandial substrate oxidation and on carbohydrate and fat balances. *J Clin Invest* 76(3) (September 1985): 1019–1024.

Gautron, L., J. K. Elmquist, and K. W. Williams. Neural control of energy balance: Translating circuits to therapies. *Cell* 161(1) (March 26, 2015): 133–145.

Gibson, A. A., R. V. Seimon, C. M. Lee, J. Ayre, J. Franklin, T. P. Markovic, I. D. Caterson, and A. Sainsbury. Do ketogenic diets really suppress appetite? A systematic review and meta-analysis. *Obes Rev* 16(1) (Janurary 2015): 64–76.

Gosby, A. K., A. D. Conigrave, N. S. Lau, M. A. Iglesias, R. M. Hall, S. A. Jebb, J. Brand-Miller et al. Testing protein leverage in lean humans: A randomised controlled experimental study. *PLoS One* 6(10) (2011): e25929.

Greenway, F. L. Physiological adaptations to weight loss and factors favouring weight regain. *Int J Obes (Lond)* 39(8) (August 2015): 1188–1196.

Hall, K. D. Mechanisms of metabolic fuel selection: Modeling human metabolism and body-weight change. *IEEE Eng Med Biol Mag* 29(1) (January–February 2010): 36–41.

Hall, K. D. Modeling metabolic adaptations and energy regulation in humans. *Annu Rev Nutr* 32 (August 21, 2012): 35–54.

Hall, K. D. Prescribing low-fat diets: Useless for long-term weight loss? *Lancet Diabetes Endocrinol* 3(12) (December 2015): 920–921.

Hall, K. D., T. Bemis, R. Brychta, K. Y. Chen, A. Courville, E. J. Crayner, S. Goodwin et al. Calorie for calorie, dietary fat restriction results in more body fat loss than carbohydrate restriction in people with obesity. *Cell Metab* 22(3) (September 1, 2015): 427–436.

Hall, K. D., J. Guo, M. Dore, and C. C. Chow. The progressive increase of food waste in America and its environmental impact. *PLoS One* 4(11) (2009): e7940.

Hall, K. D., R. A. Hammond, and H. Rahmandad. Dynamic interplay among homeostatic, hedonic, and cognitive feedback circuits regulating body weight. *Am J Public Health* 104(7) (July 2014): 1169–1175.

Hall, K. D., G. Sacks, D. Chandramohan, C. C. Chow, Y. C. Wang, S. L. Gortmaker, and B. A. Swinburn. Quantification of the effect of energy imbalance on bodyweight. *Lancet* 378(9793) (August 27, 2011): 826–837.

Hill, J. O., J. C. Peters, G. W. Reed, D. G. Schlundt, T. Sharp, and H. L. Greene. Nutrient balance in humans: Effects of diet composition. *Am J Clin Nutr* 54(1) (July 1991): 10–17.

Hilton, S., C. Patterson, and A. Teyhan. Escalating coverage of obesity in UK newspapers: The evolution and framing of the "Obesity Epidemic" from 1996 to 2010. *Obesity (Silver Spring)* 20(8) (August 2012): 1688–1695.

Hiza, H. A. B., L. Bente, and T. Fungwe. Nutrient content of the U.S. food supply, 2005. U.S. Department of Agriculture, Washington, DC, 2008.

Horton, T. J., H. Drougas, A. Brachey, G. W. Reed, J. C. Peters, and J. O. Hill. Fat and carbohydrate overfeeding in humans: Different effects on energy storage. *Am J Clin Nutr* 62(1) (July 1995): 19–29.

Hu, T., K. T. Mills, L. Yao, K. Demanelis, M. Eloustaz, W. S. Yancy Jr., T. N. Kelly, J. He, and L. A. Bazzano. Effects of low-carbohydrate diets versus low-fat diets on metabolic risk factors: A meta-analysis of randomized controlled clinical trials. *Am J Epidemiol* 176(Suppl 7) (October 1, 2012): S44–S54.

Johnston, B. C., S. Kanters, K. Bandayrel, P. Wu, F. Naji, R. A. Siemieniuk, G. D. Ball et al. Comparison of weight loss among named diet programs in overweight and obese adults: A meta-analysis. *JAMA* 312(9) (September 3, 2014): 923–933.

Johnston, C. S., S. L. Tjonn, P. D. Swan, A. White, H. Hutchins, and B. Sears. Ketogenic low-carbohydrate diets have no metabolic advantage over nonketogenic low-carbohydrate diets. *Am J Clin Nutr* 83(5) (May 2006): 1055–1061.

Keith, S. W., D. T. Redden, P. T. Katzmarzyk, M. M. Boggiano, E. C. Hanlon, R. M. Benca, D. Ruden et al. Putative contributors to the secular increase in obesity: Exploring the roads less traveled. *Int J Obes (Lond)* 30(11) (November 2006): 1585–1594.

Leidy, H. J., P. M. Clifton, A. Astrup, T. P. Wycherley, M. S. Westerterp-Plantenga, N. D. Luscombe-Marsh, S. C. Woods, and R. D. Mattes. The role of protein in weight loss and maintenance. *Am J Clin Nutr* 101 (April 29, 2015): 1320S–1329S.

Lin, B. H. and J. Guthrie. Nutritional quality of food prepared at home and away from home. U.S. Department of Agriculture, Washington, DC, 2012.

Ludwig, D. S. *Always Hungry? Conquer Cravings, Retrain Your Fat Cells, and Lose Weight Permanently.* New York: Grand Central Publishing, 2016.

Ludwig, D. S. and M. I. Friedman. Increasing adiposity: Consequence or cause of overeating? *JAMA* 311(21) (June 4, 2014): 2167–2168.

Lustig, R. H. Childhood obesity: Behavioral aberration or biochemical drive? Reinterpreting the first law of thermodynamics. *Nat Clin Pract Endocrinol Metab* 2(8) (August 2006): 447–458.

Martens, E. A., S. G. Lemmens, and M. S. Westerterp-Plantenga. Protein leverage affects energy intake of high-protein diets in humans. *Am J Clin Nutr* 97(1) (January 2013): 86–93.

Martens, E. A., S. Y. Tan, M. V. Dunlop, R. D. Mattes, and M. S. Westerterp-Plantenga. Protein leverage effects of beef protein on energy intake in humans. *Am J Clin Nutr* 99(6) (June 2014): 1397–1406.

McAllister, E. J., N. V. Dhurandhar, S. W. Keith, L. J. Aronne, J. Barger, M. Baskin, R. M. Benca et al. Ten putative contributors to the obesity epidemic. *Crit Rev Food Sci Nutr* 49(10) (November 2009): 868–913.

Moss, M. *Salt, Sugar, Fat: How the Food Giants Hooked Us*. New York: Random House, 2013.

Paoli, A., G. Bosco, E. M. Camporesi, and D. Mangar. Ketosis, ketogenic diet and food intake control: A complex relationship. *Front Psychol* 6 (2015): 27.

Pennington, A. W. Obesity. *Med Times* 80(7) (July 1952): 389–398.

Pennington, A. W. A reorientation on obesity. *N Engl J Med* 248(23) (June 4, 1953): 959–964.

Putnam, J. Major trends in the U.S. food supply, 1909–99. *Food Review* 23(1) (2000): 8–15.

Roberts, P. *The End of Food*. New York: Houghton Mifflin Harcourt Publishing Company, 2008.

Rolls, B. J. The relationship between dietary energy density and energy intake. *Physiol Behav* 97(5) (July 14, 2009): 609–615.

Rumpler, W. V., J. L. Seale, C. W. Miles, and C. E. Bodwell. Energy-intake restriction and diet-composition effects on energy expenditure in men. *Am J Clin Nutr* 53(2) (February 1991): 430–436.

Schrauwen, P., W. D. van Marken Lichtenbelt, W. H. Saris, and K. R. Westerterp. Changes in fat oxidation in response to a high-fat diet. *Am J Clin Nutr* 66(2) (August 1997): 276–282.

Schutz, Y., J. P. Flatt, and E. Jequier. Failure of dietary fat intake to promote fat oxidation: A factor favoring the development of obesity. *Am J Clin Nutr* 50(2) (August 1989): 307–314.

Shepard, T. Y., K. M. Weil, T. A. Sharp, G. K. Grunwald, M. L. Bell, J. O. Hill, and R. H. Eckel. Occasional physical inactivity combined with a high-fat diet may be important in the development and maintenance of obesity in human subjects. *Am J Clin Nutr* 73(4) (April 2001): 703–708.

Simpson, S. J. and D. Raubenheimer. Obesity: The protein leverage hypothesis. *Obes Rev* 6(2) (May 2005): 133–142.

Smith, L. P., S. W. Ng, and B. M. Popkin. Trends in us home food preparation and consumption: Analysis of national nutrition surveys and time use studies from 1965–1966 to 2007–2008. *Nutr J* 12 (2013): 45.

Smith, S. R., L. de Jonge, J. J. Zachwieja, H. Roy, T. Nguyen, J. C. Rood, M. M. Windhauser, and G. A. Bray. Fat and carbohydrate balances during adaptation to a high-fat. *Am J Clin Nutr* 71(2) (February 2000): 450–457.

Stubbs, R. J. Nutrition society medal lecture. Appetite, feeding behaviour and energy balance in human subjects. *Proc Nutr Soc* 57(3) (August 1998): 341–356.

Stubbs, R. J., C. G. Harbron, P. R. Murgatroyd, and A. M. Prentice. Covert manipulation of dietary fat and energy density: Effect on substrate flux and food intake in men eating ad libitum. *Am J Clin Nutr* 62(2) (August 1995a): 316–329.

Stubbs, R. J., P. Ritz, W. A. Coward, and A. M. Prentice. Covert manipulation of the ratio of dietary fat to carbohydrate and energy density: Effect on food intake and energy balance in free-living men eating ad libitum. *Am J Clin Nutr* 62(2) (August 1995b): 330–337.

Swinburn, B. A., G. Sacks, K. D. Hall, K. McPherson, D. T. Finegood, M. L. Moodie, and S. L. Gortmaker. The global obesity pandemic: Shaped by global drivers and local environments. *Lancet* 378(9793) (August 27, 2011): 804–814.

Taubes, G. *Good Calories, Bad Calories: Challenging the Conventional Wisdom on Diet, Weight Control, and Disease*. New York: Alfred A. Knopf, 2007.

Taubes, G. *Why We Get Fat and What to Do About It*. New York: Alfred A. Knopf, 2011.

Taubes, G. The science of obesity: What do we really know about what makes us fat? An essay by Gary Taubes. *BMJ* 346 (2013): f1050.

Thearle, M. S., N. Pannacciulli, S. Bonfiglio, K. Pacak, and J. Krakoff. Extent and determinants of thermogenic responses to 24 hours of fasting, energy balance, and five different overfeeding diets in humans. *J Clin Endocrinol Metab* 98(7) (July 2013): 2791–2799.

Tobias, D. K., M. Chen, J. E. Manson, D. S. Ludwig, W. Willett, and F. B. Hu. Effect of low-fat vs. other diet interventions on long-term weight change in adults: A systematic review and meta-analysis. *Lancet Diabetes Endocrinol* 3(12) December (2015): 968–979.

Treuth, M. S., A. L. Sunehag, L. M. Trautwein, D. M. Bier, M. W. Haymond, and N. F. Butte. Metabolic adaptation to high-fat and high-carbohydrate diets in children and adolescents. *Am J Clin Nutr* 77(2) (February 2003): 479–489.

Veldhorst, M. A., M. S. Westerterp-Plantenga, and K. R. Westerterp. Gluconeogenesis and energy expenditure after a high-protein, carbohydrate-free diet. *Am J Clin Nutr* 90(3) (September 2009): 519–526.

Walker, T. B. and M. J. Parker. Lessons from the war on dietary fat. *J Am Coll Nutr* 33(4) (2014): 347–351.

Wells, H. F. and J. C. Buzby. Dietary assessment of major trends in U.S. food consumption, 1970–2005, Economic Information Bulletin no. 33, 20, U.S. Department of Agriculture, Washington, DC, 2008.

Wells, J. C. and M. Siervo. Obesity and energy balance: Is the tail wagging the dog? *Eur J Clin Nutr* 65(11) (November 2011): 1173–1189.

Westerterp, K. R. Diet induced thermogenesis. *Nutr Metab (Lond)* 1(1) (August 18 2004): 5.

Westerterp, K. R. Metabolic adaptations to over—and underfeeding—Still a matter of debate? *Eur J Clin Nutr* 67(5) (May 2013): 443–445.

Williams, R. A., L. S. Roe, and B. J. Rolls. Comparison of three methods to reduce energy density. Effects on daily energy intake. *Appetite* 66 (July 2013): 75–83.

Woods, S. C. and D. A. D'Alessio. Central control of body weight and appetite. *J Clin Endocrinol Metab* 93(11 Suppl 1) (November 2008): S37–S50.

Wycherley, T. P., L. J. Moran, P. M. Clifton, M. Noakes, and G. D. Brinkworth. Effects of energy-restricted high-protein, low-fat compared with standard-protein, low-fat diets: A meta-analysis of randomized controlled trials. *Am J Clin Nutr* 96(6) (December 2012): 1281–1298.

Yerboeket-van de Venne, W. P. and K. R. Westerterp. Effects of dietary fat and carbohydrate exchange on human energy metabolism. *Appetite* 26(3) (June 1996): 287–300.

4 Diets for Weight Loss

George A. Bray and Patty W. Siri-Tarino

CONTENTS

ABSTRACT

This chapter has examined the use of weight loss diets in the treatment of patients with obesity. The historical background for these diets is first reviewed noting that low-fat and low-carbohydrate diets had appeared more than 100 years ago. Basic principles of energy balance are then briefly reviewed. A discussion of very-low-energy (calorie) diets is followed by a discussion of the balanced deficit diet, the low-calorie diet, the low-fat diet, the low glycemic index, and the Mediterranean-style diet. Variability of response to each diet is characteristic and considerably larger than the average weight difference between most if not all dietary comparisons. The best advice is to select a diet you can adhere to and to follow your progress by periodic recording of your body weight.

INTRODUCTION

More than 2500 years ago, Hippocrates prescribed diet and exercise in the treatment of obesity (Bray 2007). Diet was also used by Galen in Roman times and by Avicenna in the tenth century AD when Arabic medicine was the dominant medical tradition. With the dawn of the eighteenth century, we began to accumulate a scientific basis for understanding obesity. The "Oxygen Theory of Metabolism" was formulated by Lavoisier in 1787 (1789) and this was followed 50 years later by the First Law of Thermodynamics (von Helmholtz 1847) and the concept of "Energy Balance," which was shown to apply to animals and human beings during the latter part of the nineteenth century (Pettenkoffer 1861; Atwater and Benedict 1902).

Modern diets can be dated to 1863 when William Banting (1864), an undertaker, published his astounding 50-pound weight loss using a low-carbohydrate diet prescribed by his physician William Harvey (1872). At around the same time, restriction of fat along with a significant reduction in calories was espoused by the teacher and scholar von Noorden (1903). Thus, variations in macronutrient composition for weight reduction became part of medically prescribed programs for patients with obesity more than 100 years ago. Effective treatments for obesity were particularly sought after given the association of excess weight with shortened life expectancy (Bray 2007) and the shifts of patterns of disease from infection and tuberculosis in the early twentieth century to chronic diseases such as heart disease, cancer, hypertension, and diabetes by the end of World War II.

In the 1970s, the U.S. Senate Select Committee on Nutrition held hearings of "hunger" and published reports that highlighted the detrimental effects of the American diet on the rising incidence of noninfectious chronic diseases, that is, heart disease, diabetes, and cancer (U.S. Senate 1977; Bray 2007). The first Dietary Guidelines advising low-fat diets for cardiovascular health were subsequently issued in 1980. In part, the advice for low-fat diets was to reduce calorie intake given that fat contains 9 calories per gram, whereas carbohydrates and protein provide 4 calories per gram.

Although the prevalence of cardiovascular disease (CVD) has decreased over the last decades, there has been a concomitant increase in obesity and disorders related to obesity (Bray 2011; Bray and Bouchard 2014). The increase in obesity and cardiometabolic abnormalities has been due to a combination of lifestyle and environmental changes. These include decreased physical activity and increased consumption of calories largely due to increased portion sizes (Scully 2014) and heightened palatability, low cost, increased use of processed and convenience foods (Moss 2013), and sugar-sweetened soft drinks (Bray and Popkin 2013) that are energy dense but nutritionally void. Dietary approaches to combating obesity fundamentally rely on caloric restriction. Various strategies to accomplish this goal are described in this chapter. Whether and how the macronutrient composition of weight loss diets affects the magnitude of weight loss and cardiometabolic parameters is also considered.

REDUCING BODY WEIGHT IS A FUNCTION OF REDUCING CALORIE INTAKE

Reducing calorie intake below what is needed to maintain weight leads to weight loss (Bray 2011; Hall et al. 2011; Jensen et al. 2014; Apovian et al. 2015; Thomas et al. 2015). It is clear that Americans are eating more on average now compared to 25 years ago (Putnam et al. 2002; Scully 2014). In the Diabetes Prevention Program with over 1000 individuals randomized to a lifestyle program and a similar number to a placebo control group, reduction in calorie intake was the major predictor of weight loss (Diabetes Prevention Program 2004).

Effective weight loss programs can decrease body weight by 8% of baseline (Jensen et al. 2014). The rate of weight loss is initially more rapid and then falls off in a logarithmic fashion as weight is lost. Weight loss has been modeled in at least three publications and the expected weight loss over time for a predicted energy deficit of 500 kcal/day is depicted in Figure 4.1 with each of these computer-programmed weight loss patterns. Note that for the first 3–6 months, weight loss is almost "linear" but gradually tapers off until a new plateau is reached (Thomas et al. 2014).

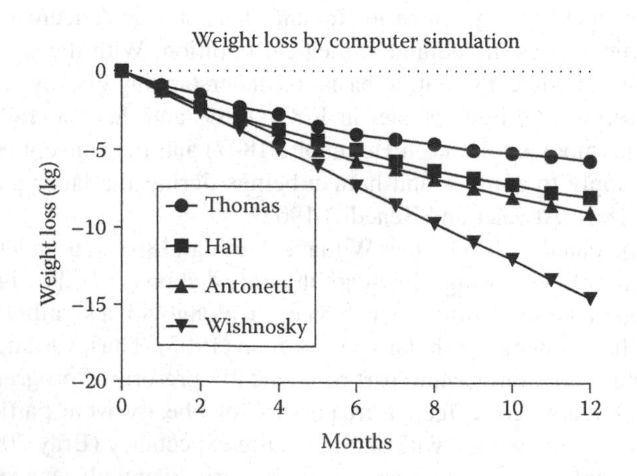

FIGURE 4.1 Rate of weight loss predicted from Computer Models.

Key Factors That Influence Weight Loss

There is a range of weight loss with all diets. This is shown for individuals in the POUNDS Lost study, one of the clinical trials of diet composition for weight loss (Sacks et al. 2009). Several factors predict this difference in response. The first is the initial rate of weight loss (Unick et al. 2015). In the Look AHEAD study, individuals in the highest tertile of weight loss at 1 and 2 months in the program had nearly twice the weight loss at 4 and 8 years as those in the lowest tertile of initial weight loss. Thus, the initial rate of weight loss is important.

A second factor predicting weight loss for any diet is the adherence to that diet. Several studies demonstrate this important factor, which is shown for the POUNDS Lost trial in Figure 4.2a (Dansinger et al. 2005; Alhassan et al. 2008; Sacks et al. 2009; Wadden et al. 2009). Another element of adherence, assessed in the Look AHEAD trial, was the degree to which individuals in the lifestyle weight loss program trial used meal replacements offered at the beginning of the program. Usage of meal replacements was positively associated with greater weight loss, as was attendance at the scheduled sessions and the amount of physical activity reported by the participants.

Genetic variation can also influence weight loss and metabolic responses to a diet. This has been shown for both the Diabetes Prevention Program (Florez et al. 2012; Papandonatos et al. 2015) and the POUNDS Lost Trial (Qi et al. 2012, 2013; Zhang 2012a,b,c; Lin et al. 2015; Xu et al. 2013, 2015; Mirzaei et al. 2014; Zheng et al. 2015). Table 4.1 summarizes the effects of the high- versus low-fat diets and high- versus average-protein diets in the POUNDS Lost study, and the effect of differing alleles of the tested genes on such factors as blood pressure, change in low-density lipoprotein–cholesterol (LDL-C), change in high-density lipoprotein–cholesterol (HDL-C), weight loss, insulin sensitivity, and energy expenditure. Using genetic profiles may be of value in the future in developing personalized medicine for the management of obesity. Several examples of genetic influences on the response to diet in the POUNDS Lost study are shown in Figure 4.3. Interestingly, both *APOA5* alleles and *LIPC* alleles affected the changes in LDL-C between individuals eating low- and high-fat diets (Zhang et al. 2012a; Xu et al. 2015). The NPY gene also influenced the response of blood pressure to the diets that were eaten (Zhang et al. 2012c).

Reduced-Calorie Regimens

Very-low-calorie diets (very-low-energy diets) have energy levels between 200 and 1000 kcal/day. The theory behind them is that the lower the energy intake, the more rapid the weight and fat loss. Most weight loss diets can produce a decline in energy expenditure with a drop in triiodothyronine

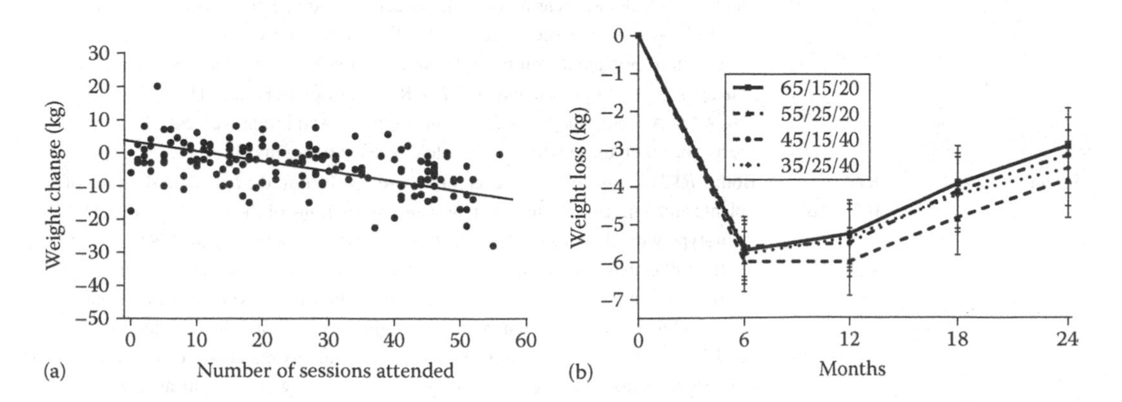

FIGURE 4.2 Effect of program attendance (a) and diet composition (b) on weight loss in the POUNDS Lost study. (a: Sacks, F.M. et al., *New Engl. J. Med.*, 360(9), 859, February 26, 2009, adherence data.)

TABLE 4.1
Genetic Markers in the POUND Lost Study That Modified Response to a Low-Carbohydrate or Low-Fat Diet

Author	Year	Gene	Changes Observed
Qi	2012	*GIPR*	The GIPR that stimulates insulin release potently in the presence of elevated glucose. The T allele (rs2287019) in those assigned the low-fat diet was associated with more weight loss and greater decreases in fasting glucose, fasting insulin, and HOMA-IR. Thus, *GIPR* rs2287019 T-allele carriers may obtain more weight loss and improvement of glucose homeostasis than those without this allele by choosing a low-fat diet.
Zhang	2012	*APOA5*	Apolipoprotein A5 is an important determinant of plasma triglyceride levels. In the low-fat (20% energy as fat) diet, carriers of the G allele exhibited greater reductions in TC and LDL-C than noncarriers. In the high-fat diet group (40% fat energy), participants with the G allele had a greater increase in HDL-C than did participants without this allele. Thus, there was more improvement in lipid profiles from long-term low-fat diet intake in the *APOA5* G-risk allele.
Zhang	2012	*FTO*	The FTO is associated with obesity. There were significant modifications of 2-year changes in fat-free mass, whole body % fat mass, total adipose tissue mass, visceral adipose tissue mass, and superficial adipose tissue mass by FTO genotype and dietary protein. Carriers of the risk allele had a greater reduction in weight, greater change in body composition, and fat distribution in response to a high-protein diet, whereas an opposite genetic effect was observed in the low-protein diet. There were also significant interactions observed at 6 months. Thus, a high-protein diet may be beneficial for weight loss and improvement of body composition and fat distribution in individuals with the risk allele of the FTO variant rs1558902 (see Figure 4.5).
Qi	2013	*IRS-1*	The IRS is a link between the insulin receptor and intracellular activity. Among participants with the A allele, the reversion rates of the metabolic syndrome were higher in the high-fat diet group than in the low-fat diet group over the 2-year intervention ($P = 0.002$), while no significant difference between diet groups was observed among those without A allele ($P = 0.27$). High-fat weight-loss diets might be more effective in the management of the metabolic syndrome.
Xu	2013	*PPM1K*	This factor is essential for the regulation and nutrient-induced activation of the branched-chain alpha-keto acid dehydrogenase complex, which catalyzes the breakdown of branched-chain amino acids (BCAA). In the high-fat diet group, the C allele was related to less weight loss and a smaller decreases in serum insulin and HOMA-IR, whereas an opposite effect of genotype on changes in insulin and HOMA-IR was observed in the low-fat diet group. At 2 years, the gene–diet interactions remained significant for weight loss ($P = 0.008$) but became null for changes in serum insulin and HOMA-IR due to weight regain. The C allele of BCAA/AAA ratio may benefit less in weight loss and improvement of insulin resistance than those without this allele when eating a high-fat diet.
Mirzaei	2014	*CRY2* *MTNR1B*	Both *CRY2* and melatonin-2 receptor 1B are involved in the circadian rhythms of plants and animals. We found significant associations of the *CRY2 rs11605924* genotype with changes of RQ, RMR, and RMR/Kg, and of the *MTNR1B rs10830963* genotype with RQ by the 2-year intervention. In addition, we observed significant modification effects of dietary fat on RQ changes for both SNPs. Our data indicate that genotype of glucose- and circadian-related loci *CRY2* and *MTNR1B might* affect long-term change in energy expenditure, and that dietary fat intake might modify the genetic effects (www.clinicaltrials.gov; NCT00072995).

(Continued)

TABLE 4.1 (*Continued*)
Genetic Markers in the POUND Lost Study That Modified Response to a Low-Carbohydrate or Low-Fat Diet

Author	Year	Gene	Changes Observed
Zheng	2015	*FTO*	FTO is associated with obesity. The A allele was associated with a greater decrease in food cravings among the participants with high-protein intake (P = 0.027), but not in those in the low-protein diet group (P = 0.384). Weight regain from 6 to 24 months attenuated the gene–protein interactions. Protein intakes did not modify the *FTO* genotype effects on other appetite measures. Individuals with the *FTO* A allele might obtain more reduction in food cravings by choosing a hypocaloric, higher-protein weight-loss diet.
Xu	2015	*LIPC*	Hepatic lipase (HL) plays a pivotal role in the metabolism of HDL-C and LDL-C. Common variants in HL gene (*LIPC*) are associated with HDL-C. After 2 years of dietary intervention, dietary fat modified the genetic effects of this gene on serum TC, LDL-C, and HDL-C. In the low-fat diet group, the A allele was related to a decrease in TC and LDL-C levels while an opposite genetic effect was found in the high-fat diet group. Additionally, the A allele was associated with less increased levels of HDL-C in the low-fat group but not in the high-fat group.
Lin	2015	*NPY*	NPY is a potent stimulator of food intake. The C allele (rs16147) was associated with a greater reduction in WC at 6 months. In addition, the genotypes showed a statistically significant interaction with dietary fat in relation to WC and subcutaneous adipose tissue: the association was stronger in individuals with high-fat intake than in those with low-fat intake. At 24 months, the association remained statistically significant for WC in the high-fat diet group (P = 0.02), although the gene–dietary fat interaction became nonsignificant. In addition, we found statistically significant genotype–dietary fat interaction on the change in total abdominal adipose tissue, visceral adipose tissue, and subcutaneous adipose tissue at 24 months: the rs16147 T allele appeared to associate with more adverse changes in the abdominal fat deposition in the high-fat diet group than in the low-fat diet group. Our data indicate that the NPY rs16147 genotypes that affect the change in abdominal adiposity in response to dietary interventions were modified by dietary fat.

Notes: GIPR, glucose-dependent insulinotropic polypeptide receptor; PPM1K, protein phosphatase Mg/Mn 1K; IRS-1, insulin receptor substrate-1; *CRY2*, cryptochrome 2; *MTNR1B*, melatonin receptor 1B; *MC4R*, melanocortin-4 receptor; *FTO*, fat mass and obesity-associated gene; *NPY*, neuropeptide Y; TC, total cholesterol; WC, waist circumference; SNP, single nucleotide polymorphism; HOMA-IR, homeostatic model assessment-insulin resistance.

and leptin (Sumithran et al. 2011). Treatment with leptin only partially corrects these changes (Rosenbaum et al. 2008), unless an individual is leptin deficient. Although these regimens result in rapid weight loss, the ability to maintain the weight loss beyond 6 months relative to counseling is attenuated (Dansinger et al. 2007). Furthermore, very-low-calorie approaches have been associated with an increased risk of gallstones compared to low-calorie approaches (Bray 2011), and therefore providers have been advised to recommend these diets in limited circumstances and under close medical supervision.

Diets that reduce carbohydrate, protein, and fat, the so-called *balanced-deficit diets or prudent diets,* have been widely used in treating obesity. These diets reduce caloric intake by 500–750 kcal/day with a lower limit of energy intake usually set at 1200 kcal/day (Avenell et al. 2004). In a meta-analysis of low-calorie diets, Avenell and colleagues (Avenell et al. 2004) found that after 12 months the difference between control and treated groups was 5.31 kg (95% CI, −5.86 to −4.77 kg) favoring the diets. In another systematic review of 16 studies that used diet and that had more than 100 subjects in each group and a duration of more than 1 year, weight loss after 2–3 years

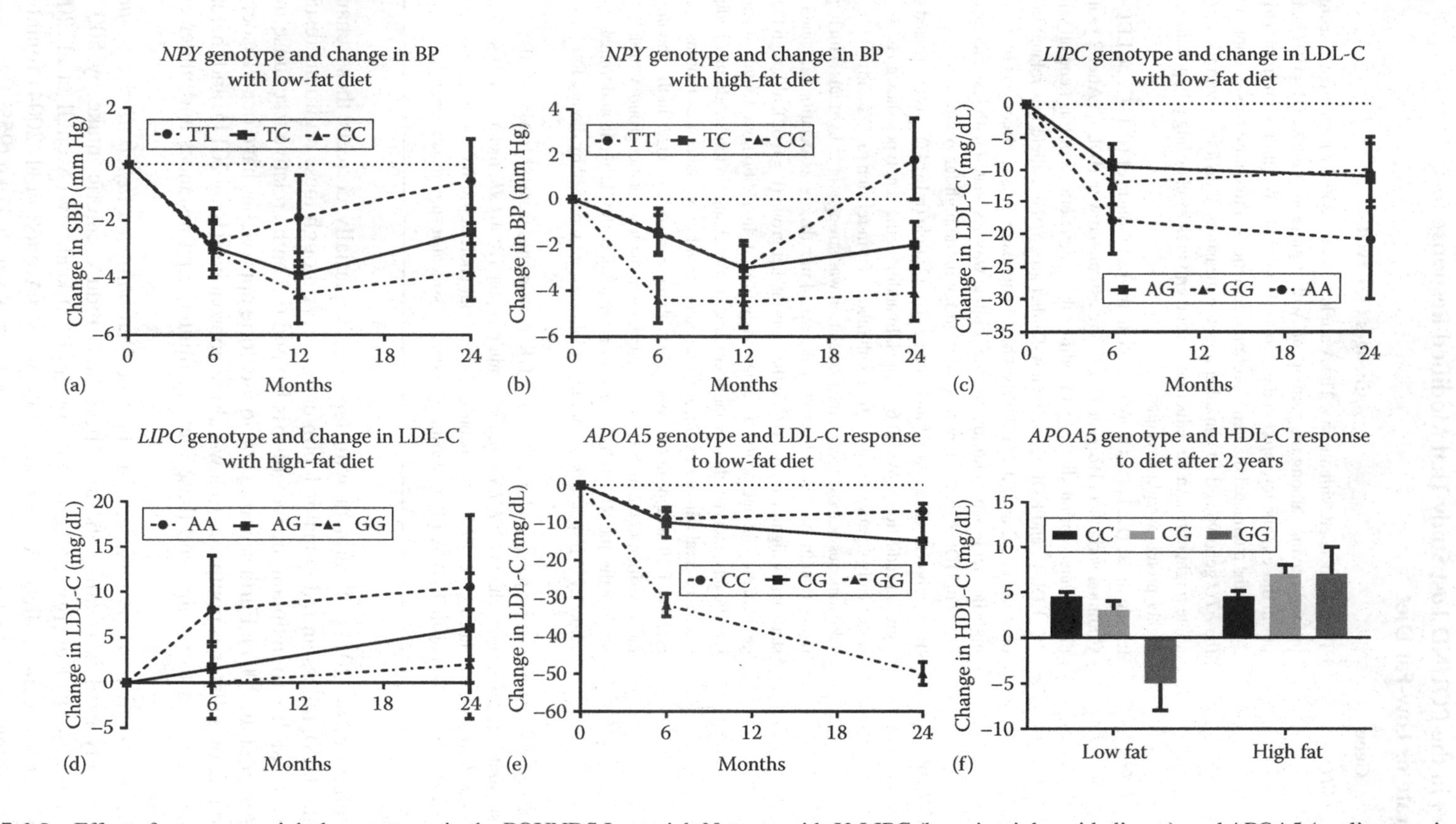

FIGURE 4.3 Effect of genes on weight loss patterns in the POUNDS Lost trial: Neuropeptide Y, LIPC (hepatic triglyceride lipase), and APOA5 (apolipoprotein A-V). (a and b) Effect of NPY genotypes Zhang et al. on systolic (a) and diastolic (b) BP in response to high- and low-fat diets; (c and d) Effect of LIPC Xu et al. on change in LDL-cholesterol in response to high- and low-fat diets; (e and f) Effect of APOA5 genotypes Zhang et al. on response of HDL-cholesterol to high- and low-fat diets.

was usually <5 kg below baseline (3.5 ± 2.4 kg; range, 0.9–10.0 kg) and after 4–7 years where there were data, it was still 3.6 ± 2.6 kg below baseline.

Portion-controlled diets or meal replacements are one way of achieving a caloric deficit (Wadden et al. 2011). This can be done most simply by using individually packaged foods. Frozen low-calorie meals containing 250–350 kcal/package can be a convenient way to do this, except for the high salt content of many of these foods. In one 4-year study, this approach resulted in early initial weight loss, which then was maintained (Flechtner-Mors and Ditschuneit 2000; Ditschuneit and Flechtner-Mors 2001).

Finally, *intermittent or alternate-day fasting regimens* (as detailed in Chapter 27) combine days of eating at "normal" consumption levels with days of caloric restriction, so that overall calorie consumption over a weeklong period is reduced. These dietary patterns represent an effective weight loss strategy, although studies to date have been limited by sample size (Varady et al. 2013). Intermittent fasting has further been shown to improve fasting triglyceride (TG) without effects on LDL-C or HDL-C concentrations. However, the TG lowering effect may not be independent of weight loss, and there have been no studies to date that have tested this effect. Studies evaluating long-term effects of alternate-day fasting regimes are also lacking.

DOES THE MACRONUTRIENT COMPOSITION OF DIETS INFLUENCE WEIGHT LOSS?

Whether the macronutrient composition of diets influences the magnitude of weight loss over a short or long term has been the subject of many research studies. In addition to their potential impact on weight loss, diets with different macronutrient composition in the context of weight loss and maintenance may also affect cardiometabolic risk parameters. This section reviews the evidence related to these topics.

Low-Fat versus Low-Carbohydrate Diets

A rationale for the potential benefit of the low-carbohydrate diet is found in the carbohydrate–insulin hypothesis (see Chapter 3). Several randomized clinical trials lasting 1 year (Brehm et al. 2003; Foster et al. 2003; Samaha et al. 2003; Stern et al. 2004; Yancy et al. 2004; Dansinger et al. 2005; Gardner et al. 2007; Brinkworth et al. 2009 [Figure 4.4a]) or 2 years (Shai et al. 2008 [Figure 4.4b]; Sacks et al. 2009 [Figure 4.3b]; Foster et al. 2010) have tested this hypothesis in head-to-head trials

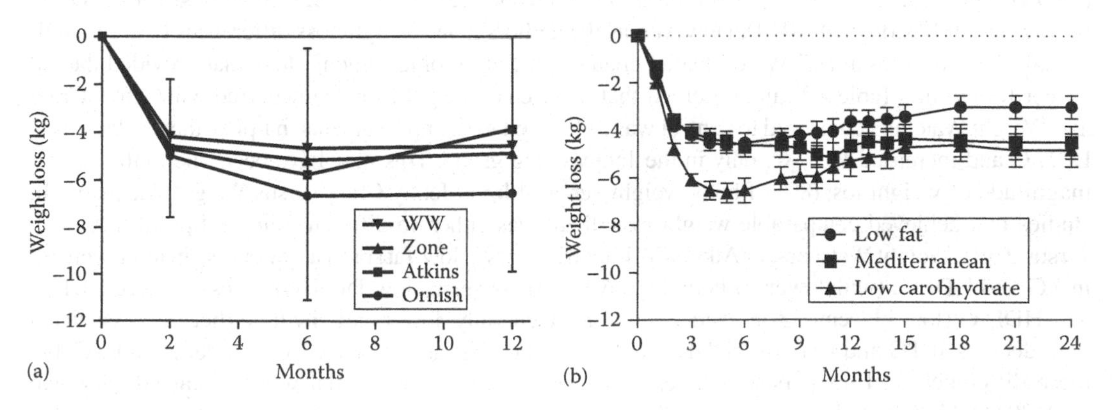

FIGURE 4.4 Comparison of diets over 1 year and 2 years. (a) Trial conducted by Dansinger et al. comparing the Atkins, Ornish, Weight Watchers, and Zone Diets; Participants were both male and females; (b) Trial comparing a low-fat diet, the Atkins diet, and a Mediterranean-style diet; The low carbohydrate diet was the Atkins Diet; participants were predominantly males. (a: Dansinger, M.L. et al., *JAMA*, 293(1), 43, 2005; b: Shai, I. et al., *New Engl. J. Med.*, 359(3), 229, 2008.)

with low-carbohydrate or low-fat diets (Figure 4.4). In the first of these comparisons, 169 obese individuals were randomized to one of four popular diets, including the Atkins Diet (2002), The Ornish Diet (1993), the Weight Watchers Diet, and the Zone Diet (Dansinger et al. 2005). At the end of 12 months, each diet produced weight loss of about 5 kg, but there was no difference between diets. Adherence to the diet was the single most important criterion of success in this trial, and the Atkins and Ornish diets were more difficult to adhere to. In a second 1-year trial, the Atkins, Zone, Ornish, and LEARN diets were compared in a group of premenopausal women (Gardner et al. 2007). This trial found that the Atkins diet produced more weight loss at 6 and 12 months compared to the other three diets, which had similar results. In this study, too, a post hoc analysis showed that adherence was the best predictor for weight loss and that the level of adherence was not very good for any diet (Alhassan et al. 2008). Two reasons are proposed for the divergent outcomes. First, the study by Gardner et al. (2007) had a more homogeneous population, including only premenopausal women. Second, the Gardner study was larger and thus had more statistical power to detect differences.

The POUNDS Lost study was conducted at two sites in the United States (Sacks et al. 2009). A total of 811 men and women were randomized to one of four diets, and 80% of them provided weights at the end of 2 years. The two-by-two factorial comparison allowed for the assessment of low versus high protein, low versus high fat, and lowest versus highest carbohydrate on body weight loss. The four diets were composed as follows: (1) 20% fat, 15% protein, 65% carbohydrate; (2) 20% fat, 25% protein, 55% carbohydrate; (3) 40% fat, 15% protein, 45%carbohydrate; or (4) 40% fat, 25%protein, 35% carbohydrate. The foods used to prepare diet plans for all four diets were the same with variation of the specific quantities. At the end of 6 months, 12 months, or 2 years, the weight loss was similar for all 4 diets (Figure 4.3b), supporting the concept that macronutrient composition is not a key determinant in weight loss success. However, two caveats should be considered when evaluating the data from POUNDS Lost and all other diet trials. These include (1) adherence to the dietary protocol is a key predictor of both the success and magnitude of weight loss and (2) the consistent inability across almost all longer-term studies to achieve the protocol-specified differential in macronutrients. The important message is that "Significant weight loss was observed with any prescribed low-carbohydrate or low-fat diet" (Johnston et al. 2014).

The technique of meta-analysis has been used to amalgamate the findings of various clinical studies evaluating popular diets. In a 2014 meta-analysis of 59 eligible articles reporting 48 unique randomized trials of "named" diets (including 7286 individuals) and compared with no diet, the largest weight losses were associated with low-carbohydrate diets (8.73 kg [95% confidence interval {CI}, 7.27–10.20 kg] at 6-month follow-up and 7.25 kg [95% CI, 5.33–9.25 kg] at 12-month follow-up) and low-fat diets (7.99 kg [95% CI, 6.01–9.92 kg] at 6-month follow-up and 7.27 kg [95% CI, 5.26–9.34 kg] at 12-month follow-up) (Johnston et al. 2014). However, as the authors note, "weight loss differences between individual diets were minimal." We evaluated changes in lipid profiles among diets that provided data at 1-year follow-up (Table 4.2) and observed that the greater weight loss that occurred with Jenny Craig and Weight Watchers compared to control was associated with improvements in lipids, that is, decreased LDL-C and increased HDL-C, only in the Jenny Craig group. This may have been due to the greater magnitude of weight lost (8% of body weight versus 4 kg in Jenny Craig versus Weight Watchers). In studies that achieved comparable weight loss, there was either no difference in lipid profiles (Ornish versus Zone, Weight Watchers, or Atkins; Volumetrics versus low-fat) or in a few cases, an improvement in TG and HDL-C (with lower-carbohydrate Atkins diets versus low-fat diets) or less reduced LDL-C and HDL-C (low glycemic Zone versus low-fat). Generally, lower-carbohydrate diets are associated with decreased TG and increased HDL-C and lower-fat diets are associated with reduced LDL-C, but these differences did not persist at 2 years, unless the weight differential was maintained (Bazzano et al. 2014). How these improvements in lipids in the context of weight loss maintenance correspond to overall improved cardiovascular health is not known. In fact, current evidence is lacking for long-term reductions in CVD or mortality from diet-induced weight loss (Look AHEAD 2013; Kritchevsky et al. 2015; Langland 2015), and benefits to all-cause and CVD mortality have only been demonstrated with improvements in cardiorespiratory fitness in obese patients (Lee et al. 2012).

TABLE 4.2
Changes in Plasma Lipids in Response to Several Popular Diets

Diet	Comparator	Achieved Weight Loss	TC	LDL-C	TG	HDL-C	TC:HDL	Non-HDL
Atkins (low carb)	Low fat	=	=	=	↓	↑		
Zone (low GI)[a]	Low fat	=		Less reduced	=	Less reduced		
Weight Watchers	Self-help	↑	=		=	=	=	
Ornish	Atkins Zone Weight Watchers	=	=	=	=	=	=	
Jenny Craig	Usual care	↑	=	↓	=	↑		
Volumetrics (low fat + FV)	Low fat	=	=	=	=	=		↓

Sources: Foster, G.D. et al., *Ann. Intern. Med.*, 153(3), 147, 2010, Ebbeling, C.B. et al., *JAMA*, 97(19), 2092, 2007; Heshka, S. et al., *JAMA*, 289(14), 1792, 2003; Dansinger, M.L. et al., *JAMA*, 293(1), 43, 2005; Rock, C.L., *Obesity (Silver Spring)*, 15(4), 939, 2007; Ello-Martin, J.A., *Am. J. Clin. Nutr.*, 85(6), 1465, 2007.

TC, total cholesterol; GI, gastrointestinal; FV, fruits and vegetables.

[a] 18-month intervention; data not reported colored in gray.

In another meta-analysis by Tobias et al. (2015), among weight loss interventions of similar intensity, low-carbohydrate interventions led to significantly greater weight loss than did low-fat interventions (18 comparisons; weighted mean difference [WMD], 1.15 kg [95% CI, 0.52 to 1.79]; *I*2 = 10%), in line with another meta-analysis by Bueno et al. (2013) that showed greater weight loss with very-low-carbohydrate ketogenic diets, that is, less than 50 g/day, compared to low-fat diets (WMD, 0.91 kg [95% CI, 0.17–1.65]). Although statistically significant, the greater weight loss observed was quite small on an absolute scale, that is, a ~1 kg weight loss corresponds to ~1% weight reduction in a 100 kg individual. When low-fat interventions were compared to higher-fat interventions, this did not lead to differences in weight change (19 comparisons; WMD, 0.36 kg [−0.66 to 1.37]). Greater weight decreases were observed only when low-fat diets were compared with a usual diet (eight comparisons; −5.41 kg [−7.29 to −3.54]). In weight loss trials, higher-fat weight loss interventions led to significantly greater weight loss than low-fat interventions when groups differed by more than 5% of calories obtained from fat at follow-up (18 comparisons; WMD, 1.04 kg [95% CI, 0.06–2.03]), and when the difference in serum TGs between the two interventions at follow-up was at least 0.06 mmol/L (~5 mg/dL) (17 comparisons; 1.38 kg [0.50–2.25]). These findings suggest that the long-term effect of low-fat diet interventions on body weight depends on the intensity of the intervention in the comparison group, which is probably a function of adherence. Similarly, in the Women's Health Initiative, a greater weight loss of ~2 kg was observed in women who adhered to the low-fat diet compared to those who did not (Howard et al. 2006). Although these study conclusions contrast with a systematic analysis by Hooper et al. (2012), which reported that low-fat diets were more effective for weight loss (1.57 kg [95% CI, 1.16–1.97]) compared to other diet interventions, the Hooper analysis included studies that were less than 1 year in duration and excluded studies designed for weight loss; their derived risk estimate was thus overweighted with trials that considered low-fat diets versus usual diets (Hooper et al. 2012). Furthermore, as with the earlier meta-analyses that showed small but statistically significant weight loss with low-carbohydrate versus low-fat diets, the absolute amount of weight loss in the Hooper analysis showing benefit of low-fat diets, that is, ~1.57 kg, was small.

A number of commercial weight loss programs have now published enough data to make comparisons possible (Gudzune et al. 2015). In a meta-analysis, Gudzune et al. reported that Weight Watchers participants achieved at least 2.6% greater weight loss at 12 months than those assigned to control/education. Jenny Craig resulted in at least 4.9% greater weight loss at 12 months than control/education and counseling. Nutrisystem resulted in at least 3.8% greater weight loss at 3 months than control/education and counseling. Very-low-calorie programs (Health Management Resources, Medifast, and OPTIFAST) resulted in at least 4.0% greater short-term weight loss than counseling, but some attenuation of effect occurred beyond 6 months when reported. Atkins resulted in 0.1%–2.9% greater weight loss at 12 months than counseling (Gudzune et al. 2015). The investigators concluded that clinicians might refer patients to Jenny Craig or Weight Watchers, the two most efficacious programs, for weight loss. Among self-directed programs, the Atkins program was the most effective for weight loss at 6 and 12 months compared to no dieting.

The impact of these commercial diets on CVD risk factors has also been examined by this group (Mehta et al. 2016). They included 27 randomized controlled trials in their analysis. At 12 months, Weight Watchers and Jenny Craig showed little difference on blood pressure or lipids as compared to control/education or counseling. In contrast, Atkins' participants achieved the same or better results than counseling with respect to blood pressure and TGs. This greater effect of the Atkins group may reflect the reduction of carbohydrate intake that will lower TGs whether or not there is weight loss and that might also reduce blood pressure through the reduction of circulating blood volume as liver glycogen is depleted. All other programs lacked long-term studies that evaluated intermediate CVD outcomes.

Nonetheless, several short-term metabolic studies lend insight into the role of dietary fat versus carbohydrate on cardiometabolic profiles in the context of weight loss and stability. In a controlled dietary intervention study, carbohydrate restriction from 54% to 26% of total energy in the context of low-saturated-fat diets was associated with a greater improvement in lipoprotein markers of CVD risk (Krauss et al. 2006). Thus, in persons who do not desire or are unable to achieve weight loss, carbohydrate restriction may represent an intervention that effectively improves these lipid parameters.

A recent randomized crossover study of 19 obese volunteers confined to a metabolic ward for 2 weeks on two occasions separated by 4–6 weeks evaluated the effects of carbohydrate versus fat restriction on fuel oxidation and total body fat loss (Hall et al. 2015). After 6 days on a balanced diet (35% fat, 15% protein, 50% carbohydrate), energy intake was reduced 30% by removing either carbohydrate or fat intake. Although it has been proposed that low-carbohydrate diets result in lower total body fat due to increased fat oxidation (Ludwig and Friedman 2014), the study by Hall et al. did not show increased fat loss, in spite of body weight reductions, when people consumed low-carbohydrate diets. The significant caveat of this study was its short duration, that is, 6 days; thus, the data provided by this study cannot be used to support or refute the hypotheses related to macronutrient intake effects on fuel oxidation. Rather, this short-term metabolic ward study highlights the energetics required to replace dietary carbohydrate with glucose and β-OH butyrate from endogenous protein and fat, respectively, during acute metabolic adaptations.

Higher-Protein Diets

Higher-protein diets may be beneficial in managing weight loss (Leidy et al. 2015). Figure 4.5a shows that individuals assigned to a high-protein diet in the POUNDS Lost study and who adhered to that diet during the 2 years of intervention lost progressively more weight (Sacks et al. 2009). A second 2-year study compared 12% and 25% protein diets eaten as part of a 30% fat diet (Skov et al. 1999; Due et al. 2008). Weight loss over 36 weeks was substantially greater with the higher-protein diet and this difference was maintained at 56 weeks but not at 104 weeks (Figure 4.5b). A meta-analysis of energy-restricted, high-protein low-fat diets compared to standard-protein low-fat diets by Wycherley et al. (2012, 2013) showed a borderline significant effect of the higher-protein diets on body weight in trials lasting over 12 weeks (−0.97 kg [95% CI, −2.07 to 0.13]) and

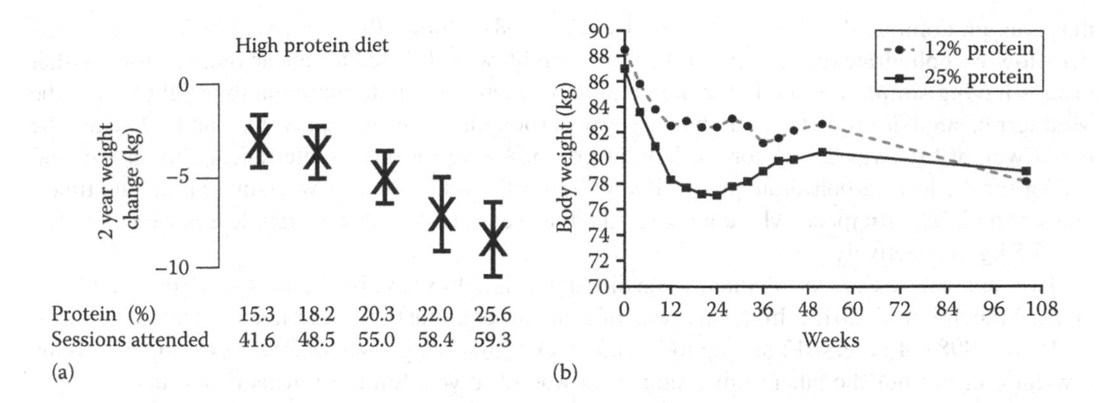

FIGURE 4.5 Effect on weight loss of adhering to a high-protein diet (a) and a high- and low-protein diet on a low-fat diet background diet (b). (a: Sacks, F.M. et al., *New Engl. J. Med.*, 360(9), 859, February 26, 2009; b: Skov, A.R. et al., *Int. J. Obes. Relat. Metab. Disord.*, 23(5), 528, 1999; Due, A. et al., *Int. J. Obes. Relat. Metab. Disord.*, 28(10), 1283, 2004.)

in trials lasting less than 12 weeks (−0.79 kg [95% CI, −1.34 to 0.37]). Fat mass, however, declined significantly more in the high-protein groups in trials lasting less than 12 weeks and in those lasting more than 12 weeks (−0.83 kg [95% CI, −1.31 to −0.34]) favoring high protein. The decrease in TGs also favored the higher-protein diets (0.23 mmol/L [95% CI, −0.36 to −0.11]) as did the increase in HDL-C (0.61 mmol/L [95% CI, 0.20–1.02]). In the trials lasting less than 12 weeks, resting energy expenditure increased more in those eating the high-protein diet (595 kJ/day [95% CI, 66.95–1124.05]). This would be similar to the effects observed with the measurement of energy expenditure during overfeeding in response to different levels of dietary protein (Bray et al. 2012). In a second meta-analysis by Schwingshackl and Hoffmann comparing low versus high glycemic index/load, fasting insulin was again the main difference in response (−0.71 μU/mL [95% CI, −1.36 to −0.05]) favoring the low–glycemic index/load diet (Schwingshackl and Hoffmann 2013a).

Low–Glycemic Index Diets

The glycemic index is based on the rise in blood glucose in response to the test food compared to the rise after a 50-g portion of white bread; glycemic load is the product of glycemic index and amount of carbohydrate in the food. The effect of low–glycemic index/load diets on weight loss has been studied in a number of randomized clinical trials in adults (Schwangshakl and Hoffman 2013b). Thomas et al. (2007) identified six studies including 202 participants that met their inclusion criteria. Three of these studies compared low–glycemic index/load diets with higher–glycemic index/load diets, while the other three compared an ad-lib low–glycemic index/load diet with a conventional energy-restricted low-fat diet, or an energy-restricted low–glycemic index/load diet with a normal energy-restricted diet. Interventions were relatively short ranging from 5 weeks to 6 months at the longest. There was a small significant difference in body weight of 1.1 kg (95% CI, −2.0 to −0.2) that favored the low–glycemic index/load diets. The body mass decreased by 1.1 kg ($P < 0.05$) and fat mass by a similar amount compared to the change of weight in the control diet group. Both total cholesterol and LDL-C fell more with the low–glycemic index/load diets (Sacks et al. 2014).

The Mediterranean Diet

The Mediterranean diet—generally characterized by high intakes of fruits, nuts, vegetables, whole-grain cereals, and olive oil, with moderate consumption of fish, poultry, and wine, and low intake of dairy, red meats, and sweets—has been compared to low-carbohydrate and low-fat diets for weight loss efficacy. One 2-year study was conducted at a single site in Israel with a worksite population that was predominantly (83%) male (Shai et al. 2008). During the rapid weight loss phase, the very-low-carbohydrate diet group lost the most weight, with the Mediterranean diet and low-fat diet groups having similar results. In the next 6 months, there was an acceleration in weight loss in the Mediterranean diet group to reach the very-low-carbohydrate diet group. At the end of 2 years, the mean weight loss was 2.9 kg for the low-fat group, 4.4 kg for the Mediterranean diet group, and 4.7 kg for the low-carbohydrate group ($P < 0.001$ for the interaction between diet group and time); among the 272 participants who completed the intervention, the mean weight losses were 3.3, 4.6, and 5.5 kg, respectively.

Two meta-analyses of the Mediterranean diet and weight loss have been published (Nordmann et al. 2011; Mancini et al. 2015). In the analysis of Mancini et al. that included five randomized clinical trials ($n = 998$) of at least 12 and up to 48 months in duration, greater weight loss compared to the low-fat diet but not the other comparator diets was observed. Similar effects of all diets on lipid levels and blood pressure were observed. The meta-analysis by Nordmann et al. (2011) identified 6 trials, including 2650 individuals (50% women). After 2 years of follow-up, individuals assigned to a Mediterranean diet had more favorable changes in WMDs of body weight (−2.2 kg; 95% CI, −3.9 to −0.6), body mass index (−0.6 kg/m^2; 95% CI, −1 to −0.1), systolic blood pressure (−1.7 mm Hg; 95% CI, −3.3 to −0.05), diastolic blood pressure (−1.5 mm Hg; 95% CI, −2.1 to −0.8), fasting plasma glucose (−3.8 mg/dL; 95% CI, −7 to −0.6), total cholesterol (−7.4 mg/dL; 95% CI, −10.3 to −4.4), and high-sensitivity C-reactive protein (−1.0 mg/L; 95% CI, −1.5 to −0.5). Thus, the Mediterranean diet is a good option available for persons seeking weight loss. Given its significant association with CVD risk reduction (see Chapter 22), this dietary pattern may be a preferred choice for dieters.

CONCLUSIONS

Diets varying in macronutrient composition have existed for over 100 years but have only more recently been systematically evaluated. In light of the current obesity epidemic, identifying effective dietary weight loss regimens is critical. Several components are key to long-term weight loss, and these include caloric restriction and adherence to the dietary regimen. All diets, as compared to usual diets, work when followed, and low-fat diets that have been traditionally recommended are no better than higher-fat diets for weight loss. Recent meta-analyses evaluating weight loss studies of similar intensity over the longer term have shown statistically significant weight reduction in persons following low-carbohydrate versus low-fat diets (Bueno et al. 2013), or vice versa (Hooper et al. 2012); the magnitude of weight loss was, however, small, that is, 1–2 kg. Similarly important to effective weight loss is the context in which it occurs; that is to say, attention to behavior modification (see also Chapter 2) and the support and structure provided by weight loss programs can provide dieters with important tools for successful weight management over the longer term (?).

In general, improvements in lipids and insulin resistance have been associated with the magnitude of weight loss. Lower-carbohydrate diets have been associated with improved TG and HDL-C, and lower-fat diets have been associated with lower LDL-C when differences in weight loss are maintained. The Mediterranean diet has been shown to reduce both weight and CVD risk (see Chapter 22), and this dietary pattern may thus be recommended assuming feasibility considerations are met.

Finally, the genes expressed during weight loss may influence both the extent of weight loss and lipid responses to diet, and knowledge of relevant genetic polymorphisms may, one day, guide diet strategies. Thus, individual responses to diets are more important than the mean weight loss achieved from a diet study, and personalization of nutrition and lifestyle regimens represents a key future direction in nutritional research. Nonetheless, the most effective interventions for weight loss and overall cardiometabolic health will incorporate diet as just one component of a multifaceted and comprehensive lifestyle regimen that includes increased physical activity, behavioral therapies, social support, and other parameters, including medical management as necessary. These topics are covered in chapters throughout this textbook.

REFERENCES

Alhassan S, Kim S, Bersamin A, King AC, Gardner CD. Dietary adherence and weight loss success among overweight women: Results from the A to Z weight loss study. *Intern J Obes* 2008; 32: 985–991.

Apovian CM, Aronne LJ, Bessesen DH, McDonnell ME, Murad MH, Pagotto U, Ryan DH, Still CD, Endocrine Society. Pharmacological management of obesity: An endocrine Society clinical practice guideline. *J Clin Endocrinol Metab* February 2015; 100(2): 342–362.

Atkins RC. *Dr. Atkins's New Diet Revolution*. New York: Avon, 2002.

Atwater WO, Benedict FG. *Experiments on the Metabolism of Matter and Energy in the Human Body, 1899–1900*. Washington, DC: Government Printing Office, U.S. Department of Agriculture, Office of experiment stations Bulletin No 109, 1902.

Avenell A, Broom J et al. Systematic review of the long-term effects and economic consequences of treatments for obesity and implications for health improvement. *Health Technol Assess* 2004; 8(21): iii–iv, 1–182.

Banting W. *A Letter on Corpulence Addressed to the Public*. London, U.K.: Harrison & Sons, 1864.

Bazzano LA, Hu T, Reynolds K, Yao L, Bunol C, Liu Y, Chen CS, Klag MJ, Whelton PK, He J. Effects of low-carbohydrate and low-fat diets: A randomized trial. *Ann Intern Med* September 2, 2014; 161(5): 309–318.

Bray GA. *The Battle of the Bulge*. Pittsburgh, PA: Dorrance Publishing, 2007.

Bray GA. *A Guide to Obesity and the Metabolic Syndrome*. Boca Raton, FL: CRC Press, 2011.

Bray GA, Bouchard C (eds.). *Handbook of Obesity*, Vol. I, 3rd edn., Vol. II 4th edn. Boca Raton, FL: Informa Publishers, 2014.

Bray GA, Popkin BM. Calorie-sweetened beverages and fructose: What have we learned 10 years later. *Pediatr Obes* August 2013; 8(4): 242–248.

Bray GA, Smith SR, de Jonge L, Xie H, Rood J, Martin CK, Most M, Brock C, Mancuso S, Redman L. Effect of dietary protein content on weight gain, energy expenditure, and body composition during overeating: A randomized controlled trial. *JAMA* 2012; 307(1): 47–55.

Brehm BJ, Seeley RJ et al. A randomized trial comparing a very low carbohydrate diet and a calorie-restricted low fat diet on body weight and cardiovascular risk factors in healthy women. *J Clin Endocrinol Metab* 2003; 88(4): 1617–1623.

Brinkworth GD, Noakes M, Buckley JD, Keogh JB, Clifton PM. Long-term effects of a very-low-carbohydrate weight loss diet compared with an isocaloric low-fat diet after 12 mo. *Am J Clin Nutr* 2009; 90: 23–32.

Bueno NB, de Melo IS, de Oliveira SL, da Rocha Ataide T. Very-low-carbohydrate ketogenic diet v. low-fat diet for long-term weight loss: A meta-analysis of randomised controlled trials. *Br J Nutr* October 2013; 110(7): 1178–1187. doi: 10.1017/S0007114513000548. Epub May 7, 2013.

Dansinger ML, Gleason JA et al. Comparison of the Atkins, Ornish, Weight Watchers, and Zone diets for weight loss and heart disease risk reduction: A randomized trial. *JAMA* 2005; 293(1): 43–53.

Dansinger ML, Tatsioni A, Wong JB, Chung M, Balk EM. Meta-analysis: The effect of dietary counseling for weight loss. *Ann Int Med* 2007; 147: 41–50.

Diabetes Prevention Program Research Group (Wing RR, Hamman RF, Bray GA, Delahanty L, Edelstein SL, Hill JO, Horton ES, Hoskin MA, Kriska A, Lachin J, Mayer-Davis EJ, Pi-Sunyer X, Regensteiner JG, Venditti B, Wylie-Rosett J). Achieving weight and activity goals among Diabetes Prevention Program lifestyle participants. *Obes Res* 2004; 12: 1426–1434.

Ditschuneit HH, Flechtner-Mors M. Value of structured meals for weight management: Risk factors and long-term weight maintenance. *Obes Res* November 2001; 9(Suppl 4): 284S–289S.

Due A, Larsen TM, Mu H, Hermansen K, Stender S, Astrup A. Comparison of 3 ad libitum diets for weight-loss maintenance, risk of cardiovascular disease, and diabetes: A 6-mo randomized controlled trial. *Am J Clin Nutr* 2008; 88: 1232–1241.

Due A, Toubro S et al. Effect of normal-fat diets, either medium or high in protein, on body weight in overweight subjects: A randomised 1-year trial. *Int J Obes Relat Metab Disord* 2004; 28(10): 1283–1290.

Ebbeling CB, Leidig MM, Feldman HA, Lovesky MM, Ludwig DS. Effects of a low-glycemic load vs low-fat diet in obese young adults: A randomized trial. *JAMA* May 16, 2007; 297(19): 2092–2102.

Ello-Martin JA, Roe LS, Ledikwe JH, Beach AM, Rolls BJ. Dietary energy density in the treatment of obesity: A year-long trial comparing 2 weight-loss diets. *Am J Clin Nutr* June 2007; 85(6): 1465–1477.

Flechtner-Mors M, Ditschuneit HH et al. Metabolic and weight loss effects of long-term dietary intervention in obese patients: Four-year results. *Obes Res* 2000; 8(5): 399–402.

Florez JC, Jablonski KA et al. Effects of genetic variants previously associated with fasting glucose and insulin in the DiabetesPrevention Program. *PLoS One* 2012; 7(9): e44424. doi: 10.1371/journal.pone.0044424.

Foster GD, Wyatt HR et al. A randomized trial of a low-carbohydrate diet for obesity. *N Engl J Med* 2003; 348(21): 2082–2090.

Foster GD, Wyatt HR et al. Weight and metabolic outcomes after 2 years on a low-carbohydrate versus low-fat diet: A randomized trial. *Ann Intern Med* August 3, 2010; 153(3): 147–157. doi: 10.7326/0003-4819-153-3-201008030-00005.

Gardner CD, Kiazand A, Alhassan S, Kim S, Stafford RS, Balise RR, Kraemer HC, King AC. Comparison of the Atkins, Zone, Ornish, and LEARN Diets for change in weight and related risk factors among overweight premenopausal women. *JAMA* 2007; 297: 969–977.

Gudzune KA, Doshi RS, Mehta AK, Chaudhry ZW, Jacobs DK, Vakil RM, Lee CJ, Bleich SN, Clark JM. Efficacy of commercial weight-loss programs: An updated systematic review. *Ann Intern Med* April 7, 2015; 162(7): 501–512.

Hall KD Bemis T et al. Calorie for calorie, dietary fat restriction results in more body fat loss than carbohydrate restriction in people with obesity. *Cell Metabol* September 1, 2015; 22(3): 427–436.

Hall KD, Sacks G et al. Quantification of the effect of energy imbalance on bodyweight. *Lancet* August 27, 2011; 378(9793): 826–837.

Harvey W. *On Corpulence in Relation to Disease: With Some Remarks on Diet*. London, U.K.: Henry Renshaw, 1872.

Heshka S, Anderson JW, Atkinson RL, Greenway FL, Hill JO, Phinney SD, Kolotkin RL, Miller-Kovach K, Pi-Sunyer FX. Weight loss with self-help compared with a structured commercial program: A randomized trial. *JAMA* April 9, 2003; 289(14): 1792–1798.

Hooper L, Abdelhamid A, Moore HJ, Douthwaite W, Skeaff CM, Summerbell CD. Effect of reducing total fat intake on body weight: Systematic review and meta-analysis of randomised controlled trials and cohort studies. *BMJ* December 6, 2012; 345: e7666. doi: 10.1136/bmj.e7666. Review.

Howard BV, Manson JE et al. Low-fat dietary pattern and weight change over 7 years: The women's health initiative dietary modification trial. *JAMA* 2006; 295(1): 39–49.

Jensen MD, Ryan DH et al. 2013 AHA/ACC/TOS guideline for the management of overweight and obesity in adults: A report of the American College of Cardiology/American Heart Association Task Force on Practice Guidelines and The Obesity Society. *J Am Coll Cardiol* July 1, 2014; 63(25 Pt B): 2985–3023. doi: 10.1016/j.jacc.2013.11.004. Epub November 12, 2013.

Johnston BC, Kanters S et al. Comparison of weight loss among named diet programs in overweight and obese adults: A meta-analysis. *JAMA* September 3, 2014; 312(9): 923–933.

Keys A. *Seven Countries. A Multivariate Analysis of Death and Coronary Heart Disease.* Cambridge, MA: Harvard University Press, 1980.

Krauss RM, Blanche PJ, Rawlings RS, Fernstrom HS, Williams PT. Separate effects of reduced carbohydrate intake and weight loss on atherogenic dyslipidemia. *Am J Clin Nutr* May 2006; 83(5): 1025–1031.

Kritchevsky SB, Beavers KM, Miller ME, Shea MK, Houston DK, Kitzman DW, Nicklas BJ. Intentional weight loss and all-cause mortality: A meta-analysis of randomized clinical trials. *PLoS One* March 20, 2015; 10(3): e0121993. doi: 10.1371/journal.pone.0121993. eCollection 2015. PMID: 25794148.

Langland JT. Efficacy of commercial weight-loss programs. *Ann Intern Med* September 1, 2015; 163(5): 398. doi: 10.7326/L15-5130. No abstract available. PMID: 26322704.

Larsen TM, Dalskov SM et al. Diets with high or low protein content and glycemic index for weight-loss maintenance. *N Engl J Med* November 25, 2010; 363(22): 2102–2113.

Lavoisier AL. *Traite elementaire de chemie, presente dan un order nouveau et d'apres les couvertes modernes*. Paris, France: Chez Cuchet, 1789.

Lee DC, Sui X, Church TS, Lavie CJ, Jackson AS, Blair SN. Changes in fitness and fatness on the development of cardiovascular disease risk factors hypertension, metabolic syndrome, and hypercholesterolemia. *J Am Coll Cardiol* February 14, 2012; 59(7): 665–672. doi: 10.1016/j.jacc.2011.11.013. PMID: 22322083.

Leidy HJ, Clifton PM, Astrup A, Wycherley TP, Westerterp-Plantenga MS, Luscombe-Marsh ND, Woods SC, Mattes RD. The role of protein in weight loss and maintenance. *Am J Clin Nutr* April 29, 2015; 101(6): 1320S–1329S. Epub ahead of print.

Lin X, Qi Q, Zheng Y, Huang T, Lathrop M, Zelenika D, Bray GA, Sacks FM, Liang L, Qi L. Neuropeptide Y genotype, central obesity and abdominal fat distribution: The POUNDS Lost trial. *Am J Clin Nutr* August 2015; 102(2): 514–519.

Look AHEAD Research Group, Wing RR et al. Cardiovascular effects of intensive lifestyle intervention in type 2 diabetes. *N Engl J Med* July 11, 2013; 369(2): 145–154. doi: 10.1056/NEJMoa1212914. Epub 2013 Jun 24. Erratum in: *N Engl J Med*. 2014 May 8;370(19):1866. PMID: 23796131.

Ludwig DS, Friedman MI. Increasing adiposity: Consequence orNordman cause of overeating? *JAMA* 2014; 311: 2167–2168.

Mancini JG, Filion KB, Atallah R, Eisenberg MJ Systematic review of the mediterranean diet for long-term weight loss. *Am J Med* December 22, 2015; 129(4): 407–415. doi: 10.1016/j.amjmed.2015.11.028. Epub ahead of print.

Mehta AK, Doshi RS, Chaudhry ZW, Jacobs DK, Vakil RM, Lee CJ, Bleich SN, Clark JM, Gudzune KA. Benefits of commercial weight-loss programs on blood pressure and lipids: A systematic review. *Prev Med* September 2016; 90: 86–99. doi: 10.1016/j.ypmed.2016.06.028. Epub June 30, 2016.

Mirzaei K, Xu M, Qibin Qi Q, Bray GA, Frank Sacks F, Qi L. Glucose and circadian related genetic variants affect response of energy expenditure to weight-loss diets: The POUNDS LOST Trial. *Am J Clin Nutr.* February 2014; 99(2): 392–399.

Moss M. *Salt Sugar Fat: How the Food Giants Hooked Us.* New York: Random House, 2013.

Nordmann AJ, Suter-Zimmermann K, Bucher HC, Shai I, Tuttle KR, Estruch R, Briel M. Meta-analysis comparing Mediterranean to low-fat diets for modification of cardiovascular risk factors. *Am J Med* September 2011; 124(9): 841–851.

Ornish D. *Eat More, Weigh Less: Dr. Dean Ornish's Life Choice Program for Losing Weight Safely while Eating Abundantly.* New York: HarperCollins, 1993.

Papandonatos GD, Pan Q et al. Genetic predisposition to weight loss & regain with lifestyle intervention: Analyses from the Diabetes Prevention Program & the Look AHEAD randomized controlled trials. *Diabetes* August 7, 2015; 64(12): 4312–4321.

Pettenkoffer M. *Ueber einem neuen Respirations-Apparat.* Munchen, Germany: Verlag der k. Akademie, 1861.

Pirozzo S, Summerbell C et al. Should we recommend low-fat diets for obesity? *Obes Rev* 2003; 4(2): 83–90.

Putnam J, Allshouse J, Kantor LS. U.S. per capita food supply trends: More calories, refined carbohydrates and fats. *Food Rev* 2002; 25 (3): 2–15.

Qi Q, Bray GA, Hu FB, Sacks FM, Qi L. Weight-loss diets modify glucose-dependent insulinotropic polypeptide receptor rs2287019 genotype effects on changes in body weight, fasting glucose, and insulin resistance: The Preventing Overweight Using Novel Dietary Strategies trial. *Am J Clin Nutr* February 2012; 95(2): 506–513.

Qi Q, Xu M, Wu H, Liang L, Champagne CM, Bray GA, Sacks FM, Qi L. IRS1 genotype modulates metabolic syndrome reversion in response to 2-year weight-loss diet intervention: The POUNDS LOST trial. *Diabetes Care* November 2013; 36(11): 3442–3447.

Rock CL, Pakiz B, Flatt SW, Quintana EL. Randomized trial of a multifaceted commercial weight loss program. *Obesity (Silver Spring)* April 2007; 15(4): 939–949.

Rosenbaum M, Sy M, Pavlovich K, Leibel RL, Hirsch J. Leptin reverses weight loss-induced changes in regional neural activity responses to visual food stimuli. *J Clin Invest* July 2008; 118(7):2583–2591.

Sacks FM, Bray GA et al. Comparison of weight-loss diets with different compositions of fat, carbohydrate and protein. *New Engl J Med* February 26, 2009; 360(9): 859–873.

Sacks FM, Carey VJ et al. Effects of high vs low glycemic index of dietary carbohydrate on cardiovascular disease risk factors and insulin sensitivity: The OmniCarb randomized clinical trial. *JAMA* December 17, 2014; 312(23): 2531–2541.

Samaha FF, Iqbal N et al. 2003. A low-carbohydrate as compared with a low-fat diet in severe obesity. *N Engl J Med* 348(21): 2074–2081.

Schwingshackl L, Hoffmann G. Long-term effects of low-fat diets either low or high in protein on cardiovascular and metabolic risk factors: A systematic review and meta-analysis. *Nutr J.* April 15, 2013a; 12: 48. doi: 10.1186/1475-2891-12-48.

Schwingshackl L, Hoffmann G. Long-term effects of low glycemic index/load vs. high glycemic index/load diets on parameters of obesity and obesity-associated risks: A systematic review and meta-analysis. *Nutr Metab Cardiovasc Dis* August 2013b; 23(8): 699–706.

Scully T. Obesity. *Nature* 2014; 508(7496): S49. doi: 10.1038/508S49a.

Shai I, Schwarzfuchs D et al. Dietary Intervention Randomized Controlled Trial (DIRECT) Group. Weight loss with a low-carbohydrate, Mediterranean, or low-fat diet. *N Engl J Med* July 17, 2008; 359(3): 229–241.

Skov AR, Toubro S et al. Randomized trial on protein vs carbohydrate in ad libitum fat reduced diet for the treatment of obesity. *Int J Obes Relat Metab Disord* 1999; 23(5): 528–536.

Stern L, Iqbal N et al. 2004. The effects of low-carbohydrate versus conventional weight loss diets in severely obese adults: One-year follow-up of a randomized trial. *Ann Intern Med* 140(10): 778–785.

Sumithran P, Prendergast LA, Delbridge E, Purcell K, Shulkes A, Kriketos A, Proietto J. Long-term persistence of hormonal adaptations to weight loss. *N Engl J Med* October 27, 2011; 365(17): 1597–1604. doi: 10.1056/NEJMoa1105816.

Thomas DE, Elliott EJ, Baur L. Low glycemic index or low glycemic load diets for overweight and obesity (Review). *Cochrane Database of Systematic Reviews* 2007; 3: CD005105. doi: 10.1002/14651858.CD005105.pub2.

Thomas DM, Gonzalez MC, Pereira AZ, Redman LM, Heymsfield SB. Time to correctly predict the amount of weight loss with dieting. *J Acad Nutr Diet* June 2014; 114(6): 857–861.

Thomas DM, Ivanescu AE et al. Predicting successful long-term weight loss from short-term weight-loss outcomes: New insights from a dynamic energy balance model (the POUNDS Lost study). *Am J Clin Nutr* March 2015; 101(3): 449–454.

Tobias DK, Chen M, Manson JE, Ludwig DS, Willett W, Hu FB. Effect of low-fat diet interventions versus other diet interventions on long-term weight change in adults: A systematic review and meta-analysis. *Lancet Diabetes Endocrinol* 2015; 3(12): 968–979.

Unick JL, Neiberg RH et al. Research Group. Weight change in the first 2 months of a lifestyle intervention predicts weight changes 8 years later. *Obesity (Silver Spring)* July 2015; 23(7): 1353–1356.

US Senate. Select Committee on Nutrition and Human Needs. *Dietary Goals for the United States*. Washington, DC: U.S. GPO, February 1977.

Varady KA, Bhutani S, Klempel MC, Kroeger CM, Trepanowski JF, Haus JM, Hoddy KK, Calvo Y. Alternate day fasting for weight loss in normal weight and overweight subjects: A randomized controlled trial. *Nutr J* 2013; 12(1): 146.

von Helmholtz H. *Uber die Erhaltung der Kraft, ein physikalische Abhandlung, vorgetragen in der Sitzung der physicalischen Gesellschaft zu Berlin am 23sten Juli 1847*. Berlin G. Reimer, 1847.

von Noorden C. *Obesity. The Indications for Reduction Cures Being Part I of Several Clinical Treatises on the Pathology and Therapy of Disorders of Metabolism and Nutrition.* Bristol, England: John Wright & Co, 1903.

Wadden TA, Neiberg RH et al. Research Group. Four-year weight losses in the Look AHEAD study: Factors associated with long-term success. *Obesity (Silver Spring)* October 2011; 19(10): 1987–1998.

Wadden TA, West DS et al. One-year weight losses in the Look AHEAD study: Factors associated with success. *Obesity (Silver Spring)* April 2009; 17(4): 713–722.

Wycherley TP, Buckley JD, Noakes M, Clifton PM, Brinkworth GD. Comparison of the effects of weight loss from a high-protein versus standard-protein energy-restricted diet on strength and aerobic capacity in overweight and obese men. *Eur J Nutr* February 2013; 52(1): 317–325.

Wycherley TP, Moran LJ, Clifton PM, Noakes M, Brinkworth GD. Effects of energy-restricted high-protein, low-fat compared with standard-protein, low-fat diets: A meta-analysis of randomized controlled trials. *Am J Clin Nutr* December 2012; 96(6): 1281–1298.

Xu M, Ng SS, Bray GA, Ryan DH, Sacks FM, Ning G, Qi L. Dietary fat intake modifies the effect of a common variant in the LIPC gene on changes in serum lipid concentrations during a long-term weight-loss intervention trial. *J Nutr* June 2015; 145(6): 1289–1294. doi: 10.3945/jn.115.212514. Epub April 29, 2015. PMID: 25926410.

Xu M, Qi Q, Liang J, Bray GA, Frank Hu F, Sacks F, Qi L. Genetic determinant for amino acid metabolites and changes in body weight and insulin resistance in response to weight-loss diets: The POUNDS LOST Trial. *Circulation* March 26, 2013; 127(12): 1283–1289.

Yancy WS, Jr, Olsen MK et al. A low-carbohydrate, ketogenic diet versus a low-fat diet to treat obesity and hyperlipidemia: A randomized, controlled trial. *Ann Intern Med* 2004; 140(10): 769–777.

Zhang X, Qi Q, Bray GA, Hu FB, Sacks FM, Qi L. APOA5 genotype modulates 2-year changes in lipid profile in response to weight-loss diet intervention: The pounds lost trial. *Am J Clin Nutr* October 2012a; 96(4): 917–922.

Zhang X, Qi Q, Liang J, Hu FB, Sacks FM, Qi L. Neuropeptide Y promoter polymorphism modifies effects of a weight-loss diet on 2-year changes of blood pressure: The preventing overweight using novel dietary strategies trial. *Hypertension* November 2012c; 60(5): 1169–1175.

Zhang X, Qi Q, Zhang C, Hu FB, Bray GA, Smith SR, Sacks FM, Qi L. FTO genotype and 2-year change in body composition and fat distribution in response to weight-loss diets: The POUNDS LOST Trial. *Diabetes* November 2012b; 61(11): 3005–3011.

Zheng Y, Huang T et al. Dietary fat modifies the effects of FTO genotype on changes in insulin sensitivity. *J Nutr* May 2015; 145(5): 977–982.

5 Weight Loss by Surgical Intervention

Nutritional Considerations and Influence on Health

Karim Kheniser and Sangeeta Kashyap

CONTENTS

ABSTRACT

Over the past several decades, the pandemic that is obesity has gone unabated and has contributed to the rise of type II diabetes and cancer. Now more than ever, therapeutic management of obesity and its associated comorbidities is needed. Traditional methods have failed to attenuate the incidence of obesity, which has given rise to more contemporary modalities. Particularly, bariatric procedures have been thrusted to the forefront, to combat obesity and its concomitant metabolic diseases. Segregated into restrictive, malabsorptive, or bypass operations, bariatric procedures have been demonstrated to be more efficacious in inducing weight loss and type II diabetes remission. Subsequently, obese patients and/or individuals with type II diabetes that are refractory to more conservative therapeutic methods, such as intensive medical therapy, have been encouraged to undergo bariatric surgery. The most popular of which is the Roux-en-y gastric bypass procedure, which reduces gastric volume and bypasses portions of the stomach, duodenum, and the initial segments of the jejunum to facilitate weight loss. Furthermore, purely restrictive procedures such as the sleeve gastrectomy have also become widely popular. The mechanisms by which the aforementioned procedures promote weight loss are primarily mediated by gastric restriction and possibly by attenuations in ghrelin secretion. This fosters early satiety and consequently reductions in food intake, which induces a negative energy balance. These procedures have shown promise, but additional research is needed to identify demographic, behavioral, and/or anthropometric characteristics that would better predict optimal outcomes after bariatric surgery.

INTRODUCTION

With the advent of laparoscopy and the concomitant reduction in perioperative complications, shorter hospital stay, quicker return to vocational status, and moderated blood loss, bariatric procedures have been catapulted to the forefront against the war on obesity (Nguyen et al. 2001; Schauer et al. 2000). Alternatively, bariatric procedures have been termed metabolic procedures because they confer positive effects on a multitude of metabolic parameters. For instance, in short- and long-term interventions, weight loss is substantial, pharmacological agents are largely discontinued, euglycemia and diabetes remission are frequently achieved, and insulin sensitivity and secretion are potentiated (Brethauer et al. 2013; Hofsø et al. 2011; Kashyap, Louis, and Kirwan 2011, 2013; Savassi-Rocha et al. 2008; Schauer et al. 2014; Sjöström et al. 2004). Comparatively, medical/lifestyle therapy has been demonstrated to induce only modest decreases in weight loss and is a requisite to improvements in high-density lipoproteins and other blood biomarkers (Ryan et al. 2010), but the positive effects are nondurable and miniscule, even with adjunct pharmacological therapy (Yanovski and Yanovski 2002), in relation to minimally invasive adjustable gastric banding procedures (Dixon et al. 2008; O'Brien et al. 2006). Unlike bariatric procedures, nonsurgical methods may be destined for failure because the homeostatic response to weight loss is dictated by unrelenting orexigenic stimuli and reciprocal changes in energy expenditure that would precipitate recidivism (Cummings et al. 2002; Cummings and Shannon 2003; Kotidis et al. 2006; Leibel, Rosenbaum, and Hirsch 1995). Moreover, even when medical therapy achieves equivalency in weight reduction, bariatric procedures prove to be more efficacious in promoting favorable alterations in insulin sensitivity (Plum et al. 2011). Above all else and unrivaled by medical therapy, bariatric procedures drastically and consistently reduce morbidity, mortality, cancer risk, and health care costs (Adams et al. 2007; Christou et al. 2004; Sjöström et al. 2007). Unequivocally, lifestyle/medical therapy has become complementary to bariatric procedures, which exert a profound moderating influence on massive obesity and provide therapeutic relief to their debilitating comorbidities.

BARIATRIC SURGERIES

Excluding adolescents who require a more diligent screening regimen and thorough collaboration between the medical team and family (Inge et al. 2004), bariatric surgeries are advocated when body mass index (BMI) exceeds 40 kg/m^2 or in the presence of comorbidities and a BMI of ≥35 kg/m^2 (National Institutes of Health 1992). Although bariatric procedures have been utilized in type II diabetics with a BMI of ≤30 kg/m^2, the research is currently sparse and has not gained widespread acceptance (Mechanick et al. 2013). Contemporary and efficacious surgical modalities that induce significant weight loss (i.e., ≥50% of excess weight loss or a BMI ≤ 35 kg/m^2 in the super-obese) are segregated into restrictive, malabsorptive, and bypass operations (Brolin 2002; Reinhold 1982; Renquist et al. 1995). Even though the latter two procedures share commonalities, in that they both bypass segments of the small intestine and facilitate malabsorption (excluding short-limb variants of Roux-en-Y gastric bypass, which has not been demonstrated to induce malabsorption), generally, bypass procedures are made in reference to Roux-en-Y gastric bypass, while malabsorptive procedures pertain to variants of biliopancreatic diversion. Restrictive procedures decrease daily caloric intake via reductions in gastric volume and the associated promotion of early satiety, while malabsorptive techniques attenuate nutrient absorption because they bypass segments of the small intestine (e.g., duodenum) and limit contact with biliopancreatic juices (Gletsu-Miller and Wright 2013). Unique to bypass and malabsorptive procedures, the circumvention of segments of the small intestine and gastric fundus play a crucial role in ameliorating diabetes, irrespective of weight loss and caloric intake (Kashyap et al. 2010; Rubino et al. 2006).

Also, in many instances, the degree and type of nutritional deficiencies that are present post-surgery are dictated by the specific surgical intervention. Generally, malabsorptive operations and possibly long-limb variants of Roux-en-Y gastric bypass reduce the absorption of lipids and patients are considered to be at higher risk for micronutrient deficiencies pre- and postoperatively (Gudzune et al. 2013). Furthermore, interindividual differences in surgical technique and intestinal morphology will also have an effect on malabsorption. In particular, the most common bariatric surgeries include Roux-en-Y gastric bypass, laparoscopic adjustable gastric banding, sleeve gastrectomy, and biliopancreatic diversion with or without duodenal switch.

ROUX-EN-Y GASTRIC BYPASS

Suited for individuals who have a propensity to ingest sweets and patients with gastroesophageal reflux disease (Buchwald 2002), the purpose of Roux-en-Y gastric bypass is to induce weight loss by reducing gastric volume to ≤30 mL and diverting ingested foods away from the distal stomach, duodenum, and minute (~initial 10 cm) segments of the jejunum (Elder and Wolfe 2007; Pories et al. 1995). The gastric pouch is created by segmenting the stomach into upper and lower quadrants, of which the lower or remnant pouch is bypassed (Moize et al. 2003). After the jejunum is transected distally from the ligament of Treitz, gastrojejunostomy and jejunojejunostomy are formed. The Roux limb, biliopancreatic limb, and common limb are denoted as representing the increments from the gastrojejunostomy to the jejunojejunostomy, from the ligament of Treitz to the jejunojejunostomy, and from the jejunojejunostomy to the ileocecal valve, respectively (Chen et al. 2013; Elder and Wolfe 2007; Gletsu-Miller and Wright 2013). Depending on the size of Roux and common limbs, the procedure can be designated as a long-limb or short-limb procedure.

Super-obese subjects (BMI ≥ 50 kg/m^2) achieve pronounced weight loss with the long-limb variant (Brolin et al. 1992; MacLean, Rhode, and Nohr 2001). The mechanism by which this occurs does not appear to be related to malabsorption, as it had a negligible contribution to the total reduction in intestinal absorption of macronutrient energy (Brolin 2002; Cummings, Overduin, and Foster-Schubert 2004; Odstrcil et al. 2010). However, standardizing biliopancreatic or Roux limb lengths, across patients, when assessing malabsorption may provide inconclusive results because it fails to account for jejunoileal length, which can improve the absorptive surface area by extending common limb length (Savassi-Rocha et al. 2008). Thus, dietary (e.g., fewer meals and less snacking) (Halmi et al. 1981), endocrine, and restrictive mechanisms appear to be the predominant mediators of weight loss.

Biliopancreatic Diversion with Duodenal Switch

Biliopancreatic diversion with duodenal switch is an invasive procedure that necessitates transection of portions of the gut and bowel and frequently requires a cholecystectomy. Initially, a sleeve gastrectomy (partitions the majority of the stomach, which leaves a "sleeve-like" stomach) is performed to reduce gastric volume to 80–100 mL, which, depending on the surgical technique, excludes the ghrelin-producing fundus (Hess and Hess 1998; Kotidis et al. 2006). Then, the duodenum is transected 4–5 cm distally from the pylorus and the distal portion of the ilium is bisected (Hess and Hess 1998). When the proximal portion of the duodenum is preserved, the incidence of ulcerations is reduced (DeMeester et al. 1987). Thereafter, the distal portion of the ileum is anastomosed to the duodenum to create a duodenoileostomy; similarly, the proximal ileum is anastomosed to the distal portion of the ileum (i.e., ileoileostomy), which is located proximally to the cecum (Hess and Hess 1998). The point from the duodenoileostomy to the ileoileostomy is denoted as representing the alimentary limb. Thus, the procedure bypasses the majority of the jejunum and duodenum and the biliopancreatic juices flow through the biliopancreatic limb into the distal portion of the ileum where the ingested food converges with and forms the common limb. The delayed mixing of biliopancreatic juices and ailments promotes malabsorption.

Its effects on weight loss are drastic and are mediated by restrictive, malabsorptive, and endocrine mechanisms. At 8 years, the majority of type II diabetics achieved remission and excess weight loss was maintained at 70%; favorable modifications to total cholesterol and low-density lipoproteins were observed (Hess and Hess 1998). Marceau et al. (1998) observed similar reductions in weight loss, as excess body weight was reduced by 73% ± 21% at 51 ± 25 months.

Biliopancreatic Diversion

Scopinaro et al. (1998) noted comparable excess weight loss outcomes in biliopancreatic diversion patients and this procedure can be applied in the non-super-obese, without the occurrence of persistent severe metabolic deficiencies (Skroubis et al. 2006). However, the main difference between biliopancreatic diversion and biliopancreatic diversion with duodenal switch is that in biliopancreatic diversion a larger gastric reservoir and the ghrelin-producing fundus are retained (Kotidis et al. 2006). Furthermore, in biliopancreatic diversion with duodenal switch, the pylorus and vagal integrity remain intact, which prevent rapid gastric emptying and increased motility (Kotidis et al. 2006); concurrently, the common limb may be more protracted in length (e.g., 100 cm), which is sensible given that it would reduce the sequela associated with malabsorption (Marceau et al. 1998).

Herein, a summation of Dr. Scopinaro's experience with biliopancreatic diversion will be discussed (Scopinaro 2012). In principal, biliopancreatic diversion is a malabsorptive procedure, but it is malleable. The pendulum can meander from a restrictive to a malabsorptive procedure, which is predicated upon the gastric volume and lengths of the alimentary and common limbs. Indeed, if gastric volume is significantly reduced to where energy intake underlies the energy absorption threshold of the alimentary and common limbs, it becomes a restrictive procedure, thus making the malabsorptive component futile (Scopinaro 2012). Conversely, if the restrictive component permits energy intake above the energy absorption threshold, then the restrictive component is undermined. Therefore, the operation cannot have dual mechanisms for weight loss (Scopinaro 2012).

Dichotomously, with respect to their side effects and complications, the effects of a small gastric volume and a large malabsorptive component become additive (Scopinaro 2012). Generally, a common limb and alimentary limb length of 50 and 250 cm is viable, respectively; however, in obese and overweight type II diabetics, the common limb can be 75 and 100 cm, respectively (Scopinaro 2012). Furthermore, a small gastric volume (e.g., 150 mL) should not be incorporated into a biliopancreatic diversion procedure because it would exacerbate nutritional deficiencies. Consequently, gastric volume should permit energy intake that exceeds the energy absorption threshold, but the overall volume of the gut (400–500 mL) should be low enough to permit rapid gastric emptying and consequently facilitate malabsorption (Scopinaro 2012; Scopinaro et al. 2011).

Laparoscopic Adjustable Gastric Banding

One of the main advantages of laparoscopic adjustable gastric banding is that normal gastrointestinal continuity is preserved and it is purely restrictive in nature. Gastric capacity is reduced to ≤30 mL by placing a collar 1–2 cm inferior to the gastroesophageal junction, and gradation in the degree of constriction can be modified by adjusting the amount of saline that is infused into the subcutaneous port, which is connected to a balloon within the collar (Elder and Wolfe 2007). The perigastric and pars flaccida surgical techniques are primarily utilized, with the latter associated with a lower rate of prolapse (Biagini and Karam 2008; O'Brien et al. 2005). At the outset, the collar confers minimal gastric restriction, but it is gradually heightened to achieve sustainable weight loss (Dixon, Dixon, and O'Brien 2005). Due to the confined gastric volume, laparoscopic adjustable gastric banding subjects will feel satiated, but this appears to be independent to alterations in leptin and the orexigenic hormone, ghrelin (Dixon, Dixon, and O'Brien 2005; Faraj et al. 2003), which has been noted to increase (Langer et al. 2005). Consequently, this may explain the myriad of excess weight loss values and poor efficacy, in some instances (Langer et al. 2005).

Sleeve Gastrectomy

Restrictive in nature, sleeve gastrectomy reduces gastric volume by resecting the greater curvature of the stomach and excluding the fundus. As such, due to reduced nutriment contact (Cummings et al. 2002), ghrelin secretion is reduced (Bohdjalian et al. 2010; Karamanakos et al. 2008; Langer et al. 2005). Also, similar to Roux-en-Y gastric bypass, the hindgut hormone glucagon-like peptide-1, which has salutary effects on glycemic control (Kashyap and Schauer 2012), and peptide YY secretions are potentiated (Karamanakos et al. 2008; Kashyap et al. 2013). Together, this will foster an anorectic state that would engender more durable weight loss. Excess weight loss of 55% has been noted at 5 years post-surgery (Bohdjalian et al. 2010). Himpens, Dobbeleir, and Peeters (2010) found similar results at 6 years, but 3-year outcomes were 77.5%. Short-term trials have demonstrated excess weight loss values of 69.7% ± 14.6% at 1 year, which was even greater than Roux-en-Y gastric bypass (60.5% ± 10.7%) (Karamanakos et al. 2008). However, in the midst of similar weight loss outcomes, Roux-en-Y gastric bypass has been shown to induce more striking effects on metabolic parameters (Kashyap et al. 2013). This data explains the increased popularity of sleeve gastrectomy as a primary therapeutic modality. Furthermore, as denoted, its efficacy has even rivaled that of Roux-en-Y gastric bypass in some instances.

Roux-en-Y Gastric Bypass vs. Laparoscopic Adjustable Gastric Banding

Roux-en-Y gastric bypass is favored by the majority of surgeons because it incurs favorable weight-independent changes to metabolic parameters. Although some evidence contraindicates the sentiment that Roux-en-Y gastric bypass has a dampening effect on ghrelin secretion (Holdstock et al. 2003; Karamanakos et al. 2008), the incurred positive effects on metabolic parameters have been shown to be partially mediated by attenuated gastroduodenal secretion of ghrelin (i.e., override inhibition), which may necessitate a vagotomy along with transection of the fundus (Williams et al. 2003). The discordant results with respect to ghrelin secretion can be due to divergent surgical techniques and/or retrograde nutriment flow through the short biliopancreatic limb (Cummings, Overduin, and Foster-Schubert 2004; Holdstock et al. 2003). Also contributory to its positive metabolic effects are increases in postprandial enteroinsular (principally glucagon-like peptide-1), peptide YY (Cummings et al. 2002; Faraj et al. 2003; Kashyap et al. 2013; Le Roux et al. 2006), and anorexigenic adipokines such as adiponectin, while the pro-lipogenic hormone, acylation-stimulating protein, is decreased (Faraj et al. 2003; Holdstock et al. 2003). Congruently, not only has Roux-en-Y gastric bypass been demonstrated to alter gut hormone and enteroinsular secretion, but the small bowel microbial milieu may be altered to where it would favor enhanced motility (Zhang et al. 2009).

Roux-en-Y gastric bypass induces definite and sustained increases in excess weight loss (Christou et al. 2004). At the 2-year mark, gastric bypass procedures were more efficacious in inducing weight loss in super-obese patients (>50 kg/m^2), in relation to laparoscopic adjustable gastric banding (Te Riele et al. 2007). Interestingly, some reports suggest that Roux-en-Y gastric bypass is less effective in inducing weight loss in the aforesaid population (Jan et al. 2005; Nguyen et al. 2009). However, this may be evident in the majority of restrictive and short-limb operations. Also, in a 4-year randomized, prospective trial, Roux-en-Y gastric bypass was superior to that of laparoscopic adjustable gastric banding in inducing weight loss, but weight loss plateaued after year 2 (Nguyen et al. 2009). Likewise, maximal weight loss was achieved within 1 or 2 years, but at 15 years there was a twofold difference in weight loss (Roux-en-Y gastric bypass = 27% $\pm$ 12%; laparoscopic adjustable gastric banding = 13% $\pm$ 14%) (Sjöström et al. 2007). Ten-year values were 25% $\pm$ 11% and 14% $\pm$ 14%, respectively. Furthermore, euglycemia was achieved in the majority of patients and demonstrated mean decrements of 70% excess weight loss at year 2, with excess weight loss stabilizing at ~50% thereafter, over a similar timespan (Pories et al. 1995).

However, with periodic follow-up and an experienced surgical team, laparoscopic adjustable gastric banding has been demonstrated to successfully ameliorate morbidities (e.g., type II diabetes, obesity, hypertension, etc.) (Biagini and Karam 2008; O'Brien et al. 2006). Furthermore, relative to bypass procedures, laparoscopic adjustable gastric banding is reversible, less invasive, and there is a lower prevalence of postoperative complications (Nguyen et al. 2009; Te Riele et al. 2007). Similar to Roux-en-Y gastric bypass, it induces remission of diabetes (73% of 30 subjects) and profound excess weight loss (62.5%) at 2 years (Dixon et al. 2008). Others obtained similar results (O'Brien et al. 1999). Furthermore, there is a contention that although Roux-en-Y gastric bypass induces profound weight loss initially, the distinction in excess weight loss between the bariatric procedures appears to be lessened after 3 years (Jan et al. 2005). Although outside the guidelines recommended by the National Institutes of Health (National Institutes of Health 1992), multiple trials have utilized the laparoscopic adjustable gastric banding or other surgeries in individuals with a BMI between 30 and 35 kg/m^2, before weight gain becomes more pronounced and morbidities unresponsive to therapy (Angrisani et al. 2004; Dixon et al. 2008; Mason et al. 1997; Parikh, Duncombe, and Fielding 2006, O'Brien et al. 2006; Rubino et al. 2006). The use of laparoscopic adjustable gastric banding in this subpopulation may abrogate the progression of obesity and undiagnosed comorbidities, thereby possibly reducing the need for more complex procedures such as long-limb Roux-en-Y gastric bypass and biliopancreatic diversion with duodenal switch, when the need for immense weight loss is required.

Nevertheless, empirical evidence indicates that Roux-en-Y gastric bypass is superior to laparoscopic adjustable gastric banding. One of the main downfalls that contributes to its inferiority is the fact that laparoscopic adjustable gastric banding patients must adhere to a more frequent pre- and postoperative visit regimen and dietary and physical activity guidelines to induce successful weight loss, in comparison to Roux-en-Y gastric bypass (Biagini and Karam 2008; El Chaar et al. 2011; Shen et al. 2004). If they fail to, weight loss will not be pronounced and consequently comorbidities will persist. Therefore, given the additional burden placed on these patients and the likelihood that they will fail to adhere to postoperative guidelines, additional research is required before the use of laparoscopic adjustable gastric banding becomes more widespread, especially in the United States where it is relatively uncommon. In conclusion, although this will need to be empirically substantiated, laparoscopic adjustable gastric banding may be relegated to a preemptive procedure where it is specifically employed to prevent morbid obesity, in patients with a BMI of $\leq$35kg/m^2 (Buchwald 2002). This does not come without caution, as imposing laparoscopic adjustable gastric banding and other procedures in this population could be problematic because surgeons with limited operative proficiency may be financially motivated to impose these procedures in poor candidates (Steinbrook 2004), which may heighten mortality risk (Flum et al. 2005). Thus, it may be advantageous to conduct high-risk (e.g., super-obese) surgeries in centers of excellence.

The invasiveness of the procedures must be counterbalanced with their safety and ability to induce remission of diabetes and successful weight loss. Ultimately, in many instances, the specific surgical intervention that is chosen is dictated by the surgeon's experience with a specific bariatric procedure and their consequent bias, pay status (i.e., private [health insurance] or government pay [e.g., Medicare and Medicaid]) (Mason et al. 1997; Renquist et al. 1996), patient risk (Jan et al. 2005), age, gender, comorbidity status, ethnicity, and the degree of weight loss that is required (Buchwald 2002; Cummings, Overduin, and Foster-Schubert 2004). For instance, patients who present with fewer comorbidities and a lower preoperative BMI may be more suited for purely restrictive procedures (Buchwald 2002). As stated by Buchwald, no gold standard procedure exists and he utilizes numerical formulas and algorithms to discern the optimal procedure for each patient (Buchwald 2002).

EATING BEHAVIOR, PROTEIN CONSUMPTION POST-SURGERY, AND RESISTANCE EXERCISE

Whether by choice, via influence from a dietician or surgeon, or stemming directly from the anatomical alterations in the gastrointestinal tract, eating behavior is significantly modified after surgery. A multitiered dietary template is employed after bariatric surgery to facilitate healing through optimal nutritional intake, minimize loss of fat-free mass (FFM), reduce gastrointestinal symptoms, and potentiate weight loss (Aills et al. 2008). At the outset, ingestion of liquid-based or soft-texture foods predominates due to inflammation and edema, which impede the passage of food (Bock 2003; Moize et al. 2003). Diets progress, in order, from a clear liquid (1–2 days [d]) to full liquid (10–14 d) to pureed (10–14 + d) to mechanically modified soft diet ($\geq$14 d), and finally a regular diet is recommended (Aills et al. 2008). Osmolality and caloric density gradually increase as diets change. To avoid dumping syndrome and facilitate weight loss, avoidance of fruit juices, liquids during meals (Halverson and Koehler 1981), sugar, and saturated fat–laden food products is recommended (Aills et al. 2008). Dumping syndrome, especially in Roux-en-Y gastric bypass, frequently occurs acutely post-surgery and represents a constellation of symptoms, which include diarrhea, bloating, abdominal pain, nausea, tachycardia, syncope, palpitations, and sweating (Laurenius et al. 2013).

Except for biliopancreatic diversion, where the gastric volume is larger, patients with preoperative binge eating disorders will be physically unable to consume large portions during one sitting in the postoperative period, as they will be inhibited by a small gastric pouch and because vomiting may ensue (De Zwaan et al. 2010); emesis is rare in laparoscopic adjustable gastric banding patients (O'Brien et al. 1999). Furthermore, manifestations of early satiety and reductions in hunger and disinhibition, especially in Roux-en-Y gastric bypass, are prerequisite to the reduction in the frequency and volume of nutriment intake (Bock 2003; Halmi et al. 1981). Preference for palatable foods is reduced, which indicates a lower impetus to eat (Ullrich et al. 2013). Moreover, eating behavior is further modified in that mastication will be methodical to avoid plugging (i.e., lodging of food), which is common when ingesting dry meat, vegetables, pasta, and bread (Mitchell et al. 2001). Dietary composition is altered in patients with the Roux-en-Y gastric bypass who should abstain from ingesting sweets (e.g., chocolate and cake), as it may lead to dumping syndrome, calorie-dense beverages, meat, dairy, and fatty foods, while sleeve gastrectomy patients avoid meat, vegetables, and fruit acutely, post-surgery (Brolin et al. 1994; Ernst et al. 2009; Halmi et al. 1981; Van De Weijgert, Ruseler, and Elte 1999). Dumping syndrome is conspicuously absent in biliopancreatic diversion and sleeve gastrectomy patients and putatively has a modest effect on excess weight loss (Bohdjalian et al. 2010; Cummings, Overduin, and Foster-Schubert 2004; Papadia et al. 2012).

Moreover, there will be marked reductions in total caloric intake, especially acutely, post-surgery (excluding biliopancreatic diversion) and consequently a greater emphasis will be placed on nutritional density to prevent malnutrition (Bavaresco et al. 2010). To give a general idea, patients with a Roux-en-Y gastric bypass will consume ~1060 ± 322 kcal/d at 6 months (Gobato, Seixas Chaves, and Chaim 2014), while sleeve gastrectomy subjects ingested between ~1163 and 1625 kcal/d at 6 months and 5 years (Moizé et al. 2013), respectively. However, caloric intake gradually increases post-surgery (Brolin et al. 1994), which may parallel weight regain. This may be a consequence to increased food tolerance, gastric expansion (Halverson and Koehler 1981), neo-fundus (proximal gastric pouch dilation with gastric stenosis) formation in sleeve gastrectomy (Himpens, Dobbeleir, and Peeters 2010), anastomotic dilation, staple line disruption, formation of gastrogastric fistula in Roux-en-Y gastric bypass, or dietary habits that emphasize calorically dense food items that do not lead to gastrointestinal distress (Mechanick et al. 2013; Van De Weijgert, Ruseler, and Elte 1999), thus prompting an endoscopy or additional diagnostic methodologies.

In the early postoperative period, patients with biliopancreatic diversion achieve weight loss through early satiety and the corresponding attenuation in food intake, which are induced by rapid gastric emptying through the expanded gastroenterostomy and distention of the post-anastomosis bowel by undigested chime (Koopmans et al. 1982; Koopmans and Sclafani 1981). About 4–6 months thereafter, weight loss is mediated by malabsorption even when eating behavior is retained (food consumption can mimic or exceed presurgery), due to the presence of a limited intestinal absorptive capacity for fat and total energy (Marceau et al. 1998; Scopinaro et al. 1998, 2000). Specifically, fat and total energy absorption decrease as total consumption increases (negative correlation) (Scopinaro et al. 2000). However, this may be modulated by increasing alimentary and common limb lengths, which purportedly increases protein and decreases fat malabsorption, respectively (Hess and Hess 1998; Scopinaro 1997). Furthermore, a positive correlation exists, with respect to protein and calcium intake and the absolute quantity that is absorbed (Scopinaro et al. 2000). Therefore, calcium and protein deficiencies may be amenable to increased caloric consumption of foods enriched in these nutrients.

Derived energy from protein (≥1 g/kg of current body weight) will be heightened to promote satiety, improve quality of life, facilitate increases in % excess weight loss, incur greater deficits in body fat percentage, and mitigate decreases in muscle mass (Raftopoulos et al. 2011). Protein supplementation may be needed to adhere to the aforesaid recommendation (Andreu et al. 2010). The importance of protein supplementation is further conveyed by the fact that Roux-en-Y gastric bypass patients will have difficulty consuming protein-rich foods (e.g., meat) and meeting the protein intake guidelines, especially acutely after surgery (Bavaresco et al. 2010; Bock 2003; Gobato, Seixas Chaves, and Chaim 2014; Moize et al. 2003). Furthermore, even when adequate intake is attained, diminished levels of pepsin and hypochlorhydria, which would reduce the incidence of ulcers (Smith et al. 1993), can inhibit protein digestion and facilitate cobalamin (vitamin B12) deficiency (Behrns, Smith, and Sarr 1994; Faria et al. 2011). Although additional research needs to be conducted, a generalized recommendation for protein intake is within the realm of 60–120 g/d (Heber et al. 2010). In particular, emphasizing whey protein intake is beneficial as it has been demonstrated to promote greater satiety and amplify protein synthesis, thereby assisting with the preservation of FFM, especially when coupled with resistance training (Hall et al. 2003; Tang et al. 2009).

However, this population may be relegated to utilizing dynamic external constant resistance devices (i.e., exercise weight machines), if they are able to fit comfortably, and/or simplistic multi-joint and single-joint free weight exercises (American College of Sports Medicine 2009). Patients who are diabetic, have orthopedic limitations, and/or have cardiovascular disease may need to have the program tailored to their needs and should proceed with caution. It is highly advisable to have a qualified exercise physiologist assist them with an exercise intervention.

DIETARY COMPLIANCE POST-SURGERY

The dissemination and prescription of vitamin supplementation without inquiring as to whether or not the patient is compliant would prove to be counterintuitive to the initial desired positive effect, which is to reduce the magnitude and prevalence of nutritional deficiencies. Limited adherence to vitamin supplementation may accentuate nutritional deficiencies, thereby highlighting the need for supplementation and patient compliance. Indeed, patients are inundated by post-bariatric nutritional deficiencies partially because they are noncompliant and due to the substandard follow-up care (Ahmad, Esmadi, and Hammad 2012; Coupaye et al. 2009; Gudzune et al. 2013; Modi et al. 2013; Shah et al. 2013). Additively, nutritional deficiencies are further accentuated by failing to prescribe prophylactic supplements from the outset (Cummings and Shannon 2003).

As such, in laparoscopic adjustable gastric banding, Roux-en-Y gastric bypass, and biliopancreatic diversion with duodenal switch, the minimal recommended dosage level is typified by 100%, 200%, and 200% of daily value for the majority (minimum of 2/3) of nutrients, respectively (Aills et al. 2008). Quantitatively, others suggest a minimum of two adult multivitamins and a mineral supplement for Roux-en-Y gastric bypass and sleeve gastrectomy patients, while laparoscopic adjustable gastric banding patients should receive one of each (Mechanick et al. 2013). However, even though the prescription of long-term vitamin and mineral therapy is vital in all bariatric patients (Donadelli et al. 2012; Heber et al. 2010), it should be emphasized that vitamin supplementation should not replace optimal dietary habits and alone will not abolish the presence of nutrient deficiencies (Donadelli et al. 2012).

INITIAL CONSULTATION

Prior to surgery, it would behoove the surgeon to discuss realistic weight loss options because many candidates have preconceived and often far-fetched assumptions about the degree of excess weight loss that they will attain (Kaly et al. 2008; Van De Weijgert, Ruseler, and Elte 1999). Even though bariatric operations have been demonstrated to induce significant weight loss, patients will rarely, if ever, achieve a BMI <25 kg/m². More importantly, it is prudent to convey that they will need to adhere to a physical activity regimen (e.g., walking, elliptical exercise machine, or cycle ergometer for a minimum of 5–10 min interspersed throughout the day [3–6 times]) (Donnelly et al. 2009), dietary guidelines, and routine physician visits to optimize weight loss. Bariatric dietary and physical activity interventions have even incurred energy deficits of ≥2000 kcal/week (Shah et al. 2011). Although postoperative physical activity confers positive effects on weight loss and overall health (Evans et al. 2007; Shah et al. 2011), many patients are not physically active or are noncompliant, although they may have good intentions (Bond et al. 2013). A lack of understanding to the aforementioned does not represent a contraindication to surgery, but it is advisable that the patient demonstrates some competency, with regard to the expected behavioral and dietary modifications that occur in tangent with surgery.

PREOPERATIVE SCREENING AND PREDICTORS OF POSTOPERATIVE OUTCOMES

Postoperative weight loss success, resolution of comorbidities, and the incidence and magnitude of perioperative complications are dictated by a plethora of variables. For example, females, especially with a history of sexual abuse (Fujioka et al. 2008; Ray et al. 2003), are associated with poorer weight loss outcomes (Coupaye et al. 2010; Ma et al. 2006; Tymitz et al. 2007). However, others contraindicate this sentiment by stating that males are more prone to attaining lower excess weight loss values (Chen et al. 2009; Melton et al. 2008; Nguyen et al. 2009). Males have more adverse outcomes (e.g., mortality at 1 year post-surgery was twofold higher) and are more prone to intestinal leaks (Fernandez et al. 2004; Flum et al. 2005; Livingston et al. 2002; Nguyen et al. 2009).

Similarly, advancing age (≥65 years), comorbidity status (e.g., sleep apnea, hypertension, diabetes), and type of procedure (revisional > laparoscopic > open surgery) are associated with a higher mortality risk and/or intestinal leaks (Fernandez et al. 2004; Flum et al. 2005; Livingston et al. 2002). The elevated risks associated with males and advancing age may be attributed to the higher prevalence of comorbidities and greater weight, which is also predictive of adverse outcomes and mortality (Fernandez et al. 2004; Livingston et al. 2002; Tymitz et al. 2007). However, evidence differs on whether preoperative weight or BMI is positively or negatively correlated with weight loss (Chen et al. 2009; Coupaye et al. 2010; Halverson and Koehler 1981; Ma et al. 2006; Melton et al. 2008). Moreover, although it has not yielded improved postoperative weight loss outcomes and reductions in perioperative complications (Alami et al. 2007; Becouarn, Topart, and Ritz 2010; Fujioka et al. 2008; Van De Weijgert, Ruseler, and Elte 1999; Van Nieuwenhove et al. 2011), advocating presurgical weight loss is advantageous because it has been demonstrated to reduce operative time, visceral fat, hepatomegaly, and surgical difficulty (Alami et al. 2007; Edholm et al. 2011; Fris 2004; Frutos et al. 2007; Van Nieuwenhove et al. 2011).

Other factors that are predictive of reduced excess weight loss outcomes include government pay status, which is associated with higher perioperative complication rates (Flum et al. 2005; Renquist et al. 1996). Furthermore, type II diabetes of greater than 10 years in duration and a $HbA_{1C} > 10$ predict reduced remission rates (Hall et al. 2010). Likewise, weight regain and insulin-dependent diabetics, which indicates long-standing diabetes, are associated with recurrence of type II diabetes (Chikunguwo et al. 2010).

The research is conflicting on whether screening for binge eating disorder should be an antecedent to surgery. One year post-surgery, well-conducted prospective studies that utilized interview-based methodologies to diagnose subjects with binge eating disorder indicated that the presence of preoperative binge eating disorder did not significantly attenuate postoperative weight loss outcomes or improvements in cardiovascular disease risk factors (Burgmer et al. 2005; Wadden et al. 2011). Similarly, others (Fujioka et al. 2008; Mitchell et al. 2001) and prospective trials that elucidated the presence of eating pathologies (e.g., binge eating disorder, loss of control over eating, etc.) via questionnaires have substantiated these findings (Bocchieri-Ricciardi et al. 2006; Chen et al. 2009; White et al. 2010). However, preoperative binge eating disorder may manifest as grazing (i.e., consuming small portions over extended periods) postoperatively, which may negate excess weight loss (Colles, Dixon, and O'Brien 2008). Concurrently, preoperative eating disorders are predictive of postoperative loss of control over eating, which may moderate weight loss outcomes, bulimic episodes, and general psychopathology (De Zwaan et al. 2010). Therefore, eating pathologies do not represent an absolute contraindication to surgery, but preoperative screening and behavioral interventions are warranted because they may result in improved postoperative weight loss outcomes by preventing the reemergence or development of postoperative aberrant eating behaviors (Ashton et al. 2011). Moreover, it may assist with preliminary patient selection, prevent distention of the gastric pouch, which may permit increased nutriment consumption, and reduce postoperative nutritional deficiencies (Royal et al. 2015; Santarpia et al. 2014; Sarwer, Dilks, and West-Smith 2011).

Especially among the morbidly obese (Aasheim et al. 2008; Gudzune et al. 2013; Kimmons et al. 2006), the etiology of micronutrient deficiencies (e.g., vitamin C, D, E, and selenium) manifests from the consumption of calorically dense and nutritionally deprived foods (Heber et al. 2010; Jastrzębska-Mierzyńska et al. 2012). Moreover, the concomitant presence of excess adiposity further exacerbates malnutrition by expanding the extracellular fluid and increasing markers of inflammation (Aasheim et al. 2008; Waki et al. 1991; Wannamethee et al. 2006). Therefore, a rigorous screening regimen in the presurgical setting is warranted not only because micronutrient deficiencies will be present, but they will be exacerbated postoperatively by the debilitating direct (e.g., malabsorption or restriction) and indirect (modify eating behavior) effects of surgery. Specifically, a preoperative comprehensive examination includes a medical history, psychosocial analysis, physical examination, and laboratory testing (Gudzune et al. 2013; Mechanick et al. 2013). With respect to the latter, clinical monitoring of complete blood counts (CBC), liver function tests, glucose, creatinine, electrolytes, iron/ferritin, vitamin B12, folate, calcium, parathyroid hormone (PTH), 1,25 dihydroxyvitamin D, albumin/prealbumin, vitamin A (Vit A), and zinc is recommended (Heber et al. 2010).

POSTOPERATIVE SCREENING

Reducing the prevalence chronic or occult nutritional deficiencies proves to be more difficult when preemptive steps are not employed and may, even, prove to be a lifelong intervention, if a screening regimen is not installed preoperatively (Santarpia et al. 2014). Indeed, in many instances, screening and nutritional counseling do not occur preoperatively, which would exacerbate postoperative nutritional deficiencies. Subsequently, postsurgical assessments become crucial to facilitate early diagnosis and treatment; assessments should not be guided by symptomatology alone, as nutritional deficiencies may only become apparent when symptoms become clinically significant. However, empirical evidence indicates that surgeons fail to adhere to the aforesaid recommendation (Brolin and Leung 1999; Gudzune et al. 2013). As a result, nutritional deficiencies and their symptomatology manifest, even in purely restrictive procedures (Gudzune et al. 2013; Santarpia et al. 2014).

Therefore, measurement of CBC, liver function tests, glucose, creatinine, and electrolyte levels are recommended at 1, 3, 6, 12, 18, and 24 months post-intervention and annually thereafter for all bariatric procedures (Heber et al. 2010). Furthermore, at 6, 12, 18, 24 months, and annually afterward, biochemical monitoring for iron/ferritin, vitamin B12, folate, calcium, 1,25 dihydroxyvitamin D, albumin/prealbumin, and PTH is advised for patients with Roux-en-Y gastric bypass, biliopancreatic diversion, or biliopancreatic diversion with duodenal switch (Heber et al. 2010).

Postoperative screening should not be relegated to the measurement of blood parameters alone, as interview-based methodologies should be utilized to screen for and diagnose pathological eating behaviors that may contribute to poor outcomes. For instance, patients with binge eating disorder or grazing tend to regain more weight and achieve lower excess weight loss (Kofman et al. 2010; Livhits et al. 2010; Mitchell et al. 2001). Likewise, loss of control over eating is predictive of weight loss at 12 and 24 months and regain at 12 months post-surgery, which may provide an indication of an imminent plateau in weight loss (White et al. 2010). Furthermore, loss of control over eating was associated with a higher prevalence of weight-related vomiting, aberrant eating behaviors, depression, and lower self-esteem (De Zwaan et al. 2010; Kofman, Lent, and Swencionis 2010). Other reports have substantiated these findings by stating that uncontrolled eaters attained lower weight loss values post-surgery, ingested more calories, and a greater proportion of energy intake was derived from fat (Colles, Dixon, and O'Brien 2008).

PRE- AND POST-INTERVENTIONS

The diminution of micro- and macronutrient deficiencies and the induction of successful excess weight loss are facilitated by an ongoing collaboration between the patient, surgeon, and dietician. Dietary and behavioral counseling and frequent follow-up scheduling may be a viable way to foster more positive outcomes after surgery. However, pre-intervention trials that have aimed to facilitate patient success have been inconclusive and scarce. In a randomized controlled trial, although 88% of gastric bypass subjects achieved successful weight loss ($\geq$50% excess weight loss), the delivery of preoperative behavioral treatment conferred no significant effect on weight loss, indices of eating habits, and physical exercise 1 year post-surgery (Lier et al. 2012). Dichotomously, in relation to those that missed >25% of their pre- and postoperative multidisciplinary team consultations, laparoscopic adjustable gastric banding patients who missed <25% lost significantly more weight (23% vs. 32% excess weight loss at 12 months, respectively), with preoperative compliance being the main determinant (El Chaar et al. 2011). Furthermore, preoperative mental health or substance abuse treatment improved postoperative excess weight loss (Clark et al. 2003). However, the latter studies were retrospective, which limits their interpretation.

A plethora of factors may confer positive effects on postoperative outcomes. In a retrospective study, social support, surgeon follow-up within the prior year, marital status, support group meeting attendance, and physical activity level inferred a positive effect on weight loss success (Livhits et al. 2010), while others have noted that adherence to postoperative follow-up consults improved excess weight loss outcomes (Shen et al. 2004). Also, the provision of bimonthly in-person or telephone-based dietary interventions (15 min) by a dietician improved short-term (6 months) weight loss outcomes, positively modified dietary composition, increased cognitive restraint, and decreased disinhibition and hunger (Sarwer et al. 2012). Similarly, adherence to a postoperative dietary program or attendance to a dietary behavioral counseling program is associated with improved dietary habits and excess weight loss; furthermore, they assist with decreasing the occurrence of premature gastric emptying, dehiscence, and pouch dilation (Halverson and Koehler 1981; Shah et al. 2013). Others have reported similar findings (Robinson et al. 2014; Win et al. 2014).

The variable effect of presurgical counseling on weight loss outcomes precludes its widespread incorporation, whereas short-term postsurgical interventions have provided the greatest benefit and warrant inclusion. Furthermore, the addition of long-term counseling during the aftermath of the initial sharp postoperative weight decline (17.9 months), when there is a propensity for weight regain, is an avenue worth considering (Kofman, Lent, and Swencionis 2010; Sarwer et al. 2012).

VITAMINS AND MINERALS

Vitamins and minerals assist with a myriad of vital functions that are associated with weight maintenance (Schrager 2005). Furthermore, many have cardioprotective (e.g., vitamin C and possibly Ca^{++}) and antiobesity effects (e.g., Ca^{++}) (Li et al. 2012; Schrager 2005). When the homeostatic milieu is disrupted, to where ingestion becomes inadequate, symptomatology associated with debilitating sequel becomes apparent. Thus, recognizing and understanding common nutritional deficiencies in bariatric patients are prudent.

Vitamin D, Parathyroid Hormone, and Calcium

The prevalence of hypovitaminosis D is heightened in the bariatric population and is common presurgery. Deficiencies in vitamin D reduce calcium uptake, which causes a rise in PTH (Johnson et al. 2006; Ybarra et al. 2005). Long-standing perturbations in vitamin D may in turn lead to metabolic bone disease, which is most common among variants of biliopancreatic diversion and long-limb (>100 cm) Roux-en-Y gastric bypass (Johnson et al. 2006). Subsequently, bone mineral density scans are recommended at 12 months, 24 months, and annually thereafter for Roux-en-Y gastric bypass and biliopancreatic diversion variants (Heber et al. 2010).

As it pertains to Roux-en-Y gastric bypass, the prevalence of vitamin D deficiency has been noted to be between 23% to 86% and 26% to 86% in the preoperative and postoperative setting, respectively (Aasheim et al. 2009; Coupaye et al. 2014; Gehrer et al. 2010; Ybarra et al. 2005). In relation, the observed deficiency rate in biliopancreatic diversion with duodenal switch and biliopancreatic diversion subjects has been documented as being as low as 29% preoperatively and high as 63% postoperatively (Aasheim et al. 2009; Homan et al. 2015; Newbury et al. 2003; Slater et al. 2004). Similarly, hypocalcemia and subsequent secondary hyperparathyroidism were prevalent in aforementioned trials (Homan et al. 2015; Newbury et al. 2003; Slater et al. 2004). Interestingly, sleeve gastrectomy patients have also been demonstrated to be deficient in vitamin D and the preoperative (23%–93%) and postoperative (32%–90%) prevalence has rivaled or exceeded Roux-en-Y gastric bypass and variants of biliopancreatic diversion (Capoccia et al. 2012; Coupaye et al. 2014;

Damms-Machado et al. 2012; Gehrer et al. 2010; Moizé et al. 2013). However, the rate tended to decrease during the aforementioned time points (Coupaye et al. 2014; Damms-Machado et al. 2012), whereas in Roux-en-Y gastric bypass and biliopancreatic diversion variants, it was largely maintained or increased. Consequently, the incidence postoperatively is largely dictated by the preoperative rate and will either be worsened or maintained, depending on screening, diagnostic, surgical, and nutritional factors.

The minimal recommended daily dosage for Roux-en-Y gastric bypass, laparoscopic adjustable gastric banding, and sleeve gastrectomy is defined as being 1200–1500 mg and 3000 international units (IU) for calcium and vitamin D, respectively; in cases of severe malabsorption, 50,000 IU 1–3 times per week may be needed (Mechanick et al. 2013). Scopinaro recommended ingestion of 2 g/d of calcium, along with monthly intramuscular vitamin D supplementation of 400,000 IU for biliopancreatic diversion patients (Scopinaro et al. 1998). Preoperative vitamin D levels should dictate the specific dosage as some subjects may require more aggressive prophylactic treatment. Goldner outlined that all subjects with baseline vitamin D levels of ≥62.5 nmol/L achieved ≥75 nmol/L postoperatively, whereas only half did with a level <62.5 nmol/L; dosage level was 800, 1200, or 5000 IU daily in Roux-en-Y gastric bypass patients (Goldner et al. 2009).

Iron

Preoperatively, subclinical inflammation and the attendant increases in hepcidin will potentiate iron malabsorption (Aeberli, Hurrell, and Zimmermann 2009; Tussing-Humphreys et al. 2010), while hypochlorhydria and the circumvention of the small bowel will further accentuate this occurrence postoperatively (Von Drygalski and Andris 2009). Therefore, iron deficiency will be most prominent in Roux-en-Y gastric bypass and malabsorptive procedures (Gehrer et al. 2010; Homan et al. 2015; Vargas-Ruiz, Hernández-Rivera, and Herrera 2008). However, sleeve gastrectomy subjects have also been shown to be deficient pre- (3%–29%) and post-surgery (18%–37.9%) (Damms-Machado et al. 2012; Gehrer et al. 2010). Indeed, anemia can also manifest and a mean corpuscular volume of <83 fentoliters is indicative of an iron-related etiology (Homan et al. 2015; Northrop-Clewes and Thurnham 2013; Vargas-Ruiz, Hernández-Rivera, and Herrera 2008). Initial and secondary-phase treatments include coadministration of 300 mg of ferrous sulfate 2–3 times/d, with vitamin C and parenteral iron administration, respectively (Heber et al. 2010).

Zinc

Relative to normal-weight individuals, obesity is associated with increased urinary zinc excretion and moderate levels of plasma and erythrocyte zinc concentrations (Marreiro, Fisberg, and Cozzolino 2004). Even prior to surgery, occult deficiencies can be present, with incidence ranging from 14% to 55% (Gehrer et al. 2010; Gobato, Seixas Chaves, and Chaim 2014). Postoperatively, the rate increased in biliopancreatic diversion variants, Roux-en-Y gastric bypass, and sleeve gastrectomy. Particularly, the prevalence ranged from 34% to 61% (Gehrer et al. 2010; Gobato, Seixas Chaves, and Chaim 2014; Homan et al. 2015; Slater et al. 2004). With respect to Roux-en-Y gastric bypass and sleeve gastrectomy, administration of zinc gluconate (30 mg/d) drastically attenuated the occurrence (Gehrer et al. 2010).

Vitamin K

Although rare, vitamin K deficiencies have been observed in biliopancreatic diversion with duodenal switch or biliopancreatic diversion patients, with the incidence and degree increasing from 1 (51%) to 4 (68%) years (Slater et al. 2004). Congruently, Homan found that 60% of the cohort were deficient at 3.5 years (Homan et al. 2015).

Vitamin A

Fat-soluble vitamin deficiencies are prominent in biliopancreatic diversion with duodenal switch and biliopancreatic diversion patients. As such, Vit A deficiency is as high as 69% and as low as 28% (Homan et al. 2015; Slater et al. 2004). Furthermore, with elapsing time, Vit A levels decrease (Aasheim et al. 2009; Slater et al. 2004). Consequently, monitoring for nyctalopia and other ocular-related symptoms of Vit A deficiency is indicated.

Vitamin B12

When co-ingested with food, cobalamin or vitamin B12 is cleaved from peptides by gastric acid and proteases, which then bind with R proteins that are abundant in saliva. Thereafter, pancreatic secretions digest the R proteins in the duodenum and allow cobalamin to bind with intrinsic factor, which is absorbed at the distal ileum (Carmel et al. 1969; Herbert 1988). However, due to the anatomical alterations to the gastrointestinal tract, this sequential system is disturbed in Roux-en-Y gastric bypass. Specifically, the etiology of cobalamin deficiency is mediated by attenuated secretions of intrinsic factor and subsequently reduced binding with cobalamin (Marcuard et al. 1989), or from reduced gastric acid secretion (Smith et al. 1993).

Preoperatively, the prevalence of vitamin 12 deficiency (<10%) has been low in biliopancreatic diversion variants, sleeve gastrectomy, and Roux-en-Y gastric bypass (Coupaye et al. 2014; Damms-Machado et al. 2012; Gehrer et al. 2010; Vargas-Ruiz, Hernández-Rivera, and Herrera 2008). Likewise, only one study with Roux-en-Y gastric bypass subjects observed a high occurrence (58%) in the postoperative setting (Gehrer et al. 2010), while others have noted a much smaller rate among the aggregate (<20%, absent, or vitamin excess) (Aasheim et al. 2009; Coupaye et al. 2014; Damms-Machado et al. 2012; Gehrer et al. 2010; Gobato, Seixas Chaves, and Chaim 2014; Vargas-Ruiz, Hernández-Rivera, and Herrera 2008). The attenuated rates are attributed to intramuscular injections of cyanocobalamin and a lower prevalence preoperatively (Aasheim et al. 2009; Gehrer et al. 2010; Gobato, Seixas Chaves, and Chaim 2014).

Congruently, patients respond well to large oral doses of cyanocobalamin therapy, in relation to parenteral administration (Kuzminski et al. 1998). Even in the presence of hypochlorhydria, crystalline vitamin 12 is absorbed effectively (Smith et al. 1993). For example, in sleeve gastrectomy and Roux-en-Y gastric bypass patients, administration of 350 μg/d crystalline vitamin 12 normalized serum vitamin 12 levels (Rhode et al. 1995, 1996).

Folate

Similar to iron, screening and supplementing for folate is recommended in menstruating women (Mechanick et al. 2013). In sleeve gastrectomy and Roux-en-Y gastric bypass subjects, folate deficiencies are less prominent pre- (3%–7%) and postoperatively (up to 22%), which are most likely attributed to dietary habits; however, the incidence was highest among sleeve gastrectomy subjects (Coupaye et al. 2014; Damms-Machado et al. 2012; Gehrer et al. 2010). Conversely, others have indicated that folate deficiencies were absent (Vargas-Ruiz, Hernández-Rivera, and Herrera 2008). Multivitamin preparations may include 400 μg of folate or up to 1000 μg/d as a secondary form of therapy (Heber et al. 2010).

Vitamin B6

Vitamin B6 deficiency may be precipitated by systemic inflammation, which is characteristic of obesity (Vasilaki et al. 2008). Deficiencies have been noted in sleeve gastrectomy subjects up to 17% postoperatively and 19% preoperatively (Coupaye et al. 2014; Damms-Machado et al. 2012). Others have observed no such deficiency pre- and postoperatively (Gehrer et al. 2010). Similarly, in biliopancreatic diversion with duodenal switch (28%–15%) and Roux-en-Y gastric bypass (16%–10%) subjects, the number of deficiencies decreased from pre- to post-surgery (Aasheim et al. 2009).

Thiamine

In a retrospective analysis, 49% of Roux-en-Y gastric bypass subjects were deficient and the authors posited that an altered microbial bowel milieu was causal, due to high serum folate levels and a positive glucose-hydrogen breath test (Lakhani et al. 2008). Dichotomously, in biliopancreatic diversion with duodenal switch (3%–0%) and Roux-en-Y gastric bypass (0%–10%) subjects, the prevalence of pre- and postoperative deficiencies was negligible (Aasheim et al. 2009).

CONCLUSION

Bariatric procedures are effective in inducing weight loss, but the specific procedure that is chosen should be predicated on the patient's goals, obesity, and comorbidity status. Alone, bariatric procedures may have limited effectiveness, especially with regard to laparoscopic adjustable gastric banding. Thus, highlighting the need for bimodal-based therapeutic interventions such as bariatric surgery and lifestyle modification is most prudent. Postoperative care encompasses dietary modification, physical activity adherence, and routine follow-up visits. However, even so, many patients will still be obese after the initial 2-year reduction in weight and should be cognizant that weight regain is common.

FUTURE RESEARCH

With the relative novelty of bariatric procedures, further research needs to discern how nutritional deficiencies that are present prior to surgery can be exacerbated post-surgery and ascertain how to effectively counteract them and their debilitating sequel. Furthermore, elucidating preoperative characteristics that predict postoperative outcomes is needed.

Differences between Bariatric Surgeries

Surgery Type and Popularity	Invasiveness	Excess Weight Loss	Nutritional Deficiencies	Effects on Metabolic Diseases (e.g., Inducing Diabetes Remission)
I. Roux-en-Y gastric bypass	4	4	4	4
II. Sleeve gastrectomy	3	3	3	3
III. Adjustable gastric banding	2	2	1	2
IV. Biliopancreatic diversion	5	5	5	5

Notes: Although Roux-en-Y gastric bypass (RYGB) is invasive, it frequently fosters diabetes remission, which may occur irrespective of weight loss outcomes (e.g., incretin effect, hormonal and neural signaling). In comparison, sleeve gastrectomy (SG) is less invasive and the achieved excess weight loss values are often similar to that noted in subjects who undergo RYGB; however, its effect on metabolic diseases is not always as drastic as that seen in RYGB. In most instances, nutritional deficiencies are equally frequent in both surgeries. Adjustable gastric banding (AGB) and biliopancreatic diversion (BPD) are less popular than SG and RYGB. BPD is highly invasive and nutritional deficiencies are common, while AGB can be described as being the antithesis (i.e., directly opposite) of BPD: although AGB is the least invasive procedure and nutritional deficiencies are not as common, it has fallen out of favor in recent years (especially in the United States). Patients who undergo AGB have difficulty achieving and sustaining significant weight loss; also, diabetes remission is least frequent. However, BPD incurs positive effects on metabolic diseases and weight loss is substantial.

1, marginal effect; 5, drastic effect; I, most popular; IV, least popular.

REFERENCES

Aasheim, E. T., S. Björkman, T. T. Søvik, M. Engström, S. E. Hanvold, T. Mala, T. Olbers, and T. Bøhmer. 2009. Vitamin status after bariatric surgery: A randomized study of gastric bypass and duodenal switch. *The American Journal of Clinical Nutrition* 90 (1): 15–22.

Aasheim, E. T., D. Hofsø, J. Hjelmesaeth, K. I. Birkeland, and T. Bøhmer. 2008. Vitamin status in morbidly obese patients: A cross-sectional study. *The American Journal of Clinical Nutrition* 87 (2): 362–369.

Adams, T. D., R. E. Gress, S. C. Smith, R. C. Halverson, S. C. Simper, W. D. Rosamond, M. J. Lamonte, A. M. Stroup, and S. C. Hunt. 2007. Long-term mortality after gastric bypass surgery. *New England Journal of Medicine* 357 (8): 753–761.

Aeberli, I., R. F. Hurrell, and M. B. Zimmermann. 2009. Overweight children have higher circulating hepcidin concentrations and lower iron status but have dietary iron intakes and bioavailability comparable with normal weight children. *International Journal of Obesity* 33 (10): 1111–1117.

Ahmad, D. S., M. Esmadi, and H. Hammad. 2012. Malnutrition secondary to non-compliance with vitamin and mineral supplements after gastric bypass surgery: What can we do about it? *The American Journal of Case Reports* 13: 209–213.

Aills, L., J. Blankenship, C. Buffington, M. Furtado, and J. Parrott. 2008. ASMBS allied health nutritional guidelines for the surgical weight loss patient. *Surgery for Obesity and Related Diseases* 4 (5): S73–S108.

Alami, R. S., J. M. Morton, R. Schuster, J. Lie, B. R. Sanchez, A. Peters, and M. J. Curet. 2007. Is there a benefit to preoperative weight loss in gastric bypass patients? A prospective randomized trial. *Surgery for Obesity and Related Diseases* 3 (2): 141–145.

American College of Sports Medicine. 2009. American College of Sports Medicine position stand. Progression models in resistance training for healthy adults. *Medicine and Science in Sports and Exercise* 41 (3): 687–708.

Andreu, A., V. Moizé, L. Rodríguez, L. Flores, and J. Vidal. 2010. Protein intake, body composition, and protein status following bariatric surgery. *Obesity Surgery* 20 (11): 1509–1515.

Angrisani, L., F. Favretti, F. Furbetta, A. Iuppa, S. B. Doldi, M. Paganelli, N. Basso, M. Lucchese, M. Zappa, and G. Lesti. 2004. Italian group for lap-band system: Results of multicenter study on patients with BMI < or =35 kg/m^2. *Obesity Surgery* 14 (3): 415–418.

Ashton, K., L. Heinberg, A. Windover, and J. Merrell. 2011. Positive response to binge eating intervention enhances postoperative weight loss. *Surgery for Obesity and Related Diseases* 7 (3): 315–320.

Bavaresco, M., S. Paganini, T. P. Lima, W. Salgado, Jr., R. Ceneviva, J. E. Dos Santos, and C. B. Nonino-Borges. 2010. Nutritional course of patients submitted to bariatric surgery. *Obesity Surgery* 20 (6): 716–721.

Becouarn, G., P. Topart, and P. Ritz. 2010. Weight loss prior to bariatric surgery is not a pre-requisite of excess weight loss outcomes in obese patients. *Obesity Surgery* 20 (5): 574–577.

Behrns, K. E., C. D. Smith, and M. G. Sarr. 1994. Prospective evaluation of gastric acid secretion and cobalamin absorption following gastric bypass for clinically severe obesity. *Digestive Diseases and Sciences* 39 (2): 315–320.

Biagini, J. and L. Karam. 2008. Ten years experience with laparoscopic adjustable gastric banding. *Obesity Surgery* 18 (5): 573–577.

Bocchieri-Ricciardi, L. E., E. Y. Chen, D. Munoz, S. Fischer, M. Dymek-Valentine, J. C. Alverdy, and D. Le Grange. 2006. Pre-surgery binge eating status: Effect on eating behavior and weight outcome after gastric bypass. *Obesity Surgery* 16 (9): 1198–1204.

Bock, M. A. 2003. Roux-En-Y gastric bypass: The dietitian's and patient's perspectives. *Nutrition in Clinical Practice* 18 (2): 141–144.

Bohdjalian, A., F. B. Langer, S. Shakeri-Leidenmühler, L. Gfrerer, B. Ludvik, J. Zacherl, and G. Prager. 2010. Sleeve gastrectomy as sole and definitive bariatric procedure: 5-Year results for weight loss and ghrelin. *Obesity Surgery* 20 (5): 535–540.

Bond, D. S., J. G. Thomas, B. A. Ryder, S. Vithiananthan, D. Pohl, and R. R. Wing. 2013. Ecological momentary assessment of the relationship between intention and physical activity behavior in bariatric surgery patients. *International Journal of Behavioral Medicine* 20 (1): 82–87.

Brethauer, S. A., A. Aminian, H. Romero-Talamás, E. Batayyah, J. Mackey, L. Kennedy, S. R. Kashyap et al. 2013. Can diabetes be surgically cured? Long-term metabolic effects of bariatric surgery in obese patients with type 2 diabetes mellitus. *Annals of Surgery* 258 (4): 628–636.

Brolin, R. E. 2002. Bariatric surgery and long-term control of morbid obesity. *JAMA* 288 (22): 2793–2796.

Brolin, R. E., H. A. Kenler, J. H. Gorman, and R. P. Cody. 1992. Long-limb gastric bypass in the superobese. A prospective randomized study. *Annals of Surgery* 215 (4): 387–395.

Brolin, R. E. and M. Leung. 1999. Survey of vitamin and mineral supplementation after gastric bypass and biliopancreatic diversion for morbid obesity. *Obesity Surgery* 9 (2): 150–154.

Brolin, R. L., L. B. Robertson, H. A. Kenler, and R. P. Cody. 1994. Weight loss and dietary intake after vertical banded gastroplasty and Roux-en-Y gastric bypass. *Annals of Surgery* 220 (6): 782–790.

Buchwald, H. 2002. A bariatric surgery algorithm. *Obesity Surgery* 12 (6): 747–750.

Burgmer, R., K. Grigutsch, S. Zipfel, A. M. Wolf, M. De Zwaan, B. Husemann, C. Albus, W. Senf, and S. Herpertz. 2005. The influence of eating behavior and eating pathology on weight loss after gastric restriction operations. *Obesity Surgery* 15 (5): 684–691.

Capoccia, D., F. Coccia, F. Paradiso, F. Abbatini, G. Casella, N. Basso, and F. Leonetti. 2012. Laparoscopic gastric sleeve and micronutrients supplementation: Our experience. *Journal of Obesity* 2012: 672162.

Carmel, R., A. H. Rosenberg, K. S. Lau, R. R. Streiff, and V. Herbert. 1969. Vitamin B12 uptake by human small bowel homogenate and its enhancement by intrinsic factor. *Gastroenterology* 56 (3): 548–555.

Chen, E., M. Roehrig, S. Herbozo, M. S. McCloskey, J. Roehrig, H. Cummings, J. Alverdy, and D. Le Grange. 2009. Compensatory eating disorder behaviors and gastric bypass surgery outcome. *International Journal of Eating Disorders* 42 (4): 363–366.

Chen, M., A. Krishnamurthy, A. R. Mohamed, and R. Green. 2013. Hematological disorders following gastric bypass surgery: Emerging concepts of the interplay between nutritional deficiency and inflammation. *BioMed Research International* 2013: 205467.

Chikunguwo, S. M., L. G. Wolfe, P. Dodson, J. G. Meador, N. Baugh, J. N. Clore, J. M. Kellum, and J. W. Maher. 2010. Analysis of factors associated with durable remission of diabetes after Roux-en-Y gastric bypass. *Surgery for Obesity and Related Diseases* 6 (3): 254–259.

Christou, N. V., J. S. Sampalis, M. Liberman, D. Look, S. Auger, A. P. McLean, and L. D. MacLean. 2004. Surgery decreases long-term mortality, morbidity, and health care use in morbidly obese patients. *Annals of Surgery* 240 (3): 416–424.

Clark, M. M., B. M. Balsiger, C. D. Sletten, K. L. Dahlman, G. Ames, D. E. Williams, H. S. Abu-Lebdeh, and M. G. Sarr. 2003. Psychosocial factors and 2-year outcome following bariatric surgery for weight loss. *Obesity Surgery* 13 (5): 739–745.

Colles, S. L., J. B. Dixon, and P. E. O'Brien. 2008. Grazing and loss of control related to eating: Two high-risk factors following bariatric surgery. *Obesity* 16 (3): 615–622.

Coupaye, M., K. Puchaux, C. Bogard, S. Msika, P. Jouet, C. Clerici, E. Larger, and S. Ledoux. 2009. Nutritional consequences of adjustable gastric banding and gastric bypass: A 1-year prospective study. *Obesity Surgery* 19 (1): 56–65.

Coupaye, M., P. Rivière, M. C. Breuil, B. Castel, C. Bogard, T. Dupré, M. Flamant, S. Msika, and S. Ledoux. 2014. Comparison of nutritional status during the first year after sleeve gastrectomy and Roux-en-Y gastric bypass. *Obesity Surgery* 24 (2): 276–283.

Coupaye, M., J. M. Sabaté, B. Castel, P. Jouet, C. Clérici, S. Msika, and S. Ledoux. 2010. Predictive factors of weight loss 1 year after laparoscopic gastric bypass in obese patients. *Obesity Surgery* 20 (12): 1671–1677.

Cummings, D. E., J. Overduin, and K. E. Foster-Schubert. 2004. Gastric bypass for obesity: Mechanisms of weight loss and diabetes resolution. *The Journal of Clinical Endocrinology and Metabolism* 89 (6): 2608–2615.

Cummings, D. E. and M. H. Shannon. 2003. Roles for ghrelin in the regulation of appetite and body weight. *Archives of Surgery* 138 (4): 389–396.

Cummings, D. E., D. S. Weigle, R. S. Frayo, P. A. Breen, M. K. Ma, E. P. Dellinger, and J. Q. Purnell. 2002. Plasma ghrelin levels after diet-induced weight loss or gastric bypass surgery. *New England Journal of Medicine* 346 (21): 1623–1630.

Damms-Machado, A., A. Friedrich, K. M. Kramer, K. Stingel, T. Meile, M. A. Küper, A. Königsrainer, and S. C. Bischoff. 2012. Pre- and postoperative nutritional deficiencies in obese patients undergoing laparoscopic sleeve gastrectomy. *Obesity Surgery* 22 (6): 881–889.

De Zwaan, M., A. Hilbert, L. Swan-Kremeier, H. Simonich, K. Lancaster, L. M. Howell, T. Monson, R. D. Crosby, and J. E. Mitchell. 2010. Comprehensive interview assessment of eating behavior 18–35 months after gastric bypass surgery for morbid obesity. *Surgery for Obesity and Related Diseases* 6 (1): 79–85.

DeMeester, T. R., K. H. Fuchs, C. S. Ball, M. Albertucci, T. C. Smyrk, and J. N. Marcus. 1987. Experimental and clinical results with proximal end-to-end duodenojejunostomy for pathologic duodenogastric reflux. *Annals of Surgery* 206 (4): 414–426.

Dixon, A. F., J. B. Dixon, and P. E. O'Brien. 2005. Laparoscopic adjustable gastric banding induces prolonged satiety: A randomized blind crossover study. *The Journal of Clinical Endocrinology and Metabolism* 90 (2): 813–819.

Dixon, J. B., P. E. O'Brien, J. Playfair, L. Chapman, L. M. Schachter, S. Skinner, J. Proietto, M. Bailey, and M. Anderson. 2008. Adjustable gastric banding and conventional therapy for type 2 diabetes: A randomized controlled trial. *Journal of the American Medical Association* 299 (3): 316–323.

Donadelli, S. P., M. V. Junqueira-Franco, C. A. De Mattos Donadelli, W. Salgado, Jr., R. Ceneviva, J. S. Marchini, J. E. Dos Santos, and C. B. Nonino. 2012. Daily vitamin supplementation and hypovitaminosis after obesity surgery. *Nutrition* 28 (4): 391–396.

Donnelly, J. E., S. N. Blair, J. M. Jakicic, M. M. Manore, J. W. Rankin, and B. K. Smith. 2009. American College of Sports Medicine Position Stand. Appropriate physical activity intervention strategies for weight loss and prevention of weight regain for adults. *Medicine and Science in Sports and Exercise* 41 (2): 459–471.

Edholm, D., J. Kullberg, A. Haenni, F. A. Karlsson, A. Ahlström, J. Hedberg, H. Ahlström, and M. Sundbom. 2011. Preoperative 4-week low-calorie diet reduces liver volume and intrahepatic fat, and facilitates laparoscopic gastric bypass in morbidly obese. *Obesity Surgery* 21 (3): 345–350.

El Chaar, M., K. McDeavitt, S. Richardson, K. S. Gersin, T. S. Kuwada, and D. Stefanidis. 2011. Does patient compliance with preoperative bariatric office visits affect postoperative excess weight loss? *Surgery for Obesity and Related Diseases* 7 (6): 743–748.

Elder, K. A. and B. M. Wolfe. 2007. Bariatric surgery: A review of procedures and outcomes. *Gastroenterology* 132 (6): 2253–2271.

Ernst, B., M. Thurnheer, B. Wilms, and B. Schultes. 2009. Differential changes in dietary habits after gastric bypass versus gastric banding operations. *Obesity Surgery* 19 (3): 274–280.

Evans, R. K., D. S. Bond, L. G. Wolfe, J. G. Meador, J. E. Herrick, J. M. Kellum, and J. W. Maher. 2007. Participation in 150 min/wk of moderate or higher intensity physical activity yields greater weight loss after gastric bypass surgery. *Surgery for Obesity and Related Diseases* 3 (5): 526–530.

Faraj, M., P. J. Havel, S. Phélis, D. Blank, A. D. Sniderman, and K. Cianflone. 2003. Plasma acylation-stimulating protein, adiponectin, leptin, and ghrelin before and after weight loss induced by gastric bypass surgery in morbidly obese subjects. *The Journal of Clinical Endocrinology and Metabolism* 88 (4): 1594–1602.

Faria, S. L., O. P. Faria, C. Buffington, M. De Almeida Cardeal, and M. K. Ito. 2011. Dietary protein intake and bariatric surgery patients: A review. *Obesity Surgery* 21 (11): 1798–1805.

Fernandez, A. Z. Jr., E. J. DeMaria, D. S. Tichansky, J. M. Kellum, L. G. Wolfe, J. Meador, and H. J. Sugerman. 2004. Experience with over 3,000 open and laparoscopic bariatric procedures: Multivariate analysis of factors related to leak and resultant mortality. *Surgical Endoscopy* 18 (2): 193–197.

Flum, D. R., L. Salem, J. A. Elrod, E. P. Dellinger, A. Cheadle, and L. Chan. 2005. Early mortality among medicare beneficiaries undergoing bariatric surgical procedures. *JAMA* 294 (15): 1903–1908.

Fris, R. J. 2004. Preoperative low energy diet diminishes liver size. *Obesity Surgery* 14 (9): 1165–1170.

Frutos, M. D., M. D. Morales, J. Luján, Q. Hernández, G. Valero, and P. Parrilla. 2007. Intragastric balloon reduces liver volume in super-obese patients, facilitating subsequent laparoscopic gastric bypass. *Obesity Surgery* 17 (2): 150–154.

Fujioka, K., E. Yan, H. J. Wang, and Z. Li. 2008. Evaluating preoperative weight loss, binge eating disorder, and sexual abuse history on Roux-en-Y gastric bypass outcome. *Surgery for Obesity and Related Diseases* 4 (2): 137–143.

Gehrer, S., B. Kern, T. Peters, C. Christoffel-Courtin, and R. Peterli. 2010. Fewer nutrient deficiencies after laparoscopic Sleeve Gastrectomy (LSG) than after laparoscopic Roux-Y-gastric bypass (LRYGB)—A prospective study. *Obesity Surgery* 20 (4): 447–453.

Gletsu-Miller, N. and B. N. Wright. 2013. Mineral malnutrition following bariatric surgery. *Advances in Nutrition* 4 (5): 506–517.

Gobato, R. C., D. F. Seixas Chaves, and E. A. Chaim. 2014. Micronutrient and physiologic parameters before and 6 months after RYGB. *Surgery for Obesity and Related Diseases* 10 (5): 944–951.

Goldner, W. S., J. A. Stoner, E. Lyden, J. Thompson, K. Taylor, L. Larson, J. Erickson, and C. McBride. 2009. Finding the optimal dose of vitamin D following Roux-En-Y gastric bypass: A prospective, randomized pilot clinical trial. *Obesity Surgery* 19 (2): 173–179.

Gudzune, K. A., M. M. Huizinga, H. Y. Chang, V. Asamoah, M. Gadgil, and J. M. Clark. 2013. Screening and diagnosis of micronutrient deficiencies before and after bariatric surgery. *Obesity Surgery* 23 (10): 1581–1589.

Hall, T. C., M. G. Pellen, P. C. Sedman, and P. K. Jain. 2010. Preoperative factors predicting remission of type 2 diabetes mellitus after Roux-En-Y gastric bypass surgery for obesity. *Obesity Surgery* 20 (9): 1245–1250.

Hall, W. L., D. J. Millward, S. J. Long, and L. M. Morgan. 2003. Casein and whey exert different effects on plasma amino acid profiles, gastrointestinal hormone secretion and appetite. *The British Journal of Nutrition* 89 (2): 239–248.

Halmi, K. A., E. Mason, J. R. Falk, and A. Stunkard. 1981. Appetitive behavior after gastric bypass for obesity. *International Journal of Obesity* 5 (5): 457–464.

Halverson, J. D. and R. E. Koehler. 1981. Gastric bypass: Analysis of weight loss and factors determining success. *Surgery* 90 (3): 446–455.

Heber, D., F. L. Greenway, L. M. Kaplan, E. Livingston, J. Salvador, and C. Still. 2010. Endocrine and nutritional management of the post-bariatric surgery patient: An Endocrine Society Clinical Practice Guideline. *The Journal of Clinical Endocrinology and Metabolism* 95 (11): 4823–4843.

Herbert, V. 1988. Vitamin B-12: Plant sources, requirements, and assay. *The American Journal of Clinical Nutrition* 48: 852–858.

Hess, D. S. and D. W. Hess. 1998. Biliopancreatic diversion with a duodenal switch. *Obesity Surgery* 8 (3): 267–282.

Himpens, J., J. Dobbeleir, and G. Peeters. 2010. Long-term results of laparoscopic sleeve gastrectomy for obesity. *Annals of Surgery* 252 (2): 319–324.

Hofsø, D., T. Jenssen, J. Bollerslev, T. Ueland, K. Godang, M. Stumvoll, R. Sandbu, J. Røislien, and J. Hjelmesæth. 2011. Beta cell function after weight loss: A clinical trial comparing gastric bypass surgery and intensive lifestyle intervention. *European Journal of Endocrinology* 164 (2): 231–238.

Holdstock, C., B. E. Engström, M. Ohrvall, L. Lind, M. Sundbom, and F. A. Karlsson. 2003. Ghrelin and adipose tissue regulatory peptides: Effect of gastric bypass surgery in obese humans. *The Journal of Clinical Endocrinology and Metabolism* 88 (7): 3177–3183.

Homan, J., B. Betzel, E. O. Aarts, K. Dogan, K. J. van Laarhoven, I. M. Janssen, and F. J. Berends. 2015. Vitamin and mineral deficiencies after biliopancreatic diversion and biliopancreatic diversion with duodenal switch—The rule rather than the exception. *Obesity Surgery* 25 (9): 1626–1632.

Inge, T. H., N. F. Krebs, V. F. Garcia, J. A. Skelton, K. S. Guice, R. S. Strauss, C. T. Albanese, M. L. Brandt, and L. D. Hammer. 2004. Bariatric surgery for severely overweight adolescents: Concerns and recommendations. *Pediatrics* 114 (1): 217–223.

Jan, J. C., D. Hong, N. Pereira, and E. J. Patterson. 2005. Laparoscopic adjustable gastric banding versus laparoscopic gastric bypass for morbid obesity: A single-institution comparison study of early results. *Journal of Gastrointestinal Surgery* 9 (1): 30–39.

Jastrzębska-Mierzyńska, M., L. Ostrowska, H. R. Hady, and J. Dadan. 2012. Assessment of dietary habits, nutritional status and blood biochemical parameters in patients prepared for bariatric surgery: A preliminary study. *Wideochir Inne Tech Maloinwazyjne* 7 (3): 156–165.

Johnson, J. M., J. W. Maher, E. J. DeMaria, R. W. Downs, L. G. Wolfe, and J. M. Kellum. 2006. The long-term effects of gastric bypass on vitamin D metabolism. *Annals of Surgery* 243 (5): 701–704.

Kaly, P., S. Orellana, T. Torrella, C. Takagishi, L. Saff-Koche, and M. M. Murr. 2008. Unrealistic weight loss expectations in candidates for bariatric surgery. *Surgery for Obesity and Related Diseases* 4 (1): 6–10.

Karamanakos, S. N., K. Vagenas, F. Kalfarentzos, and T. K. Alexandrides. 2008. Weight loss, appetite suppression, and changes in fasting and postprandial ghrelin and peptide-YY levels after Roux-en-Y gastric bypass and sleeve gastrectomy: A prospective, double blind study. *Annals of Surgery* 247 (3): 401–407.

Kashyap, S. R., D. L. Bhatt, K. Wolski, R. M. Watanabe, M. Abdul-Ghani, B. Abood, C. E. Pothier et al. 2013. Metabolic effects of bariatric surgery in patients with moderate obesity and type 2 diabetes: Analysis of a randomized control trial comparing surgery with intensive medical treatment. *Diabetes Care* 36 (8): 2175–2182.

Kashyap, S. R., S. Daud, K. R. Kelly, A. Gastaldelli, H. Win, S. Brethauer, J. P. Kirwan, and P. R. Schauer. 2010. Acute effects of gastric bypass versus gastric restrictive surgery on beta-cell function and insulinotropic hormones in severely obese patients with type 2 diabetes. *International Journal of Obesity* 34 (3): 462–471.

Kashyap, S. R., E. S. Louis, and J. P. Kirwan. 2011. Weight loss as a cure for type 2 diabetes? Fact or fantasy. *Expert Review Endocrinology & Metabolism* 6 (4): 557–561.

Kashyap, S. R. and P. Schauer. 2012. Clinical considerations for the management of residual diabetes following bariatric surgery. *Diabetes, Obesity and Metabolism* 14 (9): 773–779.

Kimmons, J. E., H. M. Blanck, B. C. Tohill, J. Zhang, and L. K. Khan. 2006. Associations between body mass index and the prevalence of low micronutrient levels among US adults. *Medscape General Medicine* 8 (4): 59.

Kofman, M. D., M. R. Lent, and C. Swencionis. 2010. Maladaptive eating patterns, quality of life, and weight outcomes following gastric bypass: Results of an Internet survey. *Obesity* 18 (10): 1938–1943.

Koopmans, H. S. and A. Sclafani. 1981. Control of body weight by lower gut signals. *International Journal of Obesity* 5 (5): 491–495.

Koopmans, H. S., A. Sclafani, C. Fichtner, and P. F. Aravich. 1982. The effects of ileal transposition on food intake and body weight loss in VMH-obese rats. *The American Journal of Clinical Nutrition* 35 (2): 284–293.

Kotidis, E. V., G. G. Koliakos, V. G. Baltzopoulos, K. N. Ioannidis, J. G. Yovos, and S. T. Papavramidis. 2006. Serum ghrelin, leptin and adiponectin levels before and after weight loss: Comparison of three methods of treatment—A prospective study. *Obesity Surgery* 16 (11): 1425–1432.

Kuzminski, A. M., E. J. Del Giacco, R. H. Allen, S. P. Stabler, and J. Lindenbaum. 1998. Effective treatment of cobalamin deficiency with oral cobalamin. *Blood* 92 (4): 1191–1198.

Lakhani, S. V., H. N. Shah, K. Alexander, F. C. Finelli, J. R. Kirkpatrick, and T. R. Koch. 2008. Small intestinal bacterial overgrowth and thiamine deficiency after Roux-en-Y gastric bypass surgery in obese patients. *Nutrition Research* 28 (5): 293–298.

Langer, F. B., M. A. Reza Hoda, A. Bohdjalian, F. X. Felberbauer, J. Zacherl, E. Wenzl, K. Schindler, A. Luger, B. Ludvik, and G. Prager. 2005. Sleeve gastrectomy and gastric banding: Effects on plasma ghrelin levels. *Obesity Surgery* 15 (7): 1024–1029.

Laurenius, A., T. Olbers, I. Näslund, and J. Karlsson. 2013. Dumping syndrome following gastric bypass: Validation of the dumping symptom rating scale. *Obesity Surgery* 23 (6): 740–755.

Le Roux, C. W., S. J. Aylwin, R. L. Batterham, C. M. Borg, F. Coyle, V. Prasad, S. Shurey, M. A. Ghatei, A. G. Patel, and S. R. Bloom. 2006. Gut hormone profiles following bariatric surgery favor an anorectic state, facilitate weight loss, and improve metabolic parameters. *Annals of Surgery* 243 (1): 108–114.

Leibel, R. L., M. Rosenbaum, and J. Hirsch. 1995. Changes in energy expenditure resulting from altered body weight. *New England Journal of Medicine* 332 (10): 621–628.

Li, K., R. Kaaks, J. Linseisen, and S. Rohrmann. 2012. Associations of dietary calcium intake and calcium supplementation with myocardial infarction and stroke risk and overall cardiovascular mortality in the Heidelberg cohort of the European Prospective Investigation into Cancer and Nutrition study (EPIC-Heidelberg). *Heart* 98 (12): 920–925.

Lier, H. Ø., E. Biringer, B. Stubhaug, and T. Tangen. 2012. The impact of preoperative counseling on postoperative treatment adherence in bariatric surgery patients: A randomized controlled trial. *Patient Education and Counseling* 87 (3): 336–342.

Livhits, M., C. Mercado, I. Yermilov, J. A. Parikh, E. Dutson, A. Mehran, C. Y. Ko, and M. M. Gibbons. 2010. Behavioral factors associated with successful weight loss after gastric bypass. *The American Surgeon* 76 (10): 1139–1142.

Livingston, E. H., S. Huerta, D. Arthur, S. Lee, S. De Shields, and D. Heber. 2002. Male gender is a predictor of morbidity and age a predictor of mortality for patients undergoing gastric bypass surgery. *Annals of Surgery* 236 (5): 576–582.

Ma, Y., S. L. Pagoto, B. C. Olendzki, A. R. Hafner, R. A. Perugini, R. Mason, and J. J. Kelly. 2006. Predictors of weight status following laparoscopic gastric bypass. *Obesity Surgery* 16 (9): 1227–1231.

MacLean, L. D., B. M. Rhode, and C. W. Nohr. 2001. Long- or short-limb gastric bypass? *Journal of Gastrointestinal Surgery* 5 (5): 525–530.

Marceau, P., F. S. Hould, S. Simard, S. Lebel, R. A. Bourque, M. Potvin, and S. Biron. 1998. Biliopancreatic diversion with duodenal switch. *World Journal of Surgery* 22 (9): 947–954.

Marcuard, S. P., D. R. Sinar, M. S. Swanson, J. F. Silverman, and J. S. Levine. 1989. Absence of luminal intrinsic factor after gastric bypass surgery for morbid obesity. *Digestive Diseases and Sciences* 34 (8): 1238–1242.

Marreiro, D. N., M. Fisberg, and S. M. Cozzolino. 2004. Zinc nutritional status and its relationships with hyperinsulinemia in obese children and adolescents. *Biological Trace Element Research* 100 (2): 137–149.

Mason, E. E., S. Tang, K. E. Renquist, D. T. Barnes, J. J. Cullen, C. Doherty, and J. W. Maher. 1997. A decade of change in obesity surgery. *Obesity Surgery* 7 (3): 189–197.

Mechanick, J. I., A. Youdim, D. B. Jones, T. Garvey, D. L. Hurley, M. McMahon, L. J. Heinberg et al. 2013. Clinical practice guidelines for the perioperative nutritional, metabolic, and nonsurgical support of the bariatric surgery patient—2013 update: Cosponsored by American Association of Clinical Endocrinologists, the Obesity Society, and American Society for Metabolic and Bariatric Surgery. *Obesity* 19 (2): 337–372.

Melton, G. B., K. E. Steele, M. A. Schweitzer, A. O. Lidor, and T. H. Magnuson. 2008. Suboptimal weight loss after gastric bypass surgery: Correlation of demographics, comorbidities, and insurance status with outcomes. *Journal of Gastrointestinal Surgery* 12 (2): 250–255.

Mitchell, J. E., K. L. Lancaster, M. A. Burgard, L. M. Howell, D. D. Krahn, R. D. Crosby, S. A. Wonderlich, and B. A. Gosnell 2001. Long-term follow-up of patients' status after gastric bypass. *Obesity Surgery* 11 (4): 464–468.

Modi, A. C., M. H. Zeller, S. A. Xanthakos, T. M. Jenkins, and T. H. Inge. 2013. Adherence to vitamin supplementation following adolescent bariatric surgery. *Obesity* 21 (3): E190–E195.

Moizé, V., A. Andreu, L. Flores, F. Torres, A. Ibarzabal, S. Delgado, A. Lacy, L. Rodriguez, and J. Vidal. 2013. Long-term dietary intake and nutritional deficiencies following sleeve gastrectomy or Roux-en-Y gastric bypass in a mediterranean population. *Journal of the Academy of Nutrition and Dietetics* 113 (3): 400–410.

Moize, V., A. Geliebter, M. E. Gluck, E. Yahav, M. Lorence, T. Colarusso, V. Drake, and L. Flancbaum. 2003. Obese patients have inadequate protein intake related to protein intolerance up to 1 year following Roux-en-Y gastric bypass. *Obesity Surgery* 13 (1): 23–28.

National Institutes of Health. 1992. Gastrointestinal surgery for severe obesity: National Institutes of Health Consensus Development Conference Statement. *American Journal of Clinical Nutrition* 5 (2 Suppl): 615S–619S.

Newbury, L., K. Dolan, M. Hatzifotis, N. Low, and G. Fielding. 2003. Calcium and vitamin D depletion and elevated parathyroid hormone following biliopancreatic diversion. *Obesity Surgery* 13 (6): 893–895.

Nguyen, N. T., C. Goldman, C. J. Rosenquist, A. Arango, C. J. Cole, S. J. Lee, and B. M. Wolfe. 2001. Laparoscopic versus open gastric bypass: A randomized study of outcomes, quality of life, and costs. *Annals of Surgery* 234 (3): 289–291.

Nguyen, N. T., J. A. Slone, X. M. Nguyen, J. S. Hartman, and D. B. Hoyt. 2009. A prospective randomized trial of laparoscopic gastric bypass versus laparoscopic adjustable gastric banding for the treatment of morbid obesity: Outcomes, quality of life, and costs. *Annals of Surgery* 250 (4): 631–641.

Northrop-Clewes, C. A. and D. I. Thurnham. 2013. Biomarkers for the differentiation of anemia and their clinical usefulness. *Journal of Blood Medicine* 4: 11–22.

O'Brien, P. E., W. A. Brown, A. Smith, P. J. McMurrick, and M. Stephens. 1999. Prospective study of a laparoscopically placed, adjustable gastric band in the treatment of morbid obesity. *The British Journal of Surgery* 86 (1): 113–118.

O'Brien, P. E., J. B. Dixon, C. Laurie, and M. Anderson. 2005. A prospective randomized trial of placement of the laparoscopic adjustable gastric band: Comparison of the perigastric and pars flaccida pathways. *Obesity Surgery* 15 (6): 820–826.

O'Brien, P. E., J. B. Dixon, C. Laurie, S. Skinner, J. Proietto, J. McNeil, B. Strauss et al. 2006. Treatment of mild to moderate obesity with laparoscopic adjustable gastric banding or an intensive medical program: A randomized trial. *Annals of Internal Medicine* 144 (9): 625–633.

Odstrcil, E. A., J. G. Martinez, C. A. Santa Ana, B. Xue, R. E. Schneider, K. J. Steffer, J. L. Porter, J. Asplin, J. A. Kuhn, and J. S. Fordtran. 2010. The contribution of malabsorption to the reduction in net energy absorption after long-limb Roux-en-Y gastric bypass. *The American Journal of Clinical Nutrition* 92 (4): 704–713.

Papadia, F. S., H. Elghadban, and A. Weiss. 2012. BPD and BPD-DS concerns and results. *Advanced Bariatric and Metabolic Surgery*. February 29. Accessed August 20, 2015. http://cdn.intechopen.com/pdfs-wm/29489.pdf.

Parikh, M., J. Duncombe, and G. A. Fielding. 2006. Laparoscopic adjustable gastric banding for patients with body mass index of < or =35 kg/m^2. *Surgery for Obesity and Related Diseases* 2 (5): 518–522.

Plum, L., L. Ahmed, G. Febres, M. Bessler, W. Inabnet, E. Kunreuther, D. J. McMahon, and J. Korner. 2011. Comparison of glucostatic parameters after hypocaloric diet or bariatric surgery and equivalent weight loss. *Obesity* 19 (11): 2149–2157.

Pories, W. J., M. S. Swanson, K. G. MacDonald, S. B. Long, P. G. Morris, B. M. Brown, H. A. Barakat, R. A. DeRamon, G. Israel, and J. M. Dolezal. 1995. Who would have thought it? An operation proves to be the most effective therapy for adult-onset diabetes mellitus. *Annals of Surgery* 222 (3): 339–350.

Raftopoulos, I., B. Bernstein, K. O'Hara, J. A. Ruby, R. Chhatrala, and J. Carty. 2011. Protein intake compliance of morbidly obese patients undergoing bariatric surgery and its effect on weight loss and biochemical parameters. *Surgery for Obesity and Related Diseases* 7 (6): 733–742.

Ray, E. C., M. W. Nickels, S. Sayeed, and H. C. Sax. 2003. Predicting success after gastric bypass: The role of psychosocial and behavioral factors. *Surgery* 134 (4): 555–563.

Reinhold, R. B. 1982. Critical analysis of long term weight loss following gastric bypass. *Surgery, Gynecology & Obstetrics* 155 (3): 385–394.

Renquist, K. E., J. J. Cullen, D. Barnes, S. Tang, C. Doherty, and E. E. Mason. 1995. The effect of follow-up on reporting success for obesity surgery. *Obesity Surgery* 5 (3): 285–292.

Renquist, K. E., E. E. Mason, S. Tang, J. J. Cullen, C. Doherty, and J. W. Maher. 1996. Pay status as a predictor of outcome in surgical treatment of obesity. *Obesity Surgery* 6 (3): 224–232.

Rhode, B. M., P. Arseneau, B. A. Cooper, M. Katz, B. M. Gilfix, and L. D. MacLean. 1996. Vitamin B-12 deficiency after gastric surgery for obesity. *The American Journal of Clinical Nutrition* 63 (1): 103–109.

Rhode, B. M., H. Tamin, B. M. Gilfix, J. S. Sampalis, C. Nohr, and L. D. MacLean. 1995. Treatment of vitamin B12 deficiency after gastric surgery for severe obesity. *Obesity Surgery* 5 (2): 154–158.

Robinson, A. H., S. Adler, H. B. Stevens, A. M. Darcy, J. M. Morton, and D. L. Safer. 2014. What variables are associated with successful weight loss outcomes for bariatric surgery after 1 year? *Surgery for Obesity and Related Diseases* 10 (4): 697–704.

Royal, S., S. Wnuk, K. Warwick, R. Hawa, and S. Sockalingam. 2015. Night eating and loss of control over eating in bariatric surgery candidates. *Journal of Clinical Psychology in Medical Settings* 22 (1): 14–19.

Rubino, F., A. Forgione, D. E. Cummings, M. Vix, D. Gnuli, G. Mingrone, M. Castagneto, and J. Marescaux. 2006. The mechanism of diabetes control after gastrointestinal bypass surgery reveals a role of the proximal small intestine in the pathophysiology of type 2 diabetes. *Annals of Surgery* 244 (5): 741–749.

Ryan, D. H., W. D. Johnson, V. H. Myers, T. L. Prather, M. M. McGlone, J. Rood, P. J. Brantley et al. 2010. Nonsurgical weight loss for extreme obesity in primary care settings: Results of the Louisiana obese subjects study. *Archives of Internal Medicine* 170 (2): 146–154.

Santarpia, L., I. Grandone, L. Alfonsi, M. Sodo, F. Contaldo, and F. Pasanisi. 2014. Long-term medical complications after malabsorptive procedures: Effects of a late clinical nutritional intervention. *Nutrition* 30 (11–12): 1301–1305.

Sarwer, D. B., R. J. Dilks, and L. West-Smith. 2011. Dietary intake and eating behavior after bariatric surgery: Threats to weight loss maintenance and strategies for success. *Surgery for Obesity and Related Diseases* 7 (5): 644–651.

Sarwer, D. B., R. H. Moore, J. C. Spitzer, T. A. Wadden, S. E. Raper, and N. N. Williams. 2012. A pilot study investigating the efficacy of postoperative dietary counseling to improve outcomes after bariatric surgery. *Surgery for Obesity and Related Diseases* 8 (5): 561–568.

Savassi-Rocha, A. L., M. T. Diniz, P. R. Savassi-Rocha, J. T. Ferreira, S. Rodrigues De Almeida Sanches, F. Diniz Mde, H. Gomes De Barros, and I. K. Fonseca. 2008. Influence of jejunoileal and common limb length on weight loss following Roux-en-Y gastric bypass. *Obesity Surgery* 18 (11): 1364–1368.

Schauer, P. R., D. L. Bhatt, J. P. Kirwan, K. Wolski, S. A. Brethauer, S. D. Navaneethan, A. Aminian et al. 2014. Bariatric surgery versus intensive medical therapy for diabetes—3-Year outcomes. *The New England Journal of Medicine* 370 (21): 2002–2013.

Schauer, P. R., S. Ikramuddin, W. Gourash, R. Ramanathan, and J. Luketich. 2000. Outcomes after laparoscopic Roux-en-Y gastric bypass for morbid obesity. *Annals of Surgery* 232 (4): 515–529.

Schrager, S. 2005. Dietary calcium intake and obesity. *Journal of the American Board of Family Medicine* 18 (3): 205–210.

Scopinaro, N. 1997. American Society for Bariatric Surgery. *14th Annual Meeting for the American Society for Bariatric Surgery* (June 4–7), Chicago, IL.

Scopinaro, N. 2012. Thirty-five years of biliopancreatic diversion: Notes on gastrointestinal physiology to complete the published information useful for a better understanding and clinical use of the operation. *Obesity Surgery* 22 (3): 427–432.

Scopinaro, N., G. F. Adami, G. M. Marinari, E. Gianetta, E. Traverso, D. Friedman, G. Camerini, G. Baschieri, and A. Simonelli. 1998. Biliopancreatic diversion. *World Journal of Surgery* 22 (9): 936–946.

Scopinaro, N., G. F. Adami, F. S. Papadia, G. Camerini, F. Carlini, L. Briatore, G. D'Alessandro et al. 2011. The effects of biliopancreatic diversion on type 2 diabetes mellitus in patients with mild obesity (BMI 30-35 kg/m^2) and simple overweight (BMI 25-30 kg/m^2): A prospective controlled study. *Obesity Surgery* 21 (7): 880–888.

Scopinaro, N., G. M. Marinari, F. Pretolesi, F. Papadia, F. Murelli, P. Marini, and G. F. Adami. 2000. Energy and nitrogen absorption after biliopancreatic diversion. *Obesity Surgery* 10 (5): 436–441.

Shah, M., B. Adams-Huet, S. Rao, P. Snell, C. Quittner, and A. Garg. 2013. The effect of dietary counseling on nutrient intakes in gastric banding surgery patients. *Journal of Investigative Medicine* 61 (8): 1165–1172.

Shah, M., P. G. Snell, S. Rao, B. Adams-Huet, C. Quittner, E. H. Livingston, and A. Garg. 2011. High-volume exercise program in obese bariatric surgery patients: A randomized, controlled trial. *Obesity* 19 (9): 1826–1834.

Shen, R., G. Dugay, K. Rajaram, I. Cabrera, N. Siegel, and C. J. Ren. 2004. Impact of patient follow-up on weight loss after bariatric surgery. *Obesity Surgery* 14 (4): 514–519.

Sjöström, L., A. K. Lindroos, M. Peltonen, J. Torgerson, C. Bouchard, B. Carlsson, S. Dahlgren et al. 2004. Lifestyle, diabetes, and cardiovascular risk factors 10 years after bariatric surgery. *New England Journal of Medicine* 351 (26): 2683–2693.

Sjöström, L., K. Narbro, C. D. Sjöström, K. Karason, B. Larsson, H. Wedel, T. Lystig et al. 2007. Effects of bariatric surgery on mortality in Swedish obese subjects. *New England Journal of Medicine* 357 (8): 741–752.

Skroubis, G., S. Anesidis, I. Kehagias, N. Mead, K. Vagenas, and F. Kalfarentzos. 2006. Roux-en-Y gastric bypass versus a variant of biliopancreatic diversion in a non-superobese population: Prospective comparison of the efficacy and the incidence of metabolic deficiencies. *Obesity Surgery* 16 (4): 488–495.

Slater, G. H., C. J. Ren, N. Siegel, T. Williams, D. Barr, B. Wolfe, K. Dolan, and G. A. Fielding. 2004. Serum fat-soluble vitamin deficiency and abnormal calcium metabolism after malabsorptive bariatric surgery. *Journal of Gastrointestinal Surgery* 8 (1): 48–55.

Smith, C. D., S. B. Herkes, K. E. Behrns, V. F. Fairbanks, K. A. Kelly, and M. G. Sarr. 1993. Gastric acid secretion and vitamin B12 absorption after vertical Roux-en-Y gastric bypass for morbid obesity. *Annals of Surgery* 218 (1): 91–96.

Steinbrook, R. 2004. Surgery for severe obesity *New England Journal of Medicine* 350 (11): 1075–1079.

Tang, J. E., D. R. Moore, G. W. Kujbida, M. A. Tarnopolsky, and S. M. Phillips. 2009. Ingestion of whey hydrolysate, casein, or soy protein isolate: Effects on mixed muscle protein synthesis at rest and following resistance exercise in young men. *Journal of Applied Physiology* 107 (3): 987–992.

Te Riele, W. W., J. M. Vogten, D. Boerma, M. J. Wiezer, and B. Van Ramshorst. 2007. Comparison of weight loss and morbidity after gastric bypass and gastric banding. A single center European experience. *Obesity Surgery* 18 (1): 11–16.

Tussing-Humphreys, L. M., E. Nemeth, G. Fantuzzi, S. Freels, A. X. Holterman, C. Galvani, S. Ayloo, J. Vitello, and C. Braunschweig. 2010. Decreased serum hepcidin and improved functional iron status 6 months after restrictive bariatric surgery. *Obesity* 18 (10): 2010–2016.

Tymitz, K., G. Kerlakian, A. Engel, and C. Bollmer. 2007. Gender differences in early outcomes following hand-assisted laparoscopic Roux-en-Y gastric bypass surgery: Gender differences in bariatric surgery. *Obesity Surgery* 17 (12): 1588–1591.

Ullrich, J., B. Ernst, B. Wilms, M. Thurnheer, and B. Schultes. 2013. Hedonic hunger is increased in severely obese patients and is reduced after gastric bypass surgery. *Obesity Surgery* 23 (1): 50–55.

Van de Weijgert, E. J., C. H. Ruseler, and J. W. Elte. 1999. Long-term follow-up after gastric surgery for morbid obesity: Preoperative weight loss improves the long-term control of morbid obesity after vertical banded gastroplasty. *Obesity Surgery* 9 (5): 426–432.

Van Nieuwenhove, Y., Z. Dambrauskas, A. Campillo-Soto, F. van Dielen, R. Wiezer, I. Janssen, M. Kramer, and A. Thorell. 2011. Preoperative very low-calorie diet and operative outcome after laparoscopic gastric bypass: A randomized multicenter study. *Archives of Surgery* 146 (11): 1300–1305.

Vargas-Ruiz, A. G., G. Hernández-Rivera, and M. F. Herrera. 2008. Prevalence of iron, folate, and vitamin B12 deficiency anemia after laparoscopic Roux-en-Y gastric bypass. *Obesity Surgery* 18 (3): 288–293.

Vasilaki, A. T., D. C. McMillan, J. Kinsella, A. Duncan, D. S. O'Reilly, and D. Talwar. 2008. Relation between pyridoxal and pyridoxal phosphate concentrations in plasma, red cells, and white cells in patients with critical illness. *The American Journal of Clinical Nutrition* 88 (1): 140–146.

Von Drygalski, A. and D. A. Andris. 2009. Anemia after bariatric surgery: More than just iron deficiency. *Nutrition in Clinical Practice* 24 (2): 217–226.

Wadden, T. A., L. F. Faulconbridge, L. R. Jones-Corneille, D. B. Sarwer, A. N. Fabricatore, J. G. Thomas, G. T. Wilson et al. 2011. Binge eating disorder and the outcome of bariatric surgery at one year: A prospective, observational study. *Obesity* 19 (6): 1220–1228.

Waki, M., J. G. Kral, M. Mazariegos, J. Wang, R. N. Pierson, Jr., and S. B. Heymsfield. 1991. Relative expansion of extracellular fluid in obese vs. nonobese women. *The American Journal of Physiology* 261 (2): E199–E203.

Wannamethee, S. G., G. D. Lowe, A. Rumley, K. R. Bruckdorfer, and P. H. Whincup. 2006. Associations of vitamin C status, fruit and vegetable intakes, and markers of inflammation and hemostasis. *The American Journal of Clinical Nutrition* 83 (3): 567–574.

White, M. A., M. A. Kalarchian, R. M. Masheb, M. D. Marcus, and C. M. Grilo. 2010. Loss of control over eating predicts outcomes in bariatric surgery patients: A prospective, 24-month follow-up study. *The Journal of Clinical Psychiatry* 71 (2): 175–184.

Williams, D. L., H. J. Grill, D. E. Cummings, and J. M. Kaplan. 2003. Vagotomy dissociates short- and long-term controls of circulating ghrelin. *Endocrinology* 144 (12): 5184–5187.

Win, A. Z., C. Ceresa, A. L. Schafer, P. Mak, and L. Stewart. 2014. Importance of nutrition visits after gastric bypass surgery for American veterans, San Francisco, 2004-2010. *Preventing Chronic Disease* 11: E226.

Yanovski, S. Z. and J. A. Yanovski. 2002. Obesity. *New England Journal of Medicine* 346 (8): 591–602.

Ybarra, J., J. Sánchez-Hernández, I. Gich, A. De Leiva, X. Rius, J. Rodríguez-Espinosa, and A. Pérez. 2005. Unchanged hypovitaminosis D and secondary hyperparathyroidism in morbid obesity after bariatric surgery. *Obesity Surgery* 15 (3): 330–335.

Zhang, H., J. K. DiBaise, A. Zuccolo, D. Kudrna, M. Braidotti, Y. Yu, P. Parameswaran et al. 2009. Human gut microbiota in obesity and after gastric bypass. *Proceedings of the National Academy of Sciences of the United States of America* 106 (7): 2365–2370.

6 Physical Activity and Cardiometabolic Health

Andrea M. Brennan and Robert Ross

CONTENTS

ABSTRACT

The inverse dose–response association between physical activity, morbidity, and mortality has been firmly established by over four decades of evidence gathered from large, prospective cohort studies. Accordingly, independent of age, sex, and ethnicity, evidence from intervention trials has established that both aerobic- and resistance-type exercises combined with a healthful diet are effective strategies for reducing cardiometabolic risk factors (abdominal obesity, insulin resistance, dyslipidemia, and hypertension) that are associated with chronic disease. The primary aim of this chapter is to review the trial evidence establishing exercise as a primary strategy for reducing cardiometabolic risk. In doing so, we consider the acute and chronic effects of exercise as well as evidence regarding the separate effects of the amount and intensity of exercise on cardiometabolic risk. We conclude with a review of recent evidence that considers the effect of sedentary behavior on cardiometabolic health that is independent of physical activity.

INTRODUCTION

Current physical activity (PA) guidelines worldwide recommend that adults accumulate 150 minutes/week of moderate-to-vigorous-intensity PA, a recommendation supported by over 60 years of scientific study based on prospective observational cohorts examining the impact of moderate-to-vigorous PA on risk for chronic disease end points (Haskell et al. 2007, Tremblay et al. 2011). While exercise guidelines stem from observational evidence, the evidence for efficacy of PA for improving intermediate risk factors for disease is derived from a large number of intervention trials that clarify the specific characteristics of an exercise program (e.g., mode, type, frequency, intensity, amount, etc.) that are most strongly associated with risk reduction. This chapter will discuss the utility of PA, including both acute and chronic effects of aerobic and resistance exercise, independent of alterations in caloric intake, as a therapeutic strategy for the reduction of cardiometabolic risk in adults. The majority of exercise interventions reviewed did not alter caloric intake. Cardiometabolic risk factors include abdominal obesity, insulin resistance, dyslipidemia, and hypertension; all factors associated with increased risk for type 2 diabetes and cardiovascular disease. Where possible, the influence of age, sex, and ethnicity will be considered.

Available evidence regarding potential dose–response relationships between the amount of exercise and its intensity on cardiometabolic risk reduction will be reviewed. Knowledge regarding dose–response relationships between exercise and cardiometabolic risk has depended largely on a comparison of groups submitted to varying doses of exercise. More recently, large-scale randomized controlled trials (RCTs) designed specifically to determine the separate effects of exercise amount and intensity (exercise dose) have emerged. Exercise amount can be defined both as total minutes of exercise prescribed and by the energy expended during an exercise session, where exercise intensity is defined relative to an individual's peak oxygen consumption during exercise (VO_2peak). Manipulating either exercise amount at a fixed intensity or exercise intensity for a fixed amount of time allows the determination of increasing exercise amount and exercise intensity on cardiometabolic risk factors.

Furthermore, opportunity for time spent in a sedentary state has increased, stemming from technological advances in the twenty-first century (Colley et al. 2011, Matthews et al. 2008). This has prompted greater scientific inquiry into the independent effects of sedentary behavior as a unique risk factor for chronic disease. This chapter will therefore summarize the existing epidemiological and intervention literature examining the relationship between sedentary behavior and risk of chronic disease, independent of moderate-to-vigorous PA.

PHYSICAL ACTIVITY AND CARDIOMETABOLIC HEALTH

Physical Activity and Abdominal Obesity

Dr. Jean Vague was the first to characterize the increased risk of chronic disease among individuals with a phenotype characterized by excess adiposity in the upper-body or abdominal region by comparison to those with a predominance of adipose tissue (AT) in the lower-body region (Vague 1956). These seminal observations have since been repeatedly confirmed leading to the well-established notion that abdominal obesity is the phenotype associated with the greatest health risk (Despres and Lemieux 2006). Abdominal obesity has traditionally been characterized using waist circumference (WC) alone (Pouliot et al. 1994), or the combination of waist-to-hip ratio (Ferland et al. 1989). The introduction of radiographic imaging modalities in the early 1980s allowed investigators to further characterize abdominal obesity by provision of direct measures of abdominal visceral and subcutaneous AT depots (Ross et al. 1992). This represented a major advance as it is now firmly established that both visceral and abdominal subcutaneous AT depots predict diabetes and cardiovascular disease risk independent of commonly measured cardiometabolic risk factors, including hypertension, dyslipidemia, and insulin resistance in addition to body mass index (BMI) (Despres and Lemieux 2006, Janiszewski, Janssen, and Ross 2007).

Aerobic Exercise and Abdominal Obesity

Evidence from RCTs has firmly established that exercise ranging from 1000 to 4000 kcal/week energy expenditure in the absence of alterations in energy intake is associated with reductions in WC (Irwin et al. 2003, Ready et al. 1995, Ross et al. 2000, 2004), visceral AT (Donnelly et al. 2003, Irwin et al. 2003, Ross et al. 2000, 2004), and abdominal subcutaneous AT (Donnelly et al. 2003, Irwin et al. 2003, Ross et al. 2000, 2004), independent of age and sex. Though the majority of participants in the preceding studies lost body weight, exercise without weight loss achieved by consuming energy to compensate for that expended through exercise has also been shown to significantly reduce abdominal adiposity (Ross et al. 2000, 2004). Although these observations are based primarily on studies in white participants, limited evidence confirms similar associations between exercise-induced reduction in components of abdominal obesity in both Hispanics and blacks (Church et al. 2007). While exercise reduces abdominal obesity in both men and women, the magnitude of response may differ. The findings from a recent meta-analysis suggest that, when examining the overall effect of aerobic exercise on abdominal obesity, the effect size for reductions in visceral AT was greater in men compared to women (Vissers et al. 2013). This may be due to higher energy expenditure in men for a given number of exercise minutes prescribed and/or higher baseline visceral AT in men compared to women (Vissers et al. 2013). However, few studies included in this review studied both men and women simultaneously (Vissers et al. 2013), precluding the ability to directly compare sex-specific responses to the exercise interventions. Further studies designed to evaluate the impact of sex on WC, visceral AT, and abdominal subcutaneous AT changes are needed.

To isolate the role of exercise intensity on cardiometabolic risk factors, the amount of exercise measured by energy expenditure is ideally held constant while intensity is manipulated. Similarly, to isolate exercise amount, intensity is held constant while amount is manipulated. Examination of Table 6.1 reveals that increasing the intensity of exercise performed does not result in further reductions in WC, visceral AT, or abdominal subcutaneous AT.

A positive dose–response relationship between the amount of exercise (energy expenditure) and reduction in the components of abdominal obesity (WC, visceral AT, and abdominal subcutaneous AT) is observed across studies varying in exercise-induced energy expenditure (Donnelly et al. 2003, Irwin et al. 2003, Kohrt et al. 1991, Ohkawara et al. 2007, Ready et al. 1995, Watkins et al. 2003). However, large discrepancies in study designs including inclusion criteria for participants and intensity of exercise performed present a limitation in defining a true dose–response relationship in this manner. Inspection of Table 6.1 reveals that in large, long-term (>6 months) RCTs specifically designed to examine the effect of increasing the amount or intensity of exercise on abdominal obesity reduction, higher exercise-induced energy expenditure does not result in greater reductions in WC. These observations are far more compelling than those observed by comparing exercise groups between studies, as the interventions' rigorously controlled and randomized design mitigates the influence of potential confounders. Thus, this evidence should be weighed more heavily and suggests that exercise reduces WC independent of the amount of exercise.

Two studies have examined the impact of increasing exercise amount on visceral and abdominal subcutaneous AT, with conflicting findings. Slentz et al. randomized 175 participants to one of four conditions: (1) low amount, moderate intensity (12 miles at 40%–55% VO_2peak/week); (2) low amount, vigorous intensity (12 miles at 65%–80% VO_2peak/week); (3) high amount, vigorous intensity (20 miles at 65%–80% VO_2peak); and (4) control (no exercise). Slentz et al. observed significant reductions in visceral and abdominal subcutaneous AT measured by computed tomography scan compared to baseline in the high amount/vigorous intensity group only, suggesting that higher amounts of exercise were necessary for reduction in visceral and abdominal subcutaneous AT (Slentz et al. 2005) (Table 6.1). However, in this study, participants were required to increase energy intake to compensate for energy expended during exercise, which limits our ability to examine effects of exercise-induced weight loss on AT depots. Keating et al. also examined the effect of the amount and intensity of exercise on visceral AT measured by magnetic resonance

TABLE 6.1
RCTs Examining Effects of Exercise Amount and/or Intensity on Abdominal Obesity

Reference	Participants	Intervention Groups	Duration (Weeks)	Change in WC	Change in ASAT	Change in VAT
Slentz et al. (2005)	Sedentary, middle-aged, overweight men and women (n = 120)	Control (no exercise) Low amount/moderate intensity (LAMI, 14 kcal/kg at 40%–55% VO_2peak) Low amount/vigorous intensity (LAVI, 14 kcal/kg at 65%–80% VO_2peak) High amount/vigorous intensity (HAVI, 23 kcal/kg at 65%–80% VO_2peak)	32		Control: +3.44 cm^2 LAMI: −3.44 cm^2 LAVI: +9.02 cm^2 HAVI: −19.18 cm^2[a] LAMI and LAVI significantly different from HAVI	Control: +14.19 cm^2 LAMI: +2.94 cm^2[a] LAVI: +3.85 cm^2[a] HAVI: −11.59 cm^2[a] LAMI and LAVI significantly different from HAVI
Slentz et al. (2005)	Sedentary, middle-aged, overweight men and women (n = 120)	Control (no exercise) Low amount/moderate intensity (LAMI, 14 kcal/kg at 40%–55% VO_2peak) Low amount/vigorous intensity (LAVI, 14 kcal/kg at 65%–80% VO_2peak) High amount/vigorous intensity (HAVI, 23 kcal/kg at 65%–80% VO_2peak)	32	Control: +0.8 LAMI: −1.6 cm[a] LAVI: −1.4 cm[a] HAVI: −3.4 cm[a] No difference between exercise groups		
Ross et al. (2015)	Sedentary, middle-aged, abdominally obese men and women (n = 300)	Control (no exercise) Low amount/low intensity (LALI; 180 and 300 kcal/session at 50% VO_2peak for women and men, respectively) High amount/low intensity (HALI; 360 and 600 kcal/session at 50% VO_2peak, respectively) High amount/high intensity (HAHI; 360 and 600 kcal/session at 75% VO_2peak, respectively)	24	Control: Not reported LALI: −3.9 cm[a] HALI: −4.6 cm[a] HAHI: −4.6 cm[a] No difference between exercise groups		

(Continued)

TABLE 6.1 (*Continued*)
RCTs Examining Effects of Exercise Amount and/or Intensity on Abdominal Obesity

Reference	Participants	Intervention Groups	Duration (Weeks)	Change in WC	Change in ASAT	Change in VAT
Church et al. (2007)	Sedentary, overweight/obese postmenopausal women, 45–75 years (n = 427)	Control (no exercise) 4 kcal/kg per week @ 50% VO_2peak 8 kcal/kg per week @ 50% VO_2peak 12 kcal/kg per week @ 50% VO_2peak	24	Control: −1.4 cm 4 kcal/kg: −1.9 cm[a] 8 kcal/kg: −2.9 cm[a] 12 kcal/kg: −1.4 cm[a] No difference between exercise groups		
Keating et al. (2015)	Sedentary, overweight/obese men and women (n = 48)	Control (no exercise) Low-to-moderate intensity, high volume (LO:HI, 50% VO_2peak, 60 minutes, 4 days/week) High intensity, low volume (HI:LO, 70% VO_2peak, 45 minutes, 3 days/week) Low-to-moderate intensity, low volume (LO:LO, 50% VO_2peak, 45 minutes, 3 days/week)	8	Control: +0.8 cm LO:HI: −2.5 cm[a] HI:LO: −2.5 cm[a] LO:LO: −0.9 cm[a] No difference between exercise groups	Control: +319.7 cm^3 LO:HI: −596.7 cm^3[a] HI:LO: −567.8 cm^3[a] LO:LO: −165.5 cm^3[a] No difference between exercise groups	Control: +92.67 cm^3 LO:HI: −386.60 cm^3[a] HI:LO: −258.38 cm^3[a] LO:LO: −212.96 cm^3[a] No difference between exercise groups

WC, waist circumference; ASAT, abdominal subcutaneous adipose tissue; VAT, visceral adipose tissue.
[a] Exercise group significantly different from control.

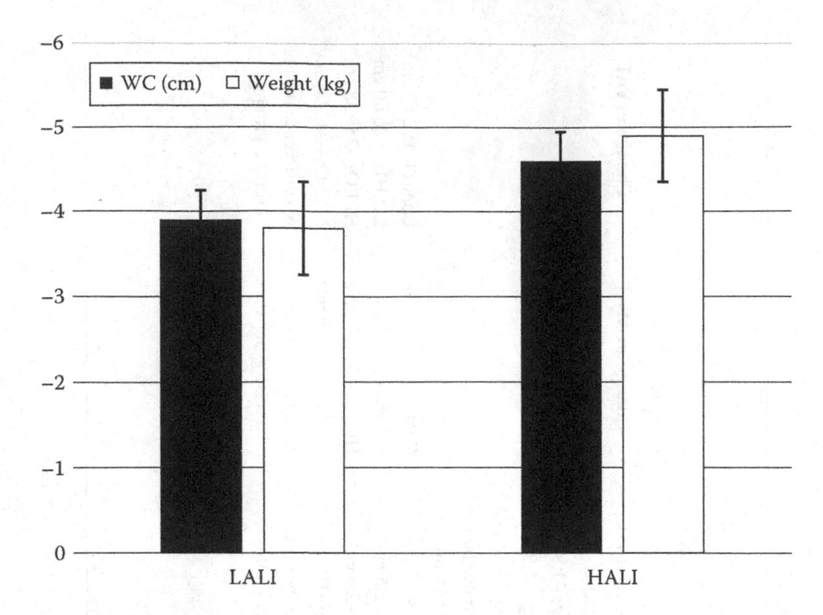

FIGURE 6.1 Effect of exercise amount on the net change in waist circumference (WC) and body weight following 24 weeks of exercise. WC, waist circumference; LALI, low amount low intensity (180 kcal and 300 kcal/session for women and men, respectively); HALI, high amount low intensity (360 kcal and 600 kcal/session for women and men, respectively). (Adapted from Ross, R. et al., *Ann. Intern. Med.*, 162(5), 325, 2015.)

imaging (Keating et al. 2015). They randomized 48 participants to one of four conditions: (1) low-to-moderate intensity, high volume (60 minutes, 4 days/week at 50% VO_2peak); (2) high intensity, low volume (45 minutes, 3 days/week at 70% VO_2peak); (3) low-to-moderate intensity, low volume (45 minutes, 3 days/week at 50% VO_2peak); and (4) control (no exercise). In contrast to Slentz et al., the authors found that while all exercise groups reduced visceral AT, there were no differences between groups, suggesting that reductions in visceral AT are independent of the amount of exercise.

As shown in Figure 6.1, the apparently limited impact of increasing energy expenditure on reduction of abdominal obesity is surprising and difficult to interpret, especially given the doubling of energy expenditure between some of the exercise conditions (Church et al. 2007, Ross et al. 2015), but suggests that individuals have a range of treatment options that are efficacious for reducing abdominal obesity. Additional RCTs that match energy expenditure between groups are needed to determine the dose–response relationships of exercise amount and intensity with abdominal obesity.

While chronic exercise reduces both visceral AT and total subcutaneous AT depots independent of sex and age, it has been suggested that a preferential mobilization of lipid from visceral adipocytes exists (Mourier et al. 1997). However, this depends on whether reductions are presented as relative to baseline AT amount or as absolute amount lost. Most individuals have a higher absolute baseline amount of subcutaneous AT compared to visceral AT. Thus, for a given exercise-induced negative energy balance, the relative reduction in visceral AT is usually greater than subcutaneous AT (Ross et al. 2000, 2004). Conversely, it is noteworthy that the absolute reduction in subcutaneous AT after exercise training is generally greater than visceral AT in middle-aged men and women (Ross et al. 2000, 2004). Therefore, whether exercise preferentially reduces visceral AT is unclear and can be interpreted differently depending on the metric used to interpret the exercise-induced response.

Resistance Exercise and Abdominal Obesity

Examination of the limited evidence in Table 6.2 reveals that resistance exercise training, without alterations in caloric intake, is effective for reducing WC across age groups in overweight or obese adult men and women without significant changes in body weight (Bateman et al. 2011, Ho et al. 2012, Stensvold et al. 2010). However, reductions appear to be smaller in magnitude compared to aerobic

TABLE 6.2
Randomized Trials Examining Effect of Aerobic and Resistance Exercise on Abdominal Obesity

Reference	Participants	Intervention Groups	Duration (Months)	Change in WC	Change in ASAT	Change in VAT
Davidson et al. (2009)	Sedentary, abdominally obese, 60–80 years old, men and women (n = 136)	Control (no exercise) Aerobic exercise (AE): 30 minutes of moderate-intensity treadmill walking (60%–75% VO_2peak) 5 times/week Resistance exercise (RE): 1 set of 9 exercises, each to volitional fatigue: chest press, shoulder raise, shoulder flexion, leg extension, leg flexion, triceps extension, biceps curl, abdominal crunches, modified push-ups, 3 times/week Combined: AE plus RE, 3 times/week	6	Control: –0.28 kg RE: –3.18 kg[a] AE: –5.08 kg[a] Combined: –4.61 kg[a] AE different from RE	Control: –0.04 kg RE: –0.21 kg AE: –0.40 kg[a] Combined: –0.40 kg[a]	Control: +0.02 kg RE: –0.21 kg AE: –0.43 kg[a] Combined: –0.35 kg[a]
Bateman et al. (2011)	Sedentary, overweight dyslipidemic men and women, aged 18–70 years (n = 196)	Resistance exercise (RE): 3 days/week, 3 sets/day of 8–12 repetitions of 8 different exercises targeting major muscle groups Aerobic exercise (AE): ~120 minutes/week at 75% VO_2max Combined: AE plus RE	8	RE: +0.25 cm AE: –1.12 cm Combined: –2.48 cm RE different from AT ($p < 0.10$), AE + RE different from RE ($p < 0.05$)		
Stensvold et al. (2010)	Middle-aged adults with metabolic syndrome (n = 43)	Control (no exercise) Aerobic interval training (AIT): Interval training as treadmill walking/running, 3 times/week Strength training (ST): 3 sets at ~80% 1-RM, target major muscle groups 3 times/week Combined: AIT 2 times/week, ST 1 time/week	3	Control: +1.7 cm AIT: –1.3 cm[a] ST: –1.4 cm[a] Combined: –0.7 cm		
Ho et al. (2012)	Sedentary, overweight or obese men and women aged 40–66 years (n = 64)	Control (no exercise) Aerobic exercise (AE): 30 minutes on a treadmill at 60% HRR Resistance exercise (RE): 30 minutes, 4 sets of 8–12 repetitions at 10-RM for major muscle groups Combined: 15-minute aerobic exercise and 15-minute RE	3	Control: –1.2 cm AE: –2.1 cm[a] RE: –2.6 cm[a] Combined: –2.6 cm[a]		

WC, waist circumference; ASAT, abdominal subcutaneous adipose tissue; VAT, visceral adipose tissue.
[a] Significantly different from control.

exercise (Davidson et al. 2009). While there seems to be a consistent effect of resistance training on reduction in WC, the effect of resistance exercise on visceral AT and abdominal subcutaneous AT is less consistent. Braith et al. summarized several RCTs that demonstrate significant reductions in visceral AT after resistance exercise training in overweight and obese middle-aged men and women (Braith and Stewart 2006). However, in a meta-analysis of RCTs that also included overweight and obese adults, Ismali et al. observed no pooled effect of resistance training on visceral AT reduction compared to controls (Ismail et al. 2012). Davidson et al. (Table 6.2) observed that while both visceral AT and abdominal subcutaneous AT were significantly reduced in the aerobic exercise and combined aerobic and resistance exercise groups, neither AT depot was significantly different from controls in the resistance exercise group (Davidson et al. 2009). The attenuated effect of resistance exercise training on abdominal obesity reduction compared to aerobic training is likely explained by the lower energy expended during resistance exercise. Discrepancies in study findings may be explained by differences in study design, differences in resistance exercise training programs, and sex-specific responses to resistance exercise.

Physical Activity and Insulin Resistance

Aerobic Exercise and Insulin Resistance

It is well established that a single bout of aerobic-type exercise is associated with marked reduction in insulin resistance, assessed by plasma glucose, oral glucose tolerance test (OGTT), and muscle glucose transporter phosphorylation, in adult men and women with normoglycemia, impaired glucose tolerance, and type 2 diabetes (Thompson et al. 2001). Improvements in insulin sensitivity ranging from 15% to 24% (Mikines et al. 1988) are observed after 1 hour of moderate-intensity exercise in healthy, normoglycemic adults (Burstein et al. 1990, Mikines et al. 1988) and in adults with insulin resistance (Perseghin et al. 1996) or type 2 diabetes (Burstein et al. 1990, Devlin et al. 1987). The acute effects of exercise on insulin resistance persist for 20–48 hours (Devlin et al. 1987, Mikines et al. 1988, Perseghin et al. 1996).

The impact of chronic aerobic exercise on insulin resistance varies depending on the method of measurement and baseline value for insulin and glucose. Among obese individuals with normal glucose levels, the findings from two reviews suggest that while exercise did not impact glucose response during an OGTT, corresponding insulin levels were reduced, suggesting a decreased insulin-to-glucose ratio and improved insulin action (Ivy 1997, Mann et al. 2014). In addition, the summary findings of several reviews suggest that aerobic exercise training directly improves insulin resistance by increasing insulin sensitivity by 40%–85% when measured by hyperinsulinemic–euglycemic clamp, independent of weight changes, in overweight or obese men and women (Dengel et al. 1996, Ross et al. 2000, 2004, Thompson et al. 2001).

The impact of aerobic exercise on blood glucose and insulin measures is more pronounced in individuals with impaired glucose tolerance and those with type 2 diabetes. The findings reported in several reviews clearly demonstrate that regular exercise improves glycemic control (HbA1c) in addition to glucose/insulin levels in individuals with type 2 diabetes (Chudyk and Petrella 2011, Hawley 2004, Hawley and Lessard 2008, Ivy 1997). Boule et al. performed a meta-analysis including 14 (12 aerobic, 2 resistance) exercise training studies and found that exercise training significantly reduced HbA1c (net change = −0.66%) among men and women with diabetes independent of weight change (Boule et al. 2005).

Overall, there appears to be a beneficial effect of increasing exercise intensity on insulin resistance. Swain et al. reviewed five clinical intervention studies comparing the effect of aerobic exercise varying in intensity on glucose control measures (Swain and Franklin 2006). These trials generally reported greater improvements after high-intensity exercise (>60% VO_2max) compared with moderate-intensity exercise (40%–55% VO_2max) in measures including fasting glucose and the insulin response to an OGTT (Swain and Franklin 2006). More recently, Ross et al. conducted an RCT examining the separate effects of exercise amount and intensity on glucose tolerance in abdominally obese adults (Ross et al. 2015). The primary finding of this trial was that in overweight or obese men and women, the benefit of reducing the 2-hour glucose response was restricted to the high intensity (75% of VO_2max) group.

The mechanisms of action by which exercise affects insulin resistance have been described in several reviews (Goodyear and Kahn 1998, Henriksen 2002, Ivy 1997). These include increased glycogen synthase, increased glucose transporter-4 protein and messenger RNA expression, including increased translocation to the plasma membrane to enhance glucose uptake, and improved muscle capillary density that enhances glucose delivery to the muscle during exercise. Additionally, changes in body composition, in particular reductions in abdominal adiposity, have been postulated to enhance exercise-related improvements in insulin sensitivity (Ross et al. 2000, 2004).

Resistance Exercise and Insulin Resistance

Evidence for an acute effect of resistance training on insulin sensitivity is scarce. However, there is limited evidence for improvements in whole-body insulin sensitivity assessed by an intravenous insulin tolerance test in healthy, sedentary, normal-weight young adult men that persists 24 hours after an acute bout of resistance exercise (Koopman et al. 2005).

The effect of chronic resistance training on glucose and insulin metabolism is equivocal. The findings reported in some studies suggest that there is no significant effect of resistance exercise training on plasma measures of insulin and glucose metabolism (e.g., fasting glucose and insulin) in both middle-aged and older adult men and women (Bateman et al. 2011, Davidson et al. 2009). However, investigations measuring changes in insulin action at the muscle (glucose uptake) show that resistance exercise training increases insulin-mediated glucose uptake in several study groups primarily including Caucasian individuals but ranging in age and health status (Tresierras and Balady 2009).

The effect of resistance training on insulin and glucose metabolism is apparent in men and women with type 2 diabetes (Tresierras and Balady 2009). The findings from several studies suggest that resistance training reduces hemoglobin A1c in diabetic men (Braith and Stewart 2006, Dunstan et al. 2002, Eriksson et al. 1997, Honkola, Forsen, and Eriksson 1997) and women (Dunstan et al. 2002, Honkola, Forsen, and Eriksson 1997), regardless of age. Two large RCTs described in Table 6.3 were designed to determine the separate impact of aerobic, resistance, and combined aerobic and resistance training on HbA1c in individuals with type 2 diabetes. The Diabetes Aerobic and Resistance Exercise study was the first controlled study with adequate power to compare changes in HbA1c after aerobic, resistance, or combined aerobic and resistance training (Sigal et al. 2007). The primary finding was that a reduction in HbA1C was observed in all exercise groups compared to controls, but the improvement was greater within the combined group compared to resistance or aerobic training alone. A limitation of this trial was that participants in the combined exercise group were required to perform both the aerobic and resistance exercise prescription, which doubled the total time for exercising for that group. Therefore, it is difficult to discern the effect of the training per se, independent of exercise time. Church et al. addressed this limitation by examining aerobic, resistance, and combined aerobic and resistance training of similar weekly training duration (Church et al. 2010) (Table 6.3). In contrast to Sigal et al., they found that only the combined aerobic and resistance training group significantly improved HbA1c compared to the control group (Church et al. 2010). This recent evidence suggests that resistance training alone is not efficacious for improving glucose control in those with type 2 diabetes. That the aerobic exercise group in this trial did not improve glycemic control may be due to participant characteristics, namely, longer duration of diabetes, higher proportions of women and nonwhite individuals, 18% of participants being treated with insulin, and the allowance for medication changes throughout the trial (Church et al. 2010).

Physical Activity and Dyslipidemia

Abnormalities in blood lipid concentrations, including hypertriglyceridemia, low high-density lipoprotein–cholesterol (HDL-C), and elevated low-density lipoprotein–cholesterol (LDL-C), are linked to other cardiometabolic risk factors such as abdominal obesity (Horton 2009) and insulin resistance

TABLE 6.3
RCTs Examining Effect of Aerobic and Resistance Exercise on Glycemic Control in T2D

Study	Participants	Study Design	Study Duration (Weeks)	Change in HgA1c
Sigal et al. (2007)	Adults aged 39–70 years with type 2 diabetes (n = 251)	Control (no exercise) Aerobic training (AT): 45 minutes at 75% HRmax, 3 times/week Resistance training (RT): 2–3 sets of 7 exercises on weight machines, 3 times/week Combined: Full aerobic training plus full RT program	22	Control: +0.07% AT: –0.43%[a] RT: –0.30%[a] Combined: –0.90%[a] Combined different from both AT and RT
Church et al. (2010)	Sedentary men and women with type 2 diabetes (n = 262)	Control (no exercise) Aerobic (AT): 12 kcal/kg per week Resistance (RT): 2 sets of 4 upper body exercises, 3 sets of 3 leg exercises, and 2 sets each of abdominal crunches and back extension, 3 days/week Combined: 10 kcal/kg per week plus RT (reduced) 2 times/week	36	Control: +0.11% AT: –0.08% RT: –0.09% Combined: –0.27%[a]

[a] Significantly different from control.

(Howard et al. 1998). Furthermore, an atherogenic lipid profile has been shown to predict cardiovascular disease and cardiovascular disease mortality in middle-aged adults with type 2 diabetes, independent of other cardiovascular disease risk factors such as fasting plasma glucose (Lehto et al. 1997).

Aerobic Exercise and Dyslipidemia

The impact of aerobic exercise on acute and chronic blood lipid responses differs. Holoszy et al. were one of the first to suggest that a single bout of exercise can significantly reduce triglycerides (TG) and increase HDL-C in hypertriglyceridemic, middle-aged sedentary men (Holoszy et al. 1965). The observations from numerous studies in both trained and untrained individuals extend these findings by illustrating that the acute effect of exercise (24–48 hours after a single exercise bout) ranges from a 10% to 25% decrease for TG levels, and a 7% to 15% increase in HDL-C (Bounds et al. 2000, Crouse et al. 1997, Grandjean, Crouse, and Rohack 2000). Not surprisingly, the greatest change is observed among individuals with higher or lower baseline levels of TG and HDL-C, respectively. Additionally, there is a positive correlation between exercise-induced energy expenditure and change in plasma TG and HDL-C, independent of weight change (Cullinane et al. 1982). However, increases in exercise intensity have not been shown to have an appreciable effect on TG or HDL-C. In contrast to TG and HDL-C, we do not observe a similar effect of acute exercise on changes in LDL-C (Crouse et al. 1997, Grandjean, Crouse, and Rohack 2000).

Several reviews and meta-analyses have summarized the relationship between chronic aerobic exercise training and blood lipid response (Durstine et al. 2001, Katzmarzyk et al. 2001, Kelley et al. 2011, Leon and Sanchez 2001). Overall, there is evidence for a beneficial effect of exercise on HDL-C and TG in adult men and women; however, observations are inconsistent. A meta-analysis of exercise training studies in adult men and women ranging in body weight and blood lipid status observed a significant 4.6% increase in HDL-C and 3.7% decrease in TG when diet was unchanged (Kelley et al. 2011). These findings are in agreement with those examining obese, overweight adults with and without dyslipidemia (Leon and Sanchez 2001). These studies differ from others wherein the effect of exercise on blood lipids was small (Katzmarzyk et al. 2001). There are several potential explanations for the disparities reported. First, there is great heterogeneity in response to exercise both between and within studies that influence the overall interpretation. This variation in response is likely due to the confounding effects of heritability on change in blood lipid levels (Katzmarzyk et al. 2001). Additionally, potential flaws including the absence of a control group, the timing of the blood measurements in relation to the last exercise session, sex differences in response (discussed in the following), and effects of simultaneous dietary intervention and weight loss may have impacted overall observations (Katzmarzyk et al. 2001). When examining exercise interventions combined with caloric restriction, stronger improvements in blood lipid levels are seen, indicating the importance of diet in regulating blood lipids (Durstine et al. 2001).

Whether men and women experience different lipid responses to exercise training is unclear, as some have shown that HDL-cholesterol changes are greater in men compared to women (Stefanick 1999), while others have not (Kokkinos and Myers 2010, Leon and Sanchez 2001). Furthermore, evidence from the HERITAGE study, wherein 675 sedentary white and black men and women participated in 20 weeks of exercise, concluded that exercise-induced changes in HDL-cholesterol, specifically, are not related to age, ethnicity, or sex (Leon et al. 2002).

While a clear dose–response relationship between the amount of exercise and intensity on lipid changes has yet to be established, overall, potential changes in lipid markers seem more related to exercise amount and not intensity (Kraus et al. 2002). Swain et al. reviewed eight clinical trials including participants ranging in age, sex, and health status that examined the impact of exercise intensity on lipid profiles (Swain and Franklin 2006). Generally, they found no effect of exercise intensity on improvements in lipid profile markers. However, the majority of reviewed studies had small sample sizes and were not adequately powered to detect an effect. Kraus et al. extended previous observations in a large RCT (described in Table 6.1) examining the effect of the amount of exercise and intensity on lipid profile markers in adult men and women with dyslipidemia (Kraus et al. 2002). They observed that individuals who exercised at a higher weekly energy expenditure saw greater improvements in lipoprotein variables including HDL-C and TG compared to those at lower energy expenditures, and these changes were not related to exercise intensity. However, this study was limited by its design, wherein the amount of exercise was not equal across low and high intensity groups (Kraus et al. 2002). Further research is needed to clarify the effect of exercise intensity on reduction in lipids.

While it appears that improvements in HDL-C and TG are correlated with weight loss, there is some evidence to suggest that improvements can occur independent of body weight changes (Carroll and Dudfield 2004, Durstine et al. 2001, Kraus et al. 2002). Exercise intervention trials designed to maintain body weight reduced TG levels by 5%–35% (Gan et al. 2003, Leon and Sanchez 2001) and increased HDL-C levels by 3%–5% (Leon and Sanchez 2001, Thomas et al. 2000). Many studies included in the preceding reviews, however, incorporate some amount of weight loss, making it difficult to separate the independent effects of PA and weight loss on blood lipid levels.

Overall, there is little evidence to suggest that aerobic exercise beneficially impacts LDL-C levels (Durstine et al. 2001). However, the benefit of PA may not be seen from the absolute improvement in lipid levels, but rather on the characteristics of lipoproteins that carry cholesterol in the blood (Kraus et al. 2002). For example, after 24 weeks of exercise in 111 sedentary overweight men and women, aerobic exercise increased LDL particle size, with larger particles shown to be less likely to contribute to cardiovascular disease (CVD) than smaller denser LDL (Krauss 2014, Kraus et al. 2002).

Resistance Exercise and Dyslipidemia

The effect of resistance exercise training on lipid profile is also unclear. While findings are inconsistent, most intervention studies in healthy adults show no improvement in lipid profiles after resistance training (Braith and Stewart 2006, Manning et al. 1991, Smutok et al. 1993). This is seen across a range of ages in both men and women. Comparing resistance training, aerobic training, and combination of aerobic and resistance training, Bateman et al. observed significant changes in TG after both aerobic and aerobic plus resistance training; however, the change in TG was not greater in aerobic plus resistance training, indicating that aerobic exercise may be the more important stimulus for change in TG (Bateman et al. 2011). It is known that greater exercise-induced weight and fat loss is associated with greater improvement in lipid profiles (Durstine et al. 2001). In this study, the aerobic training group, due to increased energy expenditure, experienced greater reduction in body weight and WC than the resistance training group, which may explain the lack of change in lipids in the latter group. Conversely, Kelley et al. conducted a meta-analysis of RCTs using resistance exercise training lasting greater than 4 weeks and found statistically significant improvement for total cholesterol (TC), LDL, and TG, but not for HDL-C (Kelley and Kelley 2009). Many of the existing studies were completed in younger individuals with normal baseline lipid levels, and this population may be less likely to show a significant response.

Physical Activity and Hypertension

Hypertension is an important predictor of CVD mortality, and relatively modest reductions in blood pressure are associated with reduced risk for cardiovascular disease morbidity and mortality (Cook et al. 1995, He and Whelton 1999).

Aerobic Exercise and Hypertension

The acute effects of aerobic exercise on blood pressure are well established (Kenney and Seals 1993). While normotensive individuals experience postexercise hypotension, the effect is more pronounced among those with hypertension, wherein reductions in systolic blood pressure (SBP) and diastolic blood pressure (DBP) of −11 and −6 mmHg, respectively, have been observed (Pescatello et al. 1999, Rueckert et al. 1996). Postexercise hypotension occurs immediately after exercise and can last for 22 hours postexercise (Brandao Rondon et al. 2002).

Reductions in blood pressure in response to chronic aerobic exercise training are also well established (Arroll and Beaglehole 1992, Cornelissen and Fagard 2005, Fagard 1999, Hagberg, Park, and Brown 2000, Kelley 1995, Kelley and Kelley 1999, Whelton et al. 2002). A recent meta-analysis summarizing observations from 93 RCTs lasting greater than 4 weeks in healthy adults showed reductions in SBP (−3.5 mmHg) and DBP (−2.5 mmHg) after endurance exercise (Cornelissen and Fagard 2005). Similar to acute exercise, BP reductions were greater in individuals with hypertension (SBP, −8.3 mmHg; DBP, −5.2). Most of the studies included in the analysis used at least 40 minutes of moderate-intensity PA 3 times/week. These observations extended seminal work by Cornelissen et al. who also observed significant reductions in SBP and DBP in response to exercise in both normotensive and hypertensive adults (Cornelissen and Fagard 2005). The beneficial effects of exercise on blood pressure were observed independent of age, sex, and BMI.

Studies examining the impact of exercise amount and intensity on blood pressure are limited. Swain et al. reviewed four aerobic exercise trials and found no overall effect of exercise intensity on SBP; however, DBP changed to a greater extent following vigorous exercise compared to moderate-intensity exercise (Swain and Franklin 2006). Cornelissen et al. also reviewed the impact of exercise intensity in training studies on blood pressure response (Cornelissen et al. 2010). The authors found no consistent effect of exercise intensity on blood pressure reduction after aerobic exercise training, with exercise intensity ranging from 40% to 70% of maximal exercise performance (Cornelissen et al. 2010). The amount of exercise does not appear to have a clear impact on the reduction in blood pressure (Kelley 1995, Kelley and Kelley 1999, Whelton et al. 2002).

There is some evidence that women with hypertension experience greater reductions in blood pressure in response to exercise training compared to men (Hagberg, Park, and Brown 2000). A recent review observed an average weighted reduction of 14.7 and 10.5 mmHg in SBP and DBP, respectively, in women, compared to 8.7 and 7.8 mmHg reduction in men in response to exercise training (Hagberg, Park, and Brown 2000). Few studies have examined ethnic differences in blood pressure response. However, a recent meta-analysis observed that, compared to Caucasian individuals, black participants experienced greater reductions in SBP and Asian participants experienced greater reductions in DBP (Whelton et al. 2002).

Resistance Exercise and Hypertension

Resistance exercise training also appears to have a beneficial effect on SBP and DBP in adult men and women (Braith and Stewart 2006, Cornelissen et al. 2011, Kelley and Kelley 2000). Two meta-analyses have been conducted to examine this relationship (Cornelissen et al. 2011, Kelley and Kelley 2000). Kelley observed a 3 mmHg decrease in SBP and DBP following progressive resistance exercise training in previously inactive adult men and women ranging in age and BMI (Kelley and Kelley 2000). Cornelissen observed similar relationships; however, while there was a significant reduction in SBP and DBP in normotensive and pre-hypertensive study groups, the effect was not significant in hypertensive groups. There was also a greater effect of resistance exercise on SBP in study groups younger than 50 years compared to those older than 50 years, as well as a larger decrease in SBP and DBP with isometric handgrip strength training compared to dynamic resistance training study groups (Cornelissen et al. 2011).

Influence of Age, Sex, and Ethnicity on PA-Induced CVD Reduction

While evidence concerning the impact of age, sex, and ethnicity on exercise-induced changes in individual cardiometabolic risk factors is scarce, a recent review summarized the influence of these factors on PA-related changes in overall cardiovascular disease risk reduction (Shiroma and Lee 2010). Overall, it appears that the inverse correlation between PA and CVD risk seen in middle-aged adults is also seen to a similar magnitude in older men and women (Shiroma and Lee 2010). Indeed, in the Women's Health Initiative, the authors categorized participants into three age groups (50–59, 60–69, and 70–79 years). All three age groups had comparable relative risks of CVD when comparing the most active with least active participants (Manson et al. 2002).

Both men and women experience inverse associations between PA and risk of developing CVD; evidence suggests that the most active women experience a 40% risk reduction compared to the least active women, whereas risk reduction is 30% in active men, suggesting that the inverse association between PA and CVD is stronger in women (Manson et al. 2002). Very few studies have examined the ethnic differences in CVD risk response to PA, as the majority of studies were conducted in white individuals. The few studies that have examined nonwhite populations observed no significant interactions among races (Gregg et al. 2003).

Efficacy and Effectiveness

The majority of the evidence reviewed from RCTs derives from tightly controlled efficacy studies. The findings from these studies support the notion that for most cardiometabolic risk factors, exercise has beneficial effects. However, while the efficacy of exercise for improving cardiometabolic health is established, the observed inability for individuals to sustain an exercise program has led some to conclude that exercise is not an effective model for sustained change in health risk (Ross et al. 2012, Wadden et al. 2011). The question then is not whether exercise will decrease cardiometabolic risk, but rather, can these changes realistically be maintained over the long term? The answer to this question remains elusive. The PROACTIVE trial investigated the effectiveness of a 2-year behaviorally based lifestyle (PA and diet) program aimed at reducing obesity and metabolic risk factors in abdominally obese adults in primary care settings (Ross et al. 2012). Participants were randomized to receive usual care, in which physicians were asked not to change their routine counseling approach for obese persons, or participate in the behavioral intervention consisting of intensive individual counseling from health educators. The authors observed significant reductions in both body weight and WC in the intervention compared with usual care group. However, only changes in WC were sustained at 24 months in men, but not women. There were no significant changes at 24 months in any of the other cardiometabolic risk factors, including lipoproteins, glucose, and blood pressure in either men or women (Ross et al. 2012). This trial and others (Wadden et al. 2011) highlight the difficulty of maintaining long-term lifestyle changes, as well as the critical gaps in knowledge concerning the most effective way to sustain behavior change.

High-Intensity Interval Training and Cardiometabolic Health

While the current national PA guidelines recommending 150 minutes of moderate-to-vigorous-intensity PA per week are evidence based and widely promoted, the majority of the adult population does not meet these guidelines (Colley et al. 2011, Matthews et al. 2008). One prominent reason is perceived lack of time to perform the activity (Reichert et al. 2007). High-intensity interval training (HIIT), which consists of brief periods of high-intensity exercise interspersed by short recovery periods, offers a potential time-efficient alternative to continuous moderate endurance activity, as the time needed to expend the same amount of calories is lower at higher intensities (Gibala, Gillen, and Percival 2014).

Mounting evidence over the last three decades has illustrated the cardiometabolic health benefits of HIIT. Recently, Kessler et al. published a systematic review that discusses the impact of HIIT on individual cardiometabolic risk factors (Kessler, Sisson, and Short 2012). The authors observed a significant improvement in insulin sensitivity, as assessed by hyperinsulinemic–euglycemic clamp, the homeostasis model assessment of fasting glucose and insulin (HOMA-IR), and an OGTT after HIIT, in addition to a significant improvement in 2-hour glucose and glucose area under the curve in studies lasting between 2 and 24 weeks' duration (Kessler, Sisson, and Short 2012). In studies that compared the efficacy of HIIT to continuous moderate-intensity aerobic exercise, the authors found similar improvements in glucose metabolism variables. For serum lipids and lipoproteins, the authors found a limited effect of HIIT on TC, HDL-C, LDL-C, or TG in the majority of studies reviewed. HIIT lasting a minimum of 12 weeks significantly improved blood pressure in those participants not currently on antihypertensive medication, and the magnitude of reduction was similar to continuous moderate-intensity exercise. At least 12 weeks of HIIT was also found to be as effective as continuous exercise for improving anthropometric markers in overweight or obese individuals (Kessler, Sisson, and Short 2012). All of the preceding cardiometabolic benefits were observed with and without changes in body weight. This suggests that HIIT is effective for improving the majority of cardiometabolic risk factors to a similar extent as continuous exercise and offers individuals who cite lack of time as a reason for inactivity a potential solution to achieve their cardiometabolic health goals.

However, there are gaps in knowledge that require further investigation. There is great inconsistency in the protocols used in interventions studying HIIT. The mode (cycling or treadmill), duration of intervals and breaks, as well as intensity prescribed all varied significantly across studies. The optimal protocol has yet to be clarified. Furthermore, while proponents of HIIT cite time efficiency as a benefit, participating in HIIT protocols can take from 20 to 60 minutes including warm-up (Kessler, Sisson, and Short 2012). Therefore, whether performing HIIT provides a time efficiency benefit is unclear. Furthermore, whether sedentary, commonly overweight, or obese adults will sustain HIIT for extended periods is not known and requires further study.

SEDENTARY TIME AS AN INDEPENDENT RISK FACTOR FOR CHRONIC DISEASE

While there is strong and unequivocal evidence that higher levels of moderate-to-vigorous PA lead to considerable improvements in cardiometabolic health, more recently, great interest has focused on studying the health risks associated with sedentary behavior (Hamilton, Hamilton, and Zderic 2007, Spanier, Marshall, and Faulkner 2006). Sedentary behavior can be defined as "any waking behavior characterized by an energy expenditure <1.5 metabolic equivalents (METs) while in a sitting or reclining posture" (Sedentary Behaviour Research Network 2012).

With increased technological advances in the twenty-first century, opportunity to be sedentary has risen. Objective data show that North American adults participate in sedentary behavior

7.5–9.5 hours per day, making up 55%–69% of their waking hours (Colley et al. 2011, Matthews et al. 2008). This has prompted greater scientific inquiry into the independent effects of sedentary behavior as a unique risk factor for chronic disease.

Much of the evidence supporting sedentary behavior as an independent risk factor is based on epidemiological studies with varying degrees of quality. Few well-designed intervention trials exist that show a cause-and-effect relationship between sedentary behavior and health across the life span. Furthermore, until recently, many of the observed relationships between health and sedentary time were based on subjective measures of activity whose validity is often poor (Atkin et al. 2012). These methodological limitations preclude the identification of sedentary behavior as an independent risk factor for disease.

Sedentary Behavior and Health Risk

Examination of Epidemiological Evidence

Several recent systematic reviews and meta-analyses have summarized epidemiological evidence describing the association between self-reported sedentary behavior and risk for chronic disease, independent of moderate-to-vigorous PA, in multiple population subgroups (Biswas et al. 2015, de Rezende et al. 2014, Ekelund et al. 2012, Gardiner et al. 2011, Lee et al. 2012). Most studies report that increased sedentary time in adults is associated with increased risk for morbidity, including CVD and incidence of type 2 diabetes, and mortality (all-cause and CVD), in addition to increased prevalence of risk factors associated with disease (Lee et al. 2012). These observations are similar in older adults (de Rezende et al. 2014). However, in most studies, after adjusting for moderate-to-vigorous PA, the magnitude of the association between sedentary time and health risk is reduced, suggesting that moderate-to-vigorous PA levels are more important for determining health risk than sedentary time (Lee et al. 2012). While evidence points to a relationship between self-reported sedentary behavior and disease, investigations using objective measures of sedentary time are less consistent. For example, Healy et al. studied the independent associations of time spent in moderate-to-vigorous PA, sedentary time, and clustered metabolic risk cross-sectionally in 169 participants from the Australian Diabetes, Obesity and Lifestyle Study (Healy et al. 2008). There were significant independent associations between sedentary time, moderate-to-vigorous PA, and clustered metabolic risk score; however, these associations disappeared after adjustment for WC (Healy et al. 2008). It is reasonable to hypothesize that individuals who spend more time in sedentary behaviors are more likely to have a greater WC due to reduced energy expenditure. The preceding observations suggest that WC explains risk to a greater degree than sedentary time.

Recent evidence has questioned traditional statistical techniques used to study sedentary behavior and cardiometabolic health in epidemiological investigations (Chaput et al. 2014, Chastin et al. 2015, Pedišić 2014). By simply adjusting for moderate-to-vigorous PA statistically, we imply that these behaviors occur in isolation from one another (Pedišić 2014). However, PA, sedentary behavior, and sleep occur along a continuum and interact with each other to influence health (Chaput et al. 2014). For example, reducing one behavior (e.g., sedentary time) necessitates an increase in another behavior (light-to-vigorous activity), which may interact to influence risk factors for disease. Chastin et al. used compositional analysis to examine relationships between PA, sedentary behavior, and cardiometabolic risk factors (Chastin et al. 2015). This type of analysis considers the interaction and co-dependence of various components of the movement continuum. Using this type of analysis on the National Health and Nutritional Examination Survey data (N = 1937), the authors observed that the distribution of behaviors as a whole was significantly associated with WC, TG, plasma glucose and insulin, SBP, and DBP. The proportion of time spent in moderate-to-vigorous-intensity PA had a stronger effect size for the majority of cardiometabolic health markers compared to sedentary behavior or light-intensity PA. Furthermore, the strongest adverse effects on cardiometabolic health outcomes occurred when time spent in moderate-to-vigorous PA was replaced with sedentary time (Chastin et al. 2015). Overall, this important study indicates that movement behaviors are dependent on each other and the overall distribution pattern may be more important and informative than examining behaviors in isolation.

TABLE 6.4
Interventions Studying Sedentary Time and Cardiometabolic Risk

Reference	Participants	Study Design	Study Duration	Outcomes	Findings
Stephens et al. (2011)	Young (26 years), nonobese, fit men and women, N = 14	Three conditions completed by each participant: (1) Active, no sitting (high energy expenditure with energy intake matched) (NO-SIT) (2) Low energy expenditure with no reduction in energy intake (SIT) (3) Sitting with energy intake reduced to match low expenditure (SIT-BAL)	24 hours	Insulin action measured by continuous infusion of [6,6-^{2}H]-glucose	Compared to NO-SIT: SIT: Insulin action reduced by 39% ($p < 0.001$) SIT-BAL: Insulin action reduced by 18% ($p = 0.07$)
Lyden et al. (2015)	Recreationally active, young (35 years), normal weight, and overweight men and women, N = 10	7-day sedentary condition, instructed to sit as much as possible, limit standing/walking, refrain from structured exercise	7 days	Fasting lipids, glucose, and insulin OGTT at baseline and immediately after sedentary condition	2-hour plasma insulin and area under insulin curve significantly elevated No change in lipid concentration
Kozey Keadle et al. (2014)	Overweight/obese, middle-aged (44 years) men and women, N = 57	Participants randomly assigned to: (1) Exercise 5 days/week for 40 minutes/session at moderate intensity (EX) (2) Reduce sedentary time and increase nonexercise PA (rST) (3) Combination of EX and rST (4) Control	12 weeks	Fasting lipids, BP, BMI, 2-hour OGTT	EX and EX-rST decreased SBP EX-rST increased insulin sensitivity index by 17.8% and decreased insulin AUC by 19.4% rST reduced BP

Examination of Intervention Studies

While epidemiological evidence points to a relationship between sedentary behavior and risk for chronic disease, evidence from intervention studies that is important for uncovering cause-and-effect relationships is lacking. Inspection of Table 6.4 reveals that studies in humans are limited by their short duration and small sample sizes. For example, evidence suggests that one day of prolonged sitting reduced insulin action in 14 young, nonobese fit men and women. However, when energy intake was matched to energy expenditure, the adverse effects of sitting were attenuated, suggesting that positive energy balance and not just sitting per se impacts insulin action (Stephens et al. 2011). In previously active individuals, 2-hour plasma insulin and insulin area under the curve following an OGTT were significantly elevated following a sedentary condition lasting 7 days compared to baseline (Lyden et al. 2015).

Interventions of longer duration also show conflicting findings. After a 12-week intervention examining four sedentary time conditions (Table 6.4), exercise combined with reductions in sedentary time significantly increased cardiorespiratory fitness, decreased SBP, increased insulin sensitivity, and decreased insulin area under the curve, while the group who only reduced sedentary time saw improvements solely in blood pressure (Kozey Keadle et al. 2014). This suggests that reducing sedentary time alone, without increasing moderate-to-vigorous-intensity PA, is not effective for improving the majority of cardiometabolic risk factors.

Overall, there is a paucity of evidence from intervention studies that links increases in sedentary behavior to increased risk for disease, independent of moderate-to-vigorous PA. The majority of evidence that points to a relationship between sedentary behavior and risk for disease, independent of activity that meets the consensus guidelines, is observational in nature. This prevents the determination of cause and effect, which can only be determined by intervention trials that involve manipulation of sedentary behavior and measurement of subsequent health changes. The few existing intervention trials described earlier show inconsistent results. Well-designed RCTs testing whether reductions in sedentary time combined with exercise training improve cardiometabolic risk more than exercise training alone are necessary to determine cause and effect and examine potential mechanisms that can explain any observed relationship. The study design should be adequately powered to detect between-group differences, and study populations should include sedentary individuals with overweight or obesity. These studies are required to determine the strength of a relationship between sedentary behavior and risk for disease.

CONCLUSION

There is strong and unequivocal evidence that regular PA is associated with improvements in cardiometabolic health across a wide range of individual risk factors. Responses to exercise may differ according to sex, age, or ethnicity, and accounting for these important factors will be a critical aspect of future research in the field. The separate effects of increasing exercise amount or intensity on cardiometabolic risk factors are unclear. It appears that increasing exercise intensity results in greater improvements in insulin resistance only. The effect of increasing exercise amount for a fixed intensity is equivocal, with some studies suggesting greater improvement in cardiometabolic risk factors, including abdominal obesity, insulin resistance, and dyslipidemia, and others showing no effect. Additionally, while aerobic exercise results in greater improvements in all cardiometabolic risk factors, resistance exercise appears to be effective only for reducing abdominal obesity, insulin resistance in individuals with type 2 diabetes, and hypertension. Notably, current evidence points to sedentary behavior as a risk factor for suboptimal cardiometabolic health. Future research is needed to determine the independent effect of sedentary behavior and how the overall distribution of PA, sedentary behavior, and sleep influence health. Notwithstanding, it remains prudent for public health practitioners to advocate for increases in PA and reductions in sedentary time.

REFERENCES

Arroll, B. and R. Beaglehole. 1992. Does physical activity lower blood pressure: A critical review of the clinical trials. *J Clin Epidemiol* 45 (5):439–447.

Atkin, A. J., T. Gorely, S. A. Clemes, T. Yates, C. Edwardson, S. Brage, J. Salmon, S. J. Marshall, and S. J. Biddle. 2012. Methods of measurement in epidemiology: Sedentary behaviour. *Int J Epidemiol* 41 (5):1460–1471.

Bateman, L. A., C. A. Slentz, L. H. Willis, A. T. Shields, L. W. Piner, C. W. Bales, J. A. Houmard, and W. E. Kraus. 2011. Comparison of aerobic versus resistance exercise training effects on metabolic syndrome (from the Studies of a Targeted Risk Reduction Intervention Through Defined Exercise-STRRIDE-AT/RT). *Am J Cardiol* 108 (6):838–844.

Biswas, A., P. I. Oh, G. E. Faulkner, R. R. Bajaj, M. A. Silver, M. S. Mitchell, and D. A. Alter. 2015. Sedentary time and its association with risk for disease incidence, mortality, and hospitalization in adults: A systematic review and meta-analysis. *Ann Intern Med* 162 (2):123–132.

Boule, N. G., S. J. Weisnagel, T. A. Lakka, A. Tremblay, R. N. Bergman, T. Rankinen, A. S. Leon et al. 2005. Effects of exercise training on glucose homeostasis: The HERITAGE Family Study. *Diabetes Care* 28 (1):108–114.

Bounds, R. G., P. W. Grandjean, B. C. O'Brien, C. Inman, and S. F. Crouse. 2000. Diet and short term plasma lipoprotein-lipid changes after exercise in trained Men. *Int J Sport Nutr Exerc Metab* 10 (2):114–127.

Braith, R. W. and K. J. Stewart. 2006. Resistance exercise training: Its role in the prevention of cardiovascular disease. *Circulation* 113 (22):2642–2650.

Brandao Rondon, M. U., M. J. Alves, A. M. Braga, O. T. Teixeira, A. C. Barretto, E. M. Krieger, and C. E. Negrao. 2002. Postexercise blood pressure reduction in elderly hypertensive patients. *J Am Coll Cardiol* 39 (4):676–682.

Burstein, R., Y. Epstein, Y. Shapiro, I. Charuzi, and E. Karnieli. 1990. Effect of an acute bout of exercise on glucose disposal in human obesity. *J Appl Physiol (1985)* 69 (1):299–304.

Carroll, S. and M. Dudfield. 2004. What is the relationship between exercise and metabolic abnormalities? A review of the metabolic syndrome. *Sports Med* 34 (6):371–418.

Chaput, J.-P., V. Carson, C. E. Gray, and M. S. Tremblay. 2014. Importance of all movement behaviors in a 24 hour period for overall health. *Int J Environ Res Public Health* 11 (12):12575–12581.

Chastin, S. F. M., J. Palarea-Albaladejo, M. L. Dontje, and D. A. Skelton. 2015. Combined effects of time spent in physical activity, sedentary behaviors and sleep on obesity and cardio-metabolic health markers: A novel compositional data analysis approach. *PloS One* 10 (10):e0139984.

Chudyk, A. and R. J. Petrella. 2011. Effects of exercise on cardiovascular risk factors in type 2 diabetes: A meta-analysis. *Diabetes Care* 34 (5):1228–1237.

Church, T. S., S. N. Blair, S. Cocreham, N. Johannsen, W. Johnson, K. Kramer, C. R. Mikus et al. 2010. Effects of aerobic and resistance training on hemoglobin A1c levels in patients with type 2 diabetes: A randomized controlled trial. *JAMA* 304 (20):2253–2262.

Church, T. S., C. P. Earnest, J. S. Skinner, and S. N. Blair. 2007. Effects of different doses of physical activity on cardiorespiratory fitness among sedentary, overweight or obese postmenopausal women with elevated blood pressure: A randomized controlled trial. *JAMA* 297 (19):2081–2091.

Colley, R. C., D. Garriguet, I. Janssen, C. L. Craig, J. Clarke, and M. S. Tremblay. 2011. Physical activity of Canadian adults: Accelerometer results from the 2007 to 2009 Canadian Health Measures Survey. *Health Rep* 22 (1):7–14.

Cook, N. R., J. Cohen, P. R. Hebert, J. O. Taylor, and C. H. Hennekens. 1995. Implications of small reductions in diastolic blood pressure for primary prevention. *Arch Intern Med* 155 (7):701–709.

Cornelissen, V. A. and R. H. Fagard. 2005. Effects of endurance training on blood pressure, blood pressure-regulating mechanisms, and cardiovascular risk factors. *Hypertension* 46 (4):667–675.

Cornelissen, V. A., R. H. Fagard, E. Coeckelberghs, and L. Vanhees. 2011. Impact of resistance training on blood pressure and other cardiovascular risk factors: A meta-analysis of randomized, controlled trials. *Hypertension* 58 (5):950–958.

Cornelissen, V. A., B. Verheyden, A. E. Aubert, and R. H. Fagard. 2010. Effects of aerobic training intensity on resting, exercise and post-exercise blood pressure, heart rate and heart-rate variability. *J Hum Hypertens* 24 (3):175–182.

Crouse, S. F., B. C. O'Brien, P. W. Grandjean, R. C. Lowe, J. J. Rohack, and J. S. Green. 1997. Effects of training and a single session of exercise on lipids and apolipoproteins in hypercholesterolemic men. *J Appl Physiol (1985)* 83 (6):2019–2028.

Cullinane, E., S. Siconolfi, A. Saritelli, and P. D. Thompson. 1982. Acute decrease in serum triglycerides with exercise: Is there a threshold for an exercise effect? *Metabolism* 31 (8):844–847.

Davidson, L. E., R. Hudson, K. Kilpatrick, J. L. Kuk, K. McMillan, P. M. Janiszewski, S. Lee, M. Lam, and R. Ross. 2009. Effects of exercise modality on insulin resistance and functional limitation in older adults: A randomized controlled trial. *Arch Intern Med* 169 (2):122–131.

Dengel, D. R., R. E. Pratley, J. M. Hagberg, E. M. Rogus, and A. P. Goldberg. 1996. Distinct effects of aerobic exercise training and weight loss on glucose homeostasis in obese sedentary men. *J Appl Physiol (1985)* 81 (1):318–325.

de Rezende, L. F., J. P. Rey-Lopez, V. K. Matsudo, and O. do Carmo Luiz. 2014. Sedentary behavior and health outcomes among older adults: A systematic review. *BMC Public Health* 14:333.

Despres, J. P. and I. Lemieux. 2006. Abdominal obesity and metabolic syndrome. *Nature* 444 (7121):881–887.

Devlin, J. T., M. Hirshman, E. D. Horton, and E. S. Horton. 1987. Enhanced peripheral and splanchnic insulin sensitivity in NIDDM men after single bout of exercise. *Diabetes* 36 (4):434–439.

Donnelly, J. E., J. O. Hill, D. J. Jacobsen, J. Potteiger, D. K. Sullivan, S. L. Johnson, K. Heelan et al. 2003. Effects of a 16-month randomized controlled exercise trial on body weight and composition in young, overweight men and women: The Midwest Exercise Trial. *Arch Intern Med* 163 (11):1343–1350.

Dunstan, D. W., R. M. Daly, N. Owen, D. Jolley, M. De Courten, J. Shaw, and P. Zimmet. 2002. High-intensity resistance training improves glycemic control in older patients with type 2 diabetes. *Diabetes Care* 25 (10):1729–1736.

Durstine, J. L., P. W. Grandjean, P. G. Davis, M. A. Ferguson, N. L. Alderson, and K. D. DuBose. 2001. Blood lipid and lipoprotein adaptations to exercise. *Sports Med* 31 (15):1033–1062.

Ekelund, U., J. Luan, L. B. Sherar, D. W. Esliger, P. Griew, and A. Cooper. 2012. Moderate to vigorous physical activity and sedentary time and cardiometabolic risk factors in children and adolescents. *JAMA* 307 (7):704–712.

Eriksson, J., S. Taimela, K. Eriksson, S. Parviainen, J. Peltonen, and U. Kujala. 1997. Resistance training in the treatment of non-insulin-dependent diabetes mellitus. *Int J Sports Med* 18 (4):242–246.

Fagard, R. H. 1999. Physical activity in the prevention and treatment of hypertension in the obese. *Med Sci Sports Exerc* 31 (11 Suppl):S624–S630.

Ferland, M., J. P. Despres, A. Tremblay, S. Pinault, A. Nadeau, S. Moorjani, P. J. Lupien, G. Theriault, and C. Bouchard. 1989. Assessment of adipose tissue distribution by computed axial tomography in obese women: Association with body density and anthropometric measurements. *Br J Nutr* 61 (2):139–148.

Gan, S. K., A. D. Kriketos, B. A. Ellis, C. H. Thompson, E. W. Kraegen, and D. J. Chisholm. 2003. Changes in aerobic capacity and visceral fat but not myocyte lipid levels predict increased insulin action after exercise in overweight and obese men. *Diabetes Care* 26 (6):1706–1713.

Gardiner, P. A., G. N. Healy, E. G. Eakin, B. K. Clark, D. W. Dunstan, J. E. Shaw, P. Z. Zimmet, and N. Owen. 2011. Associations between television viewing time and overall sitting time with the metabolic syndrome in older men and women: The Australian Diabetes, Obesity and Lifestyle study. *J Am Geriatr Soc* 59 (5):788–796.

Gibala, M. J., J. B. Gillen, and M. E. Percival. 2014. Physiological and health-related adaptations to low-volume interval training: Influences of nutrition and sex. *Sports Med* 44 (Suppl 2):S127–S137.

Goodyear, L. J. and B. B. Kahn. 1998. Exercise, glucose transport, and insulin sensitivity. *Annu Rev Med* 49:235–261.

Grandjean, P. W., S. F. Crouse, and J. J. Rohack. 2000. Influence of cholesterol status on blood lipid and lipoprotein enzyme responses to aerobic exercise. *J Appl Physiol (1985)* 89 (2):472–480.

Gregg, E. W., R. B. Gerzoff, C. J. Caspersen, D. F. Williamson, and K. M. Narayan. 2003. Relationship of walking to mortality among US adults with diabetes. *Arch Intern Med* 163 (12):1440–1447.

Hagberg, J. M., J.-J. Park, and M. D. Brown. 2000. The role of exercise training in the treatment of hypertension. *Sports Med* 30 (3):193–206.

Hamilton, M. T., D. G. Hamilton, and T. W. Zderic. 2007. Role of low energy expenditure and sitting in obesity, metabolic syndrome, type 2 diabetes, and cardiovascular disease. *Diabetes* 56 (11):2655–2667.

Haskell, W. L., I. M. Lee, R. R. Pate, K. E. Powell, S. N. Blair, B. A. Franklin, C. A. Macera, G. W. Heath, P. D. Thompson, and A. Bauman. 2007. Physical activity and public health: Updated recommendation for adults from the American College of Sports Medicine and the American Heart Association. *Circulation* 116 (9):1081–1093.

Hawley, J. A. 2004. Exercise as a therapeutic intervention for the prevention and treatment of insulin resistance. *Diabetes Metab Res Rev* 20 (5):383–393.

Hawley, J. A. and S. J. Lessard. 2008. Exercise training-induced improvements in insulin action. *Acta Physiol (Oxf)* 192 (1):127–135.

He, J. and P. K. Whelton. 1999. Elevated systolic blood pressure and risk of cardiovascular and renal disease: Overview of evidence from observational epidemiologic studies and randomized controlled trials. *Am Heart J* 138 (3 Pt 2):211–219.

Healy, G. N., K. Wijndaele, D. W. Dunstan, J. E. Shaw, J. Salmon, P. Z. Zimmet, and N. Owen. 2008. Objectively measured sedentary time, physical activity, and metabolic risk: The Australian Diabetes, Obesity and Lifestyle Study (AusDiab). *Diabetes Care* 31 (2):369–371.

Henriksen, E. J. 2002. Invited review: Effects of acute exercise and exercise training on insulin resistance. *J Appl Physiol (1985)* 93 (2):788–796.

Ho, S. S., S. S. Dhaliwal, A. P. Hills, and S. Pal. 2012. The effect of 12 weeks of aerobic, resistance or combination exercise training on cardiovascular risk factors in the overweight and obese in a randomized trial. *BMC Public Health* 12 (1):1.

Holoszy, J. O., J. S. Skinner, G. Toro, and T. J. Cureton. 1965. Effects of a six month program of endurance on the serum lipids of middle-aged men. *J Occup Environ Med* 7 (10):540.

Honkola, A., T. Forsen, and J. Eriksson. 1997. Resistance training improves the metabolic profile in individuals with type 2 diabetes. *Acta Diabetol* 34 (4):245–248.

Horton, E. S. 2009. Effects of lifestyle changes to reduce risks of diabetes and associated cardiovascular risks: Results from large scale efficacy trials. *Obesity (Silver Spring)* 17 (Suppl 3):S43–S48.

Howard, B. V., E. J. Mayer-Davis, D. Goff, D. J. Zaccaro, A. Laws, D. C. Robbins, M. F. Saad et al. 1998. Relationships between insulin resistance and lipoproteins in nondiabetic African Americans, Hispanics, and non-Hispanic whites: The Insulin Resistance Atherosclerosis Study. *Metabolism* 47 (10):1174–1179.

Irwin, M. L., Y. Yasui, C. M. Ulrich, D. Bown, R. E. Rudolph, R. S. Schwartz, M. Yukawa, E. Ajello, J. D. Potter, and A. McTiernan. 2003. Effect of exercise on total and intra-abdominal body fat in postmenopausal women: A randomized controlled trial. *JAMA* 289:323–330.

Ismail, I., S. E. Keating, M. K. Baker, and N. A. Johnson. 2012. A systematic review and meta-analysis of the effect of aerobic vs. resistance exercise training on visceral fat. *Obes Rev* 13 (1):68–91.

Ivy, J. L. 1997. Role of exercise training in the prevention and treatment of insulin resistance and non-insulin-dependent diabetes mellitus. *Sports Med* 24 (5):321–336.

Janiszewski, P. M., I. Janssen, and R. Ross. 2007. Does waist circumference predict diabetes and cardiovascular disease beyond commonly evaluated cardiometabolic risk factors? *Diabetes Care* 30 (12):3105–3109.

Katzmarzyk, P. T., A. S. Leon, T. Rankinen, J. Gagnon, J. S. Skinner, J. H. Wilmore, D. C. Rao, and C. Bouchard. 2001. Changes in blood lipids consequent to aerobic exercise training related to changes in body fatness and aerobic fitness. *Metabolism* 50 (7):841–848.

Keating, S. E., D. A. Hackett, H. M. Parker, H. T. O'Connor, J. A. Gerofi, A. Sainsbury, M. K. Baker et al. 2015. Effect of aerobic exercise training dose on liver fat and visceral adiposity. *J Hepatol* 63 (1):174–182.

Kelley, G. A. 1995. Effects of aerobic exercise in normotensive adults: A brief meta-analytic review of controlled clinical trials. *South Med J* 88 (1):42–46.

Kelley, G. A. and K. S. Kelley. 1999. Aerobic exercise and resting blood pressure in women: A meta-analytic review of controlled clinical trials. *J Womens Health Gend Based Med* 8 (6):787–803.

Kelley, G. A. and K. S. Kelley. 2000. Progressive resistance exercise and resting blood pressure a meta-analysis of randomized controlled trials. *Hypertension* 35 (3):838–843.

Kelley, G. A. and K. S. Kelley. 2009. Impact of progressive resistance training on lipids and lipoproteins in adults: A meta-analysis of randomized controlled trials. *Prev Med* 48 (1):9–19.

Kelley, G. A., K. S. Kelley, S. Roberts, and W. Haskell. 2011. Efficacy of aerobic exercise and a prudent diet for improving selected lipids and lipoproteins in adults: A meta-analysis of randomized controlled trials. *BMC Med* 9:74.

Kenney, M. J. and D. R. Seals. 1993. Postexercise hypotension. Key features, mechanisms, and clinical significance. *Hypertension* 22 (5):653–664.

Kessler, H. S., S. B. Sisson, and K. R. Short. 2012. The potential for high-intensity interval training to reduce cardiometabolic disease risk. *Sports Med* 42 (6):489–509.

Kohrt, W. M., M. T. Malley, A. R. Coggan, R. J. Spina, T. Ogawa, A. A. Ehsani, R. E. Bourey, W. H. Martin, 3rd, and J. O. Holloszy. 1991. Effects of gender, age, and fitness level on response of VO2max to training in 60–71 yr olds. *J Appl Physiol (1985)* 71 (5):2004–2011.

Kokkinos, P. and J. Myers. 2010. Exercise and physical activity clinical outcomes and applications. *Circulation* 122 (16):1637–1648.

Koopman, R., R. J. Manders, A. H. Zorenc, G. B. Hul, H. Kuipers, H. A. Keizer, and L. J. van Loon. 2005. A single session of resistance exercise enhances insulin sensitivity for at least 24 h in healthy men. *Eur J Appl Physiol* 94 (1–2):180–187.

Kozey Keadle, S., K. Lyden, J. Staudenmayer, A. Hickey, R. Viskochil, B. Braun, and P. S. Freedson. 2014. The independent and combined effects of exercise training and reducing sedentary behavior on cardiometabolic risk factors. *Appl Physiol Nutr Metab* 39 (7):770–780.

Kraus, W. E., J. A. Houmard, B. D. Duscha, K. J. Knetzger, M. B. Wharton, J. S. McCartney, C. W. Bales, S. Henes, G. P. Samsa, and J. D. Otvos. 2002. Effects of the amount and intensity of exercise on plasma lipoproteins. *N Engl J Med* 347 (19):1483–1492.

Krauss, R. M. 2014. All low-density lipoprotein particles are not created equal. *Arterioscler Thromb Vasc Biol* 34 (5):959–961.

Lee, I. M., E. J. Shiroma, F. Lobelo, P. Puska, S. N. Blair, and P. T. Katzmarzyk. 2012. Effect of physical inactivity on major non-communicable diseases worldwide: An analysis of burden of disease and life expectancy. *Lancet* 380 (9838):219–229.

Lehto, S., T. Rönnemaa, S. M. Haffher, K. Pyörälä, V. Kallio, and M. Laakso. 1997. Dyslipidemia and hyperglycemia predict coronary heart disease events in middle-aged patients with NIDDM. *Diabetes* 46 (8):1354–1359.

Leon, A. S., S. E. Gaskill, T. Rice, J. Bergeron, J. Gagnon, D. C. Rao, J. S. Skinner, J. H. Wilmore, and C. Bouchard. 2002. Variability in the response of HDL cholesterol to exercise training in the HERITAGE Family Study. *Int J Sports Med* 23 (1):1–9.

Leon, A. S. and O. A. Sanchez. 2001. Response of blood lipids to exercise training alone or combined with dietary intervention. *Med Sci Sports Exerc* 33 (6 Suppl):S502–S515.

Lyden, K., S. K. Keadle, J. Staudenmayer, B. Braun, and P. S. Freedson. 2015. Discrete features of sedentary behavior impact cardiometabolic risk factors. *Med Sci Sports Exerc* 47 (5):1079–1086.

Mann, S., C. Beedie, S. Balducci, S. Zanuso, J. Allgrove, F. Bertiato, and A. Jimenez. 2014. Changes in insulin sensitivity in response to different modalities of exercise: A review of the evidence. *Diabetes Metab Res Rev* 30 (4):257–268.

Manning, J. M., C. R. Dooly-Manning, K. White, I. Kampa, S. Silas, M. Kesselhaut, and M. Ruoff. 1991. Effects of a resistive training program on lipoprotein—Lipid levels in obese women. *Med Sci Sports Exerc* 23 (11):1222–1226.

Manson, J. E., P. Greenland, A. Z. LaCroix, M. L. Stefanick, C. P. Mouton, A. Oberman, M. G. Perri, D. S. Sheps, M. B. Pettinger, and D. S. Siscovick. 2002. Walking compared with vigorous exercise for the prevention of cardiovascular events in women. *N Engl J Med* 347 (10):716–725.

Matthews, C. E., K. Y. Chen, P. S. Freedson, M. S. Buchowski, B. M. Beech, R. R. Pate, and R. P. Troiano. 2008. Amount of time spent in sedentary behaviors in the United States, 2003–2004. *Am J Epidemiol* 167 (7):875–881.

Mikines, K. J., B. Sonne, P. A. Farrell, B. Tronier, and H. Galbo. 1988. Effect of physical exercise on sensitivity and responsiveness to insulin in humans. *Am J Physiol* 254 (3 Pt 1):E248–E259.

Mourier, A., J. F. Gautier, E. De Kerviler, A. X. Bigard, J. M. Villette, J. P. Garnier, A. Duvallet, C. Y. Guezennec, and G. Cathelineau. 1997. Mobilization of visceral adipose tissue related to the improvement in insulin sensitivity in response to physical training in NIDDM. Effects of branched-chain amino acid supplements. *Diabetes Care* 20 (3):385–391.

Ohkawara, K., S. Tanaka, M. Miyachi, K. Ishikawa-Takata, and I. Tabata. 2007. A dose–response relation between aerobic exercise and visceral fat reduction: Systematic review of clinical trials. *Int J Obes* 31 (12):1786–1797.

Pedišić, Ž. 2014. Measurement issues and poor adjustments for physical activity and sleep undermine sedentary behaviour research—The focus should shift to the balance between sleep, sedentary behaviour, standing and activity. *Kinesiology* 46 (1):135–146.

Perseghin, G., T. B. Price, K. F. Petersen, M. Roden, G. W. Cline, K. Gerow, D. L. Rothman, and G. I. Shulman. 1996. Increased glucose transport-phosphorylation and muscle glycogen synthesis after exercise training in insulin-resistant subjects. *N Engl J Med* 335 (18):1357–1362.

Pescatello, L. S., B. Miller, P. G. Danias, M. Werner, M. Hess, C. Baker, and M. Jane De Souza. 1999. Dynamic exercise normalizes resting blood pressure in mildly hypertensive premenopausal women. *Am Heart J* 138 (5 Pt 1):916–921.

Pouliot, M. C., J. P. Despres, S. Lemieux, S. Moorjani, C. Bouchard, A. Tremblay, A. Nadeau, and P. J. Lupien. 1994. Waist circumference and abdominal sagittal diameter: Best simple anthropometric indexes of abdominal visceral adipose tissue accumulation and related cardiovascular risk in men and women. *Am J Cardiol* 73 (7):460–468.

Ready, A. E., D. T. Drinkwater, J. Ducas, D. W. Fitzpatrick, D. G. Brereton, and S. C. Oades. 1995. Walking program reduces elevated cholesterol in women postmenopause. *Can J Cardiol* 11 (10):905–912.

Reichert, F. F., A. J. Barros, M. R. Domingues, and P. C. Hallal. 2007. The role of perceived personal barriers to engagement in leisure-time physical activity. *Am J Public Health* 97 (3):515–519.

Ross, R., D. Dagnone, P. J. Jones, H. Smith, A. Paddags, R. Hudson, and I. Janssen. 2000. Reduction in obesity and related comorbid conditions after diet-induced weight loss or exercise-induced weight loss in men. A randomized, controlled trial. *Ann Intern Med* 133 (2):92–103.

Ross, R., R. Hudson, P. J. Stotz, M. Lam. 2015. Effects of exercise amount and intensity on abdominal obesity and glucose tolerance in obese adults. A randomized controlled trial. *Ann Intern Med* 162 (5):325–344.

Ross, R., I. Janssen, J. Dawson, A. M. Kungl, J. L. Kuk, S. L. Wong, T. B. Nguyen-Duy, S. Lee, K. Kilpatrick, and R. Hudson. 2004. Exercise-induced reduction in obesity and insulin resistance in women: A randomized controlled trial. *Obes Res* 12 (5):789–798.

Ross, R., M. Lam, S. N. Blair, T. S. Church, M. Godwin, S. B. Hotz, A. Johnson, P. T. Katzmarzyk, L. Levesque, and S. MacDonald. 2012. Trial of prevention and reduction of obesity through active living in clinical settings: A randomized controlled trial. *Arch Intern Med* 172 (5):414–424.

Ross, R., L. Leger, D. Morris, J. de Guise, and R. Guardo. 1992. Quantification of adipose tissue by MRI: Relationship with anthropometric variables. *J Appl Physiol* 72 (2):787–795.

Rueckert, P. A., P. R. Slane, D. L. Lillis, and P. Hanson. 1996. Hemodynamic patterns and duration of post-dynamic exercise hypotension in hypertensive humans. *Med Sci Sports Exerc* 28 (1):24–32.

Sedentary Behaviour Research Network. 2012. Letter to the editor: Standardized use of the terms "sedentary" and "sedentary behaviours". *Appl Physiol Nutr Metab* 37 (3):540–542.

Shiroma, E. J. and I. M. Lee. 2010. Physical activity and cardiovascular health: Lessons learned from epidemiological studies across age, gender, and race/ethnicity. *Circulation* 122 (7):743–752.

Sigal, R. J., G. P. Kenny, N. G. Boule, G. A. Wells, D. Prud'homme, M. Fortier, R. D. Reid et al. 2007. Effects of aerobic training, resistance training, or both on glycemic control in type 2 diabetes: A randomized trial. *Ann Intern Med* 147 (6):357–369.

Slentz, C. A., L. B. Aiken, J. A. Houmard, C. W. Bales, J. L. Johnson, C. J. Tanner, B. D. Duscha, and W. E. Kraus. 2005. Inactivity, exercise, and visceral fat. STRRIDE: A randomized, controlled study of exercise intensity and amount. *J Appl Physiol* 99 (4):1613–1618.

Smutok, M. A., C. Reece, P. F. Kokkinos, C. Farmer, P. Dawson, R. Shulman, J. DeVane-Bell, J. Patterson, C. Charabogos, and A. P. Goldberg. 1993. Aerobic versus strength training for risk factor intervention in middle-aged men at high risk for coronary heart disease. *Metabolism* 42 (2):177–184.

Spanier, P. A., S. J. Marshall, and G. E. Faulkner. 2006. Tackling the obesity pandemic: A call for sedentary behaviour research. *Can J Public Health* 97 (3):255–257.

Stefanick, M. L. 1999. Physical activity for preventing and treating obesity-related dyslipoproteinemias. *Med Sci Sports Exerc* 31 (11 Suppl):S609–S618.

Stensvold, D., A. E. Tjonna, E. A. Skaug, S. Aspenes, T. Stolen, U. Wisloff, and S. A. Slordahl. 2010. Strength training versus aerobic interval training to modify risk factors of metabolic syndrome. *J Appl Physiol (1985)* 108 (4):804–810.

Stephens, B. R., K. Granados, T. W. Zderic, M. T. Hamilton, and B. Braun. 2011. Effects of 1 day of inactivity on insulin action in healthy men and women: Interaction with energy intake. *Metabolism* 60 (7):941–949.

Swain, D. P. and B. A. Franklin. 2006. Comparison of cardioprotective benefits of vigorous versus moderate intensity aerobic exercise. *Am J Cardiol* 97 (1):141–147.

Thomas, E. L., A. E. Brynes, J. McCarthy, A. P. Goldstone, J. V. Hajnal, N. Saeed, G. Frost, and J. D. Bell. 2000. Preferential loss of visceral fat following aerobic exercise, measured by magnetic resonance imaging. *Lipids* 35 (7):769–776.

Thompson, P. D., S. F. Crouse, B. Goodpaster, D. Kelley, N. Moyna, and L. Pescatello. 2001. The acute versus the chronic response to exercise. *Med Sci Sports Exerc* 33 (6 Suppl):S438–S445; discussion S452–S453.

Tremblay, M. S., D. E. Warburton, I. Janssen, D. H. Paterson, A. E. Latimer, R. E. Rhodes, M. E. Kho et al. 2011. New Canadian physical activity guidelines. *Appl Physiol Nutr Metab* 36 (1):36–46; 47–58.

Tresierras, M. A. and G. J. Balady. 2009. Resistance training in the treatment of diabetes and obesity: Mechanisms and outcomes. *J Cardiopulm Rehabil Prev* 29 (2):67–75.

Vague, J. 1956. The degree of masculine differentiation of obesities a factor determining predisposition to diabetes, atherosclerosis, gout, and uric calculous disease. *Am J Clin Nutr* 4 (1):20–34.

Vissers, D., W. Hens, J. Taeymans, J.-P. Baeyens, J. Poortmans, and L. V. Gaal. 2013. The effect of exercise on visceral adipose tissue in overweight adults: A systematic review and meta-analysis. *PloS One* 8 (2):e56415.

Wadden, T. A., S. Volger, D. B. Sarwer, M. L. Vetter, A. G. Tsai, R. I. Berkowitz, S. Kumanyika et al. 2011. A two-year randomized trial of obesity treatment in primary care practice. *N Engl J Med* 365 (21):1969–1979.

Watkins, L. L., A. Sherwood, M. Feinglos, A. Hinderliter, M. Babyak, E. Gullette, R. Waugh, and J. A. Blumenthal. 2003. Effects of exercise and weight loss on cardiac risk factors associated with syndrome X. *Arch Intern Med* 163 (16):1889–1895.

Whelton, S. P., A. Chin, X. Xin, and J. He. 2002. Effect of aerobic exercise on blood pressure: A meta-analysis of randomized, controlled trials. *Ann Intern Med* 136 (7):493–503.

7 Diet as a Potential Modulator of Body Fat Distribution

Sofia Laforest, Geneviève B. Marchand, and André Tchernof

CONTENTS

ABSTRACT

Abdominal obesity has been reported to be more closely related to cardiometabolic risk than excess adiposity *per se*. Specifically, high abdominal fat accumulation, especially in the visceral depot, is closely linked to metabolic abnormalities such as insulin resistance and hypertriglyceridemia, whereas for a similar body fat mass, subcutaneous fat accretion seems to confer a neutral/protective effect. Mechanisms regulating body fat distribution are complex and remain poorly understood. We reviewed the potential contribution of dietary components on body fat distribution independent of body weight and total adiposity. Types and amounts of fat, carbohydrates and glycemic load, proteins, as well as specific food components with bioactive functions that could affect fat accretion were examined in detail. According to available literature, there is no concrete evidence that a single nutrient directly modulates visceral fat accretion and, by extension, body fat distribution. Most available studies on diet and body fat distribution seem to point toward a nonspecific effect on total fat accumulation. Yet, some studies identified dietary components potentially linked to a detrimental fat accretion pattern (increased visceral/abdominal fat or waist circumference), including fructose, especially in the form of sugar-sweetened beverages, *trans* fatty acids, as well as high alcohol intake and refined/fast-food diets.

ABBREVIATIONS

25(OH)D	25-Hydroxyvitamin D
aP2	Adipocyte Protein 2
BCAA	Branched-chain amino acids
BCKD	Branched-chain α-keto acid dehydrogenase
BMI	Body mass index
C/EBPα	CCAAT/enhancer-binding protein alpha
CI	Confidence interval
CLA	Conjugated linoleic acid
CT	Computed tomography
DHA	Docosahexaenoic acid
DXA	Dual-energy X-ray absorptiometry
EPA	Eicosapentaenoic acid
FA	Fatty acids
GI	Glycemic index
GL	Glycemic load
GLUT4	Glucose transporter type 4
HC	Hip circumference
hsCRP	High-sensitivity C-reactive protein
LCT	Long-chain triglycerides
LPL	Lipoprotein lipase
MCT	Medium-chain triglycerides
MD	Mediterranean diet
MEDS	Mediterranean score
MRI	Magnetic resonance imaging
MUFA	Monounsaturated fatty acids
NF-κB	Nuclear factor-kappa B
PPARγ	Peroxisome proliferator-activated receptor gamma
PUFA	Polyunsaturated fatty acids
SAT	Subcutaneous adipose tissue
SFA	Saturated fatty acids
SMD	Standard mean difference
SSB	Sugar-sweetened beverages
TNFα	Tumor necrosis factor alpha
VAT	Visceral adipose tissue
WC	Waist circumference
WHR	Waist-to-hip ratio
WMD	Weighted mean difference

INTRODUCTION

Obese individuals have an increased risk of developing coronary heart disease, hypertension, type 2 diabetes, and several types of cancers (reviewed in Haslam and James (2005)). However, the risk of developing these conditions is closely related to body fat distribution patterns. More specifically, numerous studies now support the notion that excess visceral adipose tissue (VAT) accumulation is more closely related to alterations in cardiometabolic health, whereas for any given level of total adiposity, preferential subcutaneous adipose tissue (SAT) accumulation has protective or neutral effects (reviewed in Tchernof and Després (2013)). Molecular mechanisms affecting lipid storage sites have not yet been completely elucidated. Hormones, genetic or epigenetic factors, and possibly diet may all partly contribute to human body fat distribution patterns (Berry et al. 2013).

This chapter reviews scientific evidence on the modulation of body fat distribution, with visceral fat accumulation as the key indicator, by dietary factors such as macronutrients, food patterns, and other particular nutrients or food items. The major question to be addressed is whether nutritional factors can specifically modulate body fat distribution patterns or visceral fat accumulation beyond what could be accomplished solely by modulating energy intake and total body fat stores.

We have reviewed articles found in the PubMed database with search terms related to fat accumulation: body fat distribution, peripheral adiposity, visceral fat, abdominal fat, subcutaneous fat, and body composition. They were individually combined with nutritional keywords such as lipids, carbohydrates, proteins, diet, nutrients, and nutrition. A total of 224 journal articles were kept after removing duplicates. The articles were selected depending on the following specific criteria: (1) emphasis was placed on human studies; and (2) body fat distribution had to be measured by computed tomography (CT), magnetic resonance imaging (MRI), dual-energy X-ray absorptiometry (DXA), ultrasound, or waist and/or hip circumference (WC/HC). Reviews were excluded. Systematic reviews and meta-analyses were included. Relevant articles from the reference list of identified papers were added. In total, 170 studies were retained.

MACRONUTRIENTS AND THEIR RELEVANCE FOR BODY FAT DISTRIBUTION

LIPIDS

Types of Fatty Acids

Fatty acids (FA) are often classified into three broad groups, namely, saturated fatty acids (SFA), monounsaturated fatty acids (MUFA), and polyunsaturated fatty acids (PUFA). In the typical Western diet, C4 to C18 are the major SFA. They are found primarily in animal foods and oils derived from tropical fruits. MUFA are generally associated with the Mediterranean diet (MD) (see the section "Mediterranean Diet") considering that oleic acid, the major component of olive oil, is the primary MUFA in this common diet. Nuts (almonds, pecans, peanuts, cashew nuts) are also rich in MUFA. PUFA comprise a large group, including the essential FA that are, linoleic (C18:2n-6) and linolenic (C18:3n-3) acids. PUFA also refer to n-3 FA such as eicosapentaenoic acid (EPA) and docosahexaenoic acid (DHA). PUFA can be found in corn oil, sunflower oil, and seafood. *Trans* FA, usually formed by commercial incomplete hydrogenation of MUFA, are also a component of the Western diet and are known to increase cardiovascular disease risk (Mozaffarian et al. 2006).

Larson et al. reported a positive association of body fat mass with total fat, SFA, MUFA, as well as PUFA intake independent of nonfat energy intake in men and women (Larson et al. 1996). In regression analyses, SFA intake was a better predictor of body fat mass than total fat intake. VAT and SAT areas, adjusted for nonfat energy intake, were positively associated with total fat, SFA, and MUFA (Larson et al. 1996). All these associations became nonsignificant when the authors adjusted for total body fat mass (Larson et al. 1996). Their results suggest no apparent association between the FA content of the diet and body fat distribution.

In a longitudinal study in African-Americans and Hispanic-Americans, intake of SFA, MUFA, and PUFA was not associated with 5-year changes in VAT or SAT area (Hairston et al. 2012). Consistent with these results, data from a Danish cohort followed for 5 years failed to show an association between the change in WC, a surrogate measure of VAT, and total intake of fat (Halkjaer et al. 2006). In a randomized crossover study with overweight men, fat mass in both the trunk and limbs was increased in the SFA diet group and decreased in the MUFA diet group after 4 weeks, without differences in total energy intake (Piers et al. 2003). Replacement of PUFA or carbohydrates by *trans* FA increased WC in men during a 9-year follow-up, whereas there was no difference when the substitution was done with SFA or MUFA (Koh-Banerjee et al. 2003). Forouhi and collaborators found no association between intake of SFA, MUFA, or PUFA and WC (Forouhi et al. 2009). In a randomized 1-year control trial, participants were provided low-fat dietary advice from dieticians and half received 30 g of walnuts per day to increase their consumption of PUFA (Tapsell et al. 2009). Compliance was monitored by a validated diet history interview, 3-day food records coupled with an analysis of erythrocyte FA composition. The control group preferentially lost VAT at 3 months while the walnut group lost SAT (Tapsell et al. 2009). There was a trend ($p = 0.08$) at baseline for a higher SAT area in the walnut group, which can partially explain this difference (Tapsell et al. 2009). At 12 months, the walnut group had lost more body fat than the control group, but the difference did not reach statistical significance (Tapsell et al. 2009).

Taken together, the earlier mentioned studies suggest that the link between FA composition of the diet and abdominal or visceral fat accretion seems to be mediated by its association with overall adiposity levels.

Medium-Chain Triglycerides vs. Long-Chain Triglycerides

Medium-chain triglycerides (MCT) have unique properties that distinguish them from long-chain triglycerides (LCT). These characteristics seem to confer beneficial metabolic effects. MCT, after cleavage to glycerol and FA, are transported directly to the liver by the portal vein, bypassing incorporation into chylomicrons and the lymphatic system (Poppitt et al. 2010). Unlike LCT, the MCT do not require the carnitine acyltransferase enzyme to be incorporated into the mitochondria, allowing more rapid β-oxidation, a phenomenon that has been linked with greater energy expenditure and less weight gain (Bach and Babayan 1982). MCT may also increase satiety after a meal (Van Wymelbeke et al. 1998, Krotkiewski 2001, Poppitt et al. 2010). Generally, MCT comprise FA from 6 to 10 and even 12 carbons, since lauric acid (C12:0), structurally classified as an LCT, shows properties that are similar to caprylic (C8:0) and capric (C10:0) acids. MCT are found primarily in vegetable oils such as coconut (71%) and palm kernel (48%) (Health Canada 2010).

Many studies have been conducted to elucidate the effect of LCT replacement by MCT on body weight, body fat mass, WC, SAT, and VAT. Bueno and collaborators, in a recent meta-analysis, found that replacement of LCT by MCT (at least 5 g) in six randomized control trials reduces WC in both men and women (weighted mean difference [WMD]: −1.78 cm [95% confidence interval {CI}, −2.4 to −1.1]) (Bueno et al. 2015). In another meta-analysis, a similar result was reported for WC (WMD: −1.46 cm [95% CI, −2.04 to −0.87]) (Mumme and Stonehouse 2015). In addition, total SAT and VAT were also investigated. Replacement of LCT by MCT (between <1% and 24% of energy intake) in the diet led to a moderate loss of both SAT and VAT (standard mean difference [SMD]: −0.46 [95% CI, −0.64 to −0.27] and −0.55 [95% CI, −0.75 to −0.34], respectively), suggesting a greater loss of VAT in these trials. Overall, these results strongly suggest that consumption of MCT may be favorable, not only for body composition, but also toward healthier body fat distribution. Further studies are needed to confirm the relationship between MCT and reduced VAT area independent of other adiposity measurements.

n-3 Fatty Acids

Consumption of n-3 FA, namely, EPA and DHA, found principally in fatty fish and components of the MD (see the section "Mediterranean Diet") has been linked with improvements in insulin resistance and cardiovascular risk factors (Wang et al. 2006, Li 2015). Preliminary results from animal studies showed possible beneficial effects, independent of body weight. In rats, 7 weeks of a diet with 17.4% EPA and 10.1% DHA (% of total FA) reduced VAT accumulation with no difference in body weight compared to lard-fed rats (high-fat regimen used as control) (Rokling-Andersen et al. 2009). In human studies, some authors found that supplements of EPA/DHA reduce WC (Kunesova et al. 2006, Thorsdottir et al. 2007, Bays et al. 2009, DeFina et al. 2011, Crochemore et al. 2012, Munro and Garg 2012, 2013, Bender et al. 2014). In a group of 30 Japanese men and women with coronary heart disease, a supplement of 1800 mg administered over 6 months decreased SAT and VAT assessed by CT, but only the latter was also associated with the expected increase of plasma EPA level (Sato et al. 2014). However, the effect of n-3 FA was not reported to be independent of changes in body weight and fat mass in the earlier mentioned studies. Further studies are needed to confirm their effect on body fat distribution in humans.

Conjugated Linoleic Acid

Conjugated linoleic acid (CLA) supplements have been of interest following reports of their anticancer and anti-inflammatory properties as well as a potential role in modulating body fat mass (Pariza 2004, Silveira et al. 2007). CLA occurs naturally and is found primarily in ruminant meat and dairy products (Steinhart, Rickert, and Winkler 2003). It is synthetically produced from sunflower and safflower oils in supplements (Pariza, Park, and Cook 2001). The estimated daily intake of CLA is 0.36 g/day for women and 0.43 g/day for men, according to the German Nutrition Study (Steinhart, Rickert, and Winkler 2003). CLA comprises a group of 28 isomers that present two conjugated *cis* or *trans* dienes, primarily on positions C9 and C11 or C10 and C12. CLA is well absorbed in free FA form or as digested triglycerides when compared to ethyl ester (Fernie et al. 2004). Poor palatability was reported when CLA was ingested as free FA (Fernie et al. 2004). CLA has multiple effects on adipose tissue metabolism. It has been linked to decreased fat cell size and preadipocyte proliferation (Tsuboyama-Kasaoka et al. 2000, Evans, Brown, and McIntosh 2002, Brown and McIntosh 2003). Other reports showed adverse effects of CLA such as a decrease of preadipocyte differentiation via reduced peroxisome proliferator-activated receptor gamma (PPARγ) and CCAAT/enhancer-binding protein alpha activity C/EBPα (Brown et al. 2003, Kang et al. 2003), and activation of the nuclear factor-kappa B (NF-κB) pathway and subsequent expression of tumor necrosis factor alpha (TNFα) (Chung et al. 2005). Impaired insulin signaling after CLA supplementation was also reported in animal models and was linked to the impact of TNFα on the expression of key adipogenic genes such as glucose transporter type 4 (GLUT-4), lipoprotein lipase (LPL), and adipocyte Protein 2 (aP2) (Chung et al. 2005). Reports (Evans, Brown, and McIntosh 2002) suggested differential effects of the two most studied CLA isomers, *trans*10*cis*12 and *cis*9*trans*11, the latter being associated with body composition (reduction in body fat and increase of lean body mass) and the other with anticarcinogenic properties.

Some studies reported significant weight loss with CLA supplements (range, 0.59–6.8 g/day) and a fat-free mass increase (Blankson et al. 2000, Smedman and Vessby 2001, Gaullier et al. 2004, 2007, Syvertsen et al. 2007, Watras et al. 2007), while others found no effect (Berven et al. 2000, Zambell et al. 2000, Benito et al. 2001, Mougios et al. 2001, Kreider et al. 2002, Malpuech-Brugere et al. 2004, Moloney et al. 2004, Tricon et al. 2004, Whigham et al. 2004, Taylor et al. 2006, Joseph et al. 2011). WC was not significantly reduced in a meta-analysis of randomized control trials on CLA supplementation (including 534 subjects) over at least 6 months of treatment (Onakpoya et al. 2012). Accordingly, in a randomized control trial following women with the metabolic syndrome on a hypocaloric diet, women taking placebo reduced their WC, whereas women receiving CLA supplements did not (Carvalho, Uehara, and Rosa 2012). Earlier fat loss occurred in women taking the CLA supplement. However, final body fat loss was similar at the end of the 14-week trial (Carvalho, Uehara, and Rosa 2012). In obese women supplemented with 3.4 g/day of CLA, Gaullier and collaborators noted a decrease in waist-to-hip ratio (WHR) and observed that fat loss was primarily due to loss of leg fat and not abdominal fat (Gaullier et al. 2007). No change in WC was observed in another randomized control trial involving overweight and obese men and women supplemented with 3 g of CLA during 12 weeks (Laso et al. 2007). However, the investigators reported a trend toward reduced trunk fat mass assessed by DXA in the overweight group only (Laso et al. 2007). In overweight and obese men, no differences were observed in CT-assessed VAT and SAT areas after a 4-week supplementation with ~2.6 g CLA/day (Desroches et al. 2005). Similar results were obtained in men following a resistance training program, where VAT loss was not related to CLA supplementation (Adams et al. 2006).

Hence, some but not all studies show that CLA may induce fat loss, possibly by increasing lipolysis and apoptosis in adipose tissue (Pariza 2004). However, data are lacking regarding the capacity of naturally found CLA to modulate body fat distribution toward a healthier pattern. In fact, studies previously discussed used supplements including 0.59 up to 6.8 g of CLA, which is 1.3–14 times greater than general daily intake (Steinhart, Rickert, and Winkler 2003). Studies are also needed to assess the safety of CLA supplements, particularly in individuals at risk for type 2 diabetes. Since both major isomers appear to present extensive differences in functional properties, specific characterization is also required.

Carbohydrates

Percentage of Energy Intake as Carbohydrates

No cross-sectional study has reported a positive or negative association between total carbohydrate intake and VAT accumulation in either young or adult individuals (Larson et al. 1996, Stallmann-Jorgensen et al. 2007, Davis et al. 2009, Bailey et al. 2010, Lagou et al. 2011).

Glycemic Index/Load

Glycemic index (GI) and glycemic load (GL) have been extensively studied. High GI and GL diets are generally high in energy; they may be less satiating and increase insulin secretion, possibly contributing to hyperinsulinemia (Esfahani et al. 2009). In a prospective cohort study of adults, Danes Hare-Bruun and collaborators reported that individuals consuming a high GI diet had higher intakes of fat and added sugars as well as lower protein and fiber intake compared to those with a low GI. Those with a high GL diet consumed less fat and more carbohydrates such as added sugars and dietary fiber than their low GL counterparts (Hare-Bruun, Flint, and Heitmann 2006). These data suggest that high GI and GL may contribute to cardiometabolic risk.

In men, GI and GL were not associated with any of the adiposity indices measured in this prospective cohort (body weight, percent body fat, WC, and HC) (Hare-Bruun, Flint, and Heitmann 2006). In women, body weight and percent body fat changes over 6 years were positively associated with GI, whereas a trend was found with change in WC (2 cm, $p = 0.07$) (Hare-Bruun, Flint, and Heitmann 2006). Conversely, there was a borderline negative association between change in WC and GL among women (−0.5 cm for a 10% increase of GL, $p = 0.06$), suggesting a favorable effect of this diet on central adiposity (Hare-Bruun, Flint, and Heitmann 2006). On the other hand, GI and GL were not associated with WHR in either men or women in two cross-sectional studies comprising 8703 subjects (Liese et al. 2005, Rossi et al. 2010). In two other cross-sectional studies, WHR was positively associated with GI and GL in men only (Toeller et al. 2001, Mosdol et al. 2007).

A recent systematic review showed that information was insufficient to ascertain the relationship between GI, GL, and adiposity measurements in children (Rouhani et al. 2014). There is only one prospective cohort in children on this topic (DONALD study) (Buyken et al. 2008). This study found no association between GI and GL and body mass index (BMI) z-score when the entire study population was considered (Buyken et al. 2008). In fact, only one cross-sectional study reported an association between GI and waist z-score independently of age, sex, BMI, and education of the parents as well as residuals of diet variables (energy, protein, fat, carbohydrate, fiber, and GL) (Barba et al. 2012). In that study, GI was the only nutritional variable to be associated with WC (Barba et al. 2012).

Overall, there is insufficient evidence at this time to conclude on the potential benefit of a low GI/GL diet on central obesity, in either children or adults.

Discrepancy in findings among studies could be explained partially by methodology in assessing adiposity or dietary intake. Some limitations in the use of GI and GL should also be acknowledged. GI and GL are often used as commutable variables, whereas GL takes into account the amount of carbohydrates in one portion while GI does not (Venn and Green 2007). The large variation in GI measurements, individual variability, unclear impact of mixed meals, and food transformation make difficult to draw conclusions from GI and GL studies (Venn and Green 2007).

Fructose and Sugar-Sweetened Beverages

Added sweeteners and fructose have raised particular concern for public health (Lustig, Schmidt, and Brindis 2012). Hepatic fructose metabolism, which differs from that of glucose, leads to a host of metabolic alterations associated with increased plasma triglycerides and glycemia, as reviewed in (Tappy et al. 2010), and Chapters 13 through 15 of this textbook. Fructose and sugar-sweetened beverages (SSB) have also been studied in relation to visceral fat accumulation. As described in Chapter 14, Stanhope and collaborators characterized differences in central fat accumulation measured by CT in men and women consuming a fructose- or glucose-sweetened beverage providing 25% of energy for 10 weeks (Stanhope et al. 2009). For a similar weight gain in both groups, consumption of a fructose-sweetened beverage increased visceral and total fat accumulation, whereas consumption of a glucose-sweetened beverage did not. The mechanisms underlying this effect are still unclear but may involve depot-specific modulation of lipogenic enzymes (Stanhope et al. 2009). In a cross-sectional study of 791 Caucasian men and women, VAT mass and SAT mass (measured by MRI) were not associated with SSB consumption; however, their intake was positively correlated with an increased ratio of VAT to total abdominal fat area after adjustment for confounding variables (Odegaard et al. 2012). In an observational study combining the Framingham Heart Study and the Third Generation Cohort (n = 2596), men tended to consume more SSB than women (Ma et al. 2014). Of note, whereas mean BMI and fasting glycemia were not different across categories of SSB consumption (none; >1/month and <1 per week; >1/week and <1 per day; and >1 a day), the prevalence of dyslipidemia increased as SSB consumption increased (Ma et al. 2014). The association between VAT area and SSB consumption only became significant after adjustment for SAT area (Ma et al. 2014). In a 6-month, randomized control intervention study, overweight or obese men and women were given one of four drinks (sucrose-sweetened regular cola, aspartame-sweetened diet cola, 1.7% fat milk [isocaloric to the regular cola], or water) to assess changes in VAT area (Maersk et al. 2012). Whereas total fat mass did not differ across beverage groups, the increase in VAT area was higher in the regular cola group when compared to the other groups; the same was observed for total cholesterol and triglyceride levels (Maersk et al. 2012).

Davis and collaborators found no association between SSB consumption and VAT accumulation in young overweight Latino youth followed for 2 years (Davis et al. 2009). However, added sugar and SSB intakes were similar at baseline and follow-up. In a cross-sectional study in teenagers, VAT but not SAT area was associated with total fructose consumption (Pollock et al. 2012).

Available studies suggest that SSB and/or fructose may modulate body fat distribution and promote accumulation of VAT. Additional studies are required to further document this phenomenon.

Protein

Percentage of Energy Intake as Protein

Even though standard nutritional guidelines promote lower percentage of energy from protein than from fat and carbohydrate, many weight loss programs promote adherence to a moderate–high-protein intake diet (Abete et al. 2010). There is growing evidence that higher intake of protein may increase weight loss through increased satiety and thermogenesis, as reviewed in

Halton and Hu (2004) and in Chapters 4, 17, and 18 of this textbook. High-protein diets have been proposed to counteract the reduction in fat-free mass often observed in weight loss trials (Farnsworth et al. 2003, Leidy et al. 2007). Whether protein intake modulates abdominal fat accumulation will be discussed in this section.

Several randomized weight loss trials found favorable outcomes with increases in total protein intake; however, these studies often included an exercise program, which made it difficult to assess the specific nutritional impact. Arciero et al. investigated the effect of exercise and percentage of energy as protein on body composition in overweight/obese men and women (2006). They found that a 40% carbohydrate and 40% protein diet decreased abdominal fat measured by DXA by more than 25% over 3 months, whereas a standard diet (50%–55% carbohydrates, 15%–20% proteins) reduced abdominal fat by only 7.5%. Of note, the exercise training program was more vigorous in the high-protein group and included high-intensity resistance and cardiovascular training, whereas the standard diet group performed moderate cardiovascular training (Arciero et al. 2006). In a subgroup of individuals followed for 1 year, abdominal fat was not different from baseline in the high-protein group and was reduced in the standard diet group, which could reflect the difficulty of maintaining long-term lifestyle modifications such as adherence to a high-protein diet (Arciero et al. 2006). In another randomized control trial, there was no difference in abdominal fat measured by DXA in groups assigned either to high (40%–46%) or standard (15%–20%) protein diets for 12 weeks (Clifton, Bastiaans, and Keogh 2009). Interestingly, improvements in cardiometabolic risk factors were greater in those with high circulating triglyceride concentrations at baseline on the high-protein diet when compared to those on the standard-protein diet (Clifton, Bastiaans, and Keogh 2009). Similar results (no difference in fat mass measured by DXA) were obtained in obese women assigned to diets of various macronutrient distributions (15%, 50%, or 63% of energy as protein) and a training program over 14 weeks (Kerksick et al. 2010). In a recent meta-analysis comparing low/standard (<20%/20%–30%) vs. high (>30%) protein randomized weight loss clinical trials, the mean decrease in WC was 1.66 cm greater following the high-protein diets than after the low/standard-protein diets (n = 1214) (Santesso et al. 2012). Cardiometabolic risk factors such as systolic and diastolic blood pressure, total triglycerides, and fasting insulin were also significantly lower, and HDL-cholesterol levels were higher, as expected with the decrease in WC (Santesso et al. 2012).

In sum, there is little evidence to date that high protein intake is associated with reduced VAT accumulation, independent of exercise. In fact, results from six observational studies including 2393 individuals found no association between overall protein intake and VAT area measured by CT scan or MRI after adjustment for age, race, sex, baseline VAT and SAT, and energy intake (Stallmann-Jorgensen et al. 2007, Davis et al. 2009, Bailey et al. 2010, Lagou et al. 2011, Hairston et al. 2012, Kondoh et al. 2014).

Branched-Chain Amino Acids

There is growing evidence that obese individuals have a deteriorated plasma amino acid profile, including elevated levels of branched-chain amino acids (BCAA). This increase could reflect dysfunctional basic metabolism and altered catabolic pathways in adipose tissue and other sites. Newgard and collaborators reported that rats fed a protein-enriched diet had higher levels of plasma BCAA metabolites (Newgard et al. 2009). However, in a study from our group conducted on women, no direct correlation was found between dietary amino acid intake assessed by dietary records, and circulating amino acid levels (Boulet et al. 2015). There was also no association between plasma BCAA and dietary BCAA (documented by food records or as part of an intervention) in other studies (Tai et al. 2010, Piccolo et al. 2015). Available data suggest that in humans, relationships between circulating BCAA and obesity, body fat distribution, or insulin resistance are more closely related to lower activity of branched-chain α-keto acid dehydrogenase (BCKD) enzyme complex such as BCKDE1α leading to diminished tissue BCAA catabolism independent of dietary BCAA intake (Lynch and Adams 2014, Boulet et al. 2015).

DIETARY PATTERNS

Interest on diet patterns has grown over the past decades (Van Horn 2011). Dietary behavior as a whole has been suggested to contribute to a larger extent to chronic diseases than could single nutrients (Kant 2010). Grouping food into categories allows the assessment of various eating behaviors, or dietary patterns (see description in Table 7.1), which may differ according to gender, education level, ethnicity, and culture (Newby et al. 2003, McNaughton et al. 2007).This section synthesizes information on the relevance of specific dietary patterns or diets, types of foods, or other dietary indices for abdominal fat accumulation and cardiometabolic risk factors.

Villegas et al. reported that the number of men and women from south Ireland (n = 1473) with a high WC and WHR was higher in the "alcohol and convenience foods" dietary pattern than in the "prudent diet" (Villegas et al. 2004). Unexpectedly, WC and WHR were lower among those adopting the "traditional diet" (participants with the highest intake of nonalcoholic beverages, refined cereals, butter, whole milk, and sweets) than those following the "prudent diet" (Villegas et al. 2004). These associations were not significant for BMI, suggesting that being part of the "alcohol and convenience food" group relates more closely to central adiposity than to overall obesity level. In another study, African-American men with a higher "southern pattern diet" score had a higher WC and higher CT-measured VAT area; similar trends were observed between WC and the "fast-food pattern" (Liu et al. 2013). No significant association was detected between these adiposity parameters and the "prudent pattern diet." In a Brazilian study (Vilela et al. 2014), consuming a "western diet" was positively associated with WHR and WC after adjustment for BMI in women, while a positive association between WHR and a trend with WC was also observed in the "regional

TABLE 7.1
Characteristics of the Main Diet Patterns Reported

Diet Pattern	Description[a]	Studies
Prudent or healthy	High in fruits, vegetables, white meats or fish, nuts, vegetable oils, and whole grains	Villegas et al. (2004) Esmaillzadeh and Azadbakht (2008) Denova-Gutierrez et al. (2011) Amini et al. (2012) Liu et al. (2013) Vilela et al. (2014)
Western	High in refined grains, red meats, butter, eggs, hydrogenated fats, soft drinks, and sweets	Esmaillzadeh and Azadbakht (2008) Denova-Gutierrez et al. (2011) Amini et al. (2012) Vilela et al. (2014)
Alcohol and convenience foods	High intake in alcohol and meats, low consumption of fruits, vegetables, and whole grains	Villegas et al. (2004)
Southern	Traditional rural southern U.S. foods: high consumption of beans, legumes, corn products, fried fish and chicken, margarine, and butter	Liu et al. (2013)
Fast food	High in sugar, fast foods, and salty snacks	Liu et al. (2013)
Traditional (Iranian)	High consumption of grains, potato, tea, hydrogenated fats, and legumes	Esmaillzadeh and Azadbakht (2008)
Mixed diet	High consumption of fruits, vegetables, low-fat yogurt, and soy milk, but high in sweets	McNaughton et al. (2007)

[a] Description can vary according to the study and population.

traditional diet" group (high in rice, beans, tubers, meat, eggs, coffee, and sugar). In female Iranian teachers, lower total and central obesity was observed in the higher quintile of the "healthy pattern diet" while the opposite relationship was found in the "western and Iranian diet" (Esmaillzadeh and Azadbakht 2008).

Data from Iranian participants with abnormal glucose homeostasis suggest that the "western diet" is associated with central and total obesity, whereas the "high-fat dairy pattern" is associated only with total obesity level (Amini et al. 2012). A cross-sectional study in Mexican individuals identified three general dietary patterns: "westernized," "high animal protein/fat," and "prudent." The westernized and high animal protein/fat patterns were positively associated with percent total fat body and percent abdominal body fat measured by DXA while the prudent diet was related to a lower percent body fat (Denova-Gutierrez et al. 2011). Taken together, the earlier mentioned studies suggest that specific "unfavorable" dietary patterns (such as the "fast-food pattern") may influence abdominal fat but the effect seems dependent on concurrent gain in body weight or fat mass.

A small number of longitudinal studies investigated the long-term impact of various dietary patterns on body fat distribution. One study reported an inverse association between a "mixed diet pattern" (Table 7.1) and WC, but not BMI after adjustment for confounders in men, while the "fruit, vegetables and dairy pattern" (which shares similarities with the "prudent pattern" used in other studies) was associated with a decrease in both BMI and WC in women (McNaughton et al. 2007). In healthy men and women participating in the Baltimore longitudinal study (n = 459), subjects in the "white bread pattern" subgroup had a mean annual WC change of +1.32 cm, which was three times greater than that of participants in the "healthy pattern" subgroup (Newby et al. 2003).

Although many studies have reported associations between dietary patterns and obesity level, few convincingly demonstrated that they may be linked to body fat distribution profiles. Several features of these studies may underlie this conclusion. First, there are numerous differences in population characteristics consuming a particular diet (e.g., smoking status, ethnicity, sex, education level, and physical activity), some of which are strong modulators of body fat distribution (reviewed in Tchernof and Després (2013)). Moreover, the frequent use of cross-sectional designs, the variability in the populations examined, inconsistencies in the dietary patterns identified, as well as limitations and variation in the methodology used for dietary assessment make direct comparisons of available studies difficult.

Food Item Subgroups

Another method to assess the impact of diet is to segregate food items in various subgroups according to their nature or composition. The association between the relative weight of food subgroups in the diet and physiological variables can be subsequently analyzed. Several large cross-sectional studies (>1000 participants) have examined the relative distribution of food groups as a function of WC. One of these studies (McCarthy et al. 2006) including adults from Northern Ireland observed a significant increase in the risk for high WC, but not BMI, and food categories like pastries and cake, whole milk, cream and desserts (which included cream, puddings, chilled desserts, and ice cream), meat, as well as alcoholic beverages. A lower risk for high WC was also reported with higher intake of rice and pasta. Data from 1519 adults participating in the National Diet and Nutrition Survey of British adults showed positive associations between WC and portion sizes of various food groups, including whole milk, chips and processed potatoes, sweets, as well as soft drinks (Kelly et al. 2009). Portion sizes of these food groups were not associated with BMI (Kelly et al. 2009). A Swedish study including 6069 men and women examined the association between food types and WC or HC (Krachler et al. 2006). In women, a preferential fat accumulation in the hips and thighs was associated with increased consumption of vegetable oil, pasta, and 1.5% fat milk, whereas central fat accumulation was associated with higher consumption of hamburgers, potatoes, French fries, and soft drinks. In men, vegetable oil, pasta, and 1.5%–3% milk was associated with gluteofemoral fat accumulation, while central fat accumulation was positively associated with increased beer, but not wine, consumption. Results of the 12-year follow-up of the Framingham Offspring/Spouse cohort study showed that obesity-specific nutritional risk score (based on 11 components, namely total energy, energy density, carbohydrate, protein, fiber, calcium, alcohol, and total, MUFA, PUFA, and SFA) was related to abdominal obesity in women (Wolongevicz et al. 2010).

A Danish monozygotic co-twin case–control study evaluated the impact of numerous diet components on body fat distribution (Hasselbalch et al. 2010). A negative association between WC and vegetable oil intake was found in men (Hasselbalch et al. 2010). The prospective EPIC study evaluated annual WC changes in relation with food groups (Romaguera et al. 2011). A high consumption of fruits and dairy products (including milk, yogurt, and cheese; irrespective of fat content) coupled with low intake of white bread, processed meat, margarine, and soft drinks was associated with lower increases in WC for a given BMI (Romaguera et al. 2011).

Although available studies could suggest detrimental effects of a more refined or fast-food type of diet on surrogate measures of VAT, no firm conclusion can be reached about specific food items and body fat distribution. This conclusion takes into account the relative paucity of data, the heterogeneity of food patterns and populations examined, the disparities in the results, and the various adjustments that were performed (or not performed).

Mediterranean Diet

As discussed in Chapter 22, MD are characterized mainly by high consumption of vegetables, fruits, whole grains, olive oil, nuts, a moderate intake of fatty fish, dairy, and alcohol—mostly wine—as well as low consumption of red meat and sweets. This pattern received increasing scientific attention with the development of a Mediterranean score (MEDS) by Trichopoulou and collaborators, in which a diet including these components was shown to positively affect life expectancy in a prospective cohort study (Trichopoulou et al. 1995). In the growing literature of the past decades, many studies have addressed adherence to the MD and body fat distribution.

In the EPIC-PANACEA PROJECT, a cross-sectional study including 497,308 individuals from 10 European countries, a higher MEDS was associated with lower WC for a given BMI in both women and men (Romaguera et al. 2009). No significant association was found between the MEDS and BMI (Romaguera et al. 2009). In a large prospective case-cohort study in five European countries, a higher MEDS was associated with a reduction in WC, adjusted for BMI, at a 6.8-year median follow-up (Roswall et al. 2014). A longitudinal study with a mean follow-up of 7 years from the Framingham Offspring Cohort showed MEDS-related improvement in several features of the metabolic syndrome, including WC, after adjustment for BMI and change in BMI (Rumawas et al. 2009). These results are consistent with those of the SU.VI.MAX (*Supplémentation en Vitamines et Minéraux AntioXydants*) study cohort (Kesse-Guyot et al. 2013). Similarly, a 9-year follow-up of 3058 Spanish men and women showed that adherence to the MD was negatively associated with increases in WC (Funtikova et al. 2014).

In contrast to the reports mentioned earlier, a cross-sectional Lebanese study found that although the classical MEDS was associated with lower WC independent of BMI, these results were not replicated with a customized MEDS adapted for the Lebanese population. Both BMI and WC were lower with increasing values of the custom score, suggesting that the MD is associated with lower total and central adiposity (Issa et al. 2011). This result is consistent with the findings of Boghossian et al. on 258 premenopausal women (Boghossian et al. 2013). A high MEDS was, indeed, significantly associated with lower BMI, lower WC and HC, and lower body fat mass assessed by DXA (Boghossian et al. 2013). Negative associations between a higher MEDS and overall adiposity were replicated in other studies (Panagiotakos et al. 2006, Schroder et al. 2010).

Another study including 23,597 participants from the EPIC cohort showed that when energy intake was not controlled for, the MEDS was associated with a marginal increase in BMI and WC (Trichopoulou et al. 2005). For example, in the Greek cohort of the EPIC study, the MD was directly linked to increased energy intake (Ferro-Luzzi, James, and Kafatos 2002). Conversely, an Italian study reported no association between BMI or WHR and adherence to the major characteristics of the MD (Rossi et al. 2008). In a recent nutritional intervention study in a non-Mediterranean population at risk for cardiovascular diseases, both men and women significantly increased their MEDS and, as a result, decreased the energy density of their diet and thus reduced their energy intake (Leblanc et al. 2015). At the end of the intervention period (12 weeks), both genders had significantly lower WC and BMI, along with other improvements in metabolic indicators such as HDL-C (in men only) (Leblanc et al. 2015). Reports of nutritional data may need to be standardized across population studies to assess the apparent favorable impact of the MD on body fat distribution and/or overall adiposity.

One study reported lower weight gain with a higher MEDS for participants with 1 or 2 minor alleles of the *TCF7L2* gene, which has been related to diabetes (Roswall et al. 2014). In the Prevención con Dieta Mediterránea clinical trial, participants with the minor 12Ala allele of the PPARγ gene increased their WC significantly more than noncarriers of this allele, while no difference in BMI was noted. Yet, this result was only observed in the control group advised to follow a low-fat diet, not in the two Mediterranean groups. Therefore, the MD appears to protect against the detrimental effects of the 12A1a PPARγ minor allele (Razquin et al. 2009). It has been proposed that the highly concentrated MUFA and PUFA of the MD could modulate PPARγ activation (Xu et al. 1999).

While available data point toward a possible specific reduction of central adiposity with the MD, this issue is still controversial in the literature. Adaptation of the original MEDS to local populations may also complicate study comparisons. WC was generally used in large cohort studies, but additional imaging studies would be required to better assess the impact of MD on abdominal fat compartments.

OTHER NUTRIENTS OR FOOD ITEMS

A wide selection of specific nutrients or food items has been studied in relation to body fat distribution and will be briefly addressed in this section. Extensive discussion of the mechanisms underlying their possible impact on abdominal obesity is beyond the scope of this chapter.

ALCOHOL

Data on alcohol consumption and obesity are conflicting. Alcohol provides 7.1 kcal/g, yet some beverages contain active biomolecules such as polyphenols (e.g., red wine), which can positively impact cardiometabolic risk factors. Existence of the "beer belly" is a widely spread popular notion, and heavy alcohol use also leads to liver disease and other metabolic alterations. Studies on alcohol consumption and abdominal obesity are briefly reviewed here.

In Japanese men, only a trend between VAT area and alcohol intake was noted (Kondoh et al. 2014). However, a significant inverse relationship was found with abdominal subcutaneous fat along with a positive association with the VAT/SAT ratio. In age-adjusted regression analyses, alcohol intake was strongly and positively associated with VAT area (Kondoh et al. 2014). Similar results were reported by Larson and collaborators in a cohort of men and women from the United States. VAT adjusted for SAT was positively associated with alcohol intake (as a binary variable), whereas SAT adjusted for VAT was negatively associated with alcohol consumption (Larson et al. 1996). In the Framingham Heart Study, relationships between alcohol intake and VAT or SAT were studied separately in both sexes (Molenaar et al. 2009). Men whose intake was greater than 14 drinks per week (equivalent to >24 g ethanol/day) and women with intake greater than 7 drinks per week (>12 g ethanol/day) were identified as heavy drinkers, whereas the remaining individuals were classified as light and moderate drinkers (Molenaar et al. 2009). In women but not in men, SAT area was higher in light-to-moderate drinkers, whereas only in men VAT area was higher among the heavy drinkers (Molenaar et al. 2009). Another study reported that central obesity in women, assessed by DXA, was associated with low levels of alcohol consumption, which is consistent with the notion that SAT is increased preferentially in women gaining weight (Greenfield et al. 2003). In men from the Normative Aging Study, there was a trend toward a positive association between the WHR and alcohol consumption (Troisi et al. 1991). Brandhagen and collaborators reported associations between types of alcoholic beverages and measures of central adiposity in both men and women of the Swedish Obese Subjects study (Brandhagen et al. 2012). With their fully adjusted model in men, consumption of spirits was positively associated with percentage body fat, sagittal diameter, and WC, whereas beer consumption was not associated with any of these measurements (Brandhagen et al. 2012). In contrast, in women, wine and total alcohol intake were negatively associated with percent body fat (Brandhagen et al. 2012).

In overweight young adults, alcohol consumption in both sexes was not associated with, nor predictive of, VAT or SAT area (Bailey et al. 2010). However, as reported by the authors, cafeteria-based diet assessment may not reflect usual alcohol consumption in that cohort. In abdominally obese men, consumption of 40 g of ethanol (450 mL of red wine) daily over a 4-week trial did not result in increased body weight, abdominal or subcutaneous fat contents as determined by ultrasound (Beulens et al. 2006), but led to increased adiponectin secretion. Data from the EPIC study showed a 0.02 cm increase in WC per 5% increase of alcohol intake (as a proportion of total energy intake) for a given BMI only in women (Romaguera et al. 2010).

In sum, most studies show that alcohol consumption may be linked to increases in total fat mass as well as depot-specific abdominal fat storage that may be a reflection of the propensity of each sex to store fat either in central (men) or peripheral (women) compartments.

Dairy Products, Calcium, and Vitamin D

Many epidemiological findings suggest a favorable antiobesogenic effect of dairy products, likely related to high calcium and vitamin D intake (Zemel et al. 2000, Pereira et al. 2002, Jacqmain et al. 2003, Loos et al. 2004). A recent meta-analysis found that daily increase in dairy intake (550–1000 mg of additional calcium) was associated with a lower WC compared to control groups in energy restriction studies (−2.43 cm, 95% CI: −3.42, −1.44) but not in studies without energy restriction (WC: −2.19 cm, 95% CI: −8.02, 2.66) (Abargouei et al. 2012). In a randomized weight loss trial where obese men and women consumed yogurt or placebo in the form of a sugar-free gelatin snack, there was a more pronounced weight loss in the yogurt group. Furthermore, trunk fat loss was 81% higher than that of the control group, and there was a 4 cm reduction in WC. The authors proposed increased fat cell lipolysis as a potential mechanism, as supported by an increase in plasma glycerol observed only in participants who consumed yogurt (Zemel et al. 2005). In a retrospective study including overweight and obese Australians, there was an inverse relationship between total dairy food intake and WC after adjustment for age, sex, and total energy intake (Murphy et al. 2013). After adjustment for total dairy food intake, dairy protein and dairy calcium were still negatively associated with WC and DXA-measured abdominal fat (Murphy et al. 2013). In a recent randomized control trial, men and women taking calcium and vitamin D supplementation in orange juice had greater decreases in VAT area than controls treated with orange juice without supplementation after adjustment for baseline total abdominal area (SAT+VAT) to consider for baseline group differences (Rosenblum et al. 2012). Consistent with these results, Bush et al. reported that premenopausal women gained 2.7 cm^2 less visceral fat assessed by CT scan for each 100 mg/day increase of total dietary calcium over a 1-year period (Bush et al. 2010). In postmenopausal women, total dietary calcium intake was negatively associated with abdominal fat mass and percent body fat, but when adjusted for total energy intake only percent body fat was still associated with calcium intake. Nonsignificant associations were also reported between calcium intake and BMI, WHR, and WC (Heiss, Shaw, and Carothers 2008).

Vitamin D has been proposed to play a role in adipocyte differentiation, but its effects remain unclear (Kong and Li 2006). Our team reported that women with higher plasma levels of 25-Hydroxyvitamin D (25(OH)D) had smaller omental adipocytes, and lower VAT and SAT areas determined by CT (Caron-Jobin et al. 2011). In another study, overweight and obese women supplemented with 25 μg of vitamin D3 for 3 months showed no difference in WC and weight compared to controls (Salehpour et al. 2012). Wamberg and collaborators reported no difference in SAT and VAT areas (determined by MRI) in obese men and women after 26 weeks of supplementation with 175 μg of vitamin D3 compared to controls, and no difference in the cardiometabolic risk factors including the homeostasis model assessment of insulin resistance, high-sensitivity C-reactive protein (hsCRP), plasma lipids, and blood pressure (Wamberg et al. 2013). In chronic kidney disease patients, levels of 25(OH)D decreased as BMI increased and were also lower in diabetic patients. However, there was no association between vitamin D status and SAT or VAT areas as well as body fat mass (Figuiredo-Dias et al. 2012). The apparent null effect of vitamin D supplementation alone may point toward a combined action of dairy protein and/or calcium in the modulation of body fat distribution.

Soy and Isoflavones

In the Soy Health Effects study, intake of the most common isoflavone subtypes (genistein and daidzein) was assessed with a food-frequency questionnaire in 208 postmenopausal women (Goodman-Gruen and Kritz-Silverstein 2003). Women with higher genistein intake had lower BMI, fat mass, and WC than women who reported no intake of isoflavones but they were also generally more active (Goodman-Gruen and Kritz-Silverstein 2003). In two randomized control trials, postmenopausal women taking a daily shake with added soy protein and isoflavones for 3 months gained less total and SAT area than women in the casein placebo group (Sites et al. 2007, Christie et al. 2010). VAT gain was not different between the two groups (Sites et al. 2007, Christie et al. 2010). Different results were obtained in randomized control trials on exercise, isoflavones, and weight loss in postmenopausal women (Maesta et al. 2007, Choquette et al. 2011). While exercise had a favorable effect on WC, HC, and body fat mass, neither apparent additive nor synergetic effect of isoflavones was detected (Maesta et al. 2007, Choquette et al. 2011). In a weight loss trial comparing the effect of soy vs. milk protein, only those in the milk protein group experienced a reduction in BMI and body weight (Takahira et al. 2011). Decreased WC was observed in both groups but only the milk group had significant decreases in both abdominal SAT and VAT areas (Takahira et al. 2011). Overall, a specific effect of soy or isoflavones on visceral fat accumulation is improbable.

Dietary Fiber and Whole Grains

Dietary fiber and whole grain intake has been associated with body composition in many studies. McKeown and collaborators reported inverse relationships between intake of whole grain cereal fiber and percent trunk fat mass as well as percent body fat in an elderly population (60–80 years old) (McKeown et al. 2009). Of note, they did not find an association between these measurements and total fiber intake (McKeown et al. 2009). Interestingly, those in the highest quartile category of dietary fiber and/or whole grain intake were also the group with the higher energy intake (McKeown et al. 2009). Two other observational studies found no association between whole grain intake and VAT or SAT areas (Stallmann-Jorgensen et al. 2007, Davis et al. 2009).

Total fiber intake was negatively associated with VAT measured by MRI in two other studies (n = 644), but SAT was not measured (Davis et al. 2009, Parikh et al. 2012). Results from

CT scans in overweight young adults and middle-aged men and women from the United States showed no association between VAT or SAT and total fiber intake (Larson et al. 1996, Bailey et al. 2010). In U.S. Latino teenagers, VAT area was associated with insoluble fiber but not soluble fiber intake (Davis et al. 2009). On the other hand, in overweight African-American and Latino adults, soluble fiber intake was negatively associated with VAT area, whereas insoluble fiber intake was not (Hairston et al. 2012). The effects of high fiber/whole grain diet on body fat distribution do not seem to be mediated by reduced energy intake as the vast majority of the earlier mentioned studies adjusted for energy intake.

Vitamins A and C

Excess storage of fat is associated with increased FA oxidation leading to the production of larger amounts of free radicals, thus inducing a greater use of antioxidant molecules such as vitamins A and C. Therefore, low plasma levels of vitamin A and C could be associated with low-grade chronic inflammation related to obesity, especially in the visceral depot (Zulet et al. 2008).

In healthy young adults, high vitamin A intake was negatively associated with WC and WHR as well as numerous cardiometabolic risk variables such as fasting glycemia, insulin, and blood pressure (Zulet et al. 2008). However, a relationship between vitamin A intake and VAT or SAT accumulation was not found in overweight young adults (Bailey et al. 2010).

In women, higher intake of ascorbic acid was associated with lower WC (Choi et al. 2013) and lower odds ratio of having a WHR $\geq$ 0.84 (Azadbakht and Esmaillzadeh 2008). In men from the same study, no association was found between WC and vitamin C intake (Choi et al. 2013).

Probiotics and the Gut Microbiota

There is increasing evidence linking the gut microbiota to total adiposity (Rosenbaum, Knight, and Leibel 2015). A complete review of such evidence is beyond the scope of this chapter. Of note, a probiotic bacterium (LG2055) naturally present in human gut microbiota led to significant decreases of adipocyte hypertrophy in rats (Sato et al. 2008). More recently, the same team showed a reduction in VAT and SAT areas as well as WC, BMI, and body fat mass in a randomized control trial of healthy men and women supplementing their habitual diet with fermented milk containing LG2055 vs. placebo (fermented milk without LG2055) (Kadooka et al. 2010). Emerging studies on the human gut microbiota will eventually allow assessing its potential role in body fat distribution.

INFANT FEEDING PRACTICES

Other possible dietary influences on body fat distribution patterns may include early-life nutrition. Many studies have linked infant feeding practices or even maternal diet during pregnancy with the onset of obesity in the offspring, and several mechanisms were proposed to explain this association (reviewed in Lecoutre and Breton (2014, 2015) and Chapter 28 of this textbook). However, only a few studies have directly investigated infant feeding practice or maternal diet vs. body fat distribution patterns of the offspring independently of maternal BMI, socioeconomic status, and other confounding variables.

Whether breastfeeding is related to offspring adiposity later in life is still a matter of debate. Systematic reviews have concluded that exclusive breastfeeding for at least 6 months is protective against obesity (Kramer and Kakuma 2012). After adjustment for confounding variables, this relation was attenuated or abolished (Kramer and Kakuma 2012). Only a few studies have investigated duration of breastfeeding as a function of offspring body fat distribution. In a retrospective study of 442 children (EPOCH study), breastfeeding for less than 6 months or for more than 6 months had no differential impact on the accumulation of MRI-assessed VAT or SAT, sum of skinfolds, and BMI of the offspring (Crume et al. 2012). However, a protective effect of breastfeeding was apparent for those in the upper percentiles of BMI, VAT, and SAT after adjustment for confounding variables (Crume et al. 2012).

In the Generation R prospective study, children who were breastfed exclusively for at least 4 months had lower total body fat mass and peripheral fat compared to no breastfeeding at 6 months (Durmus et al. 2012). Children who were never or nonexclusively breastfed until 4 months had higher subcutaneous central fat at 24 months of age compared to exclusive breastfeeding (Durmus et al. 2012). However, there was no difference in body fat distribution related to timing of the introduction of solid foods (Durmus et al. 2012). Similarly, no difference in body fat distribution was found in the same children at 6 years of age, after adjustment for confounding variables (Durmus et al. 2014). In fact, neither timing of solid food introduction nor use of formula was associated with total skinfolds in children between 4 and 5 years of age in two other independent studies (Zive et al. 1992, Caleyachetty et al. 2013). Similar observations were made in the HELENA cohort including 3528 adolescents (Rousseaux et al. 2014). Of note, investigators of the HELENA cohort showed a trend for a protective effect of breastfeeding for those in the upper percentile of skinfold thickness and waist-to-height ratio, in line with previous results (Crume et al. 2012).

Opposite results were obtained in a Brazilian study of 185 children between 4 and 7 years. Breastfeeding duration was positively associated with percent body fat assessed by DXA, but not with WC or fat mass localized in the abdominal region (Magalhaes et al. 2012). Much like the previously cited study (Durmus et al. 2014), timing of solid food introduction was not associated with BMI, WC, total body fat mass, or central adiposity (Magalhaes et al. 2012). In young infants, introduction of cereals or meat at 5 months of age did not modulate adiposity at 9 months of age (Tang and Krebs 2014). Regarding maternal macronutrient intake, a study in a large cohort showed that fetal adiposity was highest in the abdominal region of infants from mothers with low dietary intake of protein (<16%), irrespective of carbohydrate or fat intakes, and this was caused by an increase of SAT accumulation measured by ultrasound at 19, 25, 30, and 36 weeks (Blumfield et al. 2012). Maternal diet was assessed by a validated 74-item food-frequency questionnaire during the early and late pregnancy periods. Changes in the diet was then compared to Changes in fetal adiposity. On the other hand, VAT accumulation (assessed by ultrasound) was higher when maternal calories from protein represented more than 20% energy and this was linked with carbohydrate intake, which was diminished, thereby increasing the protein-to-carbohydrate ratio. Ultrasound-measured mid-thigh fat in these fetuses was related to maternal intakes that were high in fat, low in carbohydrates, and intermediary in protein. These studies identify a plausible mechanism by which maternal protein intake can module infant body fat distribution *in utero* (Blumfield et al. 2012). In another study of pregnant adolescents, intake of total and added sugar was the best predictor of ultrasound-measured fetal abdominal fat thickness during the last trimester of pregnancy. In this cohort, a U-shaped curve was observed between energy-adjusted carbohydrate intake and abdominal fat, pointing again to an ideal maternal carbohydrate intake. Of note, gestational weight gain was not related to fat accretion in the fetus for these women (Whisner et al. 2015). A Danish study examined maternal intake of animal and vegetable protein in relation to BMI and WC of offspring at 20 years of age (Maslova et al. 2014). Offspring BMI was related to maternal protein intake during pregnancy but WC showed no significant association (Maslova et al. 2014). In the ROLO study, maternal protein intake was not associated with newborn anthropometric measurements, but SFA intake in the second and third trimesters was related to offspring WC and the waist-to-length ratio, whereas there was a negative trend between maternal PUFA intake in the third trimester and abdominal circumference at birth (Horan et al. 2014). Consistent with these results, low level of circulating PUFA in newborns was positively associated with higher central fat (Sanz et al. 2014). Finally, in a randomized control trial, modulating the ratio of n-6 to n-3 FA in the diet of pregnant women had no effect on body fat distribution in infants at birth, 6 weeks, and 4 and 12 months (Hauner et al. 2012).

Overall, there is growing evidence that maternal diet modulates body fat distribution in the offspring independently of a number of confounding factors. A moderate-protein (>16% to <20% energy) diet, and PUFA intake, appears to limit abdominal fat accretion, whereas SFA intake seems linked to detrimental adiposity profiles. However, some important facts must be acknowledged. Investigators often make statistical adjustment for energy intake in children, obliterating the fact that prenatal and postnatal nutrition may impact appetite and the desire for particular foods. Age of adiposity rebound, that is, the age between 3 and 7 years where BMI-for-age starts to increase after it reaches its lowest point, is not always considered in available studies, which could account for some differences in adiposity between groups.

CONCLUSION

Most available studies on diet and body fat distribution seem to point toward a nonspecific effect on, or protection from, fat accumulation (VAT, SAT, both, or total adiposity). Nutrients potentially linked to a detrimental fat accretion pattern (increased VAT, abdominal fat, or WC) include fructose, especially in the form of SSB, *trans* FA, as well as high alcohol consumption and refined/fast-food diets. On the other hand, some nutrients (MCT, calcium, fiber, whole grains) and dietary patterns (MD, prudent diet) have been found to reduce adiposity in epidemiological studies and there is growing evidence supporting these notions through randomized control trials. Whether these effects emerge from depot-specific impact in adipose tissue compartments remains unclear. Therefore, there is no clear evidence that a single nutrient directly modulates visceral fat accretion and, by extension, body fat distribution. However, some nutrients and/or diet patterns may affect energy balance and subsequent weight gain or loss, which will be reflected in changes in regional fat accumulation as a function of the prevailing genetic, epigenetic, and hormonal milieu (Figure 7.1).

In this context, responses to nutrients or diets present remarkable interindividual variability most likely resulting from interactions with a plethora of physiological factors. Future studies on this topic should aim to identify subpopulations of responders and nonresponders with the goal of unraveling biological modulators of the response. Considering the emerging impact of early-life nutrition, prevention strategies may also have to focus on maternal nutrition and perinatal feeding.

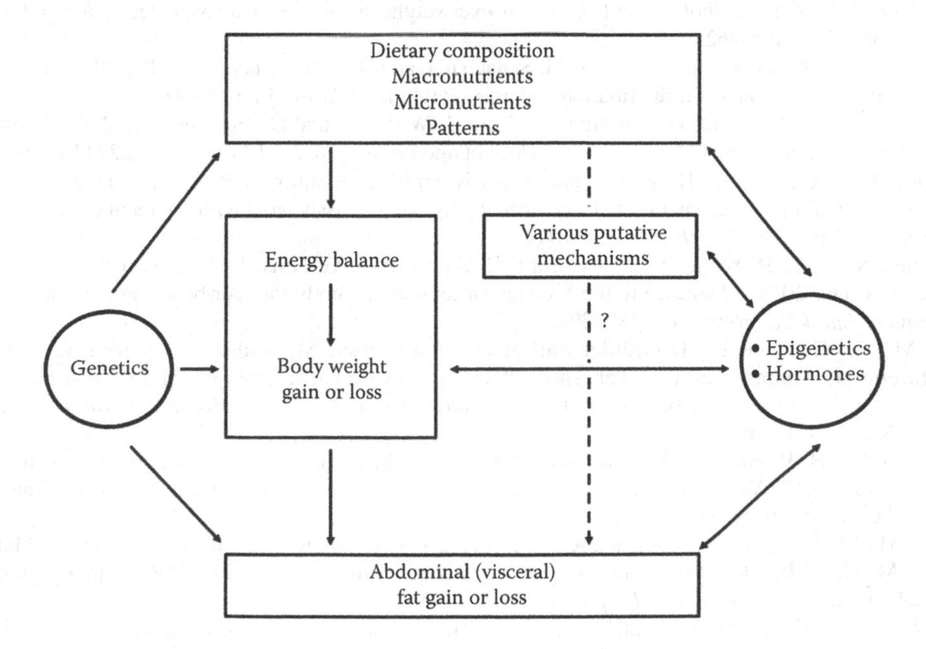

FIGURE 7.1 Potential impact of dietary factors on abdominal (visceral) fat gain or loss.

REFERENCES

Abargouei, A. S., M. Janghorbani, M. Salehi-Marzijarani, and A. Esmaillzadeh. 2012. Effect of dairy consumption on weight and body composition in adults: A systematic review and meta-analysis of randomized controlled clinical trials. *Int J Obes* 36(12):1485–1493.

Abete, I., A. Astrup, J. A. Martinez, I. Thorsdottir, and M. A. Zulet. 2010. Obesity and the metabolic syndrome: Role of different dietary macronutrient distribution patterns and specific nutritional components on weight loss and maintenance. *Nutr Rev* 68(4):214–231.

Adams, R. E., A. Hsueh, B. Alford, C. King, H. Mo, and R. Wildman. 2006. Conjugated linoleic acid supplementation does not reduce visceral adipose tissue in middle-aged men engaged in a resistance-training program. *J Int Soc Sports Nutr* 3:28–36.

Amini, M., S. Shafaeizadeh, M. Zare, H. Khosravi Boroujeni, and A. Esmaillzadeh. 2012. A cross-sectional study on food patterns and adiposity among individuals with abnormal glucose homeostasis. *Arch Iran Med* 15(3):131–135.

Arciero, P. J., C. L. Gentile, R. Martin-Pressman, M. J. Ormsbee, M. Everett, L. Zwicky, and C. A. Steele. 2006. Increased dietary protein and combined high intensity aerobic and resistance exercise improves body fat distribution and cardiovascular risk factors. *Int J Sport Nutr Exerc Metab* 16(4):373–392.

Azadbakht, L. and A. Esmaillzadeh. 2008. Dietary and non-dietary determinants of central adiposity among Tehrani women. *Public Health Nutr* 11(5):528–534.

Bach, A. C. and V. K. Babayan. 1982. Medium-chain triglycerides: An update. *Am J Clin Nutr* 36(5):950–962.

Bailey, B. W., D. K. Sullivan, E. P. Kirk, and J. E. Donnelly. 2010. Dietary predictors of visceral adiposity in overweight young adults. *Br J Nutr* 103(12):1702–1705.

Barba, G., S. Sieri, M. D. Russo, E. Donatiello, A. Formisano, F. Lauria, S. Sparano et al. 2012. Glycaemic index and body fat distribution in children: The results of the ARCA project. *Nutr Metab Cardiovasc Dis* 22(1):28–34.

Bays, H. E., K. C. Maki, R. T. Doyle, and E. Stein. 2009. The effect of prescription omega-3 fatty acids on body weight after 8 to 16 weeks of treatment for very high triglyceride levels. *Postgrad Med* 121(5):145–150.

Bender, N., M. Portmann, Z. Heg, K. Hofmann, M. Zwahlen, and M. Egger. 2014. Fish or n3-PUFA intake and body composition: A systematic review and meta-analysis. *Obes Rev* 15(8):657–665.

Benito, P., G. J. Nelson, D. S. Kelley, G. Bartolini, P. C. Schmidt, and V. Simon. 2001. The effect of conjugated linoleic acid on plasma lipoproteins and tissue fatty acid composition in humans. *Lipids* 36(3):229–236.

Berry, D. C., D. Stenesen, D. Zeve, and J. M. Graff. 2013. The developmental origins of adipose tissue. *Development* 140(19):3939–3949.

Berven, G., A. Bye, O. Hals, H. Blankson, H. Fagertun, E. Thom, J. Wadstein, and O. Gudmundsen. 2000. Safety of conjugated linoleic acid (CLA) in overweight or obese human volunteers. *Eur J Lipid Sci Technol* 102(7):455–462.

Beulens, J. W., R. M. van Beers, R. P. Stolk, G. Schaafsma, and H. F. Hendriks. 2006. The effect of moderate alcohol consumption on fat distribution and adipocytokines. *Obesity* 14(1):60–66.

Blankson, H., J. A. Stakkestad, H. Fagertun, E. Thom, J. Wadstein, and O. Gudmundsen. 2000. Conjugated linoleic acid reduces body fat mass in overweight and obese humans. *J Nutr* 130(12):2943–2948.

Blumfield, M. L., A. J. Hure, L. K. MacDonald-Wicks, R. Smith, S. J. Simpson, W. B. Giles, D. Raubenheimer, and C. E. Collins. 2012. Dietary balance during pregnancy is associated with fetal adiposity and fat distribution. *Am J Clin Nutr* 96(5):1032–1041.

Boghossian, N. S., E. H. Yeung, S. L. Mumford, C. Zhang, A. J. Gaskins, J. Wactawski-Wende, and E. F. Schisterman. 2013. Adherence to the Mediterranean diet and body fat distribution in reproductive aged women. *Eur J Clin Nutr* 67(3):289–294.

Boulet, M. M., G. Chevrier, T. Grenier-Larouche, M. Pelletier, M. Nadeau, J. Scarpa, C. Prehn, A. Marette, J. Adamski, and A. Tchernof. 2015. Alterations of plasma metabolite profiles related to adipose tissue distribution and cardiometabolic risk. *Am J Physiol Endocrinol Metab* 309(8):E736–E746.

Brandhagen, M., H. B. Forslund, L. Lissner, A. Winkvist, A. K. Lindroos, L. M. Carlsson, L. Sjostrom, and I. Larsson. 2012. Alcohol and macronutrient intake patterns are related to general and central adiposity. *Eur J Clin Nutr* 66(3):305–313.

Brown, J. M., M. S. Boysen, S. S. Jensen, R. F. Morrison, J. Storkson, R. Lea-Currie, M. Pariza, S. Mandrup, and M. K. McIntosh. 2003. Isomer-specific regulation of metabolism and PPAR gamma signaling by CLA in human preadipocytes. *J Lipid Res* 44(7):1287–1300.

Brown, J. M. and M. K. McIntosh. 2003. Conjugated linoleic acid in humans: Regulation of adiposity and insulin sensitivity. *J Nutr* 133(10):3041–3046.

Bueno, N. B., I. V. de Melo, T. T. Florencio, and A. L. Sawaya. 2015. Dietary medium-chain triacylglycerols versus long-chain triacylglycerols for body composition in adults: Systematic review and meta-analysis of randomized controlled trials. *J Am Coll Nutr* 34(2):175–183.

Bush, N. C., J. A. Alvarez, S. S. Choquette, G. R. Hunter, R. A. Oster, B. E. Darnell, and B. A. Gower. 2010. Dietary calcium intake is associated with less gain in intra-abdominal adipose tissue over 1 year. *Obesity* 18(11):2101–2104.

Buyken, A. E., G. Cheng, A. L. Gunther, A. D. Liese, T. Remer, and N. Karaolis-Danckert. 2008. Relation of dietary glycemic index, glycemic load, added sugar intake, or fiber intake to the development of body composition between ages 2 and 7 y. *Am J Clin Nutr* 88(3):755–762.

Caleyachetty, A., G. V. Krishnaveni, S. R. Veena, J. Hill, S. C. Karat, C. H. Fall, and A. K. Wills. 2013. Breastfeeding duration, age of starting solids and high BMI risk and adiposity in Indian children. *Matern Child Nutr* 9(2):199–216.

Caron-Jobin, M., A. S. Morisset, A. Tremblay, C. Huot, D. Légaré, and A. Tchernof. 2011. Elevated serum 25(OH)D concentrations, vitamin D, and calcium intakes are associated with reduced adipocyte size in women. *Obesity* 19(7):1335–1341.

Carvalho, R. F., S. K. Uehara, and G. Rosa. 2012. Microencapsulated conjugated linoleic acid associated with hypocaloric diet reduces body fat in sedentary women with metabolic syndrome. *Vasc Health Risk Manag* 8:661–667.

Choi, M. K., H. J. Song, Y. J. Paek, and H. J. Lee. 2013. Gender differences in the relationship between vitamin C and abdominal obesity. *Int J Vitam Nutr Res* 83(6):377–384.

Choquette, S., E. Riesco, E. Cormier, T. Dion, M. Aubertin-Leheudre, and I. J. Dionne. 2011. Effects of soya isoflavones and exercise on body composition and clinical risk factors of cardiovascular diseases in overweight postmenopausal women: A 6-month double-blind controlled trial. *Br J Nutr* 105(8):1199–1209.

Christie, D. R., J. Grant, B. E. Darnell, V. R. Chapman, A. Gastaldelli, and C. K. Sites. 2010. Metabolic effects of soy supplementation in postmenopausal Caucasian and African American women: A randomized, placebo-controlled trial. *Am J Obstet Gynecol* 203(2):153e1–153e9.

Chung, S., J. M. Brown, J. N. Provo, R. Hopkins, and M. K. McIntosh. 2005. Conjugated linoleic acid promotes human adipocyte insulin resistance through NFkappaB-dependent cytokine production. *J Biol Chem* 280(46):38445–38456.

Clifton, P. M., K. Bastiaans, and J. B. Keogh. 2009. High protein diets decrease total and abdominal fat and improve CVD risk profile in overweight and obese men and women with elevated triacylglycerol. *Nutr Metab Cardiovasc Dis* 19(8):548–554.

Crochemore, I. C., A. F. Souza, A. C. de Souza, and E. L. Rosado. 2012. Omega-3 polyunsaturated fatty acid supplementation does not influence body composition, insulin resistance, and lipemia in women with type 2 diabetes and obesity. *Nutr Clin Pract* 27(4):553–560.

Crume, T. L., T. M. Bahr, E. J. Mayer-Davis, R. F. Hamman, A. L. Scherzinger, E. Stamm, and D. Dabelea. 2012. Selective protection against extremes in childhood body size, abdominal fat deposition, and fat patterning in breastfed children. *Arch Pediatr Adolesc Med* 166(5):437–443.

Davis, J. N., K. E. Alexander, E. E. Ventura, C. M. Toledo-Corral, and M. I. Goran. 2009. Inverse relation between dietary fiber intake and visceral adiposity in overweight Latino youth. *Am J Clin Nutr* 90(5):1160–1166.

DeFina, L. F., L. G. Marcoux, S. M. Devers, J. P. Cleaver, and B. L. Willis. 2011. Effects of omega-3 supplementation in combination with diet and exercise on weight loss and body composition. *Am J Clin Nutr* 93(2):455–462.

Denova-Gutierrez, E., S. Castanon, J. O. Talavera, M. Flores, N. Macias, S. Rodriguez-Ramirez, Y. N. Flores, and J. Salmeron. 2011. Dietary patterns are associated with different indexes of adiposity and obesity in an urban Mexican population. *J Nutr* 141(5):921–927.

Desroches, S., P. Y. Chouinard, I. Galibois, L. Corneau, J. Delisle, B. Lamarche, P. Couture, and N. Bergeron. 2005. Lack of effect of dietary conjugated linoleic acids naturally incorporated into butter on the lipid profile and body composition of overweight and obese men. *Am J Clin Nutr* 82(2):309–319.

Durmus, B., L. Ay, L. Duijts, H. A. Moll, A. C. Hokken-Koelega, H. Raat, A. Hofman, E. A. Steegers, and V. W. Jaddoe. 2012. Infant diet and subcutaneous fat mass in early childhood: The Generation R Study. *Eur J Clin Nutr* 66(2):253–260.

Durmus, B., D. H. Heppe, O. Gishti, R. Manniesing, M. Abrahamse-Berkeveld, E. M. van der Beek, A. Hofman, L. Duijts, R. Gaillard, and V. W. Jaddoe. 2014. General and abdominal fat outcomes in school-age children associated with infant breastfeeding patterns. *Am J Clin Nutr* 99(6):1351–1358.

Esfahani, A., J. M. Wong, A. Mirrahimi, K. Srichaikul, D. J. Jenkins, and C. W. Kendall. 2009. The glycemic index: Physiological significance. *J Am Coll Nutr* 28(Suppl):439S–445S.

Esmaillzadeh, A. and L. Azadbakht. 2008. Major dietary patterns in relation to general obesity and central adiposity among Iranian women. *J Nutr* 138(2):358–363.

Evans, M., J. Brown, and M. McIntosh. 2002. Isomer-specific effects of conjugated linoleic acid (CLA) on adiposity and lipid metabolism. *J Nutr Biochem* 13(9):508.

Farnsworth, E., N. D. Luscombe, M. Noakes, G. Wittert, E. Argyiou, and P. M. Clifton. 2003. Effect of a high-protein, energy-restricted diet on body composition, glycemic control, and lipid concentrations in overweight and obese hyperinsulinemic men and women. *Am J Clin Nutr* 78(1):31–39.

Fernie, C. E., I. E. Dupont, O. Scruel, Y. A. Carpentier, J.-L. Sébédio, and C. M. Scrimgeour. 2004. Relative absorption of conjugated linoleic acid as triacylglycerol, free fatty acid and ethyl ester in a functional food matrix. *Eur J Lipid Sci Technol* 106(6):347–354.

Ferro-Luzzi, A., W. P. James, and A. Kafatos. 2002. The high-fat Greek diet: A recipe for all? *Eur J Clin Nutr* 56(9):796–809.

Figuiredo-Dias, V., L. Cuppari, M. G. Garcia-Lopes, A. B. de Carvalho, S. A. Draibe, and M. A. Kamimura. 2012. Risk factors for hypovitaminosis D in nondialyzed chronic kidney disease patients. *J Ren Nutr* 22(1):4–11.

Forouhi, N. G., S. J. Sharp, H. Du, D. L. van der A, J. Halkjaer, M. B. Schulze, A. Tjonneland et al. 2009. Dietary fat intake and subsequent weight change in adults: Results from the European Prospective Investigation into Cancer and Nutrition cohorts. *Am J Clin Nutr* 90(6):1632–1641.

Funtikova, A. N., A. A. Benitez-Arciniega, S. F. Gomez, M. Fito, R. Elosua, and H. Schroder. 2014. Mediterranean diet impact on changes in abdominal fat and 10-year incidence of abdominal obesity in a Spanish population. *Br J Nutr* 111(8):1481–1487.

Gaullier, J. M., J. Halse, H. O. Hoivik, K. Hoye, C. Syvertsen, M. Nurminiemi, C. Hassfeld, A. Einerhand, M. O'Shea, and O. Gudmundsen. 2007. Six months supplementation with conjugated linoleic acid induces regional-specific fat mass decreases in overweight and obese. *Br J Nutr* 97(3):550–560.

Gaullier, J. M., J. Halse, K. Hoye, K. Kristiansen, H. Fagertun, H. Vik, and O. Gudmundsen. 2004. Conjugated linoleic acid supplementation for 1 y reduces body fat mass in healthy overweight humans. *Am J Clin Nutr* 79(6):1118–1125.

Goodman-Gruen, D. and D. Kritz-Silverstein. 2003. Usual dietary isoflavone intake and body composition in postmenopausal women. *Menopause* 10(5):427–432.

Greenfield, J. R., K. Samaras, A. B. Jenkins, P. J. Kelly, T. D. Spector, and L. V. Campbell. 2003. Moderate alcohol consumption, dietary fat composition, and abdominal obesity in women: Evidence for gene-environment interaction. *J Clin Endocrinol Metab* 88(11):5381–5386.

Hairston, K. G., M. Z. Vitolins, J. M. Norris, A. M. Anderson, A. J. Hanley, and L. E. Wagenknecht. 2012. Lifestyle factors and 5-year abdominal fat accumulation in a minority cohort: The IRAS Family Study. *Obesity* 20(2):421–427.

Halkjaer, J., A. Tjonneland, B. L. Thomsen, K. Overvad, and T. I. Sorensen. 2006. Intake of macronutrients as predictors of 5-y changes in waist circumference. *Am J Clin Nutr* 84(4):789–797.

Halton, T. L. and F. B. Hu. 2004. The effects of high protein diets on thermogenesis, satiety and weight loss: A critical review. *J Am Coll Nutr* 23(5):373–385.

Hare-Bruun, H., A. Flint, and B. L. Heitmann. 2006. Glycemic index and glycemic load in relation to changes in body weight, body fat distribution, and body composition in adult Danes. *Am J Clin Nutr* 84(4):871–879.

Haslam, D. W. and W. P. James. 2005. Obesity. *Lancet* 366(9492):1197–1209.

Hasselbalch, A. L., B. L. Heitmann, K. O. Kyvik, and T. I. Sorensen. 2010. Associations between dietary intake and body fat independent of genetic and familial environmental background. *Int J Obes* 34(5):892–898.

Hauner, H., D. Much, C. Vollhardt, S. Brunner, D. Schmid, E. M. Sedlmeier, E. Heimberg et al. 2012. Effect of reducing the n-6:n-3 long-chain PUFA ratio during pregnancy and lactation on infant adipose tissue growth within the first year of life: An open-label randomized controlled trial. *Am J Clin Nutr* 95(2):383–394.

Health Canada. 2010. Canadian nutrient file. Found at www.food.nutrition.canada.ca/cnf-fce/index-eng.jsp.

Heiss, C. J., S. E. Shaw, and L. Carothers. 2008. Association of calcium intake and adiposity in postmenopausal women. *J Am Coll Nutr* 27(2):260–266.

Horan, M. K., C. A. McGowan, E. R. Gibney, J. M. Donnelly, and F. M. McAuliffe. 2014. Maternal low glycaemic index diet, fat intake and postprandial glucose influences neonatal adiposity—Secondary analysis from the ROLO study. *Nutr J* 13:78.

Issa, C., N. Darmon, P. Salameh, M. Maillot, M. Batal, and D. Lairon. 2011. A Mediterranean diet pattern with low consumption of liquid sweets and refined cereals is negatively associated with adiposity in adults from rural Lebanon. *Int J Obes* 35(2):251–258.

Jacqmain, M., E. Doucet, J. P. Després, C. Bouchard, and A. Tremblay. 2003. Calcium intake, body composition, and lipoprotein-lipid concentrations in adults. *Am J Clin Nutr* 77(6):1448–1452.

Joseph, S. V., H. Jacques, M. Plourde, P. L. Mitchell, R. S. McLeod, and P. J. Jones. 2011. Conjugated linoleic acid supplementation for 8 weeks does not affect body composition, lipid profile, or safety biomarkers in overweight, hyperlipidemic men. *J Nutr* 141(7):1286–1291.

Kadooka, Y., M. Sato, K. Imaizumi, A. Ogawa, K. Ikuyama, Y. Akai, M. Okano, M. Kagoshima, and T. Tsuchida. 2010. Regulation of abdominal adiposity by probiotics (*Lactobacillus gasseri* SBT2055) in adults with obese tendencies in a randomized controlled trial. *Eur J Clin Nutr* 64(6):636–643.

Kang, K., W. Liu, K. J. Albright, Y. Park, and M. W. Pariza. 2003. trans-10,cis-12 CLA inhibits differentiation of 3T3-L1 adipocytes and decreases PPAR gamma expression. *Biochem Biophys Res Commun* 303(3):795–799.

Kant, A. K. 2010. Dietary patterns: Biomarkers and chronic disease risk. *Appl Physiol Nutr Metab* 35(2):199–206.

Kelly, M. T., K. L. Rennie, J. M. Wallace, P. J. Robson, R. W. Welch, M. P. Hannon-Fletcher, and M. B. Livingstone. 2009. Associations between the portion sizes of food groups consumed and measures of adiposity in the British National Diet and Nutrition Survey. *Br J Nutr* 101(9):1413–1420.

Kerksick, C. M., J. Wismann-Bunn, D. Fogt, A. R. Thomas, L. Taylor, B. I. Campbell, C. D. Wilborn et al. 2010. Changes in weight loss, body composition and cardiovascular disease risk after altering macronutrient distributions during a regular exercise program in obese women. *Nutr J* 9:59.

Kesse-Guyot, E., N. Ahluwalia, C. Lassale, S. Hercberg, L. Fezeu, and D. Lairon. 2013. Adherence to Mediterranean diet reduces the risk of metabolic syndrome: A 6-year prospective study. *Nutr Metab Cardiovasc Dis* 23(7):677–683.

Koh-Banerjee, P., N. F. Chu, D. Spiegelman, B. Rosner, G. Colditz, W. Willett, and E. Rimm. 2003. Prospective study of the association of changes in dietary intake, physical activity, alcohol consumption, and smoking with 9-y gain in waist circumference among 16 587 US men. *Am J Clin Nutr* 78(4):719–727.

Kondoh, T., H. Takase, T. F. Yamaguchi, R. Ochiai, M. Katashima, Y. Katsuragi, and N. Sakane. 2014. Association of dietary factors with abdominal subcutaneous and visceral adiposity in Japanese men. *Obes Res Clin Pract* 8(1):e16–e25.

Kong, J. and Y. C. Li. 2006. Molecular mechanism of 1,25-dihydroxyvitamin D3 inhibition of adipogenesis in 3T3-L1 cells. *Am J Physiol Endocrinol Metab* 290(5):E916–E924.

Krachler, B., M. Eliasson, H. Stenlund, I. Johansson, G. Hallmans, and B. Lindahl. 2006. Reported food intake and distribution of body fat: A repeated cross-sectional study. *Nutr J* 5:34.

Kramer, M. S. and R. Kakuma. 2012. Optimal duration of exclusive breastfeeding. *Cochrane Database Syst Rev* 8:CD003517.

Kreider, R. B., M. P. Ferreira, M. Greenwood, M. Wilson, and A. L. Almada. 2002. Effects of conjugated linoleic acid supplementation during resistance training on body composition, bone density, strength, and selected hematological markers. *J Strength Cond Res* 16(3):325–334.

Krotkiewski, M. 2001. Value of VLCD supplementation with medium chain triglycerides. *Int J Obes Relat Metab Disord* 25(9):1393–1400.

Kunesova, M., R. Braunerova, P. Hlavaty, E. Tvrzicka, B. Stankova, J. Skrha, J. Hilgertova et al. 2006. The influence of n-3 polyunsaturated fatty acids and very low calorie diet during a short-term weight reducing regimen on weight loss and serum fatty acid composition in severely obese women. *Physiol Res* 55(1):63–72.

Lagou, V., G. Liu, H. Zhu, I. S. Stallmann-Jorgensen, B. Gutin, Y. Dong, and H. Snieder. 2011. Lifestyle and socioeconomic-status modify the effects of ADRB2 and NOS3 on adiposity in European-American and African-American adolescents. *Obesity* 19(3):595–603.

Larson, D. E., G. R. Hunter, M. J. Williams, T. Kekes-Szabo, I. Nyikos, and M. I. Goran. 1996. Dietary fat in relation to body fat and intraabdominal adipose tissue: A cross-sectional analysis. *Am J Clin Nutr* 64(5):677–684.

Laso, N., E. Brugue, J. Vidal, E. Ros, J. A. Arnaiz, X. Carne, S. Vidal, S. Mas, R. Deulofeu, and A. Lafuente. 2007. Effects of milk supplementation with conjugated linoleic acid (isomers cis-9, trans-11 and trans-10, cis-12) on body composition and metabolic syndrome components. *Br J Nutr* 98(4):860–867.

Leblanc, V., A. M. Hudon, M. M. Royer, L. Corneau, S. Dodin, C. Bégin, and S. Lemieux. 2015. Differences between men and women in dietary intakes and metabolic profile in response to a 12-week nutritional intervention promoting the Mediterranean diet. *J Nutr Sci* 4:e13.

Lecoutre, S. and C. Breton. 2014. The cellularity of offspring's adipose tissue is programmed by maternal nutritional manipulations. *Adipocyte* 3(4):256–262.

Lecoutre, S. and C. Breton. 2015. Maternal nutritional manipulations program adipose tissue dysfunction in offspring. *Front Physiol* 6:158.

Leidy, H. J., N. S. Carnell, R. D. Mattes, and W. W. Campbell. 2007. Higher protein intake preserves lean mass and satiety with weight loss in pre-obese and obese women. *Obesity* 15(2):421–429.

Li, D. 2015. Omega-3 polyunsaturated fatty acids and non-communicable diseases: Meta-analysis based systematic review. *Asia Pac J Clin Nutr* 24(1):10–15.

Liese, A. D., M. Schulz, F. Fang, T. M. Wolever, R. B. D'Agostino Jr., K. C. Sparks, and E. J. Mayer-Davis. 2005. Dietary glycemic index and glycemic load, carbohydrate and fiber intake, and measures of insulin sensitivity, secretion, and adiposity in the Insulin Resistance Atherosclerosis Study. *Diabetes Care* 28(12):2832–2838.

Liu, J., D. A. Hickson, S. K. Musani, S. A. Talegawkar, T. C. Carithers, K. L. Tucker, C. S. Fox, and H. A. Taylor. 2013. Dietary patterns, abdominal visceral adipose tissue, and cardiometabolic risk factors in African Americans: The Jackson heart study. *Obesity* 21(3):644–651.

Loos, R. J., T. Rankinen, A. S. Leon, J. S. Skinner, J. H. Wilmore, D. C. Rao, and C. Bouchard. 2004. Calcium intake is associated with adiposity in Black and White men and White women of the HERITAGE Family Study. *J Nutr* 134(7):1772–1778.

Lustig, R. H., L. A. Schmidt, and C. D. Brindis. 2012. Public health: The toxic truth about sugar. *Nature* 482(7383):27–29.

Lynch, C. J. and S. H. Adams. 2014. Branched-chain amino acids in metabolic signalling and insulin resistance. *Nat Rev Endocrinol* 10(12):723–736.

Ma, J., M. Sloan, C. S. Fox, U. Hoffmann, C. E. Smith, E. Saltzman, G. T. Rogers, P. F. Jacques, and N. M. McKeown. 2014. Sugar-sweetened beverage consumption is associated with abdominal fat partitioning in healthy adults. *J Nutr* 144(8):1283–1290.

Maersk, M., A. Belza, H. Stodkilde-Jorgensen, S. Ringgaard, E. Chabanova, H. Thomsen, S. B. Pedersen, A. Astrup, and B. Richelsen. 2012. Sucrose-sweetened beverages increase fat storage in the liver, muscle, and visceral fat depot: A 6-mo randomized intervention study. *Am J Clin Nutr* 95(2):283–289.

Maesta, N., E. A. Nahas, J. Nahas-Neto, F. L. Orsatti, C. E. Fernandes, P. Traiman, and R. C. Burini. 2007. Effects of soy protein and resistance exercise on body composition and blood lipids in postmenopausal women. *Maturitas* 56(4):350–358.

Magalhaes, T. C., S. A. Vieira, S. E. Priore, A. Q. Ribeiro, J. A. Lamounier, S. C. Franceschini, and L. F. Sant'Ana. 2012. Exclusive breastfeeding and other foods in the first six months of life: Effects on nutritional status and body composition of Brazilian children. *Scientific World Journal* 2012:468581.

Malpuech-Brugere, C., W. P. Verboeket-van de Venne, R. P. Mensink, M. A. Arnal, B. Morio, M. Brandolini, A. Saebo et al. 2004. Effects of two conjugated linoleic acid isomers on body fat mass in overweight humans. *Obes Res* 12(4):591–598.

Maslova, E., D. Rytter, B. H. Bech, T. B. Henriksen, M. A. Rasmussen, S. F. Olsen, and T. I. Halldorsson. 2014. Maternal protein intake during pregnancy and offspring overweight 20 y later. *Am J Clin Nutr* 100(4):1139–1148.

McCarthy, S. N., P. J. Robson, M. B. Livingstone, M. Kiely, A. Flynn, G. W. Cran, and M. J. Gibney. 2006. Associations between daily food intake and excess adiposity in Irish adults: Towards the development of food-based dietary guidelines for reducing the prevalence of overweight and obesity. *Int J Obes* 30(6):993–1002.

McKeown, N. M., M. Yoshida, M. K. Shea, P. F. Jacques, A. H. Lichtenstein, G. Rogers, S. L. Booth, and E. Saltzman. 2009. Whole-grain intake and cereal fiber are associated with lower abdominal adiposity in older adults. *J Nutr* 139(10):1950–1955.

McNaughton, S. A., G. D. Mishra, A. M. Stephen, and M. E. Wadsworth. 2007. Dietary patterns throughout adult life are associated with body mass index, waist circumference, blood pressure, and red cell folate. *J Nutr* 137(1):99–105.

Molenaar, E. A., J. M. Massaro, P. F. Jacques, K. M. Pou, R. C. Ellison, U. Hoffmann, K. Pencina et al. 2009. Association of lifestyle factors with abdominal subcutaneous and visceral adiposity: The Framingham Heart Study. *Diabetes Care* 32(3):505–510.

Moloney, F., T. P. Yeow, A. Mullen, J. J. Nolan, and H. M. Roche. 2004. Conjugated linoleic acid supplementation, insulin sensitivity, and lipoprotein metabolism in patients with type 2 diabetes mellitus. *Am J Clin Nutr* 80(4):887–895.

Mosdol, A., D. R. Witte, G. Frost, M. G. Marmot, and E. J. Brunner. 2007. Dietary glycemic index and glycemic load are associated with high-density-lipoprotein cholesterol at baseline but not with increased risk of diabetes in the Whitehall II study. *Am J Clin Nutr* 86(4):988–994.

Mougios, V., A. Matsakas, A. Petridou, S. Ring, A. Sagredos, A. Melissopoulou, N. Tsigilis, and M. Nikolaidis. 2001. Effect of supplementation with conjugated linoleic acid on human serum lipids and body fat. *J Nutr Biochem* 12(10):585–594.

Mozaffarian, D., M. B. Katan, A. Ascherio, M. J. Stampfer, and W. C. Willett. 2006. Trans fatty acids and cardiovascular disease. *N Engl J Med* 354(15):1601–1613.

Mumme, K. and W. Stonehouse. 2015. Effects of medium-chain triglycerides on weight loss and body composition: A meta-analysis of randomized controlled trials. *J Acad Nutr Diet* 115(2):249–263.

Munro, I. A. and M. L. Garg. 2012. Dietary supplementation with n-3 PUFA does not promote weight loss when combined with a very-low-energy diet. *Br J Nutr* 108(8):1466–1474.

Munro, I. A. and M. L. Garg. 2013. Prior supplementation with long chain omega-3 polyunsaturated fatty acids promotes weight loss in obese adults: A double-blinded randomised controlled trial. *Food Funct* 4(4):650–658.

Murphy, K. J., G. E. Crichton, K. A. Dyer, A. M. Coates, T. L. Pettman, C. Milte, A. A. Thorp et al. 2013. Dairy foods and dairy protein consumption is inversely related to markers of adiposity in obese men and women. *Nutrients* 5(11):4665–4684.

Newby, P. K., D. Muller, J. Hallfrisch, N. Qiao, R. Andres, and K. L. Tucker. 2003. Dietary patterns and changes in body mass index and waist circumference in adults. *Am J Clin Nutr* 77(6):1417–1425.

Newgard, C. B., J. An, J. R. Bain, M. J. Muehlbauer, R. D. Stevens, L. F. Lien, A. M. Haqq et al. 2009. A branched-chain amino acid-related metabolic signature that differentiates obese and lean humans and contributes to insulin resistance. *Cell Metab* 9(4):311–326.

Odegaard, A. O., A. C. Choh, S. A. Czerwinski, B. Towne, and E. W. Demerath. 2012. Sugar-sweetened and diet beverages in relation to visceral adipose tissue. *Obesity* 20(3):689–691.

Onakpoya, I. J., P. P. Posadzki, L. K. Watson, L. A. Davies, and E. Ernst. 2012. The efficacy of long-term conjugated linoleic acid (CLA) supplementation on body composition in overweight and obese individuals: A systematic review and meta-analysis of randomized clinical trials. *Eur J Nutr* 51(2):127–134.

Panagiotakos, D. B., C. Chrysohoou, C. Pitsavos, and C. Stefanadis. 2006. Association between the prevalence of obesity and adherence to the Mediterranean diet: The ATTICA study. *Nutrition* 22(5):449–456.

Parikh, S., N. K. Pollock, J. Bhagatwala, D. H. Guo, B. Gutin, H. Zhu, and Y. Dong. 2012. Adolescent fiber consumption is associated with visceral fat and inflammatory markers. *J Clin Endocrinol Metab* 97(8):E1451–E1457.

Pariza, M. W. 2004. Perspective on the safety and effectiveness of conjugated linoleic acid. *Am J Clin Nutr* 79(6 Suppl):1132s–1136s.

Pariza, M. W., Y. Park, and M. E. Cook. 2001. The biologically active isomers of conjugated linoleic acid. *Prog Lipid Res* 40(4):283–298.

Pereira, M. A., D. R. Jacobs, Jr., L. Van Horn, M. L. Slattery, A. I. Kartashov, and D. S. Ludwig. 2002. Dairy consumption, obesity, and the insulin resistance syndrome in young adults: The CARDIA Study. *JAMA* 287(16):2081–2089.

Piccolo, B. D., K. B. Comerford, S. E. Karakas, T. A. Knotts, O. Fiehn, and S. H. Adams. 2015. Whey protein supplementation does not alter plasma branched-chained amino acid profiles but results in unique metabolomics patterns in obese women enrolled in an 8-week weight loss trial. *J Nutr* 145(4):691–700.

Piers, L. S., K. Z. Walker, R. M. Stoney, M. J. Soares, and K. O'Dea. 2003. Substitution of saturated with monounsaturated fat in a 4-week diet affects body weight and composition of overweight and obese men. *Br J Nutr* 90(3):717–727.

Pollock, N. K., V. Bundy, W. Kanto, C. L. Davis, P. J. Bernard, H. Zhu, B. Gutin, and Y. Dong. 2012. Greater fructose consumption is associated with cardiometabolic risk markers and visceral adiposity in adolescents. *J Nutr* 142(2):251–257.

Poppitt, S. D., C. M. Strik, A. K. MacGibbon, B. H. McArdle, S. C. Budgett, and A. T. McGill. 2010. Fatty acid chain length, postprandial satiety and food intake in lean men. *Physiol Behav* 101(1):161–167.

Razquin, C., J. Alfredo Martinez, M. A. Martinez-Gonzalez, D. Corella, J. M. Santos, and A. Marti. 2009. The Mediterranean diet protects against waist circumference enlargement in 12Ala carriers for the PPARgamma gene: 2 years' follow-up of 774 subjects at high cardiovascular risk. *Br J Nutr* 102(5):672–679.

Rokling-Andersen, M. H., A. C. Rustan, A. J. Wensaas, O. Kaalhus, H. Wergedahl, T. H. Rost, J. Jensen, B. A. Graff, R. Caesar, and C. A. Drevon. 2009. Marine n-3 fatty acids promote size reduction of visceral adipose depots, without altering body weight and composition, in male Wistar rats fed a high-fat diet. *Br J Nutr* 102(7):995–1006.

Romaguera, D., L. Angquist, H. Du, M. U. Jakobsen, N. G. Forouhi, J. Halkjaer, E. J. Feskens et al. 2010. Dietary determinants of changes in waist circumference adjusted for body mass index—A proxy measure of visceral adiposity. *PLoS One* 5(7):e11588.

Romaguera, D., L. Angquist, H. Du, M. U. Jakobsen, N. G. Forouhi, J. Halkjaer, E. J. Feskens et al. 2011. Food composition of the diet in relation to changes in waist circumference adjusted for body mass index. *PLoS One* 6(8):e23384.

Romaguera, D., T. Norat, T. Mouw, A. M. May, C. Bamia, N. Slimani, N. Travier et al. 2009. Adherence to the Mediterranean diet is associated with lower abdominal adiposity in European men and women. *J Nutr* 139(9):1728–1737.

Rosenbaum, M., R. Knight, and R. L. Leibel. 2015. The gut microbiota in human energy homeostasis and obesity. *Trends Endocrinol Metab* 26(9):493–501.

Rosenblum, J. L., V. M. Castro, C. E. Moore, and L. M. Kaplan. 2012. Calcium and vitamin D supplementation is associated with decreased abdominal visceral adipose tissue in overweight and obese adults. *Am J Clin Nutr* 95(1):101–108.

Rossi, M., C. Bosetti, R. Talamini, P. Lagiou, E. Negri, S. Franceschi, and C. La Vecchia. 2010. Glycemic index and glycemic load in relation to body mass index and waist to hip ratio. *Eur J Nutr* 49(8):459–464.

Rossi, M., E. Negri, C. Bosetti, L. Dal Maso, R. Talamini, A. Giacosa, M. Montella, S. Franceschi, and C. La Vecchia. 2008. Mediterranean diet in relation to body mass index and waist-to-hip ratio. *Public Health Nutr* 11(2):214–217.

Roswall, N., L. Angquist, T. S. Ahluwalia, D. Romaguera, S. C. Larsen, J. N. Ostergaard, J. Halkjaer et al. 2014. Association between Mediterranean and Nordic diet scores and changes in weight and waist circumference: Influence of FTO and TCF7L2 loci. *Am J Clin Nutr* 100(4):1188–1197.

Rouhani, M. H., R. Kelishadi, M. Hashemipour, A. Esmaillzadeh, and L. Azadbakht. 2014. Glycemic index, glycemic load and childhood obesity: A systematic review. *Adv Biomed Res* 3:47.

Rousseaux, J., A. Duhamel, D. Turck, D. Molnar, J. Salleron, E. G. Artero, S. De Henauw et al. 2014. Breastfeeding shows a protective trend toward adolescents with higher abdominal adiposity. *Obes Facts* 7(5):289–301.

Rumawas, M. E., J. B. Meigs, J. T. Dwyer, N. M. McKeown, and P. F. Jacques. 2009. Mediterranean-style dietary pattern, reduced risk of metabolic syndrome traits, and incidence in the Framingham Offspring Cohort. *Am J Clin Nutr* 90(6):1608–1614.

Salehpour, A., F. Hosseinpanah, F. Shidfar, M. Vafa, M. Razaghi, S. Dehghani, A. Hoshiarrad, and M. Gohari. 2012. A 12-week double-blind randomized clinical trial of vitamin D(3) supplementation on body fat mass in healthy overweight and obese women. *Nutr J* 11:78.

Santesso, N., E. A. Akl, M. Bianchi, A. Mente, R. Mustafa, D. Heels-Ansdell, and H. J. Schunemann. 2012. Effects of higher- versus lower-protein diets on health outcomes: A systematic review and meta-analysis. *Eur J Clin Nutr* 66(7):780–788.

Sanz, N., M. Diaz, A. Lopez-Bermejo, C. Sierra, A. Fernandez, F. de Zegher, and L. Ibanez. 2014. Newborns with lower levels of circulating polyunsaturated fatty acids (PUFA) are abdominally more adipose. *Pediatr Obes* 9(3):e68–e72.

Sato, M., K. Uzu, T. Yoshida, E. M. Hamad, H. Kawakami, H. Matsuyama, I. A. Abd El-Gawad, and K. Imaizumi. 2008. Effects of milk fermented by Lactobacillus gasseri SBT2055 on adipocyte size in rats. *Br J Nutr* 99(5):1013–1017.

Sato, T., T. Kameyama, T. Ohori, A. Matsuki, and H. Inoue. 2014. Effects of eicosapentaenoic acid treatment on epicardial and abdominal visceral adipose tissue volumes in patients with coronary artery disease. *J Atheroscler Thromb* 21(10):1031–1043.

Schroder, H., M. A. Mendez, L. Ribas-Barba, M. I. Covas, and L. Serra-Majem. 2010. Mediterranean diet and waist circumference in a representative national sample of young Spaniards. *Int J Pediatr Obes* 5(6):516–519.

Silveira, M. B., R. Carraro, S. Monereo, and J. Tebar. 2007. Conjugated linoleic acid (CLA) and obesity. *Public Health Nutr* 10(10a):1181–1186.

Sites, C. K., B. C. Cooper, M. J. Toth, A. Gastaldelli, A. Arabshahi, and S. Barnes. 2007. Effect of a daily supplement of soy protein on body composition and insulin secretion in postmenopausal women. *Fertil Steril* 88(6):1609–1617.

Smedman, A. and B. Vessby. 2001. Conjugated linoleic acid supplementation in humans—Metabolic effects. *Lipids* 36(8):773–781.

Stallmann-Jorgensen, I. S., B. Gutin, J. L. Hatfield-Laube, M. C. Humphries, M. H. Johnson, and P. Barbeau. 2007. General and visceral adiposity in black and white adolescents and their relation with reported physical activity and diet. *Int J Obes* 31(4):622–629.

Stanhope, K. L., J. M. Schwarz, N. L. Keim, S. C. Griffen, A. A. Bremer, J. L. Graham, B. Hatcher et al. 2009. Consuming fructose-sweetened, not glucose-sweetened, beverages increases visceral adiposity and lipids and decreases insulin sensitivity in overweight/obese humans. *J Clin Invest* 119(5):1322–1334.

Steinhart, H., R. Rickert, and K. Winkler. 2003. Identification and analysis of conjugated linoleic acid isomers (CLA). *Eur J Med Res* 8(8):370–372.

Syvertsen, C., J. Halse, H. O. Hoivik, J. M. Gaullier, M. Nurminiemi, K. Kristiansen, A. Einerhand, M. O'Shea, and O. Gudmundsen. 2007. The effect of 6 months supplementation with conjugated linoleic acid on insulin resistance in overweight and obese. *Int J Obes* 31(7):1148–1154.

Tai, E. S., M. L. Tan, R. D. Stevens, Y. L. Low, M. J. Muehlbauer, D. L. Goh, O. R. Ilkayeva et al. 2010. Insulin resistance is associated with a metabolic profile of altered protein metabolism in Chinese and Asian-Indian men. *Diabetologia* 53(4):757–767.

Takahira, M., K. Noda, M. Fukushima, B. Zhang, R. Mitsutake, Y. Uehara, M. Ogawa, T. Kakuma, and K. Saku. 2011. Randomized, double-blind, controlled, comparative trial of formula food containing soy protein vs. milk protein in visceral fat obesity—FLAVO study. *Circ J* 75(9):2235–2243.

Tang, M. and N. F. Krebs. 2014. High protein intake from meat as complementary food increases growth but not adiposity in breastfed infants: A randomized trial. *Am J Clin Nutr* 100(5):1322–1328.

Tappy, L., K. A. Le, C. Tran, and N. Paquot. 2010. Fructose and metabolic diseases: New findings, new questions. *Nutrition* 26(11–12):1044–1049.

Tapsell, L. C., M. J. Batterham, G. Teuss, S. Y. Tan, S. Dalton, C. J. Quick, L. J. Gillen, and K. E. Charlton. 2009. Long-term effects of increased dietary polyunsaturated fat from walnuts on metabolic parameters in type II diabetes. *Eur J Clin Nutr* 63(8):1008–1015.

Taylor, J. S., S. R. Williams, R. Rhys, P. James, and M. P. Frenneaux. 2006. Conjugated linoleic acid impairs endothelial function. *Arterioscler Thromb Vasc Biol* 26(2):307–312.

Tchernof, A. and J. P. Després. 2013. Pathophysiology of human visceral obesity: An update. *Physiol Rev* 93(1):359–404.

Thorsdottir, I., H. Tomasson, I. Gunnarsdottir, E. Gisladottir, M. Kiely, M. D. Parra, N. M. Bandarra, G. Schaafsma, and J. A. Martinez. 2007. Randomized trial of weight-loss-diets for young adults varying in fish and fish oil content. *Int J Obes* 31(10):1560–1566.

Toeller, M., A. E. Buyken, G. Heitkamp, G. Cathelineau, B. Ferriss, and G. Michel. 2001. Nutrient intakes as predictors of body weight in European people with type 1 diabetes. *Int J Obes Relat Metab Disord* 25(12):1815–1822.

Trichopoulou, A., A. Kouris-Blazos, M. L. Wahlqvist, C. Gnardellis, P. Lagiou, E. Polychronopoulos, T. Vassilakou, L. Lipworth, and D. Trichopoulos. 1995. Diet and overall survival in elderly people. *BMJ* 311(7018):1457–1460.

Trichopoulou, A., A. Naska, P. Orfanos, and D. Trichopoulos. 2005. Mediterranean diet in relation to body mass index and waist-to-hip ratio: The Greek European Prospective Investigation into Cancer and Nutrition Study. *Am J Clin Nutr* 82(5):935–940.

Tricon, S., G. C. Burdge, S. Kew, T. Banerjee, J. J. Russell, E. L. Jones, R. F. Grimble, C. M. Williams, P. Yaqoob, and P. C. Calder. 2004. Opposing effects of cis-9,trans-11 and trans-10,cis-12 conjugated linoleic acid on blood lipids in healthy humans. *Am J Clin Nutr* 80(3):614–620.

Troisi, R. J., J. W. Heinold, P. S. Vokonas, and S. T. Weiss. 1991. Cigarette smoking, dietary intake, and physical activity: Effects on body fat distribution—The Normative Aging Study. *Am J Clin Nutr* 53(5):1104–1111.

Tsuboyama-Kasaoka, N., M. Takahashi, K. Tanemura, H. J. Kim, T. Tange, H. Okuyama, M. Kasai, S. Ikemoto, and O. Ezaki. 2000. Conjugated linoleic acid supplementation reduces adipose tissue by apoptosis and develops lipodystrophy in mice. *Diabetes* 49(9):1534–1542.

Van Horn, L. 2011. Eating pattern analyses: The whole is more than the sum of its parts. *J Am Diet Assoc* 111(2):203.

Van Wymelbeke, V., A. Himaya, J. Louis-Sylvestre, and M. Fantino. 1998. Influence of medium-chain and long-chain triacylglycerols on the control of food intake in men. *Am J Clin Nutr* 68(2):226–234.

Venn, B. J. and T. J. Green. 2007. Glycemic index and glycemic load: Measurement issues and their effect on diet-disease relationships. *Eur J Clin Nutr* 61(Suppl 1):S122–S131.

Vilela, A. A., R. Sichieri, R. A. Pereira, D. B. Cunha, P. R. Rodrigues, R. M. Goncalves-Silva, and M. G. Ferreira. 2014. Dietary patterns associated with anthropometric indicators of abdominal fat in adults. *Cad Saude Publica* 30(3):502–510.

Villegas, R., A. Salim, M. M. Collins, A. Flynn, and I. J. Perry. 2004. Dietary patterns in middle-aged Irish men and women defined by cluster analysis. *Public Health Nutr* 7(8):1017–1024.

Wamberg, L., U. Kampmann, H. Stodkilde-Jorgensen, L. Rejnmark, S. B. Pedersen, and B. Richelsen. 2013. Effects of vitamin D supplementation on body fat accumulation, inflammation, and metabolic risk factors in obese adults with low vitamin D levels—Results from a randomized trial. *Eur J Intern Med* 24(7):644–649.

Wang, C., W. S. Harris, M. Chung, A. H. Lichtenstein, E. M. Balk, B. Kupelnick, H. S. Jordan, and J. Lau. 2006. n-3 Fatty acids from fish or fish-oil supplements, but not alpha-linolenic acid, benefit cardiovascular disease outcomes in primary- and secondary-prevention studies: A systematic review. *Am J Clin Nutr* 84(1):5–17.

Watras, A. C., A. C. Buchholz, R. N. Close, Z. Zhang, and D. A. Schoeller. 2007. The role of conjugated linoleic acid in reducing body fat and preventing holiday weight gain. *Int J Obes* 31(3):481–487.

Whigham, L. D., M. O'Shea, I. C. Mohede, H. P. Walaski, and R. L. Atkinson. 2004. Safety profile of conjugated linoleic acid in a 12-month trial in obese humans. *Food Chem Toxicol* 42(10):1701–1709.

Whisner, C. M., B. E. Young, E. K. Pressman, R. A. Queenan, E. M. Cooper, and K. O. O'Brien. 2015. Maternal diet but not gestational weight gain predicts central adiposity accretion in utero among pregnant adolescents. *Int J Obes* 39(4):565–570.

Wolongevicz, D. M., L. Zhu, M. J. Pencina, R. W. Kimokoti, P. K. Newby, R. B. D'Agostino, and B. E. Millen. 2010. An obesity dietary quality index predicts abdominal obesity in women: Potential opportunity for new prevention and treatment paradigms. *J Obes* 2010:945987.

Xu, H. E., M. H. Lambert, V. G. Montana, D. J. Parks, S. G. Blanchard, P. J. Brown, D. D. Sternbach et al. 1999. Molecular recognition of fatty acids by peroxisome proliferator-activated receptors. *Mol Cell* 3(3):397–403.

Zambell, K. L., N. L. Keim, M. D. Van Loan, B. Gale, P. Benito, D. S. Kelley, and G. J. Nelson. 2000. Conjugated linoleic acid supplementation in humans: Effects on body composition and energy expenditure. *Lipids* 35(7):777–782.

Zemel, M. B., J. Richards, S. Mathis, A. Milstead, L. Gebhardt, and E. Silva. 2005. Dairy augmentation of total and central fat loss in obese subjects. *Int J Obes* 29(4):391–397.

Zemel, M. B., H. Shi, B. Greer, D. Dirienzo, and P. C. Zemel. 2000. Regulation of adiposity by dietary calcium. *FASEB J* 14(9):1132–1138.

Zive, M. M., H. McKay, G. C. Frank-Spohrer, S. L. Broyles, J. A. Nelson, and P. R. Nader. 1992. Infant-feeding practices and adiposity in 4-y-old Anglo- and Mexican-Americans. *Am J Clin Nutr* 55(6):1104–1108.

Zulet, M. A., B. Puchau, H. H. Hermsdorff, C. Navarro, and J. A. Martinez. 2008. Vitamin A intake is inversely related with adiposity in healthy young adults. *J Nutr Sci Vitaminol* 54(5):347–352.

8 Nutritional Considerations for Cardiometabolic Health in Childhood and Adolescent Obesity

Elizabeth Prout Parks, Jennifer Panganiban, Stephen R. Daniels, and Julie Brothers

CONTENTS

ABSTRACT

Childhood obesity develops through an interplay of genetics, environment, and behavior. Treatment of childhood obesity includes dietary modification, increasing physical activity, and, at times, medication and surgery. Obesity can lead to several comorbidities and chronic diseases, the most common include hypertension, cardiac changes, dyslipidemia, metabolic syndrome, type 2 diabetes mellitus, and nonalcoholic fatty liver disease. These diseases can serve to shorten the child's life. Our efforts should be focused on primarily reducing obesity and, when necessary, adequately treating the secondary outcomes in an effort to reduce future morbidity and mortality.

ABBREVIATIONS

ALT	Alanine aminotransferase
AST	Aspartate aminotransferase
BMI	Body mass index
CDC	Centers for Disease Control
CDO	Combined dyslipidemia of obesity
CMI	Comprehensive multidisciplinary intervention
CVD	Cardiovascular disease
DASH	Dietary approaches to stop hypertension
FDA	Food and Drug Administration
FRAGILE	Low-fructose/low glycemic index/load
GB	Gastric bypass
GI	Glycemic index
GL	Glycemic load
HbA1C	Hemoglobin A1c
HDL-C	High-density lipoprotein cholesterol
HOMA	Homeostatic Model Assessment
HOMA-IR	Homeostatic Model Assessment-Estimated Insulin Resistance
IDF	International Diabetes Federation
LDL-C	Low-density lipoprotein cholesterol
LDL-P	Low-density lipoprotein particle
LSG	Laparoscopic sleeve Gastrectomy
LVH	Left ventricular hypertrophy
METSYN	Metabolic syndrome
MC4R	Melanocortin 4 receptor
MSD	Mediterranean-style diet
NAFLD	Nonalcoholic fatty liver disease
NASH	Nonalcoholic steatohepatitis
NHANES	National Health and Nutrition Examination Survey
SWM	Structured weight management
T2DM	Type 2 diabetes mellitus
TCI	Tertiary care intervention
TG	Triglycerides
USDA	United States Department of Agriculture

DEFINITION OF OBESITY IN CHILDHOOD AND ADOLESCENCE

Obesity is caused by an energy imbalance in which individuals expend less energy than they consume. Body mass index (BMI) is an indirect measure of body fat and provides a guideline for weight in relation to height. BMI is measured as weight in kilograms divided by height in meters squared. This has become an accepted standard of measurement to classify children 2 years and older into weight categories (Deurenberg et al. 1991). Based on the Centers for Disease Control (CDC) Growth Charts, children between the ages of 2 and 20 years can be categorized as underweight, normal weight, overweight, and obese (Flegal et al. 2011). More recently, formal definitions for severe obesity with new growth charts have been developed (Gulati et al. 2012). The following are the current weight classifications for children, based on age and sex:

- Underweight: BMI percentile < 5th percentile
- Normal weight: BMI between the 5th and 85th percentiles
- Overweight: BMI between the 85th and 95th percentiles
- Obesity: BMI ≥ 95th percentile
- Severe obesity: BMI ≥ 120% of the 95th percentile or a BMI ≥ 35 kg/m^2, whichever is lower (Flegal et al. 2011, Gulati et al. 2012), which corresponds to approximately the 99th percentile or BMI z-score (standard deviations change) ≥ 2.33 (Ogden et al. 2014)

Severe obesity that exceeds the 99th percentile is tracked on a specialized percentile curve for obesity. Adult classification is used for BMI ≥ 27 kg/m^2 in adolescents over age 18 years for consideration of medication and bariatric surgery.

In adults, the classification of overweight and obesity is as follows (National Institutes of Health 1998):

- Overweight: BMI ≥ 25 kg/m^2
- Obesity: BMI ≥ 30 kg/m^2, further classified into
  - Class 1 (BMI 30–34 kg/m^2)
  - Class 2 (BMI 35–39 kg/m^2)
  - Class 3 (BMI ≥ 40 kg/m^2)

PREVALENCE AND TRENDS OF CHILDHOOD OBESITY

Based on the National Health and Nutrition Examination Survey (NHANES) analysis performed from 2011 to 2012, one-third of the U.S. childhood population is either overweight or obese (Ogden et al. 2014). The good news is that there have been no significant changes in child overweight and obesity prevalence between 2003–2004 and 2011–2012. However, the prevalence of severe obesity among children aged 2–19 years has continued to increase from 1.2% (1976–1980) to 3% (1988–1994) to 4.9% (1999–2004) and, most recently, 5.9% in 2012 (Ogden et al. 2014). Additionally, there are racial and ethnic differences in childhood obesity, with obesity being more common among American Indians, non-Hispanic blacks, and Mexican Americans when compared to non-Hispanic whites (Wang 2011, Wang et al. 2011).

CRITICAL PERIODS FOR THE ONSET OF CHILDHOOD OBESITY

Early-life risk factors for childhood obesity include the following maternal factors: gestational diabetes, depression, smoking during pregnancy, and low income (Rudolf 2011). The following factors have also been associated with the development of childhood obesity: large or small for gestational age at birth, rapid infant weight gain during the first 6 months of life, poor infant sleep, television viewing under age 24 months, more than 2 hours per day of television viewing over the age of 24 months, and early adiposity rebound, defined as follows (Blair et al. 2007).

Risk factors for an obese child becoming an obese adult include child age, parental obesity, severity of child obesity, and low-income household status (Whitaker et al. 1997, Parsons et al. 1999, CDC 2009). Longitudinal studies reveal that a substantial component of adolescent obesity is established before 5 years of age (Cunningham et al. 2014). A child with severe obesity over 12 years of age has a 75%–80% chance of becoming a Class 3 obese adult (The et al. 2010). One parent with obesity increases the risk for adult obesity in the child by 50%–80% (Whitaker et al. 1997).

Adiposity Rebound

Adiposity rebound is the period, between 3 and 6 years of age, when a child begins to lose excess infant adiposity and the BMI declines. With the decline, the BMI reaches a minimum and then begins increasing until adulthood. The earlier the age at which this minimum BMI value occurs, the more likely a child is to be overweight or obese as an adult (Williams and Goulding 2009).

CAUSES OF CHILDHOOD OBESITY

When a child or adolescent is found to be overweight or obese, it is important to differentiate between a primary cause, which is usually multifactorial, and a much rarer secondary cause. Secondary causes of obesity may be due to or associated with genetic syndromes, endocrine disorders, neurologic disorders, or medications. Table 8.1 demonstrates many of the different causes and conditions that may be associated with obesity in childhood (Gunay-Aygun et al. 1997, Speiser et al. 2005). Recently, melanocortin

TABLE 8.1
Causes of Childhood Obesity

Possible Causes	Diagnosis
Primary/simple	Multifactorial
	Environment
	Psychosocial
	Lifestyle
Genetic syndromes	Melanocortin 4 receptor (MC4R) deficiency
	Leptin deficiency
	Prader–Willi
	Turner syndrome
	Trisomy 21
	Albright hereditary osteodystrophy
	Bardet–Biedl syndrome
	Cohen syndrome
	Borjeson–Forssman–Lehmann syndrome
	Wilson–Turner syndrome
	Alstrom syndrome
	Carpenter syndrome
Endocrine disorders	Hypothyroidism
	Growth hormone deficiency
	Cortisol excess
	Hyperinsulinemia
Neurologic	Injury to the pituitary or the hypothalamus
	Brain tumor
	Cranial irradiation
	Infection
Medication	High dose and chronic glucocorticoids
	Certain antipsychotic medications
	Certain antidepressant medications
	Certain antiseizure medications
	Insulin
	Growth hormone
Psychiatric	Depression
	Eating disorder

Sources: Speiser, P.W. et al., *J. Clin. Endocrinol. Metab.*, 90, 1871, 2005; Gunay-Aygun, M. et al., *Behav. Genet.*, 27, 307, 1997.

4 receptor deficiency has been identified as the most common monogenetic cause of childhood obesity and is associated with increased linear growth and hyperinsulinism during childhood (Martinelli et al. 2011). While distinguishing between primary and secondary causes of obesity may be difficult in some instances, usually a detailed medical history, including timing of weight gain onset, developmental delays, linear growth, and diet and exercise habits; a complete review of systems; a full physical examination, notably looking for location of adipose deposition, dysmorphic facies, enlarged tonsils, undescended testis, acanthosis nigricans, striae, and/or hirsutism; and focused laboratory testing will help determine the cause (Barlow and Dietz 1998, Speiser et al. 2005). Delayed linear growth in the face of developing obesity is a major clue that there may be a secondary cause for the obesity. In addition, there may be more than one reason for the obesity, such as a medication that may cause weight gain; consuming excess calories and not exercising may also contribute to the weight gain.

TREATMENT OF CHILD AND ADOLESCENT OBESITY

Weight Management Goals in Children and Adolescents

In order to be successful, weight loss through lifestyle intervention in children requires behavioral treatment for not only the child as an individual but also the whole family as a unit (Spear et al. 2007). Target weight loss goals should be realistic and discussed at baseline and after each follow-up session as shown in Table 8.2. Epstein et al. (1994) reported that behavioral treatments that included both the parent and the child were more effective at reducing the percentage of overweight children compared to those that focused only on the child or those that had a nonspecific target. Data in adults have shown that an overall weight loss of 5%–10% reduces cardiovascular and metabolic risk. As children are still growing, and weight is based on the growth of muscle, bone, and fat mass, BMI is commonly used to estimate weight status. In children, a BMI z-score of 0.5 (reduction in the standard deviation from the norm BMI z-score = 0) reduces cardiovascular risk and is equivalent to maintaining BMI for 1 year.

As shown in Table 8.2, Barlow et al. (2007) proposed a comprehensive stepwise approach for the prevention and treatment of obesity. This includes the following stages:

- Stage 1 (prevention plus): Lifestyle intervention provided by a primary care provider
- Stage 2 (structured weight management): Monthly visits with a primary care physician and support from a registered dietitian
- Stage 3 (comprehensive multidisciplinary intervention): Intensive weight loss program composed of weekly visits for a minimum of 8–12 weeks at a pediatric weight management center
- Stage 4 (tertiary care intervention): Use of medical diets, medications, and surgery in addition to the interventions provided in Stage 3 (the approach may differ based on individual hospital protocol)

These comprehensive interventions employ a multidisciplinary team (medical provider, registered dietician, exercise specialist, mental health professional, nurse, and social worker) who focuses on behavioral therapy, dietary modification, and physical activity (Chen et al. 1997). This seems to be the most successful approach to decreasing long-term weight and risk for future comorbidities (Levine et al. 2001). The recommendations put forth that are utilized in the community focus on children receiving 5 fruits or vegetables per day, 2 hours or less of screen time, 1 hour or more of physical activity, and 0 sweetened drinks (Barlow et al. 2007).

Dietary Modification

Limited research exists for evaluating dietary treatment programs in isolation. Although the outcomes are mixed, there is evidence to support the use of a reduced energy diet as an effective component of a weight management program typically in children over age 5 years (Epstein et al. 1990, 1994).

TABLE 8.2
Weight Goals and Intervention Stages, according to Age and BMI Categories

Age (Year)	BMI Category	Weight Goal	Initial Intervention Stage	Highest Intervention Stage
<2	Weight for height	NA	Prevention counseling	Prevention counseling
2–5	5th–84th percentile or 85th –94th percentile with no health risks	Weight velocity maintenance	Prevention counseling	Prevention counseling
	85th–94th percentile with health risks	Weight maintenance or slow weight gain	Prevention plus (stage 1)	SWM (stage 2)
	≥95th percentile	Weight maintenance (weight loss of up to 1 lb/month may be acceptable if BMI is >21 or 22 kg/m^2)	Prevention plus (stage 1)	CMI (stage 3)
6–11	5th–84th percentile or 85th–94th percentile with no health risks	Weight velocity maintenance	Prevention counseling	Prevention counseling
	85th–94th percentile with health risks	Weight maintenance	Prevention plus (stage 1)	SWM (stage 2)
	95th–99th percentile	Gradual weight loss (1 lb/month or 0.5 kg/month)	Prevention plus (stage 1)	CMI (stage 3)
	≥99th percentile	Weight loss (maximum is 2 lb/week)	Prevention plus (stage 1) or stage 2 or 3 if family is motivated	TCI (stage 4), if appropriate
12–18	5th–84th percentile or 85th–94th percentile with no health risks	Weight velocity maintenance; after linear growth is complete, weight maintenance	Prevention counseling	Prevention counseling
	85th–94th percentile with health risks	Weight maintenance or gradual weight loss	Prevention plus (stage 1)	SWM (stage 2)
	95th–99th percentile	Weight loss (maximum is 2 lb/week)	Prevention plus (stage 1)	TCI (stage 4), if appropriate
	≥99th percentile	Weight loss (maximum is 2 lb/week)	Prevention plus (stage 1) or stage 2 or 3 if patient and family are motivated	TCI (stage 4), if appropriate

Source: Adapted from Barlow, S.E. and Expert Committee, *Pediatrics*, 120, S164, 2007.
SWM, structured weight management; CMI, comprehensive multidisciplinary intervention; TCI, tertiary care intervention.

Semi-Structured Diet Regimens

Semi-structured diet regimens focused on family selection of higher nutrient quality and low energy density have shown promising results (Epstein et al. 1990, 1994). Families are taught how to make healthy choices using the "traffic light" format. Foods classified as "Red" should be eaten rarely, "Yellow" eaten less often, and "Green" eaten most often (Epstein et al. 1990, 1994). The United States Department of Agriculture (USDA) MyPlate is based on the Dietary Guidelines for Americans 2010 and has replaced MyPyramid. MyPlate is a guideline for building an optimal diet for children and is aimed at the general public to provide a visual representation of the different food groups and their portion sizes. Recommendations emphasize filling half of the plate with vegetables and fruits and the other half with protein and grains, with protein having the smallest section. Protein replaces the meat category, as many protein sources are not from animals. Additionally, a separate dairy section is included. MyPlate has removed foods that have low nutritional value, such as sugar-sweetened beverages and bakery products (U.S. Department of Agriculture and U.S. Department of Health and Human Services 2011).

Meal Replacements

Meal replacements are typically composed of products such as liquid shakes, meal bars, and frozen food entrees, which provide a fixed amount of food with a known calorie content. When added to a lifestyle modification program, meal replacements have reliably increased weight losses by 2.5 and 2.4 kg, at 3 and 12 months, respectively. Berkowitz et al. (2011) studied 113 obese adolescents and demonstrated a 6.3% decrease in BMI compared with a 3.8% decrease in patients placed on a conventional diet for 4 months; however, both dietary intervention groups regained their weight at 12 months of follow-up.

Macronutrient Composition

The evidence for children and adolescents does not support any specific macronutrient or dietary strategy for BMI reduction at this time. A low-glycemic-index (GI) diet has been proposed to have beneficial metabolic effects in treatment of obesity by decreasing the postprandial rise in glucose and insulin. The GI describes how a controlled portion of carbohydrate affects blood glucose in the postprandial period. A study evaluating 22 obese children placed on a low-GI diet of 60 for 6 months (the GI for glucose = 100) found a significant decrease in BMI z-score, improved insulin resistance, and lowered triglyceride concentrations in comparison to their counterparts placed on a hypocaloric diet with a glycemic index of 90 (Parillo et al. 2012). The Mediterranean-style diet (MSD) has been shown to decrease cardiovascular events and increase life expectancy in adult populations (Grosso et al. 2014). Similarly, it has been shown to efficiently decrease metabolic syndrome (MetSyn) by 20%–43%, regardless of age, sex, physical activity, lipid levels, and blood pressure (Babio et al. 2009). This type of diet characteristically uses extra virgin olive oil, fish, wheat, olives, and grapes. A study evaluating 49 obese children with MetSyn placed on a 16-week dietary intervention found that children on the MSD had a significant decrease in BMI, lean mass, fat mass, glucose, total cholesterol, triglycerides (TG), high-density lipoprotein cholesterol (HDL-C), and low-density lipoprotein cholesterol (LDL-C) in comparison to those placed on a standard diet, which comprised 55%–60% carbohydrates (45%–50% complex and no more than 10% refined and processed sugars), 25%–30% lipids, and 15% proteins (Velázquez-López et al. 2014).

A low-fructose diet has been shown to improve LDL-C and nonalcoholic fatty liver disease (NAFLD) but does not have a significant impact on childhood BMI values (Mager et al. 2015). Fructose is a monosaccharide typically consumed in sweeteners with sucrose (50% fructose, 50% glucose) and high-fructose corn syrup (42% or 55% fructose, with the remainder glucose). Beverages with added sugar and fruit juice are the most common fructose sources in children.

Finally, low-carbohydrate diets have resulted in a significant reduction in BMI, liver enzymes, and triglyceride levels in adults with NAFLD and obesity (Foster et al. 2003, Brehm et al. 2003). These diets seem to be more efficacious than energy-restricted low-fat diets over the short term for weight loss, although there seems to be no significant difference in maintenance of decreased BMI between the diets over 1 year (Baron et al. 1986, Harvey-Berino 1998, 1999, Foster et al. 2003).

Fruits and Vegetables

Research studies have shown that children are least likely to consume adequate amounts of foods from the fruit and vegetable group. Evidence, although from cross-sectional studies, indicates that greater fruit and vegetable intake may provide modest protection against increased adiposity (Lin and Morrison 2002).

Sweetened Beverages

The consumption of sugar-sweetened beverages is a significant contributor to the development of obesity (Malik et al. 2013, DeBoer et al. 2013). Energy consumed in liquid form seems to be less regulated compared to energy consumed in solid form. According to a national survey, sugar-sweetened beverages were the sixth leading food source of energy among children, constituting 10%–15% of total caloric intake (Murphy et al. 2005). Reducing the consumption of sugar-sweetened beverages among overweight and obese adolescents is associated with a decrease in BMI (Ebbeling 2012a).

Physical and Sedentary Activity

Although energy intake is a significant portion of the energy equation, the role of energy expenditure is also important. Physical activity is the only modifiable component of the energy expenditure portion of the energy balance equation. An increase in sedentary activity along with an overall decrease in physical activity are major contributing factors to the increased prevalence of overweight and obesity in children and adolescents (Dowda et al. 2001, Berkey et al. 2003). The American Academy of Pediatrics recommends that children and adolescents participate in at least 60 minutes of moderate-intensity physical activity most days of the week, preferably daily (American Academy of Pediatrics 2000). Strategies to increase physical activity should include increases in structured and nonstructured physical activity and reduction in the amount of time spent in sedentary activities (Goran and Treuth 2001).

Screen Time

Sedentary behavior is usually in the form of screen time, which includes television, video games, computers, tablets, phones, and other media that are not used for educational activities (Falbe et al. 2013). Substantial evidence supports the importance of reducing sedentary behavior as a means of preventing and treating obesity in children (Waters et al. 2011, Braithwaite et al. 2013, Falbe et al. 2013). Reducing sedentary behavior may be more effective than increasing structured physical activity with the secondary benefit of reducing caloric intake (Epstein et al. 2008, Epstein et al. 1995).

Experts recommend screen time to be limited to less than 2 hours a day, and children under the age of 2 should have no screen time (Barlow et al. 2007). Television viewing is the most established environmental influence on the development of obesity during childhood Dietz et al. 1985, Robinson et al. 1999. The amount of time spent watching television or the presence of a television in a child's bedroom is directly related to the prevalence of obesity in children and adolescents (Gilbert-Diamond et al. 2014, Gortmaker et al. 1996, Kaur et al. 2003).

Medications for Obesity Treatment

Currently, the only medication that is approved for the treatment of obesity in adolescents under the age of 18 years is Orlistat (Yanovski and Yanovski 2014). Orlistat is a lipase inhibitor that prevents the absorption of fat and on average results in a 3% weight loss over time. It is rarely used in adolescents as it causes flatulence, abdominal pain, smelly stools, malabsorption of fat-soluble vitamins, and alteration in liver enzymes. Thus, adherence to this medication is understandably challenging for this age group. Other medications that are approved for patients over age 18 years include phentermine, phentermine plus topiramate (Qsymia), lorcaserin, and bupropion plus naltrexone (Contrave) (Yanovski and Yanovski 2014). Expected weight loss from these medications is between 5% and 10%. Topiramate is approved by the Food and Drug Administration (FDA) in children over age 10 years for seizures and migraine headaches, but not specifically for weight loss alone. The medication, however, is often used off-label for this purpose. Topiramate is a carbonic anhydrase inhibitor and binds to the GABA receptors in the brain and appears to decrease appetite, as well as alter the taste of food, resulting in decreased food consumption (Yanovski and Yanovski 2014).

Metabolic and Bariatric Surgery

Bariatric surgery combined with lifestyle management currently results in greater sustained weight loss and improvement and/or resolution of comorbidities compared with lifestyle management alone (Alqahtani and Elahmedi 2015, McGinty et al. 2015). Surgeries that are currently FDA approved for adolescents above age 13 years include the Roux-en-Y gastric bypass (GB), and the laparoscopic sleeve gastrectomy (LSG) (see criteria for surgery here). Although still available for adults, the laparoscopic adjustable band, secondary to complications in adults, was removed from FDA trials in adolescents in 2012. Both GB and LSG have shown significant improvement in obesity-related comorbidities, with 70%–100% resolution of type 2 diabetes, prediabetes (impaired glucose tolerance), insulin resistance, hypertension, dyslipidemia, and nonalcoholic steatohepatitis (NASH) (Bondada et al. 2011, Alqahtani and Elahmedi 2015). Improvements in insulin sensitivity are seen quickly, usually prior to discharge of the patient from the hospital, which implies that they are not due solely to weight loss. These changes are believed to be caused by alteration of gut hormone interactions (GLP-1, PPY, and ghrelin) with the pancreas and the brain (Lee et al. 2011). Because of these metabolic changes, the terminology "metabolic and bariatric surgery" is a more accurate description of the surgery. The LSG has very similar effects on weight loss and comorbidities to the GB but has fewer nutritional and surgical complications. Thus, the LSG is currently the most widely performed procedure in both adults and adolescents and is the surgery of choice for adolescents.

The GB is the oldest of the surgeries and is therefore considered to be the gold standard. Expected weight loss is 70%–80% of excess weight loss (weight loss over ideal body weight minus weight loss × 100%). The duodenum is bypassed and reconnected to the lower part of the jejunum, and the stomach is reduced to pouch that is able to hold 15 mm and is approximately the size of a chicken nugget. The amount of food that can be ingested is limited due to the size of the stomach. Further, because the majority of the stomach and small intestine are bypassed, the fats and simple sugars are malabsorbed, thus limiting the consumption of these foods. For the first 6 months after surgery, consuming foods high in fat or sugar results in diarrhea, a drop in blood pressure, lightheadedness, sweating, and nausea; this is called the "dumping syndrome." These symptoms may result in behavior change regarding the types of food eaten, but then decrease and often go away completely with time as the body adjusts. Unfortunately, fat-soluble vitamins (A, D, E, and K), water-soluble vitamins (B12, thiamin, and folate), and minerals (calcium, iron, zinc, and copper) are also not absorbed. Patients therefore require vitamin and mineral supplementation for life (Xanthakos 2008). Patients are also at increased risk for other surgical complications (see Chapter 5).

The LSG procedure removes the greater curve of the stomach or 80% of the stomach, leaving a narrowed gastric tube, which forms the shape of a sleeve. The reduction in the size of the stomach limits the amount of food consumed. Additionally, the hormone ghrelin, which stimulates hunger and appetite, is normally produced in the greater curvature of the stomach; removal of this section of the stomach eliminates the stimulation of hunger for at least the first 9–12 months after surgery. Nutritional complications directly related to the surgery include vitamin B12 deficiency due to the lack of the production of intrinsic factor and fluoride deficiency. Due to concerns for limited intake of food and possible rapid transit of food during digestion, additional vitamin supplementation is recommended. Further, severely obese adolescents have demonstrated an increased risk of vitamin D deficiency as well as iron-deficiency anemia prior to surgery (Xanthakos 2008, Aarts et al. 2011).

Surgical Criteria

The criteria for an adolescent to undergo metabolic and bariatric surgery are more stringent than for an adult. This surgery is considered elective with permanent and serious long-term consequences extending into adulthood. As well, there is a lack of long-term outcome data in the pediatric population.

According to Michalsky et al. (2011), the medical criteria for metabolic and bariatric surgery for an adolescent should include

- Age ≥ 13, although most facilities do not perform surgery under age 14 in the United States
- BMI ≥ 50 kg/m^2 without any comorbidities
- BMI ≥ 40 kg/m^2 with 1 serious or 2 minor comorbidities: NASH, severe psychological distress, arthropathies related to weight, hypertension, dyslipidemia, chronic venous insufficiency, panniculitis

- BMI ≥ 35 kg/m² with type 2 diabetes mellitus (T2DM), moderate-to-severe obstructive sleep apnea, pseudotumor cerebri, NASH with advanced fibrosis (Nobili et al. 2015)
- Tanner stage 4 or 5 and 95% growth completion as indicated with bone age

Additional criteria include

- Demonstrates maturity to understand risks as assessed by multiple members of the bariatric team, including the psychologist
- Attends a medical weight management program for at least 6 months
- Takes required medications, vitamins, and supplements
- Attends appointments with specialists
- Agrees not to get pregnant for at least 18 months after surgery
- Has family who will support the adolescent by providing the necessary food and materials, and supports attendance to visits and changes in the household
- Absolute contraindications include a medically correctable cause of obesity; active substance abuse problem; medical, psychiatric, or cognitive disability that impairs ability for adherence

Prior to surgery, patients are asked to demonstrate the ability to comply with behaviors that will decrease surgical complications and will allow them to be successful with surgery (Nogueira and Hrovat 2014). Patients are asked to separate eating and drinking by 20–30 minutes, which decreases the risk of vomiting early after surgery. Additionally, liquids allow for the passage of more food at a time through the sleeve. Patients must drink 64–90 fluid ounces of water daily and take sips as gulping liquid will cause chest pain. Adequate fluid intake is important in that the most common reason for hospital readmission is dehydration (Nogueira and Hrovat 2014). Patients are required to eliminate carbonated beverages to prevent bloating and gas pains with the surgery. They are asked to only drink water and soy, skim, or almond milk, because sugar-sweetened beverages have no nutritional value but have excess calories that can pass through the sleeve easily. Patients must track their protein intake to make sure they are consuming a minimum of 60 g/day to allow for sufficient wound healing, prevent hair loss, and prevent loss of muscle mass. Prior to metabolic and bariatric surgery, patients are put on a 2-week modified meal replacement diet to reduce the size of the liver. The components of this diet are not standardized but generally are comprised of 1000–1300 calories and are high in protein (Nogueira and Hrovat 2014).

CARDIOMETABOLIC COMORBIDITIES IN CHILDHOOD OBESITY

A child with a BMI at the 85th percentile or higher is at risk for medical problems affecting multiple organ systems. More than half of obese adolescents have at least one risk factor for premature cardiovascular disease (CVD) and 10% have at least three CVD risk factors, such as hypertension, dyslipidemia, and insulin resistance (Freedman et al. 1999, Daniels 2009, Steinberger et al. 2009, Power et al. 1997). This section will focus on the cardiometabolic health risks associated with childhood obesity and nutritional considerations with these risks.

Hypertension

Maintaining normal blood pressure throughout childhood and adolescence is an important aspect of pediatric cardiometabolic health. During childhood, blood pressure is strongly related to age, sex, and body size. Thus, blood pressure percentiles for children and adolescents are standardized for age, sex, and the height percentile. Normal blood pressure is defined as systolic and diastolic blood pressure below the 90th percentile (Daniels et al. 2011). Prehypertension is defined as either systolic or diastolic blood pressure between the 90th and 95th percentile or, for teenagers, above 120/80, which has been used as the definition of prehypertension in adults, but below the 95th percentile.

Stage 1 hypertension is blood pressure above the 95th percentile, but below the 99th percentile plus 5 mmHg. Stage 2 hypertension is systolic or diastolic blood pressure persistently above the 99th percentile, plus 5 mmHg. This value is generally about 12 mmHg above the 95th percentile. For a patient to have hypertension, the blood pressure must be persistently elevated on three or more occasions, days, weeks, or months apart.

Blood pressure should be measured routinely at all health maintenance visits and other health care visits after the age of 3 years. When an elevated blood pressure is detected, repeat measurements should be made within 3–6 months for prehypertension; within 1 month for stage 1; and within 1 week or sooner for Stage 2 hypertension, or if there are signs or symptoms related to hypertension.

As in adults, childhood blood pressure has many different determinants, including genetic and environmental factors. Important environmental factors include obesity, as well as diet (discussed in the following text) and physical activity. The mechanisms by which these factors raise blood pressure are often not clearly understood. However, such mechanistic knowledge is usually not necessary to implement appropriate preventive or treatment strategies.

Obesity in childhood is associated with blood pressure elevation along with a variety of other cardiometabolic alterations, as discussed elsewhere in this chapter. Weight management strategies that result in reduction of the BMI percentile have been clearly shown to reduce blood pressure, particularly when elevated blood pressure was present prior to the intervention. Haynes (1986) reviewed early studies of the impact of weight reduction on blood pressure in adults and found evidence that weight reduction resulted in lower blood pressure. Rocchini et al. (1988) demonstrated in a clinical trial that weight loss is associated with blood pressure reduction in obese adolescents. One question has been whether weight loss may be effective for blood pressure reduction because weight loss diets are often also low in sodium. Reisin et al. (1978) reported that a diet designed to reduce weight, but without restriction in sodium, results in lower blood pressure. However, the relationships may be more complex. Rocchini et al. (1989) found that adolescents with obesity were quite sensitive to sodium in their diet, such that increased sodium results in a rise in blood pressure. However, after a weight loss intervention, obese adolescents were significantly less sensitive to sodium in their diet.

For patients with severe obesity, lifestyle intervention may not be sufficient to produce adequate weight loss. For these adolescents, metabolic and bariatric surgery may be needed, as discussed earlier in this chapter. Ippisch et al. (2008) found that weight loss surgery can result in lower blood pressure, as well as decreased left ventricular mass index.

A number of dietary factors have been implicated in blood pressure elevation. These include sodium, caffeine, potassium, calcium, magnesium, folic acid, and fat content (Simons-Morton et al. 1997, Dwyer et al. 1998, Knuiman et al. 1988, Sinaiko et al. 1993, Falkner et al. 2000, He and MacGregor 2006). Sodium, caffeine, and increased fat in the diet are associated with increased blood pressure, while potassium, calcium, and magnesium have been associated with decreased blood pressure. Some evidence for these associations comes from animal studies while other evidence is derived from studies of adults, children, and adolescents. Clinical evidence may come from observational epidemiologic studies and from clinical trials. Clinical trials generally provide the best evidence, but these studies are most often focused on treatment of individuals who have already developed high blood pressure as opposed to those who are well and need preventive intervention.

Dietary sodium has attracted the most attention related to blood pressure elevation across the age span. Many studies, particularly in adults, have found a positive association between sodium intake and blood pressure. Also, some individuals are more sensitive to sodium in their diet than others (Appel et al. 2006). Unfortunately, there is no simple clinical evaluation to determine if someone has heightened sensitivity to salt, a phenomenon that may underlie the finding that the association between dietary salt and blood pressure is more evident in some groups compared to others (Falkner et al. 1986). These groups would include African Americans and those with a family history of hypertension. It is believed that sensitivity to sodium is in large part genetically determined, but specific salt sensitivity genes or polymorphisms have yet to be identified.

Most of the sodium in the diet comes from salt that is added in processing of food (canned, boxed, or frozen), not from salt that is added with cooking or at the table. This makes it more difficult for an individual or a family to lower sodium in their diet because the consumption of preprepared and packaged foods is so high compared with home-prepared foods. Most American children have a sodium intake that is well above the defined adequate intake levels, which are 1.2 g/day for children aged 4–8 years and 1.5 g/day for older children and adolescents (Appel et al. 2006, CDC 2011). This means that children and adolescents could reduce their sodium intake substantially and would have the potential benefit of lower blood pressure with no potential for adverse effects.

Studies in adults that focused on potassium supplementation have demonstrated a blood pressure–lowering effect (Weaver 2013), but there have been few studies in children. Sinaiko et al. (1993) found lower blood pressure with age in children supplemented with potassium compared to those who were not supplemented. Calcium supplementation may also be beneficial, particularly for those with a combination of elevated blood pressure and low baseline calcium intake (Dwyer et al. 1998). Calcium supplementation is associated with increased sodium excretion in the urine, which may be a potential mechanism of action related to its blood pressure–lowering effect (Lasaridis et al. 1989). Currently, there is insufficient evidence to recommend either potassium or calcium supplementation in the clinical setting.

While it is important to study dietary micro- and macronutrients, it is more useful from a clinical perspective to evaluate dietary patterns. This is because individuals and families develop their diet and purchase food related to their dietary patterns. The diet pattern that is most widely studied in adults and has emerging evidence in children is the Dietary Approaches to Stop Hypertension (DASH) diet pattern. The DASH diet has been studied extensively in adults. The DASH dietary pattern is high in fruits and vegetables and emphasizes low-fat dairy and whole grain products, while being low in simple carbohydrates, red meats, and other foods high in saturated fat (Appel et al. 1997). This dietary approach has been shown in randomized clinical feeding studies of adults to be associated with lower systolic and diastolic blood pressure that was independent of weight loss. The DASH eating pattern is not necessarily low in sodium. Subsequent studies have demonstrated that the DASH diet with the addition of sodium restriction is more effective at lowering blood pressure than the DASH diet alone in adults (Sacks et al. 2001).

There have been some studies of the DASH diet in children and adolescents. Epidemiologic studies have shown that individuals with a diet more similar to the DASH diet tend to have lower blood pressure compared to children and adolescents with a standard Western diet. The Framingham Study showed that children who had higher dietary intake of fruits and vegetables, plus low-fat dairy in their preschool years, had a smaller increase in blood pressure with age than those with lower intake of these diet components (Moore et al. 2005). Moore (2012) found similar results in a longitudinal study of adolescent girls. Couch (2008) reported the results of a clinical trial of the DASH diet compared to standard care over a 3-month period in adolescents with prehypertension or hypertension. They found that those in the DASH diet group had a significantly greater reduction in systolic blood pressure compared to those in the standard care group who received general counseling on diet and sodium reduction.

Combining the epidemiologic and clinical trial results suggests that increasing fruit and vegetable consumption, along with emphasis on low-fat dairy and whole grains with reduction in red meat, could be beneficial in both prevention of high blood pressure and management of hypertension when it occurs in children and adolescents. Further research is needed to evaluate whether additional sodium reduction may be beneficial in children and adolescents on a DASH diet. An advantage of the DASH diet is that it is a healthful diet pattern for everyone in the family. This means that it can be more easily implemented in practice and that family members can support each other in adherence over time.

It is clear that diet and nutritional factors are quite important as they relate to blood pressure elevation. Avoidance of excess weight gain and adherence to a DASH diet pattern could be beneficial in preventing blood pressure elevation in young individuals. For those who have already developed hypertension, dietary intervention should be a central aspect of any intervention plan.

Cardiovascular Risk

CVD is the leading cause of death worldwide (Mozaffarian et al. 2015). In adults, studies have demonstrated the association between obesity and the premature development of CVD (Manson et al. 1990, Ingelsson et al. 2007). Atherosclerosis begins in childhood, notably in those with overweight, obesity, and other CVD risk factors.

The Bogalusa Heart study was one of the first studies demonstrating a strong association between childhood obesity and fatty streaks and fibrous plaques located in the aorta and coronary arteries (Berenson et al. 1998). Similarly, in the Muscatine Study, Mahoney (2001) found that the greatest predictor in young adulthood of coronary calcium seen on computed tomography was being overweight during childhood. Several studies have also found that obesity in childhood and adolescence, with and without associated dyslipidemia, predisposes patients to elevated carotid intimal media thickening and endothelial dysfunction (Freedman et al. 2004, Urbina et al. 2009, Urbina et al. 2010).

In addition, obesity induces structural and hemodynamic changes in the heart, including increased blood volume and cardiac output. Pulmonary arterial hypertension from sleep apnea and hypoventilation may occur and youth with morbid obesity are at increased risk for developing a cardiomyopathy from these abnormalities (Speiser et al. 2005). Along with elevated systolic blood pressure, obesity is one of the risk factors in the development of increased left ventricular mass in the young (Yoshinaga et al. 1995, Daniels et al. 1998, Urbina et al. 1999). In adults, left ventricular hypertrophy has been found to be an independent risk factor for CVD morbidity and mortality (Flynn and Alderman 2005).

Dyslipidemia of Obesity

Nearly half of all overweight and obese children have at least one abnormal lipid value (CDC 2010). The dyslipidemia that is common in this population is called combined dyslipidemia of obesity (CDO), which consists of elevated TG, low levels of HDL-C, elevated non-HDL-C, and normal or mildly elevated LDL-C. The LDL particles (LDL-P) tend to be the small, dense subtype.

Indeed, the presence of CDO has been shown to correlate with elevated levels of insulin, overweight/obesity, and central fat deposition. In the HEALTHY study, which evaluated lipids in a large population of sixth-grade children, investigators found that one-third of overweight or obese children had a TG/HDL-C ratio > 3.0% and 11.2% had a non-HDL-C >145 mg/dL (Mietus-Snyder et al. 2013). This corroborates with the NHANES data, which found that increased levels of non-HDL-C in adolescents aged 12–19 years were associated with the MetSyn (Li et al. 2011).

In the long term, the presence of CDO appears to be the most common lipid pattern associated with clinical CVD in adulthood. In the Framingham Offspring Study, investigators found that CDO on a standard lipid profile was one predictor of early clinical CVD events, such as myocardial infarction and/or death from CVD (Robins et al. 2011). It also is a good detector of elevated small LDL-P, which is a lipid parameter that is also correlated with CVD events (Cromwell et al. 2007). Similarly, the Princeton Follow-up Study, which evaluated risk factors for early CVD during childhood and again two decades later, found that individuals with elevated TG levels and TG/HDL-C ratios at 12 years of age, and who maintained these lipid abnormalities into adulthood, were more likely to experience clinical CVD during adulthood (Morrison et al. 2012).

The treatment of obesity-related dyslipidemia is a focused change in diet and exercise habits. A referral to a registered dietitian is imperative, not just for the child but for the entire family to understand how to make appropriate dietary changes (Daniels et al. 2011). In both the pediatric and adult populations, improvement in CDO has been demonstrated with weight loss, restriction of simple carbohydrates, and increased physical activity (Nemet et al. 2005, Meyer et al. 2006, Ebbeling et al. 2007, Ebbeling et al. 2012b, Kirk et al. 2012). Changes of diet and lifestyle act to decrease TG and non-HDL-C levels, reduce TG/HDL-C ratio, and alter the LDL-P to a larger, less atherogenic subtype (Becque et al. 1988, Kang et al. 2002, Sondike et al. 2003, Watts et al. 2004, Nemet et al. 2005). In particular, restricting carbohydrates, notably simple sugars and quickly hydrolyzed starches, has been shown to decrease TG levels significantly (Pieke et al. 2000, Sondike et al. 2003, Pereira et al. 2004, Ebbeling et al. 2007). When taking a dietary history in the overweight or obese child, the amount of sweetened beverage consumed should always be assessed. Eliminating sweetened drinks (e.g., soft drinks, iced tea, lemonade, etc.) almost always results in a reduction in TGs and a simultaneous weight loss as well (Dornas et al. 2015). Along with reduction in simple sugars and carbohydrates, there should also be an increase in complex carbohydrates and fiber and consumption of low-mercury fish twice weekly.

While the majority of obese children with dyslipidemia will demonstrate evidence of CDO, there are some who may present with isolated elevation of LDL-C or with associated decreased HDL-C. While weight loss is again necessary for improvement in the cholesterol values, the dietary focus is somewhat different from those with the CDO lipid profile. In these patients, the focus is on a diet low in saturated and trans fats, ideally with 25%–30% of calories from fat, ≤7% of calories from saturated fats, and approximately 10% of calories from monounsaturated fats. There should be no dietary intake of trans fat. Food labels are required to indicate the amount of trans fat in all products. For additional LDL-C lowering, soluble fiber in the form of psyllium should be added at 6 g/day for children up to age 12 years and 12 g/day for children 12 years and older (Fletcher et al. 2005). The use of plant stanol or sterol esters, found in certain food products (e.g., special margarines, milk, oatmeal, nutrition bars, tortilla chips) as well as in pill forms, may reduce LDL-C by an additional 6%–15% at a dose of 2 g/day (Kerckhoffs et al. 2002, Fletcher et al. 2005). These are generally used in those with more significantly elevated LDL-C levels.

Metabolic Syndrome

In adults, the MetSyn is a constellation of cardiovascular and metabolic risk factors that cluster together and appear to increase the risk of premature CVD, as well as T2DM (Grundy et al. 2005, Cook et al. 2008). The risk factors include dyslipidemia (high TG, low HDL-C, increased small, dense LDL), elevated blood pressure, elevated blood glucose, excess abdominal adiposity, and pro-inflammatory and/or pro-thrombotic states (Cook et al. 2008). Over the past several years, major health organizations have proposed somewhat different criteria and cut points for the definition of MetSyn in adults (World Health Organization 1999, National Institutes of Health 2002, Alberti et al. 2005, Grundy et al. 2005), although, more recently, a joint statement from these health organizations was released in an attempt to unify the defining criteria (Alberti et al. 2009).

In the pediatric population, definition, assessment, and treatment of the MetSyn have been problematic. Part of the difficulty is that there are changes in lipid levels, blood pressure, and other metabolic measures with different ages and stages of puberty. There are also limited long-term data evaluating the tracking of the MetSyn characteristics from childhood to adulthood and the subsequent impact of these risks on premature CVD (Steinberger et al. 2009). However, it is important to identify at-risk children for MetSyn to help prevent the progression of obesity and the potentially long-term metabolic, endocrinologic, and cardiovascular ramifications. To this end, in 2007, the International Diabetes Federation (IDF) published an age-based definition of MetSyn. For children 6–9 years old, it was suggested that the term "MetSyn" not be applied, but that practitioners focus on weight reduction, especially for those children with abdominal obesity, defined as waist circumference percentile ≥90th percentile (Zimmet et al. 2007). For children 10–15 years old, MetSyn can be diagnosed with the presence of abdominal obesity, using the same definition as mentioned earlier (Zimmet et al. 2007) and at least 2 risk factors, including hypertriglyceridemia, low HDL-C, elevated blood pressure, and/or elevated fasting glucose. For those 16 years of age or older, the authors recommended using adult IDF criteria for MetSyn (Zimmet et al. 2007).

Even in children, there are identifiable risk factors for the development of MetSyn. Heredity does play a role as children of parents who have MetSyn are at increased risk of developing MetSyn, likely due to a combination of both genetics and environment (Hong et al. 1997, Steinberger et al. 2009). Ethnicity is another factor in the development of MetSyn, notably with differences in certain components of MetSyn between white, black, and Hispanic children. For example, black and Hispanic children have a higher prevalence of obesity but black youth have lower levels of TC and TG and higher HDL-C levels when compared with white children (Chen et al. 1999, Ogden et al. 2002).

While there is not a truly agreed upon definition of MetSyn in children, it does appear that focusing on lifestyle modification, especially directed toward obesity, will help to slow or even halt the development of risk factors for MetSyn. Studies have shown that modifications to both dietary composition and physical activity levels can attenuate the risk factors for MetSyn for at least 1 year (Nemet et al. 2005) and also can improve endothelial dysfunction, notably in children with excess adiposity (Woo et al. 2004). Indeed, it seems that a concentrated focus on weight control (weight stabilization or weight loss) through a combination of increased physical activity, along with a diet rich in whole grains with limited amounts of simple sugars, simple carbohydrates, and saturated fats, may help to prevent the development of MetSyn and the associated comorbidities as these children become adults.

Fructose has also been identified as a key player in MetSyn. Since fructose is unable to be regulated by insulin, fructose intake results in increased insulin resistance. Glucose and fructose are metabolized differently with the majority of fructose resulting in fat deposition in the liver, promoting fatty liver disease and increased triglyceride production. Fructose also increases inflammatory markers. Further, the by-product of metabolized fructose is uric acid, which increases blood pressure (Das 2015). In a study in obese children with MetSyn, restriction of dietary sugars from 28% to 10% in replacement for starch improved systolic blood pressure, TG, LDL-C, insulin sensitivity, and glucose tolerance after 9 days (Lustig et al. 2016).

Insulin Resistance and Type 2 Diabetes Mellitus

T2DM is a significant comorbidity of obesity in adolescents. T2DM is characterized by the development of hyperglycemia, insulin resistance, and relative impairment in insulin secretion.

Insulin resistance is a state in which a given concentration of insulin is associated with subnormal glucose response. This can be assessed using a homeostatic model assessment, which is a method used to quantify insulin resistance and beta cell function. A Homeostatic Model Assessment-Estimated Insulin Resistance ≥ 3.99 is an indicator for abnormal glucose regulation (Turchiano et al. 2012).

Impaired fasting glucose is defined as a fasting plasma glucose level of 100–125 mg/dL or hemoglobin A1c of 5.7–6.4%. Insulin resistance may develop in the early stages of childhood obesity and in very young children and has been associated with higher expression of central obesity and T2DM (Skoczen et al. 2015).

Diabetes mellitus is diagnosed by the following criteria (American Diabetes Association 2011):

- Fasting plasma glucose ≥126 mg/dL (7 mmol/L)
- Plasma glucose ≥200 mg/dL (11.1 mmol/L) measured 2 hours after an oral glucose tolerance test
- Hemoglobin A1C ≥ 6.5% (47 mmol/mL)

Multiple studies have shown that obesity can predict the development of T2DM (Freedman et al. 1999, Copeland et al. 2011, Hannon et al. 2005, Liu et al. 2010). In addition to general lifestyle management, an increase in dietary fiber, reduction in simple sugars and refined carbohydrates, and an increase in physical activity are key components to improvement in insulin and glucose regulation (Krauss et al. 2000).

For children above the age of 2, the fiber recommendation is their age + 5 g up to a maximum of 25 g daily (Williams et al. 1995), so that a 10-year-old child should consume a minimum of 15 g of fiber per day.

Nonalcoholic Fatty Liver Disease

NAFLD is the most common cause of chronic liver disease in childhood and adolescence and is found in 9.6% of children aged 2–19 (Schwimmer et al. 2006). NAFLD presents a spectrum of pathology, ranging from simple triglyceride accumulation in hepatocytes to hepatic steatosis with inflammation (steatohepatitis), fibrosis, and cirrhosis (Neuschwander-Tetri and Caldwell 2003, Chalasani et al. 2012). NAFLD is defined as macrovesicular fat accumulation in >5% of hepatocytes as assessed by liver biopsy, in the absence of excessive alcohol intake or viral, autoimmune, or drug-induced liver disease. Approximately 25% of children with NAFLD have a progressive subphenotype known as NASH (Molleston et al. 2002). An estimated 7%–10% of children with NASH will develop cirrhosis and end-stage liver disease (Rubinstein et al. 2008).

Children with NAFLD are usually asymptomatic and are found to have mildly elevated liver enzymes on screening in the setting of obesity. Elevations in alanine aminotransferase (ALT) are usually greater than aspartate aminotransferase; however, liver enzymes may be completely normal. Other forms of liver disease that cause elevations in ALT must also be ruled out (Pardee et al. 2009).

Lifestyle change with weight loss through diet and exercise remains the mainstay of therapy in NAFLD. This has proven to improve serologic markers and liver histology.

Dietary Intervention and Physical Activity

Weight loss is known to decrease delivery of free fatty acids to the liver and increase extrahepatic insulin sensitivity by means of improving peripheral glucose utilization and promoting reduction in reactive oxygen substances, as well as reducing adipose inflammation (Shah et al. 2009). Evidence to support the utility of weight loss in the treatment of pediatric NAFLD was demonstrated in a study by Nobili (2006), which evaluated the effect of lifestyle change in 84 children with biopsy-proven NAFLD. The subjects underwent a 12-month program of lifestyle advice, focusing on physical activity and dietary modifications, including a balanced, low-calorie diet (25–30 calories/kg/day; carbohydrate 50%–60%; fat 23%–30%; protein 15%–20%; fatty acid, two-thirds saturated, one-third unsaturated; ω6/ω3 ratio = 4:1) as recommended by the Italian Recommended Dietary Allowances. Patients who completed the diet and exercise program had a significant improvement in BMI, insulin sensitivity, liver enzymes, and liver echogenicity on ultrasound. They also demonstrated improved liver histology on biopsy (Nobili et al. 2008).

The role of specific dietary macronutrient composition during weight loss has not been extensively studied in children. However, low-glycemic-load diets designed to reduce postprandial rise in blood glucose and insulin either through carbohydrate restriction or low GI have shown some promise for use in treatment (Ebbeling et al. 2003). Pozzato et al. (2010) placed 26 obese children between 6 and 14 years on a normocaloric balanced diet (carbohydrates 55%–60% with <10% high glycemic index; fat 25%–30% with <10% saturated fat; protein 12%–15%) for 1 year. Mean liver fat fraction quantified by hepatic proton magnetic resonance spectroscopy declined by 8% ($p < 0.0001$) with a decrease in BMI z-score of 0.26 ($p < 0.001$). The low-GI diet, although effective in reducing NAFLD, has not been found to be more effective than a low-fat diet in children. A randomized controlled trial found an estimated 8%–10% reduction in hepatic triglyceride content quantified on proton magnetic resonance spectroscopy in obese children who underwent either a 6-month low-glycemic (low-to-moderate glycemic load of carbohydrates 40%, fat 35%–40%) or low-fat (55%–60% of carbohydrates, 20% fat, <10% saturated fat) dietary intervention with no significant difference seen between the dietary groups. BMI decreased by −1.3 kg/m^2 in the low-glycemic group (0.0007) and by 1.2 kg/m^2 in the low-fat group ($p = 0.0004$) with no significant difference between both groups (Ramon-Krauel et al. 2013).

Diets high in fructose are known to increase plasma lipids and oxidative stress. Fructose undergoes first-pass metabolism in the liver. By-products of fructose metabolism are fat deposition in the liver, increased triglyceride formation, increased uric acid formation (leading to high blood pressure), and an increase in the production but not the utilization of insulin (insulin resistance)

(Lim et al. 2010). In addition to overall weight loss, reduction in fructose intake has been proposed as a potential treatment of NAFLD (Ramon-Krauel et al. 2013). A randomized controlled 6-month pilot study of 10 children with NAFLD compared the effectiveness of a low-fructose to a low-fat diet in improving ALT levels. Patients on the low-fructose diet eliminated sugar-containing beverages, fruit juice, and food items in which high-fructose corn syrup was a primary ingredient. At the end of 6 months, oxidized LDL was significantly lower in the low-fructose group. However, ALT levels did not change in either group (Vos et al. 2009). The FRAGILE diet is a combination of low fructose/low glycemic index/low glycemic load. A study evaluated patients on a 6-month FRAGILE dietary intervention in children with NAFLD (n = 12) compared with healthy lean controls (n = 14). The investigators found that absolute fructose intake related strongly to plasma aminotransferase, systolic blood pressure, percent body fat, insulin resistance, and cholesterol level, independent of weight loss. This suggests that a modest reduction in fructose intake and glycemic index improves liver dysfunction and cardiometabolic risk (Mager et al. 2015).

Pharmacotherapy and Surgery

As in adults, pediatric pharmacotherapy of fatty liver disease has focused on treating insulin resistance and oxidative stress. Multiple drugs are being evaluated for the treatment of NAFLD, with only vitamin E demonstrating improvement in biopsy findings (Sanyal et al. 2010). Although vitamin E may have shown some benefit, it is not superior to placebo in sustained reduction in ALT (Lavine et al. 2011). The Roux-en-Y GB and the LSG are recommended for severely obese adolescents with NASH (Nobili et al. 2015).

Until the prevalence and severity of obesity improve, the prevalence of NAFLD probably will continue to rise. Unfortunately, awareness and screening for NAFLD are still lacking. There is currently no consensus on screening, diagnosis, or management of this patient population. At this time, lifestyle modification and weight loss through diet and exercise remain the mainstay of treatment. Research into the pathogenesis, risk factors, natural history, noninvasive modalities, and treatment of NAFLD is greatly needed.

SUMMARY

In conclusion, obesity in childhood and adolescence has become a major public health issue. As discussed throughout this chapter, the cardiometabolic consequences are significant and place our youth at risk of morbidity and mortality not only during childhood but into adulthood as well. We need better strategies, improved access, and more funding toward prevention and treatment at all levels of this chronic disease and the health repercussions it causes.

REFERENCES

Aarts EO, Janssen IM, Berends FJ. 2011. The gastric sleeve: Losing weight as fast as micronutrients? *Obes Surg* 21:207–211.

Alberti KG, Eckel RH, Grundy SM et al. 2009. Harmonizing the metabolic syndrome: A joint interim statement of the International Diabetes Federation Task Force on Epidemiology and Prevention; National Heart, Lung, and Blood Institute; American Heart Association; World Heart Federation; International Atherosclerosis Society; and International Association for the Study of Obesity. *Circulation* 120:1640–1645.

Alberti KG, Zimmet P, Shaw J et al. 2005. The metabolic syndrome—A new worldwide definition. *Lancet* 366:1059–1062.

Alqahtani AR, Elahmedi MO. 2015. Pediatric bariatric surgery: The clinical pathway. *Obes Surg* 25:910–921.

American Academy of Pediatrics. 2000. Physical fitness and activity in schools. *Pediatrics* 105:1156–1157.

American Diabetes Association. 2011. Standards of medical care in diabetes 2011. *Diabetes Care* 34:S11–S61.

Appel LJ, Brands MW, Daniels SR et al. 2006. Dietary approaches to prevent and treat hypertension: A scientific statement from the American Heart Association. *Hypertension* 47:296–308.

Appel LJ, Moore TJ, Obarzanek E et al. 1997. A clinical trial of the effects of dietary patterns on blood pressure. DASH Collaborative Research Group. *N Engl J Med* 336:1117–1124.

Babio N, Bulló M, Basora J et al. 2009. Adherence to the Mediterranean diet and risk of metabolic syndrome and its components. *Nutr Metab Cardiovasc Dis* 19:563–570.
Barlow SE, Dietz WH. 1998. Obesity evaluation and treatment: Expert committee recommendations. *Pediatrics* 102: e29–e39.
Barlow SE, Expert Committee. 2007. Expert committee recommendations regarding the prevention, assessment, and treatment of child and adolescents overweight and obesity: Summary report. *Pediatrics* 120:S164–S192.
Baron JA, Schori A, Crow B et al. 1986. A randomized controlled trial of low carbohydrate and low fat/high fiber diets for weight loss. *Am J Public Health* 76:1293–1296.
Becque MD, Katch VL, Rocchini AP et al. 1988. Coronary risk incidence of obese adolescents: Reduction by exercise plus diet intervention. *Pediatrics* 81:605–612.
Berenson GS, Srinivasan SR, Bao W et al. 1998. Association between multiple cardiovascular risk factors and atherosclerosis in children and young adults. The Bogalusa Heart Study. *N Engl J Med* 338:1650–1656.
Berkey CS, Rockett HR, Gillman MW et al. 2003. One-year changes in activity and in inactivity among 10- to 15-year-old boys and girls: Relationship to change in body mass index. *Pediatrics* 111:836–843.
Berkowitz RI, Wadden TA, Gehrman CA et al. 2011. Meal replacements in the treatment of adolescent obesity: A randomized controlled trial. *Obesity (Silver Spring)* 19:1193–1199.
Blair NJ, Thompson JM, Black PN et al. 2007. Risk factors for obesity in 7-year-old European children: The Auckland Birthweight Collaborative Study. *Arch Dis Child* 92:866–871.
Bondada S, Jen HC, Deugarte DA. 2011. Outcomes of bariatric surgery in adolescents. *Current Opin Pediatr* 23:552–556.
Braithwaite I, Stewart AW, Hancox RJ et al. 2013. The worldwide association between television viewing and obesity in children and adolescents: Cross sectional study. *PLoS One* 8:e74263.
Brehm BJ, Seeley RJ, Daniels SR, D'Alessio DA. 2003. A randomized trial comparing a very low carbohydrate diet and a calorie restricted low fat diet on body weight and cardiovascular risk factors in healthy women. *J Clin Endocrinol Metab* 88:1617–1623.
Centers for Disease Control and Prevention (CDC). 2009. Obesity prevalence among low-income, preschool-aged children—United States, 1998–2008. *MMWR Morb Mortal Wkly Rep* 58:769–773.
Centers for Disease Control and Prevention (CDC). 2010. Prevalence of abnormal lipid levels among youths—United States, 1999–2006. *MMWR Morb Mortal Wkly Rep* 59:29–33.
Centers for Disease Control and Prevention (CDC). 2011. Usual sodium intakes compared with current dietary guidelines—United States, 2005–2008. *MMWR Morb Mortal Wkly Rep* 60:1413–1417.
Chalasani N, Younossi Z, Lavine JE et al. 2012. The diagnosis and management of non-alcoholic fatty liver disease: Practice guideline by the American Association for the Study of Liver Diseases, American College of Gastroenterology, and the American Gastroenterological Association. *Hepatology* 55:2005–2023.
Chen W, Chen SC, Hsu HS et al. 1997. Counseling clinic for pediatric weight reduction: Program formulation and follow-up. *J Formos Med Assoc* 96:59–62.
Chen W, Srinivasan SR, Elkasabany A et al. 1999. Cardiovascular risk factors clustering features of insulin resistance syndrome (Syndrome X) in a biracial (Black-White) population of children, adolescents, and young adults: The Bogalusa Heart Study. *Am J Epidemiol* 150:667–674.
Cook S, Auinger P, Li C et al. 2008. Metabolic syndrome rates in United States adolescents, from the National Health and Nutrition Examination Survey, 1999–2002. *J Pediatr* 152:165–170.
Copeland KC, Zeitler P, Geffner M et al. 2011. Characteristics of adolescents and youth with recent-onset type 2 diabetes: The TODAY cohort at baseline. *J Clin Endocrinol Metab* 96:159–167.
Couch SC, Saelens BE, Levin L et al. 2008. The efficacy of a clinic-based behavioral nutrition intervention emphasizing a DASH-type diet for adolescents with elevated blood pressure. *J Pediatr* 152:494–501.
Cromwell WC, Otvos JD, Keyes MJ et al. 2007. LDL Particle number and risk of future cardiovascular disease in the Framingham Offspring Study—Implications for LDL management. *J Clin Lipidol* 1:583–592.
Cunningham SA, Kramer MR, Narayan KM. 2014. Incidence of childhood obesity in the United States. *N Engl J Med* 370:403–411.
Daniels SR. 2009. Complications of obesity in children and adolescents. *Int J Obes (Lond)* 33:S60–S65.
Daniels SR, Benuck I, Christakis DA et al. 2011. Expert panel on integrated guidelines for cardiovascular health and risk reduction in children and adolescents; National Heart, Lung, and Blood Institute. Expert panel on integrated guidelines for cardiovascular health and risk reduction in children and adolescents: Summary report. *Pediatrics* 128(Suppl. 5):S213–S256.
Daniels SR, Loggie JM, Khoury P et al. 1998. Left ventricular geometry and severe left ventricular hypertrophy in children and adolescents with essential hypertension. *Circulation* 97:1907–1911.
Das UN. 2015. Sucrose, fructose, glucose, and their link to metabolic syndrome and cancer. *Nutrition* 31:249–257.

DeBoer MD, Scharf RJ, Demmer RT. 2013. Sugar-sweetened beverages and weight gain in 2- to 5-year-old children. *Pediatrics* 132:413–420.
Deurenberg P, Weststrate JA, Seidell JC. 1991. Body mass index as a measure of body fatness: Age- and sex-specific prediction formulas. *Br J Nutr* 65:105–114.
Dietz WH Jr, Gortmaker SL. 1985. Do we fatten our children at the television set? Obesity and television viewing in children and adolescents. *Pediatrics* 75:807–812.
Dornas WC, de Lima WG, Pedrosa ML et al. 2015. Health implications of high-fructose intake and current research. *Adv Nutr* 6:729–737.
Dowda M, Ainsworth BE, Addy CL et al. 2001. Environmental influences, physical activity, and weight status in 8- to 16-year-olds. *Arch Pediatr Adolesc Med* 155:711–717.
Dwyer JH, Dwyer KM, Scribner RA et al. 1998. Dietary calcium, calcium supplementation, and blood pressure in African American adolescents. *Am J Clin Nutr* 68:648–655.
Ebbeling CB, Feldman HA, Chomitz VR et al. 2012a. A randomized trial of sugar-sweetened beverages and adolescent body weight. *N Engl J Med* 367:1407–1416.
Ebbeling CB, Leidig MM, Feldman HA et al. 2007. Effects of a low-glycemic load vs low-fat diet in obese young adults: A randomized trial. *JAMA* 297:2092–2102.
Ebbeling CB, Leidig MM, Sinclair KB et al. 2003. A reduced-glycemic load diet in the treatment of adolescent obesity. *Arch Pediatr Adolesc Med* 157:773–779.
Ebbeling CB, Swain JF, Feldman HA et al. 2012b. Effects of dietary composition on energy expenditure during weight-loss maintenance. *JAMA* 307:2627–2634.
Epstein LH, Roemmich JN, Robinson JL et al. 2008. A randomized trial of the effects of reducing television viewing and computer use on body mass index in young children. *Arch Pediatr Adolesc Med* 162:239–245.
Epstein LH, Valoski A, Wing RR et al. 1990. Ten-year follow-up of behavioral, family based-treatment for obese children. *JAMA* 264:2519–2523.
Epstein LH, Valoski A, Wing RR et al. 1994. Ten-year outcomes of behavioral family-based treatment for childhood obesity. *Health Psychol* 13:373–383.
Epstein LH, Valoski AM, Vara LS et al. 1995. Effects of decreasing sedentary behavior and increasing activity on weight change in obese children. *Health Psychol* 14:109–115.
Falbe J, Rosner B, Willett WC et al. 2013. Adiposity and different types of screen time. *Pediatrics* 132:e1497–e1505.
Falkner B, Kushner H, Khalsa DK et al. 1986. Sodium sensitivity, growth and family history of hypertension in young blacks. *J Hypertens Suppl* 4:S381–S383.
Falkner B, Sherif K, Michel S et al. 2000. Dietary nutrients and blood pressure in urban minority adolescents at risk for hypertension. *Arch Pediatr Adolesc Med* 154:918–922.
Flegal KM, Wei R, Ogden CL et al. 2011. Characterizing extreme values of body mass index-for-age by using the 2000 Centers for Disease Control and Prevention growth charts. *Am J Clin Nutr* 90:1314–1320.
Fletcher B, Berra K, Ades P et al. 2005. Managing abnormal blood lipids: A collaborative approach. Cosponsored by the Councils on Cardiovascular Nursing; Arteriosclerosis, Thrombosis, and Vascular Biology; Basic Cardiovascular Sciences; Cardiovascular Disease in the Young; Clinical Cardiology; Epidemiology and Prevention; Nutrition, Physical Activity, and Metabolism; Stroke; Preventive Cardiovascular Nurses Association. *Circulation* 112:3184–3209.
Flynn JT, Alderman MH. 2005. Characteristics of children with primary hypertension seen at a referral center. *Pediatr Nephrol* 20:961–966.
Foster GD, Wyatt HR, Hill JO et al. 2003. A randomized trial of a low-carbohydrate diet for obesity. *N Engl J Med* 348:2082–2090.
Freedman DS, Dietz WH, Srinivasan SR et al. 1999. The relation of overweight to cardiovascular risk factors among children and adolescents: The Bogalusa Heart Study. *Pediatrics* 103:1175–1182.
Freedman DS, Dietz WH, Tang R et al. 2004. The relation of obesity throughout life to carotid intima-media thickness in adulthood: The Bogalusa Heart Study. *Int J Obes Relat Metab Disord* 28:159–166.
Gilbert-Diamond D, Li Z, Adachi-Mejia AM et al. 2014. Association of a television in the bedroom with increased adiposity gain in a nationally representative sample of children and adolescents. *JAMA Pediatr* 168:427–434.
Goran MI, Treuth MS. 2001. Energy expenditure, physical activity, and obesity in children. *Pediatr Clin North Am* 48:931–953.
Gortmaker SL, Must A, Sobol AM et al. 1996. Television viewing as a cause of increasing obesity among children in the United States, 1986–1990. *Arch Pediatr Adolesc Med* 150:356–362.
Grosso G, Mistretta A, Marventano S et al. 2014. Beneficial effects of the Mediterranean diet on metabolic syndrome. *Curr Pharm Des* 20:5039–5044.

Grundy SM, Cleeman JI, Daniels SR et al. 2005. Diagnosis and management of the metabolic syndrome an American Heart Association/National Heart, Lung, and Blood Institute Scientific Statement. *Circulation* 112:2735–2752.
Gulati AK, Kaplan DW, Daniels SR. 2012. Clinical tracking of severely obese children: A new growth chart. *Pediatrics* 130:1136–1140.
Gunay-Aygun M, Cassidy SB, Nicholls RD. 1997. Prader-Willi and other syndromes associated with obesity and mental retardation. *Behav Genet* 27:307–324.
Hannon TS, Rao G, Arslanian SA. 2005. Childhood obesity and type 2 diabetes mellitus. *Pediatrics* 116:473–480.
Harvey-Berino J. 1998. The efficacy of dietary fat vs. total energy restriction for weight loss. *Obes Res* 6:202–207.
Harvey-Berino J. 1999. Calorie restriction is more effective for obesity treatment than dietary fat restriction. *Ann Behav Med* 21:35–39.
Haynes RB. 1986. Is weight loss an effective treatment for hypertension? The evidence against. *Can J Physiol Pharmacol* 64:825–830.
He FJ, MacGregor GA. 2006. Importance of salt in determining blood pressure in children: Meta-analysis of controlled trials. *Hypertension* 48:861–869.
Hong Y, Pedersen NL, Brismar K et al. 1997. Genetic and environmental architecture of the features of the insulin-resistance syndrome. *Am J Hum Genet* 60:143–152.
Ingelsson E, Sullivan LM, Fox CS et al. 2007. Burden and prognostic importance of subclinical cardiovascular disease in overweight and obese individuals. *Circulation* 116:375–384.
Ippisch HM, Inge TH, Daniels SR et al. 2008. Reversibility of cardiac abnormalities in morbidly obese adolescents. *J Am Coll Cardiol* 51:1342–1348.
Juonala M, Magnussen CG, Berenson GS et al. 2011. Childhood adiposity, adult adiposity, and cardiovascular risk factors. *N Engl J Med* 365:1876–1885.
Kang HS, Gutin B, Barbeau P et al. 2002. Physical training improves insulin resistance syndrome markers in obese adolescents. *Med Sci Sports Exerc* 34:1920–1927.
Kaur H, Choi WS, Mayo MS et al. 2003. Duration of television watching is associated with increased body mass index. *J Pediatr* 143:506–511.
Kerckhoffs DA, Brouns F, Hornstra G, Mensink RP. 2002. Effects on the human serum lipoprotein profile of *B*-glucan, soy protein and isoflavones, plant sterols and stanols, garlic and tocotrienols. *J Nutr* 132:2494–2505.
Kirk S, Brehm B, Saelens BE et al. 2012. Role of carbohydrate modification in weight management among obese children: A randomized clinical trial. *J Pediatr* 161:320–327.
Knuiman JT, Hautvast JG, Zwiauer KF et al. 1988. Blood pressure and excretion of sodium, potassium, calcium and magnesium in 8- and 9-year old boys from 19 European centres. *Eur J Clin Nutr* 42:847–855.
Krauss RM, Eckel RH, Howard B. 2000. AHA dietary guidelines: Revision 2000: A statement for healthcare professionals from the Nutrition Committee of the American Heart Association. *Circulation* 102:2284–2299.
Lasaridis AN, Kaisis CN, Zananiri KI et al. 1989. Increased natriuretic ability and hypotensive effect during short-term high calcium intake in essential hypertension. *Nephron* 51:517–523.
Lavine JE, Schwimmer JB, Van Natta ML, et al. 2011. Effect of vitamin E or metformin for treatment of nonalcoholic fatty liver disease in children and adolescents: The TONIC randomized controlled trial. *JAMA* 305:1659–1668.
Lee WJ, Chen CY, Chong K et al. 2011. Changes in postprandial gut hormones after metabolic surgery: A comparison of gastric bypass and sleeve gastrectomy. *Surg Obes Relat Dis* 7:683–690.
Levine MD, Ringham RM, Kalarchian MA et al. 2001. Is family-based behavioral weight control appropriate for severe pediatric obesity? *Int J Eat Disord* 30:318–328.
Li C, Ford ES, McBride PE et al. 2011. Non-high-density lipoprotein cholesterol concentration is associated with the metabolic syndrome among US youth aged 12–19 years. *J Pediatr* 158:201–207.
Lim JS, Mietus-Snyder M, Valente A et al. 2010. The role of fructose in the pathogenesis of NAFLD and the metabolic syndrome. *Nat Rev Gastroenterol Hepatol* 7:251–264.
Lin BH, Morrison RM. 2002. Higher fruit consumption linked with lower body mass index. *Food Rev* 25:28–32.
Liu LL, Lawrence JM, Davis C et al. 2010. Prevalence of overweight and obesity in youth with diabetes in USA: The SEARCH for Diabetes in Youth study. *Pediatr Diabetes* 11:4–11.
Lustig RH, Mulligan K, Noworolski SM et al. 2016. Isocaloric fructose restriction and metabolic improvement in children with obesity and metabolic syndrome. *Obesity* 24:453–460.
Mager DR, Iñiguez IR, Gilmour S et al. 2015. The effect of a low fructose and low glycemic index/load (FRAGILE) dietary intervention on indices of liver function, cardiometabolic risk factors, and body composition in children and adolescents with nonalcoholic fatty liver disease (NAFLD). *J Parenter Enteral Nutr* 39:73–84.

Mahoney LT, Burns TL, Stanford W et al. 2001. Usefulness of the Framingham risk score and body mass index to predict early coronary artery calcium in young adults (Muscatine Study). *Am J Cardiol* 88:509–515.

Malik VS, Pan A, Willett WC et al. 2013. Sugar-sweetened beverages and weight gain in children and adults: A systematic review and meta-analysis. *Am J Clin Nutr* 98:1084–1102.

Manson JE, Colditz GA, Stampfer MJ et al. 1990. A prospective study of obesity and risk of coronary heart disease in women. *N Engl J Med* 322:882–889.

Martinelli CE, Keogh JM, Greenfield JR et al. 2011. Obesity due to melanocortin 4 receptor (MC4R) deficiency is associated with increased linear growth and final height, fasting hyperinsulinemia, and incompletely suppressed growth hormone secretion. *J Clin Endocrinol Metab* 96:E181–E188.

McGinty S, Richmond TK, Desai NK. 2015. Managing adolescent obesity and the role of bariatric surgery. *Curr Opin Pediatr* 26: 434–441.

Meyer AA, Kundt G, Lenschow U et al. 2006. Improvement of early vascular changes and cardiovascular risk factors in obese children after a six-month exercise program. *J Am Coll Cardiol* 48:1865–1870.

Michalsky M, Kramer RE, Fullmer MA et al. 2011. Developing criteria for pediatric/adolescent bariatric surgery programs. *Pediatrics* 128(Suppl. 2):S65–S70.

Mietus-Snyder M, Drews KL, Otvos JD et al. 2013. Low-density lipoprotein cholesterol versus particle number in middle school children. *J Pediatr* 163:355–362.

Molleston JP, White F, Teckman J et al. 2002. Obese children with steatohepatitis can develop cirrhosis in childhood. *Am J Gastroenterol* 97:2460–2462.

Moore LL, Bradlee ML, Singer MR et al. 2012. Dietary Approaches to Stop Hypertension (DASH) eating pattern and risk of elevated blood pressure in adolescent girls. *Br J Nutr* 108:1678–1685.

Moore LL, Singer MR, Bradlee ML et al. 2005. Intake of fruits, vegetables, and dairy products in early childhood and subsequent blood pressure change. *Epidemiology* 16:4–11.

Morrison JA, Glueck CJ, Wang P. 2012. Childhood risk factors predict cardiovascular disease, impaired fasting glucose plus type 2 diabetes mellitus, and high blood pressure 26 years later at a mean age of 38 years: The Princeton-lipid research clinics follow-up study. *Metabolism* 61:531–541.

Mozaffarian D, Benjamin EJ, Go AS et al., on behalf of the American Heart Association Statistics Committee and Stroke Statistics Subcommittee. 2015. Heart disease and stroke statistics—2015 update: A report from the American Heart Association. *Circulation* 131:e29–e322.

Murphy M, Douglass J, Latulippe M, Barr S, Johnson R, Frye C. 2005. Beverages as a source of energy and nutrients in diets of children and adolescents. *FASEB J* 19:A434.

National Institutes of Health. 2002. Third report of the National Cholesterol Education Program (NCEP) expert panel on detection, evaluation, and treatment of high blood cholesterol in adults (Adult Treatment Panel III final report). Bethesda, MD: National Institutes of Health. NIH Publication No. 02-5215.

National Institutes of Health, National Heart, Lung, and Blood Institute. 1998. Clinical guidelines on the identification, evaluation, and treatment of overweight and obesity in adults: The evidence report. *Obes Res* 6(Suppl. 2):S51–S209.

Nemet D, Barkan S, Epstein Y et al. 2005. Short- and long-term beneficial effects of a combined dietary-behavioral-physical activity intervention for the treatment of childhood obesity. *Pediatrics* 115:e443–e449.

Neuschwander-Tetri BA, Caldwell SH. 2003. Nonalcholic steatohepatitis: Summary of an AASLD Single Topic Conference. *Hepatology* 37:1202–1219.

Nobili V, Manco M, Devito R et al. 2008. Lifestyle intervention and antioxidant therapy in children with nonalcoholic fatty liver disease: A randomized, controlled trial. *Hepatology* 48:119–128.

Nobili V, Marcellini M, Devito R et al. 2006. NAFLD in children: A prospective clinical-pathological study and effect of lifestyle advice. *Hepatology* 44:458–465.

Nobili V, Vajro P, Dezsofi A et al. 2015. Indications and limitations of bariatric intervention in severely obese children and adolescents with and without nonalcoholic steatohepatitis: ESPGHAN Hepatology Committee Position Statement. *J Pediatr Gastroenterol Nutr* 60:550–561.

Nogueira I, Hrovat K. 2014. Adolescent bariatric surgery: Review on nutrition considerations. *Nutr Clin Pract* 29:740–746.

Ogden CL, Carroll MD, Kit BK et al. 2014. Prevalence of childhood and adult obesity in the United States, 2011–2012. *JAMA* 311:806–814.

Ogden CL, Flegal KM, Carroll MD et al. 2002. Prevalence and trends in overweight among US children and adolescents, 1999–2000. *JAMA* 288:1728–1732.

Pardee PE, Lavine JE, Schwimmer JB. 2009. Diagnosis and treatment of pediatric nonalcoholic steatohepatitis and the implications for bariatric surgery. *Semin Pediatr Surg* 18:144–151.

Parillo M, Licenziati MR, Vacca M et al. 2012. Metabolic changes after a hypocaloric, low-glycemic-index diet in obese children. *J Endocrinol Invest* 35:629–633.

Parsons TJ, Power C, Logan S et al. 1999. Childhood predictors of adult obesity: A systematic review. *Int J Obes Relat Metab Disord* 23(Suppl. 8):S1–S107.

Pereira MA, Swain J, Goldfine AB et al. 2004. Effects of a low-glycemic load diet on resting energy expenditure and heart disease risk factors during weight loss. *JAMA* 292:2482–2490.

Pieke B, von Eckardstein A, Gülbahçe E et al. 2000. Treatment of hypertriglyceridemia by two diets rich either in unsaturated fatty acids or in carbohydrates: Effects on lipoprotein subclasses, lipolytic enzymes, lipid transfer proteins, insulin and leptin. *Int J Obes Relat Metab Disord* 24:1286—1296.

Power C, Lake JK, Cole TJ. 1997. Measurement and long-term health risks of child and adolescent fatness. *Int J Obes Relat Metab Disord* 21:507–526.

Pozzato C, Verduci E, Scaglioni S et al. 2010. Liver fat change in obese children after a 1-year nutrition-behavior intervention. *J Pediatr Gastroenterol Nutr* 51:331–335.

Ramon-Krauel M, Salsberg SL, Ebbeling CB et al. 2013. A low-glycemic-load versus low-fat diet in the treatment of fatty liver in obese children. *Child Obes* 9:252–260.

Reisin E, Abel R, Modan M et al. 1978. Effect of weight loss without salt restriction on the reduction of blood pressure in overweight hypertensive patients. *N Engl J Med* 298:1–6.

Robins SJ, Lyass A, Zachariah JP et al. 2011. Insulin resistance and the relationship of a dyslipidemia to coronary heart disease: The Framingham Heart Study. *Arterioscler Thromb Vasc Biol* 31:1208–1214.

Robinson TN. 1999. Reducing children's television viewing to prevent obesity: A randomized controlled trial. *JAMA* 282:1561–1567.

Rocchini AP, Katch V, Anderson J et al. 1988. Blood pressure and obese adolescents: Effect of weight loss. *Pediatrics* 82:16–23.

Rocchini AP, Key J, Bondie D et al. 1989. The effect of weight loss on the sensitivity of blood pressure to sodium in obese adolescents. *N Engl J Med* 321:580–585.

Rubinstein E, Lavine JE, Schwimmer JB. 2008. Hepatic, cardiovascular, and endocrine outcomes of the histological subphenotypes of nonalcoholic fatty liver disease. *Semin Liver Dis* 28:380–385.

Rudolf M. 2011. Predicting babies' risk of obesity. *Arch Dis Child* 96:995–997.

Sacks FM, Svetkey LP, Vollmer WM et al. 2001. Effects on blood pressure of reduced dietary sodium and the Dietary Approaches to Stop Hypertension (DASH) diet. DASH-Sodium Collaborative Research Group. *N Engl J Med* 344:3–10.

Sanyal AJ, Chalasani N, Kowdley KV et al. 2010. Pioglitazone, vitamin E, or placebo for nonalcoholic steatohepatitis. *N Engl J Med* 362:1675–1685.

Schwimmer JB, Deutsch R, Kahen T et al. 2006. Prevalence of fatty liver in children and adolescents. *Pediatrics* 118:1388–1393.

Shah K, Stufflebam A, Hilton TN et al. 2009. Diet and exercise interventions reduce intrahepatic fat content and improve insulin sensitivity in obese older adults. *Obesity* 17:2162–2168.

Simons-Morton DG, Hunsberger SA, Van Horn L et al. 1997. Nutrient intake and blood pressure in dietary intervention study in children. *Hypertension* 29:930–936.

Sinaiko AR, Gomez-Marin O, Prineas RJ. 1993. Effect of low sodium diet or potassium supplementation on adolescent blood pressure. *Hypertension* 21:989–994.

Skoczen S, Wojcik M, Fijorek K et al. 2015. Expression of the central obesity and type 2 diabetes mellitus genes is associated with insulin resistance in young obese children. *Exp Clin Endocrinal Diabetes* 123:252–259.

Sondike SB, Copperman N, Jacobson MS. 2003. Effects of a low-carbohydrate diet on weight loss and cardiovascular risk factor in overweight adolescents. *J Pediatr* 142:253–258.

Spear BA, Barlow SE, Ervin C et al. 2007. Recommendations for treatment of child and adolescent overweight and obesity. *Pediatrics* 120(Suppl. 4):S254–S288.

Speiser PW, Rudolf MC, Anhalt H et al., on behalf of the Obesity Consensus Working Group. 2005. Childhood obesity. *J Clin Endocrinol Metab* 90:1871–1887.

Steinberger J, Daniels SR, Eckel RH et al. 2009. Progress and challenges in metabolic syndrome in children and adolescents: A scientific statement from the American Heart Association Atherosclerosis, Hypertension, and Obesity in the Young Committee of the Council on Cardiovascular Disease in the Young; Council on Cardiovascular Nursing; and Council on Nutrition, Physical Activity, and Metabolism. *Circulation* 119:628–647.

The NS, Suchindran C, North KE et al. 2010. Association of adolescent obesity with risk of severe obesity in adulthood. *JAMA* 304:2042–2047.

Turchiano M, Sweat V, Fierman A, Convit A. 2012. Obesity, metabolic syndrome, and insulin resistance in urban high school students of minority race/ethnicity. *Arch Pediatr Adolesc Med* 166:1030–1036.

Urbina EM, Gidding SS, Bao W et al. 1999. Association of fasting blood sugar level, insulin level, and obesity with left ventricular mass in healthy children and adolescents: The Bogalusa Heart Study. *Am Heart J* 138:122–127.

Urbina EM, Kimball TR, Khoury PR et al. 2010. Increased arterial stiffness is found in adolescents with obesity or obesity-related type 2 diabetes mellitus. *J Hypertens* 28:1692–1698.

Urbina EM, Kimball TR, McCoy CE et al. 2009. Youth with obesity and obesity-related type 2 diabetes mellitus demonstrate abnormalities in carotid structure and function. *Circulation* 119:2913–2919.

U.S. Department of Agriculture and U.S. Department of Health and Human Services. 2011. *Dietary Guidelines for Americans, 2010*, 7th edn. Washington, DC: U.S. Government Printing Office. *Adv Nutr* 2:293–294.

Velázquez-López L, Santiago-Díaz G, Nava-Hernández J, Muñoz-Torres AV, Medina-Bravo P, Torres-Tamayo M. 2014. Mediterranean-style diet reduces metabolic syndrome components in obese children and adolescents with obesity. *BMC Pediatr* 14:175.

Vos MB, Weber MB, Welsh J et al. 2009. Fructose and oxidized low-density lipoprotein in pediatric nonalcoholic fatty liver disease: A pilot study. *Arch Pediatr Adolesc Med* 163:674–675.

Wang Y. 2011. Disparities in pediatric obesity in the United States. *Adv Nutr* 2:23–31.

Wang CY, Gortmaker SL, Taveras EM. 2011. Trends and racial/ethnic disparities in severe obesity among US children and adolescents, 1976–2006. *Int J Pediatr Obes* 6:12–20.

Waters E, de Silva-Sanigorski A, Burford BJ, Brown T, Campbell KJ, Gao Y, Armstrong R, Prosser L, Summerbell CD. 2011. Interventions for preventing obesity in children. *Cochrane Database Syst Rev* 2011(12): CD001871. doi: 10.1002/14651858.CD001871.pub3.

Watts K, Beye P, Siafarikas A et al. 2004. Effects of exercise training on vascular function in obese children. *J Pediatr* 144:620–625.

Weaver CM. 2013. Potassium and health. *Adv Nutr* 4:368S–377S.

Whitaker RC, Wright JA, Pepe MS et al. 1997. Predicting obesity in young adulthood from childhood and parental obesity. *N Engl J Med* 337:869–873.

Williams CL, Bollella M, Wynder EL. 1995. A new recommendation for dietary fiber in childhood. *Pediatrics* 96:985–988.

Williams SM, Goulding A. 2009. Early adiposity rebound is an important predictor of later obesity. *Obesity (Silver Spring)* 17:1310.

Woo KS, Chook P, Yu CW et al. 2004. Effects of diet and exercise on obesity-related vascular dysfunction in children. *Circulation* 109:1981–1986.

World Health Organization, Department of Noncommunicable Disease Surveillance. 1999. Report of a WHO Consultation: Definition of metabolic syndrome in definition diagnosis, and classification of diabetes mellitus and its complications: Report of a WHO Consultation, Part 1: Diagnosis and classification of diabetes mellitus. Geneva, Switzerland: World Health Organization.

Xanthakos SA. 2008. Bariatric surgery for extreme adolescent obesity: Indications, outcomes, and physiologic effects on the gut-brain axis. *Pathophysiology* 15:135–146.

Yancy WS Jr, Olsen MK, Guyton JR et al. 2004. A low-carbohydrate, ketogenic diet versus a low-fat diet to treat obesity and hyperlipidemia: A randomized, controlled trial. *Ann Intern Med* 140:769–777.

Yanovski SZ, Yanovski JA. 2014. Long-term drug treatment for obesity: A systematic and clinical review. *JAMA*. 311:74–86.

Yoshinaga M, Yuasa Y, Hatano H et al. 1995. Effect of total adipose weight and systemic hypertension on left ventricular mass in children. *Am J Cardiol* 76:785–787.

Zimmet P, Alberti KG, Kaufman F et al. 2007. The metabolic syndrome in children and adolescents—An IDF consensus report. *Pediatr Diabetes* 8:299–306.

9 Aging and Cardiovascular Disease

Lessons from Calorie Restriction

Jasper Most and Leanne M. Redman

CONTENTS

ABSTRACT

The average life expectancy of newborns in the United States is as high as never before. With advancing age, however, the incidence and prevalence of chronic diseases including cardiovascular diseases (CVDs) rise. Vice versa, poor cardiovascular health accelerates the aging process and increases mortality. Calorie restriction may decelerate both the development of CVDs and the progression of the aging process. In animal models including rodents and nonhuman primates, calorie restriction has indeed reduced the incidence of CVD and extended life span. In this book chapter, we review the available evidence for the benefit of calorie restriction on aging and CVD parameters in humans. Epidemiological data that in fact show reduced CVD mortality during food restriction are dated a century ago. More recent observational studies and data on long-term voluntary practitioners of calorie restriction offer valuable insight into the potential of calorie restriction to reduce CVD. The main focus of this chapter will be on the first clinically controlled randomized intervention studies of the CALERIE project. First, three pilot studies have investigated sustained calorie restriction by 25% for 6 or 12 months achieved through different modalities: dietary restriction, increased exercise, or a combination of both. Thereafter, in the second phase called CALERIE 2, calorie restriction by 25% was sustained for 2 years to investigate the feasibility and effects of calorie restriction beyond the initial weight loss period. Finally, we discuss alternative strategies that may achieve comparable effects of calorie restriction but may be easier to implement such as timed eating paradigms and the calorie restriction mimetic resveratrol.

AGING AND CARDIOVASCULAR DISEASE

Over the past 100 years, food supply and quality, hygiene standards, and health care have improved. As a result in 2014, the average life expectancy for an individual born in the United States was 78.8 years, 81.2 years for females and 76.4 years for males (Murphy et al. 2015), the highest estimates ever reported (Murphy et al. 2015; The Board of Trustees of the Federal Old-Age and Survivors Insurance and Federal Disability Insurance Trust Funds 2015; Xu et al. 2016). In line with this data, the age-adjusted death rate for the U.S. population in 2014 was at a record low of 725 deaths per 100,000 people (Murphy et al. 2015).

Of all the deaths reported in the United States between 2013 and 2014, 74% were accounted for by the 10 leading causes of mortality that include heart disease, cancer, chronic lower respiratory diseases, unintentional injuries, stroke, Alzheimer's disease, diabetes, influenza and pneumonia, kidney disease, and suicide (Murphy et al. 2015; Xu et al. 2016). Among these, cardiovascular diseases (CVDs), which include heart disease, hypertension, stroke, pulmonary artery disease, and diseases of the veins, accounted for approximately 31% or 800,937 deaths. As an individual advances in age, both cognitive and physical capacities decline and the susceptibility for chronic diseases including CVD increases (Lakatta and Levy 2003; Mozaffarian et al. 2015). This progressive decline of physiological integrity and body functioning with increasing age has been defined as "primary aging" (Holloszy 2000). In the United States, CVD-related deaths due to the increasing age of the population significantly increased by more than 30% (Roth et al. 2015). Even in the absence of CVD at the age of 50, the lifetime risk for men and women to develop CVD later in life is still more than 50% and ~40%, respectively (Lloyd-Jones et al. 2006).

Economically, the aging of the U.S. population has caused the total health care expenditures to rise up to $632 billion estimated in 2015 and is expected to almost double reaching $1.1 trillion over the next 10 years (Congressional Budget Office's 2015). Of the health care expenditures related to CVD, the costs in 2010 are expected to triple by 2030, from $270 billion to $820 billion (Heidenreich et al. 2011). While these estimations are based on data from 2010, the well-documented increase in risk factors for CVD such as a lack of physical activity, childhood obesity, and type II diabetes mellitus will likely contribute to a higher prevalence of CVD than anticipated, hence leading to a more significant health care burden in the future (Han, Lawlor, and Kimm 2010; Lee et al. 2012; Menke et al. 2015).

Interestingly, the increasing prevalence of these noncommunicable diseases may even outweigh the positive effect of improving health care and may cause a stagnation or even decline in life expectancy in the future (Ludwig 2016). This acceleration of aging and the increase in mortality from external factors such as the influence of lifestyle or the presence of chronic disease such as CVD has been described as "Secondary aging" (Holloszy 2000).

The progressive and detrimental interaction between aging and the development of CVD is likely being translated by their common pathologies and clinical manifestations, as summarized in Figure 9.1. With advancing age, adipose tissue mass increases and muscle mass and strength decline. The metabolic functions of these tissues including the clearance and storage of postprandial blood glucose and lipids deteriorate with age, which contributes to a disproportionate accumulation of fat in visceral and ectopic depots such as the liver and skeletal muscle (Atkins et al. 2014; Onoue et al. 2016). Ectopic fat accumulation is closely associated with disordered handling of lipids

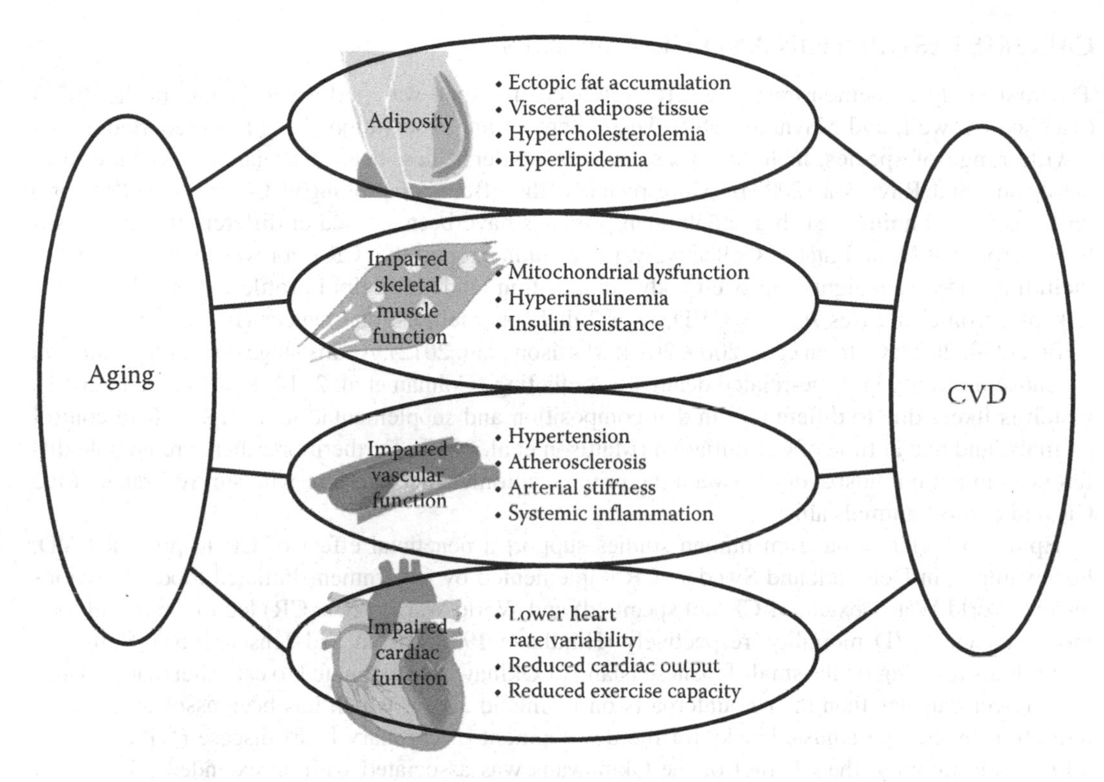

FIGURE 9.1 Overview of symptoms and risk factors of aging and CVDs. CVDs are caused by impaired functioning of the heart and the vasculature. Fat accumulation in visceral and ectopic depots is closely related to the development of CVD. They reflect an overload of healthy fat depots and are therefore associated with increased plasma concentrations of lipids, cholesterol, and inflammatory signals. Ectopic fat accumulation and inflammation impairs insulin signaling. As a consequence, cells are less responsive to the signals of insulin (insulin resistance) and take up less glucose. To compensate for this relative lack of insulin, pancreatic secretion increases and causes hyperinsulinemia. A reduced diameter of the arteries is caused by infiltration of the arterial walls by cholesterol and inflammatory signals (atherosclerosis) and by vascular resistance to dilatation. An impaired blood supply to tissues such as heart and brain can ultimately cause myocardial infarction or stroke, respectively. To maintain blood supply against a higher resistance (=smaller diameter), heart rate and blood pressure increase. Chronically elevated blood pressure and vascular resistance force the heart to pump harder. This compensation however is transient as the heart fatigues and as a consequence its capacity to pump blood into the circulation (cardiac output) and its reactivity to stimuli that would accelerate or slow its beating rate (heart rate variability) declines.

(dyslipidemia), insulin resistance, and impaired vascular and cardiac function (Lim and Meigs 2013) and is predictive of both aging (Liu and Li 2015) and CVD (Britton et al. 2013).

Because of the aging population and the increasing prevalence and costs of managing age-associated diseases, interventions to attenuate the aging process are desperately needed. The most promising nutritional intervention with the potential to counteract both primary and secondary aging in humans is calorie restriction (CR), which is defined as a sustained reduction of habitual energy intake, typically by 20%–50%, without malnutrition (Holloszy and Fontana 2007). In all animal models studied to date, including rodents and monkeys, CR has been shown to attenuate the onset of age-related chronic diseases and prolong life span (Speakman and Mitchell 2011). Evidence that CR induces a comparable effect on risk factors for CVD in humans is accumulating, giving rise to the potential for CR as an effective intervention for CVD prevention and treatment.

CALORIE RESTRICTION AND HUMAN AGING

The first study to demonstrate that CR prolonged life span was performed in rats in the 1930s (McCay, Crowell, and Maynard 1989). Thereafter, similar observations have been reported across a wide range of species, including yeast, worms, spiders, flies, fish, mice, and rats (reviewed in Heilbronn and Ravussin (2003)). More recently, the effects of prolonged CR (over 4–20 years) on longer-lived animals such as nonhuman primates have been studied at different research institutes across the United States. Collectively, these studies report that CR improves metabolic health, including reduced weight, improved body composition, and blood lipid profiles, thus reducing the risk of chronic diseases such as CVD, type 2 diabetes mellitus, and cancer (Bodkin et al. 2003; Cefalu et al. 2004; Colman et al. 2009, 2014; Mattison et al. 2012). At this stage, however, results on all-cause mortality and age-related death are conflicting (Colman et al. 2014; Mattison et al. 2012), which is likely due to differences in diet composition and supplementation, a slight CR in control animals, and age at time of CR initiation (Mattison et al. 2017). Furthermore, there are notable differences in animal husbandry between the primate colonies that interfere with survival rates of the CR and control animals alike.

Epidemiological data from human studies support a beneficial effect of CR to prevent CVD. For example, in Denmark and Sweden, CR implemented by government-initiated food restrictions during World War I (extent of CR not specified) and World War II (20% CR) led to a reduced total mortality and CVD mortality, respectively (Hindhede 1920; Strom and Jensen 1951). Similarly, individuals residing on the small Japanese island of Okinawa are estimated to eat a diet that provides 17% fewer calories than their counterparts on mainland Japan, which has been associated with a reduction in the age-adjusted risks for the development of coronary heart disease (Willcox et al. 2007). Additionally, the CR diet of the Okinawans was associated with an extended life span of 1.5 years as compared to the population of mainland Japan (Willcox et al. 2007). Sadly, an increased presence of U.S. military on Okinawa starting in 1960 led to the introduction of a Westernized diet and, consequently, the average level of CR, as well as the quality of the diet, declined. As a consequence, the life expectancy for children born today is not different between Japanese living on Okinawa and those residing on the mainland (life expectancy: girls, 87.0 vs. 86.4 years; boys, 79.4 vs. 79.5 years, respectively), whereas elderly Okinawans (>65 years) are still expected to live longer (women, 89.9 vs. 88.9 years; men, 84.5 vs. 83.8 years) (System of Social and Demographic Statistics 2016), which likely reflects their exposure to CR early in life.

Within the last decade, the first clinical controlled intervention trials to test the effect of CR on human aging have been undertaken, and while the results of these studies will not provide conclusions to the impact on life span, these trials allude to the impact of CR on mechanisms of primary and secondary aging including risk factors for age-related diseases (Das et al. 2007; Heilbronn et al. 2006; Racette et al. 2006; Ravussin et al. 2015).

PROPOSED MECHANISMS BY WHICH CR MAY AFFECT HUMAN AGING AND CVD

Extension of Life Span due to Slowing of the Rate of Aging

The ability of sustained CR to positively affect health and ameliorate aging is postulated to occur via two primary and complementary mechanisms; a reduction in energy expenditure and reduced oxidative stress.

The flux of energy through the body, or "rate of living," is a strong negative predictor for life span (Sacher and Duffy 1979). If the metabolic potential, or the energy expendable during a lifetime, is fixed per species as postulated (Sohal and Allen 1985), a reduction in energy expenditure may extend life span. During CR, a reduction in energy expenditure can be induced by lowering the metabolic mass of the individual (e.g., weight loss), by a reduction in physical activity (behavioral adaptation), or by other metabolic adaptations. CR-induced metabolic adaptations may be due to reduced oxygen requirements to produce ATP (or increased energy efficiency) or due to slowing of ATP-consuming processes (metabolic rate) (Liesa and Shirihai 2013). Despite these suggested benefits of reduced energy expenditure, it needs to be mentioned that a reduction of energy expenditure may increase the likelihood of a positive energy balance and subsequent weight regain.

Related to the rate of living theory is the oxidative damage theory of aging. Of all oxygen consumed by the electron transport chain, 1%–3% is reduced to oxygen radicals by leaking electrons. Leaking electrons are electrons that are not properly transferred along the electron transport chain and therefore diffuse back into the mitochondrial matrix. The generated oxygen radicals can accumulate in cells as toxic reactive oxygen species (ROS) (Alexeyev, Ledoux, and Wilson 2004), which in turn leads to damage to the electron transport chain and to the mitochondrial DNA. This elicits a vicious cycle, because the damaged electron transport chain leads to increased leakage of more electrons, which ultimately leads to a decline in physiological function and aging (Sohal and Weindruch 1996). Together these two theories posit that a reduction in the rate of living or metabolic rate due to CR (and hence oxygen trafficked through electron transport chain) causes fewer ROS to be accumulated. Over time, it is hypothesized that decreased accumulation of ROS yields less oxidative damage to lipids, proteins, and DNA, thereby leading to an attenuation in the rate of primary aging.

Extension of Life Span due to Prevention or Slowing of Age-Related Disease Onset

CR prevents overeating and as reviewed earlier, studies in nonhuman primates show a prevention or an attenuation of the increase in body weight and adiposity including visceral and ectopic fat accumulation in CR animals compared to the *ad libitum* fed counterparts that experience age-related increases in body weight and adiposity (Bodkin et al. 2003; Cefalu et al. 2004; Colman et al. 2009, 2014; Mattison et al. 2012). Consistently, CR animals experience less weight gain than animals on an *ad libitum* diet, yet weight trajectories within the CR groups differ between studies dependent on the study design. While some studies define CR as energy intake clamped to maintain body weight, whereas the control animals gain weight on an *ad libitum* diet (Bodkin et al. 2003), in other studies animals are fed on 30% CR and therefore lose ~10% body weight after 4 years (Cefalu et al. 2004) and 18 months (Colman et al. 1998). Over longer terms, body weight stabilizes and undergoes age-related changes yet remains lower in CR animals compared to their ad libitum (AL) fed counterparts (Mattison et al. 2005). Throughout different studies, CR induced significant reductions of dyslipidemia, hypertension, and incidence of T2DM and CVD (Bodkin et al. 2003; Cefalu et al. 2004; Colman et al. 2009, 2014; Mattison et al. 2012). If CR is similarly effective in humans as in primates (e.g., there is no age-induced increase in the prevalence of obesity, the age-related decline in physical activity is no more than 10%, blood pressure is ~25% lower, and there is no evidence of diabetes mellitus), the American Heart Association and World Heart Federation estimate that 2 million premature deaths due to CVD among men and women could be prevented by CR diets (Sacco et al. 2016).

Since mortality and longevity are not typically obtainable endpoints in human studies, an understanding of the influence of antiaging therapies such as CR on human aging is reliant on the measurement of aging biomarkers. Proposed and well-studied biomarkers indicative of advanced aging are high body core temperature and high insulin concentrations (Roth et al. 2002). High body temperature likely reflects a high metabolic rate (rate of living) and hence a shortened life span (Keil, Cummings, and de Magalhaes 2015). Chronically elevated concentrations of insulin may favor CVD by promoting age-induced increases of adiposity and insulin resistance (Zhang and Liu 2014). The Baltimore Longitudinal Study of Aging (Shock 1984) investigated the validity of these biomarkers through their study of mortality in healthy men. A comparison of core body temperature and insulin levels between those individuals with values in the upper versus lower half of the cohort for these measures showed that mortality was indeed positively associated with increased core temperature and insulin concentrations (Roth et al. 2002). The study of these two biomarkers in nonhuman primate colonies provided additional evidence of the impact of CR diets on the attenuation of aging. Nonhuman primates consuming a CR diet had reduced rates of mortality and an attenuation of the age-associated changes in both core body temperature and insulin in comparison to the animals maintained *ad libitum* (Roth et al. 2002).

EVIDENCE FOR THE ANTIAGING EFFECTS OF CR IN HUMANS

An Unintended Study of CR from the Biosphere 2 Experiment

Biosphere 2 is a 3.15-acre ecological enclosure that unintentionally provided an opportunity to study the effects of CR in humans under controlled conditions (Walford, Harris, and Gunion 1992). A group of eight nonobese individuals between the ages of 25 and 67 entered the Biosphere 2 enclosure for 6 months. Due to unanticipated agricultural problems with the growing and harvesting of food inside the enclosure, the energy intake of the inhabitants was restricted by ~29%. The diet composition was diverse, largely vegetarian, and provided adequate protein, high fiber, and low fat. Over the 6-month observational period, the CR diet resulted in a 15% weight loss.

In line with the hypothesis that CR may reduce the rate of living, 24-h energy expenditure in the Biosphere inhabitants assessed 1 week and 6 months after exiting the Biosphere enclosure was less than energy expenditure in 152 non-CR free-living subjects with similar heights and weights, with appropriate statistical adjustment for age, sex, fat-free mass, and fat mass (Weyer et al. 1999, 2000). The CR diet produced a subtle yet nonsignificant reduction in core temperature; however, this observation may have been underestimated because the thermostats were not calibrated for temperatures <96°F (Walford et al. 1999). Moreover, a rapid increase in insulin levels within a month after exiting the enclosure suggested that the CR experienced during the enclosure decreased insulin concentrations (Walford et al. 2002). The increase in insulin concentrations was accompanied by an increase in body mass index (BMI) of 1.4 kg/m^2. As proposed in previous studies, the CR diet of the Biosphere inhabitants significantly improved the CVD risk. The 6-month CR diet (~29% reduction in energy intake from baseline levels) decreased the percentage of body fat, plasma triglycerides, serum cholesterol, low-density lipoprotein (LDL)-cholesterol, as well as systolic and diastolic blood pressures during the first 3 months of weight loss, but not further when body weight was maintained after 3 months within the enclosure (Walford, Harris, and Gunion 1992; Walford et al. 2002). Furthermore, a reduction in white blood cell count by 30%–40% may indicate a reduced state of systemic inflammation.

Self-Administered CR in the Calorie Restriction Optimal Nutrition Society

Members of the Calorie Restriction Optimal Nutrition (CRON) Society report self-prescribing and administering CR diets for 3–15 years, on a voluntary basis. Observational studies in these individuals have allowed for the long-term effects of CR in weight-stable humans to be better understood (Fontana et al. 2004; Holloszy and Fontana 2007; Yang et al. 2016). As compared to a group of individuals (matched for age and socioeconomic status) consuming a regular Western diet, members of the CRON Society consume 30% less energy and their CR diets meet all recommended levels for essential nutrients (Fontana et al. 2004). They have a low BMI (<20 kg/m^2) and a low percent of body fat (<10%), and none of the 50 men and women (age range 30–82 years) practicing long-term CR, who have been extensively studied, report taking any medication or show evidence of any chronic disease.

While data on longevity, or mortality, are not yet available for the CRON Society members, as compared to body fat–matched athletes consuming Western diets, these self-prescribing CR individuals have significantly lower core body temperature and slightly lower insulin concentrations, which could reflect an attenuated rate of primary and secondary aging (Fontana, Klein, and Holloszy 2010; Soare et al. 2011). As to be expected due to the higher volume of training, the group of athletes consumed more than double the amount of energy, whereas macronutrient composition of the diets is comparable between groups (Fontana, Klein, and Holloszy 2010). With regard to CVD, clinical outcome measures for cardiac and vascular function such as carotid artery intima-media thickness, left ventricular diastolic function, and heart rate variability are significantly improved in the CRON group compared to age- and socioeconomic status–matched control subjects (Fontana et al. 2007; Meyer et al. 2006; Stein et al. 2012). Furthermore, systolic and diastolic blood pressures, total cholesterol, LDL-cholesterol, and plasma triglycerides were significantly lower, whereas high-density lipoprotein (HDL)-cholesterol and free fatty acid concentrations were higher as compared to control subjects (Fontana et al. 2004, 2007). Reduced concentrations of tumor necrosis factor alpha (TNF alpha), C-reactive protein (CRP), platelet-derived growth factor AB, resistin, and interleukin 6 in the CRON group also suggest that CR diets may induce anti-inflammatory mechanisms as well as ameliorate dyslipidemia and insulin resistance (Fontana, Klein, and Holloszy 2010; Fontana et al. 2004; Meyer et al. 2006).

Short-Duration Interventions with Calorie Restriction

In a randomized, controlled 10-week intervention study, the effects of 20% CR (with adequate nutritional intake and micronutrient levels "approaching recommended daily allowances") on energy metabolism have been investigated. Contrary to the oxidative damage theory of aging, a reduction in metabolic rate in the CR subjects did not lead to a concomitant reduction of indicators of oxidative stress such as malondialdehyde, LDL-oxidation or 8-hydroxy-2-deoxyguanosine, catalase, and superoxide dismutase (Loft et al. 1995; Velthuis-te Wierik et al. 1995). However, CR for 10 weeks significantly reduced body weight (Velthuis-te Wierik et al. 1994) and improved CVD risk factors including a reduction in systolic and diastolic blood pressure and increased fibrinolytic activity (Loft et al. 1995; Velthuis-te Wierik et al. 1995). Importantly, after 10 weeks of intervention, body weight was not stabilized yet, thus no distinction can be made between the effects of weight loss and CR itself.

Longer-Duration Interventions with Calorie Restriction

The Comprehensive Assessment of Long-Term Effects of Reducing Intake of Energy (CALERIE) trials were initiated by the U.S. National Institute of Aging to provide the first randomized controlled clinical trials of longer-duration CR in healthy, nonobese humans. The CALERIE trials were conducted in two phases. The overall purpose of the first three individual studies in Phase 1 (CALERIE 1) was to inform the design and clinical endpoints in a larger, randomized controlled trial of CR for longer duration in Phase 2 (CALERIE 2).

CALERIE 1

In CALERIE 1, three pilot studies evaluated the feasibility and effects of different modalities of CR on biomarkers of aging, and metabolic health after 6 months (Heilbronn et al. 2006) or 12 months (Das et al. 2007; Racette et al. 2006). Compliance to the CR regimen, or calculation of CR, was determined by the energy-intake balance method, in which the First Law of Thermodynamics is applied to human physiology. This states that the amount of energy intake is equal to the amount of energy expenditure plus the changes in body energy stores (de Jonge et al. 2007). In the CALERIE studies, body composition (vis-à-vis energy stores) and total daily energy expenditure were measured by means of dual-energy x-ray absorptiometry and doubly labeled water before and after the intervention, which equate to energy intake throughout the intervention. CR was then the ratio of actual energy intake to baseline energy requirements. These data and calculations were not available in real time throughout the trials, and therefore body weight was used as a proxy for CR. The study participants followed a strict behavioral intervention that required frequent individual meetings with the behavioral counselors and meetings with the whole CR group at the study center. In addition, foods were provided to participants at regular intervals and this required a visit to the center twice per day during these periods so that breakfast and dinner meals were eaten under supervision by the dieticians and the lunch and weekend meals were packaged to go. Any unconsumed foods were returned and weighed. These strategies helped study participants comply with the CR diets throughout the trials.

CALERIE 1 at Pennington Biomedical Research Center (PBRC) in Baton Rouge compared a reduction of energy intake alone (25% CR) for 6 months to a group that had a combined reduction in energy intake and an increase in energy expenditure through exercise (−12.5% energy intake + 12.5% energy expenditure = 25% CR+EX), to a group that achieved a 15 kg weight loss through a low-calorie diet, and to a control group eating an *ad libitum* diet (Heilbronn et al. 2006). Participants were provided with their food during baseline assessments until week 12 and for 2 weeks prior to post measurements.

The 25% CR group achieved an actual CR of 18% and lost 10% of body mass, 24% fat mass, and 5% fat-free mass over the 6-month intervention (Heilbronn et al. 2006). Indicated by steady negative slopes of weekly body weight measurements, weight maintenance was not achieved during the 6-month study. In support of the rate of living hypothesis, all components of energy expenditure—sleep (Heilbronn et al. 2006), rest (Martin et al. 2007), 24-h sedentary (Heilbronn et al. 2006), and free-living (Redman et al. 2009)—were reduced below baseline levels after 6 months of 25% CR. The observed reduction in sedentary energy expenditure (sleep and 24 h) was ~6% lower than the energy expenditure that was expected on the basis of the metabolic mass of the individuals at the end of the study, indicating metabolic adaptation. Interestingly, thyroid hormone (T3 and T4) and leptin concentrations were significantly reduced after 6 months and were significantly related to this metabolic adaptation (Heilbronn et al. 2006; Lecoultre, Ravussin, and Redman 2011). In line with this suggested antiaging effect, core body temperature (assessed over 24 h) and fasting insulin concentrations were also reduced by the 25% CR diet (Heilbronn et al. 2006). Importantly, despite the observed decline in physical activity (total energy expenditure) in the CR group, thigh muscle mass, lower body skeletal muscle strength (knee flexor and extensor strength), and physical functioning (VO_{2peak}/VO_{2max} on a treadmill, expressed per kilogram of body mass) were preserved or even increased during CR (Larson-Meyer et al. 2010; Weiss et al. 2007). Since strength and physical functioning decline with age, it is important that CR does not accelerate these effects that can lead to increased susceptibility to falls, frailty, and fractures. Interestingly, whether CR was achieved by diet alone (CR group) or diet in conjunction with exercise (CR+EX group), it had no effect on body composition outcomes or effects on cardiometabolic risk factors. However, aerobic fitness, which is also a risk factor for CVD, was notably improved to a greater extent in the CR+EX group. Since longer-term studies comparing CR and CR+EX have not been undertaken, it is difficult to know if the outcomes of these two different modalities would remain consistent with each other over time or if one intervention would prevail with greater CR benefits.

The individuals consuming the 25% CR diet for 6 months had a significant reduction in subcutaneous adipocyte size, visceral adipose tissue (multislice computed tomography), and reduced intrahepatic lipid content (magnetic resonance spectroscopy) (Larson-Meyer et al. 2006; Redman et al. 2007). In line with these improvements in overall adiposity and fat distribution, plasma triglyceride concentrations and hemostatic Factor VIIc were significantly reduced with the 25% CR diet (Lefevre et al. 2009). Surprisingly, the 6 months of CR did not affect various other risk factors that are associated with CVD such as concentrations of lipoproteins (LDL-cholesterol and HDL-cholesterol), fibrinogen, homocysteine, CRP, or blood pressure (Lefevre et al. 2009). Also, flow-mediated dilatation as a measure of endothelial function was not changed. The lack of an effect of CR on these latter measures may have been related to the younger age of the study participants (<50 years) as well as their impeccable health status even before beginning the CR intervention. Nevertheless, this 6-month study of 25% CR estimated that based on the changes in total and HDL cholesterol (expressed as their ratio), systolic blood pressure, as well as participants age and gender (Anderson et al. 1991), the 10-year risk for CVD was attenuated by 29% (Lefevre et al. 2009). The reduction in CVD risk by CR is further supported by significant improvements in insulin sensitivity and β-cell function (assessed by frequently sampled intravenous glucose tolerance test [FSIGTT]), which may suggest that CR interventions over the longer term may also mediate downstream effects on the development of type 2 diabetes mellitus (Larson-Meyer et al. 2006).

For the CALERIE 1 study at Washington University in St. Louis, 48 individuals who were not obese and between 50 and 60 years of age were randomly assigned to either 20% CR, or a 20% increase in energy expenditure through endurance exercise or a control group following a healthy lifestyle (Racette et al. 2006). Noteworthy, the achieved degree of CR was lower as compared to the 6-month study at PBRC (13% as compared to 18%), which can be explained by the lower initiated CR, a lower level of compliance to the dietary intervention throughout the study, and because the estimated energy intake was based on energy requirements at baseline and was not adjusted throughout the study as participants lost weight. Interestingly, despite this lower CR, the observed reductions in weight (10.7%) were similar to those measured at PBRC. While in the study at PBRC (Heilbronn et al. 2006), reductions in thyroid hormone levels were associated with the reduction in metabolic rate in both the CR and CR+EX groups, no effect on T3 concentrations was observed after weight loss that was exclusively exercise induced (achieved calorie deficit of 12.8%), suggesting that exercise ameliorates the weight loss–induced decline of T3 (Fontana et al. 2006; Weiss et al. 2008). The 12-month CR intervention reduced concentrations of LDL-cholesterol and CRP indicative of a reduced metabolic risk profile (Fontana et al. 2007). In line with these improvements, fat accumulation in visceral adipose tissue was reduced by 37% as assessed by magnetic resonance imaging and adipose tissue endocrine function was improved as reflected by increased adiponectin and reduced leptin concentrations after 1 year of CR. In addition, insulin sensitivity, measured during an oral glucose tolerance test (OGTT), was improved after 1 year of CR (Villareal et al. 2006; Weiss et al. 2006). Additionally, a CR diet–induced improvement of left ventricular diastolic function and reductions of oxidative stress to DNA and RNA in white blood cells suggested a preventive effect of CR on aging and CVD (Hofer et al. 2008; Riordan et al. 2008). Despite the longer duration of the study in St. Louis as compared to PBRC, the participants of both weight loss groups did not achieve a weight maintenance status after a year and thus, as we have mentioned before, a distinction between the effects of weight loss and CR is not possible (Racette et al. 2006).

In the CALERIE 1 study at Tufts University in Boston, 46 young (24–42 years old) men and women who were overweight (BMI, 25–29.9 kg/m^2) were assigned to either a high- or a low-glycemic-load diet at 30% CR for 1 year (Das et al. 2007). The degree of CR achieved by the 2 CR groups did not differ significantly (15% CR), and therefore the 8% loss of body weight and 15% loss of body fat were also similar. CR-induced reductions of the resting metabolic rate and plasma insulin concentrations are in line with previously mentioned studies (Pittas et al. 2006). As in the other two pilot studies, CR lowered risk factors for CVD including reduced concentrations of plasma triglycerides, cholesterol, and CRP (Ahmed et al. 2009; Das et al. 2007; Pittas et al. 2006). Insulin sensitivity and first-phase acute insulin secretion, assessed by an OGTT and a FSIGTT, improved and may contribute to a reduced risk of type 2 diabetes mellitus and hence to reduced secondary aging. Contrary to the hypothesis of this pilot, all effects of CR were independent of the glycemic load of the diet.

CALERIE 2

Most recently, the CALERIE 2 trial was completed and the first results from the trial are starting to emerge. The goal of the CALERIE 2 trial was to investigate the safety and efficacy of a 25% CR diet for 2 years compared to an *ad libitum* diet. Unlike the individual trials in Phase 1,

CALERIE 2 was conducted as a single protocol across the three CALERIE 1 study sites (PBRC, Washington University, Tufts University), and 220 healthy individuals of normal weight between 21 and 51 years old were enrolled in the 2-year study (Rochon et al. 2011). Adherence to CR was supported by a number of intervention enhancements including the supervised delivery of the CR intervention, and individual and group counseling through the intervention by psychologists and nutritionists (Rickman et al. 2011). Moreover, the meals for the first 4 weeks were provided as guidance by example. Participants were exposed to 3 different diet patterns (Western, Mediterranean, low glycemic) to be educated on food selection and portion sizes. In addition, participants received training on food record-keeping because diets were continually monitored by daily self-monitoring reports (recorded on PDA devices) and by 6-day food records every 6 months. Provided meals were fully adequate in all essential nutrients and for self-selected meals, participants were guided to consume macronutrients as advised by the Dietary Reference Intakes (i.e., 45%–65%, 20%–35%, and 10%–35% for carbohydrate, fat, and protein, respectively). In addition, all participants received a daily multivitamin and mineral supplement and additional calcium to ensure that participants in both treatment arms met the current recommendations for these nutrients (Rochon et al. 2011). Participants in the AL received no specific intervention or counseling (Rochon et al. 2011). As planned in the study design, the reduction in body weight (−11.5%) was achieved at 12 months and maintained thereafter for the rest of the study. Total fat mass was also significantly reduced by CR (−23%) and maintained over the 2 years (Ravussin et al. 2015; Villareal et al. 2016). Similar to CALERIE 1, the 25% CR induced a metabolic adaptation in resting metabolic rate at 12 months. After 24 months, metabolic adaptation was still significant within the CR group, however not significantly different from the group adhering to the *ad libitum* diet any more (Ravussin et al. 2015). In a similar fashion, reductions in core temperatures after 12 and 24 months were significantly reduced from baseline with 25% CR, but not significantly different between the CR and control groups (Ravussin et al. 2015). A diminishing level of CR across the 2 years might explain the lack of significance at the 24-month assessment (CALERIE 1, 18% during 6 months; CALERIE 2, 19.5% ± 0.8% during the first 6 months and 9.1% ± 0.7% on average for the remainder of the study). Importantly, in an ancillary study of CALERIE 2 at one center and in a subset of participants (ClinicalTrials.gov Identifier: NCT02695511) that were more compliant (14.8% vs. 11.7% CR during the 2 years), metabolic adaptation in both 24 h and sleeping energy expenditure (measured in a room calorimeter) was significant after both 1 and 2 years of intervention in the CR group (Redman et al. 2014). As in CALERIE 1, metabolic adaptation in sleeping energy expenditure was associated with decreased leptin and thyroid hormone concentrations (Redman et al. 2014).

In line with previous but mostly shorter-duration studies of CR, 24 months of 25% CR in CALERIE 2 improved numerous markers of CVD risk. Blood pressure, total cholesterol, LDL-cholesterol, triglycerides, CRP, and TNF alpha decreased significantly and HDL-cholesterol increased in the CR group, whereas no changes were observed in the control group (Ravussin et al. 2015). Similarly, the CR group had a significant improvement in insulin sensitivity (HOMA-IR, 1.2–0.9), which was also not observed in the control group. These effects are remarkable considering that the participants were screened on the basis of their health status and blood pressure, plasma glucose, insulin, and lipids were all required to be in the normal range at enrollment, prior to the initiation of the CR intervention.

The safety of CR as well as the quality of life of CR participants was closely monitored in the Phase 2 study, and measured indicators suggest little concern toward longer-term implementation of CR, at least in healthy individuals (Ravussin et al. 2015). Monitored safety concerns in the CR group were low BMI (<18.5 kg/m^2, n = 1; resolved and intervention continued), treatment-resistant anemia (n = 4; 2 resolved and intervention continued), and decreased bone mineral density (≥5% from baseline, n = 3; 2 resolved [returned to <5% from baseline] and intervention continued). A decline in average bone mineral density (lumbar spine, −1.2%, and femoral neck, −1.7%) was observed in the CR group but this was found to occur in proportion to the loss of body mass, suggesting that the risk of bone injury was not increased. The intraindividual variability in bone loss however suggests that regular, close monitoring of bone health is important for individuals following CR diets (Villareal et al. 2016). Quality of life evaluated by validated measures of mood, self-reported hunger, sexual function, and cognitive function remained unchanged or improved (mood) after CR for 2 years (Martin et al. 2016).

Taken together, the epidemiological studies as well as the controlled clinical trials of CR indicate that a reduction in usual calorie intake when sustained for a long period of time can induce favorable effects on the normal mechanisms of human aging. In particular, the age-induced weight gain and partitioning of energy in adipose tissues including visceral and ectopic depots are attenuated with CR diets. Furthermore, circulating levels of insulin, plasma lipids, and inflammatory markers are improved alongside a slowing of the metabolic rate. Provided that CR interventions preserve strength and physical function and do not accelerate the age-induced loss of bone, this nutritional intervention might be impactful to the World Health Organization target to reduce noncommunicable diseases worldwide by 25% in the next 10 years.

ALTERNATIVE STRATEGIES FOR CR

While evidence for the benefit of CR in humans is accumulating, one of the greatest pitfalls of this nutritional intervention is the difficulty to maintain adherence to CR over a longer period of time, especially in the current obesogenic environment that is characteristic of energy-dense foods and sedentary lifestyles. Further research is needed to test whether alternative strategies to CR that are easier to implement achieve equivalent health benefits.

Timed Eating Paradigms

An emerging approach to dietary interventions is timed eating that follows the idea that meal times and calorie intake should be more closely linked with circadian rhythms of hormones rather than just following the traditional 3-meal per day paradigm. It is hypothesized that when there is a misalignment between eating patterns and circadian rhythms such as secretion of metabolic hormones (leptin, insulin, and thyroid hormones), there is a greater propensity for metabolic disorders like insulin resistance, dyslipidemia, and hence development and mortality of CVD (Gu et al. 2015). This phenomenon also termed as "metabolic jetlag" is commonly observed, for example, in shift workers, individuals who have been shown to have increased prevalence of CVD (Copertaro et al. 2008; Gu et al. 2015). Interestingly, in a recent study, a reduction in erratic eating behavior and eating duration (time between the first and last calorie intake of the day was 4 h 35 min less than during an observational control period of 3 weeks at baseline) induced an unintentional CR of 20%, which resulted in a 3 kg reduction in body weight after 16 weeks (Gill and Panda 2015). To date, altered calorie intake with timed eating paradigms has not been directly compared to traditional CR diets, and therefore it remains to be investigated whether timed eating can attenuate biomarkers of human aging or incidences of age-related diseases (Froy and Miskin 2010).

Alternate-Day Fasting

The first human clinical intervention study on CR (without malnutrition) implemented CR by alternate-day fasting for 3 years (Vallejo 1957). As the name implies, alternate-day fasting paradigms involve a day of normal eating followed by a day of either complete fasting or a significantly reduced level of dietary intake such as <20%. In the Vallejo study, 60 out of 120 men received 900 and 2300 kcal on alternate days for 3 years, estimated to be equivalent to 35% CR overall, whereas the 60 others were fed *ad libitum*. Strikingly, the death rate (6 vs. 13) and hospital admissions (123 vs. 219) were ~50% lower in the individuals fed CR through an alternate-day fasting diet (Stunkard 1976). A more recent study that imposed a complete day of fasting followed by a day of *ad libitum* eating for 3 weeks reduced participants' body weight by 2.5% (Heilbronn et al. 2005). This suggests that CR can be achieved with these kinds of time-restricted eating paradigms. In this 3-week study, the alternate-day fasting did not reduce oxidative stress, resting metabolic rate, or body core temperature. However, a scientific conundrum noted by the authors is when to collect follow-up measurements, following a day of fasting or a day of feeding. The ability to sustain these kinds of eating paradigms for longer-term studies is questioned because lightheadedness, constipation, and irritability (on fast days) were frequently reported (Heilbronn et al. 2005). Longer-duration studies of alternative-day eating paradigms are lacking, especially those with a direct comparison to traditional CR diets. The reader is referred to Chapter 27 of this textbook for a more detailed review of the effects of alternate-day fasting on measures of cardiometabolic health.

CR Mimetics

Given the long-standing quest for the fountain of youth and development of an antiaging remedy in a single pill, scientists are screening plants and their bioactive components for potential antiaging effects. Probably, the most promising compounds with the ability to mimic the effects of CR diets are activators of the sirtuin-AMPK-PGC1α cascade, which can stimulate glucose uptake, substrate oxidation, and mitochondrial biogenesis (Bonkowski and Sinclair 2016). To date, the most potent one is resveratrol, a polyphenolic antioxidant of grapes and red wine. In the past decade, resveratrol has been added to various diets including high-fat diets administered to numerous rodent models. Consistently, these studies reported improvements in metabolic health (attenuation or protection of the negative effects of a high-fat diet on body composition, insulin sensitivity, and dyslipidemia) and the induction of cellular antiaging pathways (Baur et al. 2006; Lagouge et al. 2006; Pearson et al. 2008). However, despite these improvements, an extension of life span has not yet been achieved (Marchal, Pifferi, and Aujard 2013). In humans, resveratrol supplementation has induced remarkably similar effects to the 25% CR diet in the CALERIE trials. Supplementation with a daily dose of 80 mg resveratrol reduced sleeping metabolic rate (with no alterations in body mass), improved mitochondrial capacity (ex vivo respirometry on vastus lateralis), and lowered fasting insulin concentrations, blood pressure and intrahepatic lipid content after 30 days in a placebo-controlled crossover study with 11 obese men (Timmers et al. 2011). Conversely, a study in healthy, nonobese women reported no effect of resveratrol supplementation on metabolic health, which questions the efficacy of resveratrol in healthier populations (Yoshino et al. 2012). Supplementation studies similar to those of CR are difficult to compare given the differences in dosage and also trial lengths. The effect of resveratrol and other CR mimetics on human aging remains to be determined. Moreover, the added benefit of resveratrol to CR diets or the effect of CR diets that provide high levels of polyphenols is not yet known.

CONCLUSION

Based on the cumulative data of CR on human aging from epidemiological, observational, and clinical intervention studies to date, we can conclude that moderate CR (>10% reduction in energy intake below baseline levels) sustained for at least several months induces significant improvements in the metabolic health profile. The slowing of metabolic processes and a reduction in risk factors for the development of age-related diseases including CVD are hypothesized to be key mediators for the antiaging effects of CR on longevity in nonhuman primates. While data on longevity does not yet exist in human trials of CR, the ability of CR to ameliorate these factors in shorter-duration studies has been shown consistently.

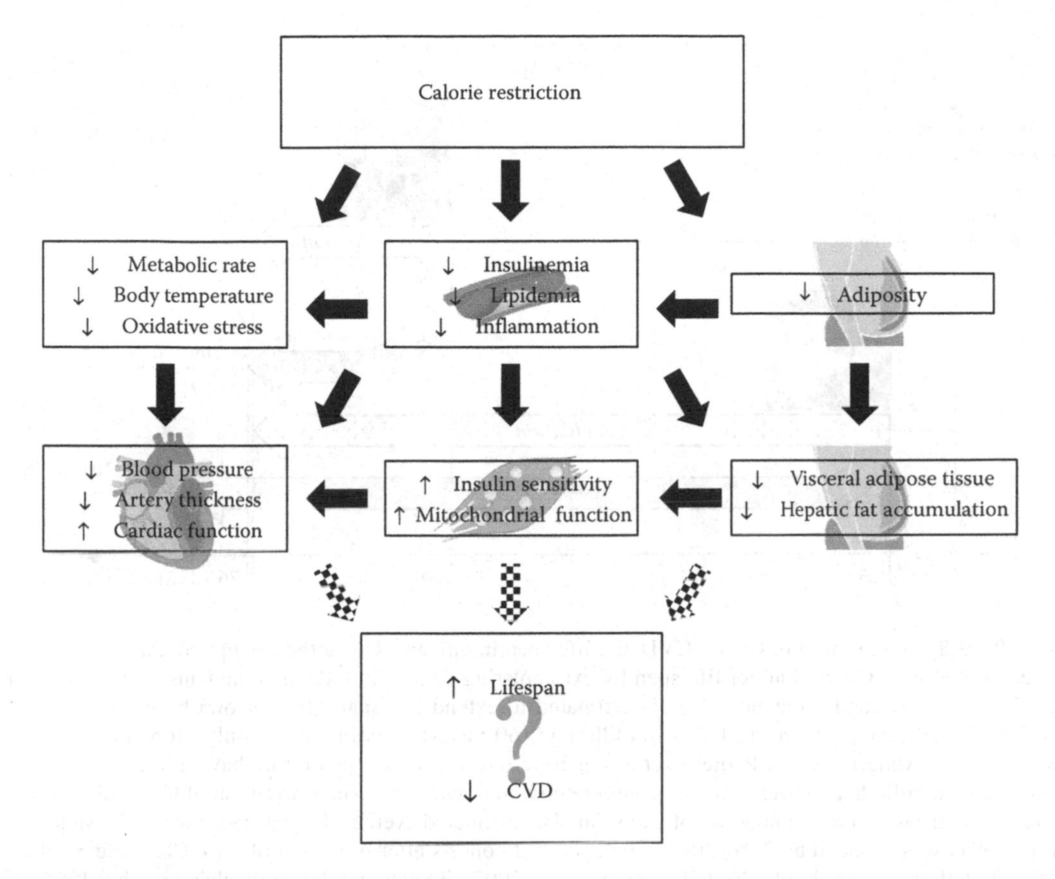

FIGURE 9.2 A proposed hierarchical model for the effects of CR on parameters of aging and CVDs. CR reduces metabolic rate through a reduction in body mass, physical activity, and metabolic adaptation. In line with hypotheses on the progression of aging, a reduction in metabolic rate coincided with less oxidative stress, assessed in skeletal muscle and plasma cells, and may cause reduced body temperature. In addition, the prolonged restriction in energy intake significantly reduces whole-body adiposity and induced a healthier plasma profile with lower concentrations of insulin, triglycerides, LDL, cholesterol, and inflammatory markers. In line with these results, visceral and ectopic (hepatic) fat accumulation decreases during CR and skeletal muscle metabolic function such as insulin sensitivity and mitochondrial function improve. An amelioration of oxidative stress, inflammation, and an improvement in mitochondrial function may contribute to reductions in blood pressure and artery thickness and thus reduced the risk of atherosclerosis and improved cardiac function. In concert, these improvements suggest that CR may significantly attenuate the progression of aging and the development of CVD.

We have proposed a hierarchical model (Figure 9.2) for these well-documented effects of CR on common parameters of aging and CVD. Future studies need to investigate whether the reductions in the rate of living and the cardiovascular risk profile indeed translate into prolonged health span and life span. It has been estimated that if 20% CR is sustained for 50 years, life span could be prolonged by ~5 years (Figure 9.3). This number may be even higher, because a possible reduction in CVD mortality is not depicted in this mathematical model because the only data available on the effects of CR on CVD-specific mortality is from the government-induced food restriction in Norway during World War II (Strom and Jensen 1951). Because adherence to sustained CR is challenging especially in the current obesogenic environment, investigation of more plausible eating regimens to induce CR including alternate-day fasting or the use of nutritional supplements that mimic CR effects may reveal valuable alternatives to the traditional CR diets.

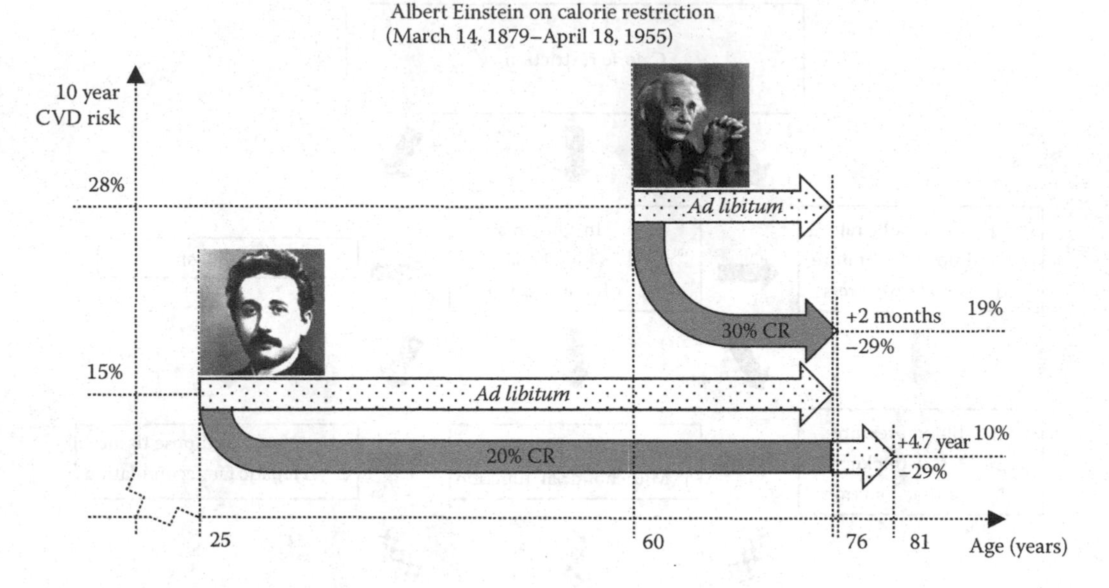

FIGURE 9.3 The impact of CR on CVD and life span in humans. Using the example of Albert Einstein, we estimated how CR may affect life span by extrapolating data from rodents to humans. Early-onset (at age 25) CR, sustained throughout life, is estimated to extend life span (gray arrow) by almost 5 years (white, dotted peak). Initiating CR at middle age (60 years) is estimated to only elongate life span by 2 months. Adhering to a CR diet over a longer period of time may therefore have a larger impact on human's metabolic health over time and consequently on human life span. Prevention of CVD might additionally contribute to a prolongation of life span. The estimated average 10-year risk for CVD (Anderson et al. 1991) was reduced by 25%–30% in independent cohorts after 6 months of 25% CR (Lefevre et al. 2009) and after 12 months of 20% CR (Fontana et al. 2007). To date, no data is available on the effects of CR on CVD-specific mortality, but a 50% lower CVD incidence in nonhuman primates on young-onset CR shows that CR has a significant impact on CVD and thus likely on CVD mortality. (From Colman, R.J. et al., *Science*, 325(5937), 201, 2009.)

REFERENCES

Ahmed, T., S. K. Das, J. K. Golden et al. 2009. Calorie restriction enhances T-cell-mediated immune response in adult overweight men and women. *J Gerontol A Biol Sci Med Sci* 64(11):1107–1113.

Alexeyev, M. F., S. P. Ledoux, and G. L. Wilson. 2004. Mitochondrial DNA and aging. *Clin Sci (Lond)* 107(4):355–364.

Anderson, K. M., P. W. Wilson, P. M. Odell, and W. B. Kannel. 1991. An updated coronary risk profile. A statement for health professionals. *Circulation* 83(1):356–362.

Atkins, J. L., P. H. Whincup, R. W. Morris et al. 2014. Sarcopenic obesity and risk of cardiovascular disease and mortality: A population-based cohort study of older men. *J Am Geriatr Soc* 62(2):253–260.

Baur, J. A., K. J. Pearson, N. L. Price et al. 2006. Resveratrol improves health and survival of mice on a high-calorie diet. *Nature* 444(7117):337–342.

Bodkin, N. L., T. M. Alexander, H. K. Ortmeyer, E. Johnson, and B. C. Hansen. 2003. Mortality and morbidity in laboratory-maintained Rhesus monkeys and effects of long-term dietary restriction. *J Gerontol A Biol Sci Med Sci* 58(3):212–219.

Bonkowski, M. S. and D. A. Sinclair. 2016. Slowing ageing by design: The rise of NAD+ and sirtuin-activating compounds. *Nat Rev Mol Cell Biol* 17(11):679–690.

Britton, K. A., J. M. Massaro, J. M. Murabito et al. 2013. Body fat distribution, incident cardiovascular disease, cancer, and all-cause mortality. *J Am Coll Cardiol* 62(10):921–925.

Cefalu, W. T., Z. Q. Wang, A. D. Bell-Farrow et al. 2004. Caloric restriction and cardiovascular aging in cynomolgus monkeys (*Macaca fascicularis*): Metabolic, physiologic, and atherosclerotic measures from a 4-year intervention trial. *J Gerontol A Biol Sci Med Sci* 59(10):1007–1014.

Colman, R. J., R. M. Anderson, S. C. Johnson et al. 2009. Caloric restriction delays disease onset and mortality in rhesus monkeys. *Science* 325 (5937):201–204.

Colman, R. J., T. M. Beasley, J. W. Kemnitz et al. 2014. Caloric restriction reduces age-related and all-cause mortality in rhesus monkeys. *Nat Commun* 5:3557.

Colman, R. J., E. B. Roecker, J. J. Ramsey, and J. W. Kemnitz. 1998. The effect of dietary restriction on body composition in adult male and female rhesus macaques. *Aging (Albany NY)* 10(2):83–92.

Congressional Budget Office's. 2015. Medicare Baseline. https://www.cbo.gov/sites/default/files/recurringdata/51302-2015-03-medicare.pdf, accessed on July 21, 2017.

Copertaro, A., M. Bracci, M. Barbaresi, and L. Santarelli. 2008. Assessment of cardiovascular risk in shift healthcare workers. *Eur J Cardiovasc Prevent Rehabil* 15(2):224–229.

Das, S. K., C. H. Gilhooly, J. K. Golden et al. 2007. Long-term effects of 2 energy-restricted diets differing in glycemic load on dietary adherence, body composition, and metabolism in CALERIE: A 1-y randomized controlled trial. *Am J Clin Nutr* 85(4):1023–1030.

de Jonge, L., J. P. DeLany, T. Nguyen et al. 2007. Validation study of energy expenditure and intake during calorie restriction using doubly labeled water and changes in body composition. *Am J Clin Nutr* 85(1):73–79.

Fontana, L., S. Klein, and J. O. Holloszy. 2010. Effects of long-term calorie restriction and endurance exercise on glucose tolerance, insulin action, and adipokine production. *Age (Dordr)* 32(1):97–108.

Fontana, L., S. Klein, J. O. Holloszy, and B. N. Premachandra. 2006. Effect of long-term calorie restriction with adequate protein and micronutrients on thyroid hormones. *J Clin Endocrinol Metab* 91(8):3232–3235.

Fontana, L., T. E. Meyer, S. Klein, and J. O. Holloszy. 2004. Long-term calorie restriction is highly effective in reducing the risk for atherosclerosis in humans. *Proc Natl Acad Sci USA* 101(17):6659–6663.

Fontana, L., D. T. Villareal, E. P. Weiss et al. 2007. Calorie restriction or exercise: Effects on coronary heart disease risk factors. A randomized, controlled trial. *Am J Physiol Endocrinol Metab* 293(1):E197–E202.

Froy, O. and R. Miskin. 2010. Effect of feeding regimens on circadian rhythms: Implications for aging and longevity. *Aging (Albany NY)* 2(1):7–27.

Gill, S. and S. Panda. 2015. A smartphone app reveals erratic diurnal eating patterns in humans that can be modulated for health benefits. *Cell Metab* 22(5):789–798.

Gu, F., J. Han, F. Laden et al. 2015. Total and cause-specific mortality of U.S. nurses working rotating night shifts. *Am J Prevent Med* 48(3):241–252.

Han, J. C., D. A. Lawlor, and S. Y. Kimm. 2010. Childhood obesity. *Lancet* 375(9727):1737–1748.

Heidenreich, P. A., J. G. Trogdon, O. A. Khavjou et al. 2011. Forecasting the future of cardiovascular disease in the United States: A policy statement from the American Heart Association. *Circulation* 123(8):933–944.

Heilbronn, L. K., L. de Jonge, M. I. Frisard et al. 2006. Effect of 6-month calorie restriction on biomarkers of longevity, metabolic adaptation, and oxidative stress in overweight individuals: A randomized controlled trial. *JAMA* 295(13):1539–1548.

Heilbronn, L. K. and E. Ravussin. 2003. Calorie restriction and aging: Review of the literature and implications for studies in humans. *Am J Clin Nutr* 78(3):361–369.

Heilbronn, L. K., S. R. Smith, C. K. Martin, S. D. Anton, and E. Ravussin. 2005. Alternate-day fasting in nonobese subjects: Effects on body weight, body composition, and energy metabolism. *Am J Clin Nutr* 81(1):69–73.

Hindhede, M. 1920. The effect of food restriction during war on mortality in Copenhagen. *JAMA* 74:381–382.

Hofer, T., L. Fontana, S. D. Anton et al. 2008. Long-term effects of caloric restriction or exercise on DNA and RNA oxidation levels in white blood cells and urine in humans. *Rejuvenation Res* 11(4):793–799.

Holloszy, J. O. 2000. The biology of aging. *Mayo Clin Proc* 75(Suppl):S3–S8; discussion S8–S9.

Holloszy, J. O. and L. Fontana. 2007. Caloric restriction in humans. *Exp Gerontol* 42(8):709–712.

Keil, G., E. Cummings, and J. P. de Magalhaes. 2015. Being cool: How body temperature influences ageing and longevity. *Biogerontology* 16(4):383–397.

Lagouge, M., C. Argmann, Z. Gerhart-Hines et al. 2006. Resveratrol improves mitochondrial function and protects against metabolic disease by activating SIRT1 and PGC-1alpha. *Cell* 127(6):1109–1122.

Lakatta, E. G. and D. Levy. 2003. Arterial and cardiac aging: Major shareholders in cardiovascular disease enterprises: Part I: Aging arteries: A "set up" for vascular disease. *Circulation* 107(1):139–146.

Larson-Meyer, D. E., L. K. Heilbronn, L. M. Redman et al. 2006. Effect of calorie restriction with or without exercise on insulin sensitivity, beta-cell function, fat cell size, and ectopic lipid in overweight subjects. *Diabetes Care* 29(6):1337–1344.

Larson-Meyer, D. E., L. Redman, L. K. Heilbronn, C. K. Martin, and E. Ravussin. 2010. Caloric restriction with or without exercise: The fitness versus fatness debate. *Med Sci Sports Exerc* 42(1):152–159.

Lecoultre, V., E. Ravussin, and L. M. Redman. 2011. The fall in leptin concentration is a major determinant of the metabolic adaptation induced by caloric restriction independently of the changes in leptin circadian rhythms. *J Clin Endocrinol Metab* 96(9):E1512–E1516.

Lee, I. M., E. J. Shiroma, F. Lobelo et al. 2012. Effect of physical inactivity on major non-communicable diseases worldwide: An analysis of burden of disease and life expectancy. *Lancet* 380(9838):219–229.

Lefevre, M., L. M. Redman, L. K. Heilbronn et al. 2009. Caloric restriction alone and with exercise improves CVD risk in healthy non-obese individuals. *Atherosclerosis* 203(1):206–213.

Liesa, M. and O. S. Shirihai. 2013. Mitochondrial dynamics in the regulation of nutrient utilization and energy expenditure. *Cell Metab* 17(4):491–506.

Lim, S. and J. B. Meigs. 2013. Ectopic fat and cardiometabolic and vascular risk. *Int J Cardiol* 169(3):166–176.

Liu, H. H. and J. J. Li. 2015. Aging and dyslipidemia: A review of potential mechanisms. *Ageing Res Rev* 19:43–52.

Lloyd-Jones, D. M., E. P. Leip, M. G. Larson et al. 2006. Prediction of lifetime risk for cardiovascular disease by risk factor burden at 50 years of age. *Circulation* 113(6):791–798.

Loft, S., E. J. Velthuis-te Wierik, H. van den Berg, and H. E. Poulsen. 1995. Energy restriction and oxidative DNA damage in humans. *Cancer Epidemiol Biomarkers Prev* 4(5):515–519.

Ludwig, D. S. 2016. Lifespan weighed down by diet. *JAMA* 315(21):2269–2270.

Marchal, J., F. Pifferi, and F. Aujard. 2013. Resveratrol in mammals: Effects on aging biomarkers, age-related diseases, and life span. *Ann N Y Acad Sci* 1290:67–73.

Martin, C. K., M. Bhapkar, A. G. Pittas et al. 2016. Effect of calorie restriction on mood, quality of life, sleep, and sexual function in healthy nonobese adults: The CALERIE 2 randomized clinical trial. *JAMA Intern Med.* 176(6):743–752.

Martin, C. K., L. K. Heilbronn, L. de Jonge et al. 2007. Effect of calorie restriction on resting metabolic rate and spontaneous physical activity. *Obesity (Silver Spring)* 15(12):2964–2973.

Mattison, J. A., A. Black, J. Huck et al. 2005. Age-related decline in caloric intake and motivation for food in rhesus monkeys. *Neurobiol Aging* 26(7):1117–1127.

Mattison, J. A., R. J. Colman, T. M. Beasley et al. 2017. Caloric restriction improves health and survival of rhesus monkeys. *Nat Commun* 8:14063.

Mattison, J. A., G. S. Roth, T. M. Beasley et al. 2012. Impact of caloric restriction on health and survival in rhesus monkeys from the NIA study. *Nature* 489(7415):318–321.

McCay, C. M., M. F. Crowell, and L. A. Maynard. 1989. The effect of retarded growth upon the length of life span and upon the ultimate body size. 1935. *Nutrition* 5(3):155–171; discussion 172.

Menke, A., S. Casagrande, L. Geiss, and C. C. Cowie. 2015. Prevalence of and trends in diabetes among adults in the United States, 1988–2012. *JAMA* 314(10):1021–1029.

Meyer, T. E., S. J. Kovacs, A. A. Ehsani et al. 2006. Long-term caloric restriction ameliorates the decline in diastolic function in humans. *J Am Coll Cardiol* 47(2):398–402.

Mozaffarian, D., E. J. Benjamin, A. S. Go et al. 2015. Heart disease and stroke statistics—2015 update: A report from the American Heart Association. *Circulation* 131(4):e29–e322.

Murphy, S. L., K. D. Kochanek, J. Xu, and E. Arias. 2015. Mortality in the United States, 2014. NCHS data brief, no. 229. Hyattsville, MD: National Center for Health Statistics.

Onoue, Y., Y. Izumiya, S. Hanatani et al. 2016. A simple sarcopenia screening test predicts future adverse events in patients with heart failure. *Int J Cardiol* 215:301–306.

Pearson, K. J., J. A. Baur, K. N. Lewis et al. 2008. Resveratrol delays age-related deterioration and mimics transcriptional aspects of dietary restriction without extending life span. *Cell Metab* 8(2):157–168.

Pittas, A. G., S. B. Roberts, S. K. Das et al. 2006. The effects of the dietary glycemic load on type 2 diabetes risk factors during weight loss. *Obesity (Silver Spring)* 14(12):2200–2209.

Racette, S. B., E. P. Weiss, D. T. Villareal et al. 2006. One year of caloric restriction in humans: Feasibility and effects on body composition and abdominal adipose tissue. *J Gerontol A Biol Sci Med Sci* 61 (9):943–950.

Ravussin, E., L. M. Redman, J. Rochon et al. 2015. A 2-year randomized controlled trial of human caloric restriction: Feasibility and effects on predictors of health span and longevity. *J Gerontol A Biol Sci Med Sci* 70(9):1097–1104.

Redman, L. M., L. K. Heilbronn, C. K. Martin et al. 2007. Effect of calorie restriction with or without exercise on body composition and fat distribution. *J Clin Endocrinol Metab* 92(3):865–872.

Redman, L. M., L. K. Heilbronn, C. K. Martin et al. 2009. Metabolic and behavioral compensations in response to caloric restriction: Implications for the maintenance of weight loss. *PLoS One* 4(2):e4377.

Redman, L. M., S. R. Smith, V. Dixit, and E. Ravussin. 2014. Evidence of metabolic adaptation after 2 years of 25% calorie restriction in non-obese humans. In *The Obesity Week Conference*, Boston, MA, Abstract T-3032-OR.

Rickman, A. D., D. A. Williamson, C. K. Martin et al. 2011. The CALERIE Study: Design and methods of an innovative 25% caloric restriction intervention. *Contemp Clin Trials* 32(6):874–881.

Riordan, M. M., E. P. Weiss, T. E. Meyer et al. 2008. The effects of caloric restriction- and exercise-induced weight loss on left ventricular diastolic function. *Am J Physiol Heart Circ Physiol* 294(3):H1174–H1182.

Rochon, J., C. W. Bales, E. Ravussin et al. 2011. Design and conduct of the CALERIE study: Comprehensive assessment of the long-term effects of reducing intake of energy. *J Gerontol A Biol Sci Med Sci* 66(1):97–108.

Roth, G. A., M. D. Huffman, A. E. Moran et al. 2015. Global and regional patterns in cardiovascular mortality from 1990 to 2013. *Circulation* 132(17):1667–1678.

Roth, G. S., M. A. Lane, D. K. Ingram et al. 2002. Biomarkers of caloric restriction may predict longevity in humans. *Science* 297(5582):811.

Sacco, R. L., G. A. Roth, K. S. Reddy et al. 2016. The heart of 25 by 25: Achieving the goal of reducing global and regional premature deaths from cardiovascular diseases and stroke: A modeling study from the American Heart Association and World Heart Federation. *Circulation* 133(23):e674–e690.

Sacher, G. A. and P. H. Duffy. 1979. Genetic relation of life span to metabolic rate for inbred mouse strains and their hybrids. *Fed Proc* 38(2):184–188.

Shock, N. W. 1984. Normal human aging: The Baltimore longitudinal study of aging. U.S. G. P. O. Superintendent of documents. Washington, DC: National Institute on Aging (DHHS/NIH), Bethesda, MD.

Soare, A., R. Cangemi, D. Omodei, J. O. Holloszy, and L. Fontana. 2011. Long-term calorie restriction, but not endurance exercise, lowers core body temperature in humans. *Aging (Albany NY)* 3(4):374–379.

Sohal, R. S. and R. G. Allen. 1985. Relationship between metabolic rate, free radicals, differentiation and aging: A unified theory. *Basic Life Sci* 35:75–104.

Sohal, R. S. and R. Weindruch. 1996. Oxidative stress, caloric restriction, and aging. *Science* 273(5271):59–63.

Speakman, J. R. and S. E. Mitchell. 2011. Caloric restriction. *Mol Aspects Med* 32(3):159–221.

Stein, P. K., A. Soare, T. E. Meyer et al. 2012. Caloric restriction may reverse age-related autonomic decline in humans. *Aging Cell* 11(4):644–650.

Strom, A. and R. A. Jensen. 1951. Mortality from circulatory diseases in Norway 1940–1945. *Lancet* 1(6647):126–129.

Stunkard, A. J. 1976. Nutrition, aging and obesity. In Rockstein, M. and Sussman, M. L., eds. *Nutrition, Longevity, and Aging*. New York: Academic Press, pp. 253–284.

System of Social and Demographic Statistics. 2016. Health and Medical Care. Ministry of Internal Affairs and Communications, Tokyo, Japan.

The Board of Trustees of the Federal Old-Age and Survivors Insurance and Federal Disability Insurance Trust Funds. 2015. The 2015 annual report of the board of trustees of the federal old-age and survivors insurance and federal disability insurance trust funds. Washington, DC: U.S Government Publishing Office.

Timmers, S., E. Konings, L. Bilet et al. 2011. Calorie restriction-like effects of 30 days of resveratrol supplementation on energy metabolism and metabolic profile in obese humans. *Cell Metab* 14(5):612–622.

Vallejo, E. A. 1957. Hunger diet on alternate days in the nutrition of the aged. *Prensa Med Argent* 44(2):119–120.

Velthuis-te Wierik, E. J., P. Meijer, C. Kluft, and H. van den Berg. 1995. Beneficial effect of a moderately energy-restricted diet on fibrinolytic factors in non-obese men. *Metabolism* 44(12):1548–1552.

Velthuis-te Wierik, E. J., H. van den Berg, G. Schaafsma, H. F. Hendriks, and A. Brouwer. 1994. Energy restriction, a useful intervention to retard human ageing? Results of a feasibility study. *Eur J Clin Nutr* 48(2):138–148.

Villareal, D. T., L. Fontana, S. K. Das et al. 2016. Effect of two-year caloric restriction on bone metabolism and bone mineral density in non-obese younger adults: A randomized clinical trial. *J Bone Miner Res* 31(1):40–51.

Villareal, D. T., L. Fontana, E. P. Weiss et al. 2006. Bone mineral density response to caloric restriction-induced weight loss or exercise-induced weight loss: A randomized controlled trial. *Arch Intern Med* 166(22):2502–2510.

Walford, R. L., S. B. Harris, and M. W. Gunion. 1992. The calorically restricted low-fat nutrient-dense diet in Biosphere 2 significantly lowers blood glucose, total leukocyte count, cholesterol, and blood pressure in humans. *Proc Natl Acad Sci USA* 89(23):11533–11537.

Walford, R. L., D. Mock, T. MacCallum, and J. L. Laseter. 1999. Physiologic changes in humans subjected to severe, selective calorie restriction for two years in biosphere 2: Health, aging, and toxicological perspectives. *Toxicol Sci* 52(2 Suppl):61–65.

Walford, R. L., D. Mock, R. Verdery, and T. MacCallum. 2002. Calorie restriction in biosphere 2: Alterations in physiologic, hematologic, hormonal, and biochemical parameters in humans restricted for a 2-year period. *J Gerontol A Biol Sci Med Sci* 57(6):B211–B224.

Weiss, E. P., S. B. Racette, D. T. Villareal et al. 2006. Improvements in glucose tolerance and insulin action induced by increasing energy expenditure or decreasing energy intake: A randomized controlled trial. *Am J Clin Nutr* 84(5):1033–1042.

Weiss, E. P., S. B. Racette, D. T. Villareal et al. 2007. Lower extremity muscle size and strength and aerobic capacity decrease with caloric restriction but not with exercise-induced weight loss. *J Appl Physiol* 102(2):634–640.

Weiss, E. P., D. T. Villareal, S. B. Racette et al. 2008. Caloric restriction but not exercise-induced reductions in fat mass decrease plasma triiodothyronine concentrations: A randomized controlled trial. *Rejuvenation Res* 11(3):605–609.

Weyer, C., S. Snitker, R. Rising, C. Bogardus, and E. Ravussin. 1999. Determinants of energy expenditure and fuel utilization in man: Effects of body composition, age, sex, ethnicity and glucose tolerance in 916 subjects. *Int J Obes Relat Metab Disord* 23(7):715–722.

Weyer, C., R. L. Walford, I. T. Harper et al. 2000. Energy metabolism after 2 y of energy restriction: The biosphere 2 experiment. *Am J Clin Nutr* 72(4):946–953.

Willcox, B. J., D. C. Willcox, H. Todoriki et al. 2007. Caloric restriction, the traditional Okinawan diet, and healthy aging: The diet of the world's longest-lived people and its potential impact on morbidity and life span. *Ann N Y Acad Sci* 1114:434–455.

Xu, J. Q., S. L. Murphy, K. D. Kochanek, and B. A. Bastian. 2016. Deaths: Final data for 2013. National vital statistics reports. Hyattsville, MD: National Center for Health Statistics.

Yang, L., D. Licastro, E. Cava et al. 2016. Long-term calorie restriction enhances cellular quality-control processes in human skeletal muscle. *Cell Rep* 14(3):422–428.

Yoshino, J., C. Conte, L. Fontana et al. 2012. Resveratrol supplementation does not improve metabolic function in nonobese women with normal glucose tolerance. *Cell Metab* 16(5):658–664.

Zhang, J. and F. Liu. 2014. Tissue-specific insulin signaling in the regulation of metabolism and aging. *IUBMB Life* 66(7):485–495.

Section II

Dietary Fats and Cardiometabolic Health

10 Omega-3 and Omega-6 Fatty Acids*

Roles in Cardiometabolic Disease

William S. Harris

CONTENTS

ABSTRACT

Omega-3 and omega-6 FAs both have beneficial roles to play in reducing risk for cardiovascular disease (CVD). Although this is largely noncontroversial for the former FA family, some researchers have cautioned that the latter family may actually increase risk for CVD. This review will summarize the relevant human evidence, which shows that, in fact, both FA families are protective. The presumed "pro-inflammatory" nature of the omega-6 FAs (which is the basis for their hypothetical adverse effects) is not supported in a wide variety of human observational and interventional studies. The individual members of the omega-6 FA family can have completely opposing associations with risk; therefore there is no rational basis for summing all of the omega-6 FAs into a single metric and ascribing some health effect to the whole group. The primary omega-6 FA in the diet, linoleic acid, is associated with lower risk for both coronary heart disease and type 2 diabetes, hence lowering intakes (and thus blood levels) would be expected to raise, not lower, risk. Recommended intakes of linoleic acid in the 5%–10% range still apply. Most studies support the view that replacing saturated and trans fats in the diet with both the omega-6 and omega-3 FAs is the best overall strategy for reducing cardiometabolic risk.

* Disclosures: WSH is the President of OmegaQuant Analytics, LLC, a laboratory that offers fatty acid testing. He is also a scientific advisor for the Global Organization for EPA and DHA (fish oil trade association).

INTRODUCTION

Long-held dogmas regarding the roles of essentially all of the classes of dietary fatty acids (FAs) vis-à-vis coronary heart disease (CHD) are being challenged. Saturated FAs, the perennial "bad" fats, may not be as bad as we've thought (see Chapter 11), and the monounsaturated FA oleic acid, which predominates in olive oil (an important component of the Mediterranean diet), may not be as cardioprotective as once believed based on the results of recent meta-analyses (Chowdhury et al., 2014) and animal feeding studies (Brown, Shelness, and Rudel, 2007). Similarly, the marine-derived omega-3 polyunsaturated fatty acids (PUFAs), which have historically found a place among the "healthiest" of all dietary fats, have fallen on hard times following the publication of several null randomized trials (Rizos et al., 2012). A suspicious eye is now being cast on linoleic acid (LA), the principal vegetable-oil-derived omega-6 PUFA—once taken almost as a medicine using the tablespoon to lower cholesterol—with some proposing that, instead of preventing, it may be contributing to CHD (Cunnane and Guesnet, 2011; Ramsden et al., 2013). Even with the *trans* FAs, which are almost universally seen as detrimental, there is a controversy regarding the potentially differential effects of "natural" (i.e., ruminant) derived species versus the industrially produced species (Bendsen et al., 2011; Gebauer et al., 2015) (see Chapter 12). Understandably, the public is becoming skeptical of official proclamations of what constitutes a "healthy fat."

The purpose of this chapter is to consider the evidence for and against a cardioprotective role for the omega-3 and omega-6 FAs. The reader is referred to several prior reviews on omega-3 (De Caterina, 2011; Mozaffarian and Wu, 2011; Khawaja, Gaziano, and Djousse, 2014; Kromhout and de Goede, 2014) and omega-6 (Harris et al., 2009b; Czernichow, Thomas, and Bruckert, 2010) that have tread similar ground. These two families comprise all of the PUFAs (those containing at least 2 double bonds) in the diet and, for the most part, in the body. One member of each is classically considered to be an "essential" FA because, like vitamins, humans cannot live without them in the diet. These are LA and its omega-3 counterpart alpha-linolenic acid (ALA), although the relative essentiality—indeed, even the term "essential"—of each has come under scrutiny (as noted by Cunnane who enumerates many problems with the current paradigm) (e.g., essentiality may apply to only some stages of the life cycle, LA needs may be lower in the presence of sufficient ALA, etc.) (Cunnane, 2003). The structures of these two FA classes and their most important members are shown in Figure 10.1.

As it constitutes by far the largest amount in the diet, the omega-6 class will be considered first. Special emphasis will be placed on the pro/anti-inflammatory effects of these FA families.

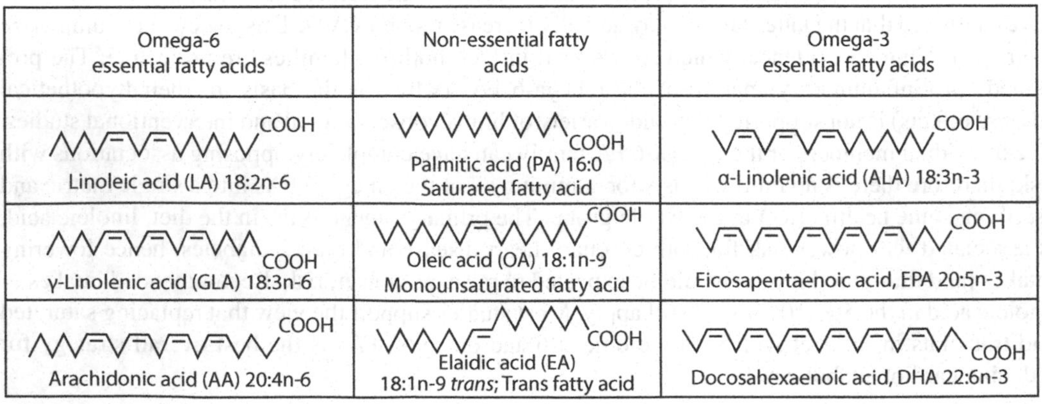

Omega-6 essential fatty acids	Non-essential fatty acids	Omega-3 essential fatty acids
COOH Linoleic acid (LA) 18:2n-6	COOH Palmitic acid (PA) 16:0 Saturated fatty acid	COOH α-Linolenic acid (ALA) 18:3n-3
COOH γ-Linolenic acid (GLA) 18:3n-6	COOH Oleic acid (OA) 18:1n-9 Monounsaturated fatty acid	COOH Eicosapentaenoic acid, EPA 20:5n-3
COOH Arachidonic acid (AA) 20:4n-6	COOH Elaidic acid (EA) 18:1n-9 *trans*; Trans fatty acid	COOH Docosahexaenoic acid, DHA 22:6n-3

FIGURE 10.1 The two essential FA families, omega-6 (n-6) and omega-3 (n-3), are shown with important representative members on the left and right. In the center are three examples of FAs that are not dietary essentials. The molecular structures assume a carbon atom at each inflection point with 1–3 hydrogen atoms not shown.

OMEGA-6 FATTY ACIDS

Effects on Lipids

The cholesterol-lowering effect of LA is well established from human trials. In a meta-analysis of 60 feeding studies including 1672 volunteers, the substitution of PUFA (the vast majority of which was LA, varying from 0.6% to 28.8% energy) for carbohydrates had more favorable effects on the ratio of total cholesterol to high-density lipoprotein (HDL) cholesterol than any class of FAs (Siguel, 1996; Mensink et al., 2003). Epidemiologically, the replacement of 10% of calories from saturated FAs with omega-6 PUFA is associated with an 18 mg/dL decrease in low-density lipoprotein cholesterol (LDL-C), greater than that observed with similar replacement with carbohydrate (Mensink and Katan, 1992). These findings confirm an LDL-lowering effect of omega-6 PUFA beyond that produced by a lower saturated FA intake. Both baseline and 6-year follow-up changes in serum omega-6 FA levels, which reflect changes in dietary LA (Bradbury et al., 2010), were inversely related to the size of very-low-density lipoprotein (VLDL) particles, and directly related to LDL and HDL particle size (Mantyselka et al., 2014). Others reported that higher serum concentrations of LA were significantly associated with lower concentrations of total LDL particles, and higher concentrations of serum LA and arachidonic acid (AA) were significantly associated with lower levels of large VLDL particles and higher levels of large HDL particles (Choo et al., 2010). Favorable effects of LA on cholesterol levels are thus well documented and would predict significant reductions in CHD risk.

Effects on Inflammatory Markers

As noted earlier, some investigators have proposed that LA intakes in America are excessive (Blasbalg et al., 2011), and far from reducing risk for inflammatory diseases like CHD, they may actually be increasing risk for them (Ramsden et al., 2013). This perspective builds upon the following logic: (1) LA is the precursor for AA; therefore, higher LA intakes will lead to higher AA tissue levels; (2) AA is the substrate for the production of certain pro-inflammatory eicosanoids, so higher AA levels would lead to a greater production of these molecules; (3) AA levels in membranes are rate-limiting for the production of eicosanoids; and (4) CHD is a disease with major inflammatory components and so the more pro-inflammatory eicosanoids produced, the more inflammation should be present that should translate into more CHD. Thus, higher intakes of LA may increase risk for CHD.

Although not intrinsically illogical, this perspective fails to consider several important findings. First, a systematic review of 36 studies reported that variations in dietary LA, either reduced by up to 90% or increased by as much as sixfold, did not affect plasma phospholipid AA levels (Rett and Whelan, 2011). The authors concluded, "Our results do not support the concept that modifying current intakes of dietary linoleic acid has an effect on changing levels of arachidonic acid in plasma, serum or erythrocytes in adults consuming Western-type diets." On the other hand, a recent feeding study that aimed to provide a low-LA diet (i.e., 2.4% energy vs. 7.4% energy) for 12 weeks reported reductions in plasma AA levels (Taha et al., 2014). It is difficult, however, to determine how much AA levels fell since whole plasma AA was not reported, but only AA in isolated lipid fractions. In addition, the intake of AA was reduced by about 50% in the low-LA diet. Thus, it is unclear whether the reduction in circulating LA was the cause of the reduced AA levels.

Second, studies testing the effect of LA on inflammatory status in humans have routinely found no increase in marker levels. In a recent review (Johnson and Fritsche, 2012), 15 trials were examined that met inclusion criteria, and the authors concluded that "virtually no evidence is available from randomized, controlled intervention studies among healthy, non-infant human beings to show that addition of LA to the diet increases the concentration of inflammatory markers."

Another potential concern with increasing LA intakes is that it will lower blood levels of the long-chain omega-3 FAs eicosapentaenoic acid (EPA) and docosahexaenoic acid (DHA)

(Cleland et al., 1992) presumably by slowing conversion of ALA to EPA, and/or by competing with these two FAs for esterification sites in membrane phospholipids. To the extent that EPA/DHA is cardioprotective, such an effect would be counterproductive. The evidence in this regard is mixed. For example, one study (Liou et al., 2007) increased the LA intake from 3.8% to 10.5% of total energy in the diets of 22 men for 4 weeks. The high-LA diet did lower plasma phospholipid EPA levels slightly (from 1% to 0.6%), but it raised DHA levels by the same amount (from 3% to 3.4%), leaving the sum of EPA + DHA (4%) unaffected. They also observed no effects on inflammatory markers or platelet aggregation with the high-LA diet. Another study tested the effects of increasing amounts of omega-6 FAs in the diet on cardiac tissue omega-3 levels in rats fed various levels of fish oil (Slee et al., 2010). The authors reported that the omega-6 intake did not affect the uptake of omega-3 in the heart.

Linoleic Acid Metabolites

As noted, the "LA is harmful" hypothesis depends heavily on the view that an LA metabolite, AA, is converted to potent pro-inflammatory signaling molecules. While this is partly true, what is often overlooked is that AA also gives rise to *anti*-inflammatory metabolites (e.g., lipoxin A4), as well as anti-aggregatory, vasodilative molecules like prostacyclin. Indeed, the epoxyeicosatrienoic acids synthesized from AA produce vasodilation, stimulate angiogenesis, have anti-inflammatory actions, and protect the heart against ischemia–reperfusion injury (Spector, 2009). AA can be converted into an ever-expanding list of bioactive compounds via cyclooxygenase, lipoxygenases, and cytochrome P450 monooxygenases (Figure 10.2a). But AA is not the only omega-6 FA with potential effects on CHD—LA itself can be converted to a wide variety of bioactive molecules by these enzymes (Figure 10.2a). Not shown in this figure is nitrated LA (LNO_2), an LA metabolite that has been shown to have cardioprotective effects (Baker et al., 2009). In addition, LNO_2 is a powerful ligand for peroxisome proliferator activator receptor-gamma (PPAR-γ) (Schopfer et al., 2005), a nuclear transcription factor that controls cell differentiation as well as production of metabolic and anti-inflammatory signaling molecules. At physiologically relevant levels, LNO_2 rivals the effects of the thiazolidinediones on PPAR-γ (Schopfer et al., 2005). LA can also be converted to a growing number of oxygenated metabolites (i.e., oxylipins) by cyclooxygenase, lipoxygenases, and/or cytochrome P-450 epoxygenases (Figure 10.2a), the individual and aggregate effects of which have not been systematically examined.

LA can also be metabolized to dihomo-gamma-linolenic acid from which other bioactive lipids can be produced including prostaglandins of the 1-series (Wang, Lin, and Gu, 2012). Within the LA "metabolome," one finds a constellation of products including a variety of prostaglandins, leukotrienes, ligands for endocannabinoid receptors, lipoxins, isoprostanes, nitrated AA, and epoxides, among others. Considering only the cyclooxygenase, lipoxygenase, and cytochrome P450 pathways, Tam lists 8 metabolites of LA and 41 from AA (Tam, 2013) (Figure 10.2a). Some are "pro-inflammatory" but some are "anti-inflammatory" or promote the resolution of inflammatory insults. Often these effects have only been observed in certain cell/tissue types and under potentially non-physiological conditions, and their effects or those of other metabolites in normal physiology remain to be discovered. The net impact on human metabolism (and CHD risk) of this multitude of products will ultimately be determined by their interaction among themselves (and with their omega-3 FA analogs), and is virtually impossible to predict. Hence, to label the entire class of omega-6 FA metabolites as "proinflammatory" is far too simplistic.

Associations with CHD Events in Prospective Observational Studies

The classic tool of nutritional epidemiology has been the prospective cohort study in which large numbers of healthy subjects are recruited, their diets analyzed by a variety of techniques [24-h recall, 3-day food record, food frequency questionnaire, etc. (Shim, Oh, and Kim, 2014)], and a wide range

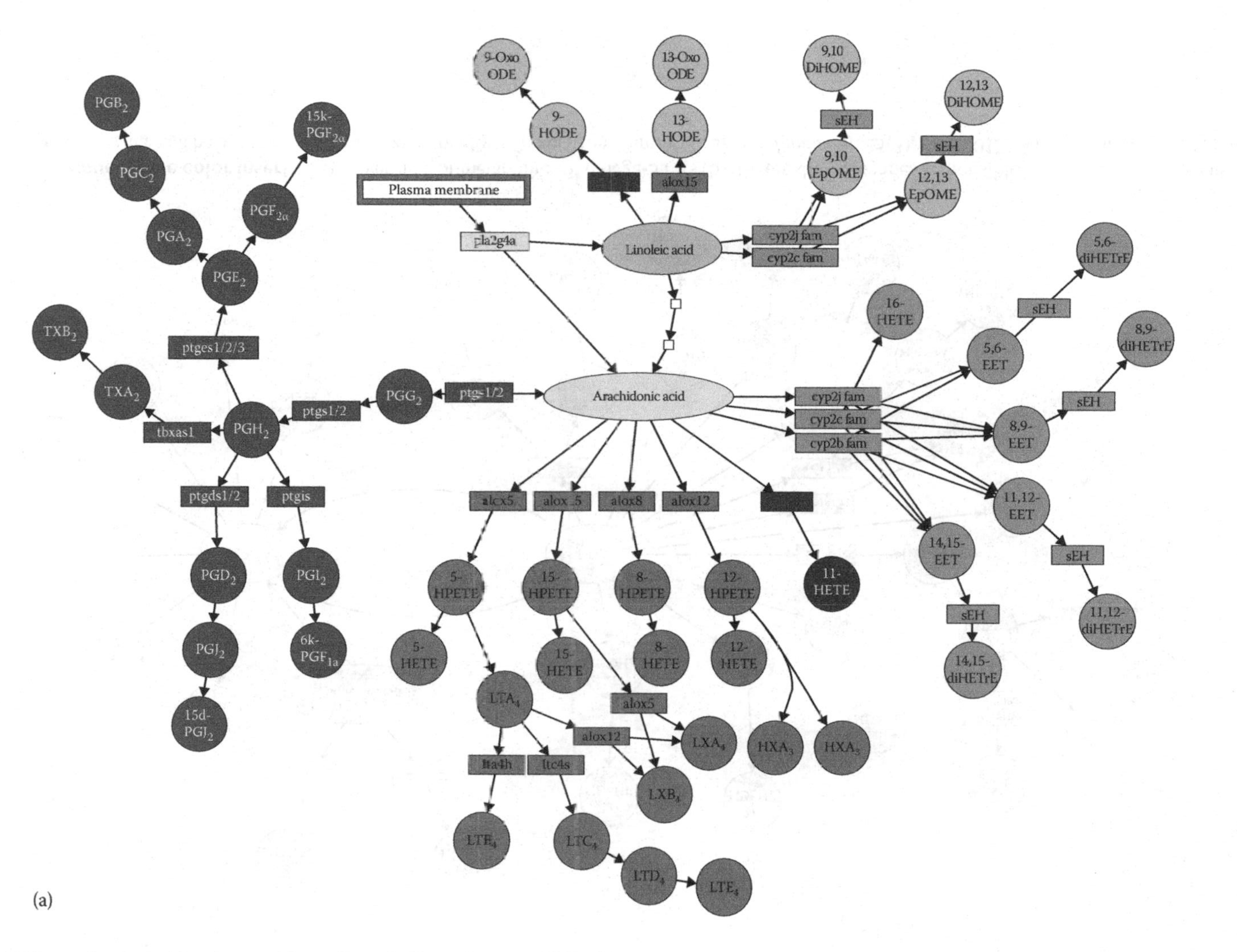

FIGURE 10.2 (See color insert.) An overview of metabolites of omega-6 FAs (a).

(*Continued*)

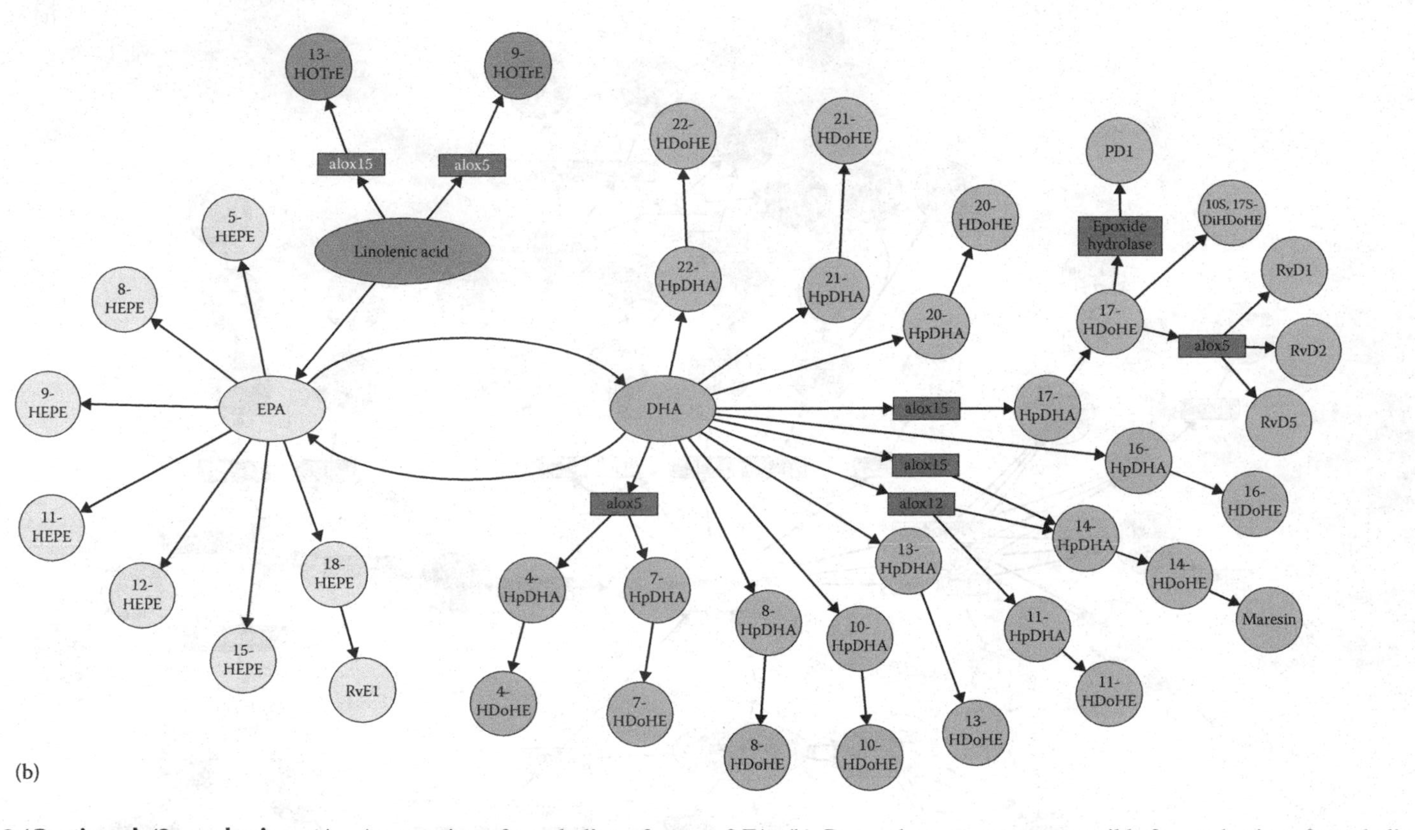

FIGURE 10.2 (*Continued*) (See color insert.) An overview of metabolites of omega-3 FAs (b). Boxes show enzymes responsible for production of metabolites (brown boxes designate processes that can be accomplished nonenzymatically). (Taken from Tam, V.C., *Semin. Immunol.*, 25(3), 240, 2013. With permission; Abbreviations given in the original paper.)

of biometric and health-related measures are collected. In some studies, biological samples are taken for biomarker measurement. The cohort is then followed without any prescribed interventions for a number of years, and the incidence of different diseases is tracked. With these data, sophisticated statistical analysis is applied to explore the question of how food/nutrient/pattern is associated with an outcome of interest. The strengths of such studies are their "real world" setting and the ability to include many thousands of subjects. Their weaknesses include not being able to control every aspect of a person's life, and the very real possibility that, even though nutrient X (whether from dietary data or biomarker level) is strongly associated with incident disease, it may be other factors that track with nutrient X that are the real reason for the observed relationships. This "unmeasured confounding" makes it impossible to conclude that a cause and effect relationship exists between the nutrient and the disease outcome. Nevertheless, such associations (if they are seen in multiple studies conducted under a variety of conditions) build a strong circumstantial case for a link between nutrient and disease.

Many studies have been performed in the area of FAs and cardiovascular disease (CVD). They are best summarized in meta-analyses. The most comprehensive meta-analysis in recent years examined the relations between *dietary* and *circulating* levels of all major FAs and CHD outcomes (Chowdhury et al., 2014). Here, contra the "omega-6-are-harmful" hypothesis, there was no association between LA levels when replacing saturated fat and CHD in the full analysis, and a favorable association when the controversial Sydney Heart Study (Ramsden et al., 2013) was excluded. Even more contra was the finding, based on 10 studies including some 23,000 individuals with over 3,700 CHD events, that higher levels of circulating AA—the presumed toxic omega-6 mediator—were associated with *lower* risk for CHD events (HR, 0.83, 95% confidence interval [CI], 0.74–0.92).

Farvid et al. have published the largest and most recent (as of December 2015) meta-analysis that specifically addressed the relations between omega-6 FAs (primarily LA and AA) when replacing either carbohydrates or saturated fat and CHD morbidity and mortality (Farvid et al., 2014). Utilizing data from both published and unpublished studies (via direct investigator contact), 13 cohort studies involving about 310,000 individuals with over 12,000 CHD events and about 5,900 CHD deaths were examined. The primary outcome was myocardial infarction, ischemic heart disease, sudden cardiac arrest, acute coronary syndrome, and CHD deaths. Intakes of LA were estimated by a variety of types of dietary intake instruments, and follow-up ranged from 5 to 30 years. Comparing the highest to the lowest intake groups (10th to 90th percentiles for LA intake ranged from 1.1% to 9.5% energy) and risk for CHD events was lower by 15% (0.85 (0.78, 0.92)), and for CHD death by 21% (0.79 (0.71, 0.89)), both statistically significant. Viewed another way, risk for events was *increased* by 18% and death by 27% in the lowest intake group compared to the highest.

The fact that these relations were observed using such blunt instruments as dietary questionnaires could suggest that the findings are robust. However, as noted earlier, unmeasured confounding factors could be influencing the outcomes. The observation that replacing either saturated fats or carbohydrates with vegetable oils produced essentially the same CHD benefit suggests that it is not the reduced intake of the nutrient being replaced by LA that affords the benefit, but LA itself. Finally, since the LA effect was independent of the intake of ALA (the omega-3 FA found primarily in soybean oil where it constitutes about 6% of total FAs compared with 54% as LA), the benefit observed cannot easily be attributed to co-consumption of the ALA as some have hypothesized (Ramsden et al., 2013).

Randomized Trials

Of course, the most direct way to test the hypothesis that higher LA intakes reduce risk for CHD is to perform a randomized controlled trial (RCT). This has been attempted many times, and nearly as many meta-analyses have been employed to summarize their findings. Depending on which trials one includes, there is either a significant reduction in risk (Mozaffarian, Micha, and Wallace, 2010) or no effect (Chowdhury et al., 2014; Ramsden et al., 2013; Schwingshackl and Hoffmann, 2014) of higher omega-6 intakes. In a meta-analysis including only the four trials utilizing soybean oil (which contains about 50% LA and 7% ALA), there was a significant 22% reduction in CHD events (Ramsden et al., 2010). In these trials, omega-6 PUFA consumption was often raised to very high levels (far exceeding the currently recommended 5%–10% energy from PUFA and producing, in three trials, omega-6:omega-3 PUFA ratios ranging from 7 to 21) and demonstrated CHD benefit, not detriment. Thus, these results directly contradict the view that high omega-6 PUFA intakes or "high" omega-6:omega-3 PUFA ratios increase the risk of CHD (Hibbeln et al., 2006). Ramsden examined the effects on CHD events in two other trials utilizing corn oil (no ALA) and found no significant effects (Ramsden et al., 2010). The findings from this study stand in contrast to the authors' statement that "advice to specifically increase omega-6 PUFA intake is unlikely to provide the intended benefits, and may actually increase the risk of CHD and death."

All this being said, this is a difficult hypothesis to properly test in large-scale, multiyear intervention trials because one major dietary component like LA is (must be) substituted for another potentially active (vis-à-vis CHD) component. Hence, interpretation is challenging. Because of these concerns, it has been argued that prospective cohort data should be given the same evidentiary weight as RCTs in nutrition because each has relevant strengths and weaknesses (Harris et al., 2009a). When these two types of data (and others) are viewed in the aggregate, a strong case for a protective effect of LA on CHD can be made (Harris et al., 2009b).

OMEGA-3 FATTY ACIDS

Effects on Lipids

The first and most well-characterized effect of the marine omega-3 FAs was triglyceride lowering. This effect was first summarized in 1989 (Harris, 1989) and has been confirmed in more recent meta-analyses (Leslie et al., 2015). Reductions ranging from 10% to 50% can be achieved with "pharmacological" doses of EPA+DHA (e.g., 3–4 g/day) with the variability largely associated with the degree of hypertriglyceridemia (Harris et al., 1997; Davidson et al., 2007). In patients with very elevated triglyceride levels, LDL-C levels have been observed to rise (Jacobson, 2008), an effect attributed to the DHA component of marine oils (Wei and Jacobson, 2011). Whether the small increase in LDL-C impacts risk for CHD in the patient taking 3–4 g of EPA+DHA per day is unknown, but in the view of the author, it seems unlikely given the fact that the mechanisms responsible for the reduction in risk for CVD may have little to do with reducing serum triglyceride levels as discussed in the following text.

Beneficial effects on CVD endpoints have been observed with long-term dietary intakes of <1 g/day of EPA+DHA, and the doses used in major clinical CVD trials (typically 1–2 g) have little or no impact on serum triglyceride levels (Radack, Deck, and Huster, 1990; Roche and Gibney, 1996; Investigators, 1999; Schwellenbach et al., 2006). It is beyond the scope of this review to cover in detail the proposed nonlipoprotein-related mechanisms of omega-3 FAs (besides inflammation; see as follows). Briefly, however, these include increased myocardial resistance to arrhythmias (Reiffel and McDonald, 2006), enhanced plaque stability (Thies et al., 2003), reduction in heart rate (Mozaffarian et al., 2005b), improved endothelial function (Nestel et al., 2002; Xin, Wei, and Li, 2012), increased heart rate variability (Xin, Wei, and Li, 2013), and a variety of other antiatherosclerotic and antithrombotic processes (Robinson and Stone, 2006). The cellular and molecular bases for these effects of omega-3 FAs are multiple. The interested reader is referred to recent reviews (De Caterina, 2011; Poudyal et al., 2011; Serhan and Petasis, 2011; Rangel-Huerta et al., 2012; Shearer, Savinova, and Harris, 2012; Calder, 2013).

Effect on Inflammatory Markers

The anti-inflammatory and inflammation-resolving properties of the omega-3 FAs are relatively well documented (Calder, 2013). Such documentation comes from observational studies and randomized trials, and mechanistic insights have been obtained from cell culture work. With respect to the former, a recent report from the Framingham Offspring Study documented the significant inverse correlations between erythrocyte EPA+DHA levels [the Omega-3 Index (Harris and von Schacky, 2004)] and eight different biomarkers of inflammatory processes across a wide spectrum of systems (Fontes et al., 2015). As summarized in Fontes et al., 6 of 8 prior studies using dietary omega-3 PUFA data found a significant inverse association between at least one inflammatory biomarker and intakes. In addition, in 10 of 12 biomarker-based studies, significant inverse relations for at least one inflammatory marker with EPA and/or DHA levels were observed. Similarly, a recent meta-analysis of 68 trials in patients with chronic, non-autoimmune diseases found overall significant reductions in C-reactive protein and interleukin 6 and marginally significant reductions in tumor necrosis factor alpha after omega-3 PUFA supplementation (Li et al., 2014). Another marker of inflammation more directly tied to vascular inflammation is lipoprotein-associated phospholipase A2 (LpPLA-2), which has been linked closely with CVD events and is localized in atherosclerotic plaques (Mallat, Lambeau, and Tedgui, 2010). Levels of LpPLA-2 were reduced by treatment with 4 g/day of EPA (Bays et al., 2013) and with 3.4 g/day of EPA+DHA (Davidson et al., 2009). Hence, there is support both from observational and from interventional studies for an anti-inflammatory effect of omega-3 FA. The extent to which this is the basis for the cardioprotective effects of these long-chain marine FAs is unclear.

The mechanisms by which EPA and/or DHA exert their anti-inflammatory effects appear to ultimately derive from their effects on membrane biophysics. By altering lipid raft composition (Williams et al., 2012; Turk and Chapkin, 2013), the long-chain omega-3 FAs can alter endocytic activity (Pinot et al., 2014), L-type calcium channels, the Na^+–Ca^{2+} exchanger, and other signaling pathways involving activation of phospholipases, synthesis of eicosanoids, and regulation of receptor-associated enzymes and protein kinases (Siddiqui, Harvey, and Zaloga, 2008). Like AA, EPA and DHA can be metabolized into resolvins, protectins, and a number of other oxylipins (Figure 10.2b), which can impede inflammatory processes. By serving as a ligand for transcription factors such as PPAR-γ, they can interfere with the production of nuclear factor kappa B (NFκB) that is the transcription factor that ultimately controls the synthesis of a variety of cytokines and adhesion molecules as well as cyclooxygenase 2, inducible nitric oxide synthase, and matrix metalloproteinases (Figure 10.3).

NFκB synthesis is also inhibited by activation of transcription factor I kappa B, the production of which is stimulated by activation of GPR120 by these same FAs [as summarized in (Calder, 2013)]. Higher levels of EPA and DHA also reduce membrane phospholipid levels of AA, thereby reducing the pro-inflammatory cytokines and oxylipins derived from this important omega-6 FA. It is by these interacting and concerted mechanisms that fish oil exerts its anti-inflammatory effects across many cell types.

Associations with CHD Events in Prospective Observational Studies

While prospective cohort studies also have significant limitations, the relations between nutrient intakes (or, better, nutrient biomarker levels) and disease outcomes should be considered complementary to, and equally important as, RCT data. There have been at least 16 cohort studies that have used dietary estimates of EPA+DHA intake as the exposure marker for CHD endpoints, and 13 studies that have used circulating EPA+DHA levels. These have been included in a major meta-analysis that examined all FAs, not just the omega-3 FAs (Chowdhury et al., 2014). In this analysis,

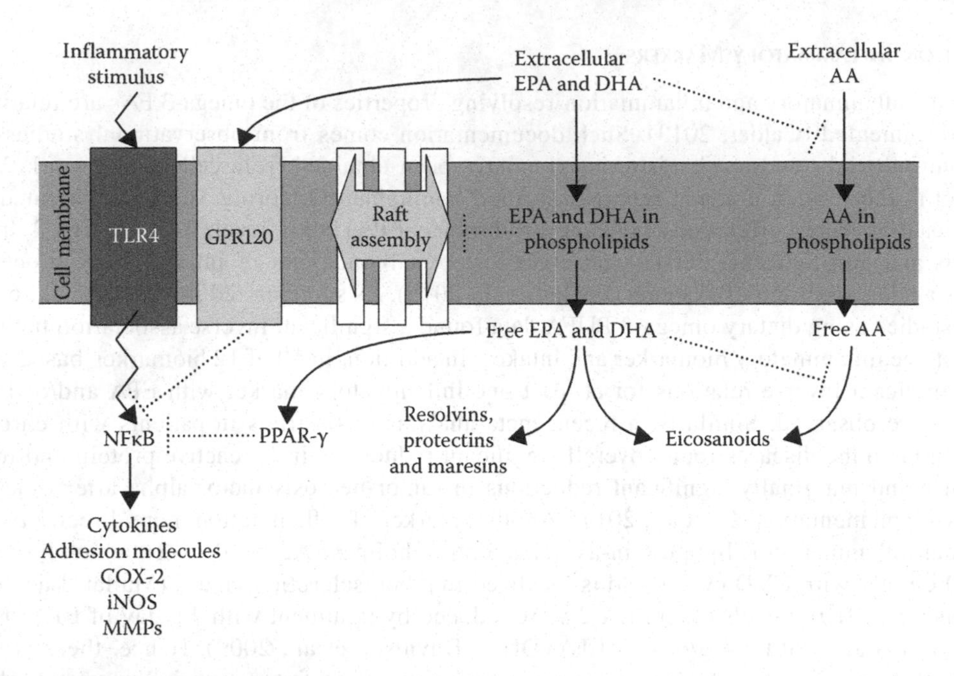

FIGURE 10.3 Summary of the anti-inflammatory actions of marine omega-3 PUFAs. COX, cyclooxygenase; GPR, G-protein coupled receptor; iNOS, inducible nitric oxide synthase; MMP, matrix metalloproteinase. Dotted lines indicate inhibition. (Taken from Calder, P.C., *Br. J. Clin. Pharmacol.*, 75(3), 645, 2013. With permission.)

upper tertile (vs. lower) intakes of long-chain omega-3 FA were associated with a 13% (95% CI, 3%–22%) reduction in CHD events, and this class of FAs was the only one linked to a lower risk of events. Consistent with this, higher circulating levels of these two omega-3 FAs (and levels of docosapentaenoic acid) were significantly associated with reduced risk for CHD events. This indicates that, in the long run and in more "natural" settings outside of clinical trials, long-chain omega-3 FAs are consistently and directly associated with better cardiac health. Of course as alluded to in the omega-6 FA section, unmeasured confounding should always be considered as a possible contributing explanation for the "benefits" of omega-3 FA. That is, there are many lifestyle, medical, and social factors associated with higher omega-3 levels (Harris et al., 2016). It is always possible that benefits seen in "association" studies may not be attributable to EPA+DHA per se but to other behaviors or factors found in people who have higher blood levels of these FAs.

Randomized Trials

As summarized earlier, there are a wealth of data from population (He et al., 2004), case-control (Siscovick et al., 1995), prospective cohort (Albert et al., 2002; Iso et al., 2006), and RCTs (Burr et al., 1989; Marchioli et al., 2002; Yokoyama et al., 2007; Investigators, 2008) supporting a cardioprotective effect of omega-3 FAs. With respect to the latter study designs, there have been eight major RCTs (each including at least 2000 patients) examining the effects of omega-3 FAs and risk for cardiovascular endpoints and/or death. These have been widely reviewed and summarized (Saravanan et al., 2010; De Caterina, 2011; Mozaffarian and Wu, 2011; Kromhout et al., 2012). This extensive literature has generated multiple meta-analyses over the years, with four being published in 2012 alone (Kotwal et al., 2012; Kwak et al., 2012; Rizos et al., 2012; Trikalinos et al., 2012). The report by Rizos et al. garnered the greatest attention as it was published in *JAMA* (Rizos et al., 2012). This group concluded that there was insufficient evidence to conclude that omega-3 FA supplements reduced risk for CVD. This was a surprising conclusion given that they reported a significant 9% reduction in risk for cardiac death ($p = 0.01$). The authors took the position that the alpha (normally 0.05) should be adjusted for multiple testing (to <0.006). This highly unusual (and controversial) statistical maneuver in a meta-analysis converted a positive finding to a null finding and injected considerable confusion into the omega-3 and CVD issue (Harris, 2013). Other recent meta-analyses have reached different conclusions (Musa-Veloso et al., 2011; Delgado-Lista et al., 2012; Trikalinos et al., 2012; Casula et al., 2013) finding overall benefit for omega-3 FAs (as also was found in the data, if not the interpretation, in Rizos et al. (2012)).

ASSESSING OMEGA-6 AND OMEGA-3 FATTY ACID STATUS

Whether in reference to dietary FA intakes or blood-based biomarker FA levels, there are many ways to express what is sometimes called "omega status." Our bias over the last 12 years has been to use the Omega-3 Index (erythrocyte EPA+DHA, expressed as a percent of total FAs) (Harris and von Schacky, 2004; von Schacky, 2014). This marker has gained widespread use in the FA research community owing to its ease of analysis, intuitive meaning, low within-person variability (Harris and Thomas, 2010), insensitivity to acute omega-3 FA loads (Harris et al., 2013), strong correlation with cardiac EPA+DHA levels (Harris et al., 2004), responsiveness to omega-3 supplementation (Flock et al., 2013), and utility as both a biomarker and risk factor for CHD (Harris, 2009). An alternate expression of "omega status" is the omega-6/omega-3 ratio. This pools all omega-6 FAs and all omega-3 FAs, regardless of chain length or double bond number, and then divides the former by the latter. In the author's opinion, this metric is of little to no use for reasons previously outlined (Harris, 2006). Among the theoretical weaknesses of this ratio are (1) the failure to distinguish among the specific FA species within each class, effectively allowing ALA to "count" as equivalent metabolically to EPA, DPA, and DHA, and LA as equivalent to AA (or gamma-linolenic or adrenic acid); (2) the imprecision that arises from the fact that a virtually endless array of FA levels can all produce the same ratio; (3) the implicit presumption that the omega-6 FAs are "bad" and the omega-3 FAs are "good"; and (4) that lowering a "high" ratio (which is presumably bad) can be accomplished in five ways, at least one of which involves actually lowering omega-3 levels. In a workshop sponsored by the UK Food Standards Agency that addressed the utility of the omega-6/omega-3 ratio, the panel concluded, "On the basis of this review of the experimental evidence and on theoretical grounds, it was concluded that the n-6:n-3 FA ratio is not a useful concept and that it distracts attention away from increasing absolute intakes of long-chain n-3 FAs which have been shown to have beneficial effects on cardiovascular health" (Stanley et al., 2007).

SUMMARY

Omega-3 and omega-6 FAs may be viewed as "partners in prevention" as they relate to cardiometabolic diseases (Harris, 2010). Synthesizing evidence from a wide variety of investigations supports the view that higher versus lower intakes of both LA and EPA+DHA have favorable cardiometabolic effects (Mozaffarian et al., 2005a). While opposing views remain regarding LA (Ramsden et al., 2012, 2013; Bazinet and Chu, 2014), the consensus in this author's view continues to support the recommendation of many health authorities for 3%–11% of energy as LA (Harris et al., 2009b; FAO, 2010; Vannice and Rasmussen, 2014). Given the safety record of EPA+DHA (Villani et al., 2013), recommendations for the marine omega-3 FAs of between 250 and 1000 mg/day (Kris-Etherton, Harris, and Appel, 2002; Harris, Kris-Etherton, and Harris, 2008; Vannice and Rasmussen, 2014) or even higher as suggested from Japanese studies (Sekikawa, Doyle, and Kuller, 2015) are reasonable for reducing the risk for cardiometabolic diseases.

REFERENCES

Albert, C.M., H. Campos, M.J. Stampfer, P.M. Ridker, J.E. Manson, W.C. Willett, and J. Ma. 2002. Blood levels of long-chain n-3 fatty acids and the risk of sudden death. *N Engl J Med* 346:1113–1118.

Baker, P.R., F.J. Schopfer, V.B. O'Donnell, and B.A. Freeman. 2009. Convergence of nitric oxide and lipid signaling: Anti-inflammatory nitro-fatty acids. *Free Radic Biol Med* 46 (8):989–1003.

Bays, H.E., C.M. Ballantyne, R.A. Braeckman, W.G. Stirtan, and P.N. Soni. 2013. Icosapent ethyl, a pure ethyl ester of eicosapentaenoic acid: Effects on circulating markers of inflammation from the MARINE and ANCHOR studies. *Am J Cardiovasc Drugs* 13:37–46.

Bazinet, R.P. and M.W. Chu. 2014. Omega-6 polyunsaturated fatty acids: Is a broad cholesterol-lowering health claim appropriate? *CMAJ* 186 (6):434–439.

Bendsen, N.T., S. Stender, P.B. Szecsi, S.B. Pedersen, S. Basu, L.I. Hellgren, J.W. Newman, T.M. Larsen, S.B. Haugaard, and A. Astrup. 2011. Effect of industrially produced trans fat on markers of systemic inflammation: Evidence from a randomized trial in women. *J Lipid Res* 52:1821–1828.

Blasbalg, T.L., J.R. Hibbeln, C.E. Ramsden, S.F. Majchrzak, and R.R. Rawlings. 2011. Changes in consumption of omega-3 and omega-6 fatty acids in the United States during the 20th century. *Am J Clin Nutr* 93 (5):950–962.

Bradbury, K.E., C. Murray Skeaff, T.J. Green, A.R. Gray, and F.L. Crowe. 2010. The serum fatty acids myristic acid and linoleic acid are better predictors of serum cholesterol concentrations when measured as molecular percentages rather than as absolute concentrations. *Am J Clin Nutr* 91 (2):398–405.

Brown, J.M., G.S. Shelness, and L.L. Rudel. 2007. Monounsaturated fatty acids and atherosclerosis: Opposing views from epidemiology and experimental animal models. *Curr Atheroscler Rep* 9:494–500.

Burr, M.L., A.M. Fehily, J.F. Gilbert, S. Rogers, R.M. Holliday, P.M. Sweetnam, P.C. Elwood, and N.M. Deadman. 1989. Effects of changes in fat, fish, and fibre intakes on death and myocardial reinfarction: Diet and reinfarction trial (DART). *Lancet* 2:757–761.

Calder, P.C. 2013. Omega-3 polyunsaturated fatty acids and inflammatory processes: Nutrition or pharmacology? *Br J Clin Pharmacol* 75 (3):645–662.

Casula, M., D. Soranna, A.L. Catapano, and G. Corrao. 2013. Long-term effect of high dose omega-3 fatty acid supplementation for secondary prevention of cardiovascular outcomes: A meta-analysis of randomized, double blind, placebo controlled trials. *Atheroscler Suppl* 14 (2):243–251.

Choo, J., H. Ueshima, J.D. Curb, C. Shin, R.W. Evans, A. El-Saed, T. Kadowaki et al. 2010. Serum n-6 fatty acids and lipoprotein subclasses in middle-aged men: The population-based cross-sectional ERA-JUMP study. *Am J Clin Nutr* 91 (5):1195–1203.

Chowdhury, R., S. Warnakula, S. Kunutsor, F. Crowe, H.A. Ward, L. Johnson, O.H. Franco et al. 2014. Association of dietary, circulating, and supplement fatty acids with coronary risk: A systematic review and meta-analysis. *Ann Intern Med* 160 (6):398–406.

Cleland, L.G., M.J. James, M.A. Neumann, M. D'Angelo, and R.A. Gibson. 1992. Linoleate inhibits EPA incorporation from dietary fish-oil supplements in human subjects. *Am J Clin Nutr* 55:395–399.

Cunnane, S.C. 2003. Problems with essential fatty acids: Time for a new paradigm? *Prog Lipid Res* 42 (6):544–568.

Cunnane, S.C. and P. Guesnet. 2011. Linoleic acid recommendations—A house of cards. *Prostaglandins Leukot Essent Fatty Acids* 85:399–402.

Czernichow, S., D. Thomas, and E. Bruckert. 2010. n-6 Fatty acids and cardiovascular health: A review of the evidence for dietary intake recommendations. *Br J Nutr* 104:788–796.

Davidson, M.H., K.C. Maki, H. Bays, R. Carter, and C.M. Ballantyne. 2009. Effects of prescription omega-3-acid ethyl esters on lipoprotein particle concentrations, apolipoproteins AI and CIII, and lipoprotein-associated phospholipase A(2) mass in statin-treated subjects with hypertriglyceridemia. *J Clin Lipidol* 3:332–340.

Davidson, M.H., E.A. Stein, H.E. Bays, K.C. Maki, R.T. Doyle, R.A. Shalwitz, C.M. Ballantyne, and H.N. Ginsberg. 2007. Efficacy and tolerability of adding prescription omega-3 fatty acids 4 g/d to simvastatin 40 mg/d in hypertriglyceridemic patients: An 8-week, randomized, double-blind, placebo-controlled study. *Clin Ther* 29:1354–1367.

De Caterina, R. 2011. n-3 fatty acids in cardiovascular disease. *N Engl J Med* 364:2439–2450.

Delgado-Lista, J., P. Perez-Martinez, J. Lopez-Miranda, and F. Perez-Jimenez. 2012. Long chain omega-3 fatty acids and cardiovascular disease: A systematic review. *Br J Nutr* 107 (Suppl 2):S201–S213.

FAO. 2010. Fats and fatty acids in human nutrition: Report of an expert consultation. FAO Food and Nutrition Paper. Rome, Italy.

Farvid, M.S., M. Ding, A. Pan, Q. Sun, S.E. Chiuve, L.M. Steffen, W.C. Willett, and F.B. Hu. 2014. Dietary linoleic acid and risk of coronary heart disease: A systematic review and meta-analysis of prospective cohort studies. *Circulation* 130 (18):1568–1578.

Flock, M.R., A.C. Skulas-Ray, W.S. Harris, T.D. Etherton, J.A. Fleming, and P.M. Kris-Etherton. 2013. Determinants of erythrocyte omega-3 fatty acid content in response to fish oil supplementation: A dose-response randomized controlled trial. *J Am Heart Assoc* 2 (6):e000513.

Fontes, J.D., F. Rahman, S. Lacey, M.G. Larson, R.S. Vasan, E.J. Benjamin, W.S. Harris, and S.J. Robins. 2015. Red blood cell fatty acids and biomarkers of inflammation: A cross-sectional study in a community-based cohort. *Atherosclerosis* 240 (2):431–436.

Gebauer, S.K., F. Destaillats, F. Dionisi, R.M. Krauss, and D.J. Baer. 2015. Vaccenic acid and trans fatty acid isomers from partially hydrogenated oil both adversely affect LDL cholesterol: A double-blind, randomized controlled trial. *Am J Clin Nutr* 102 (6):1339–1346.

Harris, W. 2010. Omega-6 and omega-3 fatty acids: Partners in prevention. *Curr Opin Clin Nutr Metab Care* 13 (2):125–129.

Harris, W.S. 1989. Fish oils and plasma lipid and lipoprotein metabolism in humans: A critical review. *J Lipid Res* 30:785–807.

Harris, W.S. 2006. The omega-6/omega-3 ratio and cardiovascular disease risk: Uses and abuses. *Curr Atheroscler Rep* 8:453–459.

Harris, W.S. 2009. The omega-3 index: From biomarker to risk marker to risk factor. *Curr Atheroscler Rep* 11:411–417.

Harris, W.S. 2013. Are n-3 fatty acids still cardioprotective? *Curr Opin Clin Nutr Metab Care* 16 (2):141–149.

Harris, W.S., K.F. Kennedy, T.M. Maddox, S. Kutty, and J.A. Spertus. 2016. Multiple differences between patients who initiate fish oil supplementation post-myocardial infarction and those who do not: The TRIUMPH study. *Nutr Res* 36 (1):65–71.

Harris, W.S., H.N. Ginsberg, N. Arunakul, N.S. Shachter, S.L. Windsor, M. Adams, L. Berglund, and K. Osmundsen. 1997. Safety and efficacy of Omacor in severe hypertriglyceridemia. *J Cardiovasc Risk* 4:385–392.

Harris, W.S., P.M. Kris-Etherton, and K.A. Harris. 2008. Intakes of long-chain omega-3 fatty acid associated with reduced risk for death from coronary heart disease in healthy adults. *Curr Atheroscler Rep* 10 (6):503–509.

Harris, W.S., D. Mozaffarian, M. Lefevre, C.D. Toner, J. Colombo, S.C. Cunnane, J.M. Holden, D.M. Klurfeld, M.C. Morris, and J. Whelan. 2009a. Towards establishing dietary reference intakes for eicosapentaenoic and docosahexaenoic acids. *J Nutr* 139:804S-819S.

Harris, W.S., D. Mozaffarian, E.B. Rimm, P.M Kris-Etherton, L.L. Rudel, L.J. Appel, M.M. Engler, M.B. Engler, and F.M. Sacks. 2009b. Omega-6 fatty acids and risk for cardiovascular disease: A science advisory from the American Heart Association Nutrition Committee. *Circulation* 119:902–907.

Harris, W.S., S.A. Sands, S.L. Windsor, H.A. Ali, T.L. Stevens, A. Magalski, C.B. Porter, and A.M. Borkon. 2004. Omega-3 fatty acids in cardiac biopsies from heart transplant patients: Correlation with erythrocytes and response to supplementation. *Circulation* 110:1645–1649.

Harris, W.S. and R.M. Thomas. 2010. Biological variability of blood omega-3 biomarkers. *Clin Biochem* 43 (3):338–340.

Harris, W.S., S.A. Varvel, J.V. Pottala, G.R. Warnick, and J.P. McConnell. 2013. Comparative effects of an acute dose of fish oil on omega-3 fatty acid levels in red blood cells versus plasma: Implications for clinical utility. *J Clin Lipidol* 7 (5):433–440.

Harris, W.S. and C. von Schacky. 2004. The omega-3 index: A new risk factor for death from coronary heart disease? *Prev Med* 39:212–220.

He, K., Y. Song, M.L. Daviglus, K. Liu, L. Van Horn, A.R. Dyer, and P. Greenland. 2004. Accumulated evidence on fish consumption and coronary heart disease mortality: A meta-analysis of cohort studies. *Circulation* 109:2705–2711.

Hibbeln, J.R., L.R. Nieminen, T.L. Blasbalg, J.A. Riggs, and W.E. Lands. 2006. Healthy intakes of n-3 and n-6 fatty acids: Estimations considering worldwide diversity. *Am J Clin Nutr* 83:1483S–1493S.

Investigators, GISSI-HF. 2008. Effect of n-3 polyunsaturated fatty acids in patients with chronic heart failure (the GISSI-HF trial): A randomised, double-blind, placebo-controlled trial. *Lancet* 372:1223–1230.

Investigators, GISSI-Prevenzione. 1999. Dietary supplementation with n-3 polyunsaturated fatty acids and vitamin E in 11,324 patients with myocardial infarction: Results of the GISSI-Prevenzione trial. *Lancet* 354:447–455.

Iso, H., M. Kobayashi, J. Ishihara, S. Sasaki, K. Okada, Y. Kita, Y. Kokubo, and S. Tsugane. 2006. Intake of fish and n3 fatty acids and risk of coronary heart disease among Japanese: The Japan Public Health Center-Based (JPHC) Study Cohort I. *Circulation* 113:195–202.

Jacobson, T.A. 2008. Role of n-3 fatty acids in the treatment of hypertriglyceridemia and cardiovascular disease. *Am J Clin Nutr* 87 (6):1981S–1990S.

Johnson, G.H. and K. Fritsche. 2012. Effect of dietary linoleic acid on markers of inflammation in healthy persons: A systematic review of randomized controlled trials. *J Acad Nutr Diet* 112 (7):1029–1041.e1-15.

Khawaja, O.A., J.M. Gaziano, and L. Djousse. 2014. N-3 fatty acids for prevention of cardiovascular disease. *Curr Atheroscler Rep* 16 (11):450.

Kotwal, S., M. Jun, D. Sullivan, V. Perkovic, and B. Neal. 2012. Omega 3 Fatty acids and cardiovascular outcomes: Systematic review and meta-analysis. *Circ Cardiovasc Qual Outcomes* 5 (6):808–818.

Kris-Etherton, P.M., W.S. Harris, and L.J. Appel. 2002. Fish consumption, fish oil, omega-3 fatty acids, and cardiovascular disease. *Circulation* 106:2747–2757.

Kromhout, D. and J. de Goede. 2014. Update on cardiometabolic health effects of omega-3 fatty acids. *Curr Opin Lipidol* 25 (1):85–90.

Kromhout, D., S. Yasuda, J.M. Geleijnse, and H. Shimokawa. 2012. Fish oil and omega-3 fatty acids in cardiovascular disease: Do they really work? *Eur Heart J* 33:436–443.

Kwak, S.M., S.K. Myung, Y.J. Lee, and H.G. Seo. 2012. Efficacy of omega-3 fatty acid supplements (eicosapentaenoic acid and docosahexaenoic acid) in the secondary prevention of cardiovascular disease: A meta-analysis of randomized, double-blind, placebo-controlled trials. *Arch Intern Med* 172:686–694.

Leslie, M.A., D.J. Cohen, D.M. Liddle, L.E. Robinson, and D.W. Ma. 2015. A review of the effect of omega-3 polyunsaturated fatty acids on blood triacylglycerol levels in normolipidemic and borderline hyperlipidemic individuals. *Lipids Health Dis* 14:53.

Li, K., T. Huang, J. Zheng, K. Wu, and D. Li. 2014. Effect of marine-derived n-3 polyunsaturated fatty acids on C-reactive protein, interleukin 6 and tumor necrosis factor alpha: A meta-analysis. *PLoS One* 9 (2):e88103.

Liou, Y.A., D.J. King, D. Zibrik, and S.M. Innis. 2007. Decreasing linoleic acid with constant alpha-linolenic acid in dietary fats increases (n-3) eicosapentaenoic acid in plasma phospholipids in healthy men. *J Nutr* 137:945–952.

Mallat, Z., G. Lambeau, and A. Tedgui. 2010. Lipoprotein-associated and secreted phospholipases A(2) in cardiovascular disease: Roles as biological effectors and biomarkers. *Circulation* 122 (21):2183–2200.

Mantyselka, P., L. Niskanen, H. Kautiainen, J. Saltevo, P. Wurtz, P. Soininen, A.J. Kangas, M. Ala-Korpela, and M. Vanhala. 2014. Cross-sectional and longitudinal associations of circulating omega-3 and omega-6 fatty acids with lipoprotein particle concentrations and sizes: Population-based cohort study with 6-year follow-up. *Lipids Health Dis* 13:28.

Marchioli, R., F. Barzi, E. Bomba, C. Chieffo, D. Di Gregorio, R. Di Mascio, M.G. Franzosi et al. 2002. Early protection against sudden death by n-3 polyunsaturated fatty acids after myocardial infarction: Time-course analysis of the results of the Gruppo Italiano per lo Studio della Sopravvivenza nell'Infarto Miocardico (GISSI)-Prevenzione. *Circulation* 105:1897–1903.

Mensink, R.P. and M.B. Katan. 1992. Effect of dietary fatty acids on serum lipids and lipoproteins. A meta-analysis of 27 trials. *Arterioscler Thromb* 12:911–919.

Mensink, R.P., P.L. Zock, A.D. Kester, and M.B. Katan. 2003. Effects of dietary fatty acids and carbohydrates on the ratio of serum total to HDL cholesterol and on serum lipids and apolipoproteins: A meta-analysis of 60 controlled trials. *Am J Clin Nutr* 77:1146–1155.

Mozaffarian, D., A. Ascherio, F.B. Hu, M.J. Stampfer, W.C. Willett, D.S. Siscovick, and E.B. Rimm. 2005a. Interplay between different polyunsaturated fatty acids and risk of coronary heart disease in men. *Circulation* 111:157–164.

Mozaffarian, D., A. Geelen, I.A. Brouwer, J.M. Geleijnse, P.L. Zock, and M.B. Katan. 2005b. Effect of fish oil on heart rate in humans: A meta-analysis of randomized controlled trials. *Circulation* 112:1945–1952.

Mozaffarian, D., R. Micha, and S. Wallace. 2010. Effects on coronary heart disease of increasing polyunsaturated fat in place of saturated fat: A systematic review and meta-analysis of randomized controlled trials. *PLoS Med* 7:e1000252.

Mozaffarian, D. and J.H. Wu. 2011. Omega-3 fatty acids and cardiovascular disease: Effects on risk factors, molecular pathways, and clinical events. *J Am Coll Cardiol* 58 (20):2047–2067.

Musa-Veloso, K., M.A. Binns, A. Kocenas, C. Chung, H. Rice, H. Oppedal-Olsen, H. Lloyd, and S. Lemke. 2011. Impact of low v. moderate intakes of long-chain n-3 fatty acids on risk of coronary heart disease. *Br J Nutr* 106:1129–1141.

Nestel, P., H. Shige, S. Pomeroy, M. Cehun, M. Abbey, and D. Raederstorff. 2002. The n-3 fatty acids eicosapentaenoic acid and docosahexaenoic acid increase systemic arterial compliance in humans. *Am J Clin Nutr* 76:326–330.

Pinot, M., S. Vanni, S. Pagnotta, S. Lacas-Gervais, L.A. Payet, T. Ferreira, R. Gautier, B. Goud, B. Antonny, and H. Barelli. 2014. Lipid cell biology. Polyunsaturated phospholipids facilitate membrane deformation and fission by endocytic proteins. *Science* 345 (6197):693–697.

Poudyal, H., S.K. Panchal, V. Diwan, and L. Brown. 2011. Omega-3 fatty acids and metabolic syndrome: Effects and emerging mechanisms of action. *Prog Lipid Res* 50 (4):372–387.

Radack, K.L., C.C. Deck, and G.A. Huster. 1990. n-3 Fatty acid effects on lipids, lipoproteins, and apolipoproteins at very low doses: Results of a randomized controlled trial in hypertriglyceridemic subjects. *Am J Clin Nutr* 51:599–605.

Ramsden, C.E., J.R. Hibbeln, S.F. Majchrzak, and J.M. Davis. 2010. n-6 Fatty acid-specific and mixed polyunsaturate dietary interventions have different effects on CHD risk: A meta-analysis of randomised controlled trials. *Br J Nutr* 104:1586–1600.

Ramsden, C.E., A. Ringel, A.E. Feldstein, A.Y. Taha, B.A. MacIntosh, J.R. Hibbeln, S.F. Majchrzak-Hong et al. 2012. Lowering dietary linoleic acid reduces bioactive oxidized linoleic acid metabolites in humans. *Prostaglandins Leukot Essent Fatty Acids* 87 (4–5):135–141.

Ramsden, C.E., D. Zamora, B. Leelarthaepin, S.F. Majchrzak-Hong, K.R. Faurot, C.M. Suchindran, A. Ringel, J.M. Davis, and J.R. Hibbeln. 2013. Use of dietary linoleic acid for secondary prevention of coronary heart disease and death: Evaluation of recovered data from the Sydney Diet Heart Study and updated meta-analysis. *BMJ* 346:e8707.

Rangel-Huerta, O.D., C.M. Aguilera, M.D. Mesa, and A. Gil. 2012. Omega-3 long-chain polyunsaturated fatty acids supplementation on inflammatory biomakers: A systematic review of randomised clinical trials. *Br J Nutr* 107 (Suppl 2):S159–S170.

Reiffel, J.A. and A. McDonald. 2006. Antiarrhythmic effects of omega-3 fatty acids. *Am J Cardiol* 98:50i–60i.

Rett, B.S. and J. Whelan. 2011. Increasing dietary linoleic acid does not increase tissue arachidonic acid content in adults consuming Western-type diets: A systematic review. *Nutr Metab (Lond)* 8:36.

Rizos, E.C., E.E. Ntzani, E. Bika, M.S. Kostapanos, and M.S. Elisaf. 2012. Association between omega-3 fatty acid supplementation and risk of major cardiovascular disease events: A systematic review and meta-analysis. *JAMA* 308:1024–1033.

Robinson, J.G. and N.J. Stone. 2006. Antiatherosclerotic and antithrombotic effects of omega-3 fatty acids. *Am J Cardiol* 98:39i–49i.

Roche, H.M. and M.J. Gibney. 1996. Postprandial triacylglycerolaemia: The effect of low-fat dietary treatment with and without fish oil supplementation. *Eur J Clin Nutr* 50:617–624.

Saravanan, P., N.C. Davidson, E.B. Schmidt, and P.C. Calder. 2010. Cardiovascular effects of marine omega-3 fatty acids. *Lancet* 376:540–550.

Schopfer, F.J., Y. Lin, P.R. Baker, T. Cui, M. Garcia-Barrio, J. Zhang, K. Chen, Y.E. Chen, and B.A. Freeman. 2005. Nitrolinoleic acid: An endogenous peroxisome proliferator-activated receptor gamma ligand. *Proc Natl Acad Sci USA* 102:2340–2345.

Schwellenbach, L.J., K.L. Olson, K.J. McConnell, R.S. Stolcpart, J.D. Nash, and J.A. Merenich. 2006. The triglyceride-lowering effects of a modest dose of docosahexaenoic acid alone versus in combination with low dose eicosapentaenoic acid in patients with coronary artery disease and elevated triglycerides. *J Am Coll Nutr* 25:480–485.

Schwingshackl, L. and G. Hoffmann. 2014. Dietary fatty acids in the secondary prevention of coronary heart disease: A systematic review, meta-analysis and meta-regression. *BMJ Open* 4 (4):e004487.

Sekikawa, A., M.F. Doyle, and L.H. Kuller. 2015. Recent findings of long-chain n-3 polyunsaturated fatty acids (LCn-3 PUFAs) on atherosclerosis and coronary heart disease (CHD) contrasting studies in Western countries to Japan. *Trends Cardiovasc Med* 25 (8):717–723.

Serhan, C.N. and N.A. Petasis. 2011. Resolvins and protectins in inflammation resolution. *Chem Rev* 111:5922–5943.

Shearer, G.C., O.V. Savinova, and W.S. Harris. 2012. Fish oil - How does it reduce plasma triglycerides? *Biochim Biophys Acta* 1821:843–851.

Shim, J.S., K. Oh, and H.C. Kim. 2014. Dietary assessment methods in epidemiologic studies. *Epidemiol Health* 36:e2014009.

Siddiqui, R.A., K.A. Harvey, and G.P. Zaloga. 2008. Modulation of enzymatic activities by n-3 polyunsaturated fatty acids to support cardiovascular health. *J Nutr Biochem* 19:417–437.

Siguel, E. 1996. A new relationship between total/high density lipoprotein cholesterol and polyunsaturated fatty acids. *Lipids* 31 (Suppl):S51–S56.

Siscovick, D.S., T.E. Raghunathan, I. King, S. Weinmann, K.G. Wicklund, J. Albright, V. Bovbjerg et al. 1995. Dietary intake and cell membrane levels of long-chain n-3 polyunsaturated fatty acids and the risk of primary cardiac arrest. *J Am Med Assoc* 274:1363–1367.

Slee, E.L., P.L. McLennan, A.J. Owen, and M.L. Theiss. 2010. Low dietary fish-oil threshold for myocardial membrane n-3 PUFA enrichment independent of n-6 PUFA intake in rats. *J Lipid Res* 51 (7):1841–1848.

Spector, A.A. 2009. Arachidonic acid cytochrome P450 epoxygenase pathway. *J Lipid Res* 50 (Suppl):S52–S56.

Stanley, J.C., R.L. Elsom, P.C. Calder, B.A. Griffin, W.S. Harris, S.A. Jebb, J.A. Lovegrove, C.S. Moore, R.A. Riemersma, and T.A. Sanders. 2007. UK Food Standards Agency Workshop Report: The effects of the dietary n-6:n-3 fatty acid ratio on cardiovascular health. *Br J Nutr* 98:1305–1310.

Taha, A.Y., Y. Cheon, K.F. Faurot, B. Macintosh, S.F. Majchrzak-Hong, J.D. Mann, J.R. Hibbeln, A. Ringel, and C.E. Ramsden. 2014. Dietary omega-6 fatty acid lowering increases bioavailability of omega-3 polyunsaturated fatty acids in human plasma lipid pools. *Prostaglandins Leukot Essent Fatty Acids* 90 (5):151–157.

Tam, V.C. 2013. Lipidomic profiling of bioactive lipids by mass spectrometry during microbial infections. *Semin Immunol* 25 (3):240–248.

Thies, F., J.M. Garry, P. Yaqoob, K. Rerkasem, J. Williams, C.P. Shearman, P.J. Gallagher, P.C. Calder, and R.F. Grimble. 2003. Association of n-3 polyunsaturated fatty acids with stability of atherosclerotic plaques: A randomised controlled trial. *Lancet* 361:477–485.

Trikalinos, T.A., J. Lee, D. Moorthy, W.W. Yu, J. Lau, A.H. Lichtenstein, and M. Chung. 2012. *Effects of Eicosapentaenoic Acid and Docosahexaenoic Acid on Mortality Across Diverse Settings: Systematic Review and Meta-Analysis of Randomized Trials and Prospective Cohorts*. Rockville, MD: Department of Health and Human Services, Agency for Healthcare Research and Quality.

Turk, H.F. and R.S. Chapkin. 2013. Membrane lipid raft organization is uniquely modified by n-3 polyunsaturated fatty acids. *Prostaglandins Leukot Essent Fatty Acids* 88 (1):43–47.

Vannice, G. and H. Rasmussen. 2014. Position of the academy of nutrition and dietetics: Dietary Fatty acids for healthy adults. *J Acad Nutr Diet* 114 (1):136–153.

Villani, A.M., M. Crotty, L.G. Cleland, M.J. James, R.J. Fraser, L. Cobiac, and M.D. Miller. 2013. Fish oil administration in older adults with cardiovascular disease or cardiovascular risk factors: Is there potential for adverse events? A systematic review of the literature. *Int J Cardiol* 168 (4):4371–4375.

von Schacky, C. 2014. Omega-3 index and cardiovascular health. *Nutrients* 6 (2):799–814.

Wang, X., H. Lin, and Y. Gu. 2012. Multiple roles of dihomo-gamma-linolenic acid against proliferation diseases. *Lipids Health Dis* 11:25.

Wei, M.Y. and T.A. Jacobson. 2011. Effects of eicosapentaenoic acid versus docosahexaenoic acid on serum lipids: A systematic review and meta-analysis. *Curr Atheroscler Rep* 13:474–483.

Williams, J.A., S.E. Batten, M. Harris, B.D. Rockett, S.R. Shaikh, W. Stillwell, and S.R. Wassall. 2012. Docosahexaenoic and eicosapentaenoic acids segregate differently between raft and nonraft domains. *Biophys J* 103 (2):228–237.

Xin, W., W. Wei, and X. Li. 2012. Effect of fish oil supplementation on fasting vascular endothelial function in humans: A meta-analysis of randomized controlled trials. *PLoS One* 7 (9):e46028.

Xin, W., W. Wei, and X.Y. Li. 2013. Short-term effects of fish-oil supplementation on heart rate variability in humans: A meta-analysis of randomized controlled trials. *Am J Clin Nutr* 97 (5):926–935.

Yokoyama, M., H. Origasa, M. Matsuzaki, Y. Matsuzawa, Y. Saito, Y. Ishikawa, S. Oikawa et al. 2007. Effects of eicosapentaenoic acid on major coronary events in hypercholesterolaemic patients (JELIS): A randomised open-label, blinded endpoint analysis. *Lancet* 369:1090–1098.

11 Evolving Role of Saturated Fatty Acids

Patty W. Siri-Tarino and Ronald M. Krauss

CONTENTS

ABSTRACT

Given their cholesterol-raising ability and (like other fats) higher caloric content per gram compared to proteins or carbohydrates, saturated fatty acids (SFAs) have been a focus of dietary guidelines for cardiovascular health since their inception. Restriction of this class of fatty acids was advised, however, without reference to the replacement nutrient, in part contributing to food formulations high in sugars and refined carbohydrates that can adversely affect cardiometabolic health. Moreover, in light of more recent research highlighting factors that modulate the effects of SFAs on cardiometabolic risk, including the heterogeneity of SFAs themselves, food sources of SFAs, and variation in individual responsiveness to diet, a foods-based approach that moves away from targeting restriction of SFAs as a whole is warranted. A reevaluation of how nutritional science is communicated to the public is further informed by recent research demonstrating diets high in SFAs and low in carbohydrate as an effective therapeutic regimen for some individuals with obesity and/or diabetes. Future dietary recommendations should emphasize individualized approaches that consider both the context of the SFAs consumed and the individuals consuming them.

PRIMER ON SFA BIOCHEMISTRY AND PHYSIOLOGY

Saturated fatty acids (SFAs) contain no double bonds as a result of having all of their carbons "saturated" with hydrogen molecules. The most abundant SFAs contain between 12 and 22 carbons (Chow 2000). SFAs between 12 and 18 carbons in chain length can be desaturated to their respective monounsaturated products via stearoyl-CoA-desaturase, with increasingly more efficient conversion of SFAs of longer chain length according to cellular studies conducted in rats (Legrand and Rioux 2010). Tracer studies in humans have also documented greater rates of desaturation of C18:0 versus

TABLE 11.1
Common SFAs and Their Typical Food Sources

Common Name	Carbon Chain Length	Typical Food Sources
Butyric acid	C4:0	Butter and dairy fat
Lauric acid	C12:0	Coconut oil
Myristic acid	C14:0	Coconut oil and dairy fat
Palmitic acid	C16:0	Palm oil, meat, and dairy fats
Stearic acid	C18:0	Meat fat and cocoa butter

C16:0 (Rhee et al. 1997), although on an absolute level, the rates of conversion are relatively small, that is, 14% and 2%, respectively. It is unclear whether the biological desaturation of SFAs affects their hypercholesterolemic properties (Rhee et al. 1997).

SFAs are structural components of sphingolipids and ceramides, which are contained in cell membranes, skin, and myelin. SFAs have specific physiological functions, including protein fatty acid acylation, specifically N-terminal myristoylation and side chain palmitoylation (Nettleton, Legrand, and Mensink 2015). The myristoyl moiety mediates protein subcellular localization and protein–protein or protein–membrane interactions that enable the biological functions of the myristoylated proteins. Further, various SFAs have different cellular and biological functions. Myristic acid may enhance the bioavailability of docosahexaenoic acid and eicosapentaenoic acid at an optimal level of 1.2% of total energy (at 1.8%, it reduced bioavailability); butyric acid may protect against early tumorigenic events; and medium-chain fatty acids appear to be differentially metabolized, resulting in less adipose tissue deposition compared to long-chain fatty acids (Legrand and Rioux 2010). More recent evidence suggests that very-long-chain saturated fatty acids (C20:0–C24:0) may also have metabolic benefits (Mozaffarian 2016).

Because humans can synthesize them *de novo*, there is no dietary requirement for SFAs. Further, it is important to note that plasma concentrations of even-chained SFAs do not accurately reflect their dietary consumption given endogenous metabolic pathways. In fact, SFAs present in blood are not strongly associated with dietary SFA consumption (Ma et al. 2015, Morio et al. 2016). Rather, dietary carbohydrates appear to be an important determinant of plasma SFA concentrations by driving *de novo* lipogenesis (Forsythe et al. 2010).

The major dietary sources of SFAs in the U.S. diet are red meat and dairy foods (Table 11.1). Palmitic acid (C16:0) is the most abundant SFA in both categories, along with stearic acid in meat, and myristic acid in dairy. Tropical oils, including palm and coconut oils, are also sources of SFAs, specifically lauric and myristic acids as well as palmitic acid.

EVOLVING HISTORY OF STUDIES OF SFA EFFECTS ON LIPIDS, LIPOPROTEINS, AND CVD RISK

In 1909, as reviewed in Steinberg (2004), the St. Petersburg-based pathologist Alexander Ignatowski fed rabbits high-protein diets containing meat, eggs, and milk and showed that such diets induced arterial lesions that resembled human atherosclerosis (Ignatowski 1909). Several years later, Nikolai Anichkov at the same institute showed that the same phenomenon could be induced by feeding rabbits purified cholesterol (Anitschkow 1913). Anichkov would subsequently conduct an elaborate series of experiments using various animal models over the next decades to establish a role for blood cholesterol in the pathogenesis of atherosclerosis as reviewed in Konstantinov, Mejevoi, and Anichkov (2006), a finding that would set the stage for the many experimental studies to follow that were aimed at understanding atherosclerotic progression and the dietary and pharmacological therapies that could effectively modulate it.

Metabolic Studies Evaluating Diet and Lipid Profiles

Experimental studies in humans during the mid-twentieth century showed that blood cholesterol level was increased by dietary SFAs relative to other macronutrients as reviewed in Konstantinov, Mejevoi, and Anichkov (2006). Substituting plant foods for animal foods led to a significant decrease in blood cholesterol levels (Kinsell et al. 1952), an effect found to be due to the unsaturation of vegetable fats (Ahrens, Blankenhorn, and Tsaltas 1954). Metabolic studies in men conducted by Ancel Keys evaluated effects on blood cholesterol concentrations of varying quantities of dietary saturated and polyunsaturated fats (Keys, Anderson, and Grande 1957). Consistent with the earlier findings, increases in serum cholesterol were a function of higher dietary saturated fat and lower polyunsaturated fat content of the diets (Keys, Anderson, and Grande 1957). The effects of monounsaturated fats were estimated to be neutral. Further, the investigators noted that these relationships were based on group averages, whereas the reliability of individual prediction of change in cholesterol level was low due to significant variations in dietary response (Keys, Anderson, and Grande 1957). Hegsted et al. subsequently reported that SFAs with chain lengths of 14 and 16 carbons, but not those with 10, 12, and 18 carbons, raised total serum cholesterol and also considered a role for dietary cholesterol (Hegsted et al. 1965).

A more recent meta-analysis of data from 27 controlled diet trials published between 1970 and 1991 that evaluated effects of replacing SFAs with other macronutrients on total cholesterol (TC), low density lipoprotein-cholesterol (LDL-C), and high density lipoprotein-cholesterol (HDL-C) was in good agreement with the Keys and Hegsted equations, with changes in total serum cholesterol increased by C14:0 and C10:0 SFAs and decreased by polyunsaturated fats (Mensink and Katan 1992). Notably, Mensink and Katan showed that the replacement of fat with carbohydrate led to increases in plasma triglycerides independent of the type of fat replaced (Mensink and Katan 1992). Further, replacement of saturated fats with unsaturated fats decreased the LDL to HDL ratio, whereas replacement with carbohydrates had no effect. Thus, it was concluded that under isocaloric, metabolic ward conditions, the most favorable lipoprotein profiles were achieved when saturated fats were replaced with unsaturated fat, without decreasing the total fat intake. A similar evaluation by the same investigators showed that replacement of SFAs and *trans* fatty acids with unsaturated fatty acids was associated with decreases in the TC:HDL-C ratio, whereas replacement with carbohydrate was associated with no change (Mensink et al. 2003). Of note, LDL-C may only be increased with SFAs when polyunsaturated fatty acid (PUFA) intake is below ~5% (Hayes et al. 1997). As for specific SFAs, when replacing carbohydrate, lauric acid (C12:0) raised LDL-C, the most compared to myristic (C14:0) and palmitic (C16:0) acids. However, lauric acid also raised HDL-C significantly, thus resulting in the largest reduction in the TC:HDL-C ratio (Mensink et al. 2003).

Diet and CVD Studies

Clinical trials evaluating the effect of replacing saturated fats with polyunsaturated fats on cardiovascular disease (CVD) events, for example, myocardial infarction and CHD death, in the 1960s and 1970s, generally showed reduced CVD risk (Dayton and Pearce 1969, Leren 1970, Turpeinen et al. 1979), although there were also trials, including some completed nearly 20 years later, that showed no effects on CVD of this replacement scenario (Burr et al. 1989, Frantz et al. 1989, Watts et al. 1992).

Positive associations of dietary SFAs with CVD were observed in an epidemiological study across seven countries conducted by Keys around the same time (Keys et al. 1966). More recently, the Seven Countries Study has been criticized for including only those data that supported a positive linear relationship between SFAs and CVD (Lustig 2012, Taubes 2007). As with all epidemiological studies, associations are not evidence of causality. It is also important to note that consideration of a single macronutrient in isolation, that is, not in relation to what is being replaced, is necessarily limiting. Nonetheless, the findings from the Seven Countries Study among other epidemiological studies along with the aforementioned metabolic trials formed the basis for the "diet-heart" hypothesis, which pointed to SFAs as a major dietary determinant of the increasing CVD rates that were occurring in the United States in the decades after the Second World War.

Based on epidemiological, metabolic, and clinical trial evidence available at the time, restriction of both SFAs and total fats was advised in the first U.S. dietary guidelines (United States Department of Agriculture and Department of Health and Human Services 1980). The advice to reduce total fats in the diet was thought to be a pragmatic approach that would enable the reduction of SFAs. Since these guidelines were issued, an increasing body of research, as described in the following, speaks to the newly appreciated complexity of the SFA–CVD relationship, including a refinement in lipoprotein measures as biomarkers of CVD, the importance of specifying the replacement nutrient, the heterogeneity of SFAs, variable effects of different SFA food sources, and interindividual variability in response to diets (Siri-Tarino et al. 2015). Further, the epidemics of obesity and diabetes have pushed to the forefront the need for appropriate lifestyle therapies for their management, and diets lower in carbohydrates, and higher in SFAs, provide an option. These developments support a shift in dietary guidance toward foods and dietary patterns rather than macronutrients.

Refined CVD Risk Assessment

The concept that LDL particles provide a better assessment of risk than cholesterol alone dates to the 1950s and has been carried through to current investigations (Krauss 2014). LDL particles exist along a spectrum of sizes and densities with differing cholesterol content and associations with CVD risk. The distribution of the LDL particle subclasses varies between individuals, with medium particles generally the most abundant in healthy individuals and smaller and more dense LDL (sdLDL) particles associated with increased CVD risk compared to larger LDL. Recent large prospective cohort studies have shown that levels of sdLDL predict CVD risk in various populations independently of LDL-C concentrations (Hoogeveen et al. 2014, Tsai et al. 2014). Smaller LDL have reduced LDL receptor affinity, and hence slower plasma clearance, as well as greater binding to arterial proteoglycans and greater oxidative susceptibility (Berneis and Krauss 2002). sdLDL particles may also contain more apoCIII and be subject to increased nonenzymatic glycation, features that have been associated with greater atherogenicity (Siri-Tarino et al. 2015).

LDL-C concentrations can misrepresent the number of LDL particles in persons with a predominance of sdLDL. Thus, in two individuals with a similar LDL cholesterol concentration, there may be differential CVD risk based on the number and quality of LDL particles, with persons with increased particle numbers and/or increased smaller and more dense LDL particles at increased CVD risk. Half of the general population demonstrates discordance between LDL-C and LDL particle number, where discordance is defined as a differential in the population percentile of 12% or more, and in such cases, LDL particle number more accurately predicts CVD risk (Davidson et al. 2011). Of note, discordance occurs in as many as 75% of persons with type 2 diabetes mellitus (T2DM) or metabolic syndrome or in people taking statins (Davidson et al. 2011).

Importantly, diet can shift LDL particle distribution and composition as reviewed in Siri-Tarino et al. (2015), such that dietary carbohydrate, which increases triglycerides, is associated with a shift in distribution toward sdLDL particles. In contrast, higher saturated fat content of diets has been associated with larger and more buoyant particles (Dreon et al. 1998, Krauss et al. 2006). Self-reported changes in intake of total SFAs from 6%E to 18%E in the context of high-fat, moderate-carbohydrate diets and lower-fat, higher-carbohydrate diets (46% fat:39% carbohydrate vs. 24% fat:59% carbohydrate, respectively) were positively associated with increases in the mass of large LDL particles, but not with changes in LDL-C concentrations (Dreon et al. 1998). In a carefully executed feeding intervention, high versus low levels (15% and 8%, respectively) of SFAs in the context of a lower carbohydrate (26%) diet showed that the increase in LDL-C on the higher SFA diet was attributable to an increase in larger and medium LDL particles without effects on small, dense particles (Krauss et al. 2006). In contrast, in the context of a diet whose primary protein source was beef (Mangravite et al. 2011) versus mixed protein sources, for example, chicken, fish, and tofu, as provided in the aforementioned dietary intervention trial (Krauss et al. 2006), effects of higher saturated fat (15% vs. 8%) led to increases in sdLDL particles as well as increases in apoB, total, LDL, and non-HDL cholesterol, thus suggesting that very high red meat intake may modify the effects of SFAs on lipid and lipoprotein profiles (Mangravite et al. 2011). Finally, a recent study in persons with pattern B—defined as lipoprotein profiles with a preponderance of sdLDL—showed that very high concentrations of SFAs (18%E vs. 8% E), provided mostly from dairy fat in the context of moderate carbohydrate intake (40% E), resulted in significant increases in the concentrations of small and medium LDL (Chiu et al. 2016b). Thus, the preferential effect of SFAs on larger, more buoyant LDL particles likely depends on context, including but not limited to the food sources of SFAs, the total carbohydrate content of the diet, the metabolic characteristics of the individuals consuming the diet, and/or possible threshold effects for SFAs above which LDL particles of all sizes are affected.

SFAs in Context

Replacement Nutrient

The effects of SFAs on CVD risk in weight-stable individuals are intrinsically a function of the nutrient that replaces it. Although this premise dates back to early metabolic studies conducted in the 1950s, dietary recommendations and public health messaging have generally focused on reducing SFAs without specifying appropriate replacement nutrients (DGAC 2015, Eckel et al. 2014). In meta-analyses summarizing the effects of prospective cohort studies evaluating diet–CVD relationships, SFAs *per se* have not been associated with CVD (Mente et al. 2009, Siri-Tarino et al. 2010, Skeaff and Miller 2009). In part, the lack of association may have been due to the inability to discern from the component studies the effects of the replacement nutrient. In particular, it would be relevant to assess the adverse effects of *trans* fatty acids and refined carbohydrates versus the potential for beneficial effects of PUFAs on CVD risk (Mente et al. 2009, Skeaff and Miller 2009). Importantly, the replacement of SFAs with refined carbohydrates—as commonly occurs in practice—has been associated with no improvement, or a worsening, of CVD risk (Hu 2010).

A meta-analysis of RCTs that specifically considered PUFA replacement of SFAs showed CVD benefit of this replacement scenario at a level comparable to what would have been predicted based on changes in lipid profiles (Micha and Mozaffarian 2010). More recent meta-analyses that included different sets of component studies have presented inconsistent results, with neutral (Chowdhury et al. 2014, Ramsden et al. 2013) or even adverse effects (Ramsden et al. 2010) of PUFAs reported. However, these analyses were compromised by the inclusion of component studies that used *trans* fats in either the control or intervention arms (Willett, Stampfer, and Sacks 2014). *Trans* fats were often used to replace SFAs in food products, but have since been shown to increase LDL-C and triglyceride and decrease HDL-C, and thus increase CVD risk, relative to SFAs (see Chapter 12). A reanalysis of one of the aforementioned meta-analyses with the confounded study excluded showed significant benefit when SFAs were replaced with PUFAs, that is, relative risk for CVD = 0.81 (0.68–0.98) (Chowdhury et al. 2014), in line with a Cochrane review that showed modest but significant benefit on CVD events of this replacement scenario (Hooper et al. 2015).

The type of PUFAs, that is, omega-3 fatty acids and omega-6 fatty acids, used to replace SFAs can differentially affect CVD risk (Ramsden et al. 2013). Omega-3 fatty acids have been associated with CVD benefit in observational studies, although these results have not been supported by recent clinical trials in higher-risk populations (Siri-Tarino et al. 2015). The role of omega-3 fatty acids in primary prevention is currently being investigated. Epidemiological data also support beneficial effects of omega-6 fatty acids (Farvid et al. 2014). Further, plasma biomarkers for omega-6 fatty acids, which can be used to assess their consumption since they cannot be synthesized in vivo, have been associated with improved cardiometabolic risk (Chapter 10).

Given the adverse effects of dietary carbohydrates on components of atherogenic dyslipidemia as described in the following, monounsaturated fatty acids (MUFAs) were shown to be a better replacement for SFAs than carbohydrates in persons at high cardiometabolic risk (Berglund et al. 2007). However, there are observational data in a Finnish population that suggest that MUFA replacement of SFAs, *trans* fats, or carbohydrates is associated with increased CHD risk (Virtanen et al. 2014). There are also intervention studies in African green monkeys on high-cholesterol diets that indicate comparable effects of dietary MUFAs and SFAs on aortic atherosclerosis when compared to PUFAs (Rudel, Parks, and Sawyer 1995). These results, as well as similar findings in hypercholesterolemic mouse models (Degirolamo, Shelness, and Rudel 2009), have been attributed to a more rigid cholesteryl ester structure with MUFAs and SFAs than with PUFAs.

Atherogenic Dyslipidemia and the Obesity and Diabetes Epidemics

As reviewed elsewhere (Siri-Tarino et al. 2015), both excess calories and dietary carbohydrates, particularly refined and processed carbohydrates, can induce or amplify atherogenic dyslipidemia, a trait characterized by a cluster of interrelated lipid and lipoprotein changes, namely elevated triglyceride, reduced HDL-C, and increased sdLDL. Importantly, each of these components has been associated with increased CVD risk (Ballantyne et al. 2001, Manninen et al. 1992, Sarwar et al. 2007). Of note, nonfasting triglyceride, representing in part remnant lipoproteins derived from chylomicron and VLDL triglyceride hydrolysis, can be more strongly predictive of CVD than fasting triglyceride (Bansal et al. 2007, Nordestgaard et al. 2007).

Food Sources of SFAs and Dietary Patterns

The food source of SFAs can modulate their association with CVD risk. In the Multi-Ethnic Study of Atherosclerosis, SFAs from meat were associated with increased CVD risk, whereas consumption of comparable amounts of SFAs from dairy sources was associated with decreased CVD risk (de Oliveira Otto et al. 2012). Epidemiological studies have suggested that red meat intake is more strongly associated with CVD risk than other sources of protein (Bernstein et al. 2012, Sinha et al. 2009) and that the major determinant of this association may be processed red meats (Micha, Wallace, and Mozaffarian 2010). More recently, a carefully controlled feeding trial that compared cheese and meats as food sources matched for SFA content in the context of a diet with 36% of energy from fat relative to a lower-fat (23%E), higher-carbohydrate diet showed a 5% increase in HDL-C and an 8% increase in apoAI in both the cheese and meat groups relative to a lower-fat (23%E), higher-carbohydrate diet (Thorning et al. 2015). However, effects of the high SFAs in the context of either meat or cheese were not observed for LDL or total cholesterol as would have been expected, a finding that may have been due to the high MUFA content of both the cheese and meat diets. Thus, SFA effects on lipoprotein profiles in the context of meat were no different than those for cheese, and these two diets led to less atherogenic profiles compared to a lower-fat, higher-carbohydrate diet (26% energy).

Food sources of dairy have been shown to be relevant, with several studies showing that the consumption of full-fat cheese relative to butter and other nondairy sources of SFAs resulted in lower total and LDL cholesterol (Siri-Tarino et al. 2015). Further, specific evaluation of the SFA content of dairy has not been shown to have adverse effects on lipid and lipoprotein profiles in several recent metabolic studies (Raziani et al. 2016, Thorning et al. 2015). Full-fat versus regular-fat cheese did not adversely alter LDL-C, triglyceride, insulin, glucose, blood pressure, or waist circumference in a real-world study in which these foods were substituted for components of habitual diets (Raziani et al. 2016), suggesting that SFAs in the context of full-fat cheese can be consumed as part of a healthy diet. However, possible attenuation of a cholesterol-raising effect could have been related to weaknesses in study compliance, statistical power, and/or unspecified food replacement scenarios (Siri-Tarino and Krauss 2016). Nonetheless, the neutral or beneficial effects of dairy foods on cardiometabolic profiles irrespective of SFA content may be due to other components of the food source, including vitamin D, calcium, magnesium, potassium, and whey protein. Fermented dairy products, such as yogurt, may be particularly effective at improving cardiometabolic profiles (Astrup 2014, St-Onge, Farnworth, and Jones 2000), possibly through effects on the gut microbiome.

Although tropical oils such as coconut and palm do not represent a major source of SFA consumption in the United States, there is some evidence that lauric acid, the main SFA contained in these foods, does not adversely affect the TC:HDL ratio or other CVD biomarkers (Mensink et al. 2003, Voon et al. 2011).

Variations in SFA content have also been examined in the context of established heart-healthy dietary patterns such as the Dietary Approaches to Stop Hypertension (DASH) diet, which emphasizes fruits, vegetables, low-fat dairy products, whole grains, poultry, fish, and nuts (Appel et al. 1997).

SFA EFFECTS ON OTHER CARDIOMETABOLIC HEALTH RISK FACTORS

Studies of dietary SFAs relative to other macronutrients in the context of weight stability have generally not shown an association with insulin sensitivity and T2DM (Forouhi et al. 2014, Ma et al. 2015, Morio et al. 2016, Siri-Tarino et al. 2015). In particular, replacing SFAs with MUFAs (Chiu et al. 2014, Jebb et al. 2010, Tierney et al. 2011), PUFAs (Tierney et al. 2011), or carbohydrates (Jebb et al. 2010) had no or only modest (Vessby et al. 2001) effects on insulin sensitivity. Dictary SFA intake was not associated with incident diabetes in a meta-analysis (Micha and Mozaffarian 2010).

Plasma concentrations of SFAs have also been evaluated in relation to diabetes risk. Several studies have documented associations of levels of even-chain-length SFAs, that is, C14:0 (myristic), C16:0 (palmitic), and C18:0 (stearic) with increased T2DM risk (Forouhi et al. 2014, Ma et al. 2015). However, it is not clear to what extent these reflect dietary SFA intake as opposed to *de novo* lipogenesis, which is driven by dietary carbohydrates.

In contrast, blood concentrations of odd-chained SFAs have been inversely associated with T2DM. These SFAs (C15:0 and C17:0) reflect the consumption of dairy fats as does the plasma biomarker C16:1n-7, trans-palmitoleic acid, which has also been shown to be inversely associated with insulin resistance (Mozaffarian et al. 2010). As covered in Chapter 25, an emerging literature suggests that dairy foods are neutrally or inversely associated with T2DM (Sluijs et al. 2012). Although some studies point to low-fat, fermented dairy products as being most beneficial (O'Connor et al. 2014), recent studies have suggested that the effects on insulin sensitivity of full-fat dairy are just as beneficial as low-fat dairy products (Benatar, Sidhu, and Stewart 2013). In addition to other components of dairy foods such as calcium, magnesium, and other nutrients that have been associated with improved cardiometabolic risk, dairy foods also contain short- and medium-chain SFAs that have different biological properties and affect health differently (inverse) compared to long-chain SFAs. Thus, the diversity of foods containing SFAs and the heterogeneity of SFAs themselves may modulate insulin sensitivity and provide further substantiation for the concept that consideration for total SFA content of the diet does not provide a meaningful measure of the overall quality of the diet.

Cellular and animal data suggest that diets high in SFAs adversely affect inflammation, but data supporting effects of SFAs on inflammatory markers in humans are more limited (Siri-Tarino et al. 2015). Although one study showed a decrease in two inflammatory markers, interleukin-6 (IL-6) and E-selectin, when oleic acid was replaced with stearic acid or a combination of lauric, myristic, and palmitic acids (Baer et al. 2004), other studies have not demonstrated such effects. Diets high in SFAs, that is, lauric, myristic, and palmitic, did not alter the inflammatory biomarkers TNF-α, IL-1β, IL-6, IL-8, high-sensitivity C-reactive protein (hs-CRP), or interferon-γ (Voon et al. 2011). There was also no effect of high SFAs in the context of a very-low-carbohydrate diet on hs-CRP, IL-6, IL-8, TNFα, or MCP-1 (Forsythe et al. 2010).

Keogh et al. reported impaired flow-mediated dilation (FMD) with administration of diets high in SFAs versus PUFAs, MUFAs, or carbohydrates (Keogh et al. 2005) as did de Roos and Fuentes (de Roos, Bots, and Katan 2001, Fuentes et al. 2001). Sanders et al. showed no changes in FMD with diets high in SFAs (~15% total energy) compared to diets high in MUFAs or carbohydrates with SFAs at ~9% of total energy in 121 insulin-resistant men and women (Sanders et al. 2013). Notably, in the latter study, SFAs were provided by palm oil and milk fat rather than meat fats, and refined high oleic sunflower oil rather than extra-virgin olive oil was used as a source of MUFAs.

In the context of weight loss, very-low-carbohydrate diets high in SFAs were associated with lower concentrations of inflammatory markers compared to a low-fat diet (Forsythe et al. 2008); although weight loss was consistently greater with the very-low-carbohydrate diet, changes in inflammatory markers were not associated with the magnitude of weight loss.

Some evidence exists for modest but significant adverse effects of meals high in SFAs on postprandial inflammatory responses compared to meals rich in PUFAs, MUFAs, or carbohydrates (Masson and Mensink 2011, Nappo et al. 2002, Raz et al. 2013). In contrast, several studies have shown no differences in postprandial inflammatory markers in response to meals of varying food and macronutrient composition (Jimenez-Gomez et al. 2009, Manning et al. 2008, Teng et al. 2015). High versus low PUFA:SFA ratios also did not affect postprandial inflammatory responses (Poppitt et al. 2008). Differences in study population or meal composition may explain the inconsistent results, but overall, no strong evidence in humans is available for SFA effects on inflammation.

As regards blood pressure, while one trial showed a decrease with MUFA, but not SFA (Rasmussen et al. 2006), and another showed a decrease with PUFA or MUFA replacement of SFAs (Lahoz et al. 1997), seven other trials showed no effects of replacing SFAs with PUFAs, MUFAs, or carbohydrates on blood pressure (Micha and Mozaffarian 2010). Importantly, high saturated fat (14% of energy) in the context of the DASH diet was shown to lead to comparable reductions in blood pressure compared to a DASH diet with low saturated fat (8% of energy) (Chiu et al. 2016a), emphasizing the role of dietary pattern over macronutrients in the determination of cardiometabolic health.

VARIABILITY IN RESPONSE OF LDL-C TO SATURATED FAT

Persons with a higher baseline LDL-C have been shown to respond to reductions in SFAs with greater reductions in LDL-C (Denke 1995). In addition, overweight (Chiu et al. 2014) and insulin-resistant (Lefevre et al. 2005) individuals have been reported to be less responsive to the effects of SFAs on LDL-C, as have women versus men (Weggemans et al. 1999).

A number of genetic variants have been reported to be associated with LDL-C response to SFA intake. Among the most consistent of these is the relation of the apoE4 isoform with a greater LDL-C response (Dreon et al. 1995). Similarly, the presence of serine to threonine at position 347 in the apoAIV gene was associated with a greater LDL response to a change from a higher SFA diet to a National Cholesterol Education Program Step 1 diet (Jansen et al. 1997). Replacement of dietary SFAs with PUFAs was associated with no changes in LDL-C but greater decreases in dense LDL-C in persons with a glutamine to histidine substitution at position 360 (Wallace et al. 2000). Polymorphisms in apoB have also been shown to modulate effects of changes in dietary fat on LDL-C, although none of these were specifically related to changes in dietary SFAs (Masson, McNeill, and Avenell 2003). Cumulatively, however, the effect sizes for these genetic influences on dietary LDL-C are small and account for only a minimal portion of interindividual variation in response.

APPLYING NEW KNOWLEDGE TO DIETARY GUIDELINES

The message to reduce SFAs has been an oversimplified one, which may have unintentionally led to the increased consumption of refined and processed carbohydrates, a replacement scenario that has been associated with no benefit or even a worsening of CVD risk, at least in part through its induction of atherogenic dyslipidemia. In light of the current epidemics of obesity and insulin resistance, reduction of sugars and refined carbohydrates as sources of high calories but also for their specific adverse metabolic effects may be more effective in improving cardiometabolic health. Of note, processed food formulations that combine high sugars and high SFAs and are stripped of nutritional content may represent a different category of "foods" and may be particularly detrimental.

The 2015 Dietary Guidelines for Americans have moved toward recommending foods and dietary patterns, but the specification of a limitation on SFAs is retained (DGAC 2015). In contrast, the Dutch have recently moved away from nutrient recommendations as first issued in 1986 toward guidelines that are exclusively food based (Kromhout et al. 2016). In France, dietary guidelines advise the limitation of total SFAs to less than 12% of energy, but also consider SFA subtypes, with a specific limitation of lauric, myristic, and palmitic to less than 8% (Nettleton, Legrand, and Mensink 2015). Thus, an appreciation for the complexity and subtleties of the SFA–CVD relationship is now beginning to shape recommendations for public health.

CONCLUSIONS

Investigation of the effects of dietary SFAs on cardiometabolic risk over the last half century has revealed the complexity and nuances of this relationship. Although it is clear that SFAs in relation to other macronutrients can affect lipid and lipoprotein profiles, the evidence for effects of dietary SFAs on other CVD risk factors such as blood pressure, insulin sensitivity, inflammation, and endothelial function is equivocal. The diversity of SFAs and the variable food sources and dietary patterns in which they are consumed modulate their effects.

REFERENCES

Ahrens, E. H., Jr., D. H. Blankenhorn, and T. T. Tsaltas. 1954. Effect on human serum lipids of substituting plant for animal fat in diet. *Proc Soc Exp Biol Med* 86 (4):872–878.

Anitschkow, N. 1913. Ueber die Veranderungen der Kaninchenaorta bei experimenteller Cholesterinsteatose. *Beitr Pathol Anat* 56:379–404.

Appel, L. J., T. J. Moore, E. Obarzanek, W. M. Vollmer, L. P. Svetkey, F. M. Sacks, G. A. Bray et al. 1997. A clinical trial of the effects of dietary patterns on blood pressure. DASH Collaborative Research Group. *N Engl J Med* 336 (16):1117–1124. doi: 10.1056/NEJM199704173361601.

Astrup, A. 2014. Yogurt and dairy product consumption to prevent cardiometabolic diseases: Epidemiologic and experimental studies. *Am J Clin Nutr* 99 (5 Suppl):1235S–1242S. doi: 10.3945/ajcn.113.073015.

Baer, D. J., J. T. Judd, B. A. Clevidence, and R. P. Tracy. 2004. Dietary fatty acids affect plasma markers of inflammation in healthy men fed controlled diets: A randomized crossover study. *Am J Clin Nutr* 79 (6):969–973.

Ballantyne, C. M., A. G. Olsson, T. J. Cook, M. F. Mercuri, T. R. Pedersen, and J. Kjekshus. 2001. Influence of low high-density lipoprotein cholesterol and elevated triglyceride on coronary heart disease events and response to simvastatin therapy in 4S. *Circulation* 104 (25):3046–3051.

Bansal, S., J. E. Buring, N. Rifai, S. Mora, F. M. Sacks, and P. M. Ridker. 2007. Fasting compared with nonfasting triglycerides and risk of cardiovascular events in women. *JAMA* 298 (3):309–316. doi: 10.1001/jama.298.3.309.

Benatar, J. R., K. Sidhu, and R. A. Stewart. 2013. Effects of high and low fat dairy food on cardio-metabolic risk factors: A meta-analysis of randomized studies. *PLoS One* 8 (10):e76480. doi: 10.1371/journal.pone.0076480.

Berglund, L., M. Lefevre, H. N. Ginsberg, P. M. Kris-Etherton, P. J. Elmer, P. W. Stewart, A. Ershow et al. 2007. Comparison of monounsaturated fat with carbohydrates as a replacement for saturated fat in subjects with a high metabolic risk profile: Studies in the fasting and postprandial states. *Am J Clin Nutr* 86 (6):1611–1620.

Berneis, K. K. and R. M. Krauss. 2002. Metabolic origins and clinical significance of LDL heterogeneity. *J Lipid Res* 43 (9):1363–1379.

Bernstein, A. M., A. Pan, K. M. Rexrode, M. Stampfer, F. B. Hu, D. Mozaffarian, and W. C. Willett. 2012. Dietary protein sources and the risk of stroke in men and women. *Stroke* 43 (3):637–644. doi: 10.1161/STROKEAHA.111.633404.

Burr, M. L., A. M. Fehily, J. F. Gilbert, S. Rogers, R. M. Holliday, P. M. Sweetnam, P. C. Elwood, and N. M. Deadman. 1989. Effects of changes in fat, fish, and fibre intakes on death and myocardial reinfarction: Diet and reinfarction trial (DART). *Lancet* 2 (8666):757–761.

Chiu, S., N. Bergeron, P. T. Williams, G. A. Bray, B. Sutherland, and R. M. Krauss. 2016a. Comparison of the DASH (Dietary Approaches to Stop Hypertension) diet and a higher-fat DASH diet on blood pressure and lipids and lipoproteins: A randomized controlled trial. *Am J Clin Nutr* 103 (2):341–347. doi: 10.3945/ajcn.115.123281.

Chiu, S., P. T. Williams, T. Dawson, R. N. Bergman, D. Stefanovski, S. M. Watkins, and R. M. Krauss. 2014. Diets high in protein or saturated fat do not affect insulin sensitivity or plasma concentrations of lipids and lipoproteins in overweight and obese adults. *J Nutr* 144 (11):1753–1759. doi: 10.3945/jn.114.197624.

Chiu, S., P. T. Williams, and R. M. Krauss, 2016b. Effects of a high saturated fat diet on LDL particles in adults with atherogenic dyslipidemia: A randomized controlled trial. *PLoS One* 12 (2):e0170664. doi: 10.1371/journal.pone.0170664.

Chow, C. K., ed. 2000. *Fatty Acids in Foods and their Health Implications*. New York: Marcel Dekker, Inc.

Chowdhury, R., S. Warnakula, S. Kunutsor, F. Crowe, H. A. Ward, L. Johnson, O. H. Franco et al. 2014. Association of dietary, circulating, and supplement fatty acids with coronary risk: A systematic review and meta-analysis. *Ann Intern Med* 160 (6):398–406. doi: 10.7326/M13-1788.

Davidson, M. H., C. M. Ballantyne, T. A. Jacobson, V. A. Bittner, L. T. Braun, A. S. Brown, W. V. Brown et al. 2011. Clinical utility of inflammatory markers and advanced lipoprotein testing: Advice from an expert panel of lipid specialists. *J Clin Lipidol* 5 (5):338–367. doi: 10.1016/j.jacl.2011.07.005.

Dayton, S. and M. L. Pearce. 1969. Diet high in unsaturated fat. A controlled clinical trial. *Minn Med* 52 (8):1237–1242.

de Oliveira Otto, M. C., D. Mozaffarian, D. Kromhout, A. G. Bertoni, C. T. Sibley, D. R. Jacobs, Jr., and J. A. Nettleton. 2012. Dietary intake of saturated fat by food source and incident cardiovascular disease: The Multi-Ethnic Study of Atherosclerosis. *Am J Clin Nutr* 96 (2):397–404. doi: 10.3945/ajcn.112.037770.

de Roos, N. M., M. L. Bots, and M. B. Katan. 2001. Replacement of dietary saturated fatty acids by trans fatty acids lowers serum HDL cholesterol and impairs endothelial function in healthy men and women. *Arterioscler Thromb Vasc Biol* 21 (7):1233–1237.

Degirolamo, C., G. S. Shelness, and L. L. Rudel. 2009. LDL cholesteryl oleate as a predictor for atherosclerosis: Evidence from human and animal studies on dietary fat. *J Lipid Res* 50 (Suppl):S434–S439. doi: 10.1194/jlr.R800076-JLR200.

Denke, M. A. 1995. Review of human studies evaluating individual dietary responsiveness in patients with hypercholesterolemia. *Am J Clin Nutr* 62 (2):471S–477S.

DGAC. 2015. *Scientific Report of the 2015 Dietary Guidelines Advisory Committee*. Accessed July 18, 2017. https://health.gov/dietaryguidelines/2015-scientific-report/pdfs/scientific-report-of-the-2015-dietary-guidelines-advisory-committee.pdf.

Dreon, D. M., H. A. Fernstrom, H. Campos, P. Blanche, P. T. Williams, and R. M. Krauss. 1998. Change in dietary saturated fat intake is correlated with change in mass of large low-density-lipoprotein particles in men. *Am J Clin Nutr* 67 (5):828–836.

Dreon, D. M., H. A. Fernstrom, B. Miller, and R. M. Krauss. 1995. Apolipoprotein E isoform phenotype and LDL subclass response to a reduced-fat diet. *Arterioscler Thromb Vasc Biol* 15 (1):105–111.

Eckel, R. H., J. M. Jakicic, J. D. Ard, J. M. de Jesus, N. Houston Miller, V. S. Hubbard, I. M. Lee et al., Guidelines American College of Cardiology/American Heart Association Task Force on Practice. 2014. 2013 AHA/ACC guideline on lifestyle management to reduce cardiovascular risk: A report of the American College of Cardiology/American Heart Association Task Force on Practice Guidelines. *J Am Coll Cardiol* 63 (25 Pt B):2960–2984. doi: 10.1016/j.jacc.2013.11.003.

Farvid, M. S., M. Ding, A. Pan, Q. Sun, S. E. Chiuve, L. M. Steffen, W. C. Willett, and F. B. Hu. 2014. Dietary linoleic acid and risk of coronary heart disease: A systematic review and meta-analysis of prospective cohort studies. *Circulation* 130 (18):1568–1578. doi: 10.1161/CIRCULATIONAHA.114.010236.

Forouhi, N. G., A. Koulman, S. J. Sharp, F. Imamura, J. Kroger, M. B. Schulze, F. L. Crowe et al. 2014. Differences in the prospective association between individual plasma phospholipid saturated fatty acids and incident type 2 diabetes: The EPIC-InterAct case-cohort study. *Lancet Diabetes Endocrinol* 2 (10):810–818. doi: 10.1016/S2213-8587(14)70146-9.

Forsythe, C. E., S. D. Phinney, R. D. Feinman, B. M. Volk, D. Freidenreich, E. Quann, K. Ballard et al. 2010. Limited effect of dietary saturated fat on plasma saturated fat in the context of a low carbohydrate diet. *Lipids* 45 (10):947–962. doi: 10.1007/s11745-010-3467-3.

Forsythe, C. E., S. D. Phinney, M. L. Fernandez, E. E. Quann, R. J. Wood, D. M. Bibus, W. J. Kraemer, R. D. Feinman, and J. S. Volek. 2008. Comparison of low fat and low carbohydrate diets on circulating fatty acid composition and markers of inflammation. *Lipids* 43 (1):65–77. doi: 10.1007/s11745-007-3132-7.

Frantz, I. D., Jr., E. A. Dawson, P. L. Ashman, L. C. Gatewood, G. E. Bartsch, K. Kuba, and E. R. Brewer. 1989. Test of effect of lipid lowering by diet on cardiovascular risk. The Minnesota Coronary Survey. *Arteriosclerosis* 9 (1):129–135.

Fuentes, F., J. Lopez-Miranda, E. Sanchez, F. Sanchez, J. Paez, E. Paz-Rojas, C. Marin et al. 2001. Mediterranean and low-fat diets improve endothelial function in hypercholesterolemic men. *Ann Intern Med* 134 (12):1115–1119.

Hayes, K. C., P. Khosla, T. Hajri, and A. Pronczuk. 1997. Saturated fatty acids and LDL receptor modulation in humans and monkeys. *Prostaglandins Leukot Essent Fatty Acids* 57 (4–5):411–418.

Hegsted, D. M., R. B. McGandy, M. L. Myers, and F. J. Stare. 1965. Quantitative effects of dietary fat on serum cholesterol in man. *Am J Clin Nutr* 17 (5):281–295.

Hoogeveen, R. C., J. W. Gaubatz, W. Sun, R. C. Dodge, J. R. Crosby, J. Jiang, D. Couper et al. 2014. Small dense low-density lipoprotein-cholesterol concentrations predict risk for coronary heart disease: The Atherosclerosis Risk In Communities (ARIC) study. *Arterioscler Thromb Vasc Biol* 34 (5):1069–1077. doi: 10.1161/ATVBAHA.114.303284.

Hooper, L., N. Martin, A. Abdelhamid, and G. Davey Smith. 2015. Reduction in saturated fat intake for cardiovascular disease. *Cochrane Database Syst Rev* 6:CD011737. doi: 10.1002/14651858.CD011737.

Hu, F. B. 2010. Are refined carbohydrates worse than saturated fat? *Am J Clin Nutr* 91 (6):1541–1542. doi: 10.3945/ajcn.2010.29622.

Ignatowski, A. 1909. Uber die Wirkung des Tierischen Eiweisses auf die Aorta und die paerenchymatosen Organe der Kaninchen. *Virchows Arch Pathol Anat* 198:248–270.

Jansen, S., J. Lopez-Miranda, J. Salas, J. M. Ordovas, P. Castro, C. Marin, M. A. Ostos et al. 1997. Effect of 347-serine mutation in apoprotein A-IV on plasma LDL cholesterol response to dietary fat. *Arterioscler Thromb Vasc Biol* 17 (8):1532–1538.

Jebb, S. A., J. A. Lovegrove, B. A. Griffin, G. S. Frost, C. S. Moore, M. D. Chatfield, L. J. Bluck, C. M. Williams, and T. A. Sanders. 2010. Effect of changing the amount and type of fat and carbohydrate on insulin sensitivity and cardiovascular risk: The RISCK (Reading, Imperial, Surrey, Cambridge, and Kings) trial. *Am J Clin Nutr* 92 (4):748–758. doi: 10.3945/ajcn.2009.29096.

Jimenez-Gomez, Y., J. Lopez-Miranda, L. M. Blanco-Colio, C. Marin, P. Perez-Martinez, J. Ruano, J. A. Paniagua, F. Rodriguez, J. Egido, and F. Perez-Jimenez. 2009. Olive oil and walnut breakfasts reduce the postprandial inflammatory response in mononuclear cells compared with a butter breakfast in healthy men. *Atherosclerosis* 204 (2):e70–e76. doi: 10.1016/j.atherosclerosis.2008.09.011.

Keogh, J. B., J. A. Grieger, M. Noakes, and P. M. Clifton. 2005. Flow-mediated dilatation is impaired by a high-saturated fat diet but not by a high-carbohydrate diet. *Arterioscler Thromb Vasc Biol* 25 (6):1274–1279. doi: 10.1161/01.ATV.0000163185.28245.a1.

Keys, A., J. T. Anderson, and F. Grande. 1957. Prediction of serum-cholesterol responses of man to changes in fats in the diet. *Lancet* 273 (7003):959–966.

Keys, A., C. Aravanis, H. W. Blackburn, F. S. Van Buchem, R. Buzina, B. D. Djordjevic, A. S. Dontas et al. 1966. Epidemiological studies related to coronary heart disease: Characteristics of men aged 40–59 in seven countries. *Acta Med Scand Suppl* 460:1–392.

Kinsell, L. W., J. Partridge, L. Boling, S. Margen, and G. Michaels. 1952. Dietary modification of serum cholesterol and phospholipid levels. *J Clin Endocrinol Metab* 12 (7):909–913. doi: 10.1210/jcem-12-7-909.

Konstantinov, I. E., N. Mejevoi, and N. M. Anichkov. 2006. Nikolai N. Anichkov and his theory of atherosclerosis. *Tex Heart Inst J* 33 (4):417–423.

Krauss, R. M. 2014. All low-density lipoprotein particles are not created equal. *Arterioscler Thromb Vasc Biol* 34 (5):959–961. doi: 10.1161/ATVBAHA.114.303458.

Krauss, R. M., P. J. Blanche, R. S. Rawlings, H. S. Fernstrom, and P. T. Williams. 2006. Separate effects of reduced carbohydrate intake and weight loss on atherogenic dyslipidemia. *Am J Clin Nutr* 83 (5):1025–1031.

Kromhout, D., C. J. Spaaij, J. de Goede, and R. M. Weggemans. 2016. The 2015 Dutch food-based dietary guidelines. *Eur J Clin Nutr* 70 (8):869–878. doi: 10.1038/ejcn.2016.52.

Lahoz, C., R. Alonso, J. M. Ordovas, A. Lopez-Farre, M. de Oya, and P. Mata. 1997. Effects of dietary fat saturation on eicosanoid production, platelet aggregation and blood pressure. *Eur J Clin Invest* 27 (9):780–787.

Lefevre, M., C. M. Champagne, R. T. Tulley, J. C. Rood, and M. M. Most. 2005. Individual variability in cardiovascular disease risk factor responses to low-fat and low-saturated-fat diets in men: Body mass index, adiposity, and insulin resistance predict changes in LDL cholesterol. *Am J Clin Nutr* 82 (5):957–963.

Legrand, P. and V. Rioux. 2010. The complex and important cellular and metabolic functions of saturated fatty acids. *Lipids* 45 (10):941–946. doi: 10.1007/s11745-010-3444-x.

Leren, P. 1970. The Oslo diet-heart study. Eleven-year report. *Circulation* 42 (5):935–942.

Lustig, R. H. 2012. *Fat Chance: Beating the Odds against Sugar, Processed Food, Obesity and Disease*. Plume (Penguin Random House, New York).

Ma, W., J. H. Wu, Q. Wang, R. N. Lemaitre, K. J. Mukamal, L. Djousse, I. B. King et al. 2015. Prospective association of fatty acids in the *de novo* lipogenesis pathway with risk of type 2 diabetes: The Cardiovascular Health Study. *Am J Clin Nutr* 101 (1):153–163. doi: 10.3945/ajcn.114.092601.

Mangravite, L. M., S. Chiu, K. Wojnoonski, R. S. Rawlings, N. Bergeron, and R. M. Krauss. 2011. Changes in atherogenic dyslipidemia induced by carbohydrate restriction in men are dependent on dietary protein source. *J Nutr* 141 (12):2180–2185. doi: 10.3945/jn.111.139477.

Manninen, V., L. Tenkanen, P. Koskinen, J. K. Huttunen, M. Manttari, O. P. Heinonen, and M. H. Frick. 1992. Joint effects of serum triglyceride and LDL cholesterol and HDL cholesterol concentrations on coronary heart disease risk in the Helsinki Heart Study. Implications for treatment. *Circulation* 85 (1):37–45.

Manning, P. J., W. H. Sutherland, M. M. McGrath, S. A. de Jong, R. J. Walker, and M. J. Williams. 2008. Postprandial cytokine concentrations and meal composition in obese and lean women. *Obesity (Silver Spring)* 16 (9):2046–2052. doi: 10.1038/oby.2008.334.

Masson, C. J. and R. P. Mensink. 2011. Exchanging saturated fatty acids for (n-6) polyunsaturated fatty acids in a mixed meal may decrease postprandial lipemia and markers of inflammation and endothelial activity in overweight men. *J Nutr* 141 (5):816–821. doi: 10.3945/jn.110.136432.

Masson, L. F., G. McNeill, and A. Avenell. 2003. Genetic variation and the lipid response to dietary intervention: A systematic review. *Am J Clin Nutr* 77 (5):1098–1111.

Mensink, R. P. and M. B. Katan. 1992. Effect of dietary fatty acids on serum lipids and lipoproteins. A meta-analysis of 27 trials. *Arterioscler Thromb* 12 (8):911–919.

Mensink, R. P., P. L. Zock, A. D. Kester, and M. B. Katan. 2003. Effects of dietary fatty acids and carbohydrates on the ratio of serum total to HDL cholesterol and on serum lipids and apolipoproteins: A meta-analysis of 60 controlled trials. *Am J Clin Nutr* 77 (5):1146–1155.

Mente, A., L. de Koning, H. S. Shannon, and S. S. Anand. 2009. A systematic review of the evidence supporting a causal link between dietary factors and coronary heart disease. *Arch Intern Med* 169 (7):659–669. doi: 10.1001/archinternmed.2009.38.

Micha, R. and D. Mozaffarian. 2010. Saturated fat and cardiometabolic risk factors, coronary heart disease, stroke, and diabetes: A fresh look at the evidence. *Lipids* 45 (10):893–905. doi: 10.1007/s11745-010-3393-4.

Micha, R., S. K. Wallace, and D. Mozaffarian. 2010. Red and processed meat consumption and risk of incident coronary heart disease, stroke, and diabetes mellitus: A systematic review and meta-analysis. *Circulation* 121 (21):2271–2283. doi: 10.1161/CIRCULATIONAHA.109.924977.

Morio, B., A. Fardet, P. Legrand, and J. M. Lecerf. 2016. Involvement of dietary saturated fats, from all sources or of dairy origin only, in insulin resistance and type 2 diabetes. *Nutr Rev* 74 (1):33–47. doi: 10.1093/nutrit/nuv043.

Mozaffarian, D. 2016. Dietary and policy priorities for cardiovascular disease, diabetes, and obesity: A comprehensive review. *Circulation* 133 (2):187–225. doi: 10.1161/CIRCULATIONAHA.115.018585.

Mozaffarian, D., H. Cao, I. B. King, R. N. Lemaitre, X. Song, D. S. Siscovick, and G. S. Hotamisligil. 2010. Trans-palmitoleic acid, metabolic risk factors, and new-onset diabetes in U.S. adults: A cohort study. *Ann Intern Med* 153 (12):790–799. doi: 10.1059/0003-4819-153-12-201012210-00005.

Nappo, F., K. Esposito, M. Cioffi, G. Giugliano, A. M. Molinari, G. Paolisso, R. Marfella, and D. Giugliano. 2002. Postprandial endothelial activation in healthy subjects and in type 2 diabetic patients: Role of fat and carbohydrate meals. *J Am Coll Cardiol* 39 (7):1145–1150.

Nettleton, J. A., P. Legrand, and R. P. Mensink. 2015. ISSFAL 2014 debate: It is time to update saturated fat recommendations. *Ann Nutr Metab* 66 (2–3):104–108. doi: 10.1159/000371585.

Nordestgaard, B. G., M. Benn, P. Schnohr, and A. Tybjaerg-Hansen. 2007. Nonfasting triglycerides and risk of myocardial infarction, ischemic heart disease, and death in men and women. *JAMA* 298 (3):299–308. doi: 10.1001/jama.298.3.299.

O'Connor, L. M., M. A. Lentjes, R. N. Luben, K. T. Khaw, N. J. Wareham, and N. G. Forouhi. 2014. Dietary dairy product intake and incident type 2 diabetes: A prospective study using dietary data from a 7-day food diary. *Diabetologia* 57 (5):909–917. doi: 10.1007/s00125-014-3176-1.

Poppitt, S. D., G. F. Keogh, F. E. Lithander, Y. Wang, T. B. Mulvey, Y. K. Chan, B. H. McArdle, and G. J. Cooper. 2008. Postprandial response of adiponectin, interleukin-6, tumor necrosis factor-alpha, and C-reactive protein to a high-fat dietary load. *Nutrition* 24 (4):322–329. doi: 10.1016/j.nut.2007.12.012.

Ramsden, C. E., J. R. Hibbeln, S. F. Majchrzak, and J. M. Davis. 2010. n-6 fatty acid-specific and mixed polyunsaturate dietary interventions have different effects on CHD risk: A meta-analysis of randomised controlled trials. *Br J Nutr* 104 (11):1586–1600. doi: 10.1017/S0007114510004010.

Ramsden, C. E., D. Zamora, B. Leelarthaepin, S. F. Majchrzak-Hong, K. R. Faurot, C. M. Suchindran, A. Ringel, J. M. Davis, and J. R. Hibbeln. 2013. Use of dietary linoleic acid for secondary prevention of coronary heart disease and death: Evaluation of recovered data from the Sydney Diet Heart Study and updated meta-analysis. *BMJ* 346:e8707. doi: 10.1136/bmj.e8707.

Rasmussen, B. M., B. Vessby, M. Uusitupa, L. Berglund, E. Pedersen, G. Riccardi, A. A. Rivellese, L. Tapsell, and K. Hermansen. 2006. Effects of dietary saturated, monounsaturated, and n-3 fatty acids on blood pressure in healthy subjects. *Am J Clin Nutr* 83 (2):221–226.

Raz, O., A. Steinvil, S. Berliner, T. Rosenzweig, D. Justo, and I. Shapira. 2013. The effect of two iso-caloric meals containing equal amounts of fats with a different fat composition on the inflammatory and metabolic markers in apparently healthy volunteers. *J Inflamm (Lond)* 10 (1):3. doi: 10.1186/1476-9255-10-3.

Raziani, F., T. Tholstrup, M. D. Kristensen, M. L. Svanegaard, C. Ritz, A. Astrup, and A. Raben. 2016. High intake of regular-fat cheese compared with reduced-fat cheese does not affect LDL cholesterol or risk markers of the metabolic syndrome: A randomized controlled trial. *Am J Clin Nutr* 104 (4):973–981. doi: 10.3945/ajcn.116.134932.

Rhee, S. K., A. J. Kayani, A. Ciszek, and J. T. Brenna. 1997. Desaturation and interconversion of dietary stearic and palmitic acids in human plasma and lipoproteins. *Am J Clin Nutr* 65 (2):451–458.

Rudel, L. L., J. S. Parks, and J. K. Sawyer. 1995. Compared with dietary monounsaturated and saturated fat, polyunsaturated fat protects African green monkeys from coronary artery atherosclerosis. *Arterioscler Thromb Vasc Biol* 15 (12):2101–2110.

Sanders, T. A., F. J. Lewis, L. M. Goff, P. J. Chowienczyk, and Risck Study Group. 2013. SFAs do not impair endothelial function and arterial stiffness. *Am J Clin Nutr* 98 (3):677–683. doi: 10.3945/ajcn.113.063644.

Sarwar, N., J. Danesh, G. Eiriksdottir, G. Sigurdsson, N. Wareham, S. Bingham, S. M. Boekholdt, K. T. Khaw, and V. Gudnason. 2007. Triglycerides and the risk of coronary heart disease: 10,158 incident cases among 262,525 participants in 29 Western prospective studies. *Circulation* 115 (4):450–458. doi: 10.1161/CIRCULATIONAHA.106.637793.

Sinha, R., A. J. Cross, B. I. Graubard, M. F. Leitzmann, and A. Schatzkin. 2009. Meat intake and mortality: A prospective study of over half a million people. *Arch Intern Med* 169 (6):562–571. doi: 10.1001/archinternmed.2009.6.

Siri-Tarino, P. W., S. Chiu, N. Bergeron, and R. M. Krauss. 2015. Saturated fats versus polyunsaturated fats versus carbohydrates for cardiovascular disease prevention and treatment. *Annu Rev Nutr* 35:517–543. doi: 10.1146/annurev-nutr-071714-034449.

Siri-Tarino, P. W. and R. M. Krauss. 2016. Which cheese to choose? *Am J Clin Nutr* 104 (4):953–954. doi: 10.3945/ajcn.116.143305.

Siri-Tarino, P. W., Q. Sun, F. B. Hu, and R. M. Krauss. 2010. Meta-analysis of prospective cohort studies evaluating the association of saturated fat with cardiovascular disease. *Am J Clin Nutr* 91 (3):535–546. doi: 10.3945/ajcn.2009.27725.

Skeaff, C. M. and J. Miller. 2009. Dietary fat and coronary heart disease: Summary of evidence from prospective cohort and randomised controlled trials. *Ann Nutr Metab* 55 (1–3):173–201. doi: 10.1159/000229002.

Sluijs, I., N. G. Forouhi, J. W. Beulens, Y. T. van der Schouw, C. Agnoli, L. Arriola, B. Balkau et al. 2012. The amount and type of dairy product intake and incident type 2 diabetes: Results from the EPIC-InterAct Study. *Am J Clin Nutr* 96 (2):382–390. doi: 10.3945/ajcn.111.021907.

Steinberg, D. 2004. Thematic review series: The pathogenesis of atherosclerosis. An interpretive history of the cholesterol controversy: Part I. *J Lipid Res* 45 (9):1583–1593. doi: 10.1194/jlr.R400003-JLR200.

St-Onge, M. P., E. R. Farnworth, and P. J. Jones. 2000. Consumption of fermented and nonfermented dairy products: Effects on cholesterol concentrations and metabolism. *Am J Clin Nutr* 71 (3):674–681.

Taubes, G. 2007. *Good Calories, Bad Calories*. New York: Knopf Doubleday Publishing Group.

Teng, K. T., C. Y. Chang, M. S. Kanthimathi, A. T. Tan, and K. Nesaretnam. 2015. Effects of amount and type of dietary fats on postprandial lipemia and thrombogenic markers in individuals with metabolic syndrome. *Atherosclerosis* 242 (1):281–287. doi: 10.1016/j.atherosclerosis.2015.07.003.

Thorning, T. K., F. Raziani, N. T. Bendsen, A. Astrup, T. Tholstrup, and A. Raben. 2015. Diets with high-fat cheese, high-fat meat, or carbohydrate on cardiovascular risk markers in overweight postmenopausal women: A randomized crossover trial. *Am J Clin Nutr* 102 (3):573–581. doi: 10.3945/ajcn.115.109116.

Tierney, A. C., J. McMonagle, D. I. Shaw, H. L. Gulseth, O. Helal, W. H. Saris, J. A. Paniagua et al. 2011. Effects of dietary fat modification on insulin sensitivity and on other risk factors of the metabolic syndrome—LIPGENE: A European randomized dietary intervention study. *Int J Obes (Lond)* 35 (6):800–809. doi: 10.1038/ijo.2010.209.

Tsai, M. Y., B. T. Steffen, W. Guan, R. L. McClelland, R. Warnick, J. McConnell, D. M. Hoefner, and A. T. Remaley. 2014. New automated assay of small dense low-density lipoprotein cholesterol identifies risk of coronary heart disease: The Multi-ethnic Study of Atherosclerosis. *Arterioscler Thromb Vasc Biol* 34 (1):196–201. doi: 10.1161/ATVBAHA.113.302401.

Turpeinen, O., M. J. Karvonen, M. Pekkarinen, M. Miettinen, R. Elosuo, and E. Paavilainen. 1979. Dietary prevention of coronary heart disease: The Finnish Mental Hospital Study. *Int J Epidemiol* 8 (2):99–118.

United States Department of Agriculture and Department of Health and Human Services. 1980. Nutrition and your health: Dietary guidelines for Americans. Accessed on July 18, 2017. https://health.gov/dietaryguidelines/1980thin.pdf?_ga=1.154075386.374455698.1466036773.

Vessby, B., M. Uusitupa, K. Hermansen, G. Riccardi, A. A. Rivellese, L. C. Tapsell, C. Nalsen et al. 2001. Substituting dietary saturated for monounsaturated fat impairs insulin sensitivity in healthy men and women: The KANWU Study. *Diabetologia* 44 (3):312–319.

Virtanen, J. K., J. Mursu, T. P. Tuomainen, and S. Voutilainen. 2014. Dietary fatty acids and risk of coronary heart disease in men: The Kuopio Ischemic Heart Disease Risk Factor Study. *Arterioscler Thromb Vasc Biol* 34 (12):2679–2687. doi: 10.1161/ATVBAHA.114.304082.

Voon, P. T., T. K. Ng, V. K. Lee, and K. Nesaretnam. 2011. Diets high in palmitic acid (16:0), lauric and myristic acids (12:0 + 14:0), or oleic acid (18:1) do not alter postprandial or fasting plasma homocysteine and inflammatory markers in healthy Malaysian adults. *Am J Clin Nutr* 94 (6):1451–1457. doi: 10.3945/ajcn.111.020107.

Wallace, A. J., S. E. Humphries, R. M. Fisher, J. I. Mann, A. Chisholm, and W. H. Sutherland. 2000. Genetic factors associated with response of LDL subfractions to change in the nature of dietary fat. *Atherosclerosis* 149 (2):387–394.

Watts, G. F., B. Lewis, J. N. Brunt, E. S. Lewis, D. J. Coltart, L. D. Smith, J. I. Mann, and A. V. Swan. 1992. Effects on coronary artery disease of lipid-lowering diet, or diet plus cholestyramine, in the St Thomas' Atherosclerosis Regression Study (STARS). *Lancet* 339 (8793):563–569.

Weggemans, R. M., P. L. Zock, R. Urgert, and M. B. Katan. 1999. Differences between men and women in the response of serum cholesterol to dietary changes. *Eur J Clin Invest* 29 (10):827–834.

Willett, W. C., M. J. Stampfer, and F. M. Sacks. 2014. Association of dietary, circulating, and supplement fatty acids with coronary risk. *Ann Intern Med* 161 (6):453. doi: 10.7326/L14-5018.

12 Effects of Dietary *Trans* Fatty Acids on Cardiovascular Risk

Ronald P. Mensink

CONTENTS

ABSTRACT

Most double bonds of the unsaturated fatty acids in the diet have the so-called *cis* configuration, but fatty acids with double bonds in the *trans* configuration also exist. These so-called *trans* fatty acids (TFA) are mainly produced by the industry during the partial hydrogenation of vegetable oils rich in *cis*-polyunsaturated fatty acids (linoleic acid and α-linolenic acid) like sunflower oil and soybean oil. However, TFA are also formed by the bacterial transformation of polyunsaturated fatty acids in the first stomach of ruminant animals. This chapter first summarizes the effects of TFA intake on the serum lipoprotein profile and other markers related to cardiometabolic health. Then, relationships with cardiovascular risk are discussed.

ABBREVIATIONS

CHD Coronary heart disease
CLA Conjugated linoleic acid
CVD Cardiovascular disease
HDL High-density lipoproteins
iTFA Industrially produced *trans* fatty acids
LDL Low-density lipoproteins
rTFA Ruminant *trans* fatty acids
TFA *Trans* fatty acids

INTRODUCTION

Most double bonds of the unsaturated fatty acids in the diet have the so-called *cis* configuration, but fatty acids with double bonds in the *trans* configuration also exist. These so-called *trans* fatty acids (TFA) are mainly produced during the partial hydrogenation of vegetable oils rich in *cis*-polyunsaturated fatty acids (linoleic acid and α-linolenic acid) like sunflower oil and soybean oil. Through partial hydrogenation, the liquid oils are converted into fats with increased functionality and stability that can be used for frying and baking and for the manufacturing of foods such as biscuits, shortening, and margarines with longer shelf life. Fats rich in these industrially produced TFA (iTFA) were mainly used as substitutes for natural fats rich in saturated fatty acids such as butter, lard, and tropical oils. Typically, these iTFA have 18 carbon atoms and one double bond, mainly located between the (n-5)-carbon and the (n-12)-carbon atom. When the double bond is located at the (n-9)-position, this specific TFA isomer is called elaidic acid (*trans*-C18:1n-9). In contrast to partial hydrogenation, the full hydrogenation of vegetables oils does not result in the production of TFA but of stearic acid (Figure 12.1). However, TFA are also formed by the bacterial transformation of polyunsaturated fatty acids in the first stomach of ruminant animals. In ruminant fats, *trans* isomers with 18 carbon atoms and one double bond also dominate, but *trans* isomers with 14 and 16 carbon atoms are present as well. As bacterial transformation is a more selective process, the double bond in ruminant TFA (rTFA) is mainly, but not exclusively, located at the (n-7)-carbon atom. This TFA is called *trans*-vaccenic acid or briefly vaccenic acid (*trans*-C18:1n-7). Most rTFA in the diet are from dairy origin. Though most TFA in the diet have one double bond, TFA isomers of linoleic acid and α-linolenic acid also exist. In this respect, conjugated linoleic acid (CLA) is well known. CLA refers to a mixture of positional and geometric isomers of linoleic acid, whose double bounds can be in either *trans* or *cis* configuration. CLA differs from most natural polyunsaturated fatty acids in that the double bounds are not separated by a methylene carbon but are conjugated. One common CLA isomer has a *cis* double bond at the (n-9) carbon atom and a *trans* double bond at the (n-7) position and is present in ruminant fat. However, it can also be formed in the human body by the desaturation of vaccenic acid.

In this chapter the effects of TFA on cardiovascular risk in humans will be reviewed. The focus will be on dietary intervention studies and meta-analyses as related to the intakes of TFA with 18 carbon atoms and one double bond.

Trans-MUFA:
Elaidic acid and its
positional isomers
Trans-C18:1n-9
Linoleic acid
C18:2n-6
Stearic acid
C18:0
Cis-MUFA:
Oleic acid and its
positional isomers
Cis-C18:1n-9

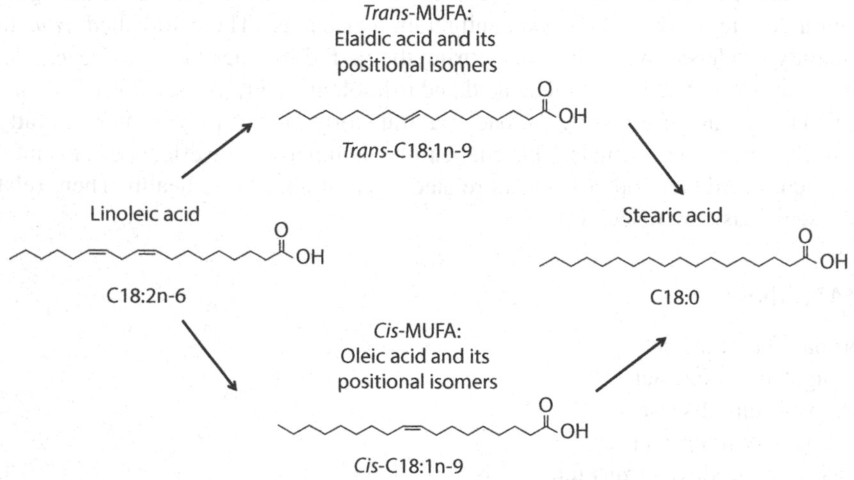

FIGURE 12.1 Simplified scheme of partial and full hydrogenation. Partial hydrogenation of linoleic acid leads to the formation of *trans*- and *cis*-monounsaturated fatty acids (MUFA), while full hydrogenation leads to the formation of stearic acid.

TFA AND RISK MARKERS FOR CARDIOVASCULAR DISEASE

Numerous human intervention studies have addressed the effects of iTFA on risk markers for cardiovascular disease (CVD). Typical intakes of iTFA in these studies were >4% of energy. In most of these studies, the distribution of the double bond over the TFA molecule was not reported. Therefore, it is not known if the different isomers of the iTFA molecule exert different metabolic effects. Further, TFA from dairy origin have been studied less extensively and generally at intakes <3% of energy. Only more recent studies have specifically focused on rTFA. As already described, TFA from dairy origin have predominantly the double bond at the (n-7)-position. It should be kept in mind, however, that iTFA also include isomers with the double bond at this position. Thus, iTFA and rTFA are composed of a mixture of different positional isomers that partly overlap.

Serum Lipids and Lipoproteins

More than 40 years ago, a few studies addressed the effects of iTFA on serum total cholesterol concentrations. Results, however, were conflicting. In one study, it was reported that the cholesterolemic effects of iTFA were comparable to those of oleic acid (Mattson, Hollenback, and Kligman 1975), the most common *cis*-monounsaturated fatty acid in the diet. Two other studies, however, suggested that these *trans*-isomers increased serum total cholesterol concentrations, but less than saturated fatty acids did (Vergroesen 1972, Vergroesen and Gottenbos 1975). In these studies, effects on lipoproteins were not reported. About 25 years ago, a paper was published reporting the results of a well-controlled dietary intervention study with 59 healthy subjects who received three mixed natural diets in random order for three weeks each (Mensink and Katan 1990). The nutrient composition of the diets was similar, except for 10% of the daily energy intake, which was provided as oleic acid, as *trans* isomers of oleic acid (iTFA), or as a mixture of saturated fatty acids. It was reported that iTFA increased the concentration of cholesterol in the atherogenic low-density lipoproteins (LDL) as compared with oleic acid. Effects of iTFA on LDL-cholesterol, however, were slightly less than those of a mixture of saturated fatty acids. More importantly, however, was the finding that iTFA lowered high-density lipoprotein (HDL) cholesterol concentrations as compared with the other two diets. Together, these changes resulted in the most unfavorable lipoprotein profile following a diet high in iTFA. This study was criticized, also because the intake of iTFA exceeded habitual intakes at that time, which were typically less than 4% of daily energy intake (De Vries et al. 1997). Later studies, however, using lower intakes of iTFA largely confirmed these effects.

In 2010, Brouwer, Wanders, and Katan (2010) published a meta-analysis describing the effects of TFA on plasma lipoproteins. Effects were expressed relative to those of an isocaloric amount of *cis*-monounsaturated fatty acids. In the end, 23 trials were identified, which provided 28 data points that were used to estimate the effects of iTFA. It was calculated that LDL-cholesterol increased by 0.048 mmol/L and HDL-cholesterol decreased by 0.010 mmol/L for each 1% of energy from iTFA replacing *cis*-monounsaturated fatty acids (Figure 12.2). For the plasma LDL-cholesterol to HDL-cholesterol ratio, this estimate was 0.055. A high plasma LDL-cholesterol to HDL-cholesterol is strongly associated with coronary heart disease (CHD). Effects of iTFA on other plasma lipids and lipoproteins were not estimated. However, an earlier meta-analysis including eight studies reported that iTFA increased concentrations of serum triacylglycerol and apoB100 and decreased those of apoA-I as compared with *cis*-monounsaturated fatty acids (Mensink et al. 2003). Thus, it is evident that the effects of iTFA have adverse effects on the serum lipoprotein profile.

The question then arises if TFA from ruminants have comparable effects. Five trials were identified that provided six data points that could be used to calculate the effects of rTFA on plasma lipids (Brouwer, Wanders, and Katan 2010). It was estimated that increasing the intake of 1% of energy from rTFA at the expense of *cis*-monounsaturated fatty acids increased LDL-cholesterol by 0.045 mmol/L, decreased HDL-cholesterol by 0.009 mmol/L, and increased the LDL-cholesterol to

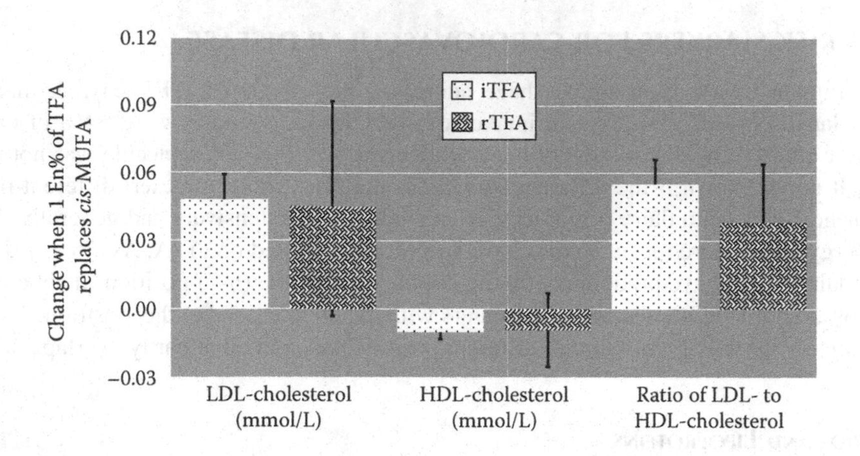

FIGURE 12.2 Effects on serum lipids when 1% of energy (En%) of industrially produced *trans* fatty acids (iTFA) or of *trans* fatty acids from ruminant fats (rTFA) in the diets replaces *cis*-monounsaturated fatty acids (*cis*-MUFA). Data are means (±95% confidence intervals) and are derived from Brouwer, Wanders, and Katan (2010).

HDL-cholesterol ratio by 0.038. These effects were slightly less than those of iTFA, although differences did not reach statistical significance. It should be noted, however, that the confidence intervals for the estimates of rTFA were very wide and estimates for LDL-cholesterol and HDL-cholesterol were not significantly different from zero (Figure 12.2). The wide confidence intervals for rTFA are, at least partly, due to the fact that intakes in the various intervention studies were in general quite low, which makes it difficult to obtain precise estimates for their effects. Based on their meta-analysis, however, Gayet-Boyer et al. (2014) reported that rTFA does not affect the LDL-cholesterol to HDL-cholesterol ratio. Thus, earlier reports on the effects of iTFA and rTFA on the serum lipoprotein profile were controversial. Recently, however, Gebauer et al. (2015) published the results of a double-blind randomized crossover trial involving 106 healthy subjects. In that well-designed and controlled study, diets differed by about 3.0%–3.5% of daily energy intakes from iTGA, rTFA, or stearic acid. Compared with the diet rich in iTFA, the diet rich in rTFA increased concentrations of total cholesterol, LDL-cholesterol, HDL-cholesterol, triacylglycerol, apoA-I, and apoB. Effects on the total cholesterol to HDL-cholesterol ratio were comparable between the diet rich in iTFA and that rich in rTFA. The diet high in stearic acid had a more favorable effect on total cholesterol, LDL-cholesterol, the total cholesterol to HDL cholesterol ratio, and apoB than either the diet rich in rTFA or rich in iTFA. Stearic acid and rTFA had comparable effects on HDL-cholesterol, triacylglycerol, and apoA-I concentrations. Finally, the effects of stearic acid and rTFA on triacylglycerol concentrations were comparable. Thus, this adequately powered study shows that effects of rTFA on the serum lipoprotein profile are not favorable as compared with those of iTFA.

Mechanistic Studies

To explain the effects of iTFA on the lipoprotein profile, several mechanistic studies have been carried out. Effects of rTFA are less well documented. Several studies have focused on cholesteryl ester transfer protein (CETP). CETP is a plasma protein that is involved in the exchange of cholesteryl esters from HDL for triacylglycerols from very-low-density lipoproteins (VLDL) and LDL. Thus, a high-CETP activity could lead to decreases in HDL-cholesterol and increases in LDL-cholesterol and VLDL-cholesterol. Indeed, iTFA increased CETP activity as compared with saturated fatty acids, *cis*-monounsaturated fatty acids and linoleic acid (Abbey and Nestel 1994, Lichtenstein et al. 2001, van Tol et al. 1995). Chardigny et al. (2008), however, did not observe any changes in CETP activity after consumption of diets rich in iTFA or rTFA. In other studies, milk fat rich in rTFA had comparable effects on CETP activity as compared with milk fat with lower levels of rTFA (Malpuech-Brugère et al. 2010, Lacroix et al. 2012). Thus, these findings suggest that iTFA increases CETP activity, especially at high intakes. Further, Sundram, French, and Clandinin (2003) have reported that iTFA increases endogenous cholesterol synthesis as compared with a mixture of palmitic acid and oleic acid. In contrast, no specific effects of iTFA on cholesterol synthesis were observed in another study (Matthan et al. 2000). Finally, Matthan et al. (2004) concluded that the catabolism of apoA-I from HDL was increased and that of LDL apoB-100 was decreased after intake of iTFA. Thus, the underlying mechanism by which iTFA and rTFA affect lipoprotein metabolism remains to be elucidated, but it is likely that multiple, interrelated pathways are involved.

LDL Particle Size

LDL particles vary in size, density, and composition. It is thought that small and dense LDLs are more atherogenic than larger, less dense LDLs. Studies relating TFA intake to LDL particle size are equivocal. Mauger et al. (2003) have reported that increasing the intake of iTFA at the expense of a mixture of other fatty acids dose-dependently decreased LDL particle size. Chardigny et al. (2008) showed that iTFA and rTFA do not have different effects on the concentrations of small, dense LDL particles. Finally, Tricon et al. (2006) concluded that dairy products naturally enriched in rTFA have comparable effects on small, dense LDL concentrations as regular dairy products.

LDL Oxidation

Oxidation of polyunsaturated fatty acids in the LDL particle may lead to the formation of oxidized LDL (oxLDL) or minimally modified LDL (mmLDL). These are pro-inflammatory and proatherogenic lipoprotein particles that can activate pathways involved in the development of atherosclerotic lesions. However, there is no generally accepted method to examine *in vivo* susceptibility of LDL to oxidation. Resistance of LDL toward an oxidative challenge can be determined *in vitro* by measuring the lag-phase, which is the time before oxidized products of fatty acids within the LDL particle start to arise. Also, the rate of oxidation and the amount of oxidative products formed can be measured. Copper ions are frequently used to initiate the oxidation process. Using this approach, effects of diets rich in saturated fatty acids, *cis*-monounsaturated fatty acids, and *cis*-polyunsaturated fatty acids had comparable effects on *in vitro* LDL oxidizability to iTFA (Cuchel et al. 1996, Halvorsen et al. 1996, Nestel et al. 1992). In addition, the uptake of LDL by macrophages or the relative electrophoretic mobility of LDL was not changed (Halvorsen et al. 1996). These latter two parameters may be affected by the degree of modification of the LDL particle. Smit et al. (2011), however, showed that consumption of iTFA increased urinary 8-iso-$PGF_{2\alpha}$ levels, which is an isoprostane produced by the nonenzymatic peroxidation of arachidonic acid and serves as an *in vivo* marker for free radical–induced lipid peroxidation and may be increased in patients with CHD. It was, however, discussed that increased urinary 8-iso-$PGF_{2\alpha}$ levels may also be the result of a shift from a decreased endogenous breakdown of 8-iso-$PGF_{2\alpha}$ to an increased urinary excretion of this isoprostane. At much lower intakes, Tholstrup et al. (2006) did not, however, observe any effects of butter rich in rTFA on urinary 8-iso-$PGF_{2\alpha}$ levels as compared with regular butter. Also, *in vitro* LDL oxidizability did not change when subjects were fed diets with dairy products naturally enriched in rTFA (Tricon et al. 2006). Taken together, these studies suggest that iTFA and rTFA do exert adverse effects on *in vitro* LDL oxidation or *in vivo* lipid peroxidation.

Lipoprotein(a)

Lipoprotein(a) [Lp(a)] is an LDL particle with an apolipoprotein (a) molecule covalently bound to apoB100. Serum concentrations of Lp(a), which have a very strong genetic component, are positively related with cardiovascular risk. The effects of iTFA have been examined in many intervention studies. In most of these studies, Lp(a) concentrations were increased after consumption of diets rich in iTFA, as compared with diets rich in saturated or *cis*-unsaturated fatty acids (Almendingen et al. 1995, Aro et al.

1997, Clevidence et al. 1997, Judd et al. 1998, Mensink et al. 1992, Nestel et al. 1992). Larger increases were observed in subjects with higher baseline Lp(a) (Clevidence et al. 1997, Mensink et al. 1992). In three other studies, Lp(a) concentrations were not significantly increased after iTFA intake (Lichtenstein et al. 1999, 2006, Müller et al. 1998). Effects of rTFA have been studied less extensively. Chardigny et al. (2008) have reported that iTFA and rTFA had comparable effects on Lp(a) concentrations after the consumption of iTFA or rTFA. In contrast, Gebauer et al. (2015) found that rTFA increased Lp(a) as compared with iTFA and stearic acid.

Glucose Homeostasis

Aronis, Khan, and Mantzoros (2012) carried out a systematic review on the effects of iTFA on fasting glucose and insulin concentrations. In total, seven randomized controlled trials were identified. Diets were provided for 4–16 weeks, and a total of 208 subjects were included. Intake of TFA varied between 2.6% and 9.0% of energy. In all studies, iTFA were replaced by other fatty acids and total fat intake within a study was therefore constant. Even at these relatively high intakes, no effects were observed on fasting plasma glucose or insulin concentrations. Studies that specifically focused on dairy products also do not suggest that this source of TFA affects glucose metabolism (Tholstrup et al. 2006, Tricon et al. 2006, Werner et al. 2013). Thus, there is no evidence that the effects of iTFA or rTFA on glucose homeostasis are different from those of saturated fatty acids, oleic acid, or linoleic acid.

Blood Pressure

No intervention studies have been carried out that were specifically designed to examine the effects of TFA on blood pressure. However, blood pressure has been measured in several randomized controlled trials as a secondary outcome. In these trials, iTFA were exchanged for an isocaloric amount of saturated fatty acids, oleic acid, or linoleic acid. No effects on systolic or diastolic blood pressure were reported (Lichtenstein et al. 2003, Mensink, de Louw, and Katan 1991, Zock et al. 1993). Likewise, studies focusing on dairy products naturally enriched in TFA did not demonstrate effects on blood pressure (Chardigny et al. 2008, Lacroix et al. 2012, Malpuech-Brugère et al. 2010). In all these studies, subjects were normotensive. It is therefore still possible that TFA may increase blood pressure in hypertensive subjects, but effects—if any—are likely to be small.

Hemostatic Function

A proper hemostatic function is the result of a complex interplay between molecules derived and secreted from the endothelium, platelets, and leukocytes and from factors that are part of the coagulation and fibrinolytic pathways. If disturbed, a thrombus may be formed within the blood stream, which may lead to a myocardial infarction or stroke. In contrast, impaired hemostasis can lead to excessive bleeding.

Only a few intervention studies have examined the effects of TFA on markers for hemostatic function. Almendingen et al. (1996) reported that a diet rich in partially hydrogenated soybean oil unfavorably affected plasminogen activator inhibitor type 1 (PAI-1) antigen and PAI-1 activity as compared with a diet high in butter fat. PAI-1 is part of the fibrinolytic system, which breaks down clots. However, other markers related to platelet activation (β-thromboglobulin), the coagulation cascade (factor VIIc, fibrinopeptide A), and the fibrinolytic system (D-dimers, tissue plasminogen activator) were not affected. Mutanen and Aro (1997) concluded that stearic acid and iTFA had similar effects on markers of coagulation and fibrinolysis. Collagen-induced platelet aggregation, however, was reduced in the diet rich in TFA, as compared with the diet rich in stearic acid. Other parameters related to platelet function or to endothelial function did not change. Finally, Louheranta et al. (1999) reported that oleic acid and iTFA have comparable effects on factor VII, a coagulation factor. These three studies were carried out in the fasted state. Effects of a single meal rich in elaidic acid on activated FVII concentrations (FVIIa) during the postprandial phase were studied by Sanders et al. (2000). However, no evidence was found that the meal rich in elaidic acid had a different impact on postprandial changes in FVIIa compared with meals enriched with oleic acid, stearic acid, or medium-chain triglycerides. In a later study, coagulant and fibrinolytic markers were also not different during the fasting and postprandial phase, when subjects had consumed a diet rich in iTFA or oleic acid for 2 weeks (Sanders et al. 2003). For rTFA, no difference in effects on FVIIc and PAI-1 was found between butter rich in rTFA and regular butter (Tholstrup et al. 2006). Gebauer et al. (2015), however, reported that rTFA lowered fibrinogen concentrations as compared with iTFA and stearic acid, while no effects on factor VII were observed. Overall, these intervention studies do not provide clear evidence that iTFA or rTFA have an adverse effect on hemostatic function as compared with other fatty acids.

Vascular Function

Many markers exist to investigate the different aspects of the vasculature. One frequently used method is flow-mediated vasodilation (FMD) of the brachial artery, which is considered as the noninvasive gold standard technique to measure vascular endothelial function. Brachial FMD is inversely associated with future cardiovascular events (Ras et al. 2012). Plasma biomarkers are also used to assess vascular function such as the soluble forms of vascular cell adhesion molecule 1, intercellular adhesion molecule 1, and endothelial selectin (sE-selectin). Increased concentrations of these molecules, which are involved in the binding of white blood cells to the vascular endothelium, are positively related to future cardiovascular events (Blankenberg, Barbaux, and Tiret 2003).

In one of the few studies on the effects of iTFA on FMD, de Roos, Bots, and Katan (2001) reported impaired fasting FMD as compared with an isocaloric amount of saturated fatty acids. In contrast, no postprandial impairment in FMD was found after the intake of a meal rich in iTFA (de Roos et al. 2002). Five weeks of iTFA consumption increased plasma sE-selectin levels as compared with saturated and *cis*-monounsaturated fatty acids (Baer et al. 2004). These detrimental effects of iTFA on sE-selectin, however, were not confirmed by Smit et al. (2011). In the study of Gebauer et al. (2015), sE-selectin concentrations were comparable after the consumption of diets rich in iTFA, rTFA, or stearic acid.

Inflammation

Inflammatory signals play a major role in all stages of atherosclerosis and evoke many other responses. Vascular inflammation, for example, stimulates the generation of vascular cell adhesion molecules. In addition, the inflammatory network is complex. Frequently measured markers used to measure low-grade systemic inflammation include TNFα, interleukin-6 (IL-6), and C-reactive protein (CRP). Baer et al. (2004) have reported that a diet high in iTFA significantly increased IL-6 and CRP concentrations as compared with oleic acid. These effects were not specific for iTFA as diets rich in stearic acid and a mixture of saturated fatty acids had similar effects on IL-6. Surprisingly, when part of the iTFA was replaced by stearic acid (C18:0), effects were no longer evident. Smit et al. (2011), however, found no effects of a diet rich in iTFA (7.3% of energy) on various inflammatory markers—including IL-6 and CRP—as compared with a control diet rich in oleic acid. Other studies also reported no effect of either iTFA or rTFA on plasma CRP or IL-6 concentrations (Gebauer et al. 2015, Lichtenstein et al. 2006, Motard-Bélanger et al. 2008, Tardy et al. 2009, Tholstrup et al. 2006, Werner et al. 2013).

TFA AND CARDIOVASCULAR DISEASE

In addition to effects on cardiovascular risk markers, the relationship between TFA intake and CVD itself has also been studied. It is clear that, for evident reasons, no randomized controlled trials have been carried out in this field and one has to rely on prospective cohort studies. In these studies, TFA intake has been assessed in two ways. First, TFA consumption was estimated using recorded food intake using, for example, food frequency questionnaires or food records. One disadvantage of this approach is that it is difficult to obtain precise estimates of nutrient intakes, in particular, at the individual level. For example, the composition of food products between different batches and different brands can be highly variable, fatty acid composition in nutrient databases are not complete, and people do not remember accurately what—and how much—was actually consumed. Such sources of errors may attenuate possible relationships between TFA intake and CVD risk. For the second approach, TFA levels can be assessed in plasma or fat tissue. As the majority of TFA in the human body are derived from dietary sources, this biomarker approach may provide a good estimate for TFA intakes over the past weeks or even years.

Chowdhury et al. (2014) identified five prospective cohort studies that examined the relationship between TFA intake and coronary risk. These studies were from the United States and Europe, and among the 155,270 participants, 4,662 coronary events were recorded. It was estimated that subjects in the top tertile of TFA intake had a 16% higher risk for coronary events compared to those in the bottom tertile of TFA intake (RR: 1.16, 95% CI: 1.06–1.27). In an earlier meta-analysis using data from four prospective cohort studies, including 4,965 coronary events among 139,836 participants, it was estimated that a 2% higher energy intake from TFA as an isocaloric replacement for carbohydrate was associated with a RR of 1.23 (95% CI: 1.11–1.37) (Mozaffarian and Clarke 2009). In another meta-analysis, Bendsen et al. (2011) estimated the effects of total TFA, iTFA, and rTFA on total CHD. For total TFA (6 cohorts; 186,531 participants; 6,135 cases for total CHD), the RR was 1.22 (95% CI: 1.08–1.38). Similar calculations were done for iTFA (3 cohorts; 91,778 participants; 1,089 cases). The RR for CHD events was 1.21 (95% CI: 0.97–1.50). For rTFA (4 cohorts; 95,464 participants; 1,463 cases), the RR was 0.92 (95% CI: 0.76–1.11). These findings, however, do not prove that the source of TFA is important for CHD risk. First of all, the RR estimates for iTFA and rTFA were not significantly different from one and overlapped. Secondly, at the time the study was performed, the intake of iTFA and its range was much larger than that of rTFA, which may have affected estimates. A comparison of the RR at similar ranges of intakes would therefore be very informative. In fact, Weggemans, Rudrum, and Trautwein (2004) concluded that no differences in the risk of CHD were evident between total, ruminant, and industrial TFA when the intake is below 2.5 g per day.

In the meta-analyses discussed earlier, the focus was on the relationship between the intakes of TFA with 18 carbon atoms and one single double bond. However, as discussed earlier, diets also provide minor amounts of other TFA. These intakes are even more difficult to estimate. Therefore, the most reliable estimate of intakes due to the low levels in the diet is to estimate levels in tissue lipid fractions. Still, it has to be acknowledged that TFA are metabolized in the human body and one TFA molecule can be converted into another TFA molecule. Vaccenic acid, for example, can be desaturated by a Δ9-desaturase (stearoyl-CoA desaturase-1), giving rise to the formation of a specific CLA isomer. Relationships between TFA in plasma lipids on CVD risk have been examined in several prospective cohort studies. In the Multi-Ethnic Study of Atherosclerosis cohort of 2837 U.S. adults, the proportion of *trans*-palmitoleic acid (*trans*-C16:1n-7) in the plasma phospholipid fraction was not related to incident CVD or CHD (de Oliveira Otto et al. 2013). In the Cardiovascular Health Study, a prospective cohort of older U.S. citizens, *trans*-isomers of linoleic acid in plasma phospholipids with two double bonds in the *trans* configuration were adversely related with total mortality, especially with CVD (Wang et al. 2014). The study cohort consisted of 2742 elderly individuals. No associations were observed for *trans*-monounsaturated fatty acids with 16 or 18 carbon atoms. Thus, these studies suggested that differences between the various TFA might exist, although further investigation and confirmation of these findings is needed.

INTAKES AND RECOMMENDATIONS

A very detailed report on worldwide fatty acid intake was published a few years ago (Micha et al. 2014). It was estimated that in 2010, the mean global TFA intake was 1.4% of energy with the highest intakes in Egypt (6.5% of energy) and the lowest intakes in the Caribbean region (0.2% of energy). Only 12 of the 187 countries included had mean intakes below 0.5% of energy, while 12 countries had intakes above 2% of energy. For the U.S. population, mean daily iTFA intake in 2006 was estimated to be 1.3 g per person with a 90th percentile of 2.6 g. Assuming a daily energy intake of about 2000 kcal, this would equal 0.6% and 1.2% of energy, respectively (Doell et al. 2012). Trends in TFA intakes between the 1980–1982 and 2007–2009 periods have been reported for the Minnesota Heart Survey (Honors et al. 2014). It was estimated that for women, intakes decreased gradually during this period from 2.9% to 1.9% of energy and for men, from 2.7% to 1.7% of energy. Also, results among the Framingham Heart Study participants showed that between the 1991–1995 and 2005–2008 periods, TFA intake had decreased from 1.5% to 1.2% of energy (Vadiveloo et al. 2014).

Various governmental agencies have issued recommendations for the intake of TFA. Although different wordings are used, the general consensus is that intakes should be as low as possible. If an upper limit is formulated, it is frequently mentioned that intakes should not exceed 1% of energy, as a zero-TFA diet is virtually impossible, due to the presence of naturally occurring TFA. Despite decreases in iTFA intake, also due to the reformulation of fats used for food formulations, it is evident that a large part of the global population still consumes levels above recommended intakes.

CONCLUSION

Prospective epidemiological cohort studies consistently support the finding that iTFA intake is associated with an increased risk of CHD. Evidence from many controlled human intervention studies suggests that these effects are mediated, at least in part, through adverse effects on the serum lipoprotein profile. Intakes show a linear-dose response with serum LDL-cholesterol, demonstrating that effects are proportional to the amounts of iTFA consumed. Elevated LDL-cholesterol has been causally linked to CHD. Although a protective causal role for HDL in CHD has not been established, iTFA also dose-dependently decrease HDL-cholesterol concentrations as compared with other fatty acids. Diets rich in iTFA also increase fasting triacylglycerol concentrations, which are also positively related to CHD risk. Therefore, there is a solid, evidence-based basis to minimize the use of iTFA and to keep intakes as low as possible. Finally, there is evidence indicating that iTFA increase Lp(a), especially in people with elevated concentrations, but the significance of this finding for CVD risk is unclear. At least for LDL-cholesterol, effects of iTFA and rTFA are comparable. Relationships between the intakes TFA with CVD risk are less clear, also due to lower intakes of rTFA than of iTFA at the time the studies were performed. However, while differences in effects of iTFA and rTFA are of interest scientifically, this may not be a critical public health issue as long as intakes of rTFA remain at current low levels.

REFERENCES

Abbey, M. and P. J. Nestel. 1994. Plasma cholesteryl ester transfer protein activity is increased when trans-elaidic acid is substituted for cis-oleic acid in the diet. *Atherosclerosis* 106 (1):99–107.

Almendingen, K., O. Jordal, P. Kierulf, B. Sandstad, and J. I. Pedersen. 1995. Effects of partially hydrogenated fish oil, partially hydrogenated soybean oil, and butter on serum lipoproteins and Lp[a] in men. *J Lipid Res* 36 (6):1370–1384.

Almendingen, K., I. Seljeflot, B. Sandstad, and J. I. Pedersen. 1996. Effects of partially hydrogenated fish oil, partially hydrogenated soybean oil, and butter on hemostatic variables in men. *Arterioscler Thromb Vasc Biol* 16 (3):375–380.

Aro, A., M. Jauhiainen, R. Partanen, I. Salminen, and M. Mutanen. 1997. Stearic acid, trans fatty acids, and dairy fat: Effects on serum and lipoprotein lipids, apolipoproteins, lipoprotein(a), and lipid transfer proteins in healthy subjects. *Am J Clin Nutr* 65 (5):1419–1426.

Aronis, K. N., S. M. Khan, and C. S. Mantzoros. 2012. Effects of trans fatty acids on glucose homeostasis: A meta-analysis of randomized, placebo-controlled clinical trials. *Am J Clin Nutr* 96 (5):1093–1099. doi: 10.3945/ajcn.112.040576.

Baer, D. J., J. T. Judd, B. A. Clevidence, and R. P. Tracy. 2004. Dietary fatty acids affect plasma markers of inflammation in healthy men fed controlled diets: A randomized crossover study. *Am J Clin Nutr* 79 (6):969–973.

Bendsen, N. T., R. Christensen, E. M. Bartels, and A. Astrup. 2011. Consumption of industrial and ruminant trans fatty acids and risk of coronary heart disease: A systematic review and meta-analysis of cohort studies. *Eur J Clin Nutr* 65 (7):773–783. doi: 10.1038/ejcn.2011.34.

Blankenberg, S., S. Barbaux, and L. Tiret. 2003. Adhesion molecules and atherosclerosis. *Atherosclerosis* 170 (2):191–203.

Brouwer, I. A., A. J. Wanders, and M. B. Katan. 2010. Effect of animal and industrial trans fatty acids on HDL and LDL cholesterol levels in humans—A quantitative review. *PLoS One* 5 (3):e9434. doi: 10.1371/journal.pone.0009434.

Chardigny, J. M., F. Destaillats, C. Malpuech-Brugere, J. Moulin, D. E. Bauman, A. L. Lock, D. M. Barbano et al. 2008. Do trans fatty acids from industrially produced sources and from natural sources have the same effect on cardiovascular disease risk factors in healthy subjects? Results of the trans Fatty Acids Collaboration (TRANSFACT) study. *Am J Clin Nutr* 87 (3):558–566.

Chowdhury, R., S. Warnakula, S. Kunutsor, F. Crowe, H. A. Ward, L. Johnson, O. H. Franco et al. 2014. Association of dietary, circulating, and supplement fatty acids with coronary risk: A systematic review and meta-analysis. *Ann Intern Med* 160 (9):398–406. doi: 10.7326/M13-1788.

Clevidence, B. A., J. T. Judd, E. J. Schaefer, J. L. Jenner, A. H. Lichtenstein, R. A. Muesing, J. Wittes, and M. E. Sunkin. 1997. Plasma lipoprotein (a) levels in men and women consuming diets enriched in saturated, cis-, or trans-monounsaturated fatty acids. *Arterioscler Thromb Vasc Biol* 17 (9):1657–1661.

Cuchel, M., U. S. Schwab, P. J. Jones, S. Vogel, C. Lammi-Keefe, Z. Li, J. Ordovas, J. R. McNamara, E. J. Schaefer, and A. H. Lichtenstein. 1996. Impact of hydrogenated fat consumption on endogenous cholesterol synthesis and susceptibility of low-density lipoprotein to oxidation in moderately hypercholesterolemic individuals. *Metabolism* 45 (2):241–247.

de Oliveira Otto, M. C., J. A. Nettleton, R. N. Lemaitre, L. M. Steffen, D. Kromhout, S. S. Rich, M. Y. Tsai, D. R. Jacobs, and D. Mozaffarian. 2013. Biomarkers of dairy fatty acids and risk of cardiovascular disease in the multi-ethnic study of atherosclerosis. *J Am Heart Assoc* 2 (4):e000092. doi: 10.1161/JAHA.113.000092.

de Roos, N. M., M. L. Bots, and M. B. Katan. 2001. Replacement of dietary saturated fatty acids by trans fatty acids lowers serum HDL cholesterol and impairs endothelial function in healthy men and women. *Arterioscler Thromb Vasc Biol* 21 (7):1233–1237.

de Roos, N. M., E. Siebelink, M. L. Bots, A. van Tol, E. G. Schouten, and M. B. Katan. 2002. Trans monounsaturated fatty acids and saturated fatty acids have similar effects on postprandial flow-mediated vasodilation. *Eur J Clin Nutr* 56 (7):674–679. doi: 10.1038/sj.ejcn.1601377.

De Vries, J. H. M., A. M. Jansen, D. Kromhout, P. van de Bovenkamp, W. A. van Staveren, R. P. Mensink, and M. B. Katan. 1997. The fatty acid and sterol content of food composites of middle-aged men in seven countries. *J Food Compos Anal* 10 (2):115–141.

Doell, D., D. Folmer, H. Lee, M. Honigfort, and S. Carberry. 2012. Updated estimate of trans fat intake by the US population. *Food Addit Contam Part A Chem Anal Control Expo Risk Assess* 29 (6):861–874. doi: 10.1080/19440049.2012.664570.

Gayet-Boyer, C., F. Tenenhaus-Aziza, C. Prunet, C. Marmonier, C. Malpuech-Brugere, B. Lamarche, and J. M. Chardigny. 2014. Is there a linear relationship between the dose of ruminant trans-fatty acids and cardiovascular risk markers in healthy subjects: Results from a systematic review and meta-regression of randomised clinical trials. *Br J Nutr* 112 (12):1914–1922. doi: 10.1017/S0007114514002578.

Gebauer, S. K., F. Destaillats, F. Dionisi, R. M. Krauss, and D. J. Baer. 2015. Vaccenic acid and trans fatty acid isomers from partially hydrogenated oil both adversely affect LDL cholesterol: A double-blind, randomized controlled trial. *Am J Clin Nutr* 102 (6):1339–1346. doi: 10.3945/ajcn.115.116129.

Halvorsen, B., K. Almendingen, M. S. Nenseter, J. I. Pedersen, and E. N. Christiansen. 1996. Effects of partially hydrogenated fish oil, partially hydrogenated soybean oil and butter on the susceptibility of low density lipoprotein to oxidative modification in men. *Eur J Clin Nutr* 50 (6):364–370.

Honors, M. A., L. J. Harnack, X. Zhou, and L. M. Steffen. 2014. Trends in fatty acid intake of adults in the Minneapolis-St Paul, MN Metropolitan Area, 1980–1982 through 2007–2009. *J Am Heart Assoc* 3 (5):e001023. doi: 10.1161/JAHA.114.001023.

Judd, J. T., D. J. Baer, B. A. Clevidence, R. A. Muesing, S. C. Chen, J. A. Weststrate, G. W. Meijer et al. 1998. Effects of margarine compared with those of butter on blood lipid profiles related to cardiovascular disease risk factors in normolipemic adults fed controlled diets. *Am J Clin Nutr* 68 (4):768–777.

Lacroix, E., A. Charest, A. Cyr, L. Baril-Gravel, Y. Lebeuf, P. Paquin, P. Y. Chouinard, P. Couture, and B. Lamarche. 2012. Randomized controlled study of the effect of a butter naturally enriched in trans fatty acids on blood lipids in healthy women. *Am J Clin Nutr* 95 (2):318–325. doi: 10.3945/ajcn.111.023408.

Lichtenstein, A. H., L. M. Ausman, S. M. Jalbert, and E. J. Schaefer. 1999. Effects of different forms of dietary hydrogenated fats on serum lipoprotein cholesterol levels. *N Engl J Med* 340 (25):1933–1940. doi: 10.1056/NEJM199906243402501.

Lichtenstein, A. H., A. T. Erkkila, B. Lamarche, U. S. Schwab, S. M. Jalbert, and L. M. Ausman. 2003. Influence of hydrogenated fat and butter on CVD risk factors: Remnant-like particles, glucose and insulin, blood pressure and C-reactive protein. *Atherosclerosis* 171 (1):97–107.

Lichtenstein, A. H., M. Jauhiainen, S. McGladdery, L. M. Ausman, S. M. Jalbert, M. Vilella-Bach, C. Ehnholm, J. Frohlich, and E. J. Schaefer. 2001. Impact of hydrogenated fat on high density lipoprotein subfractions and metabolism. *J Lipid Res* 42 (4):597–604.

Lichtenstein, A. H., N. R. Matthan, S. M. Jalbert, N. A. Resteghini, E. J. Schaefer, and L. M. Ausman. 2006. Novel soybean oils with different fatty acid profiles alter cardiovascular disease risk factors in moderately hyperlipidemic subjects. *Am J Clin Nutr* 84 (3):497–504.

Louheranta, A. M., A. K. Turpeinen, H. M. Vidgren, U. S. Schwab, and M. I. Uusitupa. 1999. A high-trans fatty acid diet and insulin sensitivity in young healthy women. *Metabolism* 48 (7):870–875.

Malpuech-Brugère, C., J. Mouriot, C. Boue-Vaysse, N. Combe, J. L. Peyraud, P. LeRuyet, G. Chesneau, B. Morio, and J. M. Chardigny. 2010. Differential impact of milk fatty acid profiles on cardiovascular risk biomarkers in healthy men and women. *Eur J Clin Nutr* 64 (7):752–759. doi: 10.1038/ejcn.2010.73.

Matthan, N. R., L. M. Ausman, A. H. Lichtenstein, and P. J. Jones. 2000. Hydrogenated fat consumption affects cholesterol synthesis in moderately hypercholesterolemic women. *J Lipid Res* 41 (5):834–839.

Matthan, N. R., F. K. Welty, P. H. Barrett, C. Harausz, G. G. Dolnikowski, J. S. Parks, R. H. Eckel, E. J. Schaefer, and A. H. Lichtenstein. 2004. Dietary hydrogenated fat increases high-density lipoprotein apoA-I catabolism and decreases low-density lipoprotein apoB-100 catabolism in hypercholesterolemic women. *Arterioscler Thromb Vasc Biol* 24 (6):1092–1097. doi: 10.1161/01.ATV.0000128410.23161.be.

Mattson, F. H., E. J. Hollenbach, and A. M. Kligman. 1975. Effect of hydrogenated fat on the plasma cholesterol and triglyceride levels of man. *Am J Clin Nutr* 28 (7):726–731.

Mauger, J. F., A. H. Lichtenstein, L. M. Ausman, S. M. Jalbert, M. Jauhiainen, C. Ehnholm, and B. Lamarche. 2003. Effect of different forms of dietary hydrogenated fats on LDL particle size. *Am J Clin Nutr* 78 (3):370–375.

Mensink, R. P., M. H. de Louw, and M. B. Katan. 1991. Effects of dietary trans fatty acids on blood pressure in normotensive subjects. *Eur J Clin Nutr* 45 (8):375–382.

Mensink, R. P. and M. B. Katan. 1990. Effect of dietary trans fatty acids on high-density and low-density lipoprotein cholesterol levels in healthy subjects. *N Engl J Med* 323 (7):439–445. doi: 10.1056/NEJM199008163230703.

Mensink, R. P., P. L. Zock, M. B. Katan, and G. Hornstra. 1992. Effect of dietary cis and trans fatty acids on serum lipoprotein[a] levels in humans. *J Lipid Res* 33 (10):1493–1501.

Mensink, R. P., P. L. Zock, A. D. Kester, and M. B. Katan. 2003. Effects of dietary fatty acids and carbohydrates on the ratio of serum total to HDL cholesterol and on serum lipids and apolipoproteins: A meta-analysis of 60 controlled trials. *Am J Clin Nutr* 77 (5):1146–1155.

Micha, R., S. Khatibzadeh, P. Shi, S. Fahimi, S. Lim, K. G. Andrews, R. E. Engell, J. Powles, M. Ezzati, and D. Mozaffarian. 2014. Global, regional, and national consumption levels of dietary fats and oils in 1990 and 2010: A systematic analysis including 266 country-specific nutrition surveys. *BMJ* 348:g2272. doi: 10.1136/bmj.g2272.

Motard-Bélanger, A., A. Charest, G. Grenier, P. Paquin, Y. Chouinard, S. Lemieux, P. Couture, and B. Lamarche. 2008. Study of the effect of trans fatty acids from ruminants on blood lipids and other risk factors for cardiovascular disease. *Am J Clin Nutr* 87 (3):593–599.

Mozaffarian, D. and R. Clarke. 2009. Quantitative effects on cardiovascular risk factors and coronary heart disease risk of replacing partially hydrogenated vegetable oils with other fats and oils. *Eur J Clin Nutr* 63 (Suppl. 2):S22–S33. doi: 10.1038/sj.ejcn.1602976.

Müller, H., O. Jordal, P. Kierulf, B. Kirkhus, and J. I. Pedersen. 1998. Replacement of partially hydrogenated soybean oil by palm oil in margarine without unfavorable effects on serum lipoproteins. *Lipids* 33 (9):879–887.

Mutanen, M. and A. Aro. 1997. Coagulation and fibrinolysis factors in healthy subjects consuming high stearic or trans fatty acid diets. *Thromb Haemost* 77 (1):99–104.

Nestel, P., M. Noakes, B. Belling, R. McArthur, P. Clifton, E. Janus, and M. Abbey. 1992. Plasma lipoprotein lipid and Lp[a] changes with substitution of elaidic acid for oleic acid in the diet. *J Lipid Res* 33 (7):1029–1036.

Ras, R. T., M. T. Streppel, R. Draijer, and P. L. Zock. 2012. Flow-mediated dilation and cardiovascular risk prediction: A systematic review with meta-analysis. *Int J Cardiol* 168 (1):344–351. doi: 10.1016/j.ijcard.2012.09.047.

Sanders, T. A., T. de Grassi, G. J. Miller, and J. H. Morrissey. 2000. Influence of fatty acid chain length and cis/trans isomerization on postprandial lipemia and factor VII in healthy subjects (postprandial lipids and factor VII). *Atherosclerosis* 149 (2):413–420.

Sanders, T. A., F. R. Oakley, D. Crook, J. A. Cooper, and G. J. Miller. 2003. High intakes of trans monounsaturated fatty acids taken for 2 weeks do not influence procoagulant and fibrinolytic risk markers for CHD in young healthy men. *Br J Nutr* 89 (6):767–776. doi: 10.1079/BJN2003850.

Smit, L. A., M. B. Katan, A. J. Wanders, S. Basu, and I. A. Brouwer. 2011. A high intake of trans fatty acids has little effect on markers of inflammation and oxidative stress in humans. *J Nutr* 141 (9):1673–1678. doi: 10.3945/jn.110.134668.

Sundram, K., M. A. French, and M. T. Clandinin. 2003. Exchanging partially hydrogenated fat for palmitic acid in the diet increases LDL-cholesterol and endogenous cholesterol synthesis in normocholesterolemic women. *Eur J Nutr* 42 (4):188–194. doi: 10.1007/s00394-003-0411-9.

Tardy, A. L., S. Lambert-Porcheron, C. Malpuech-Brugere, C. Giraudet, J. P. Rigaudiere, B. Laillet, P. Leruyet et al. 2009. Dairy and industrial sources of trans fat do not impair peripheral insulin sensitivity in overweight women. *Am J Clin Nutr* 90 (1):88–94. doi: 10.3945/ajcn.2009.27515.

Tholstrup, T., M. Raff, S. Basu, P. Nonboe, K. Sejrsen, and E. M. Straarup. 2006. Effects of butter high in ruminant trans and monounsaturated fatty acids on lipoproteins, incorporation of fatty acids into lipid classes, plasma C-reactive protein, oxidative stress, hemostatic variables, and insulin in healthy young men. *Am J Clin Nutr* 83 (2):237–243.

Tricon, S., G. C. Burdge, E. L. Jones, J. J. Russell, S. El-Khazen, E. Moretti, W. L. Hall et al. 2006. Effects of dairy products naturally enriched with cis-9,trans-11 conjugated linoleic acid on the blood lipid profile in healthy middle-aged men. *Am J Clin Nutr* 83 (4):744–753.

Vadiveloo, M., M. Scott, P. Quatromoni, P. Jacques, and N. Parekh. 2014. Trends in dietary fat and high-fat food intakes from 1991 to 2008 in the Framingham Heart Study participants. *Br J Nutr* 111 (4):724–734. doi: 10.1017/S0007114513002924.

van Tol, A., P. L. Zock, T. van Gent, L. M. Scheek, and M. B. Katan. 1995. Dietary trans fatty acids increase serum cholesterylester transfer protein activity in man. *Atherosclerosis* 115 (1):129–134.

Vergroesen, A. J. 1972. Dietary fat and cardiovascular disease: Possible modes of action of linoleic acid. *Proc Nutr Soc* 31 (3):323–329.

Vergroesen, A. J. and J. J. Gottenbos. 1975. *The Role of Fats in Human Nutrition*. New York: Academic Press.

Wang, Q., F. Imamura, R. N. Lemaitre, E. B. Rimm, M. Wang, I. B. King, X. Song, D. Siscovick, and D. Mozaffarian. 2014. Plasma phospholipid trans-fatty acids levels, cardiovascular diseases, and total mortality: The cardiovascular health study. *J Am Heart Assoc* 3 (4):e000914. doi: 10.1161/JAHA.114.000914.

Weggemans, R. M., M. Rudrum, and E. A. Trautwein. 2004. Intake of ruminant versus industrial trans fatty acids and risk of coronary heart disease—What is the evidence? *Eur J Lipid Sci Technol* 106 (6):390–397. doi: 10.1002/ejlt.200300932.

Werner, L. B., L. I. Hellgren, M. Raff, S. K. Jensen, R. A. Petersen, T. Drachmann, and T. Tholstrup. 2013. Effects of butter from mountain-pasture grazing cows on risk markers of the metabolic syndrome compared with conventional Danish butter: A randomized controlled study. *Lipids Health Dis* 12:99. doi: 10.1186/1476-511X-12-99.

Zock, P. L., R. A. Blijlevens, J. H. de Vries, and M. B. Katan. 1993. Effects of stearic acid and trans fatty acids versus linoleic acid on blood pressure in normotensive women and men. *Eur J Clin Nutr* 47 (6):437–444.

Section III

Dietary Carbohydrates and Cardiometabolic Health

13 Epidemiologic and Mechanistic Studies of Sucrose and Fructose in Beverages and Their Relation to Obesity and Cardiovascular Risk

George A. Bray

CONTENTS

ABSTRACT

Consumption of calorie-sweetened beverages has continued to increase and plays a role in the epidemic of obesity, the metabolic syndrome, and fatty liver disease. Data from the Global Burden of Disease Study, NHANES, and USDA dietary surveys are used to understand changes in sugar and fructose consumption in beverages. Meta-analyses, randomized clinical trials, and clinical studies were used to evaluate outcomes of beverage and fructose intake. About 75% of all foods and beverages contain added sugar in a large array of forms. Consumption of soft drinks has increased five-fold since 1950. Meta-analyses suggest that consumption of sugar-sweetened beverages is related to the risk of obesity, diabetes, cardiovascular risk factors, and the metabolic syndrome. Drinking two 16 ounce sugar-sweetened beverages per day for 6 months induced features of the metabolic syndrome and fatty liver in healthy human beings. Fructose increases blood pressure and serum lipids. Randomized, controlled trials in children and adults lasting 6 months to 2 years have shown that replacing the intake of sugar-sweetened soft drinks with low-energy drinks reduces weight gain or induces weight loss. Recent studies suggest a gene-SSB relationship in modulating weight gain.

INTRODUCTION

The rapid and steady increase of sugar-sweetened beverage intake of the past 50 years of the twentieth century appears to have declined recently, but overall the level of intake is still very high (Ng et al. 2012; Ford and Dietz 2013; Kit et al. 2013; Ludwig 2013). This chapter will argue that the amount of sugar (sucrose), and the fructose which it contains, poses a significant health risk for many Americans and that something needs to be done about it (Nestle 2015). A major source of sucrose in our diet is in the beverages we drink, and this will be a principal focus of this chapter. These sugar-sweetened beverages have several components. The first is the "energy" that is provided when the sucrose (or high fructose corn syrup, HFCS) is metabolized to glucose and fructose and then to water and carbon dioxide in the body. The second is the fructose moiety of the sucrose molecule (or HFCS), which seems to have detrimental effects independent of the energy that it provides. The third component of many beverages is caffeine, which heightens alertness and may be mildly addictive, leading to increased consumption of sugar-sweetened beverages. Finally, there are the other components of SSB including flavorings, sodium, potassium, and other additives that may have metabolic and/or clinical effects.

Sugar is sweet, and the fructose it contains even sweeter. There is an innate human desire for sweetness. If sugar, HFCS, and fructose were not sweet there would be little or no debate about their risk because their consumption would undoubtedly be less. A preference for sweet taste is present in newborn infants and increases in intensity throughout childhood. It may even be that the "craving" for sweets can be enhanced further by early exposure to intense sweeteners. Human beings have consumed almost all of the sugar that has been produced, which drives increasing production. At the time of the American Revolution in 1776, Americans consumed about 4 pounds of sugar per person each year. By 1850, this had risen to 20 pounds per capita and by 1994 to 120 pounds each year (Johnson et al. 2007). The food industry has used sugar as a major sweetener for delivery of increasing amounts of beverages and food over the past half century (Moss 2013). The result has been that the consumption of sugar-sweetened beverages rose by a startling 38.5 gallons per person between 1950 and 2000 (10.8 gallons per person in 1950 to 49.3 gallons per person in 2000) (Putnam and Allshouse 2003a,b). We have seen small declines since then. Between 2001–2002 and 2009–2010, total daily beverage consumption (excluding water) decreased from 24.4% to 21.1% of energy intake. Significant decreases occurred in sugar-sweetened sodas (13.5%–10.2% energy), whole milk (2.7%–1.6% energy), fruit juices with sugar added (2.3%–2.1% energy), and fruit-flavored drinks (1.6%–0.8% energy). Significant increases occurred for sweetened coffees/teas, energy drinks, sport drinks, and unsweetened juices though the contribution of each to total energy intake remained <1% (Nielsen et al. 2002). Low-/no-calorie drink consumption also increased, rising from 0.2 to 1.3 oz/d (Mesirow and Welsh 2015).

Food manufacturers continue to find new ways to increase sugar consumption by constantly manufacturing new food and beverage products, be they in fruit juice, energy drinks, vitamin waters, protein waters, or sports drinks (Moss 2013). This chapter concludes that sugar and related caloric sweeteners provide nutritionally invisible calories that in the amounts now consumed pose a health risk to many Americans (Bray 2013).

My research interest in the role of sugar and fructose in human health was stimulated by a quotation from John Yudkin, professor of nutrition at Queen's college, London: "If then there is reason to be concerned about a dietary cause of a widespread disease [obesity], one should look for some constituent of man's diet that has been introduced recently or has increased considerably, recently" (Yudkin 1972). There is clear evidence that dietary factors are driving weight up, but genetic variation also plays a key role. Some genes such as the *OB* gene and the *MC4R* gene have a major effect on obesity (Loos 2012), while others contribute only a small amount individually but collectively provide the background for individual responses to diet (Speliotes et al. 2010; Locke et al. 2015). A gene–environment interaction has been demonstrated for soft drinks and weight gain (Qi et al. 2012). We might state the relation of diet and genes this way: "Genetic variability loads the gun; the diet and environment pull the trigger" (Bray 2015).

A key paper about fructose and health was published in 2004 showing a correlation between rising consumption of HFCS and obesity just as Yudkin had predicted (Bray et al. 2004). Although correlation does not prove causation, the data presaged an increasing body of scholarly work that has highlighted the important relation between sucrose and HFCS (and the fructose they contain) and the risk of obesity and several diseases. The decade of the 1980s began quietly enough for obesity research and for the sugar industry. The prevalence of obesity, though rising slowly through the first half of the twentieth century, was still only 14% in 1960–1962 (Ogden et al. 2007, 2014). Sugar had received a relatively clean bill of health from the National Academy of Science in the *Diet and Health Report*—its only health problem according to this authoritative book was its role in dental caries (National Research Council 1989). The metabolic syndrome was yet to be clearly defined (Reaven 1988); we did not know that calories in sweetened beverages were nutritionally invisible and were not adequately compensated by a reduction in food intake. Finally, the concept of non-alcoholic fatty liver disease was only beginning to emerge (Abdelmalek et al. 2010; Vernon et al. 2011); up to that time it was "alcohol" that was the major nutritional factor producing liver disease. This was the calm before the storm. What a difference 25 years can make! As I look back it is clear that the increasing consumption of sugar of HFCS and the fructose that they both contain has dramatically increased the health risks for many people (Bray et al. 2004; Bray 2013; Bray and Popkin 2013). This chapter focuses on this issue.

In the 1960s and 1970s, sugar from beverages represented only a third of our total added sugar intake, but this rose to two-thirds of our sugar intake by the year 2000 and has subsequently been declining to about 40% of total added sugar intake (Duffey and Popkin 2008; Slining and Popkin 2013). Finally after a long period of refusing to put an upper limit on sugar intake, the 2015 Dietary Guidelines Advisory Committee has recommended a 10% upper level. This is the level recommended by the American Heart Association (AHA) and the Food and Agriculture Organization (FAO).

EFFECTS ATTRIBUTABLE TO THE ENERGY IN BEVERAGES

EPIDEMIOLOGY

Several meta-analyses have shown a strong relationship between sugar-sweetened beverages and obesity. One of the earliest of these was by Vartanian et al. (2007). This meta-analysis showed a clear relationship between beverage intake and obesity and weight gain, which was largely eliminated with adjustment for energy intake. That is, the effect of the beverages could be largely attributed to the extra sugar energy that they provided. The results of their meta-analysis are summarized in Table 13.1.

Other meta-analyses followed, almost all of which showed a relationship between sugar-sweetened beverage consumption and obesity. Another meta-analysis by Olesen and Heitman (2009) included 14 prospective and 5 experimental studies, which found a positive association between intake of calorically sweetened beverages and obesity. Three experimental studies also found positive effects of calorically sweetened beverages and changes in body fat, but two did not find these effects; none were negative. Eight prospective studies adjusted for energy intake and seven of these found essentially the same associations. Olesen and Heitman concluded that a high intake of calorically sweetened beverages can be regarded as a determinant for obesity. Other reviews and meta-analyses have reached generally similar conclusions (Malik et al. 2006, 2010a,b, 2013; TeMorenga et al. 2012, 2014). In addition to increasing the risk of obesity, sugar and sugar-sweetened beverages enhance the risk of diabetes (Malik et al. 2010a) and cardiovascular disease (Yang et al. 2014).

In contrast to this consistent body of data, a recent meta-analysis concluded that the relationship between sweetened beverage intake and obesity was incorrect since adjustment for energy intake and physical activity removed the effect (Trumbo and Rivers 2014). If it is the "energy" in the beverage that is the culprit, their conclusion could not have been otherwise because they eliminated

TABLE 13.1
Effect Size for Energy Intake and Body Weight in the Meta-Analysis by Vartanian et al. (2007)

Research Design	Energy Intake	Body Weight
Cross-sectional studies	0.13 (0.12, 0.14)	0.06 (0.03, 0.08)
Longitudinal studies	0.24 (0.23, 0.26	0.03 (0.00, 0.06)
Short experimental studies	0.24 (0.16, 0.31)	0.24 (0.18, 0.28)
Overall effects	0.16 (0.15, 0.16)	0.06 (0.05, 0.08)

Data are effect size and 95% CI for the effect size.

"calories" by their adjustment for this central factor in the relationship (Trumbo and Rivers 2014). This study was supported by industry, and as Bes-Rastrollo et al. (2013) point out nearly 90% of papers supported by industry that studied the relation of beverages to obesity found no relationship whereas nearly 90% of those with independent funding did find this relationship. The importance of calorie intake, but not physical activity, on the effect of sugar-sweetened beverages on body was shown by Tucker et al. (2015). In this 4-year study of 170 non-smoking women, 4-year weight gain was significantly greater (2.7 kg) in the women drinking sugar-sweetened beverages than in the women who consumed artificially sweetened beverages (−0.1 kg) or no soft drinks (0.5 kg). Adjusting for energy intake weakened the effect as one would expect if these invisible "calories" were the driving force. Adjusting for physical activity had no effect on risk (Tucker et al. 2015).

Clinical Studies and Randomized Clinical Trials

Clinical studies have also shown that over a period of 10 weeks, subjects drinking a set amount of sugar-sweetened beverages gained weight compared to subjects drinking a comparable amount of artificially sweetened beverages who lost weight. In this trial, 41 overweight men and women entered a 10-week parallel arm study. One group (n = 21) received 3.4 MJ (813 kcal) of sugar-containing beverages and the other group (n = 20) received artificially sweetened beverages containing about 1 MJ (240 kcal) and no sugar. After 10 weeks, energy intake had increased by 1.6 MJ/d (382 kcal/d) and sucrose to 28% of energy intake. Protein and fat intake declined in the sugar group. Body weight and fat mass increased by 1.6 and 1.3 kg, respectively, in the sugar group and decreased by 1.0 and 0.3 kg in the group drinking aspartame-sweetened beverages. Blood pressure increased by 3.8/4.1 mmHg in the sugar-consuming group (Raben et al. 2002). Concentrations of several inflammatory markers were also changed. Haptoglobin rose by 13%, transferrin by 5%, and C-reactive protein by 6% in the sucrose group, but fell by 16%, 2%, and 26%, respectively, in the aspartame-sweetened beverage group (Sørensen et al. 2005).

In a study by Maersk et al. (2012), 47 overweight men and women completed a 6-month trial. Participants were randomized to receive 1 of 4 treatments: 1 liter/d of sugar-sweetened cola (≈ two 16 oz beverages), 1 liter/d of diet cola, 1 liter/d of milk, or 1 liter/d of water. Carbohydrate was 100 g/d from cola (1/2 fructose) and 47 g/d from milk (no fructose). During this 6-month period, visceral, liver, and muscle fat increased in those drinking the sugar-sweetened cola beverage even though total fat and subcutaneous fat did not. Systolic blood pressure, plasma triglycerides, and total cholesterol were also higher in those drinking the sugar-sweetened cola beverage than in those receiving one of the other beverages.

A series of randomized, controlled trials in children and adults lasting 6 months to 2 years have shown that weight gain is slowed by replacing sugar-sweetened beverages with alternative beverages. The two most noteworthy were done by a group from Boston (Ebbeling et al. 2012) and by a group from Amsterdam (de Ruyter et al. 2012). After 1 year, the group drinking artificially sweetened beverages in the Boston study gained significantly less weight than the group receiving the sugar-sweetened beverages. The Amsterdam study went further and provided either 250 mL of an artificially sweetened beverage or a sugar-containing beverage providing 104 kcal to 641 youth over an 18-month period. The BMI, weight, and skinfold-thickness and fat mass increased significantly less in the low-caloric beverage group.

In a post hoc analysis of the Amsterdam study, the authors examined the predicted weight change from computer models with the actual changes to calculate the energy deficit. They found that the heavier children (the upper half of the group) in terms of weight category failed to compensate adequately. That is, they ate more calories than predicted for their age, sex, and size. These "invisible" calories are a major concern for the problem of weight gain with sugar-sweetened beverages.

Mechanisms for Weight Gain Associated with Soft Drinks

One of the detrimental consequences of ingesting the nutritionally invisible calories in beverages is that the mechanisms that regulate caloric intake do not recognize them, and they thus become add-on calories (Rolls et al. 1990; Mattes 1996, 2006). Beverages do not suppress the intake of other food calories to an appropriate degree to prevent weight gain. Thus, beverage calories can be viewed as "add-on" calories enhancing the risk of obesity. The ground-breaking works of Mattes and his associates and Rolls and her colleagues have led to dozens of replications highlighting this relationship (Rolls et al. 1990; DiMeglio and Mattes 2000; DellaValle et al. 2005; Flood et al. 2006; Mattes 2006; Mourao et al. 2007). A recent meta-analysis confirmed the relationship between intake of low-energy beverages versus sugar-containing beverages on energy intake and body weight (Rogers et al. 2016). Rogers et al. (2016) examined both animal and human studies where a low-energy substitute was compared to a control that included sugar-containing beverages or water. In the 129 human studies of short-term interventions, energy intake from a preload + ad-libitum meal was significantly lower with the low-energy drink than a sugar-sweetened drink. Among 10 sustained intervention studies, the absolute value for total or change in energy intake was lower with the low-energy beverage than a sugar-sweetened beverage. Finally, in studies lasting more than 4 weeks (12 comparisons), difference in weight loss or weight gain favored the low-energy drink by 1.41 kg in adults and 1.04 kg in children, comparing the low-energy drink to a sugar-sweetened one. They conclude that both single-meal and longer-term studies consistently showed a reduction in energy intake and/or body weight in the low energy intake group compared to the group with sugar-sweetened beverages (Rogers et al. 2016).

Studies of the brain response to fructose and glucose have added to our understanding of the problem (Page et al. 2013). A study of adolescents who were either lean or obese showed important differences in the brain's response to oral fructose or glucose. In the adolescents who were lean, both glucose and fructose increased perfusion of brain areas involved in "executive function and control" (prefrontal cortex) but did not activate the "homeostatic" appetite control areas (hypothalamus) (Jastreboff et al. 2016). A very different picture was seen in the adolescents with obesity where ingestion of either fructose or glucose reduced perfusion of the executive region of the brain (prefrontal cortex) and increased activity in the "reward" or "pleasure" centers. This suggests that obese adolescents may lack the ability to downregulate the hedonic and homeostatic regions of the brain after oral ingestion of fructose or glucose. In addition, the ingestion of fructose produced a greater increase in perfusion of the pleasure or reward centers in the adolescents with obesity—something not seen in the lean adolescents. The authors speculate that the reduced response of the executive centers to fructose/glucose may reduce their ability to control intake of sugar-sweetened beverages (Jastreboff et al. 2016; Bray 2016).

CARDIOMETABOLIC EFFECTS ATTRIBUTABLE TO THE SUCROSE (SUGAR) AND FRUCTOSE IN BEVERAGES

Epidemiology

In addition to the data consistently showing that the energy intake of sugar-sweetened beverages can increase body fatness, there is a body of studies showing that these same beverages have detrimental effects on cardiometabolic risk (Malik et al. 2010). A recent meta-analysis showed that adding fructose to the diet in controlled studies produced weight gain unless calories were reduced somewhere else in the diet, that is, a hypercaloric diet produced by adding fructose produced weight gain as one would expect. However, when the fructose was substituted for starch isocalorically, there was no weight gain as one would anticipate (Ng et al. 2012; Sievenpiper et al. 2012). In addition, this group showed that substituting fructose for starch in the diet did not appear to have the detrimental effects noted above for sugar-sweetened beverages. Addition of fructose to the diet or in foods independent of its presence in sugar or HFCS represents only a small amount of fructose. By focusing only on studies with fructose replacing other carbohydrate, the authors appear to me to have overlooked the importance of the invisible calories from sugar that are provided by sugar-sweetened beverages.

In an analysis of worldwide burden of diseases related to consumption of sugar-sweetened beverages, Singh et al. (2015) estimated that there were 184,000 deaths/y attributable to the consumption of sugar-sweetened beverages, another 133,000 attributable to diabetes mellitus, 45,000 to cardiovascular disease, and 6,450 to cancers.

Malik et al. evaluated sugar-sweetened beverage intake and body weight and cardiometabolic disease in a meta-analysis of 8 prospective cohort studies of weight gain and 10 prospective cohort studies of cardiometabolic disease risk. They showed a clear and consistent positive association between sugar-sweetened beverage intake and weight gain. Among the 294,617 participants in the meta-analysis, the highest level of intake had a 24% greater risk of cardiometabolic diseases than those in the lowest group. They concluded that higher consumption of calorically sweetened beverages is associated with both the risk of weight gain and the risk of cardiometabolic diseases (Malik et al. 2010a).

Data from the Health Professionals Follow-up study have added to evidence for the detrimental effects of beverages on risk for CVD. This cohort provides a prospective group for analyzing the 3683 CHD cases over 22 years of follow-up in 42,883 men. Participants in the top quartile of sugar-sweetened beverage intake had a 20% higher relative risk of CHD than those in the bottom quartile after adjustment for age, smoking, physical activity, alcohol, multivitamins, family history, diet quality, energy intake, body mass index, preenrollment weight change, and dieting. Artificially sweetened beverage consumption was not significantly associated with CHD. Adjustment for self-reported high cholesterol, high triglycerides, high blood pressure, and diagnosed type 2 diabetes mellitus slightly attenuated these associations. Intake of sugar-sweetened but not artificially sweetened beverages was significantly associated with increased plasma triglycerides, C-reactive protein, interleukin-6, and tumor necrosis factor receptors 1 and 2 and decreased high-density lipoprotein cholesterol, lipoprotein(a), and leptin ($P < 0.02$) (de Koning et al. 2012).

Data from the National Center for Health Statistics has also been used to examine the trends in sugar consumption and its impact on cardiovascular mortality. Among US adults, the adjusted mean percentage of daily calories from added sugar increased from 15.7% in 1988–1994 to 16.8% ($P = 0.02$) in 1999–2004 and decreased to 14.9% in 2005–2010. Most adults consumed 10% or more of calories from added sugar (71.4%), and approximately 10% of adults consumed 25% or more in 2005–2010. This rise and then stabilization or decrease is consistent with the observations of Mesirow and Welsh noted elsewhere (2015). During 14.6 years of follow-up, 831 CVD deaths were identified during 163,039 person-years. The adjusted hazard ratios (HRs) for CVD mortality across quintiles of the percentage of daily calories consumed from added sugar were 1.00, 1.09, 1.23, 1.49, and 2.43 ($P < 0.001$), respectively (Yang et al. 2014). Adjusted HRs were 1.30 and

2.75 (P = 0.004), respectively, comparing participants who consumed 10.0%–24.9% or 25.0% or more calories from added sugar with those who consumed less than 10.0% of calories from added sugar. These findings were largely consistent across age groups, sex, race/ethnicity (except among non-Hispanic blacks), educational attainment, physical activity, health eating index, and body mass index (Yang et al. 2014).

Sweetened beverage consumption was significantly positively associated with risk of total stroke and cerebral infarction but not with hemorrhagic stroke (Larsson et al. 2014). The multivariable RRs comparing ≥2 (median: 2.1) servings/d (200 mL/serving) with 0.1 to <0.5 (median: 0.3) servings/d were 1.19 for total stroke and 1.22 for cerebral infarction. These findings suggest that sweetened beverage consumption is positively associated with the risk of stroke (Larsson et al. 2014).

In addition to cardiovascular disease, consumption of sugar and sugar-sweetened beverages increases the incidence of diabetes mellitus (Bazzano et al.2008). In a meta-analysis of 17 cohorts (38,253 cases/10,126,754 person-years), higher consumption of sugar-sweetened beverages was associated with a greater incidence of type 2 diabetes (Imamura et al. 2015). An increase of one serving per day increased the risk of diabetes by 18% (95% confidence interval 9%–28%, and 13% after adjustment for adiposity) and for artificially sweetened beverages, 25% and 8% (respectively) and for fruit juice, 5% and 7% (respectively). Potential sources of heterogeneity or bias were not evident for sugar-sweetened beverages. However, for artificially sweetened beverages, publication bias and residual confounding were indicated. For fruit juice, the finding was nonsignificant in studies ascertaining type 2 diabetes objectively (P for heterogeneity = 0.008). Under specified assumptions for population attributable fraction, 20.9 million events of type 2 diabetes were predicted to occur over 10 years in the USA (absolute event rate 11.0%), 1.8 million would be attributable to consumption of sugar-sweetened beverages (population attributable fraction 8.7%), and of 2.6 million events in the UK (absolute event rate 5.8%), 79,000 would be attributable to consumption of sugar-sweetened beverages (population attributable fraction 3.6%). Imamura et al. (2015) conclude that habitual consumption of sugar-sweetened beverages was associated with a greater incidence of type 2 diabetes, independently of adiposity measured as BMI. Although artificially sweetened beverages and fruit juice also showed positive associations with incidence of type 2 diabetes, the findings were likely to involve publication bias and residual confounding. Nonetheless, both artificially sweetened beverages and fruit juice are unlikely to be healthy alternatives to sugar-sweetened beverages for the prevention of type 2 diabetes (Imamura et al. 2015).

Although the intake of sugar-sweetened soft drinks has been reported to be associated with an increased risk of type 2 diabetes, it is unclear whether this is because of the sugar content or related lifestyle factors, whether similar associations hold for artificially sweetened soft drinks, and how these associations are related to BMI. Greenwood et al. (2014) conducted a systematic literature review and dose-response meta-analysis of evidence from prospective cohorts to explore these issues. They found 11 publications on 9 cohorts. Consumption values were converted to mL/d, permitting the exploration of linear and nonlinear dose-response trends. The summary relative risks for sugar-sweetened beverages were 1.20/330 mL per d (P = X), and 1.13/330 mL per d (P = 0.02) for artificially sweetened soft drinks. The association with sugar-sweetened soft drinks was slightly lower in studies adjusting for BMI, consistent with BMI being involved in the causal pathway. There was no evidence of effect modification, though both these comparisons lacked statistical power. Heterogeneity between studies was high. The included studies were observational, so their results should be interpreted cautiously, but findings indicate a positive association between sugar-sweetened soft drink intake and type 2 diabetes risk, attenuated by adjustment for BMI. The trend was less consistent for artificially sweetened soft drinks.

Finally, fructose intake clearly influences the prevalence of gout. The prevalence of gout was studied in the 49,166 men from the Health Professionals Follow-up Study using the Food Frequency Measures of beverage intake and the incidence of gout. The men in the top quintile of fructose intake had an approximately 80% increased risk compared to men is the lowest quintile of fructose intake (Choi and Curran 2008).

Mechanisms for the Effects of Sucrose and Fructose

Sucrose and fructose increase blood pressure in acute and longer-term studies. Acute ingestion of fructose orally increased blood pressure in healthy volunteers compared to the same quantity of glucose or saline. Fifteen healthy men drank 500 mL volumes of water (placebo) alone or with 60 g of fructose or glucose on three occasions and blood pressure, metabolic rate, and autonomic nervous system activity were measured for 2 hours (Brown et al. 2008). Fructose, but not water or glucose, increased diastolic blood pressure by 4 mmHg within 20 minutes.

In longer-term studies, Raben et al. (2002) showed that weight gain over 10 weeks in individuals drinking sugar-sweetened beverages was associated with increased blood pressure, but not in the group drinking the artificially sweetened beverages who actually lost weight. An increase in blood pressure was also evident in the study by Maersk et al. (2012) where those drinking the sugar-sweetened cola beverage for 6 months had an increase in systolic blood pressure without any significant change in body fat or body weight.

Sucrose and fructose also affect lipid metabolism (Teff et al. 2009). In an early clinical study comparing the effect of 50 g of glucose, 50 g of fructose, and 100 g of sucrose on plasma triglycerides, Cohen and Schall (1988) found that both fructose in the amount found in sucrose *and* sucrose increased plasma triglycerides following a meal, but that glucose did not, leading them to conclude that the rise in triglycerides was due to the fructose either alone or as part of sucrose (table sugar), and not glucose.

A 10-week study comparing beverages providing 25% of calories from fructose with a beverage providing 25% of calories from glucose showed that fructose increased postprandial triglycerides, particularly at night. This study also showed that de novo fat synthesis was increased in those consuming fructose-containing drinks. Most importantly, visceral fat, a depot which has the strongest association with cardiovascular risks, increased with only 10 weeks of drinking a fructose beverage compared to the glucose beverage (Stanhope and Havel 2009; Stanhope et al. 2011; Stanhope 2012). In this study, 32 men and women were randomly assigned to either 25% of calories as fructose in beverages or glucose in beverages for 10 weeks along with ad-lib intake of a weight maintenance diet. Subjects were studied before and after ingesting their respective beverages (Stanhope and Havel 2009). Triglycerides at night were significantly higher in those receiving the beverages with fructose than glucose.

In a somewhat-longer clinical study, the daily intake of 1 liter per day (approximately two 16 oz servings) of cola, diet cola, milk, or water were compared in parallel study groups. The sugar-sweetened cola consumed for 6 months increased liver fat, visceral fat, muscle fat, and plasma triglycerides compared to the other beverages (Maersk et al. 2012). From a public health perspective it is concerning that drinking as little as two sugar-sweetened beverages per day for 6 months can increase risk of fatty liver and induce features of the metabolic syndrome. These studies certainly need to be repeated, but if replicated, the public should be warned about the hazards of drinking sugar-sweetened beverages in much the same way as the Food and Drug Administration warns people about risk of taking medications.

Fructose also has interesting effects at the cellular level by inducing inflammatory markers in human kidney cells (Cirillo et al. 2009). Incubation of HK-2 (human kidney cells) with fructose increases monocyte chemotactic protein-1. Knock-down of ketohexokinase, the enzyme that phosphorylates fructose, blocks this effect as do antioxidants. Fructose also increased intracellular uric acid (Johnson et al. 2010).

Fructose is a sweet-tasting sugar that is found naturally in fruits and some vegetables. In modest amounts, it has been part of the human diet for eons (Wolf et al. 2008). It has the highest sweetness taste of all natural components of sugar. It is the dramatic increase in its consumption over the past 30 years that has led to concerns of its detrimental health effect (Bray 2013). It is not the only caloric sweetener found in our food supply. As noted above, about 75% of all U.S. foods and beverages contain added sugars (Ng et al. 2012). The large increase in added sugar intake has led to a major increase in total fructose intake, an increase that has occurred since about 1980

(Bray et al. 2004; Duffey and Popkin 2008). While many health problems are linked with this increase in fructose intake, fatty liver disease is one whose increase is noted in both the United States and Europe and may be linked with the rising fructose intake (Dekker et al. 2010; Ouyang et al. 2008).

SCHEMATIC MODEL OF THE RELATION OF SUGAR, CAFFEINE, AND FRUCTOSE TO CARDIOMETABOLIC DISORDERS

A schematic representation of the health consequences of the sucrose and fructose in soft drinks is shown in Figure 13.1 (Bray and Popkin 2014). This figure pulls together the findings from the studies described above into a single model. The high levels of consumption of sugar-sweetened beverages and other sugary beverages (Duffey and Popkin 2008; Marriott et al. 2009; Popkin 2010; Welsh et al. 2010; Bray 2013) is viewed as the driver for the increase in energy and fructose intake, which play a role in the development of obesity and the metabolic consequences depicted in Figure 13.1 (Bray 2013). The caffeine present in these beverages may serve as a positive feedback signal for continuing ingestion due to its ability to stimulate the central nervous system. Interestingly, the FDA is currently reviewing use of caffeine, a drug which some consider to be mildly addictive. Even 3 weeks of sugar-sweetened beverage ingestion was sufficient to alter lipid metabolism by increasing low-density and decreasing high-density lipoprotein cholesterol, which is a marker of increased CVD risk (Aeberli et al. 2011; Bray 2013). This and other research by

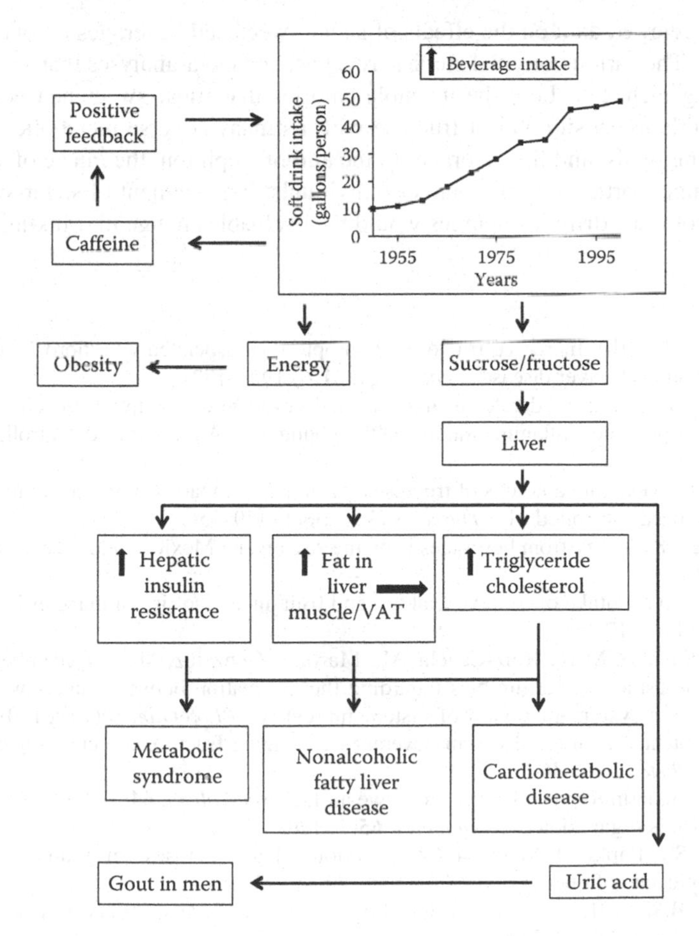

FIGURE 13.1 Model showing some potential consequences of increasing fructose and energy intake from sugar or high fructose corn syrup in beverages.

Aeberli et al. (2013) provide insights into the unique role of fructose in initiating liver dysfunction and possibly leading to non-alcoholic fatty liver disease and the metabolic syndrome, which have become increasingly prevalent (Dekker et al. 2010; Bray 2013).

One key question that Aeberli et al. (2013) began to address is whether the detrimental effects of fructose are simply the result of a linear dose-response to our increasing dietary intake of fructose, or whether there is a threshold below which fructose is without harm. Stanhope et al. (2015) have addressed this question and found a linear response to increasing fructose intake. Consuming beverages containing 10%, 17.5%, or 25% of daily energy requirement from HFCS produced significant linear dose-response increases of lipid/lipoprotein risk factors for CVD and uric acid. Compared with beverages containing 0% HFCS, all 3 doses of HFCS-containing beverages increased concentrations of postprandial triglyceride, and the 2 higher doses increased fasting and/or postprandial concentrations of non-HDL cholesterol, LDL cholesterol, apolipoprotein B, apolipoprotein CIII, and uric acid (Stanhope et al. 2015). This increase in CVD risk factors with increasing amounts of HFCS is particularly important as many studies have shown that there is a group of adolescents and young adults that consume large amounts of sugar-sweetened beverages both in the US as well as other countries (Barquera et al. 2008; Duffey and Popkin 2008; Ng et al. 2011). In fact, it appears that a major push toward marketing sugar-sweetened beverages exists in low- and middle-income countries (Kleiman et al. 2011).

CONCLUSIONS AND RECOMMENDATIONS

This chapter has reviewed data on the effects of sugar-sweetened beverages on obesity and cardiometabolic disease. The various original studies, reviews, and meta-analyses that have been included provide a damning picture of both the invisible calories that sugar-sweetened beverages provide to people susceptible to obesity and of fructose with its many adverse metabolic effects on blood pressure, circulating lipids, and lipid storage. In the author's opinion, the intake of sugar-sweetened beverages is too high, particularly in younger individuals. Replacement of sugar-sweetened beverages with water from safe drinking sources would be a valuable change in drinking patterns.

REFERENCES

Abdelmalek, M.F. et al., 2010. Increased fructose consumption is associated with fibrosis severity in patients with nonalcoholic fatty liver disease. *Hepatology*, **51**(6):1961–1971.

Aeberli, I. et al., 2011. Low to moderate sugar-sweetened beverage consumption impairs glucose and lipid metabolism and promotes inflammation in healthy young men: A randomized controlled trial. *Am J Clin Nutr*, **94**(2):479–485.

Aeberli, I. et al., 2013. Moderate amounts of fructose consumption impair insulin sensitivity in healthy young men: A randomized controlled trial. *Diabetes Care*, **36**(1):150–156.

Barquera, S. et al., 2008. Energy from beverages is on the rise among Mexican adolescents and adults. *J Nutr*, **138**:2454–2461.

Bazzano, L.A. et al., 2008. Intake of fruit, vegetables, and fruit juices and risk of diabetes in women. *Diabetes Care*, **31**(7):1311–1317.

Bes-Rastrollo, M., Schulze, M.B., Ruiz-Canela, M., Martinez-Gonzalez, M.A., December 2013. Financial conflicts of interest and reporting bias regarding the association between sugar-sweetened beverages and weight gain: A systematic review of systematic reviews. *PLoS One*, **10**(12):e1001578.

Bray, G.A., 2013. Potential health risks from beverages containing fructose found in sugar or high-fructose corn syrup. *Diabetes Care*, **36**:11–12.

Bray, G.A., 2015. From farm to fat cell: Why aren't we all fat? *Metabolism*, **64**(3):349–353.

Bray, G.A., July 2016. Is sugar addictive? *Diabetes*, **65**(7):1797–1799.

Bray, G.A., Nielsen, S.J., Popkin, B.M., 2004. Consumption of high-fructose corn syrup in beverages may play a role in the epidemic of obesity. *Am J Clin Nutr*, **79**(4):537–543.

Bray, G.A., Popkin, B.M., 2013. Calorie-sweetened beverages and fructose: What have we learned 10 years later. *Pediatr Obes*, **8**(4):242–248.

Bray, G.A., Popkin, B.M., 2014. Dietary sugar and body weight: Have we reached a crisis in the epidemic of obesity and diabetes? Health be damned! Pour on the sugar. *Diabetes Care*, **37**:950–956.

Brown, C.M., Dulloo, A.G., Yepuri, G., Montani, J.P., 2008. Fructose ingestion acutely elevated blood pressure in healthy young humans. *Am J Physiol Regul Integr Comp Physiol*, **294**(3):R730–R737.

Choi, H.K., Curhan, G., 2008. Soft drinks, fructose consumption, and the risk of gout in men: Prospective cohort study. *BMJ*, **336**(7639):309–312.

Cirillo, P., Gersch, M.S., Mu, W., Scherer, P.M., Kim, K.M., Gesualdo, L., Henderson, G.N., Johnson, R.J., Sautin, Y.Y., 2009. Ketohexokinase-dependent metabolism of fructose induces proinflammatory mediators in proximal tubular cells. *J Am Soc Nephrol*, **20**(3):545–553.

Cohen, J.C., Schall, R., 1988. Reassessing the effects of simple carbohydrates on the serum triglyceride responses to fat meals. *Am J Clin Nutr*, **48**(4):1031–1034.

Dekker, M.J. et al., 2010. Fructose: A highly lipogenic nutrient implicated in insulin resistance, hepatic steatosis, and the metabolic syndrome. *Am J Physiol Endocrinol Metab*, **299**(5):E685–E694.

de Koning, L., Malik, V.S., Kellogg, M.D., Rimm, E.B., Willett, W.C., Hu, F.B., 2012. Sweetened beverage consumption, incident coronary heart disease, and biomarkers of risk in men. *Circulation*, **125**(14):1735–1741.

DellaValle, D.M., Roe, L.S., Rolls, B.J., 2005. Does the consumption of caloric and non-caloric beverages with a meal affect energy intake? *Appetite*, **44**(2):187–193.

de Ruyter, J.C. et al., 2012. A trial of sugar-free or sugar-sweetened beverages and body weight in children. *N Engl J Med*, **367**(15):1397–1406.

DiMeglio, D.P., Mattes, R.D., 2000. Liquid versus solid carbohydrate: Effects on food intake and body weight. *Int J Obes Relat Metab Disord*, **24**(6):794–800.

Duffey, K.J., Popkin, B.M., 2008. High-fructose corn syrup: Is this what's for dinner? *Am J Clin Nutr*, **88**(6):1722S–1732S.

Ebbeling, C.B. et al., 2012. A randomized trial of sugar-sweetened beverages and adolescent body weight. *N Engl J Med*, **367**(15):1407–1416.

Flood, J., Roe, L., Rolls, B., 2006. The effect of increased beverage portion size on energy intake at a meal. *J Am Diet Assoc*, **106**(12):1984–1990.

Ford, E.S., Dietz, W.H., 2013. Trends in energy intake among adults in the United States: Findings from NHANES. *Am J Clin Nutr*, **97**(4):848–853.

Greenwood, D.C., Threapleton, D.E., Evans, C.E., Cleghorn, C.L., Nykjaer, C., Woodhead, C., Burley, V.J., 2014. Association between sugar-sweetened and artificially sweetened soft drinks and type 2 diabetes: Systematic review and dose-response meta-analysis of prospective studies. *Br J Nutr*, **112**(5):725–734.

Imamura, F., O'Connor, L., Ye, Z., Mursu, J., Hayashino, Y., Bhupathiraju, S.N., Forouhi, N.G., 2015. Consumption of sugar sweetened beverages, artificially sweetened beverages, and fruit juice and incidence of type 2 diabetes: Systematic review, meta-analysis, and estimation of population attributable fraction. *BMJ*, **351**:h3576.

Jastreboff, A.M., Sinha, R., Arora, J., et al., 2016. Altered brain response to drinking glucose and fructose in obese adolescents. *Diabetes*, **65**:1929–1939.

Johnson, R.J., Sanchez-Lozada, L.G., Nakagawa, T., 2010. The effect of fructose on renal biology and disease. *J Am Soc Nephrol*, **21**(12):2036–2039.

Johnson, R.J., Segal, M.S., Sautin, Y., Nakagawa, T., Feig, D.I., Kang, D.H., Gersch, M.S., Benner, S., Sánchez-Lozada, L.G., 2007. Potential role of sugar (fructose) in the epidemic of hypertension, obesity and the metabolic syndrome, diabetes, kidney disease, and cardiovascular disease. *Am J Clin Nutr*, **86**(4):899–906.

Kit, B.K. et al., 2013. Trends in sugar-sweetened beverage consumption among youth and adults in the United States: 1999–2010. *Am J Clin Nutr*, **98**(1):180–188.

Kleiman, S., Ng, S.W., Popkin, B., 2011. Drinking to our health: Can beverage companies cut calories while maintaining profits? *Obes Rev*, **13**(3):258–274.

Larsson, S.C., Akesson, A., Wolk, A., 2014. Sweetened beverage consumption is associated with increased risk of stroke in women and men. *J Nutr*, **144**(6):856–860.

Locke, A.E. et al., 2015. Genetic studies of body mass index yield new insights for obesity biology. *Nature*, **518**(7538):197–206.

Loos, R.J., 2012. Genetic determinants of common obesity and their value in prediction. *Best Pract Res Clin Endocrinol Metab*, **26**(2):211–226.

Ludwig, D.S., 2013. Examining the health effects of fructose. *JAMA*, **310**(1):33–34.

Maersk, M., Belza, A., Stødkilde-Jørgensen, H., Ringgaard, S., Chabanova, E., Thomsen, H., Pedersen, S.B., Astrup, A., Richelsen, B., 2012. Sucrose-sweetened beverages increase fat storage in the liver, muscle, and visceral fat depot: A 6-mo randomized intervention study. *Am J Clin Nutr*, **95**(2):283–289.

Malik, V.S. et al., 2010b. Sugar-sweetened beverages and risk of metabolic syndrome and type 2 diabetes: A meta-analysis. *Diabetes Care*, **33**(11):2477–2483.
Malik, V.S., Popkin, B.M., Bray, G.A., Després, J.P., Hu, F.B., 2010a. Sugar-sweetened beverages, obesity, type 2 diabetes mellitus, and cardiovascular disease risk. *Circulation*, **121**(11):1356–1364.
Malik, V.S., Schulze, M.B., Hu, F.B., 2006. Intake of sugar-sweetened beverages and weight gain: A systematic review. *Am J Clin Nutr*, **84**(2):274–288.
Malik, V.S., Willett, W.C., Hu, F.B., 2013. Global obesity: Trends, risk factors and policy implications. *Nat Rev Endocrinol*, **9**(1):13–27.
Marriott, B.P., Cole, N., Lee, E., 2009. National estimates of dietary fructose intake increased from 1977 to 2004 in the United States. *J Nutr*, **139**(6):1228S–1235S.
Mattes, R., 2006. Fluid calories and energy balance: The good, the bad, and the uncertain. *Physiol Behav*, **89**(1):66–70.
Mattes, R.D., 1996. Dietary compensation by humans for supplemental energy provided as ethanol or carbohydrate in fluids. *Physiol Behav*, **59**(1):179–187.
Mesirow, M.S., Welsh, J.A., 2015. Changing beverage consumption patterns have resulted in fewer liquid calories in the diets of US children: National Health and Nutrition Examination Survey 2001–2010. *J Acad Nutr Diet*, **115**(4):559–566.
Moss, M., 2013. *Salt Sugar Fat: How the Food Giants Hooked Us*. New York: Random House.
Mourao, D.M., Bressan, J., Campbell, W.W., Mattes, R.D., 2007. Effects of food form on appetite and energy intake in lean and obese young adults. *Int J Obes (Lond)*, **31**(11):1688–1695.
National Research Council, 1989, *Diet and Health, Implications for Reducing Chronic Disease Risk*. Washington, DC: National Academy Press.
Nestle, M., 2015. *Soda Politicss: Taking on Big Soda (and Winning)*. New York: Oxford University Press.
Ng, S.W. et al., 2011. Patterns and trends of beverage consumption among children and adults in Great Britain, 1986–2009. *Br J Nutr* **20**:1–16.
Ng, S.W., Slining, M.M., Popkin, B.M., 2012. Use of caloric and noncaloric sweeteners in US consumer packaged foods, 2005–2009. *J Acad Nutr Diet*, **112**(11):1828–1834.e6.
Nielsen, S.J., Siega-Riz, A.M., Popkin, B.M., 2002. Trends in food locations and sources among adolescents and young adults. *Prev Med*, **35**(2):107–113.
Ogden, C.L. et al., 2007. The epidemiology of obesity. *Gastroenterology*, **132**:1087–1102.
Ogden, C.L., Carroll, M.D., Kit, B.K., Flegal, K.M., 2014. Prevalence of childhood and adult obesity in the United States, 2011–2012. *JAMA*, **311**(8):806–814.
Olsen, N.J., Heitmann, B.L., 2009. Intake of calorically sweetened beverages and obesity. *Obes Rev*, **10**(1):68–75.
Ouyang, X. et al., 2008. Fructose consumption as a risk factor for non-alcoholic fatty liver disease. *J Hepatol*, **48**(6):993–999.
Page Ka, C.O.A.J. et al., 2013. Effects of fructose vs glucose on regional cerebral blood flow in brain regions involved with appetite and reward pathways. *JAMA*, **309**(1):63–70.
Popkin, B.M., 2010. Patterns of beverage use across the lifecycle. *Physiol Behav*, **100**(1):4–9.
Putnam, J., Allshouse, J., 2003a. Trends in U.S. per capita consumption of dairy products, 1909 to 2001. *Amber Waves*, **1**:12–13.
Putnam, J.J., Allshouse, J.E., 2003b. 1970–1997 Food consumption, prices, and expenditures. Economic Research Service Bull. No. 965. USDA Food & Rural Economic Division, p. 34.
Qi, Q. et al., 2012. Sugar-sweetened beverages and genetic risk of obesity. *N Engl J Med*, **367**(15):1387–1396.
Raben, A. et al., 2002. Sucrose compared with artificial sweeteners: Different effects on ad libitum food intake and body weight after 10 wk of supplementation in overweight subjects. *Am J Clin Nutr*, **76**(4):721–729.
Reaven, G.M., 1988. Banting lecture 1988. Role of insulin resistance in human disease. *Diabetes*, **37**(12):1595–1607.
Rogers, P.J. et al., 2016. Does low-energy consumption affect energy intake and bodyweight? A systematic review, including meta-analyses, of the evidence from human and animal studies. *Int J Obes (Lond)*, **40**(3):381–394.
Rolls, B.J., Kim, S., Fedoroff, I.C., 1990. Effects of drinks sweetened with sucrose or aspartame on hunger, thirst and food intake in men. *Physiol Behav*, **48**(1):19–26.
Sievenpiper, J.L. et al., 2012. Effect of fructose on body weight in controlled feeding trials: A systematic review and meta-analysis. *Ann Intern Med*, **156**(4):291–304.

Singh, G.M., Micha, R., Khatibzadeh, S., Lim, S., Ezzati, M., Mozaffarian, D., 2015. Global Burden of Diseases Nutrition and Chronic Diseases Expert Group (NutriCoDE). Estimated global, regional, and national disease burdens related to sugar-sweetened beverage consumption in 2010. *Circulation*, **132**(8):639–666.

Slining, M.M., Popkin, B.M., 2013. Trends in intakes and sources of solid fats and added sugars among U.S. children and adolescents: 1994–2010. *Pediatr Obes*, **8**(4):307–324.

Sørensen, L.B., Raben, A., Stender, S., Astrup, A., 2005. Effect of sucrose on inflammatory markers in overweight humans. *Am J Clin Nutr*, **82**(2):421–427.

Speliotes, E.K. et al., 2010. Association analyses of 249,796 individuals reveal 18 new loci associated with body mass index. *Nat Genet*, **42**(11):937–948.

Stanhope, K.L., 2012. Role of fructose-containing sugars in the epidemics of obesity and metabolic syndrome. *Annu Rev Med*, **63**:329–343.

Stanhope, K.L. et al., 2011. Consumption of fructose and high fructose corn syrup increase postprandial triglycerides, LDL-cholesterol, and apolipoprotein-B in young men and women. *J Clin Endocrinol Metabol*, **96**(10):E1596–E1605.

Stanhope, K.L., Havel, P.J., 2009. Fructose consumption: Considerations for future research on its effects on adipose distribution, lipid metabolism, and insulin sensitivity in humans. *J Nutr*, **139**(6):1236S–1241S.

Stanhope, K.L., Medici, V., Bremer, A.A., Lee, V., Lam, H.D., Nunez, M.V., Chen, G.X., Keim, N.L., Havel, P.J., 2015. A dose-response study of consuming high-fructose corn syrup-sweetened beverages on lipid/lipoprotein risk factors for cardiovascular disease in young adults. *Am J Clin Nutr* **101**(6):1144–1154.

Teff, K.L. et al., 2009. Endocrine and metabolic effects of consuming fructose- and glucose-sweetened beverages with meals in obese men and women: Influence of insulin resistance on plasma triglyceride responses. *J Clin Endocrinol Metab*, **94**(5):1562–1569.

Te Morenga, L., Simonette, M., Mann, J., 2012. Dietary sugars and body weight: Systematic review and meta-analyses of randomised controlled trials and cohort studies. *BMJ*, **346**:e7492. doi: 10.1136/bmj.e7492.

Te Morenga, L.A., Howatson, A.J., Jones, R.M., Mann, J., 2014. Dietary sugars and cardiometabolic risk: Systematic review and meta-analyses of randomized controlled trials of the effects on blood pressure and lipids. *Am J Clin Nutr*, **100**(1):65–79.

Trumbo, P.R., Rivers, C.R., 2014. Systematic review of the evidence for an association between sugar-sweetened beverage consumption and risk of obesity. *Nutr Rev*, **72**(9):566–574.

Tucker, L.A., Tucker, J.M., Bailey, B.W., Le Ceminant, J.D., 2015. A 4-year prospective study of soft drink consumption and weight gain: The role of calorie intake and physical activity. *Am J Health Promot*, **29**:262–265.

Vartanian, L.R., Schwartz, M.B., Brownell, K.D., 2007. Effects of soft drink consumption on nutrition and health: A systematic review and meta-analysis. *Am J Public Health*, **97**(4):667–675.

Vernon, G., Baranova, A., Younossi, Z.M., 2011. Systematic review: The epidemiology and natural history of non-alcoholic fatty liver disease and non-alcoholic steatohepatitis in adults. *Aliment Pharmacol Ther*, **34**(3):274–285.

Welsh, J.A. et al., 2010. Caloric sweetener consumption and dyslipidemia among US adults. *JAMA*, **303**(15):1490–1497.

Wolf, A., Bray, G.A., Popkin, B.M., 2008. A short history of beverages and how our body treats them. *Obes Rev*, **9**:151–164.

Yang, Q., Zhang, Z., Gregg, E.W., Flanders, W.D., Merritt, R., Hu, F.B., 2014. Added sugar intake and cardiovascular diseases mortality among US adults. *JAMA Intern Med*, **174**(4):516–524.

Yudkin, J., 1972. *Sweet and Dangerous: The New Facts about the Sugar You Eat as a Cause of Heart Disease, Diabetes, and Other Killers*. London, U.K.: David McKay Co.

14 Effects and Mechanisms of Fructose-Containing Sugars in the Pathophysiology of Metabolic Syndrome

Kimber L. Stanhope and Peter J. Havel

CONTENTS

ABSTRACT

The objective of this chapter is to present the mechanisms and evidence that support the hypothesis that increased consumption of added sugars contributes to the development of metabolic syndrome (MetS). MetS is described along with its formally defined diagnostic criteria and less well-recognized risk factors. The amount and types of sugar consumed in the United States are discussed. The mechanistic scenario by which consumption of fructose or fructose-containing sugar may promote the development of components of MetS and how this scenario differs from the established paradigm are described. We cite the epidemiological studies that demonstrate associations between sugar consumption and all the formally defined, and some of the less well-recognized, risk factors for MetS. Results from dietary intervention studies showing that many of these risk factors are adversely affected when sugar intake is increased and beneficially affected when sugar intake is decreased are presented. We conclude that specific recommendations to reduce consumption of added sugars to the levels recommended by the 2015–2020 Dietary Guidelines for American, or to the even lower levels recommended by the American Heart Association, may be beneficial in the prevention and management of MetS.

INTRODUCTION

The objective of this chapter is to present the mechanisms and evidence that support the hypothesis that increased consumption of added sugars contributes to the development of metabolic syndrome (MetS). MetS is described along with its formally defined diagnostic criteria and less well-recognized risk factors. The amount and types of sugar consumed in the United States are discussed. The term *added sugars* in this chapter refers to sugars not naturally occurring in foods, and these consist mainly of the fructose-containing sugars (sucrose) and high-fructose corn syrup (HFCS). It also refers to the sugars added to both beverages and solid foods, even though as previously detailed (Stanhope 2016), it cannot be assumed that sugar in solid food and sugar in beverage have equivalent effects. We describe the mechanistic scenario by which consumption of fructose or fructose-containing sugar may promote the development of components of MetS and how this scenario differs from the established paradigm. We present the epidemiological and the direct experimental evidence concerning the effects of fructose or added sugar consumption on each of the formally defined and some of the less well-recognized risk factors for MetS. We conclude with consideration of whether prevention and treatment of MetS should include specific nutrition advice to reduce the consumption of added sugars.

DESCRIPTION OF METABOLIC SYNDROME

MetS is well described by the MetS concepts that were affirmed and recently reported by the Cardiometabolic Think Tank (Sperling et al. 2015). This group of individual experts representing more than 20 professional organizations convened in June, 2014, to focus on a new care model for the MetS (Sperling et al. 2015).

AFFIRMED CONCEPTS

The six affirmed concepts (AC.) presented below represent the evidence-based consensus of the group (Sperling et al. 2015):

AC.1. MetS is a progressive pathophysiological state associated with substantially increased risk for development of type 2 diabetes (T2D) and atherosclerotic cardiovascular disease.

AC.2. MetS is clinically manifested by a cluster of risk factors that are causally interrelated (not aggregating by chance alone).

AC.3. Risk for adverse health outcomes increases substantially with the accumulation of component MetS risk factors, in addition to unmeasured ("residual risk") factors. The timely recognition of MetS risk factors helps to identify individuals at high risk for ASCVD and T2D and to initiate preventive strategies before end-organ damage occurs.

AC.4. Obesity is a MetS risk factor that is imperfectly gauged by body mass index and/or waist circumference and is modulated by adipocyte distribution, size, and function, as well as race, behavior, and lifestyle. Excess ectopic and/or visceral adiposity is fundamental to the pathophysiology of MetS.

AC.5. Treatment of MetS should prioritize therapeutic lifestyle changes, including a healthy diet and regular physical activity, to address all risk factors. Treatment should also continue to be focused on specific interventions for component MetS risk factors.

AC.6. The term "MetS" will be used to designate a portfolio of descriptors that have previously included the terms *cardioMetS, insulin resistance syndrome, syndrome X*, and others.

MetS Risk Factors

A key finding of the Cardiometabolic Think Tank is that MetS is a cluster of risk factors that include those that are formally defined and those that are less well-recognized (Sperling et al. 2015).

Formally Defined Diagnostic Criteria

The formally defined risk factors, shown in Table 14.1, are included in the MetS diagnostic criteria. The current criteria were proposed in a joint interim statement of the International Diabetes Federation Task Force on Epidemiology and Prevention; National Heart, Lung, and Blood Institute; American Heart Association; World Heart Federation; International Atherosclerosis Society; and International Association for the Study of Obesity (Alberti et al. 2009). A person with 3 out of the 5 formally defined risk factors included in Table 14.1 qualifies for a diagnosis of MetS. The formally defined risk factors are easily measured in clinical practice.

Other Risk Factors That Are Not Formally Recognized

Insulin resistance is a critical feature of MetS, which associates with all five of the formally defined criteria (Sperling et al. 2015). It is not included in Table 14.1 because it is not formally defined or easy to measure in clinical practice. Also not included in Table 14.1 are other less well-recognized risk factors that include elevated levels of apolipoprotein B, small dense LDL, C-reactive protein, fibrinogen, and microalbuminuria (Grundy et al. 2005, Sperling et al. 2015). The Cardiometabolic Think Tank did not include fatty liver (Fan and Peng 2007, Fabbrini et al. 2009, Bremer, Mietus-Snyder, and Lustig 2012, Gaharwar et al. 2015, Marino and Jornayvaz 2015) or uric acid (Chaudhary et al. 2013, Yadav et al. 2013, Billiet et al. 2014, Liu et al. 2015, Nejatinamini et al. 2015) on this list; however, recent evidence and reviews of the literature support their inclusion.

TABLE 14.1
Criteria for Clinical Diagnosis[a] of the Metabolic Syndrome

Risk Factor	Categorical Cut Points
Elevated triglycerides (or drug treatment for elevated triglycerides)	≥150 mg/dL (1.7 mmol/L)
Reduced HDL-C (or drug treatment for reduced HDL-C)	<40 mg/dL (1.0 mmol/L) in males, <50 mg/dL (1.3 mmol/L) in females
Elevated blood pressure (antihypertensive drug treatment)	Systolic ≥130 and/or diastolic ≥85 mm Hg
Increased waist circumference	Population- and country-specific definitions Previous cutoffs: ≥102 cm for males, ≥88 cm for females
Elevated fasting glucose (or drug treatment of elevated glucose)	≥100 mg/dL (5.6 mmol/L)

[a] Metabolic syndrome is diagnosed by a co-occurrence of three of the above risk factors.

Residual Risk Factors

The Cardiometabolic Think Tank also recognized the existence of residual risk indicators. These can include low birth weight, birth from a mother with gestational diabetes, parental history of MetS, and low socioeconomic status (Sperling et al. 2015). Not only do these add to the risk burden, they can impose an increased risk very early in life. Both of these, total risk burden (Berry et al. 2012) and early life risk exposure (DeBoer et al. 2015a,b), markedly increase the risk of adverse health outcomes (e.g., T2D and CVD) later in life.

Lifestyle Risk Factors

The Cardiometabolic Think Tank recognizes that lifestyle, specifically physical activity and nutrition, are modifiable factors crucial to prevent and treat MetS and its consequences (Sperling et al. 2015). For nutrition, it is recommended that emphasis should be placed on dietary patterns such as the Dietary Approaches to Stop Hypertension (DASH) and Mediterranean-style diets rather than specific macronutrients (Sperling et al. 2015). This lack of focus on specific macronutrients contrasts with the key recommendation of the 2015–2020 Dietary Guidelines for Americans (United States Department of Health and Human Services and U.S. Department of Agriculture 2015) and the World Health Organization guideline (World Health Organization 2015) that added sugar consumption be limited to less than 10% of daily calories. However, for both the US Dietary Guidelines and the World Health Organization, the main rationale for the recommendation to limit added sugars relates to meeting food group and nutrient needs within calorie limits rather than the possibility that consumption of added sugars may specifically contribute to the development of MetS or chronic disease compared with other macronutrients.

ADDED SUGARS

The remainder of this chapter will address the questions of whether consumption of added sugars should be considered a modifiable risk factor for MetS and whether the nutrition emphasis proposed by the Cardiometabolic Think Tank (Sperling et al. 2015) should be expanded to include a specific recommendation to reduce consumption of added sugars.

Consumption Levels of Added Sugars

Americans consume more than three times more energy as processed sugar, 368 kcal/day, than naturally occurring sugars. Sugar-sweetened beverages (SSBs) contribute 33% of these calories, solid sugar and candy contribute 16%, cakes and other baked goods contribute 13%, and ice cream and other dairy desserts contribute 9% (Johnson et al. 2009). Self-reported food intake data suggests that 13% of the U.S. population consume 25% or more of their daily energy as added, processed sugar (Marriott et al. 2010). The average level of added sugars intake in the U.S. is approximately 13%–15% of daily calories for adults 20–60 years of age (Ervin and Ogden 2013, Yang et al. 2014) and 16% for children and adolescents (Ervin et al. 2012). These figures may underestimate consumption of added sugars, as self-reported food intake is often underreported (Livingstone and Black 2003), and sugar is one of the foods most likely to be underreported (Rangan et al. 2014). The United States leads the world in sugar consumption with levels more than double the world average. Sugar consumption in Brazil, Australia, Argentina, and Mexico is close to the U.S. level, while it is 75% lower in China and much of Africa (Suisse Research Institute Credit 2013).

Sources of Added Sugars

The predominant source of dietary added sugars throughout the world is sucrose, which is extracted and purified from sugarcane and sugar beets. However, in the United States, a significant amount of the added sugars energy is provided by HFCS. HFCS is derived from the hydrolysis of cornstarch, which produces glucose syrup, and then isomerization of the glucose syrup to produce syrup containing 42% fructose. The fructose in this syrup can be extracted to produce syrup that has 90% fructose. The proportion of fructose to glucose in the final HFCS product is variable depending on how much of the 90% fructose syrup is added to the 42% fructose syrup. Food nutrition labels do not provide information regarding the proportion or amount of fructose in the HFCS that is contained in the product. Information from the Corn Refiners Association (The Corn Refiners Association n.d.) states that HFCS comes in two formulations—HFCS-42, which has 42% fructose, and HFCS-55, which has 55% fructose. However, analyses of popular SSB showed the mean fructose content in the HFCS used was 59% (range 47%–65%), and several major brands appear to be produced with HFCS that is 65% fructose (Ventura, Davis, and Goran 2011). Therefore, while consumers can be certain that sucrose always contains 50% fructose and 50% glucose, they cannot determine from the food label the fructose content of the HFCS used.

Plausible Mechanisms by Which Consumption of Fructose-Containing Sugar May Promote the Development of MetS

The proportion of fructose in added sugars is an important issue because a large body of scientific evidence from studies in animals and humans indicates that consumption of fructose results in more adverse changes in components of MetS than consumption of glucose. This includes a study from our group in which subjects consuming 25% of their energy requirement (Ereq) as fructose-sweetened beverages for 10 weeks exhibited increases of *de novo* lipogenesis (DNL), visceral adipose tissue deposition, dyslipidemia, and circulating uric acid and markers of inflammation and reductions of fatty acid oxidation and insulin sensitivity, while subjects consuming glucose-sweetened beverages did not, despite comparable body weight gain (Stanhope et al. 2009, Cox et al. 2011, 2012a,b). These results, our more recent reports (Stanhope et al. 2011a, 2015), and the findings from a number of other investigators support the plausibility of the mechanisms, described below and illustrated in Figure 14.1, by which consumption of added, fructose-containing sugars may mediate or contribute to MetS.

Unregulated Hepatic Uptake and Metabolism of Fructose

Hepatic glucose metabolism is regulated by insulin and hepatic energy needs, and this allows most of the ingested glucose, from starch or a glucose-sweetened beverage, arriving via the portal vein to bypass the liver and reach the systemic circulation. In contrast, the initial phosphorylation of dietary fructose is largely catalyzed by fructokinase, which is not regulated by hepatic energy status (Mayes 1993, Havel 2005). This results in unregulated fructose uptake by the liver, with most of the ingested fructose being metabolized in the liver and very little reaching the systemic circulation (Teff et al. 2009). The excess substrate generated from the unregulated metabolism of fructose in the liver leads to increased DNL (Stanhope et al. 2009). Recent evidence from the research group of Schwarz and colleagues demonstrates that fructose consumption can increase DNL more than isocaloric complex carbohydrates even in subjects consuming energy-balanced, weight-maintaining diets (Schwarz et al. 2015).

DNL, Hepatic Lipids, and Hepatic Insulin Resistance

DNL increases the hepatic lipid supply directly (Maersk et al. 2012, Sevastianova et al. 2012, Schwarz et al. 2015), via synthesis of fatty acids, and indirectly, by inhibiting fatty acid oxidation (Cox et al. 2012a, Schwarz et al. 2015). Increased levels of hepatic lipids may also promote hepatic insulin resistance (Schwarz et al. 2015), possibly by increasing levels of diacylglycerol (DAG), which activates protein kinase C epsilon (PKCε) leading to increased serine rather than tyrosine

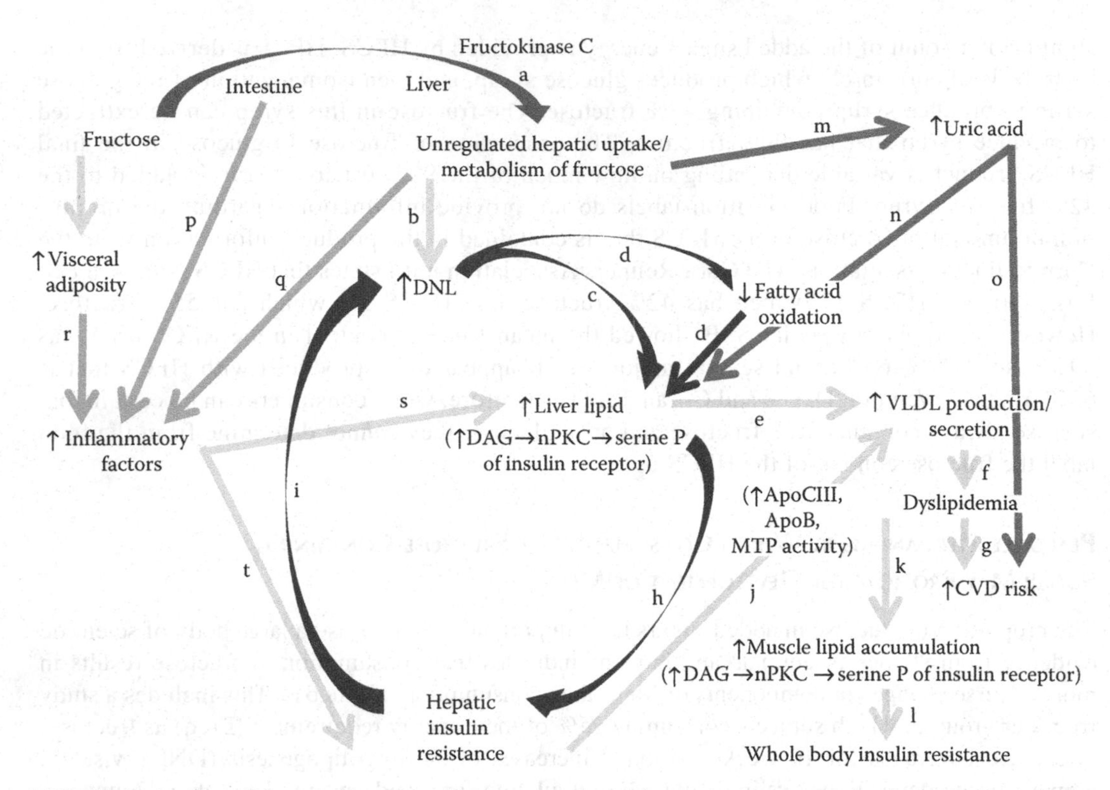

FIGURE 14.1 Potential mechanisms by which consumption of fructose promotes the development of metabolic syndrome: The initial phosphorylation of dietary fructose in the liver is largely catalyzed by fructokinase C (a), which is not regulated by hepatic energy status. This results in unregulated fructose uptake and metabolism by the liver. The excess substrate leads to increased DNL (b). DNL increases the intrahepatic lipid supply directly via synthesis of fatty acids (c) and indirectly by inhibiting fatty acid oxidation (d). Increased levels of intrahepatic lipid content promote very low–density lipoprotein (VLDL) production and secretion (e). This leads to increased levels of circulating TG and low-density lipoprotein cholesterol (dyslipidemia [f]), risk factors for CVD (g). Increased levels of hepatic lipid may also promote hepatic insulin resistance by increasing levels of diacylglycerol, which may activate novel protein kinase C (nPKC) and lead to serine phosphorylation (serine P) of the insulin receptor and insulin receptor substrate 1 (IRS-1) and impaired insulin action (h). Due to selective insulin resistance, DNL is even more strongly activated in the insulin-resistant liver DNL (i), which has the potential to generate a vicious cycle (circular arrows). This cycle would be expected to further exacerbate VLDL production and secretion via increased intrahepatic lipid supply. Hepatic insulin resistance also exacerbates VLDL production/secretion (j) by increasing apolipoprotein (apo)B availability and apoCIII synthesis and by upregulating microsomal triglyceride transfer protein expression. This exacerbates and sustains exposure to circulating TG, leading to muscle lipid accumulation (k), impaired insulin signaling, and whole-body insulin resistance (l). The fructokinase-catalyzed phosphorylation of fructose to fructose-1-phosphate, which results in the conversion of ATP to AMP and a depletion of inorganic phosphate, leads to uric acid production via the purine degradation pathway (m). High levels of uric acid are associated and may contribute to increased risk for development of fatty liver (n), CVD (o), and MetS. Fructose exposure in the intestine (p) and liver (q) and fructose-induced increases of visceral adipose (r) may promote inflammatory responses that further promote liver lipid accumulation (s) and/or impair hepatic insulin signaling (t). (Reprinted from Stanhope, K.L. and Havel, P.J., Mechanisms by which dietary sugars influence lipid metabolism, circulating lipids and lipoproteins, and cardiovascular risk, in M. Goran and L. Tappy, Eds., *Dietary Sugars and Health*, Taylor & Francis Group, LLC., Boca Raton, FL, pp. 267–282, 2014. With permission.)

phosphorylation of the insulin receptor and insulin receptor substrate 1 (IRS-1) and, thus, impaired insulin action (Jornayvaz and Shulman 2012). Due to selective insulin resistance, DNL is even more strongly activated in the insulin-resistant liver (Lewis et al. 2002). This has the potential to generate a vicious cycle: DNL increases liver lipid, which increases hepatic insulin resistance, which further increases DNL (Figure 14.1—circular arrows).

Very Low–Density Lipoprotein Production and Secretion

Increased intrahepatic lipid content promotes very low–density lipoprotein 1 (VLDL1) production and secretion (Adiels et al. 2006), which leads to increased circulating levels of postprandial triglyceride (TG) and dyslipidemia (Adiels et al. 2008). Our short-term studies demonstrate that postprandial levels of TG are increased within 1 day of fructose, HFCS or sucrose consumption at 25% Ereq (Teff et al. 2004, 2009, Stanhope and Havel 2008a). The vicious cycle described above would be expected to further exacerbate VLDL production and secretion by increasing the hepatic lipid supply (Adiels et al. 2006). Hepatic insulin resistance, however, may also indirectly increase VLDL production and secretion by (1) increasing the availability of apolipoprotein B (apoB) (Fisher 2012, Christian, Sacco, and Adeli 2013), the protein component of VLDL; (2) upregulating microsomal triglyceride transfer protein expression (Lewis et al. 2002), which catalyzes the assembly of TG and apoB into VLDL; and (3) increasing the production of apolipoprotein CIII (apoCIII) (Yao and Wang 2012). There is evidence to suggest that apoCIII plays a critical role in promoting the second-step incorporation of lipid into VLDL, which converts VLDL2 (smaller, TG-poor particles) into larger, TG-rich VLDL1 particles (Sundaram et al. 2010, Qin et al. 2011). Both fructose-fed rhesus monkeys (Bremer et al. 2014) and young adults consuming HFCS-sweetened beverages (Stanhope et al. 2015) exhibit increased levels of fasting and/or postprandial apoCIII.

Dyslipidemia

The overproduction of VLDL1 has been described as the underlying defect that leads to the dyslipidemia that is characteristic of patients with T2D and MetS: high blood concentrations of TG and small dense LDL and low blood concentrations of HDL (Adiels et al. 2008). A possible mechanism for this relationship is that as levels of VLDL1 increase, this lipoprotein subclass becomes the preferred substrate of cholesteryl ester transfer protein (CETP) (Chapman et al. 2010). CETP exchanges the cholesterol in LDL and HDL with the TG in VLDL1. The resulting TG-enriched LDL can undergo hepatic lipase-mediated lipolysis, yielding smaller, denser LDL. Small dense LDL is considered to be more atherogenic than larger, more buoyant LDL in part due to its reduced affinity for the LDL receptor, thus increasing its retention time in the circulation (Diffenderfer and Schaefer 2014). The TG-enriched HDL resulting from CETP remodeling is more likely to be degraded by the kidney rather than continue participation in reverse cholesterol transport (Packard 2003, Chapman et al. 2010). This scenario is proatherogenic as opposed to the antiatherogenic scenario that occurs when VLDL1 levels are low and LDL and HDL are the preferred substrates of CETP. In the antiatherogenic scenario, CETP catalyzes the transfer of cholesterol from HDL to LDL. The cholesterol-enriched LDL is then cleared by hepatic LDL receptors, and the cholesterol-depleted HDL continues participation in reverse cholesterol transport (Chapman et al. 2010).

It has also been suggested that apolipoprotein CIII (apoCIII) is the primary mediator of the relationship between VLDL and small dense LDL (Sacks 2015) and CVD (Wyler von Ballmoos, Haring, and Sacks 2015). VLDL can contain apoE or apoCIII or both. ApoCIII inhibits the clearance of TG-rich lipoproteins from the circulation (Boren et al. 2015), while apoE binds to high-affinity hepatic receptors and allows for clearance of lipoproteins (Sacks 2015). In hypertriglyceridemia, excessive production of a VLDL subspecies that does not contain apoE, but is relatively enriched in apoCIII, results in an accumulation of TG-rich VLDL that is metabolized by lipolytic enzymes to small dense LDL (Sacks 2015).

Intramyocellular Lipid Accumulation and Whole-Body Insulin Resistance

Increased exposure of skeletal muscle to high circulating postprandial TG concentrations, along with decreased fat oxidation (Cox et al. 2012a) during fructose consumption, may lead to intramyocellular lipid accumulation (Maersk et al. 2012). Intramyocellular lipid concentrations are correlated with reduced whole-body insulin sensitivity in humans (Krssak et al. 1999). It is possible, but not definitive (Watt and Hoy 2012), that this relationship is mediated by the same mechanism described for the development of hepatic insulin resistance: DAG-mediated activation of PKCε resulting in serine phosphorylation of the insulin receptor, IRS-1, and other downstream insulin signaling proteins (Samuel and Shulman 2012). It is also possible that other factors such as inflammation and oxidative stress (Anderson et al. 2009) contribute to muscle insulin resistance (Coen and Goodpaster 2012). While the mechanisms that lead to muscle insulin resistance are not established, two short-term (9 and 21 days) studies in which subjects consuming fructose exhibited reduced hepatic insulin sensitivity during hyperinsulinemic euglycemic clamps, but not reduced whole-body insulin sensitivity (Aeberli et al. 2013, Schwarz et al. 2015), suggest that whole-body insulin resistance occurs subsequently to hepatic insulin resistance.

Hyperuricemia

The unregulated hepatic uptake and metabolism of fructose also leads to increased concentrations of circulating uric acid (Cox et al. 2012b, Bruun et al. 2015, Stanhope et al. 2015). The fructokinase-catalyzed phosphorylation of fructose to fructose 1-phosphate, which results in the conversion of adenosine triphosphate (ATP) to adenosine monophosphate (AMP) and a depletion of inorganic phosphate, leads to uric acid production via the purine degradation pathway (Mayes 1993). Uric acid is a potential mediator of metabolic disease, with most but not all (Zalawadiya et al. 2015) recent studies reporting that it is strongly associated with and predictive of MetS, fatty liver, and CVD (Cai et al. 2013, Billiet et al. 2014, Viazzi et al. 2014). High uric acid levels resulting from fructose consumption may also explain the association between sugar consumption and increased blood pressure (Johnson et al. 2015). Studies performed in rodents suggest that the mechanisms involve the uric acid–dependent activation of the rennin–angiotensin system via the induction of oxidative stress and development of endothelial dysfunction due to reduction in endothelial nitric oxide levels (Feig et al. 2013).

Visceral Adipose Accumulation

There is little evidence in human subjects upon which to base a mechanism by which fructose may preferentially promote fat accumulation into visceral adipose tissue (VAT) over subcutaneous adipose tissue (SAT). We have hypothesized that reduced lipoprotein lipase (LPL) activity during consumption of fructose may be involved (Stanhope et al. 2009, Stanhope 2012). LPL activity is an important determinant of TG storage in the adipocyte (Eckel 1989). However, the LPL in SAT is markedly more sensitive to activation by insulin than the LPL in VAT (Fried et al. 1993), which in the insulin-sensitive individual would favor the storage of TG in SAT instead of VAT. Fructose consumption, however, reduces insulin sensitivity and also postmeal insulin responses, unlike glucose or starch consumption (Stanhope et al. 2011b), thus lowering LPL activity (Stanhope et al. 2009). This would preferentially lower TG uptake by SAT, thereby increasing the availability of TG for uptake into VAT. Recently, it has been reported that VAT accumulation is positively associated with the amount of apoCIII in apoB-containing lipoproteins (Wang et al. 2014). While the author suggests that VAT accumulation increases the amount of apoCIII in apoB-containing lipoproteins, it is interesting to speculate whether apoCIII may be involved in mediating fructose-induced VAT accumulation. Circulating apoCIII concentrations are increased by fructose consumption (Bremer et al. 2014, Stanhope et al. 2015), and apoCIII has been demonstrated to inhibit LPL *in vitro* (Wang et al. 1985).

Inflammation

A chronic state of inflammation may also be an important contributor to the pathophysiology underlying MetS (Khodabandeloo et al. 2016, Welty, Alfaddagh, and Elajami 2016). Fructose may promote inflammatory responses by several pathways.

Fructose exposure, compared with glucose exposure, results in the activation of c-jun NH_2-terminal kinase (JNK) in isolated hepatocytes (Wei et al. 2007). In nonparenchymal liver cells, such as hepatic macrophages and hepatic stellate cells, JNK is involved in inflammation and fibrosis (Seki, Brenner, and Karin 2012). JNK activation may also be involved in fructose-induced hepatic insulin resistance via increased serine phosphorylation of IRS-1 and reduced insulin-stimulated tyrosine phosphorylation of IRS-1 and IRS-2 (Wei et al. 2007, 2013).

Studies in mice and nonhuman primates show that direct exposure of the intestine to fructose increases the intestinal translocation of endotoxin, which appears to produce hepatic toxicity (Bergheim et al. 2008, Kavanagh et al. 2013). Specifically, in nonhuman primates fed weight-maintaining diets with fructose for 6 weeks, biochemical indicators of liver injury and inflammation were markedly increased compared with control diet, and these changes were highly correlated to indices of microbial translocation (Kavanagh et al. 2013). In mice consuming fructose, administration of antibiotics prevented endotoxemia and reduced lipid accumulation and peroxidation in the liver (Bergheim et al. 2008).

The increase in visceral fat resulting from overconsumption of fructose (Stanhope et al. 2009, Maersk et al. 2012) could also lead to chronic, low-grade inflammation that can alter lipolysis, insulin sensitivity, fibrinolysis, and possibly macrophage infiltration (Tchernof and Despres 2013).

Fructose Overload versus the Established Paradigm

As discussed in detail above, the delivery of elevated amounts of fructose to the intestine and liver results in a cascade of events that promote the development of MetS. This sequence of events differs from the more established paradigm described for the development of MetS (Asrih and Jornayvaz 2015). In this scenario, VAT accumulation due to overnutrition and a sedentary lifestyle leads to large, insulin-resistant, and more lipolytic adipocytes and increased circulating levels of free fatty acids (FFA). In the liver, the FFA promote liver lipid accumulation and VLDL production/secretion. In muscle, the FFA interfere with insulin signaling. We have suggested that this pathway (Asrih and Jornayvaz 2015) does not explain the metabolic dysregulation resulting from excess consumption of fructose and fructose-containing sugars (Stanhope and Havel 2008b, Stanhope 2012). Subjects consuming fructose for 10 weeks had significantly lower 24-hour circulating FFA concentrations than subjects consuming glucose (Stanhope et al. 2009). Overall, the results from this study (Stanhope et al. 2009) support the hypothesis that in a setting of positive energy balance (~1.5 kg weight gain in 8 weeks), the hepatic substrate overload and upregulation of DNL induced by fructose consumption represents a much faster route to metabolic dysregulation than the modest increases of circulating FFA induced by glucose consumption. Furthermore, the results of Schwarz et al. demonstrate that fructose can induce metabolic dysregulation even in the absence of weight gain (Schwarz et al. 2015). In this study, men consuming 25% Ereq from fructose-sweetened beverages as part of an energy-balanced diet exhibited increased DNL, inhibition of whole-body fat oxidation, increased liver lipid content, and decreased liver insulin sensitivity in only 9 days, without an increase of body weight (Schwarz et al. 2015).

DIETARY SUGAR CONSUMPTION AS A MODIFIABLE RISK FACTOR FOR METS: SCIENTIFIC EVIDENCE

Results from both observational and dietary intervention studies support the suggestion that added sugars consumption is a modifiable risk factor for MetS.

Observational Studies

Epidemiological studies report positive associations between the consumption of added sugars or SSB and MetS in both children (Bremer, Auinger, and Byrd 2009, Wang et al. 2013, Eloranta et al. 2014, Mirmiran et al. 2015) and adults (Dhingra et al. 2007, Denova-Gutierrez et al. 2010, Hostmark 2010, Mattei et al. 2012, Barrio-Lopez et al. 2013, Green et al. 2014, Ejtahed et al. 2015). Interestingly, in the Framingham Heart Study Offspring and Third Generation cohorts, the odds ratios for having at least one MetS risk factor (excluding waist circumference) in SSB consumers versus non-SSB consumers were comparable in normal-weight (1.9 odd ratio, CI: 1.4–2.6), overweight (2.0, 1.4–2.9), and obese individuals (1.9, 1.1–3.4) [85], suggesting the effects of SSB consumption on MetS risk factors is not mainly dependent on body weight/adiposity. It was recently reported that SSB consumption increased the risk of MetS in Korean women ($n = 8540$) but not in men ($n = 5432$) (Chung et al. 2015). However, less than 25% of these participants consumed ≥1 SSB/week. The total added sugars consumption of the SSB consumers averaged 9% and 12% of daily energy for men and women, respectively (Chung et al. 2015), which is below the 13%–15% estimates for all U.S. adults (Ervin and Ogden 2013, Yang et al. 2014).

The formally defined individual components of MetS: hypertriglyceridemia (Duffey et al. 2010, Welsh et al. 2010, 2011, de Koning et al. 2012, Ambrosini et al. 2013), low HDL (Welsh et al. 2010, 2011, de Koning et al. 2012, Kosova, Auinger, and Bremer 2013, Hert et al. 2014), increased waist circumference/VAT (Collison et al. 2010, Odegaard et al. 2012, Pollock et al. 2012, Kosova, Auinger, and Bremer 2013, Chan et al. 2014, Ma et al. 2014, Mollard et al. 2014), elevated blood pressure (Brown et al. 2011, Cohen, Curhan, and Forman 2012, Kell et al. 2014, Xi et al. 2015), and high fasting glucose/homeostatic model assessment of insulin resistance (HOMA-IR) (Bremer, Auinger, and Byrd 2009, Perichart-Perera et al. 2010, Wang et al. 2013, Lana, Rodriguez-Artalejo, and Lopez-Garcia 2014, Wang 2014, Santiago-Torres et al. 2016) have all been shown to be associated with sugar consumption in observational studies. Some of the components of MetS that are not formally defined have also been reported to be associated with sugar consumption: insulin resistance (indexed by parameters other than HOMA-IR) (Yoshida et al. 2007, Wang 2014), fatty liver (Zelber-Sagi et al. 2007, Assy et al. 2008, Ouyang et al. 2008, Ma et al. 2015), and elevated circulating uric acid (Choi et al. 2008, Bomback et al. 2010, Chang 2011, Zgaga et al. 2012, Lin et al. 2013), small dense LDL (Aeberli et al. 2007), C-reactive protein (Kosova, Auinger, and Bremer 2013, Hert et al. 2014, Gonzalez-Gil et al. 2015), and fibrinogen (Miura et al. 2006) concentrations.

Dietary Intervention Studies

Numerous studies in which added sugars have been added to or removed from the diets of human subjects show effects on the formally defined and not formally defined risk factors for MetS.

Effects of Sugar Consumption on the Formally Defined Components of MetS

TG, HDL, blood pressure, waist circumference/VAT, and fasting glucose concentrations.

TG

The diagnostic criterion for MetS is a fasting TG concentration ≥150 mg/dL. However, our laboratory has conducted three dietary intervention studies in which participants were provided with beverages sweetened with fructose or HFCS, and all three demonstrated that the effects of fructose-containing sugars on fasting TG concentrations were minimal compared with the effects on circulating postprandial TG profiles (Swarbrick et al. 2008, Stanhope et al. 2009, 2015). Fasting TG concentrations were unchanged in the two 10-week studies in which subjects consumed 25% Ereq as fructose (Swarbrick et al. 2008, Stanhope et al. 2009). In the 2-week dose–response study (Stanhope et al. 2015), we observed a modest increase of fasting TG in subjects consuming beverages containing 25% Ereq as HFCS that was significant compared with baseline (+11.2 ± 3.4 mg/dL (mean ± SEM), $P < 0.01$) but not compared with the aspartame-consuming control group ($P = 0.11$). In contrast, consumption of these beverages induced highly significant increases in postprandial TG, particularly 4–6 hours after dinner, the final meal of the day (+65–70 mg/dL for 25% Ereq fructose-sweetened beverages [Swarbrick et al. 2008, Stanhope et al. 2009], +37 ± 5 mg/dL for 25% Ereq HFCS-sweetened beverages [Stanhope et al. 2015]). Subjects consuming the lowest dose of HFCS-sweetened beverages in the dose–response study, 10% Ereq, also exhibited increased postprandial TG concentrations (+22 ± 8 mg/dL) that were significant compared with baseline ($P < 0.05$) and with the aspartame-consuming control group ($P < 0.001$). The previously cited study by Schwarz et al. also reported no effect on fasting TG (102 ± 7 vs 100 ± 7 mg/dL; $P = 0.67$) and a marked effect on mean postprandial TG concentrations (172 ± 29 vs 140 ± 28 mg/dL; $P = 0.002$) when men consumed energy-balanced, weight-maintaining diets that included fructose-sweetened beverages compared with when they consumed isocaloric complex carbohydrate diets (Schwarz et al. 2015).

However, despite the less marked effects on fasting TG, a recent meta-analysis of 38 randomized trials (total *n* of 1660) comparing the effects of altered sugar consumption (either di- or monosaccharide) with a control arm on fasting TG concentrations reported an increase of 10 mg/dL (95% CI: 6, 13 mg/dL; $P < 0.0001$) with high sugar consumption (Te Morenga et al. 2014). These studies (Te Morenga et al. 2014) and the studies conducted by our laboratory (Swarbrick et al. 2008, Stanhope et al. 2009, 2011a, 2015) also support an effect of sugar to increase total cholesterol and LDL-cholesterol.

HDL

The diagnostic criterion for MetS is a fasting HDL concentration <50 mg/dL for women and <40 mg/dL for men. In our recently completed study of 187 men and women, age 18–40 years and BMI 18–35 kg/m^2, low HDL was the most prevalent MetS criteria at baseline, occurring in more than 50% of the study group. High TG, the 2nd most prevalent MetS criterion, occurred in 15% of the group. The published dietary intervention studies do not support a mechanism by which sugar-induced overproduction of VLDL1 leads to TG enrichment of HDL, followed by degradation in the kidneys and a lowering of circulating HDL levels. We have reported that fructose and/or HFCS consumption do not affect HDL concentrations (Stanhope et al. 2011a, 2009, 2015, Swarbrick et al. 2008). Te Morenga et al. pooled the results of 29 studies (total *n* of 1515) and observed a small but significant effect of dietary sugars, an increase in HDL by 0.8 mg/dL (95% CI: 0.0, 1.2 mg/dL; $P = 0.02$) (Te Morenga et al. 2014). However, in a recent 6-week crossover study, Maki et al. reported a lowering of HDL concentrations when subjects consumed sucrose-sweetened beverage and dessert compared with when they consumed 2% fat milk and yogurt (Maki et al. 2015). It is also worth noting that post hoc analyses of our previous 10-week study (Stanhope et al. 2009) and our recently published 2-week study (Stanhope et al. 2015) show an HDL-lowering effect of sugar consumption in subjects with higher compared with lower plasma HDL concentrations at baseline. Specifically, when we divided 80 subjects who consumed 25% Ereq as fructose-, HFCS-, or sucrose-sweetened beverages for 2 weeks into two groups based on baseline HDL concentrations ≥ or < than 45 mg/dL, the subjects with the higher HDL levels exhibited a lowering of HDL (−3.4 ± 1.0 mg/dL) that was significant compared with their baseline levels ($P = 0.002$) and compared with the change in subjects with lower HDL concentrations (+0.5 ± 0.5 mg/dL, $P = 0.0006$ higher vs lower HDL at basline). Research is needed to examine HDL function and HDL subspecies in response to sugar consumption. Interestingly, it has recently been suggested (Taskinen and Boren 2015) that low HDL-C may simply be a long-term marker of persistently elevated circulating TG and therefore not directly involved in the pathophysiology of CVD.

Blood Pressure

Either systolic blood pressure ≥130 mm Hg or diastolic blood pressure ≥85 mm Hg represents a diagnostic criterion for MetS. While none of our intervention studies with dietary sugars have demonstrated an effect of sugar consumption on blood pressure (Swarbrick et al. 2008, Stanhope et al. 2009, 2011a, 2015), Te Morenga et al. reported that sugar consumption increased diastolic blood pressure by 1.4 mm Hg (95% CI: 0.3, 2.5 mm Hg; $P < 0.02$) in 324 subjects pooled from 12 published clinical studies (Te Morenga et al. 2014). There was a significant interaction between study length and the change of blood pressure, with diastolic blood pressure increasing by 5.6 mm Hg (95% CI: 2.5, 8.8 mm Hg; $P = 0.0005$) in subjects pooled from three trials lasting longer than 8 weeks (Te Morenga et al. 2014). It is important to note, however, that in these three longer trials, subjects consumed sucrose (+20% of daily calories) with *ad libitum* diets and their change in body weight was 1.8–4.0 kg higher than the control groups provided with starch, aspartame-sweetened snacks, and/or beverages. In the eight trials in which energy-balanced diets were provided or recommended, diastolic blood pressure increased by 0.65 (95% CI: −0.31, 1.61 mm Hg; $P = 0.18$). Marked reductions of blood pressure have been reported when the intervention consisted of reducing sugar consumption. Diastolic blood pressure decreased by 5 mm Hg (95% CI: −8.1 to −1.8 mm

Hg; $P = 0.003$) in only 9 days in 43 Latino and African-American children with MetS receiving controlled, energy-balanced diets that decreased their added sugars consumption from their usual 27% to 10% Ereq (Lustig et al. 2016). In another study, children with nonalcoholic fatty liver disease (NAFLD) who reduced consumption of fructose from beverages and refined foods exhibited a significant lowering of systolic blood pressure by approximately 12 mm Hg at 3 and 6 months (Mager et al. 2015). These blood pressure reductions, however, could have been mediated by decreased body weight in the 9-day study (-0.9 ± 0.2 kg; $P < 0.001$) (Lustig et al. 2016) and decreased body fat in the 6-month study (36.4 ± 6.4 vs $29.9 \pm 8.4\%$; $P = 0.04$) (Mager et al. 2015). Thus, studies that show a weight- or body fat–independent effect of increased or reduced sugar consumption on blood pressure are lacking.

Waist Circumference/VAT

The Cardiometabolic Think Tank states that visceral adiposity is fundamental to the pathophysiology of MetS (Sperling et al. 2015); however, the diagnostic criterion for visceral adiposity is waist circumference. Waist circumference is easy and inexpensive to measure in both clinical and research settings. However, unlike assessment of VAT and SAT by magnetic resonance or computed tomography imaging, it does not distinguish between intra- and extra-abdominal fat. Three studies of varying length, 6 months (Maersk et al. 2012), 10 weeks (Stanhope et al. 2009), and 4 weeks (Silbernagel et al. 2011), have assessed the effects of sugar consumption on VAT and SAT accumulation with imaging of the abdominal region. The 6-month study was conducted in Denmark and subjects consumed 1 L/day of sucrose-sweetened cola (~20% Ereq), isocaloric amounts of low-fat milk, 1 L/day aspartame-sweetened beverages, or 1 L/day water for 6 months (Maersk et al. 2012). Body weight at the end of the intervention period was not significantly different from the baseline in any group. Subjects consuming sucrose exhibited increased VAT, while the other three groups did not. The increase of VAT in subjects consuming sucrose was significantly greater than in the subjects who consumed low-fat milk, despite comparable changes of body weight (Sucrose: +1.3%; Milk: +1.4%) (Maersk et al. 2012). The 10-week study conducted by our laboratory reported that, despite comparable increases of body weight (~1.5 kg; $P = 0.47$, between group difference) and waist circumference (~1.8 cm; $P = 0.86$, between group difference), subjects consuming fructose-sweetened beverages preferentially accumulated fat in VAT, while subjects consuming glucose exhibited a significant increase of fat in SAT (Stanhope et al. 2009). While the fructose-induced increase in VAT ($P < 0.01$ compared with baseline) was nearly statistically significant compared to that of glucose ($P = 0.059$ between group difference), it was significant in men consuming fructose compared with men consuming glucose ($P < 0.05$) (Stanhope et al. 2009). In contrast, a 4-week study found no differences in VAT and SAT accumulation in subjects consuming high levels of fructose or glucose (Silbernagel et al. 2011). This may be related to the shorter duration, but it may also be due to the nearly significant difference in body weight gain between the two groups ($P = 0.056$). Glucose consumption resulted in weight gain ($+1.7 \pm 0.4$ kg, $P = 0.001$ within group), and fructose consumption did not ($+0.2$ kg ± 0.6 kg, $P = 0.40$). More studies that (1) utilize imaging to differentiate SAT and VAT, (2) utilize intervention periods longer than 4 weeks, and (3) are not confounded by differential weight gain between groups are needed to clarify the effects of added sugar intake on visceral adiposity.

Fasting Glucose Concentrations

The final MetS diagnostic criterion is impaired fasting glucose, defined as a fasting blood glucose concentration $\geq$100 mg/dL. High fasting blood glucose was the least prevalent (5%) MetS criterion in our recent study population of 187 young men and women. Impaired fasting glucose is associated with increased risk of future T2D and is indicative of insulin resistance, specifically hepatic insulin resistance (Abdul-Ghani and DeFronzo 2009). Impaired glucose tolerance, indexed as a 2-hour glucose concentration between 140 and 199 mg/dL during an oral glucose tolerance test (OGTT), is indicative of whole-body insulin resistance, and is an even stronger predictor of future T2D (Abdul-Ghani and DeFronzo 2009). In two separate studies, we observed increases of fasting glucose concentrations in older, overweight adults consuming 25% Ereq fructose-sweetened beverages for 10 weeks (Swarbrick et al. 2008, Stanhope et al. 2009). Reiser et al. reported increases of fasting glucose and impaired glucose tolerance when insulin-resistant subjects consumed standardized 6-week crossover diets containing 18% or 33% Ereq as sucrose compared with a diet providing 5% Ereq sucrose (Reiser et al. 1981). In contrast to these studies, fasting glucose concentrations were not changed in subjects consuming fructose- or HFCS-sweetened beverages for 2 weeks (Stanhope et al. 2011a) or sucrose-sweetened beverages for 6 months (Maersk et al. 2012). Fasting glucose was reduced (−5.4 mg/dL, 95% CI: −7.2, −3.6 mm Hg; $P < 0.001$), and glucose tolerance was improved in the 43 Latino and African-American children with MetS who lost weight when consuming controlled, energy-balanced meals that decreased their consumption of added sugars from their usual 27% to 10% Ereq for 9 days (Lustig et al. 2016). Fasting glucose concentrations were also decreased in overweight/obese adults who were provided with four servings of water/day as replacements for caloric beverages for 6 months (Tate et al. 2012). They exhibited reduced fasting glucose concentrations (~ −3 mg/dL) compared with their baseline levels ($P = 0.0027$) and compared with the control group who received general dietary instructions and no water ($P = 0.019$). During the 6-month intervention, both the group consuming water and the control group lost significant amounts of body weight (−2.0% ± 0.4% and −1.8% ± 0.4%, respectively) (Tate et al. 2012). Effects of sugar consumption on fasting blood glucose may prove to be more discernable and consistent in intervention studies that reduce sugar consumption rather than increase it.

Effects of Sugar Consumption on Components of MetS That Are Not Formally Defined: Liver Lipid Accumulation, Insulin Resistance, and other Biomarkers of MetS.

Liver Lipid Accumulation

NAFLD has been described as an important comorbidity of MetS (Marchesini et al. 2001), and it has been suggested that it be included as a criterion for the diagnosis of MetS (Tarantino and Finelli 2013). Fatty liver also plays a prominent role in the mechanism by which we propose that consumption of added sugars promotes the development of MetS, particularly insulin resistance and dyslipidemia. Measuring hepatic lipid content noninvasively via imaging (magnetic resonance imaging and magnetic resonance spectroscopy) is a fairly new technique. Accordingly, there are only a few intervention studies that have reported the effect of sugar consumption on liver fat content. In the previously discussed 6-month intervention, subjects consuming 1 L/day sucrose-sweetened cola exhibited increased liver fat compared with those consuming isocaloric amounts of milk, or isovolumetric amounts of water or aspartame-sweetened beverages (Maersk et al. 2012). Consumption of 25% Ereq as fructose-sweetened beverages increased liver fat in 9 days compared with isocaloric complex carbohydrate in men consuming energy-balanced diets that prevented weight gain (Schwarz et al. 2015). In another study, 14 overweight adults who normally consumed about three cans of soda per day were provided and asked to replace the soda with aspartame-beverages for 12 weeks (Campos et al. 2015). The reduction in liver fat content in the subjects who switched to consuming aspartame was 53% greater than that of the control group that continued to consume the SSBs ($P < 0.05$). Importantly, the eight subjects with higher levels of liver fat (>5%) exhibited more marked decreases of hepatic lipid content than the six subjects with lower amounts of liver fat prior to intervention (−57% vs −17%, $P < 0.05$) (Campos et al. 2015).

Insulin Resistance

Insulin resistance is a critical feature of MetS and has been proposed to be an important link between liver fat accumulation and MetS (Asrih and Jornayvaz 2015). As previously stated, it is not a diagnostic criterion for MetS because it is not formally defined or easy to measure in clinical practice. Numerous methods have been employed to assess insulin sensitivity in research studies, and the advantages and limitations of these methods have been recently described (Dube et al. 2013).

The easiest and least expensive method is HOMA-IR, which requires only the measurement of fasting glucose and insulin. Its main advantage is its utility for large population studies (Dube et al. 2013); however, it is frequently used in intervention studies with limited sample sizes. Shaibi et al. compared the sensitivity of HOMA-IR to detect changes of insulin sensitivity to more laborious methods in adolescents participating in two separate lifestyle interventions (Shaibi et al. 2011). Boys in a 16-week exercise intervention study exhibited a 45% improvement of insulin sensitivity measured by frequently sampled intravenous glucose tolerance tests that was not detected by HOMA-IR. Young females participating in a 12-week study testing a nutrition education program exhibited a 34% improvement in an index of whole-body insulin sensitivity assessed during an OGTT with multiple sampling that failed to be detected by HOMA-IR (Shaibi et al. 2011).

Unfortunately, most of the dietary intervention studies testing the effects of sugar consumption on insulin sensitivity have utilized HOMA-IR. While Johnston et al. did observe an increase in HOMA-IR in overweight men consuming an isocaloric diet containing 25% Ereq as fructose-sweetened beverage compared with men consuming the same diet with glucose-sweetened beverage (Johnston et al. 2013), most studies have failed to detect effects on HOMA-IR. For example, as noted above, subjects consuming 1 L of sucrose-sweetened beverage/day exhibited increased liver fat compared to all three control groups and also an increase in intramyocellular fat compared with baseline levels (Maersk et al. 2012). These changes would be expected to be associated with a decrease of insulin sensitivity; however, the changes in insulin sensitivity as assessed by HOMA-IR were highly variable (i.e., -5.0 ± 24.0 for the group consuming diet cola; 13.7 ± 23.5 for group consuming water [mean ± SEM]) and not different among the four groups. Subjects who consumed aspartame-sweetened beverages in place of SSB also exhibited significant decreases of liver fat; however, insulin sensitivity assessed by HOMA-IR was not significantly affected (Campos et al. 2015). In contrast, Schwarz and colleagues measured both hepatic and whole-body insulin sensitivity with hyperinsulinemic euglycemic clamps, along with an assessment of endogenous glucose production (Schwarz et al. 2015). In addition to significant increases of DNL and liver fat content, they also observed a significant decrease of hepatic insulin sensitivity (nonfasting endogenous glucose production rate 30% higher during fructose consumption compared with complex carbohydrate consumption, $P < 0.01$), while whole-body sensitivity was unchanged (Schwarz et al. 2015). Hepatic insulin sensitivity, assessed by endogenous glucose production, was also decreased during 3 weeks of moderate (80 g/day, ~13% Ereq) fructose consumption compared with glucose consumption, while whole-body insulin sensitivity was not different (Aeberli et al. 2013). As already stated, these two short-term studies support the sequence of events described in our proposed mechanism, in which whole-body insulin resistance occurs downstream of hepatic insulin resistance. In our longer 10-week study, we observed a 17% decrease of whole-body insulin sensitivity in subjects consuming fructose using deuterated glucose to measure glucose disposal through the glycolytic pathway during an OGTT (Stanhope et al. 2009). Studies assessing the changes in insulin sensitivity during sucrose and HFCS consumption utilizing techniques more sensitive than HOMA-IR are needed.

Other Biomarkers of MetS

Several studies have demonstrated that consumption of fructose and fructose-containing sugars increase circulating uric acid (Cox et al. 2012b, Johnston et al. 2013, Bruun et al. 2015, Stanhope et al. 2015), apolipoprotein B (Swarbrick et al. 2008, Stanhope et al. 2009, 2011a, 2015), and small dense LDL (Stanhope et al. 2009, 2011a, Aeberli et al. 2011). Our recent data (Stanhope et al. 2015) also demonstrate that apoCIII is increased by HFCS consumption and that both uric acid and apoCIII are strong biomarkers, and possibly mediators, of independent pathways by which consumption of HFCS increases risk factors for CVD. C-reactive protein (CRP), a general marker of inflammation, was increased in young healthy men after both fructose and glucose consumption (40 or 80 g/day for 3 weeks) (Aeberli et al. 2011) and in older subjects with impaired glucose tolerance after sucrose, HFCS, or honey consumption (50 g/day for 2 weeks) (Raatz, Johnson, and Picklo 2015). Our group has not detected increases of CRP during sugar consumption in humans but have observed increases of monocyte chemotactic protein-1 (MCP-1) and plasminogen activator inhibitor-1 (Cox et al. 2011). In rhesus monkeys consuming fructose-sweetened beverages for 1 year, MCP-1 and CRP were increased after 6 and 12 months (Bremer et al. 2011).

CONCLUSION

Evidence from epidemiological studies suggest that consumption of fructose-containing sugars is associated with the prevalence and/or development of MetS and all of the established components of the MetS, plus features of MetS that are not formally defined, such as insulin resistance, fatty liver, and hyperuricemia. Results from dietary intervention studies showing that many of these components and features are adversely affected when sugar intake is increased and beneficially affected when sugar intake is decreased corroborate the epidemiological evidence. There are plausible and interconnected mechanisms by which consumption of fructose-containing sugars may lead to the development of the clustered, interrelated risk factors that constitute MetS. Therefore, we believe that consumption of added sugars should be considered a modifiable risk factor for MetS. The recommendation of the Cardiometabolic Think Tank to emphasize dietary patterns such as the DASH and Mediterranean diets (Sperling et al. 2015) is sound. However, specific recommendations to reduce consumption of added sugars to the levels recommended by the 2015–2020 Dietary Guidelines for American (United States Department of Health and Human Services and U.S. Department of Agriculture 2015) or to the even lower levels recommended by the American Heart Association (Johnson et al. 2009) may be beneficial in the prevention and management of MetS.

ACKNOWLEDGMENTS

The studies conducted by Drs. Havel and Stanhope's research group were supported with funding from NIH grants R01 HL-075675, 1R01 HL-091333, and 1R01 HL-107256 and a multicampus award from the University of California, Office of the President (UCOP #142691). These projects also received support from Grant Number UL1 RR024146 from the National Center for Research Resources (NCRR), a component of the National Institutes of Health (NIH), and NIH Roadmap for Medical Research. Dr. Stanhope is UC Davis School of Medicine Dean's Scholar in Women's Health supported by the Office of the Dean, UC Davis School of Medicine.

CONFLICTS OF INTEREST

Drs. Stanhope and Havel have no conflicts of interest to report.

REFERENCES

Abdul-Ghani, M. A. and R. A. DeFronzo. 2009. Pathophysiology of prediabetes. *Curr Diab Rep* 9(3):193–199.

Adiels, M., S. O. Olofsson, M. R. Taskinen, and J. Boren. 2008. Overproduction of very low-density lipoproteins is the hallmark of the dyslipidemia in the metabolic syndrome. *Arterioscler Thromb Vasc Biol* 28(7):1225–1236. doi: 10.1161/ATVBAHA.107.160192.

Adiels, M., M. R. Taskinen, C. Packard, M. J. Caslake, A. Soro-Paavonen, J. Westerbacka, S. Vehkavaara et al. 2006. Overproduction of large VLDL particles is driven by increased liver fat content in man. *Diabetologia* 49(4):755–765. doi: 10.1007/s00125-005-0125-z.

Aeberli, I., P. A. Gerber, M. Hochuli, S. Kohler, S. R. Haile, I. Gouni-Berthold, H. K. Berthold, G. A. Spinas, and K. Berneis. 2011. Low to moderate sugar-sweetened beverage consumption impairs glucose and lipid metabolism and promotes inflammation in healthy young men: A randomized controlled trial. *Am J Clin Nutr* 94(2):479–485. doi: 10.3945/ajcn.111.013540.

Aeberli, I., M. Hochuli, P. A. Gerber, L. Sze, S. B. Murer, L. Tappy, G. A. Spinas, and K. Berneis. 2013. Moderate amounts of fructose consumption impair insulin sensitivity in healthy young men: A randomized controlled trial. *Diabetes Care* 36(1):150–156. doi: 10.2337/dc12-0540.

Aeberli, I., M. B. Zimmermann, L. Molinari, R. Lehmann, D. l'Allemand, G. A. Spinas, and K. Berneis. 2007. Fructose intake is a predictor of LDL particle size in overweight schoolchildren. *Am J Clin Nutr* 86(4):1174–1178.

Alberti, K. G., R. H. Eckel, S. M. Grundy, P. Z. Zimmet, J. I. Cleeman, K. A. Donato, J. C. Fruchart et al. 2009. Harmonizing the metabolic syndrome: A joint interim statement of the International Diabetes Federation Task Force on Epidemiology and Prevention; National Heart, Lung, and Blood Institute; American Heart Association; World Heart Federation; International Atherosclerosis Society; and International Association for the Study of Obesity. *Circulation* 120(16):1640–1645. doi: 10.1161/CIRCULATIONAHA.109.192644.

Ambrosini, G. L., W. H. Oddy, R. C. Huang, T. A. Mori, L. J. Beilin, and S. A. Jebb. 2013. Prospective associations between sugar-sweetened beverage intakes and cardiometabolic risk factors in adolescents. *Am J Clin Nutr* 98(2):327–334. doi: 10.3945/ajcn.112.051383.

Anderson, E. J., M. E. Lustig, K. E. Boyle, T. L. Woodlief, D. A. Kane, C. T. Lin, J. W. Price, 3rd et al. 2009. Mitochondrial H_2O_2 emission and cellular redox state link excess fat intake to insulin resistance in both rodents and humans. *J Clin Invest* 119(3):573–581. doi: 10.1172/JCI37048.

Asrih, M. and F. R. Jornayvaz. 2015. Metabolic syndrome and nonalcoholic fatty liver disease: Is insulin resistance the link? *Mol Cell Endocrinol.* 418 (Pt 1):55–65.

Assy, N., G. Nasser, I. Kamayse, W. Nseir, Z. Beniashvili, A. Djibre, and M. Grosovski. 2008. Soft drink consumption linked with fatty liver in the absence of traditional risk factors. *Can J Gastroenterol* 22(10):811–816.

Barrio-Lopez, M. T., M. A. Martinez-Gonzalez, A. Fernandez-Montero, J. J. Beunza, I. Zazpe, and M. Bes-Rastrollo. 2013. Prospective study of changes in sugar-sweetened beverage consumption and the incidence of the metabolic syndrome and its components: The SUN cohort. *Br J Nutr* 110(9):1722–1731. doi: 10.1017/S0007114513000822.

Bergheim, I., S. Weber, M. Vos, S. Kramer, V. Volynets, S. Kaserouni, C. J. McClain, and S. C. Bischoff. 2008. Antibiotics protect against fructose-induced hepatic lipid accumulation in mice: Role of endotoxin. *J Hepatol* 48(6):983–992. doi: 10.1016/j.jhep.2008.01.035.

Berry, J. D., A. Dyer, X. Cai, D. B. Garside, H. Ning, A. Thomas, P. Greenland, L. Van Horn, R. P. Tracy, and D. M. Lloyd-Jones. 2012. Lifetime risks of cardiovascular disease. *N Engl J Med* 366(4):321–329. doi: 10.1056/NEJMoa1012848.

Billiet, L., S. Doaty, J. D. Katz, and M. T. Velasquez. 2014. Review of hyperuricemia as new marker for metabolic syndrome. *ISRN Rheumatol* 2014:852954. doi: 10.1155/2014/852954.

Bomback, A. S., V. K. Derebail, D. A. Shoham, C. A. Anderson, L. M. Steffen, W. D. Rosamond, and A. V. Kshirsagar. 2010. Sugar-sweetened soda consumption, hyperuricemia, and kidney disease. *Kidney Int* 77(7):609–616. doi: 10.1038/ki.2009.500.

Boren, J., G. F. Watts, M. Adiels, S. Soderlund, D. C. Chan, A. Hakkarainen, N. Lundbom et al. 2015. Kinetic and related determinants of plasma triglyceride concentration in abdominal obesity: Multicenter tracer kinetic tudy. *Arterioscler Thromb Vasc Biol* 35(10):2218–2224. doi: 10.1161/ATVBAHA.115.305614.

Bremer, A. A., P. Auinger, and R. S. Byrd. 2009. Relationship between insulin resistance-associated metabolic parameters and anthropometric measurements with sugar-sweetened beverage intake and physical activity levels in US adolescents: Findings from the 1999–2004 National Health and Nutrition Examination Survey. *Arch Pediatr Adolesc Med* 163(4):328–335.

Bremer, A. A., M. Mietus-Snyder, and R. H. Lustig. 2012. Toward a unifying hypothesis of metabolic syndrome. *Pediatrics* 129(3):557–570. doi: 10.1542/peds.2011-2912.

Bremer, A. A., K. L. Stanhope, J. L. Graham, B. P. Cummings, S. B. Ampah, B. R. Saville, and P. J. Havel. 2014. Fish oil supplementation ameliorates fructose-induced hypertriglyceridemia and insulin resistance in adult male rhesus macaques. *J Nutr* 144(1):5–11. doi: 10.3945/jn.113.178061.

Bremer, A. A., K. L. Stanhope, J. L. Graham, B. P. Cummings, W. Wang, B. R. Saville, and P. J. Havel. 2011. Fructose-fed rhesus monkeys: A nonhuman primate model of insulin resistance, metabolic syndrome, and type 2 diabetes. *Clin Transl Sci* 4(4):243–252. doi: 10.1111/j.1752-8062.2011.00298.x.

Brown, I. J., J. Stamler, L. Van Horn, C. E. Robertson, Q. Chan, A. R. Dyer, C. C. Huang et al. 2011. Sugar-sweetened beverage, sugar intake of individuals, and their blood pressure: International study of macro/micronutrients and blood pressure. *Hypertension* 57(4):695–701. doi: 10.1161/HYPERTENSIONAHA.110.165456.

Bruun, J. M., M. Maersk, A. Belza, A. Astrup, and B. Richelsen. 2015. Consumption of sucrose-sweetened soft drinks increases plasma levels of uric acid in overweight and obese subjects: A 6-month randomised controlled trial. *Eur J Clin Nutr* 69(8):949–953. doi: 10.1038/ejcn.2015.95.

Cai, W., X. Wu, B. Zhang, L. Miao, Y. P. Sun, Y. Zou, and H. Yao. 2013. Serum uric acid levels and non-alcoholic fatty liver disease in Uyghur and Han ethnic groups in northwestern China. *Arq Bras Endocrinol Metabol* 57(8):617–622.

Campos, V., C. Despland, V. Brandejsky, R. Kreis, P. Schneiter, A. Chiolero, C. Boesch, and L. Tappy. 2015. Sugar- and artificially sweetened beverages and intrahepatic fat: A randomized controlled trial. *Obesity (Silver Spring)* 23(12):2335–2339. doi: 10.1002/oby.21310.

Chan, T. F., W. T. Lin, H. L. Huang, C. Y. Lee, P. W. Wu, Y. W. Chiu, C. C. Huang, S. Tsai, C. L. Lin, and C. H. Lee. 2014. Consumption of sugar-sweetened beverages is associated with components of the metabolic syndrome in adolescents. *Nutrients* 6(5):2088–2103. doi: 10.3390/nu6052088.

Chang, W. C. 2011. Dietary intake and the risk of hyperuricemia, gout and chronic kidney disease in elderly Taiwanese men. *Aging Male* 14(3):195–202. doi: 10.3109/13685538.2010.512372.

Chapman, M. J., W. Le Goff, M. Guerin, and A. Kontush. 2010. Cholesteryl ester transfer protein: At the heart of the action of lipid-modulating therapy with statins, fibrates, niacin, and cholesteryl ester transfer protein inhibitors. *Eur Heart J* 31(2):149–164. doi: 10.1093/eurheartj/ehp399.

Chaudhary, K., K. Malhotra, J. Sowers, and A. Aroor. 2013. Uric Acid - key ingredient in the recipe for cardiorenal metabolic syndrome. *Cardiorenal Med* 3(3):208–220. doi: 10.1159/000355405.

Choi, J. W., E. S. Ford, X. Gao, and H. K. Choi. 2008. Sugar-sweetened soft drinks, diet soft drinks, and serum uric acid level: The Third National Health and Nutrition Examination Survey. *Arthritis Rheum* 59(1):109–116. doi: 10.1002/art.23245.

Christian, P., J. Sacco, and K. Adeli. 2013. Autophagy: Emerging roles in lipid homeostasis and metabolic control. *Biochim Biophys Acta* 1831(4):819–824. doi: 10.1016/j.bbalip.2012.12.009.

Chung, S., K. Ha, H. S. Lee, C. I. Kim, H. Joung, H. Y. Paik, and Y. Song. 2015. Soft drink consumption is positively associated with metabolic syndrome risk factors only in Korean women: Data from the 2007–2011 Korea National Health and Nutrition Examination Survey. *Metabolism* 64(11):1477–1484. doi: 10.1016/j.metabol.2015.07.012.

Coen, P. M. and B. H. Goodpaster. 2012. Role of intramyocelluar lipids in human health. *Trends Endocrinol Metab* 23(8):391–398. doi: 10.1016/j.tem.2012.05.009.

Cohen, L., G. Curhan, and J. Forman. 2012. Association of sweetened beverage intake with incident hypertension. *J Gen Intern Med* 27(9):11271134. doi: 10.1007/s11606-012-2069-6.

Collison, K. S., M. Z. Zaidi, S. N. Subhani, K. Al-Rubeaan, M. Shoukri, and F. A. Al-Mohanna. 2010. Sugar-sweetened carbonated beverage consumption correlates with BMI, waist circumference, and poor dietary choices in school children. *BMC Public Health* 10:234. doi: 10.1186/1471-2458-10-234.

Cox, C. L., K. L. Stanhope, J. M. Schwarz, J. L. Graham, B. Hatcher, S. C. Griffen, A. A. Bremer et al. 2011. Circulating concentrations of monocyte chemoattractant protein-1, plasminogen activator inhibitor 1, and soluble leukocyte adhesion molecule-1 in overweight/obese men and women consuming fructose- or glucose-sweetened beverages for 10 weeks. *J Clin Endocrinol Metab* 96(12):E2034–E2038. doi: 10.1210/jc.2011-1050.

Cox, C. L., K. L. Stanhope, J. M. Schwarz, J. L. Graham, B. Hatcher, S. C. Griffen, A. A. Bremer et al. 2012a. Consumption of fructose-sweetened beverages for 10 weeks reduces net fat oxidation and energy expenditure in overweight/obese men and women. *Eur J Clin Nutr* 66(2):201–208. doi: 10.1038/ejcn.2011.159.

Cox, C. L., K. L. Stanhope, J. M. Schwarz, J. L. Graham, B. Hatcher, S. C. Griffen, A. A. Bremer et al. 2012b. Consumption of fructose- but not glucose-sweetened beverages for 10 weeks increases circulating concentrations of uric acid, retinol binding protein-4, and gamma-glutamyl transferase activity in overweight/obese humans. *Nutr Metab (Lond)* 9(1):68. doi: 10.1186/1743-7075-9-68.

de Koning, L., V. S. Malik, M. D. Kellogg, E. B. Rimm, W. C. Willett, and F. B. Hu. 2012. Sweetened beverage consumption, incident coronary heart disease, and biomarkers of risk in men. *Circulation* 125(14):1735–1741. doi: 10.1161/CIRCULATIONAHA.111.067017.

DeBoer, M. D., M. J. Gurka, J. G. Woo, and J. A. Morrison. 2015a. Severity of metabolic syndrome as a predictor of cardiovascular disease between childhood and adulthood: The Princeton Lipid Research Cohort Study. *J Am Coll Cardiol* 66(6):755–757. doi: 10.1016/j.jacc.2015.05.061.

DeBoer, M. D., M. J. Gurka, J. G. Woo, and J. A. Morrison. 2015b. Severity of the metabolic syndrome as a predictor of type 2 diabetes between childhood and adulthood: The Princeton Lipid Research Cohort Study. *Diabetologia*. 58(12):2745–2752.

Denova-Gutierrez, E., J. O. Talavera, G. Huitron-Bravo, P. Mendez-Hernandez, and J. Salmeron. 2010. Sweetened beverage consumption and increased risk of metabolic syndrome in Mexican adults. *Public Health Nutr* 13(6):835–842. doi: 10.1017/S1368980009991145.

Dhingra, R., L. Sullivan, P. F. Jacques, T. J. Wang, C. S. Fox, J. B. Meigs, R. B. D'Agostino, J. M. Gaziano, and R. S. Vasan. 2007. Soft drink consumption and risk of developing cardiometabolic risk factors and the metabolic syndrome in middle-aged adults in the community. *Circulation* 116(5):480–488.

Diffenderfer, M. R. and E. J. Schaefer. 2014. The composition and metabolism of large and small LDL. *Curr Opin Lipidol* 25(3):221–226. doi: 10.1097/MOL.0000000000000067.

Dube, S., I. Errazuriz, C. Cobelli, R. Basu, and A. Basu. 2013. Assessment of insulin action on carbohydrate metabolism: Physiological and non-physiological methods. *Diabet Med* 30(6):664–670. doi: 10.1111/dme.12189.

Duffey, K. J., P. Gordon-Larsen, L. M. Steffen, D. R. Jacobs, Jr., and B. M. Popkin. 2010. Drinking caloric beverages increases the risk of adverse cardiometabolic outcomes in the Coronary Artery Risk Development in Young Adults (CARDIA) Study. *Am J Clin Nutr* 92(4):954–959. doi: 10.3945/ajcn.2010.29478.

Eckel, R. H. 1989. Lipoprotein lipase. A multifunctional enzyme relevant to common metabolic diseases. *N Engl J Med* 320(16):1060–1068. doi: 10.1056/NEJM198904203201607.

Ejtahed, H. S., Z. Bahadoran, P. Mirmiran, and F. Azizi. 2015. Sugar-sweetened beverage consumption is associated with metabolic syndrome in iranian adults: Tehran lipid and glucose study. *Endocrinol Metab (Seoul)* 30(3):334–342. doi: 10.3803/EnM.2015.30.3.334.

Eloranta, A. M., V. Lindi, U. Schwab, S. Kiiskinen, T. Venalainen, H. M. Lakka, D. E. Laaksonen, and T. A. Lakka. 2014. Dietary factors associated with metabolic risk score in Finnish children aged 6–8 years: The PANIC study. *Eur J Nutr* 53(6):1431–1439. doi: 10.1007/s00394-013-0646-z.

Ervin, R. B., B. K. Kit, M. D. Carroll, and C. L. Ogden. 2012. Consumption of added sugar among U.S. children and adolescents, 2005–2008. *NCHS Data Brief* (87):1–8.

Ervin, R. B. and C. L. Ogden. 2013. Consumption of added sugars among U.S. adults, 2005–2010. *NCHS Data Brief* (122):1–8.

Fabbrini, E., F. Magkos, B. S. Mohammed, T. Pietka, N. A. Abumrad, B. W. Patterson, A. Okunade, and S. Klein. 2009. Intrahepatic fat, not visceral fat, is linked with metabolic complications of obesity. *Proc Natl Acad Sci USA* 106(36):15430–15435. doi: 10.1073/pnas.0904944106.

Fan, J. G. and Y. D. Peng. 2007. Metabolic syndrome and non-alcoholic fatty liver disease: Asian definitions and Asian studies. *Hepatobiliary Pancreat Dis Int* 6(6):572–578.

Feig, D. I., M. Madero, D. I. Jalal, L. G. Sanchez-Lozada, and R. J. Johnson. 2013. Uric acid and the origins of hypertension. *J Pediatr* 162(5):896–902. doi: 10.1016/j.jpeds.2012.12.078.

Fisher, E. A. 2012. The degradation of apolipoprotein B100: Multiple opportunities to regulate VLDL triglyceride production by different proteolytic pathways. *Biochim Biophys Acta* 1821(5):778–781. doi: 10.1016/j.bbalip.2012.02.001.

Fried, S. K., C. D. Russell, N. L. Grauso, and R. E. Brolin. 1993. Lipoprotein lipase regulation by insulin and glucocorticoid in subcutaneous and omental adipose tissues of obese women and men. *J Clin Invest* 92(5):2191–2198.

Gaharwar, R., S. Trikha, S. L. Margekar, O. P. Jatav, and P. D. Ganga. 2015. Study of clinical profile of patients of non alcoholic fatty liver disease and its association with metabolic syndrome. *J Assoc Physicians India* 63(1):12–16.

Gonzalez-Gil, E. M., J. Santabarbara, P. Russo, W. Ahrens, M. Claessens, L. Lissner, C. Bornhorst et al. 2015. Food intake and inflammation in European children: The IDEFICS study. *Eur J Nutr.* doi: 10.1007/s00394-015-1054-3.

Green, A. K., P. F. Jacques, G. Rogers, C. S. Fox, J. B. Meigs, and N. M. McKeown. 2014. Sugar-sweetened beverages and prevalence of the metabolically abnormal phenotype in the Framingham Heart Study. *Obesity (Silver Spring)* 22(5):E157–E163. doi: 10.1002/oby.20724.

Grundy, S. M., J. I. Cleeman, S. R. Daniels, K. A. Donato, R. H. Eckel, B. A. Franklin, D. J. Gordon et al. 2005. Diagnosis and management of the metabolic syndrome: An American Heart Association/National Heart, Lung, and Blood Institute Scientific Statement. *Circulation* 112(17):2735–2752. doi: 10.1161/CIRCULATIONAHA.105.169404.

Havel, P. J. 2005. Dietary fructose: Implications for dysregulation of energy homeostasis and lipid/carbohydrate metabolism. *Nutr Rev* 63(5):133–157.

Hert, K. A., P. S. Fisk, 2nd, Y. S. Rhee, and A. R. Brunt. 2014. Decreased consumption of sugar-sweetened beverages improved selected biomarkers of chronic disease risk among US adults: 1999 to 2010. *Nutr Res* 34(1):58–65. doi: 10.1016/j.nutres.2013.10.005.

Hostmark, A. T. 2010. The Oslo health study: Soft drink intake is associated with the metabolic syndrome. *Appl Physiol Nutr Metab* 35(5):635–642. doi: 10.1139/H10-059.

Johnson, R. J., M. A. Lanaspa, L. Gabriela Sanchez-Lozada, and B. Rodriguez-Iturbe. 2015. The discovery of hypertension: Evolving views on the role of the kidneys, and current hot topics. *Am J Physiol Renal Physiol* 308(3):F167–F178. doi: 10.1152/ajprenal.00503.2014.

Johnson, R. K., L. J. Appel, M. Brands, B. V. Howard, M. Lefevre, R. H. Lustig, F. Sacks, L. M. Steffen, and J. Wylie-Rosett. 2009. Dietary sugars intake and cardiovascular health: A scientific statement from the American Heart Association. *Circulation* 120(11):1011–1020. doi: 10.1161/CIRCULATIONAHA.109.192627.

Johnston, R. D., M. C. Stephenson, H. Crossland, S. M. Cordon, E. Palcidi, E. F. Cox, M. A. Taylor, G. P. Aithal, and I. A. Macdonald. 2013. No difference between high-fructose and high-glucose diets on liver triacylglycerol or biochemistry in healthy overweight men. *Gastroenterology* 145(5):1016–1025.e2. doi: 10.1053/j.gastro.2013.07.012.

Jornayvaz, F. R. and G. I. Shulman. 2012. Diacylglycerol activation of protein kinase Cepsilon and hepatic insulin resistance. *Cell Metab* 15(5):574–584. doi: 10.1016/j.cmet.2012.03.005.

Kavanagh, K., A. T. Wylie, K. L. Tucker, T. J. Hamp, R. Z. Gharaibeh, A. A. Fodor, and J. M. Cullen. 2013. Dietary fructose induces endotoxemia and hepatic injury in calorically controlled primates. *Am J Clin Nutr* 98(2):349–357. doi: 10.3945/ajcn.112.057331.

Kell, K. P., M. I. Cardel, M. M. Bohan Brown, and J. R. Fernandez. 2014. Added sugars in the diet are positively associated with diastolic blood pressure and triglycerides in children. *Am J Clin Nutr* 100(1):46–52. doi: 10.3945/ajcn.113.076505.

Khodabandeloo, H., S. Gorgani-Firuzjaee, S. Panahi, and R. Meshkani. 2016. Molecular and cellular mechanisms linking inflammation to insulin resistance and beta-cell dysfunction. *Transl Res.* 167(1):228–256.

Kosova, E. C., P. Auinger, and A. A. Bremer. 2013. The relationships between sugar-sweetened beverage intake and cardiometabolic markers in young children. *J Acad Nutr Diet* 113(2):219–227. doi: 10.1016/j.jand.2012.10.020.

Krssak, M., K. Falk Petersen, A. Dresner, L. DiPietro, S. M. Vogel, D. L. Rothman, M. Roden, and G. I. Shulman. 1999. Intramyocellular lipid concentrations are correlated with insulin sensitivity in humans: A 1H NMR spectroscopy study. *Diabetologia* 42(1):113–116.

Lana, A., F. Rodriguez-Artalejo, and E. Lopez-Garcia. 2014. Consumption of sugar-sweetened beverages is positively related to insulin resistance and higher plasma leptin concentrations in men and nonoverweight women. *J Nutr* 144(7):1099–1105. doi: 10.3945/jn.114.195230.

Lewis, G. F., A. Carpentier, K. Adeli, and A. Giacca. 2002. Disordered fat storage and mobilization in the pathogenesis of insulin resistance and type 2 diabetes. *Endocr Rev* 23(2):201–229.

Lin, W. T., H. L. Huang, M. C. Huang, T. F. Chan, S. Y. Ciou, C. Y. Lee, Y. W. Chiu et al. 2013. Effects on uric acid, body mass index and blood pressure in adolescents of consuming beverages sweetened with high-fructose corn syrup. *Int J Obes (Lond)* 37(4):532–539. doi: 10.1038/ijo.2012.121.

Liu, Z., S. Que, L. Zhou, and S. Zheng. 2015. Dose-response relationship of serum uric acid with metabolic syndrome and non-alcoholic fatty liver disease incidence: A meta-analysis of prospective studies. *Sci Rep* 5:14325. doi: 10.1038/srep14325.

Livingstone, M. B. and A. E. Black. 2003. Markers of the validity of reported energy intake. *J Nutr* 133(Suppl 3):895S–920S.

Lustig, R. H., K. Mulligan, S. M. Noworolski, V. W. Tai, M. J. Wen, A. Erkin-Cakmak, A. Gugliucci, and J. M. Schwarz. 2016. Isocaloric fructose restriction and metabolic improvement in children with obesity and metabolic syndrome. *Obesity (Silver Spring)* 24(2):453–460.

Ma, J., C. S. Fox, P. F. Jacques, E. K. Speliotes, U. Hoffmann, C. E. Smith, E. Saltzman, and N. M. McKeown. 2015. Sugar-sweetened beverage, diet soda, and fatty liver disease in the Framingham Heart Study cohorts. *J Hepatol* 63(2):462–469. doi: 10.1016/j.jhep.2015.03.032.

Ma, J., M. Sloan, C. S. Fox, U. Hoffmann, C. E. Smith, E. Saltzman, G. T. Rogers, P. F. Jacques, and N. M. McKeown. 2014. Sugar-sweetened beverage consumption is associated with abdominal fat partitioning in healthy adults. *J Nutr* 144(8):1283–1290. doi: 10.3945/jn.113.188599.

Maersk, M., A. Belza, H. Stodkilde-Jorgensen, S. Ringgaard, E. Chabanova, H. Thomsen, S. B. Pedersen, A. Astrup, and B. Richelsen. 2012. Sucrose-sweetened beverages increase fat storage in the liver, muscle, and visceral fat depot: A 6-mo randomized intervention study. *Am J Clin Nutr* 95(2):283–289. doi: 10.3945/ajcn.111.022533.

Mager, D. R., I. R. Iniguez, S. Gilmour, and J. Yap. 2015. The effect of a low fructose and low glycemic index/load (FRAGILE) dietary intervention on indices of liver function, cardiometabolic risk factors, and body composition in children and adolescents with nonalcoholic fatty liver disease (NAFLD). *JPEN J Parenter Enteral Nutr* 39(1):73–84. doi: 10.1177/0148607113501201.

Maki, K. C., K. M. Nieman, A. L. Schild, V. N. Kaden, A. L. Lawless, K. M. Kelley, and T. M. Rains. 2015. Sugar-sweetened product consumption alters glucose homeostasis compared with dairy product consumption in men and women at risk of type 2 diabetes mellitus. *J Nutr* 145(3):459–466. doi: 10.3945/jn.114.204503.

Marchesini, G., M. Brizi, G. Bianchi, S. Tomassetti, E. Bugianesi, M. Lenzi, A. J. McCullough, S. Natale, G. Forlani, and N. Melchionda. 2001. Nonalcoholic fatty liver disease: A feature of the metabolic syndrome. *Diabetes* 50(8):1844–1850.

Marino, L. and F. R. Jornayvaz. 2015. Endocrine causes of nonalcoholic fatty liver disease. *World J Gastroenterol* 21(39):11053–11076. doi: 10.3748/wjg.v21.i39.11053.

Marriott, B. P., L. Olsho, L. Hadden, and P. Connor. 2010. Intake of added sugars and selected nutrients in the United States, National Health and Nutrition Examination Survey (NHANES) 2003–2006. *Crit Rev Food Sci Nutr* 50(3):228–258. doi: 10.1080/10408391003626223.

Mattei, J., V. Malik, F. B. Hu, and H. Campos. 2012. Substituting homemade fruit juice for sugar-sweetened beverages is associated with lower odds of metabolic syndrome among Hispanic adults. *J Nutr* 142(6):1081–1087. doi: 10.3945/jn.111.149344.

Mayes, P. A. 1993. Intermediary metabolism of fructose. *Am J Clin Nutr* 58(5 Suppl):754S–765S.

Mirmiran, P., E. Yuzbashian, G. Asghari, S. Hosseinpour-Niazi, and F. Azizi. 2015. Consumption of sugar sweetened beverage is associated with incidence of metabolic syndrome in Tehranian children and adolescents. *Nutr Metab (Lond)* 12:25. doi: 10.1186/s12986-015-0021-6.

Miura, K., H. Nakagawa, H. Ueshima, A. Okayama, S. Saitoh, J. D. Curb, B. L. Rodriguez et al. 2006. Dietary factors related to higher plasma fibrinogen levels of Japanese-americans in hawaii compared with Japanese in Japan. *Arterioscler Thromb Vasc Biol* 26(7):1674–1679. doi: 10.1161/01.ATV.0000225701.20965.b9.

Mollard, R. C., M. Senechal, A. C. MacIntosh, J. Hay, B. A. Wicklow, K. D. Wittmeier, E. A. Sellers et al. 2014. Dietary determinants of hepatic steatosis and visceral adiposity in overweight and obese youth at risk of type 2 diabetes. *Am J Clin Nutr* 99(4):804–812. doi: 10.3945/ajcn.113.079277.

Nejatinamini, S., A. Ataie-Jafari, M. Qorbani, S. Nikoohemat, R. Kelishadi, H. Asayesh, and S. Hosseini. 2015. Association between serum uric acid level and metabolic syndrome components. *J Diabetes Metab Disord* 14:70. doi: 10.1186/s40200-015-0200-z.

Odegaard, A. O., A. C. Choh, S. A. Czerwinski, B. Towne, and E. W. Demerath. 2012. Sugar-sweetened and diet beverages in relation to visceral adipose tissue. *Obesity (Silver Spring)* 20(3):689–691. doi: 10.1038/oby.2011.277.

Ouyang, X., P. Cirillo, Y. Sautin, S. McCall, J. L. Bruchette, A. M. Diehl, R. J. Johnson, and M. F. Abdelmalek. 2008. Fructose consumption as a risk factor for non-alcoholic fatty liver disease. *J Hepatol* 48(6):993–999. doi: 10.1016/j.jhep.2008.02.011.

Packard, C. J. 2003. Triacylglycerol-rich lipoproteins and the generation of small, dense low-density lipoprotein. *Biochem Soc Trans* 31(Pt 5):1066–1069.

Perichart-Perera, O., M. Balas-Nakash, A. Rodriguez-Cano, C. Munoz-Manrique, A. Monge-Urrea, and F. Vadillo-Ortega. 2010. Correlates of dietary energy sources with cardiovascular disease risk markers in Mexican school-age children. *J Am Diet Assoc* 110(2):253–260. doi: 10.1016/j.jada.2009.10.031.

Pollock, N. K., V. Bundy, W. Kanto, C. L. Davis, P. J. Bernard, H. Zhu, B. Gutin, and Y. Dong. 2012. Greater fructose consumption is associated with cardiometabolic risk markers and visceral adiposity in adolescents. *J Nutr* 142(2):251–257. doi: 10.3945/jn.111.150219.

Qin, W., M. Sundaram, Y. Wang, H. Zhou, S. Zhong, C. C. Chang, S. Manhas et al. 2011. Missense mutation in APOC3 within the C-terminal lipid binding domain of human ApoC-III results in impaired assembly and secretion of triacylglycerol-rich very low density lipoproteins: Evidence that ApoC-III plays a major role in the formation of lipid precursors within the microsomal lumen. *J Biol Chem* 286(31):27769–27780. doi: 10.1074/jbc.M110.203679.

Raatz, S. K., L. K. Johnson, and M. J. Picklo. 2015. Consumption of honey, sucrose, and high-fructose corn syrup produces similar metabolic effects in glucose-tolerant and -intolerant individuals. *J Nutr* 145(10):2265–2272. doi: 10.3945/jn.115.218016.

Rangan, A., M. Allman-Farinelli, E. Donohoe, and T. Gill. 2014. Misreporting of energy intake in the 2007 Australian Children's Survey: Differences in the reporting of food types between plausible, under- and over-reporters of energy intake. *J Hum Nutr Diet* 27(5):450–458.

Reiser, S., E. Bohn, J. Hallfrisch, O. E. Michaelis, 4th, M. Keeney, and E. S. Prather. 1981. Serum insulin and glucose in hyperinsulinemic subjects fed three different levels of sucrose. *Am J Clin Nutr* 34(11):2348–2358.

Sacks, F. M. 2015. The crucial roles of apolipoproteins E and C-III in apoB lipoprotein metabolism in normolipidemia and hypertriglyceridemia. *Curr Opin Lipidol* 26(1):56–63. doi: 10.1097/MOL.0000000000000146.

Samuel, V. T. and G. I. Shulman. 2012. Mechanisms for insulin resistance: Common threads and missing links. *Cell* 148(5):852–871. doi: 10.1016/j.cell.2012.02.017.

Santiago-Torres, M., Y. Cui, A. K. Adams, D. B. Allen, A. L. Carrel, J. Y. Guo, A. Delgado-Rendon, T. L. LaRowe, and D. A. Schoeller. 2016. Familial and individual predictors of obesity and insulin resistance in urban Hispanic children. *Pediatr Obes* 11(1):54–60.

Schwarz, J. M., S. M. Noworolski, M. J. Wen, A. Dyachenko, J. L. Prior, M. E. Weinberg, L. A. Herraiz et al. 2015. Effect of a high-fructose weight-maintaining diet on lipogenesis and liver fat. *J Clin Endocrinol Metab* 100(6):2434–2442. doi: 10.1210/jc.2014-3678.

Seki, E., D. A. Brenner, and M. Karin. 2012. A liver full of JNK: Signaling in regulation of cell function and disease pathogenesis, and clinical approaches. *Gastroenterology* 143(2):307–320. doi: 10.1053/j.gastro.2012.06.004.

Sevastianova, K., A. Santos, A. Kotronen, A. Hakkarainen, J. Makkonen, K. Silander, M. Peltonen et al. 2012. Effect of short-term carbohydrate overfeeding and long-term weight loss on liver fat in overweight humans. *Am J Clin Nutr* 96(4):727–734. doi: 10.3945/ajcn.112.038695.

Shaibi, G. Q., J. N. Davis, M. J. Weigensberg, and M. I. Goran. 2011. Improving insulin resistance in obese youth: Choose your measures wisely. *Int J Pediatr Obes* 6(2–2):e290–e296. doi: 10.3109/17477166.2010.528766.

Silbernagel, G., J. Machann, S. Unmuth, F. Schick, N. Stefan, H. U. Haring, and A. Fritsche. 2011. Effects of 4-week very-high-fructose/glucose diets on insulin sensitivity, visceral fat and intrahepatic lipids: An exploratory trial. *Br J Nutr* 106(1):79–86.

Sperling, L. S., J. I. Mechanick, I. J. Neeland, C. J. Herrick, J. P. Despres, C. E. Ndumele, K. Vijayaraghavan et al. 2015. The CardioMetabolic Health Alliance: Working toward a new care model for the metabolic syndrome. *J Am Coll Cardiol* 66(9):1050–1067. doi: 10.1016/j.jacc.2015.06.1328.

Stanhope, K. L. 2012. Role of fructose-containing sugars in the epidemics of obesity and metabolic syndrome. *Annu Rev Med* 63:329–343.

Stanhope, K. L. 2016. Sugar consumption, metabolic disease and obesity: The state of the controversy. *Crit Rev Clin Lab Sci* 53(1):52–67. doi: 10.3109/10408363.2015.1084990.

Stanhope, K. L., A. A. Bremer, V. Medici, K. Nakajima, Y. Ito, T. Nakano, G. Chen et al. 2011a. Consumption of fructose and high fructose corn syrup increase postprandial triglycerides, LDL-cholesterol, and apolipoprotein-B in young men and women. *J Clin Endocrinol Metab* 96(10):E1596–E1605. doi: 10.1210/jc.2011-1251.

Stanhope, K. L., S. C. Griffen, A. A. Bremer, R. G. Vink, E. J. Schaefer, K. Nakajima, J. M. Schwarz et al. 2011b. Metabolic responses to prolonged consumption of glucose- and fructose-sweetened beverages are not associated with postprandial or 24-h glucose and insulin excursions. *Am J Clin Nutr* 94(1):112–119. doi: 10.3945/ajcn.110.002246.

Stanhope, K.L. and Havel, P.J., *Dietary Sugars and Health*, Taylor & Francis Group, LLC, Boca Raton, FL, 2014.

Stanhope, K. L. and P. J. Havel. 2008a. Endocrine and metabolic effects of consuming beverages sweetened with fructose, glucose, sucrose, or high-fructose corn syrup. *Am J Clin Nutr* 88(6):1733S–1737S. doi: 10.3945/ajcn.2008.25825D.

Stanhope, K. L. and P. J. Havel. 2008b. Fructose consumption: Potential mechanisms for its effects to increase visceral adiposity and induce dyslipidemia and insulin resistance. *Curr Opin Lipidol* 19(1):16–24.

Stanhope, K. L. and Havel, P. J. 2014. Mechanisms by which dietary sugars influence lipid metabolism, circulating lipids and lipoproteins, and cardiovascular risk. In M. Goran and L. Tappy (Eds.), *Dietary Sugars and Health*, Taylor & Francis Group, LLC., Boca Raton, FL, pp. 267–282.

Stanhope, K. L., V. Medici, A. A. Bremer, V. Lee, H. D. Lam, M. V. Nunez, G. X. Chen, N. L. Keim, and P. J. Havel. 2015. A dose-response study of consuming high-fructose corn syrup-sweetened beverages on lipid/lipoprotein risk factors for cardiovascular disease in young adults. *Am J Clin Nutr* 101(6):1144–1154. doi: 10.3945/ajcn.114.100461.

Stanhope, K. L., J. M. Schwarz, N. L. Keim, S. C. Griffen, A. A. Bremer, J. L. Graham, B. Hatcher et al. 2009. Consuming fructose-sweetened, not glucose-sweetened, beverages increases visceral adiposity and lipids and decreases insulin sensitivity in overweight/obese humans. *J Clin Invest* 119(5):1322–1334. doi: 10.1172/JCI37385.

Suisse Research Institute Credit. 2013. Sugar consumption at a crossroads. Version September 2013. Available at: https://publications.credit-suisse.com/tasks/render/file/index.cfm?fileid=780BF4A8-B3D1-13A0-D2514E21EFFB0479.

Sundaram, M., S. Zhong, M. Bou Khalil, H. Zhou, Z. G. Jiang, Y. Zhao, J. Iqbal et al. 2010. Functional analysis of the missense APOC3 mutation Ala23Thr associated with human hypotriglyceridemia. *J Lipid Res* 51(6):1524–1534. doi: 10.1194/jlr.M005108.

Swarbrick, M. M., K. L. Stanhope, S. S. Elliott, J. L. Graham, R. M. Krauss, M. P. Christiansen, S. C. Griffen, N. L. Keim, and P. J. Havel. 2008. Consumption of fructose-sweetened beverages for 10 weeks increases postprandial triacylglycerol and apolipoprotein-B concentrations in overweight and obese women. *Br J Nutr* 100(5):947–952.

Tarantino, G. and C. Finelli. 2013. What about non-alcoholic fatty liver disease as a new criterion to define metabolic syndrome? *World J Gastroenterol* 19(22):3375–3384. doi: 10.3748/wjg.v19.i22.3375.

Taskinen, M. R. and J. Boren. 2015. New insights into the pathophysiology of dyslipidemia in type 2 diabetes. *Atherosclerosis* 239(2):483–495. doi: 10.1016/j.atherosclerosis.2015.01.039.

Tate, D. F., G. Turner-McGrievy, E. Lyons, J. Stevens, K. Erickson, K. Polzien, M. Diamond, X. Wang, and B. Popkin. 2012. Replacing caloric beverages with water or diet beverages for weight loss in adults: Main results of the Choose Healthy Options Consciously Everyday (CHOICE) randomized clinical trial. *Am J Clin Nutr* 95(3):555–563. doi: 10.3945/ajcn.111.026278.

Tchernof, A. and J. P. Despres. 2013. Pathophysiology of human visceral obesity: An update. *Physiol Rev* 93(1):359–404. doi: 10.1152/physrev.00033.2011.

Te Morenga, L. A., A. J. Howatson, R. M. Jones, and J. Mann. 2014. Dietary sugars and cardiometabolic risk: Systematic review and meta-analyses of randomized controlled trials of the effects on blood pressure and lipids. *Am J Clin Nutr* 100(1):65–79. doi: 10.3945/ajcn.113.081521.

Teff, K. L., S. S. Elliott, M. Tschop, T. J. Kieffer, D. Rader, M. Heiman, R. R. Townsend, N. L. Keim, D. D'Alessio, and P. J. Havel. 2004. Dietary fructose reduces circulating insulin and leptin, attenuates postprandial suppression of ghrelin, and increases triglycerides in women. *J Clin Endocrinol Metab* 89(6):2963–2972.

Teff, K. L., J. Grudziak, R. R. Townsend, T. N. Dunn, R. W. Grant, S. H. Adams, N. L. Keim, B. P. Cummings, K. L. Stanhope, and P. J. Havel. 2009. Endocrine and metabolic effects of consuming fructose- and glucose-sweetened beverages with meals in obese men and women: Influence of insulin resistance on plasma triglyceride responses. *J Clin Endocrinol Metab* 94(5):1562–1659. doi: 10.1210/jc.2008-2192.

The Corn Refiners Association. The facts about high fructose corn syrup. Accessed December 16, 2015. http://sweetsurprise.com/comparing-hfcs-and-other-sweeteners.

United States Department of Health and Human Services and U.S. Department of Agriculture. December 2015. *2015–2020 Dietary Guidelines for Americans*, 8th edn. Accessed December 28, 2016. Available at: http://health.gov/dietaryguidelines/2015/guidelines/.

Ventura, E. E., J. N. Davis, and M. I. Goran. 2011. Sugar content of popular sweetened beverages based on objective laboratory analysis: Focus on fructose content. *Obesity (Silver Spring)* 19(4):868–874. doi: 10.1038/oby.2010.255.

Viazzi, F., D. Garneri, G. Leoncini, A. Gonnella, M. L. Muiesan, E. Ambrosioni, F. V. Costa et al. 2014. Serum uric acid and its relationship with metabolic syndrome and cardiovascular risk profile in patients with hypertension: Insights from the I-DEMAND study. *Nutr Metab Cardiovasc Dis* 24(8):921–927.

Wang, C. S., W. J. McConathy, H. U. Kloer, and P. Alaupovic. 1985. Modulation of lipoprotein lipase activity by apolipoproteins. Effect of apolipoprotein C-III. *J Clin Invest* 75(2):384–390. doi: 10.1172/JCI111711.

Wang, J. 2014. Consumption of added sugars and development of metabolic syndrome components among a sample of youth at risk of obesity. *Appl Physiol Nutr Metab* 39(4):512. doi: 10.1139/apnm-2013-0456.

Wang, J. W., S. Mark, M. Henderson, J. O'Loughlin, A. Tremblay, J. Wortman, G. Paradis, and K. Gray-Donald. 2013. Adiposity and glucose intolerance exacerbate components of metabolic syndrome in children consuming sugar-sweetened beverages: QUALITY cohort study. *Pediatr Obes* 8(4):284–293. doi: 10.1111/j.2047-6310.2012.00108.x.

Wang, L., F. M. Sacks, J. D. Furtado, M. Ricks, A. B. Courville, and A. E. Sumner. 2014. Racial differences between African-American and white women in insulin resistance and visceral adiposity are associated with differences in apoCIII containing apoAI and apoB lipoproteins. *Nutr Metab (Lond)* 11(1):56. doi: 10.1186/1743-7075-11-56.

Watt, M. J. and A. J. Hoy. 2012. Lipid metabolism in skeletal muscle: Generation of adaptive and maladaptive intracellular signals for cellular function. *Am J Physiol Endocrinol Metab* 302(11):E1315–E1328. doi: 10.1152/ajpendo.00561.2011.

Wei, Y., D. Wang, G. Moran, A. Estrada, and M. J. Pagliassotti. 2013. Fructose-induced stress signaling in the liver involves methylglyoxal. *Nutr Metab (Lond)* 10(1):32. doi: 10.1186/1743-7075-10-32.

Wei, Y., D. Wang, F. Topczewski, and M. J. Pagliassotti. 2007. Fructose-mediated stress signaling in the liver: Implications for hepatic insulin resistance. *J Nutr Biochem* 18(1):1–9.

Welsh, J. A., A. Sharma, J. L. Abramson, V. Vaccarino, C. Gillespie, and M. B. Vos. 2010. Caloric sweetener consumption and dyslipidemia among US adults. *JAMA* 303(15):1490–1497. doi: 10.1001/jama.2010.449.

Welsh, J. A., A. Sharma, S. A. Cunningham, and M. B. Vos. 2011. Consumption of added sugars and indicators of cardiovascular disease risk among US adolescents. *Circulation* 123(3):249–257. doi: 10.1161/CIRCULATIONAHA.110.972166.

Welty, F. K., A. Alfaddagh, and T. K. Elajami. 2016. Targeting inflammation in metabolic syndrome. *Transl Res* 167(1):257–280.

World Health Organization. 2015. Guideline: Sugars intake for adults and children. Accessed December 28, 2016. Available at: http://apps.who.int/iris/bitstream/10665/149782/1/9789241549028_eng.pdf.

Wyler von Ballmoos, M. C., B. Haring, and F. M. Sacks. 2015. The risk of cardiovascular events with increased apolipoprotein CIII: A systematic review and meta-analysis. *J Clin Lipidol* 9(4):498–510. doi: 10.1016/j.jacl.2015.05.002.

Xi, B., Y. Huang, K. H. Reilly, S. Li, R. Zheng, M. T. Barrio-Lopez, M. A. Martinez-Gonzalez, and D. Zhou. 2015. Sugar-sweetened beverages and risk of hypertension and CVD: A dose-response meta-analysis. *Br J Nutr* 113(5):709–717. doi: 10.1017/S0007114514004383.

Yadav, D., E. S. Lee, H. M. Kim, E. Y. Lee, E. Choi, and C. H. Chung. 2013. Hyperuricemia as a potential determinant of metabolic syndrome. *J Lifestyle Med* 3(2):98–106.

Yang, Q., Z. Zhang, E. W. Gregg, W. D. Flanders, R. Merritt, and F. B. Hu. 2014. Added sugar intake and cardiovascular diseases mortality among US adults. *JAMA Intern Med* 174(4):516–524. doi: 10.1001/jamainternmed.2013.13563.

Yao, Z. and Y. Wang. 2012. Apolipoprotein C-III and hepatic triglyceride-rich lipoprotein production. *Curr Opin Lipidol* 23(3):206–212. doi: 10.1097/MOL.0b013e328352dc70.

Yoshida, M., N. M. McKeown, G. Rogers, J. B. Meigs, E. Saltzman, R. D'Agostino, and P. F. Jacques. 2007. Surrogate markers of insulin resistance are associated with consumption of sugar-sweetened drinks and fruit juice in middle and older-aged adults. *J Nutr* 137(9):2121–2127.

Zalawadiya, S. K., V. Veeranna, S. Mallikethi-Reddy, C. Bavishi, A. Lunagaria, A. Kottam, and L. Afonso. 2015. Uric acid and cardiovascular disease risk reclassification: Findings from NHANES III. *Eur J Prev Cardiol* 22(4):513–518.

Zelber-Sagi, S., D. Nitzan-Kaluski, R. Goldsmith, M. Webb, L. Blendis, Z. Halpern, and R. Oren. 2007. Long term nutritional intake and the risk for non-alcoholic fatty liver disease (NAFLD): A population based study. *J Hepatol* 47(5):711–717. doi: 10.1016/j.jhep.2007.06.020.

Zgaga, L., E. Theodoratou, J. Kyle, S. M. Farrington, F. Agakov, A. Tenesa, M. Walker et al. 2012. The association of dietary intake of purine-rich vegetables, sugar-sweetened beverages and dairy with plasma urate, in a cross-sectional study. *PLoS One* 7(6):e38123. doi: 10.1371/journal.pone.0038123.

15 Dietary Carbohydrate Restriction in the Management of NAFLD and Metabolic Syndrome

Grace Marie Jones, Kathleen Mulligan, and Jean-Marc Schwarz

CONTENTS

ABSTRACT

Nonalcoholic fatty liver disease (NAFLD) and metabolic syndrome (MetS), which are influenced by diet and genetics, contribute individually to the increased risk for cardiovascular disease and type 2 diabetes. Understanding the etiology of these diseases is paramount to the development of effective preventive steps and treatments. Here, we focus on NAFLD as MetS has been covered elsewhere. NAFLD is a cluster of diseases that ranges from accumulation of fat in the liver to inflammation and to cirrhosis of the liver. Currently, the worldwide incidence of NAFLD is 24% and affects both adults and children. The specific mechanisms by which the liver accumulates fat are unknown but involve an imbalance in the flow of lipids entering and exiting the liver. Obesity plays a central role, as adipose tissue is involved in many pathways that directly impact the pathology of NAFLD. Interestingly, risk factors for NAFLD and its progression have been linked to specific polymorphisms in genes that encode for proteins involved in the metabolism of hepatic lipids. Currently, the primary treatment for NAFLD is weight loss and lifestyle changes. A hypocaloric diet and reductions in carbohydrate intake have been shown to reduce the accumulation of hepatic fat in NAFLD patients. Our recommendations for treating this patient population include not only the restriction of carbohydrates but also a specific reduction in the intake of simple sugars. Pharmacological agents such as vitamins, bile acid analogs, and probiotics and prebiotics are often prescribed in the presence of other comorbidities such as type 2 diabetes.

INTRODUCTION

Nonalcoholic steatohepatitis (NASH) was first described in 20 patients at the Mayo Clinic in 1980 (Ludwig, Viggiano et al. 1980). Since then, our understanding of nonalcoholic fatty liver disease (NAFLD) and NASH has evolved, and many efforts have gone into elucidating its etiology, diagnosis, progression, and treatment. NAFLD is an umbrella term that describes a full spectrum of diseases ranging from hepatic fat accumulation to cirrhosis of the liver (Kleiner, Brunt et al. 2005). NAFLD is defined by histological analysis of liver biopsies showing fat infiltration in ≥5% hepatic cells (Figure 15.1) of people consuming no more than one or two servings of alcohol per day in women and men, respectively (Chalasani, Younossi et al. 2012). NAFLD is associated with other prevalent chronic diseases such as obesity and metabolic syndrome (MetS) (Kang, Greenson et al. 2006, Masuoka and Chalasani 2013), the symptoms of which include elevated fasting blood glucose, hypertension, dyslipidemia, and increased waist circumference. Together, these comorbid conditions increase the risk for cardiovascular disease and type 2 diabetes (Targher, Bertolini et al. 2007, Siddiqui, Fuchs et al. 2015). In this chapter, we focus on the effectiveness of carbohydrate restriction as a dietary intervention for NAFLD. Additionally, we briefly discuss the progression of NAFLD, theories of etiology, risk factors, and treatments, followed by dietary recommendations for NAFLD treatment.

SCOPE OF DISEASE

Hepatic Triglyceride Accumulation

The liver plays a central role in lipid metabolism, and hepatic triglyceride accumulation is the result of an imbalance between the hepatic influx and efflux of fatty acids (FAs). On one hand, the liver takes up circulating nonesterified fatty acids (NEFAs) and fat from triglyceride-rich lipoprotein remnants and synthesizes FAs (*de novo* lipogenesis [DNL]) from carbohydrates, while on the other hand, it secretes FAs as triglycerides in very-low-density lipoproteins (VLDL) and produces energy from FAs through β-oxidation (Figure 15.2) (Liu, Bengmark et al. 2010). Triglyceride accumulation in the liver is a disruption in the delicate balance of the uptake, synthesis, and export of FAs as VLDL or hepatic oxidation (Fabbrini, Sullivan et al. 2010).

A proposed mechanism of NAFLD or ectopic fat accumulation is the presence of a positive energy balance and limited adipose tissue storage capacity, leading to increased circulating NEFAs and spillover into ectopic tissues including the liver (Mittendorfer, Magkos et al. 2009). In this situation of large FA input, the liver is unable to oxidize or secrete the increased FAs and lipid droplets accumulate. Obesity with adipose tissue insulin resistance can also increase lipolysis owing to diminished suppression of hormone-sensitive lipase by insulin, thus resulting in increased free FA flux to the liver. In addition, acute hyperinsulinemia inhibits the formation and secretion of VLDL (Lewis, Uffelman et al. 1995), while the stimulation of DNL by insulin continues to produce new fat from carbohydrate. Together, these factors can lead to FA accumulation in the liver (Tessari, Coracina et al. 2009). A 2005 study reported that DNL accounted for 26% of the FAs present in the livers of individuals with NAFLD (Donnelly, Smith et al. 2005). Additionally, it has been demonstrated that DNL is significantly elevated in insulin-resistant states (Tappy, Schwarz et al. 1998, Tappy, Berger et al. 1999, Schwarz, Chiolero et al. 2000, Lo, Mulligan et al. 2001,

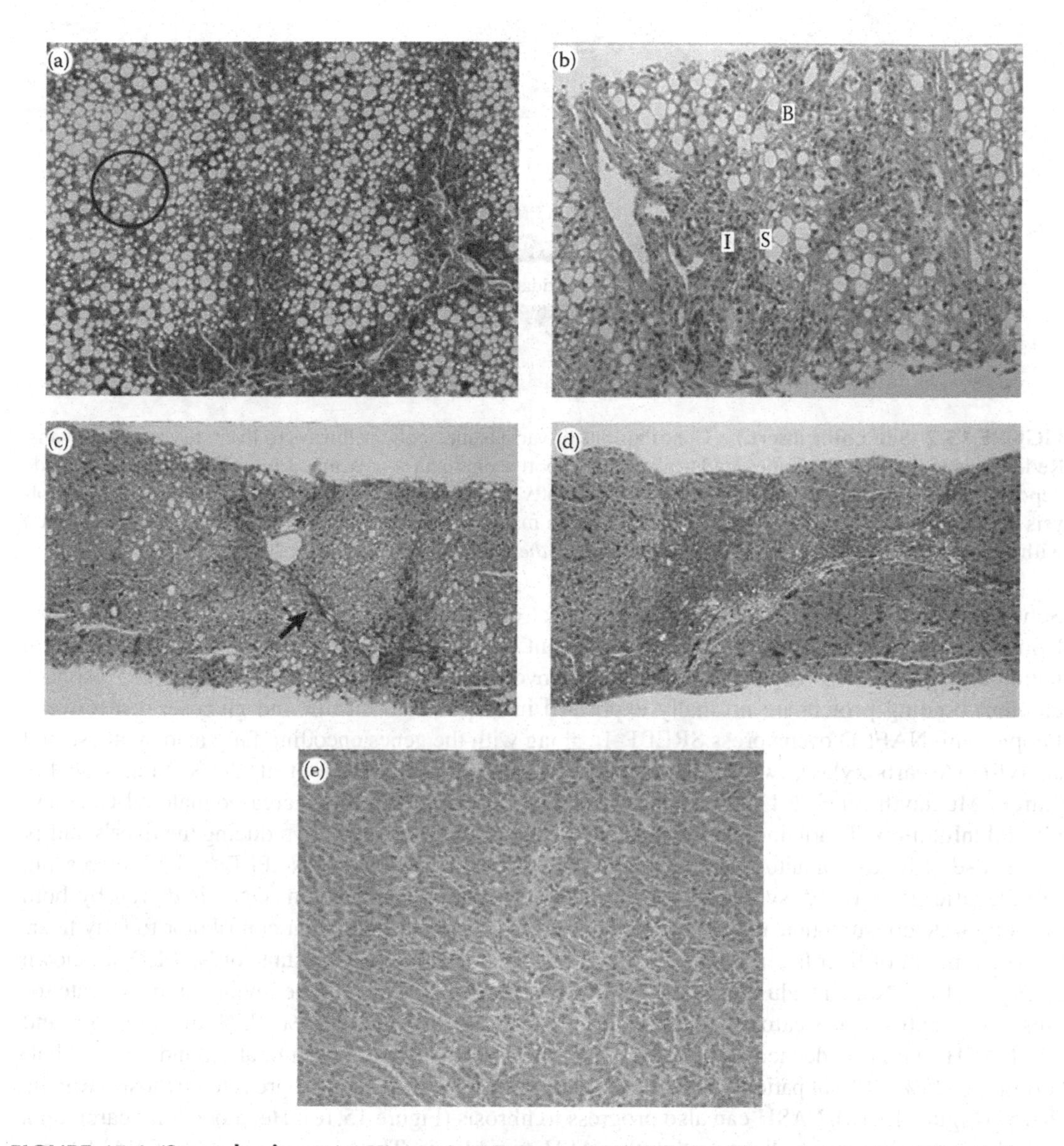

FIGURE 15.1 (See color insert.) Histological features of NAFLD. (a) Marked steatosis without inflammation, hepatocytes injury (ballooning), or fibrosis. Steatosis is concentrated in acinar zone 3, the microcirculatory unit through which blood exists the liver around the terminal hepatic venule (in circle) and shows sparing of the periportal, zone 1 hepatocytes, the microcirculatory unit through which portal and systemic blood enter and mix. This is the adult pattern of nonalcoholic fatty liver disease (NAFLD) (trichrome staining). (b) Steatohepatitis with marked steatosis (S), ballooning (B), lobular and portal inflammation (I) and extensive bridging fibrosis (hematoxylin and eosin staining). (c) Fibrosis in the perisinusoidal spaces of zone 3 is detected by trichrome stain; bridging fibrosis (arrow) is noted between two central veins. Hepatocytes with steatosis are seen, but no ballooned hepatocytes are present. (d) Nonalcoholic steatohepatisis (NASH) with cirrhosis, but no active lesions remain. One would only know this was a case of NASH-related cirrhosis by having had a prior biopsy with the diagnosis of active NASH. (e) Hepatocellular carcinoma after the development of NASH and cirrhosis. (Reprinted by permission from Macmillian Publishers Ltd.: *Nat. Rev. Dis. Primers*, (Brunt 2015) Copyright, 2015.)

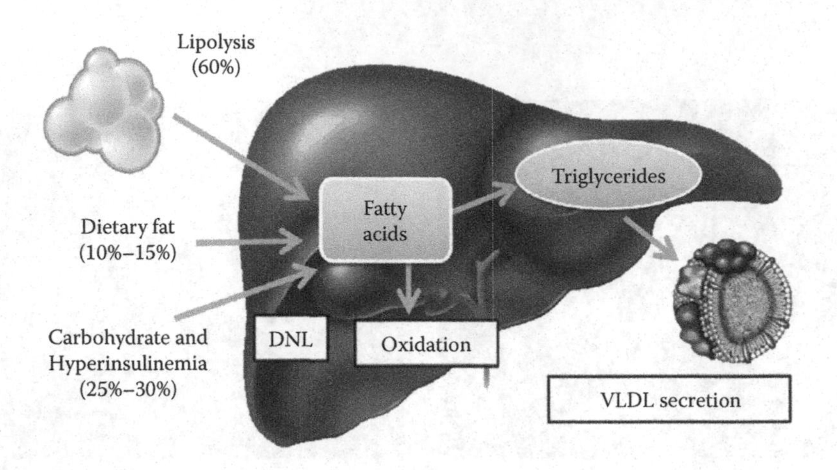

FIGURE 15.2 (See color insert.) Contributions of various metabolic pathways to liver steatosis in humans. Reductions in fatty acid oxidation and triglyceride export seem to have only minor roles in hepatic triglyceride deposition. By contrast, the increased availability of fatty acids from the adipose tissue through unabated lipolysis and *de novo* lipogenesis (DNL) from glucose are major providers of lipids in steatotic livers. (Reprinted with permission from Taskinen, M.R. and Boren, J., *Atherosclerosis*, 239(2), 483, 2015.)

Schwarz, Mulligan et al. 2002, Schwarz, Linfoot et al. 2003) and in NAFLD (Lambert, Ramos-Roman et al. 2014). The sterol regulatory element binding protein 1c (SREBP-1c), a transcription factor essential for the expression of proteins involved in glycolysis, and carbohydrate response element binding protein are normally expressed in response to insulin and glucose, respectively. People with NAFLD overexpress SREBP-1c along with the genes encoding fatty acid synthase and acetyl-CoA carboxylase, two key lipogenic enzymes (Higuchi, Kato et al. 2008, Lima-Cabello, Garcia-Mediavilla et al. 2011). Importantly, expression of ACC leads to increased malonyl-CoA levels and inhibition of carnitine palmitoyltransferase-1 (CPT-1), effectively reducing the liver's ability to dispose of lipids via mitochondrial β-oxidation. Thus, DNL impacts NAFLD by both increasing intrahepatic *de novo* FA synthesis and decreasing hepatic FA oxidation. DNL is driven by both carbohydrate consumption and hyperinsulinemia and may be a significant contributor to fatty liver.

The amount of liver fat, inflammation, and scar tissue determines the stage of NAFLD, as shown in Figure 15.1 (Nalbantoglu and Brunt 2014, Brunt 2015). NAFLD can be divided into two categories: (1) steatosis or steatosis with inflammation (approximately 70%–75% of patients), and (2) NASH, which is defined by the combination of steatosis with inflammation and cellular ballooning (~25%–30% of patients). Nearly 20% of patients with NASH progress to cirrhosis (Rinella 2015) (Figure 15.1d). NASH can also progress to fibrosis (Figure 15.1c). Hepatocellular carcinoma can also occur in patients diagnosed with NASH or cirrhosis. The beginning stages of NAFLD are asymptomatic; the initial diagnosis can be dependent on abnormal liver function tests, specifically alanine aminotransferase (ALT) and aspartate aminotransferase (AST) levels (Maximos, Bril et al. 2015); histological analysis of a liver biopsy sample, which is the standard for NAFLD diagnosis (Nalbantoglu and Brunt 2014); or radiologic imaging (Charatcharoenwitthaya and Lindor 2007). Radiologic imaging includes (1) ultrasound (Dasarathy, Dasarathy et al. 2009), (2) noncontrast computed tomography (CT) (Rofsky and Fleishaker 1995), and (3) magnetic resonance spectroscopy (MRS) and/or imaging (MRI) (Reeder, Cruite et al. 2011).

Risk Factors and Etiology

Factors that play a role in the development and progression of NAFLD include metabolic and genetic influences (Romeo, Kozlitina et al. 2008, Makkonen, Pietilainen et al. 2009), nutrition, inflammatory bowel disease, HIV status (Cassol, Misra et al. 2013), infection with the hepatitis C virus (Patel and

Harrison 2012), the gut microbiota (Machado and Cortez-Pinto 2012, Mouzaki, Comelli et al. 2013), adipose tissue, and the immune system. NAFLD is a multifactorial disease that has many mechanisms that regulate its establishment and progression. A central factor is obesity (Hsiao, Kuo et al. 2007), which is impacted by diet, genetic predisposition, level of physical activity, and the gut microbiota (Greenhill 2015). Moreover, adipose tissue plays a role in increased circulation of free FAs (Donnelly, Smith et al. 2005), insulin resistance, and proinflammatory mediators (Catalan, Gomez-Ambrosi et al. 2015). Each of these factors has separate downstream effects that directly impact the entire spectrum of NAFLD from steatosis to fibrosis to cirrhosis and hepatocellular cancer. Additionally, disruptions in the intestinal lining, caused by small intestinal bacterial overgrowth, can lead to the presence of endotoxins in the bloodstream, which enter the liver via the portal vein, contributing to the inflammatory response and steatohepatitis (Cani, Amar et al. 2007, Miele, Valenza et al. 2009).

Genome-wide association studies have identified loss-of-function gene variants that are involved in hepatic lipid metabolism and play a major role in the pathogenesis of NAFLD (Dongiovanni, Romeo et al. 2015). The I148M variant of the *patatin-like phospholipase domain-containing 3* gene, *PNPLA3* or adiponutrin, a lipase involved in the hydrolysis of triglycerides (Pingitore, Pirazzi et al. 2014), was strongly associated with increased fat levels and inflammation in the liver. Interestingly, Hispanics as a group are more susceptible to NAFLD and are more likely to have the I148M variant than African- or European-Americans (Romeo, Kozlitina et al. 2008). A second variant, E167K of the *transmembrane 6 superfamily member 2* gene, was found in two separate studies (Holmen, Zhang et al. 2014, Kozlitina, Smagris et al. 2014) and has been shown to regulate hepatic lipid metabolism via VLDL secretion (Mahdessian, Taxiarchis et al. 2014). Additionally, the *glucokinase regulator* P446L polymorphism has a significant association with NAFLD and has been shown to increase *DNL*, liver fibrosis, and triglyceride levels (Speliotes, Yerges-Armstrong et al. 2011, Wu, Lemaitre et al. 2013, Petta, Miele et al. 2014, Aguilar-Olivos, Almeda-Valdes et al. 2015, Santoro, Caprio et al. 2015). Other genes involved in hepatic lipid metabolism, including *FATP5*, *LYPLAL1*, *NCAN*, *PPAR*, *PPP1R3B*, *LPIN1*, *TRIB1*, and *UCP2*,* have been implicated in the pathogenesis of NAFLD. However, further research is needed to clarify their suspected roles (Speliotes, Yerges-Armstrong et al. 2011, Kitamoto, Kitamoto et al. 2014).

A handful of clinical studies on NAFLD and the gut microbiota have shown a change in the abundances of particular phyla in people with NAFLD and NASH when compared with healthy controls. While a direct role of the gut microbiota has not been demonstrated, evidence for its role in insulin resistance and obesity, two risk factors for NAFLD, has been suggested (Ley, Turnbaugh et al. 2006, Cani and Delzenne 2009, Caricilli and Saad 2013). Emerging data will elucidate the role of the gut microbiota and its interaction with diet in the development of CVD, obesity, type 2 diabetes, and NAFLD. Other comorbid conditions in which NAFLD has been described include polycystic ovary syndrome (Karoli, Fatima et al. 2013, Vassilatou, Vassiliadi et al. 2015), hypothyroidism (Sert, Pirgon et al. 2013, Ludwig, Holzner et al. 2015), obstructive sleep apnea (Chou, Liang et al. 2015, Qi, Huang et al. 2015), hypopituitarism and hypogonadism (Hazlehurst and Tomlinson 2013), Hepatitis C (Bondini and Younossi 2006), and HIV (Guaraldi, Squillace et al. 2008).

Epidemiology

A recent meta-analysis reported that the global prevalence of NAFLD was 24% (Zhu, Dai et al. 2015). This number, however, might be misleadingly low in that the reported prevalence of NAFLD varies widely and is highly dependent on the method of diagnosis and the population studied. Estimated prevalence is 20%–30% in Western countries and 5%–18% in Asia (Satapathy and Sanyal 2015). The prevalence of NAFLD in different studies in Asian countries has ranged from 27% in China (264 of 922 randomly selected subjects via MRS; [Wong, Chu et al. 2012]), 18% in Japan (in 47 of 263 living liver donors via

* *FATP5*, fatty acid transport protein 5; *LYPLAL1*, lysophospholipase-like 1; *NCAN*, neurocan; *PPAR*, peroxisome proliferator-activated receptor; *PPP1R3B*, protein phosphatase 1 regulatory subunit 3B; *LPIN1*, lipin 1; *TRIB1*, tribbles homologue 1; and *UCP2*, uncoupling protein 2.

biopsy) (Yamamoto, Takada et al. 2007), 51% in Korea (303 of 589 living liver donors via biopsy, ultrasound, and/or CT) (Lee, Kim et al. 2007), and in India, depending on the region, between 9% and 35% via ultrasound and/or CT (Singh, Nayak et al. 2004, Amarapurkar, Kamani et al. 2007, Mohan, Farooq et al. 2009, Das, Das et al. 2010). Conversely, studies performed in western countries have reported the prevalence of NAFLD to be 20%–25% in Italy (57 of 287 subjects without suspected liver diseases versus 78 of 311 subjects with suspected liver disease via ultrasound) (Bedogni, Miglioli et al. 2005), 26% in Spain (198 of 766 subjects in a cross-sectional population study via ultrasound) (Caballeria, Pera et al. 2010), and 26% in the United Kingdom (295 of 1118 primary care patients with abnormal liver function tests via ultrasound) (Armstrong, Houlihan et al. 2012). In the large U.S. Dallas Heart Study that used MRS, the prevalence of hepatic steatosis was 34% (Browning, Szczepaniak et al. 2004). The prevalence in this study varied based on ethnicity: 45% in Hispanics, 33% in Whites, and 24% in Blacks. There were no differences between males and females among Hispanics or Blacks; however, the prevalence of steatosis in white men was greater than that in white women (42% versus 24%, respectively).

NAFLD in Children

The prevalence of NAFLD in the pediatric population is increasing in parallel with the rise in childhood obesity. Children are susceptible to the same risk factors for NAFLD as adults, including influences of race/ethnicity, family history, and genetic and environmental factors. One environmental factor unique to this population is the feeding regimen during infancy. A 2009 study showed that children breastfed 0.5–17 months (median = 8 months, n = 91) were less likely to develop NASH and fibrosis compared to formula-fed children (Nobili, Bedogni et al. 2009). Furthermore, longer duration of breastfeeding, up to 17 months, was associated with lower risk of NASH. Presently, the treatment of NAFLD in children is focused on reducing obesity through weight loss and negative-energy balance/energy restriction diets (Nobili, Alkhouri et al. 2015).

Treatment

Presently, weight loss and lifestyle changes are the primary NAFLD-specific treatments recommended. Other approaches, which will be discussed later, include use of insulin-sensitizing agents, antioxidants, and other agents. Current weight loss methods used to treat NAFLD/NASH can be categorized as follows: (1) behavior therapy/lifestyle modification, (2) anti-obesity drugs, and (3) weight loss surgery. The magnitude of weight loss has a proportional relationship with disease improvement (Promrat, Kleiner et al. 2010). Behavioral therapy (Centis, Marzocchi et al. 2010, Moscatiello, Di Luzio et al. 2011), increased physical activity (Bae, Suh et al. 2012), and dietary recommendations should lead to a decrease in caloric intake, increase in energy expenditure, and consequent weight reduction (Chalasani, Younossi et al. 2012). While specific exercises and diets have not been identified to treat NAFLD, high-intensity exercise (Oh, Shida et al. 2015) and carbohydrate restriction (40% CHO versus 60% CHO) (Ryan, Abbasi et al. 2007, Browning, Baker et al. 2011) (<10% CHO versus low-fat diet, 45%–65% CHO) (Ryan, Abbasi et al. 2007, Browning, Baker et al. 2011) when compared to other diets with similar weight loss have been shown to significantly reduce the level of hepatic fat. Interestingly, a recent meta-analysis of 28 randomized trials (n = 1644 randomized patients) showed that exercise alone was associated with reductions of hepatic lipids (standardized mean difference, −0.69), AST and ALT levels, and weighted mean difference, −4.85 IU/L and −3.30 IU/L, respectively (Orci, Gariani et al. 2016). Additionally, Orci et al. found that subjects with a higher baseline BMI benefitted from physical activity with respect to lowering liver fat. Orlistat, a proven weight loss aid, functions to reduce dietary fat absorption and is used to manage people with obesity (Rucker, Padwal et al. 2007). However, it is currently not recommended as a stand-alone treatment for NAFLD as studies have shown no histologic improvements with its use (Chalasani, Younossi et al. 2012). Finally, bariatric surgery, which leads to significant weight loss, includes Roux-en-Y gastric bypass, laparoscopic adjustable banding, sleeve gastrectomy, or biliopancreatic diversion with duodenal switch, has been shown to improve AST and ALT levels and liver histology (Bower, Toma et al. 2015). However, controlled studies have not evaluated bariatric surgery as a treatment for NAFLD, and therefore, this procedure is not a primary treatment (Chalasani, Younossi et al. 2012, Aguilar-Olivos, Almeda-Valdes et al. 2015).

EFFECT OF CARBOHYDRATE RESTRICTION ON NAFLD

A central factor in the pathophysiology of NAFLD is obesity, and therefore the primary component of NAFLD treatment is through weight loss and lifestyle modification, including diet and physical activity. As described earlier, many studies have shown weight loss to promote the reduction of hepatic fat in NAFLD patients. Furthermore, the association of NAFLD with other chronic diseases, such as type 2 diabetes and cardiovascular disease, has led to investigations that include the redistribution of macronutrients, increased macronutrient quality, or specific dietary patterns (i.e., Mediterranean diet). Here we focus on the studies that sought to assess the effect of carbohydrate (CHO) restriction, with or without weight loss, on NAFLD.

Low-Carbohydrate Diets in NAFLD (See Table 15.1)

Based on the USDA guidelines, the current recommended distribution of macronutrient intake ranges from 45% to 65% of calories from carbohydrates, 5% to 35% of calories from protein, and 20% to 35% of calories from fat (U.S. Department of Health and Human Services and U.S. Department of Agriculture 2015). A low-carbohydrate or carbohydrate-restricted diet would typically limit the calories from carbohydrate to less than 35% (Sedlacek, Playdon et al. 2011, Tay, Luscombe-Marsh et al. 2015), whereas a high-carbohydrate diet generally consists of a minimum of 45% of calories derived from carbohydrates (Krebs, Elley et al. 2012, Masters, Aarabi et al. 2012). Several studies have examined the effect of carbohydrate restriction on NAFLD and other associated risk factors such as weight, liver enzyme levels, and glucose metabolism (Table 15.1). Table 15.2 summarizes the macronutrient content in these studies.

In 2005, Huang et al. conducted a pilot study that investigated the impact of intense 1-year nutritional counseling and moderate carbohydrate intake in overweight and obese people with liver biopsy–diagnosed NASH. They found that 60% of participants responded favorably to the intervention. In patients with an improved histological score, there were significant mean reductions in weight (7%), BMI (−2.25 kg/m^2), waist circumference (−6.94 cm), and aminotransferase levels (−15.44 IU/L AST and −33.11 IU/L ALT) (Huang, Greenson et al. 2005). Additionally, these individuals demonstrated reductions in liver fat and total NASH score. This study suggested that intense nutritional education is an important aspect of weight loss and improvement in NASH scoring. However, they did not address how the modification of macronutrient content, in conjunction with nutritional education, affected features of NAFLD/NASH as there was no control group. To that end, two groups examined the effect of dietary counseling combined with either a hypocaloric low-carbohydrate diet (<90 g CHO) versus a hypocaloric low-fat diet (Haufe, Engeli et al. 2011) or an isocaloric low-fat, high-carbohydrate diet versus an ad libitum Mediterranean diet (Ryan, Itsiopoulos et al. 2013). The study by Haufe et al. aimed to assess whether reducing overall caloric intake by 30% decreased liver fat or whether the specific reduction of either carbohydrate or fat calories caused a decline in ectopic liver fat. In this randomized study of overweight and obese subjects, some with a high liver fat content (assessed by MRS), both the low-carbohydrate and low-fat diets had similar effects on weight loss and reductions in liver fat. The authors concluded that these improvements were due to the reduction in caloric intake and not to a shift in relative percentages of macronutrients (Haufe, Engeli et al. 2011). Ryan et al. utilized a randomized crossover intervention study design to evaluate how insulin sensitivity and liver fat are impacted by a low-fat, high-carbohydrate diet (30% calories from fat, 50% from carbohydrate, and 20% from protein) versus the Mediterranean diet (40% calories from fat, 40% from carbohydrate, and 20% from protein) in subjects with NAFLD. This study found

TABLE 15.1
Characteristics and Results of Dietary Intervention Studies in Subjects with NAFLD, NASH, or High Liver Fat

First Author, Pub Year	Subjects	n	BMI (kg/m²)	Assessments	Measure Liver Fat	Intervention/Protocol	Results
Browning et al. (2011)	NAFLD (MRS)	18 9-CRD 9-CaloricRest.	35.7 ± 7	Hepatic TG, weight	MRS	2 weeks: <20 CHO g/day (CRD) or 1200–1500 calories/day (caloric rest.)	Both diets: ↓ liver fat (42%) and ↓ weight (4.3%), greater loss with CRD diet.
Duarte et al. (2014)	NAFLD (biopsy), overweight or obese	48	31.8 ± 4.7	AST, ALT, BMI, lipids, HOMA, HbA1c. insulin, body composition	N/A	75 days: high-protein, hypocaloric diet, 25% kcal Fat. 35% protein. 40% CHO. 20 g fiber/day	Improvements in lipid profile, glucose homeostasis, and liver enzymes.
Haufe et al. (2011)	Overweight and obese, some with high liver fat content	102	28–40.6	Liver fat, SAT, VAT Lipids, Glucose metabolism, ALT, AST, biochemical parameters	MRS	6 months: weekly group meetings + hypocaloric diet (reduced by 3 0%): ≤90 g CHO, 0.8 g protein/kg weight, ≥3 0% fat (Low CHO) or ≤20% fat,0.8 g protein/kg weight, remaining kcal from CHO (low fat)	Both diets resulted in similar ↓ liver fat, ↓SAT, ↓VAT, ↓ weight loss. Low CHO greater ↑ insulin sensitivity, ↓ total and LDL cholesterol, ↓ TGF-β1.
Huang et al. (2005)	Overweight/ obese with NASH (biopsy)	15	34 ± 7	Hepatichistological improvement, insulin resistance, SAT, VAT,	Biopsy	1 year: 40%–45%CHO (complex + Fiber), 35%–40% fat (MUFAs and PUFAs), and 15%–20% protein	Improvements in HOMA, liver histology ↓ weight, ↓ BMI, ↓ TAT, ↓ VAT, ↓ AST, ↓ ALT (reductions not significant).

(*Continued*)

TABLE 15.1 (*Continued*)
Characteristics and Results of Dietary Intervention Studies in Subjects with NAFLD, NASH, or High Liver Fat

First Author, Pub Year	Subjects	n	BMI (kg/m²)	Assessments	Measure Liver Fat	Intervention/Protocol	Results
Kani et al. (2014)	NAFLD (sonography)	45 low kcal, 15, low kcal- CHO, 15, low kcal CHO, soy, 15	45.6 ± 2.6 low kcal, 49.3 ± 3.5 low kcal- CHO,48.5 ± 3.7 low kcal-CHC, soy	Liver enzymes, coagulating factors, lip id profiles, EMI, weight,	N/A	8 weeks: low kcal diet, 55% CHO: 15% protein: 30% fat or low kcalCHO, 45%CHO: 20% protein: 35% Fat, 30 g red meat or Low kcal-CHO, 45% CHO: 20% protein: 35% Fat with 30 g soy nut	All three groups improved, greatest improvement of assessments in Low kcal-CHO with 30 g soy nut group.
Perez-Guisado et al. (2011a)	Overweight with metabolic syndrome (MetS) and NAFLD	14	36.5 ± 0.54	Steatosis, weight, BMI, LDLc, ALT, AST, glycemia, blood pressure, TAGs	Ultrasound	12 weeks: Spanich Ketogenic Mediterranean Diet (SKMD): unlimited kcal, ≤30 green vegetable CHO, ≥30 mL virgin olive oil, 200–300 mL wine	All subjects cured of MS, significant reduction in all measured assessments.
Ryan et al. (2013)	NAFLD (biopsy), nondiabetic	12	32.0 ± 4.2	Hepatic steatosis and Insulin sensitivity	^{1}H-MRS	6 weeks: dietary counseling, low-fat, high-CHO (LF-HCD) and 5 weeks: dietary counseling, Mediterranean diet(MD)	LF-HCD: ↓, liver fat (7%), no change in insulin sensitivity, MD: ↓ liver fat (39%), ↑ insulin Sensitivity

TABLE 15.2
Macronutrient Composition of Dietary Intervention Studies in Subjects with NAFLD, NASH, or High Liver Fat

1st Author, Pub Year	Macronutrient Composition
Browning et al. (2011)	*50% carbohydrate:* 16% protein: 34% fat *versus* *8% carbohydrate:* 33% protein: 59% fat
Duarte et al. (2014)	*40% carbohydrate:* 35% protein: 25% fat plus 20 g fiber/day
Haufe et al. (2011)	*≤90 g carbohydrates,* 0.8 g protein per kg body weight, and a minim urn of 30% fat *versus* Fat content of ≤20% of total energy intake, 0.8 g protein per kg body weight, and the remaining energy content provided by carbohydrates
Huang et al. (2005)	*40%–45% of daily calories from carbohydrates* with an emphasis on complex carbohydrates with fiber, 35%–40% fat (emphasized mono-and polyunsaturated fats), and 15%–20% protein
Kani et al. (2014)	*55% carbohydrate:*15% protein: 30% Fat *versus* *45% carbohydrate:* 20% protein: 35% Fat, 30 g red meat *versus* *45% carbohydrate:* 20% protein: 35% Fat with 30 g soy nut
Perez-Guisado et al. (2011)	*<30 g of carbohydrates* in the form of green vegetables and salad, a minimum of 30 mL of virgin olive oil, 200–400 mL of red wine, unlimited protein
Ryan et al. (2013)	*40% carbohydrate:* 40% fat (mono- and polyunsaturated fats): 20% protein *versus* *50% carbohydrate:* 30% fat: 20% protein

that the low-fat, high-carbohydrate diet reduced liver fat by 7% (assessed by MRS) and did not change insulin sensitivity (assessed by hyperinsulinemic-euglycemic clamp), whereas the moderate carbohydrate restriction diet (Mediterranean diet) resulted in a 39% decrease in liver fat and increased insulin sensitivity, both without weight loss (Ryan, Itsiopoulos et al. 2013). Together, these studies show that while nutritional education is important (education included group and individual nutrition counseling emphasizing healthy choices by a nutritionist and the promotion of gradual weight loss by a registered dietician), two of the three studies show that macronutrient content, particularly the reduced carbohydrate, results in improved NAFLD features. However, one study suggested that the reduction of calories plays a greater role in the reduction of liver fat than the reduction of carbohydrate.

This latter issue was addressed in part by Browning et al. (Browning, Baker et al. 2011) and Kani et al. (Kani, Alavian et al. 2014) by evaluating whether carbohydrate restriction or caloric restriction reduces hepatic triglycerides and whether a low-carbohydrate, low-calorie diet has a beneficial role in NAFLD. The Browning study found both a 2-week very low–carbohydrate diet (8% calories from CHO) and a caloric restriction diet (1200–1500 kcal/day, 50% calories from CHO) resulted in a 4.3% weight loss and a 42% reduction of hepatic triglycerides as measured by MRS. However, when the effects on liver fat, measured by MRS, were examined for each diet, the reduction of liver fat was considerably greater with the CHO-restricted diet (55% versus 28% for the caloric restriction diet) (Browning, Baker et al. 2011). The second study controlled for caloric intake, with a 200–500 kcal/day reduction of required intake, and randomized subjects to: (1) low-calorie diet, 55% CHO:15% protein:30% fat, or (2) a low-calorie, high-carbohydrate diet, 45% CHO:20% protein:35% fat, or (3) low-calorie, low-carbohydrate diet + soy, 45% CHO:20% protein:35% fat plus 30 g soy protein and 30 g red meat. This 8-week study found that a low-calorie, high-carbohydrate, soy-containing diet significantly reduced ALT levels and serum fibrinogen levels, markers of liver function and inflammation, respectively, as compared to a low-calorie diet or a low-calorie, moderate-carbohydrate diet (Kani, Alavian et al. 2014). Taken together, these studies show that hypocaloric diets improved features of NAFLD. However, a hypocaloric diet combined with a CHO-restricted diet resulted in greater improvements in a short-term study of both 2 and 8 weeks.

Interestingly, Kani et al. found that a moderately high protein intake of 20% of calories supplemented with or without 30 g of soy was beneficial to weight reduction and lipid and metabolic markers. While the inclusion of soy in the diet tended to be associated with greater improvements, the differences were not statistically significant compared to the diet without soy. The researchers hypothesized that the components of soy might reduce NAFLD-induced inflammation. It is unclear whether these effects resulted from higher protein intake *per se* or reduction in carbohydrate calories by substitution of protein. In the liver, protein is important for hepatocyte regeneration, lipoprotein assembly, and lipid export. While research on the effect of high-protein diets and NAFLD has not been done, early studies demonstrate a positive effect. Duarte et al. showed that a hypocaloric high-protein, low-carbohydrate diet (35% calories from protein and 40% calories from CHO) in NAFLD patients resulted in improvements in lipid profile, glucose homeostasis, and liver enzymes compared to baseline (Bezerra Duarte, Faintuch et al. 2014). A prospective study that investigated the effect of the Spanish Ketogenic Mediterranean Diet (SKMD), a very low–carbohydrate (≤30 g of carbohydrate), high-protein diet, in overweight Spanish men found that the 12-week intervention caused significant reductions in body weight and aminotransferase levels (Perez-Guisado and Munoz-Serrano 2011a). Importantly, 21.4% of subjects experienced total regression of fatty liver as measured by abdominal ultrasonography (Perez-Guisado and Munoz-Serrano 2011a). The SKMD has also been used to successfully treat risk factors for NAFLD, such as MetS and obesity (Perez-Guisado, Munoz-Serrano et al. 2008, Perez-Guisado and Munoz-Serrano 2011b). Although further studies are needed to verify these results, a high-protein, low-carbohydrate diet may be beneficial to NAFLD patients.

Carbohydrate Quality

Recent studies have suggested that not only carbohydrate quantity but also carbohydrate quality (simple versus complex) can play a role in influencing liver fat content. In a pilot study, eight healthy adults hospitalized in a metabolic ward for 19 days were given two weight-maintaining isocaloric diets with the same macronutrient distribution (15% protein, 35% fat, 50% carbohydrate) for consecutive 9-day periods. During one dietary period, 25% of energy came from fructose; during the other periods, complex carbohydrate was substituted for fructose (Schwarz, Noworolski et al. 2015). While weight was stable on both diets, the high-fructose diet resulted in higher levels of DNL (18.6% ± 1.4% versus 11.0% ± 1.4%, complex carbohydrate; P = 0.001) and higher liver fat, measured by MRS, in all participants (137% of values with complex carbohydrate). In an outpatient feeding study in obese children who reported high levels of sugar intake (>15% sugar and >5% fructose of daily caloric intake), 9 days of fructose restriction with isocaloric substitution of complex carbohydrate resulted in reductions in fasting glucose, insulin, and lipids (Lustig, Mulligan et al. 2016). Importantly, these same subjects had a 56% decrease in DNL-Area Under the Curve (n = 40) and 22% reduction in liver fat (n = 36) (Schwarz, Noworolski et al. 2017). Although the individuals in each of these studies were not selected for liver fat levels (≥5%), these carefully controlled dietary studies suggest that carbohydrate quality, simple carbohydrates, specifically fructose, plays an important role in liver fat accumulation and that DNL is a contributor to liver fat.

The relationship between fructose, lipogenesis, and liver fat is notable. Fructose is a potent stimulator of DNL in that its metabolism bypasses the first regulatory enzyme of the glycolytic pathway. Because the enzymes for fructose metabolism are entirely hepatic, it is essentially metabolized in the liver and provides lipogenic precursors such as acetyl-CoA for DNL. Animal studies have shown that fructose is converted to FAs at rates of up to 18.9 times greater than glucose (Mayes and Laker 1986) and produces increased hepatic triglyceride levels (Thorburn, Storlien et al. 1989). A 2005 study in healthy humans showed that fructose is a potent lipogenic substrate and that it significantly increases hepatic triglyceride levels (Faeh, Minehira et al. 2005). Therefore, an increase in fructose providing lipogenic precursors and an increase in DNL can contribute to hepatic FA accumulation or NAFLD (Fabbrini, Sullivan et al. 2010); conversely, a reduction in dietary fructose intake can lead to decreases in liver fat content.

Recommendations

Many studies have evaluated the effects of low-carbohydrate versus low-fat diets for the prevention of cardiovascular disease, type 2 diabetes, and MetS on liver function but not specifically in the context of NAFLD. A meta-analysis of randomized controlled clinical trials found that both diets reduced body weight and other risk factors for NAFLD (Hu, Mills et al. 2012). Based on human studies and the known mechanisms that promote accumulation of liver fat, we recommend the following nutritional measures to reduce the risk for cardiovascular disease, type 2 diabetes, and hyperlipidemia in NAFLD patients:

- Intense nutritional education and lifestyle support group.
- If weight loss is indicated, a hypocaloric diet, to improve aminotransferase levels and promote weight reduction (Andersen, Gluud et al. 1991, Petersen, Dufour et al. 2005, Ryan, Abbasi et al. 2007).
- A diet with a total carbohydrate intake of less than 45% (Huang, Greenson et al. 2005, Browning, Baker et al. 2011, Haufe, Engeli et al. 2011, Perez-Guisado and Munoz-Serrano 2011, Ryan, Itsiopoulos et al. 2013, Bezerra Duarte, Faintuch et al. 2014, Kani, Alavian et al. 2014).
- A diet with reduced simple sugar intake, especially fructose, to less than 10% of caloric intake (Volynets, Machann et al. 2013, Schwarz, Noworolski et al. 2015, Gugliucci, Lustig et al. 2016, Lustig, Mulligan et al. 2016).
- Dietary fats should be high in mono- and polyunsaturated FAs (Bjermo, Iggman et al. 2012, Bozzetto, Prinster et al. 2012, Rosqvist, Iggman et al. 2014).

OTHER DIETARY TREATMENTS

Antioxidants

Oxidative stress is thought to play a key role in the development of NAFLD (Satapati, Kucejova et al. 2016). Because of this, antioxidants, specifically vitamin E, a free-radical scavenger, have been the focus of several randomized clinical trials. The results of the adult Pioglitazone versus Vitamin E versus Placebo for the Treatment of Non-diabetic Patients with Nonalcoholic Steatohepatitis (PIVENS) trial, which investigated the potential therapeutic effect of vitamin E (800 IU/day) or pioglitazone (30 mg/day) or placebo over 96 weeks, showed that treatment with vitamin E resulted in an improvement in histologic scoring compared to placebo and pioglitazone (Sanyal, Chalasani et al. 2010). Both vitamin E and pioglitazone resulted in significant reductions in AST and ALT levels compared to placebo. Additionally in a meta-analysis of nine trials (n = 119), vitamin E was found to reduce the levels of AST and ALT, markers of disease status in patients with NAFLD, NASH, and chronic hepatitis C (Ji, Sun et al. 2014). Interestingly, the results of the Treatment of Nonalcoholic Fatty Liver Disease in Children study, in which Vitamin E, metformin, and placebo were tested, significant reductions in both hepatocellular ballooning and NAFLD activity score* were observed in all test groups (Lavine, Schwimmer et al. 2011), similar to the adult PIVENS study that tested pioglitazone, vitamin E, and placebo. Additionally, there was no difference between the groups in ALT levels. While vitamin E continues to be considered a NAFLD/NASH therapeutic, its exact mechanism and benefit need further investigation (Chalasani, Younossi et al. 2012).

Polyphenols are naturally occurring antioxidants found in a range of foods including onions, broccoli, apples, grapes, milk thistle, and curry (Salomone, Godos et al. 2015). Several randomized clinical trials in people with NAFLD examined the efficacy of polyphenols and have shown

* The NAFLD activity score assessed on a scale of 0–8, with higher scores indicating more disease. The components of this measure includes steatosis (0–3), lobular inflammation (0–3), and hepatocellular ballooning (0–2) (Lavine, Schwimmer et al. 2011).

beneficial effects such as significant reductions in ALT, AST, and insulin resistance with resveratrol, found in red grapes, mulberries, peanuts, and cocoa (Faghihzadeh, Adibi et al. 2014, Chen, Zhao et al. 2015). Additionally, silymarin alone, a component of milk thistle, resulted in reductions in AST and ALT levels (Solhi, Ghahremani et al. 2014). While these results are promising, further clinical trials are needed to understand dosage, bioavailability, and potential toxicities, as well as the impact of polyphenols on inflammation and fibrosis, and the role of polyphenols in NAFLD treatment.

Probiotics and Prebiotics

The gut microbiota has recently gained much attention due to new techniques that allow for its characterization and investigations into its modulation. The liver is directly linked to the intestines by the portal vein and is therefore influenced by the nature of the bacterial population, such as LPS, or by its effects, increased gut permeability (Cani, Amar et al. 2007). Together, these might contribute to the pathogenesis of NAFLD. There is much interest in the potential of probiotics and prebiotics in the management of NAFLD. However, pending clinical trials in humans and the need to identify a clear mechanism of action leave many questions unanswered (Aller, De Luis et al. 2011, Kirpich, Marsano et al. 2015, Lambert, Parnell et al. 2015).

PHARMACEUTICAL APPROACHES TO THE MANAGEMENT OF NAFLD

Currently, there are no approved pharmacological treatments for the management of NAFLD. However, there are emerging agents that have promise, including insulin-sensitizing agents, glucagon-like peptide-1 (GLP-1) agonists, and bile acid analogs.

Insulin-Sensitizing Agents

Insulin resistance is thought to play a critical role in the pathogenesis of NAFLD and is strongly associated with an increased risk for type 2 diabetes and cardiovascular disease (Eguchi, Eguchi et al. 2006). Accordingly, many have studied the effectiveness of the biguanide metformin and thiazolidinediones such as pioglitazone, two classes of insulin sensitizers, for the management of NAFLD. Metformin, an antidiabetic drug, is believed to function primarily by reducing hepatic gluconeogenesis, stimulating glucose uptake by muscle, and increasing FA oxidation in both skeletal muscle and liver to increase insulin sensitivity. Several trials that examined the effectiveness of metformin in NAFLD showed reductions in ALT and insulin resistance (Marchesini, Brizi et al. 2001, Schwimmer, Behling et al. 2005, Nobili, Marcellini et al. 2006, Duseja, Das et al. 2007, Loomba, Lutchman et al. 2009, Nadeau, Ehlers et al. 2009); some have also shown histologic improvements and lower AST levels (Nair, Diehl et al. 2004, Bugianesi, Gentilcore et al. 2005). However, a meta-analysis (Rakoski, Singal et al. 2010) of three controlled trials (n = 96) in which aminotransferase levels and/or histology were measured demonstrated that there were no differences between the metformin versus control groups (Uygun, Kadayifci et al. 2004, Haukeland, Konopski et al. 2009). As such, metformin is not currently recommended as a NAFLD-specific treatment but is used for patients with concurrent diabetes and insulin resistance (Chalasani, Younossi et al. 2012, Spengler and Loomba 2015). The thiazolidinedione drug class, to which Pioglitazone belongs, binds peroxisome proliferator-activated receptor gamma (PPARγ), a transcription factor that activates genes involved in regulating FA storage and glucose metabolism. Pioglitazone acts as an insulin sensitizer by promoting adipocyte differentiation and the redistribution of liver and muscle fat to adipose tissue (Miyazaki, Mahankali et al. 2002). The aforementioned PIVENS study (Sanyal, Chalasani et al. 2010) and Belfort et al. (Belfort, Harrison et al. 2006) showed pioglitazone improved AST and ALT serum levels, steatosis, and steatohepatitis (assessed by biopsy and MRS). While long-term use is required, the safety and efficacy of pioglitazone has not been evaluated. Finally, the double-blind, randomized liraglutide safety and efficacy in patients with non-alcoholic steatohepatitis (LEAN) study tested the effect of daily liraglutide injections for 48 weeks in overweight patients with biopsy-proven NASH (Armstrong, Gaunt et al. 2016). The LEAN study found that 39% (n = 9/23) of patients taking liraglutide showed resolution of NASH compared to 9% (n = 2/22) of the control group. Overall, the liraglutide group was more likely to have improvements in steatosis, 83% versus 45% of the control group. Interestingly, the patients that received liraglutide had significant reductions in weight, BMI, and HbA1c levels as compared to the placebo group. Together, these improvements show the effectiveness of liraglutide and the need for longer and larger randomized controlled trials. Other classes of drugs that need further investigation include dipeptidyl peptidase-4 inhibitors, other GLP-1 receptor agonists (Li, Zhao et al. 2015), and renal sodium glucose transporter blockers (Jung, Jang et al. 2014).

Bile Acid Analogs

Obeticholic acid, a synthetic variant of chenodeoxycholic acid, functions to activate the farnesoid X receptor (Cariou, van Harmelen et al. 2006, Porez, Prawitt et al. 2012). Activation of this receptor results in improved insulin sensitivity and decreases in hepatic gluconeogenesis and plasma triglyceride levels (Cariou, van Harmelen et al. 2006, Porez, Prawitt et al. 2012). A randomized controlled study evaluated the efficacy of obeticholic acid in 283 diabetic and nondiabetic volunteers with NASH (farnesoid X nuclear receptor ligand obeticholic acid for non-cirrhotic, non-alcoholic steatohepatitis study). After 72 weeks, twice the number of subjects treated with obeticholic acid had histological improvements compared to the placebo group (n = 50 [45%] versus n = 23 [21%]) (Neuschwander-Tetri, Loomba et al. 2015). Additionally, the NAFLD activity score and ALT were both reduced and significantly different between the two groups, favoring the treated group. The results of this study show obeticholic acid to be a promising treatment for NASH. However, 23% (n = 33 of 141) of the treatment group suffered from pruritus as compared to 6% (n = 9 of 142) in the placebo-controlled group and an increase in LDL and total cholesterol in the treatment group as compared to the control group. The long-term safety profile and efficacy of the drug requires further study.

A second synthetic molecule, aramchol, composed of cholic acid, a bile acid, and arachidic acid, a saturated FA, functions to inhibit stearoyl coenzyme A desaturase 1 (SCD1). SCD1 is an enzyme involved in the biosynthesis of FAs, and preclinical studies have shown that its inhibition decreases the synthesis of FAs and increases β-oxidation in the liver and brown adipose tissue (Dobrzyn, Dobrzyn et al. 2004, Dobrzyn and Ntambi 2005). Recently, a randomized 3-month trial demonstrated the efficacy and short-term safety of aramchol in people with NAFLD (n = 20) (Safadi, Konikoff et al. 2014). Specifically, there was an average 12.6% decrease in liver fat in those randomized to aramchol compared to a 6.4% increase in liver fat in the control group. While these results are promising, the long-term effects of aramchol have not yet been evaluated.

Pentoxifylline

The efficacy of pentoxifylline, a nonspecific TNFα inhibitor, as an NAFLD therapeutic has been studied in several trials yielding mixed results. Adams et al. and Satapathy et al. reported improvements in AST and ALT levels (Adams, Zein et al. 2004, Satapathy, Garg et al. 2004). Additionally, Satapathy et al. showed significant serum TNFα reduction and improved insulin resistance, measured by the homeostatic metabolic assessment insulin resistance index. Conversely, in other placebo-controlled studies pentoxifylline treatment resulted in no change in aminotransferase levels (Van Wagner, Koppe et al. 2011) or improved histology (Zein, Yerian et al. 2011). Interestingly, two independent meta-analyses with overlap in datasets, (1) three randomized studies and two prospective studies, n = 147 and (2) five randomized placebo-controlled trials, n = 147, showed pentoxifylline not only reduced aminotransferase levels but also reduced body weight, BMI, blood glucose, lobular inflammation, TNFα, and fibrosis (Du, Ma et al. 2014, Zeng, Zhang et al. 2014). At this time, further studies are necessary to clarify the potential of pentoxifylline as a therapeutic.

SUMMARY

Currently, NAFLD is a hidden epidemic. Although the disease is asymptomatic, the risk factors, such as MetS, central obesity, hypertension, dyslipidemia, or type 2 diabetes (Rinella 2015), can be readily determined and are used to screen patients that are suspected to have NAFLD. As of now, there is no standard of treatment besides moderate weight loss. While multiple clinical trials have evaluated the effectiveness of pharmaceutical and dietary treatments on the improvement of steatosis, standard recommendations promote weight loss through diet and lifestyle changes. Successful weight loss and improvement in liver histology have been demonstrated in subjects that reduced carbohydrate intake to less than 45% of total caloric intake. Attention toward carbohydrate quality as well as quantity is recommended, with particular attention to reducing simple carbohydrate consumption. Dietary fat intake should consist primarily of mono- and polyunsaturated fats.

REFERENCES

Adams, L. A., C. O. Zein, P. Angulo, and K. D. Lindor (2004). A pilot trial of pentoxifylline in nonalcoholic steatohepatitis. *Am J Gastroenterol* **99**(12): 2365–2368.

Aguilar-Olivos, N. E., P. Almeda-Valdes, C. A. Aguilar-Salinas, M. Uribe, and N. Mendez-Sanchez (2015). The role of bariatric surgery in the management of nonalcoholic fatty liver disease and metabolic syndrome. *Metabolism* **65**(8): 1196–1207.

Aller, R., D. A. De Luis, O. Izaola, R. Conde, M. Gonzalez Sagrado, D. Primo, B. De La Fuente, and J. Gonzalez (2011). Effect of a probiotic on liver aminotransferases in nonalcoholic fatty liver disease patients: A double blind randomized clinical trial. *Eur Rev Med Pharmacol Sci* **15**(9): 1090–1095.

Amarapurkar, D., P. Kamani, N. Patel, P. Gupte, P. Kumar, S. Agal, R. Baijal, S. Lala, D. Chaudhary, and A. Deshpande (2007). Prevalence of non-alcoholic fatty liver disease: Population based study. *Ann Hepatol* **6**(3): 161–163.

Andersen, T., C. Gluud, M. B. Franzmann, and P. Christoffersen (1991). Hepatic effects of dietary weight loss in morbidly obese subjects. *J Hepatol* **12**(2): 224–229.

Armstrong, M. J., P. Gaunt, G. P. Aithal, D. Barton, D. Hull, R. Parker, J. M. Hazlehurst et al. (2016). Liraglutide safety and efficacy in patients with non-alcoholic steatohepatitis (LEAN): A multicentre, double-blind, randomised, placebo-controlled phase 2 study. *Lancet* **387**(10019): 679–690.

Armstrong, M. J., D. D. Houlihan, L. Bentham, J. C. Shaw, R. Cramb, S. Olliff, P. S. Gill, J. M. Neuberger, R. J. Lilford, and P. N. Newsome (2012). Presence and severity of non-alcoholic fatty liver disease in a large prospective primary care cohort. *J Hepatol* **56**(1): 234–240.

Bae, J. C., S. Suh, S. E. Park, E. J. Rhee, C. Y. Park, K. W. Oh, S. W. Park et al. (2012). Regular exercise is associated with a reduction in the risk of NAFLD and decreased liver enzymes in individuals with NAFLD independent of obesity in Korean adults. *PLoS One* **7**(10): e46819.

Bedogni, G., L. Miglioli, F. Masutti, C. Tiribelli, G. Marchesini, and S. Bellentani (2005). Prevalence of and risk factors for nonalcoholic fatty liver disease: The Dionysos nutrition and liver study. *Hepatology* **42**(1): 44–52.

Belfort, R., S. A. Harrison, K. Brown, C. Darland, J. Finch, J. Hardies, B. Balas et al. (2006). A placebo-controlled trial of pioglitazone in subjects with nonalcoholic steatohepatitis. *N Engl J Med* **355**(22): 2297–2307.

Bezerra Duarte, S. M., J. Faintuch, J. T. Stefano, M. B. Sobral de Oliveira, D. F. de Campos Mazo, F. Rabelo, D. Vanni, M. A. Nogueira, F. J. Carrilho, and C. P. Marques Souza de Oliveira (2014). Hypocaloric high-protein diet improves clinical and biochemical markers in patients with nonalcoholic fatty liver disease (NAFLD). *Nutr Hosp* **29**(1): 94–101.

Bjermo, H., D. Iggman, J. Kullberg, I. Dahlman, L. Johansson, L. Persson, J. Berglund et al. (2012). Effects of n-6 PUFAs compared with SFAs on liver fat, lipoproteins, and inflammation in abdominal obesity: A randomized controlled trial. *Am J Clin Nutr* **95**(5): 1003–1012.

Bondini, S. and Z. M. Younossi (2006). Non-alcoholic fatty liver disease and hepatitis C infection. *Minerva Gastroenterol Dietol* **52**(2): 135–143.

Bower, G., T. Toma, L. Harling, L. R. Jiao, E. Efthimiou, A. Darzi, T. Athanasiou, and H. Ashrafian (2015). Bariatric surgery and non-alcoholic fatty liver disease: A systematic review of liver biochemistry and histology. *Obes Surg* **25**(12): 2280–2289.

Bozzetto, L., A. Prinster, G. Annuzzi, L. Costagliola, A. Mangione, A. Vitelli, R. Mazzarella et al. (2012). Liver fat is reduced by an isoenergetic MUFA diet in a controlled randomized study in type 2 diabetic patients. *Diabetes Care* **35**(7): 1429–1435.

Browning, J. D., J. A. Baker, T. Rogers, J. Davis, S. Satapati, and S. C. Burgess (2011). Short-term weight loss and hepatic triglyceride reduction: Evidence of a metabolic advantage with dietary carbohydrate restriction. *Am J Clin Nutr* **93**(5): 1048–1052.

Browning, J. D., L. S. Szczepaniak, R. Dobbins, P. Nuremberg, J. D. Horton, J. C. Cohen, S. M. Grundy, and H. H. Hobbs (2004). Prevalence of hepatic steatosis in an urban population in the United States: Impact of ethnicity. *Hepatology* **40**(6): 1387–1395.

Brunt, E. M. (2015). Nonalcoholic fatty liver disease. *Nat Rev Dis Primers* **1**: 15080.

Bugianesi, E., E. Gentilcore, R. Manini, S. Natale, E. Vanni, N. Villanova, E. David, M. Rizzetto, and G. Marchesini (2005). A randomized controlled trial of metformin versus vitamin E or prescriptive diet in nonalcoholic fatty liver disease. *Am J Gastroenterol* **100**(5): 1082–1090.

Caballeria, L., G. Pera, M. A. Auladell, P. Toran, L. Munoz, D. Miranda, A. Aluma et al. (2010). Prevalence and factors associated with the presence of nonalcoholic fatty liver disease in an adult population in Spain. *Eur J Gastroenterol Hepatol* **22**(1): 24–32.

Cani, P. D., J. Amar, M. A. Iglesias, M. Poggi, C. Knauf, D. Bastelica, A. M. Neyrinck et al. (2007). Metabolic endotoxemia initiates obesity and insulin resistance. *Diabetes* **56**(7): 1761–1772.

Cani, P. D. and N. M. Delzenne (2009). Interplay between obesity and associated metabolic disorders: New insights into the gut microbiota. *Curr Opin Pharmacol* **9**(6): 737–743.

Caricilli, A. M. and M. J. Saad (2013). The role of gut microbiota on insulin resistance. *Nutrients* **5**(3): 829–851.

Cariou, B., K. van Harmelen, D. Duran-Sandoval, T. H. van Dijk, A. Grefhorst, M. Abdelkarim, S. Caron et al. (2006). The farnesoid X receptor modulates adiposity and peripheral insulin sensitivity in mice. *J Biol Chem* **281**(16): 11039–11049.

Cassol, E., V. Misra, A. Holman, A. Kamat, S. Morgello, and D. Gabuzda (2013). Plasma metabolomics identifies lipid abnormalities linked to markers of inflammation, microbial translocation, and hepatic function in HIV patients receiving protease inhibitors. *BMC Infect Dis* **13**: 203.

Catalan, V., J. Gomez-Ambrosi, A. Rodriguez, B. Ramirez, P. Andrada, F. Rotellar, V. Valenti et al. (2015). Expression of S6K1 in human visceral adipose tissue is upregulated in obesity and related to insulin resistance and inflammation. *Acta Diabetol* **52**(2): 257–266.

Centis, E., R. Marzocchi, S. Di Domizio, M. F. Ciaravella, and G. Marchesini (2010). The effect of lifestyle changes in non-alcoholic fatty liver disease. *Dig Dis* **28**(1): 267–273.

Chalasani, N., Z. Younossi, J. E. Lavine, A. M. Diehl, E. M. Brunt, K. Cusi, M. Charlton et al. (2012). The diagnosis and management of non-alcoholic fatty liver disease: Practice guideline by the American Gastroenterological Association, American Association for the Study of Liver Diseases, and American College of Gastroenterology. *Gastroenterology* **142**(7): 1592–1609.

Charatcharoenwitthaya, P. and K. D. Lindor (2007). Role of radiologic modalities in the management of non-alcoholic steatohepatitis. *Clin Liver Dis* **11**(1): 37–54, viii.

Chen, S., X. Zhao, L. Ran, J. Wan, X. Wang, Y. Qin, F. Shu et al. (2015). Resveratrol improves insulin resistance, glucose and lipid metabolism in patients with non-alcoholic fatty liver disease: A randomized controlled trial. *Dig Liver Dis* **47**(3): 226–232.

Chou, T. C., W. M. Liang, C. B. Wang, T. N. Wu, and L. W. Hang (2015). Obstructive sleep apnea is associated with liver disease: A population-based cohort study. *Sleep Med* **16**(8): 955–960.

Das, K., K. Das, P. S. Mukherjee, A. Ghosh, S. Ghosh, A. R. Mridha, T. Dhibar et al. (2010). Nonobese population in a developing country has a high prevalence of nonalcoholic fatty liver and significant liver disease. *Hepatology* **51**(5): 1593–1602.

Dasarathy, S., J. Dasarathy, A. Khiyami, R. Joseph, R. Lopez, and A. J. McCullough (2009). Validity of real time ultrasound in the diagnosis of hepatic steatosis: A prospective study. *J Hepatol* **51**(6): 1061–1067.

Dobrzyn, A. and J. M. Ntambi (2005). Stearoyl-CoA desaturase as a new drug target for obesity treatment. *Obes Rev* **6**(2): 169–174.

Dobrzyn, P., A. Dobrzyn, M. Miyazaki, P. Cohen, E. Asilmaz, D. G. Hardie, J. M. Friedman, and J. M. Ntambi (2004). Stearoyl-CoA desaturase 1 deficiency increases fatty acid oxidation by activating AMP-activated protein kinase in liver. *Proc Natl Acad Sci USA* **101**(17): 6409–6414.

Dongiovanni, P., S. Romeo, and L. Valenti (2015). Genetic factors in the pathogenesis of nonalcoholic fatty liver and steatohepatitis. *Biomed Res Int* **2015**: 460190.

Donnelly, K. L., C. I. Smith, S. J. Schwarzenberg, J. Jessurun, M. D. Boldt, and E. J. Parks (2005). Sources of fatty acids stored in liver and secreted via lipoproteins in patients with nonalcoholic fatty liver disease. *J Clin Invest* **115**(5): 1343–1351.

Du, J., Y. Y. Ma, C. H. Yu, and Y. M. Li (2014). Effects of pentoxifylline on nonalcoholic fatty liver disease: A meta-analysis. *World J Gastroenterol* **20**(2): 569–577.

Duseja, A., A. Das, R. K. Dhiman, Y. K. Chawla, K. T. Thumburu, S. Bhadada, and A. Bhansali (2007). Metformin is effective in achieving biochemical response in patients with nonalcoholic fatty liver disease (NAFLD) not responding to lifestyle interventions. *Ann Hepatol* **6**(4): 222–226.

Eguchi, Y., T. Eguchi, T. Mizuta, Y. Ide, T. Yasutake, R. Iwakiri, A. Hisatomi et al. (2006). Visceral fat accumulation and insulin resistance are important factors in nonalcoholic fatty liver disease. *J Gastroenterol* **41**(5): 462–469.

Fabbrini, E., S. Sullivan, and S. Klein (2010). Obesity and nonalcoholic fatty liver disease: Biochemical, metabolic, and clinical implications. *Hepatology* **51**(2): 679–689.

Faeh, D., K. Minehira, J. M. Schwarz, R. Periasamy, S. Park, and L. Tappy (2005). Effect of fructose overfeeding and fish oil administration on hepatic de novo lipogenesis and insulin sensitivity in healthy men. *Diabetes* **54**(7): 1907–1913.

Faghihzadeh, F., P. Adibi, R. Rafiei, and A. Hekmatdoost (2014). Resveratrol supplementation improves inflammatory biomarkers in patients with nonalcoholic fatty liver disease. *Nutr Res* **34**(10): 837–843.

Greenhill, C. (2015). Obesity: Gut microbiota, host genetics and diet interact to affect the risk of developing obesity and the metabolic syndrome. *Nat Rev Endocrinol* **11**(11): 630.

Guaraldi, G., N. Squillace, C. Stentarelli, G. Orlando, R. D'Amico, G. Ligabue, F. Fiocchi et al. (2008). Nonalcoholic fatty liver disease in HIV-infected patients referred to a metabolic clinic: Prevalence, characteristics, and predictors. *Clin Infect Dis* **47**(2): 250–257.

Gugliucci, A., R. H. Lustig, R. Caccavello, A. Erkin-Cakmak, S. M. Noworolski, V. W. Tai, M. J. Wen, K. Mulligan, and J. M. Schwarz (2016). Short-term isocaloric fructose restriction lowers apoC-III levels and yields less atherogenic lipoprotein profiles in children with obesity and metabolic syndrome. *Atherosclerosis* **253**: 171–177.

Haufe, S., S. Engeli, P. Kast, J. Bohnke, W. Utz, V. Haas, M. Hermsdorf et al. (2011). Randomized comparison of reduced fat and reduced carbohydrate hypocaloric diets on intrahepatic fat in overweight and obese human subjects. *Hepatology* **53**(5): 1504–1514.

Haukeland, J. W., Z. Konopski, H. B. Eggesbo, H. L. von Volkmann, G. Raschpichler, K. Bjoro, T. Haaland, E. M. Loberg, and K. Birkeland (2009). Metformin in patients with non-alcoholic fatty liver disease: A randomized, controlled trial. *Scand J Gastroenterol* **44**(7): 853–860.

Hazlehurst, J. M. and J. W. Tomlinson (2013). Non-alcoholic fatty liver disease in common endocrine disorders. *Eur J Endocrinol* **169**(2): R27–R37.

Higuchi, N., M. Kato, Y. Shundo, H. Tajiri, M. Tanaka, N. Yamashita, M. Kohjima et al. (2008). Liver X receptor in cooperation with SREBP-1c is a major lipid synthesis regulator in nonalcoholic fatty liver disease. *Hepatol Res* **38**(11): 1122–1129.

Holmen, O. L., H. Zhang, Y. Fan, D. H. Hovelson, E. M. Schmidt, W. Zhou, Y. Guo et al. (2014). Systematic evaluation of coding variation identifies a candidate causal variant in TM6SF2 influencing total cholesterol and myocardial infarction risk. *Nat Genet* **46**(4): 345–351.

Hsiao, P. J., K. K. Kuo, S. J. Shin, Y. H. Yang, W. Y. Lin, J. F. Yang, C. C. Chiu, W. L. Chuang, T. R. Tsai, and M. L. Yu (2007). Significant correlations between severe fatty liver and risk factors for metabolic syndrome. *J Gastroenterol Hepatol* **22**(12): 2118–2123.

Hu, T., K. T. Mills, L. Yao, K. Demanelis, M. Eloustaz, W. S. Yancy, Jr., T. N. Kelly, J. He, and L. A. Bazzano (2012). Effects of low-carbohydrate diets versus low-fat diets on metabolic risk factors: A meta-analysis of randomized controlled clinical trials. *Am J Epidemiol* **176** (Suppl 7): S44–S54.

Huang, M. A., J. K. Greenson, C. Chao, L. Anderson, D. Peterman, J. Jacobson, D. Emick, A. S. Lok, and H. S. Conjeevaram (2005). One-year intense nutritional counseling results in histological improvement in patients with non-alcoholic steatohepatitis: A pilot study. *Am J Gastroenterol* **100**(5): 1072–1081.

Ji, H. F., Y. Sun, and L. Shen (2014). Effect of vitamin E supplementation on aminotransferase levels in patients with NAFLD, NASH, and CHC: Results from a meta-analysis. *Nutrition* **30**(9): 986–991.

Jung, C. H., J. E. Jang, and J. Y. Park (2014). A novel therapeutic agent for type 2 diabetes mellitus: SGLT2 inhibitor. *Diabetes Metab J* **38**(4): 261–273.

Kang, H., J. K. Greenson, J. T. Omo, C. Chao, D. Peterman, L. Anderson, L. Foess-Wood, M. A. Sherbondy, and H. S. Conjeevaram (2006). Metabolic syndrome is associated with greater histologic severity, higher carbohydrate, and lower fat diet in patients with NAFLD. *Am J Gastroenterol* **101**(10): 2247–2253.

Kani, A. H., S. M. Alavian, A. Esmaillzadeh, P. Adibi, and L. Azadbakht (2014). Effects of a novel therapeutic diet on liver enzymes and coagulating factors in patients with non-alcoholic fatty liver disease: A parallel randomized trial. *Nutrition* **30**(7–8): 814–821.

Karoli, R., J. Fatima, A. Chandra, U. Gupta, F. U. Islam, and G. Singh (2013). Prevalence of hepatic steatosis in women with polycystic ovary syndrome. *J Hum Reprod Sci* **6**(1): 9–14.

Kirpich, I. A., L. S. Marsano, and C. J. McClain (2015). Gut-liver axis, nutrition, and non-alcoholic fatty liver disease. *Clin Biochem* **48**(13–14): 923–930.

Kitamoto, A., T. Kitamoto, T. Nakamura, Y. Ogawa, M. Yoneda, H. Hyogo, H. Ochi et al. (2014). Association of polymorphisms in GCKR and TRIB1 with nonalcoholic fatty liver disease and metabolic syndrome traits. *Endocr J* **61**(7): 683–689.

Kleiner, D. E., E. M. Brunt, M. Van Natta, C. Behling, M. J. Contos, O. W. Cummings, L. D. Ferrell et al. (2005). Design and validation of a histological scoring system for nonalcoholic fatty liver disease. *Hepatology* **41**(6): 1313–1321.

Kozlitina, J., E. Smagris, S. Stender, B. G. Nordestgaard, H. H. Zhou, A. Tybjaerg-Hansen, T. F. Vogt, H. H. Hobbs, and J. C. Cohen (2014). Exome-wide association study identifies a TM6SF2 variant that confers susceptibility to nonalcoholic fatty liver disease. *Nat Genet* **46**(4): 352–356.

Krebs, J. D., C. R. Elley, A. Parry-Strong, H. Lunt, P. L. Drury, D. A. Bell, E. Robinson, S. A. Moyes, and J. I. Mann (2012). The Diabetes Excess Weight Loss (DEWL) Trial: A randomised controlled trial of high-protein versus high-carbohydrate diets over 2 years in type 2 diabetes. *Diabetologia* **55**(4): 905–914.

Lambert, J. E., J. A. Parnell, B. Eksteen, M. Raman, M. R. Bomhof, K. P. Rioux, K. L. Madsen, and R. A. Reimer (2015). Gut microbiota manipulation with prebiotics in patients with non-alcoholic fatty liver disease: A randomized controlled trial protocol. *BMC Gastroenterol* **15**: 169.

Lambert, J. E., M. A. Ramos-Roman, J. D. Browning, and E. J. Parks (2014). Increased de novo lipogenesis is a distinct characteristic of individuals with nonalcoholic fatty liver disease. *Gastroenterology* **146**(3): 726–735.

Lavine, J. E., J. B. Schwimmer, M. L. Van Natta, J. P. Molleston, K. F. Murray, P. Rosenthal, S. H. Abrams et al. (2011). Effect of vitamin E or metformin for treatment of nonalcoholic fatty liver disease in children and adolescents: The TONIC randomized controlled trial. *JAMA* **305**(16): 1659–1668.

Lee, J. Y., K. M. Kim, S. G. Lee, E. Yu, Y. S. Lim, H. C. Lee, Y. H. Chung, Y. S. Lee, and D. J. Suh (2007). Prevalence and risk factors of non-alcoholic fatty liver disease in potential living liver donors in Korea: A review of 589 consecutive liver biopsies in a single center. *J Hepatol* **47**(2): 239–244.

Lewis, G. F., K. D. Uffelman, L. W. Szeto, B. Weller, and G. Steiner (1995). Interaction between free fatty acids and insulin in the acute control of very low density lipoprotein production in humans. *J Clin Invest* **95**(1): 158–166.

Ley, R. E., P. J. Turnbaugh, S. Klein, and J. I. Gordon (2006). Microbial ecology: Human gut microbes associated with obesity. *Nature* **444**(7122): 1022–1023.

Li, C. L., L. J. Zhao, X. L. Zhou, H. X. Wu, and J. J. Zhao (2015). Review on the effect of glucagon-like peptide-1 receptor agonists and dipeptidyl peptidase-4 inhibitors for the treatment of non-alcoholic fatty liver disease. *J Huazhong Univ Sci Technolog Med Sci* **35**(3): 333–336.

Lima-Cabello, E., M. V. Garcia-Mediavilla, M. E. Miquilena-Colina, J. Vargas-Castrillon, T. Lozano-Rodriguez, M. Fernandez-Bermejo, J. L. Olcoz, J. Gonzalez-Gallego, C. Garcia-Monzon, and S. Sanchez-Campos (2011). Enhanced expression of pro-inflammatory mediators and liver X-receptor-regulated lipogenic genes in non-alcoholic fatty liver disease and hepatitis C. *Clin Sci (Lond)* **120**(6): 239–250.

Liu, Q., S. Bengmark, and S. Qu (2010). The role of hepatic fat accumulation in pathogenesis of non-alcoholic fatty liver disease (NAFLD). *Lipids Health Dis* **9**: 42.

Lo, J. C., K. Mulligan, M. A. Noor, J. M. Schwarz, R. A. Halvorsen, C. Grunfeld, and M. Schambelan (2001). The effects of recombinant human growth hormone on body composition and glucose metabolism in HIV-infected patients with fat accumulation. *J Clin Endocrinol Metab* **86**(8): 3480–3487.

Loomba, R., G. Lutchman, D. E. Kleiner, M. Ricks, J. J. Feld, B. B. Borg, A. Modi et al. (2009). Clinical trial: Pilot study of metformin for the treatment of non-alcoholic steatohepatitis. *Aliment Pharmacol Ther* **29**(2): 172–182.

Ludwig, J., T. R. Viggiano, D. B. McGill, and B. J. Oh (1980). Nonalcoholic steatohepatitis: Mayo Clinic experiences with a hitherto unnamed disease. *Mayo Clin Proc* **55**(7): 434–438.

Ludwig, U., D. Holzner, C. Denzer, A. Greinert, M. M. Haenle, S. Oeztuerk, W. Koenig et al. (2015). Subclinical and clinical hypothyroidism and non-alcoholic fatty liver disease: A cross-sectional study of a random population sample aged 18 to 65 years. *BMC Endocr Disord* **15**(1): 41.

Lustig, R. H., K. Mulligan, S. M. Noworolski, V. W. Tai, M. J. Wen, A. Erkin-Cakmak, A. Gugliucci, and J. M. Schwarz (2016). Isocaloric fructose restriction and metabolic improvement in children with obesity and metabolic syndrome. *Obesity (Silver Spring)* **24**(2): 453–460.

Machado, M. V. and H. Cortez-Pinto (2012). Gut microbiota and nonalcoholic fatty liver disease. *Ann Hepatol* **11**(4): 440–449.

Mahdessian, H., A. Taxiarchis, S. Popov, A. Silveira, A. Franco-Cereceda, A. Hamsten, P. Eriksson, and F. van't Hooft (2014). TM6SF2 is a regulator of liver fat metabolism influencing triglyceride secretion and hepatic lipid droplet content. *Proc Natl Acad Sci USA* **111**(24): 8913–8918.

Makkonen, J., K. H. Pietilainen, A. Rissanen, J. Kaprio, and H. Yki-Jarvinen (2009). Genetic factors contribute to variation in serum alanine aminotransferase activity independent of obesity and alcohol: A study in monozygotic and dizygotic twins. *J Hepatol* **50**(5): 1035–1042.

Marchesini, G., M. Brizi, G. Bianchi, S. Tomassetti, M. Zoli, and N. Melchionda (2001). Metformin in non-alcoholic steatohepatitis. *Lancet* **358**(9285): 893–894.

Masters, B., S. Aarabi, F. Sidhwa, and F. Wood (2012). High-carbohydrate, high-protein, low-fat versus low-carbohydrate, high-protein, high-fat enteral feeds for burns. *Cochrane Database Syst Rev* **1**: CD006122.

Masuoka, H. C. and N. Chalasani (2013). Nonalcoholic fatty liver disease: An emerging threat to obese and diabetic individuals. *Ann N Y Acad Sci* **1281**: 106–122.

Maximos, M., F. Bril, P. Portillo Sanchez, R. Lomonaco, B. Orsak, D. Biernacki, A. Suman, M. Weber, and K. Cusi (2015). The role of liver fat and insulin resistance as determinants of plasma aminotransferase elevation in nonalcoholic fatty liver disease. *Hepatology* **61**(1): 153–160.

Mayes, P. A. and M. E. Laker (1986). Effects of acute and long-term fructose administration on liver lipid metabolism. *Prog Biochem Pharmacol* **21**: 33–58.

Miele, L., V. Valenza, G. La Torre, M. Montalto, G. Cammarota, R. Ricci, R. Masciana et al. (2009). Increased intestinal permeability and tight junction alterations in nonalcoholic fatty liver disease. *Hepatology* **49**(6): 1877–1887.

Mittendorfer, B., F. Magkos, E. Fabbrini, B. S. Mohammed, and S. Klein (2009). Relationship between body fat mass and free fatty acid kinetics in men and women. *Obesity (Silver Spring)* **17**(10): 1872–1877.

Miyazaki, Y., A. Mahankali, M. Matsuda, S. Mahankali, J. Hardies, K. Cusi, L. J. Mandarino, and R. A. DeFronzo (2002). Effect of pioglitazone on abdominal fat distribution and insulin sensitivity in type 2 diabetic patients. *J Clin Endocrinol Metab* **87**(6): 2784–2791.

Mohan, V., S. Farooq, M. Deepa, R. Ravikumar, and C. S. Pitchumoni (2009). Prevalence of non-alcoholic fatty liver disease in urban south Indians in relation to different grades of glucose intolerance and metabolic syndrome. *Diabetes Res Clin Pract* **84**(1): 84–91.

Moscatiello, S., R. Di Luzio, E. Bugianesi, A. Suppini, I. J. Hickman, S. Di Domizio, R. Dalle Grave, and G. Marchesini (2011). Cognitive-behavioral treatment of nonalcoholic Fatty liver disease: A propensity score-adjusted observational study. *Obesity (Silver Spring)* **19**(4): 763–770.

Mouzaki, M., E. M. Comelli, B. M. Arendt, J. Bonengel, S. K. Fung, S. E. Fischer, I. D. McGilvray, and J. P. Allard (2013). Intestinal microbiota in patients with nonalcoholic fatty liver disease. *Hepatology* **58**(1): 120–127.

Nadeau, K. J., L. B. Ehlers, P. S. Zeitler, and K. Love-Osborne (2009). Treatment of non-alcoholic fatty liver disease with metformin versus lifestyle intervention in insulin-resistant adolescents. *Pediatr Diabetes* **10**(1): 5–13.

Nair, S., A. M. Diehl, M. Wiseman, G. H. Farr, Jr., and R. P. Perrillo (2004). Metformin in the treatment of non-alcoholic steatohepatitis: A pilot open label trial. *Aliment Pharmacol Ther* **20**(1): 23–28.

Nalbantoglu, I. L. and E. M. Brunt (2014). Role of liver biopsy in nonalcoholic fatty liver disease. *World J Gastroenterol* **20**(27): 9026–9037.

Neuschwander-Tetri, B. A., R. Loomba, A. J. Sanyal, J. E. Lavine, M. L. Van Natta, M. F. Abdelmalek, N. Chalasani et al. (2015). Farnesoid X nuclear receptor ligand obeticholic acid for non-cirrhotic, non-alcoholic steatohepatitis (FLINT): A multicentre, randomised, placebo-controlled trial. *Lancet* **385**(9972): 956–965.

Nobili, V., N. Alkhouri, A. Alisi, C. Della Corte, E. Fitzpatrick, M. Raponi, and A. Dhawan (2015). Nonalcoholic fatty liver disease: A challenge for pediatricians. *JAMA Pediatr* **169**(2): 170–176.

Nobili, V., G. Bedogni, A. Alisi, A. Pietrobattista, A. Alterio, C. Tiribelli, and C. Agostoni (2009). A protective effect of breastfeeding on the progression of non-alcoholic fatty liver disease. *Arch Dis Child* **94**(10): 801–805.

Nobili, V., M. Marcellini, R. Devito, P. Ciampalini, F. Piemonte, D. Comparcola, M. R. Sartorelli, and P. Angulo (2006). NAFLD in children: A prospective clinical-pathological study and effect of lifestyle advice. *Hepatology* **44**(2): 458–465.

Oh, S., T. Shida, K. Yamagishi, K. Tanaka, R. So, T. Tsujimoto, and J. Shoda (2015). Moderate to vigorous physical activity volume is an important factor for managing nonalcoholic fatty liver disease: A retrospective study. *Hepatology* **61**(4): 1205–1215.

Orci, L. A., K. Gariani, G. Oldani, V. Delaune, P. Morel, and C. Toso (2016). Exercise-based interventions for non-alcoholic fatty liver disease: A meta-analysis and meta-regression. *Clin Gastroenterol Hepatol* **14**(10): 1398–1411.

Patel, A. and S. A. Harrison (2012). Hepatitis C virus infection and nonalcoholic steatohepatitis. *Gastroenterol Hepatol (N Y)* **8**(5): 305–312.

Perez-Guisado, J. and A. Munoz-Serrano (2011a). The effect of the Spanish Ketogenic Mediterranean Diet on nonalcoholic fatty liver disease: A pilot study. *J Med Food* **14**(7–8): 677–680.

Perez-Guisado, J. and A. Munoz-Serrano (2011b). A pilot study of the Spanish Ketogenic Mediterranean Diet: An effective therapy for the metabolic syndrome. *J Med Food* **14**(7–8): 681–687.

Perez-Guisado, J., A. Munoz-Serrano, and A. Alonso-Moraga (2008). Spanish Ketogenic Mediterranean diet: A healthy cardiovascular diet for weight loss. *Nutr J* **7**: 30.

Petersen, K. F., S. Dufour, D. Befroy, M. Lehrke, R. E. Hendler, and G. I. Shulman (2005). Reversal of nonalcoholic hepatic steatosis, hepatic insulin resistance, and hyperglycemia by moderate weight reduction in patients with type 2 diabetes. *Diabetes* **54**(3): 603–608.

Petta, S., L. Miele, E. Bugianesi, C. Camma, C. Rosso, S. Boccia, D. Cabibi et al. (2014). Glucokinase regulatory protein gene polymorphism affects liver fibrosis in non-alcoholic fatty liver disease. *PLoS One* **9**(2): e87523.

Pingitore, P., C. Pirazzi, R. M. Mancina, B. M. Motta, C. Indiveri, A. Pujia, T. Montalcini, K. Hedfalk, and S. Romeo (2014). Recombinant PNPLA3 protein shows triglyceride hydrolase activity and its I148M mutation results in loss of function. *Biochim Biophys Acta* **1841**(4): 574–580.

Porez, G., J. Prawitt, B. Gross, and B. Staels (2012). Bile acid receptors as targets for the treatment of dyslipidemia and cardiovascular disease. *J Lipid Res* **53**(9): 1723–1737.

Promrat, K., D. E. Kleiner, H. M. Niemeier, E. Jackvony, M. Kearns, J. R. Wands, J. L. Fava, and R. R. Wing (2010). Randomized controlled trial testing the effects of weight loss on nonalcoholic steatohepatitis. *Hepatology* **51**(1): 121–129.

Qi, J. C., J. C. Huang, Q. C. Lin, J. M. Zhao, X. Lin, L. D. Chen, J. F. Huang, and X. Chen (2015). Relationship between obstructive sleep apnea and nonalcoholic fatty liver disease in nonobese adults. *Sleep Breath* **20**(2): 529–535.

Rakoski, M. O., A. G. Singal, M. A. Rogers, and H. Conjeevaram (2010). Meta-analysis: Insulin sensitizers for the treatment of non-alcoholic steatohepatitis. *Aliment Pharmacol Ther* **32**(10): 1211–1221.

Reeder, S. B., I. Cruite, G. Hamilton, and C. B. Sirlin (2011). Quantitative assessment of liver fat with magnetic resonance imaging and spectroscopy. *J Magn Reson Imaging* **34**(4): 729–749.

Rinella, M. E. (2015). Nonalcoholic fatty liver disease: A systematic review. *JAMA* **313**(22): 2263–2273.

Rofsky, N. M. and H. Fleishaker (1995). CT and MRI of diffuse liver disease. *Semin Ultrasound CT MR* **16**(1): 16–33.

Romeo, S., J. Kozlitina, C. Xing, A. Pertsemlidis, D. Cox, L. A. Pennacchio, E. Boerwinkle, J. C. Cohen, and H. H. Hobbs (2008). Genetic variation in PNPLA3 confers susceptibility to nonalcoholic fatty liver disease. *Nat Genet* **40**(12): 1461–1465.

Rosqvist, F., D. Iggman, J. Kullberg, J. Cedernaes, H. E. Johansson, A. Larsson, L. Johansson et al. (2014). Overfeeding polyunsaturated and saturated fat causes distinct effects on liver and visceral fat accumulation in humans. *Diabetes* **63**(7): 2356–2368.

Rucker, D., R. Padwal, S. K. Li, C. Curioni, and D. C. Lau (2007). Long term pharmacotherapy for obesity and overweight: Updated meta-analysis. *BMJ* **335**(7631): 1194–1199.

Ryan, M. C., F. Abbasi, C. Lamendola, S. Carter, and T. L. McLaughlin (2007). Serum alanine aminotransferase levels decrease further with carbohydrate than fat restriction in insulin-resistant adults. *Diabetes Care* **30**(5): 1075–1080.

Ryan, M. C., C. Itsiopoulos, T. Thodis, G. Ward, N. Trost, S. Hofferberth, K. O'Dea, P. V. Desmond, N. A. Johnson, and A. M. Wilson (2013). The Mediterranean diet improves hepatic steatosis and insulin sensitivity in individuals with non-alcoholic fatty liver disease. *J Hepatol* **59**(1): 138–143.

Safadi, R., F. M. Konikoff, M. Mahamid, S. Zelber-Sagi, M. Halpern, T. Gilat, R. Oren, and FLORA Group (2014). The fatty acid-bile acid conjugate Aramchol reduces liver fat content in patients with nonalcoholic fatty liver disease. *Clin Gastroenterol Hepatol* **12**(12): 2085–2091 e2081.

Salomone, F., J. Godos, and S. Zelber-Sagi (2015). Natural antioxidants for non-alcoholic fatty liver disease: Molecular targets and clinical perspectives. *Liver Int* **36**(1): 5–20.

Santoro, N., S. Caprio, B. Pierpont, M. Van Name, M. Savoye, and E. J. Parks (2015). Hepatic de novo lipogenesis in obese youth is modulated by a common variant in the GCKR gene. *J Clin Endocrinol Metab* **100**(8): E1125–E1132.

Sanyal, A. J., N. Chalasani, K. V. Kowdley, A. McCullough, A. M. Diehl, N. M. Bass, B. A. Neuschwander-Tetri et al. (2010). Pioglitazone, vitamin E, or placebo for nonalcoholic steatohepatitis. *N Engl J Med* **362**(18): 1675–1685.

Satapathy, S. K., S. Garg, R. Chauhan, P. Sakhuja, V. Malhotra, B. C. Sharma, and S. K. Sarin (2004). Beneficial effects of tumor necrosis factor-alpha inhibition by pentoxifylline on clinical, biochemical, and metabolic parameters of patients with nonalcoholic steatohepatitis. *Am J Gastroenterol* **99**(10): 1946–1952.

Satapathy, S. K. and A. J. Sanyal (2015). Epidemiology and natural history of nonalcoholic fatty liver disease. *Semin Liver Dis* **35**(3): 221–235.

Satapati, S., B. Kucejova, J. A. Duarte, J. A. Fletcher, L. Reynolds, N. E. Sunny, T. He et al. (2016). Mitochondrial metabolism mediates oxidative stress and inflammation in fatty liver. *J Clin Invest* **126**(4): 1605.

Schwarz, J. M., R. Chiolero, J. P. Revelly, C. Cayeux, P. Schneiter, E. Jequier, T. Chen, and L. Tappy (2000). Effects of enteral carbohydrates on de novo lipogenesis in critically ill patients. *Am J Clin Nutr* **72**(4): 940–945.

Schwarz, J. M., P. Linfoot, D. Dare, and K. Aghajanian (2003). Hepatic de novo lipogenesis in normoinsulinemic and hyperinsulinemic subjects consuming high-fat, low-carbohydrate and low-fat, high-carbohydrate isoenergetic diets. *Am J Clin Nutr* **77**(1): 43–50.

Schwarz, J. M., K. Mulligan, J. Lee, J. C. Lo, M. Wen, M. A. Noor, C. Grunfeld, and M. Schambelan (2002). Effects of recombinant human growth hormone on hepatic lipid and carbohydrate metabolism in HIV-infected patients with fat accumulation. *J Clin Endocrinol Metab* **87**(2): 942.

Schwarz, J. M., S. M. Noworolski, M. J. Wen, A. Dyachenko, J. L. Prior, M. E. Weinberg, L. A. Herraiz et al. (2015). Effect of a High-Fructose Weight-Maintaining Diet on Lipogenesis and Liver Fat. *J Clin Endocrinol Metab* **100**(6): 2434–2442.

Schwarz, J. M., S. M. Noworolski, A. Erkin-Cakmak, N. J., Korn, M. J. Wen, V. W. Tai, G. M. Jones et al. (2017). Effects of dietary fructose restriction on liver sat, de novo lipogenesis, and insulin kinetics in children with obesity. *Gastroenterology* **153**(3): 743–752.

Schwimmer, J. B., C. Behling, R. Newbury, R. Deutsch, C. Nievergelt, N. J. Schork, and J. E. Lavine (2005). Histopathology of pediatric nonalcoholic fatty liver disease. *Hepatology* **42**(3): 641–649.

Sedlacek, S. M., M. C. Playdon, P. Wolfe, J. N. McGinley, M. R. Wisthoff, E. A. Daeninck, W. Jiang, Z. Zhu, and H. J. Thompson (2011). Effect of a low fat versus a low carbohydrate weight loss dietary intervention on biomarkers of long term survival in breast cancer patients ('CHOICE'): Study protocol. *BMC Cancer* **11**: 287.

Sert, A., O. Pirgon, E. Aypar, H. Yilmaz, and D. Odabas (2013). Subclinical hypothyroidism as a risk factor for the development of cardiovascular disease in obese adolescents with nonalcoholic fatty liver disease. *Pediatr Cardiol* **34**(5): 1166–1174.

Siddiqui, M. S., M. Fuchs, M. O. Idowu, V. A. Luketic, S. Boyett, C. Sargeant, R. T. Stravitz et al. (2015). Severity of nonalcoholic fatty liver disease and progression to cirrhosis are associated with atherogenic lipoprotein profile. *Clin Gastroenterol Hepatol* **13**(5): 1000–1008 e1003.

Singh, S. P., S. Nayak, M. Swain, N. Rout, R. N. Mallik, O. Agrawal, C. Meher, and M. Rao (2004). Prevalence of nonalcoholic fatty liver disease in coastal eastern India: A preliminary ultrasonographic survey. *Trop Gastroenterol* **25**(2): 76–79.

Solhi, H., R. Ghahremani, A. M. Kazemifar, and Z. Hoseini Yazdi (2014). Silymarin in treatment of non-alcoholic steatohepatitis: A randomized clinical trial. *Caspian J Intern Med* **5**(1): 9–12.

Speliotes, E. K., L. M. Yerges-Armstrong, J. Wu, R. Hernaez, L. J. Kim, C. D. Palmer, V. Gudnason et al. (2011). Genome-wide association analysis identifies variants associated with nonalcoholic fatty liver disease that have distinct effects on metabolic traits. *PLoS Genet* **7**(3): e1001324.

Spengler, E. K. and R. Loomba (2015). Recommendations for diagnosis, referral for liver biopsy, and treatment of nonalcoholic fatty liver disease and nonalcoholic steatohepatitis. *Mayo Clin Proc* **90**(9): 1233–1246.

Tappy, L., M. Berger, J. M. Schwarz, M. McCamish, J. P. Revelly, P. Schneiter, E. Jequier, and R. Chiolero (1999). Hepatic and peripheral glucose metabolism in intensive care patients receiving continuous high- or low-carbohydrate enteral nutrition. *JPEN J Parenter Enteral Nutr* **23**(5): 260–267; discussion 267–268.

Tappy, L., J. M. Schwarz, P. Schneiter, C. Cayeux, J. P. Revelly, C. K. Fagerquist, E. Jequier, and R. Chiolero (1998). Effects of isoenergetic glucose-based or lipid-based parenteral nutrition on glucose metabolism, de novo lipogenesis, and respiratory gas exchanges in critically ill patients. *Crit Care Med* **26**(5): 860–867.

Targher, G., L. Bertolini, R. Padovani, S. Rodella, R. Tessari, L. Zenari, C. Day, and G. Arcaro (2007). Prevalence of nonalcoholic fatty liver disease and its association with cardiovascular disease among type 2 diabetic patients. *Diabetes Care* **30**(5): 1212–1218.

Taskinen, M. R. and J. Boren (2015). New insights into the pathophysiology of dyslipidemia in type 2 diabetes. *Atherosclerosis* **239**(2): 483–495.

Tay, J., N. D. Luscombe-Marsh, C. H. Thompson, M. Noakes, J. D. Buckley, G. A. Wittert, W. S. Yancy, Jr., and G. D. Brinkworth (2015). Response to comment on Tay et al. A very low-carbohydrate, low-saturated fat diet for type 2 diabetes management: A randomized trial. *Diabetes Care* 2014;37:2909–2918. *Diabetes Care* **38**(4): e65–e66.

Tessari, P., A. Coracina, A. Cosma, and A. Tiengo (2009). Hepatic lipid metabolism and non-alcoholic fatty liver disease. *Nutr Metab Cardiovasc Dis* **19**(4): 291–302.

Thorburn, A. W., L. H. Storlien, A. B. Jenkins, S. Khouri, and E. W. Kraegen (1989). Fructose-induced in vivo insulin resistance and elevated plasma triglyceride levels in rats. *Am J Clin Nutr* **49**(6): 1155–1163.

U.S. Department of Health and Human Services and U.S. Department of Agriculture December (2015). Dietary guidelines for Americans. 2015-2020. Retrieved December 2015, from http://health.gov/dietaryguidelines/2015/guidelines/.

Uygun, A., A. Kadayifci, A. T. Isik, T. Ozgurtas, S. Deveci, A. Tuzun, Z. Yesilova, M. Gulsen, and K. Dagalp (2004). Metformin in the treatment of patients with non-alcoholic steatohepatitis. *Aliment Pharmacol Ther* **19**(5): 537–544.

Van Wagner, L. B., S. W. Koppe, E. M. Brunt, J. Gottstein, K. Gardikiotes, R. M. Green, and M. E. Rinella (2011). Pentoxifylline for the treatment of non-alcoholic steatohepatitis: A randomized controlled trial. *Ann Hepatol* **10**(3): 277–286.

Vassilatou, E., D. A. Vassiliadi, K. Salambasis, H. Lazaridou, N. Koutsomitopoulos, N. Kelekis, D. Kassanos, D. J. Hadjidakis, and G. Dimitriadis (2015). Increased prevalence of polycystic ovary syndrome in premenopausal women with nonalcoholic fatty liver disease. *Eur J Endocrinol* **173**(6): 739–747.

Volynets, V., J. Machann, M. A. Kuper, I. B. Maier, A. Spruss, A. Konigsrainer, S. C. Bischoff, and I. Bergheim (2013). A moderate weight reduction through dietary intervention decreases hepatic fat content in patients with non-alcoholic fatty liver disease (NAFLD): A pilot study. *Eur J Nutr* **52**(2): 527–535.

Wong, V. W., W. C. Chu, G. L. Wong, R. S. Chan, A. M. Chim, A. Ong, D. K. Yeung et al. (2012). Prevalence of non-alcoholic fatty liver disease and advanced fibrosis in Hong Kong Chinese: A population study using proton-magnetic resonance spectroscopy and transient elastography. *Gut* **61**(3): 409–415.

Wu, J. H., R. N. Lemaitre, A. Manichaikul, W. Guan, T. Tanaka, M. Foy, E. K. Kabagambe et al. (2013). Genome-wide association study identifies novel loci associated with concentrations of four plasma phospholipid fatty acids in the de novo lipogenesis pathway: Results from the Cohorts for Heart and Aging Research in Genomic Epidemiology (CHARGE) consortium. *Circ Cardiovasc Genet* **6**(2): 171–183.

Yamamoto, K., Y. Takada, Y. Fujimoto, H. Haga, F. Oike, N. Kobayashi, and K. Tanaka (2007). Nonalcoholic steatohepatitis in donors for living donor liver transplantation. *Transplantation* **83**(3): 257–262.

Zein, C. O., L. M. Yerian, P. Gogate, R. Lopez, J. P. Kirwan, A. E. Feldstein, and A. J. McCullough (2011). Pentoxifylline improves nonalcoholic steatohepatitis: A randomized placebo-controlled trial. *Hepatology* **54**(5): 1610–1619.

Zeng, T., C. L. Zhang, X. L. Zhao, and K. Q. Xie (2014). Pentoxifylline for the treatment of nonalcoholic fatty liver disease: A meta-analysis of randomized double-blind, placebo-controlled studies. *Eur J Gastroenterol Hepatol* **26**(6): 646–653.

Zhu, J. Z., Y. N. Dai, Y. M. Wang, Q. Y. Zhou, C. H. Yu, and Y. M. Li (2015). Prevalence of Nonalcoholic Fatty Liver Disease and Economy. *Dig Dis Sci* **60**(11): 3194–3202.

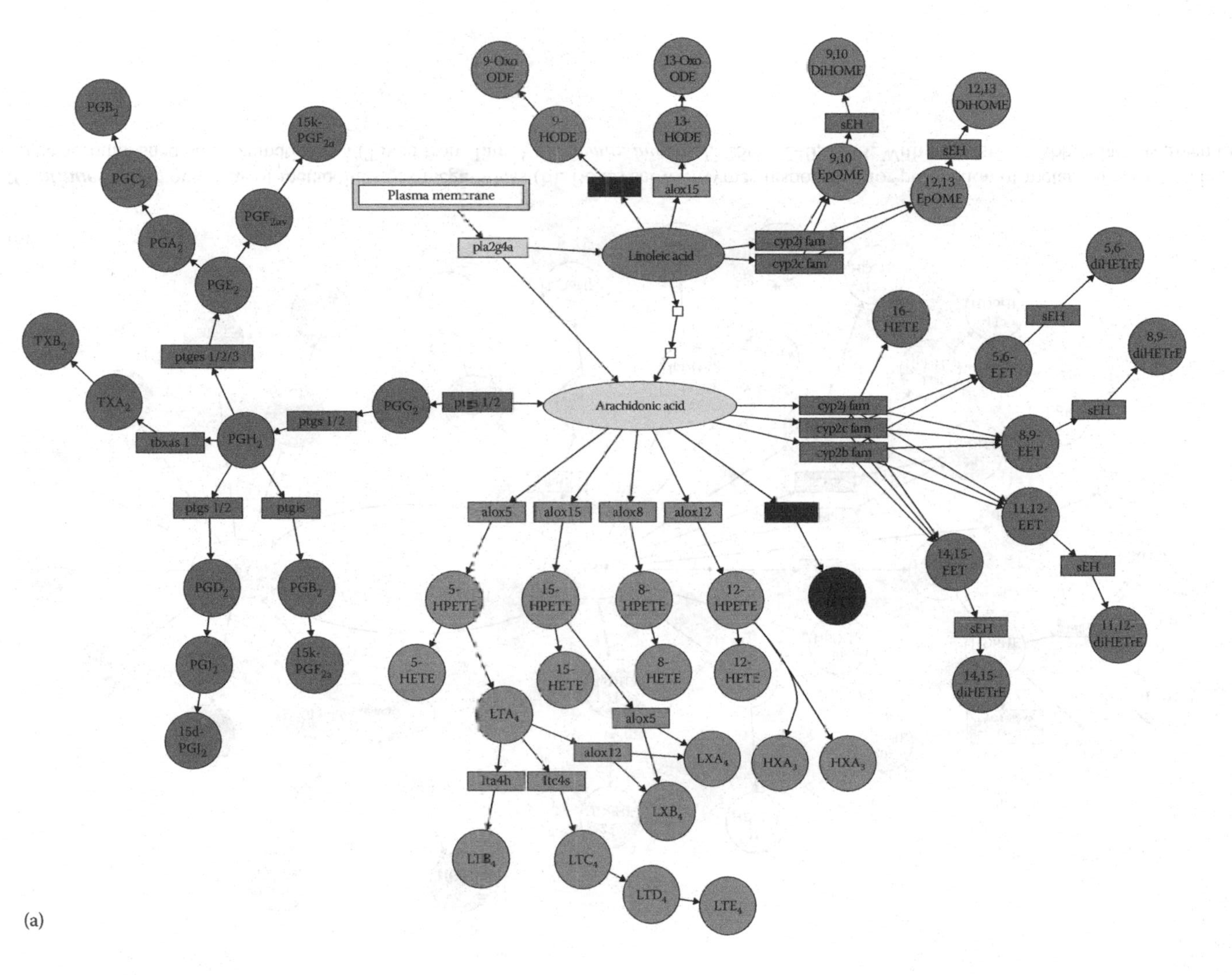

FIGURE 10.2 An overview of metabolites of omega-6 FAs (a). (*Continued*)

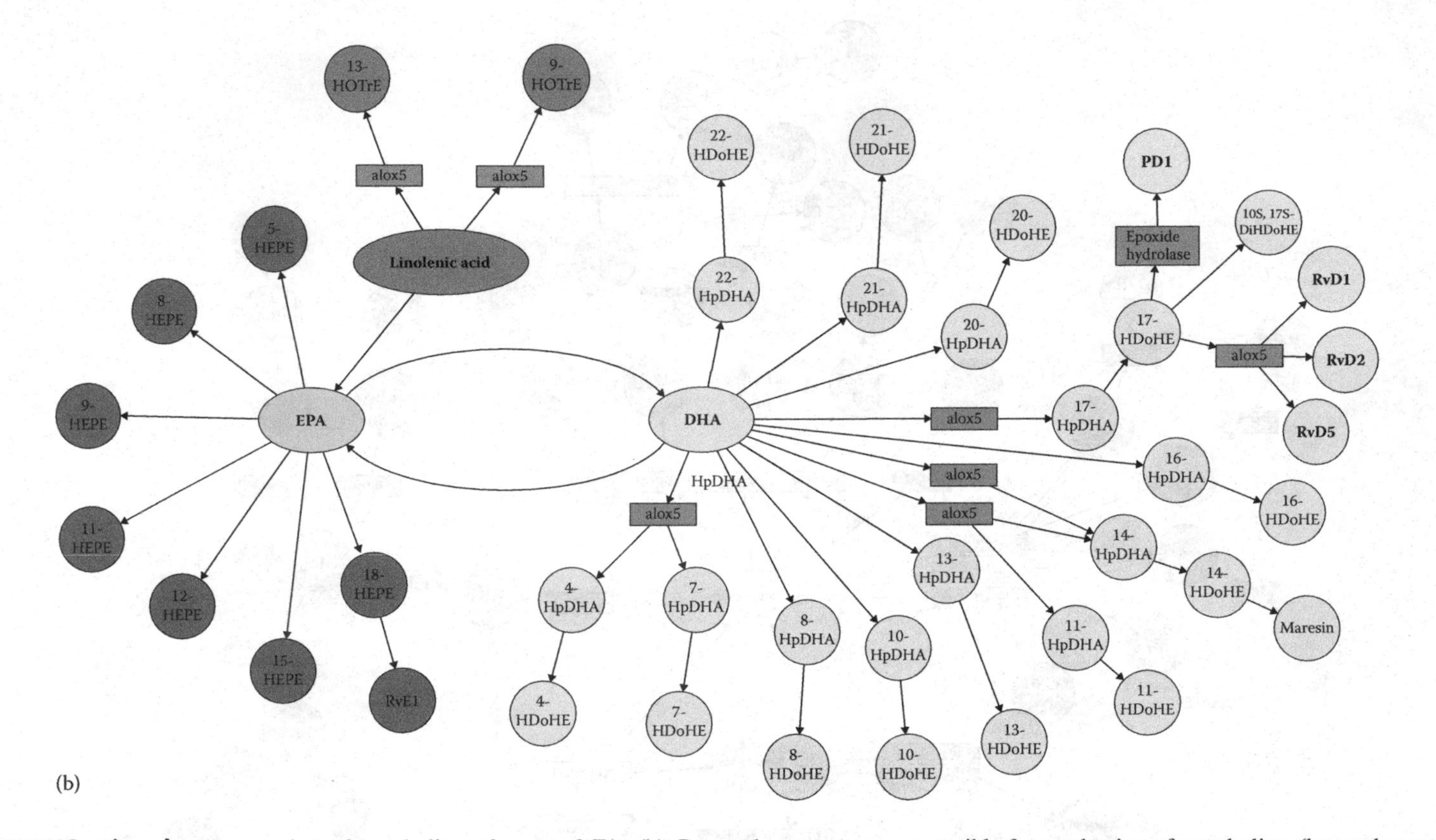

FIGURE 10.2 (*Continued*) An overview of metabolites of omega-3 FAs (b). Boxes show enzymes responsible for production of metabolites (brown boxes designate processes that can be accomplished nonenzymatically). (Taken from Tam, V.C., *Semin. Immunol.*, 25(3), 240, 2013. With permission; Abbreviations given in the original paper.)

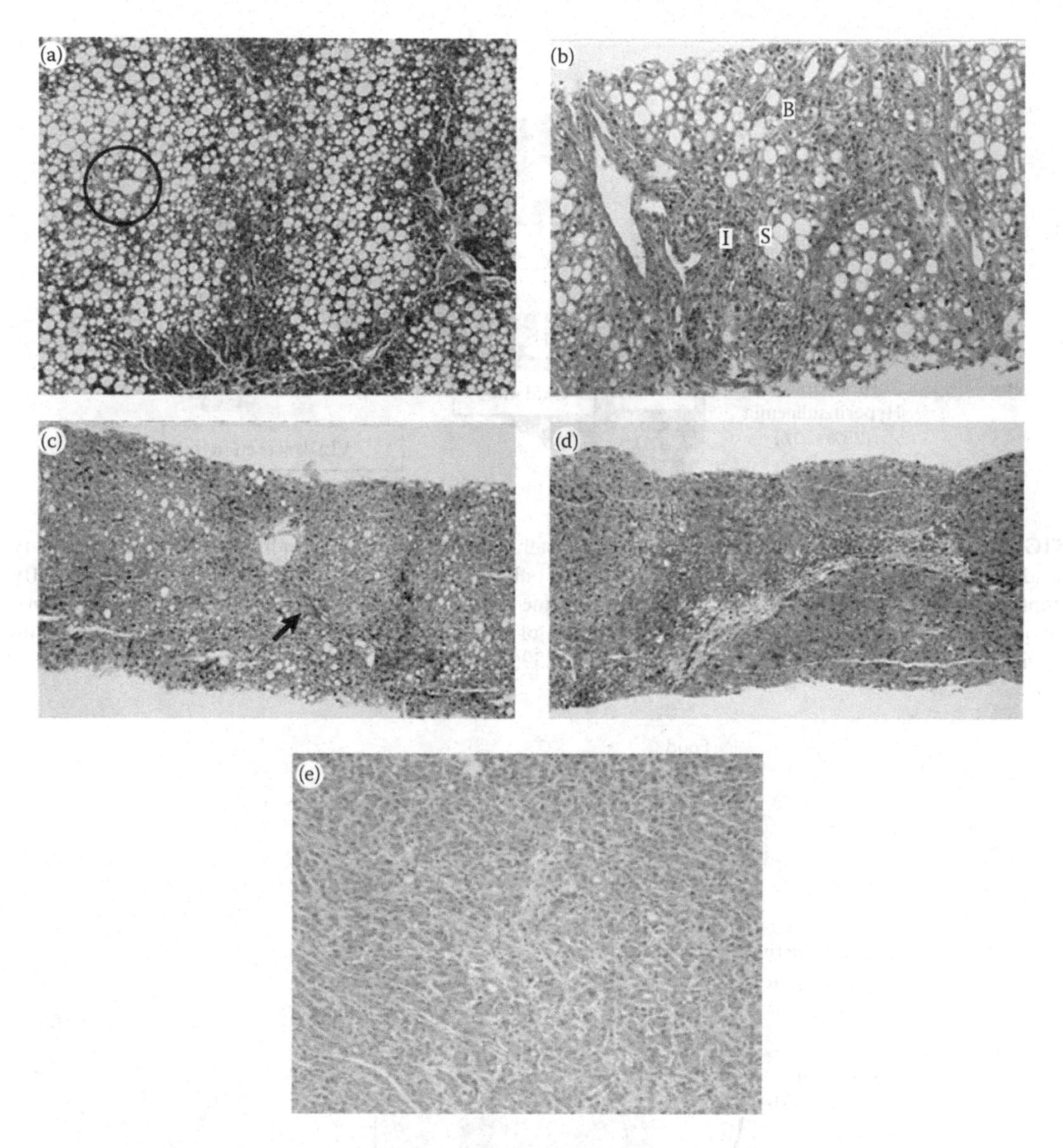

FIGURE 15.1 Histological features of NAFLD. (a) Marked steatosis without inflammation, hepatocytes injury (ballooning), or fibrosis. Steatosis is concentrated in acinar zone 3, the microcirculatory unit through which blood exists the liver around the terminal hepatic venule (in circle) and shows sparing of the periportal, zone 1 hepatocytes, the microcirculatory unit through which portal and systemic blood enter and mix. This is the adult pattern of nonalcoholic fatty liver disease (NAFLD) (trichrome staining). (b) Steatohepatitis with marked steatosis (S), ballooning (B), lobular and portal inflammation (I) and extensive bridging fibrosis (hematoxylin and eosin staining). (c) Fibrosis in the perisinusoidal spaces of zone 3 is detected by trichrome stain; bridging fibrosis (arrow) is noted between two central veins. Hepatocytes with steatosis are seen, but no ballooned hepatocytes are present. (d) Nonalcoholic steatohepatisis (NASH) with cirrhosis, but no active lesions remain. One would only know this was a case of NASH-related cirrhosis by having had a prior biopsy with the diagnosis of active NASH. (e) Hepatocellular carcinoma after the development of NASH and cirrhosis. (Reprinted by permission from Macmillian Publishers Ltd.: *Nat. Rev. Dis. Primers*, (Brunt 2015) Copyright, 2015.)

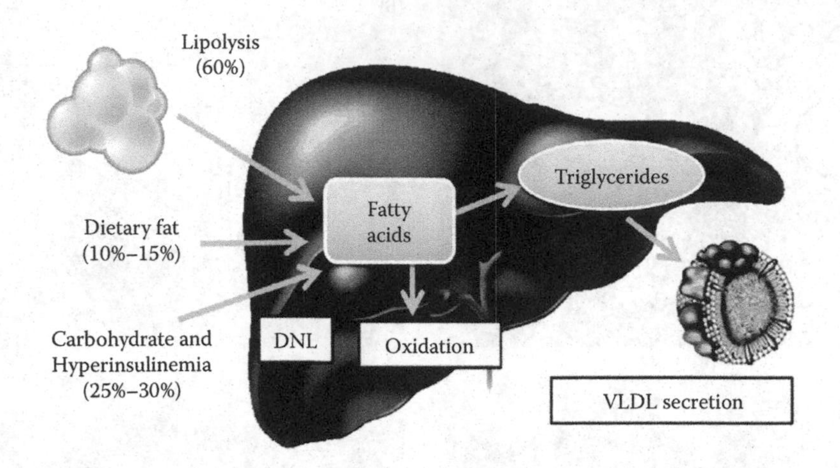

FIGURE 15.2 Contributions of various metabolic pathways to liver steatosis in humans. Reductions in fatty acid oxidation and triglyceride export seem to have only minor roles in hepatic triglyceride deposition. By contrast, the increased availability of fatty acids from the adipose tissue through unabated lipolysis and *de novo* lipogenesis (DNL) from glucose are major providers of lipids in steatotic livers. (Reprinted with permission from Taskinen, M.R. and Boren, J., *Atherosclerosis*, 239(2), 483, 2015.)

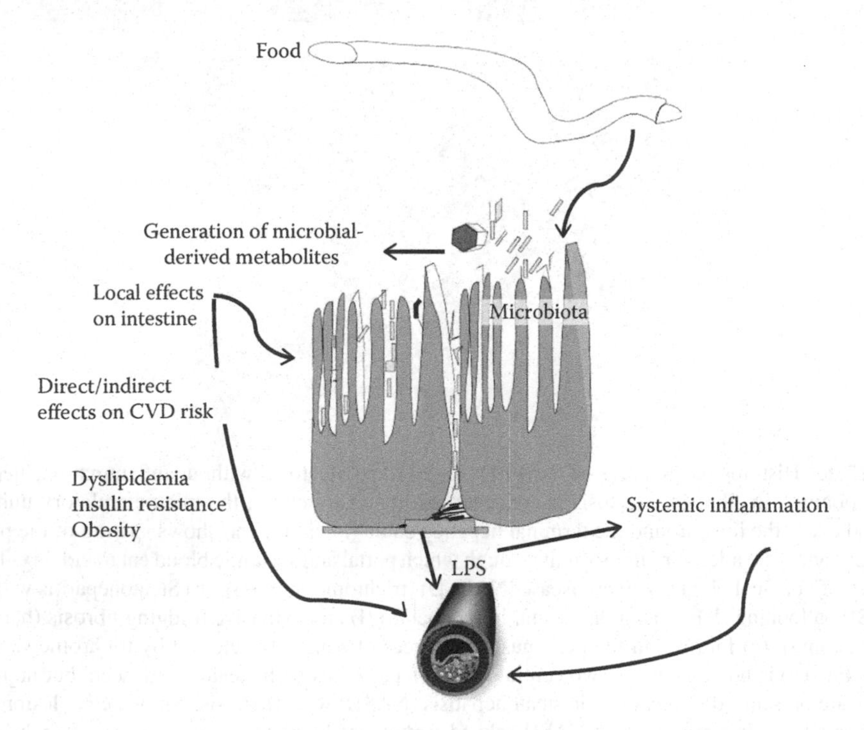

FIGURE 30.1 Potential mechanisms by which the gut microbiota affects cardiovascular risk. Changes in microbial community structure can change gut permeability and allow microbes to enter the bloodstream (Leaky gut syndrome). *Lps* or other bacterial products can induce low-grade systemic inflammation. Alternatively, the microbiota can metabolize nutrients in food to specific metabolites that either increase or decrease susceptibility to cardiometabolic disease.

16 Dietary Starches and Grains
Effects on Cardiometabolic Risk

Nathalie Bergeron and Ronald M. Krauss

CONTENTS

ABSTRACT

The 2015 Dietary Guidelines Advisory Committee is the first to recommend an upper limit for added sugars, based on adverse effects of excess intake on adiposity and cardiometabolic risk. Although there has been continued guidance to replace added sugars with healthy carbohydrates, no specific recommendations regarding intake of dietary starch and total carbohydrates have been made. In this chapter, we review evidence from randomized controlled trials and prospective cohort studies of the effects of dietary carbohydrates on cardiometabolic health, taking into consideration the quantity of dietary carbohydrates consumed and their quality described in terms of their glycemic index/glycemic load and their degree of processing (e.g., whole vs. refined grains). Replacement of refined grains with whole grain products has been shown to improve features of atherogenic dyslipidemia and glycemic control. Overall, the evidence to date suggests that limiting total carbohydrate intake and emphasizing minimally or unprocessed whole grains (~3 servings/day) is associated with reduced risk for CVD and type 2 diabetes.

INTRODUCTION

Dietary carbohydrates are the main energy (E) source in the diet, representing an average of 48% and 51% of daily calories in U.S. males and females, respectively (DGAC 2015), and ~63% of daily E intake worldwide (ChartsBin.com 2016). In the United States, it is estimated that ~15%

of daily calories are derived from added sugars (Yang et al. 2014), with the remainder of carbohydrates (33%E–36%E) consumed as naturally occurring sugars and starches. As we continue to contend with obesity, insulin resistance, and their associated risk for type 2 diabetes (T2DM) and cardiovascular disease (CVD), concerns over the amount and quality of carbohydrates that are consumed have come to the forefront of nutrition policy documents, in recognition of the view that higher-carbohydrate diets may contribute to deterioration of metabolic variables associated with cardiometabolic risk.

Carbohydrates are commonly categorized as sugars, oligosaccharides (indigestible carbohydrates comprising 2–10 monosaccharide units), and polysaccharides (i.e., starches) on the basis of their chemical structure. More relevant to cardiometabolic health are properties that take into account how carbohydrates are digested and absorbed in the small intestine and how they affect glycemia, insulinemia, and ensuing metabolic responses. When categorized in this way, carbohydrates that are not digested and absorbed in the human small intestine, namely, dietary fiber and oligosaccharides, are separated from "glycemic/available" carbohydrates. As such, carbohydrate-rich foods are often classified on the basis of their blood glucose-raising effects in comparison to glucose or white bread (glycemic index, GI) and their glycemic load (GL), which considers both the GI of a food and its total carbohydrate content, thus reflecting both carbohydrate quality and quantity (Jenkins et al. 1981, Salmerón et al. 1997b). Carbohydrate-rich foods can also be classified based on their degree of processing (whole vs. refined grains). While a standard definition is still lacking, whole grain foods are generally referred to as those made from the entire grain and consisting of the endosperm, germ, and bran, the outer layer of the whole grain that protects the starchy endosperm from digestive enzymes (this definition, however, remains imperfect as it fails to take into consideration the extent of processing of the product, i.e., milled vs. whole kernel grains). Conversely, in refined grain products, only the endosperm remains after removal of the bran and germ.

In this chapter, we review evidence from randomized controlled trials and prospective cohort studies, focused mainly on the effects of complex carbohydrates (i.e., starches) on risk factors and clinical outcomes for CVD and diabetes. We take into consideration the *quantity* of dietary carbohydrates consumed and, importantly, their *quality* described in terms of their GI/GL and their degree of processing (e.g., whole vs. refined grains). These properties affect the rate of digestion of carbohydrate-containing foods and are more strongly related to measures of cardiometabolic health than is categorization based on the chemical structure of carbohydrates (Mozaffarian 2016). Readers are referred to Chapters 13 through 15 for comprehensive reviews of the effects of added sugars and the value of their restriction on cardiometabolic health.

CARBOHYDRATE QUANTITY

Lipid and Lipoprotein Risk Factors

In 1977, the Senate Select Committee on Nutrition and Human Needs issued dietary goals for the American people that recommended reduction in total fat intake to no more than 30%E, reduction of saturated fat to 10%E, and an increase in dietary carbohydrate consumption to 58%E (48%E as complex carbohydrate and naturally occurring sugars; 10%E as refined/processed sugars) to reduce CVD risk, and for prevention of overweight, obesity, and diabetes. Less often appreciated is the recognition that Americans have generally followed the nutrition advice promulgated by the USDA and the American Heart Association, with a recent report showing a reduction in intake of total fat from 45%E to 34%E, saturated fat from 13.5%E to 10.7%E, and a reciprocal increase in total carbohydrate intake from 39%E to 51%E from 1971 to 2011 (Cohen et al. 2015). While restriction of saturated fat is a well-established and effective strategy for LDL-cholesterol (C) lowering, it is increasingly recognized that the concurrent increase in carbohydrates that has accompanied the adoption of low-fat diets (Cohen et al. 2015) promotes features of atherogenic dyslipidemia including elevated plasma triglycerides (TG), reduced HDL-C, and increased concentrations of small dense LDL particles (Dreon et al.

1994, 1997, 1999), an effect that is independent of starch quality (Bergeron et al. 2016, Sacks et al. 2014). Notably, whereas hepatic lipogenesis has been implicated in the triglyceride-raising effects of added sugars/fructose (see Chapters 14 and 15), we and others have shown that high carbohydrate intake increases levels of apoCIII in apoB-containing lipoproteins (Furtado et al. 2008, Shin and Krauss 2010). This may contribute to the atherogenic effects of these particles both by retarding their plasma clearance and directly promoting inflammation (Sacks 2015).

The earlier findings are generally consistent with numerous clinical trials comparing effects on lipids and lipoproteins of diets varying in carbohydrate amount, namely, low-carbohydrate vs. low-fat diets, without consideration for carbohydrate quality. In a meta-analysis of 23 longer-term (6–24 months) randomized controlled trials (N = 2788) in which lower-carbohydrate (≤45%E; weighted mean 23%E) and low-fat higher-carbohydrate diets (fat ≤30%E; weighted mean 26%E; carbohydrates ≥46%E) were compared, the lower-carbohydrate diets resulted in a greater decrease in plasma TG (pooled mean net change, −14 mg/dL; 95% CI −19.4, −8.7) and greater increase in HDL-C (3.3 mg/dL; 95% CI 1.9, 4.7) from baseline, but a lesser reduction in LDL-C levels (3.7 mg/dL; 95% CI 1.0, 6.4) compared to higher-carbohydrate low-fat diets (Hu et al. 2012). While these effects occurred in the context of comparable reductions in body weight across diets, one must consider the likelihood that changes in plasma lipids may, at least in part, have been mediated by weight loss. In an earlier meta-analysis of 30 short-term feeding studies (2–12 weeks) conducted under weight maintenance conditions (N = 1213), low-fat high-carbohydrate diets (fat, 18%E–30%E; carbohydrates, 53%E–65%E) were compared with moderate-fat diets (fat, 34%E–50%E; carbohydrates, 35%E–50%E) in which carbohydrates were partially replaced with monounsaturated fats, whereas saturated fat was on average comparable across diets (8%E–9%E) (Cao et al. 2009). Under these isoenergetic conditions, there was a significant increase in HDL-C (2.28 mg/dL) and a reduction in plasma TG (−9.36 mg/dL) with the moderate-fat lower-carbohydrate diets compared to low-fat diets, and similar reductions in LDL-C across diets. Based on these lipid changes, predicted CVD risk was calculated and estimated to be 6.4% lower in men and 9.3% lower in women consuming moderate-fat lower-carbohydrate diets compared to low-fat diets (Cao et al. 2009).

Although LDL-C remains the clinical benchmark for assessing efficacy of lipid-lowering therapy, information about LDL particle subclass concentrations, particularly small vs. larger LDL, may more accurately reflect effects on CVD risk (Krauss 2010, 2014). In a 13-week dietary intervention in moderately overweight men, a low-carbohydrate diet (26%E) reduced small dense LDL (P = 0.03) and increased LDL peak particle diameter (P = 0.007), a measure of the diameter of the most abundant class of LDL particles, compared to a higher-carbohydrate diet (54%E) (Krauss et al. 2006), also suggesting a benefit of carbohydrate restriction on measures of CVD risk. A very-low-carbohydrate weight maintenance ketogenic diet (8%E) consumed for 6 weeks has also been shown to significantly increase LDL peak particle diameter and the percentage of larger LDL-I in comparison to a habitual lower-fat (32%E) higher-carbohydrate (47%E) diet (Sharman et al. 2002).

CVD Risk

Because evidence from randomized trials with clinical outcome data is lacking, we rely on epidemiological evidence to study the relationship of diet composition to CVD risk. Several large prospective cohort studies have evaluated the association of low-carbohydrate diets with CVD risk and mortality. In most instances, dietary intake was assessed with food frequency questionnaires and translated into an overall low-carbohydrate diet score that also considered energy from protein and fat (Fung et al. 2010, Halton et al. 2006, Nakamura et al. 2014) or only protein (Lagiou et al. 2012, Trichopoulou et al. 2007). (Note that the lowest decile low-carbohydrate diet score reflected higher carbohydrate intake and, conversely, the highest decile score reflected lower carbohydrate intake.) Comparison of the highest vs. lowest deciles of the low-carbohydrate diet score showed no association with coronary heart disease (CHD) risk (relative risk [RR] 0.94, 95% CI 0.74–1.19) (Halton et al. 2006) or CVD mortality (HR 1.00, 95% CI 0.84–1.2) (Fung et al. 2010) in women from the

Nurses' Health Study (NHS; N > 82,000 women followed for 20–26 years). However, in men from the Health Professionals Follow-up Study cohort (HPFS; N = 44,548; 20 years follow-up), a low-carbohydrate diet was associated with an increase in CVD mortality (HR 1.15, 95% CI 0.96–1.37) which was largely attributed to concurrent intake of animal-based foods. By contrast, low-carbohydrate vegetable-based diets were associated with reduced CVD mortality in both cohorts (pooled HR 0.77, 95% CI 0.68–0.87) (Fung et al. 2010). Together the earlier findings differ from what has been reported for Swedish women (N ≥ 42,000; mean follow-up 12–15.7 years) (Lagiou et al. 2007, 2012), and Greek men and women of the European Prospective Investigation into Cancer and Nutrition (EPIC) study (N = 22,944; follow-up 10 years), in whom a low-carbohydrate high-protein diet was associated with increased cardiovascular mortality (Lagiou et al. 2007, Trichopoulou et al. 2007) and increased incidence of cardiovascular events (Lagiou et al. 2012).

The discrepancies in findings across cohorts, that is, showing an increase in CVD risk and mortality with low carbohydrate intake in cohorts from Sweden and Greece but no effect in U.S. women, may reflect differences in the quality of carbohydrate-containing foods that are displaced with carbohydrate restriction. It has indeed been argued that in Swedish women, replacement of mostly whole grains with protein may have had detrimental effects on measures of CVD, whereas among U.S. women (NHS), replacement of mostly refined starches and sugars with any other nutrient would be less likely to adversely affect risk (Willett 2007). Notably, in the NHS cohort (Halton et al. 2006), subgroup analysis of the relationship of individual macronutrients revealed that whereas total carbohydrate intake was marginally associated with CVD risk (RR 1.22, 95% CI 0.95–1.56), glycemic load (the product of GI and the amount of carbohydrate in a given food) was significantly associated with increased risk (RR 1.90, 95% CI 1.15–3.15), emphasizing the importance of considering both the quantity and quality of carbohydrates consumed.

Glycemic Control

Acute postprandial glucose and insulin responses to test meals are commonly used as indicators of whole-body insulin sensitivity. It is generally believed that over time, chronically high levels of glucose and, thereby, insulin can lead to pancreatic ß-cell dysfunction and the development of insulin resistance, a predisposing condition to T2DM and increased CVD risk (Blaak et al. 2012). Because carbohydrate is the main macronutrient affecting insulin secretion and ensuing blood glucose levels, many studies have focused on either dietary carbohydrate restriction or the manipulation of carbohydrate quality and the relationship of these dietary strategies to measures of glycemic control and diabetes risk.

Many randomized controlled trials testing effects of carbohydrate quantity on measures of glycemic control have, by design, been conducted under weight loss conditions, precluding inference to weight stable conditions. In the earlier referenced meta-analysis of 23 longer-term randomized controlled trials (N = 2788) that compared low-carbohydrate diets to low-fat diets (Hu et al. 2012), pooled mean net changes from baseline in fasting blood glucose did not differ for low-carbohydrate (−10.4 mg/dL) vs. low-fat diets (−10.1 mg/dL), likely due to weight loss, which was comparable across diets (−6.1 kg and −5.0 kg, respectively). Notably, however, a series of small studies conducted in eight men with untreated T2DM showed that improvements in glycemic control through dietary modification can occur under conditions where body weight is unchanged. In these 5–10-week trials, a low-carbohydrate diet (achieved primarily by restriction of dietary starches and providing 30%E carbohydrate, 30% protein, 40% fat) in replacement for a higher-carbohydrate lower-fat diet (55%E carbohydrate, 15% protein, 30% fat) reduced fasting glucose levels and 24 h total glucose area by ≥28% and ≥35%, respectively, with no change in fasting insulin levels (Nuttall et al. 2008, Gannon et al. 2010). Mean glycated hemoglobin (HbA1c, a measure of glycemic control over a 2 to 3-month period) was also decreased by 25% after 10 weeks (Gannon et al. 2010), in overall agreement with a 12-month study in obese patients (80% men) that showed a greater reduction in glycated hemoglobin (−0.7%) in a subgroup of 54 diabetic patients assigned to a low-carbohydrate diet vs. low-fat diet, even after adjustment for weight loss (Stern et al. 2004). While the earlier findings suggest a beneficial effect of carbohydrate restriction *per se* on glycemic control, larger studies in more diverse patient populations are warranted before definitive conclusions can be drawn.

Diabetes Risk

Data linking total carbohydrate intake to risk of T2DM is derived largely from cohorts where low carbohydrate scores were used to characterize dietary intake. During 20 years of follow-up of the NHS and HPFS cohorts, there was no association of extreme deciles of the low-carbohydrate diet score with diabetes risk among women (Halton et al. 2008), but there was an increased risk associated with reduced carbohydrate intake among men, the latter driven largely by concurrent high intake of red and processed meat (de Koning et al. 2011); after adjustment for these dietary variables, the association of the low carbohydrate score with diabetes was no longer significant. In a Japanese cohort of 64,674 men and women (5 years follow-up), the risk of T2DM was reduced for the lowest vs. highest quintile of carbohydrate intake among women (RR 0.63, 95% CI 0.46–0.84), but this effect became nonsignificant after adjustment for GL, illustrating the importance of carbohydrate quality in diabetes risk (Nanri et al. 2015). A number of epidemiological studies found no association of total carbohydrate intake with predicted risk of diabetes (Hu et al. 2001). These observations are in general agreement with a meta-analysis of 22 cohort studies that showed a greater association with diabetes risk for glucose (RR 1.77, 95% CI 1.06–2.65) and fructose (RR 1.68, 95% CI 1.01–2.59) than for total carbohydrate intake (RR 1.23, 95% CI 1.09–1.39) in trials ≥10 years of follow-up (Alhazmi et al. 2012).

In summary, observational studies among U.S., European, and Asian cohorts using "low-carbohydrate diet scores" to qualify dietary consumption show mostly no association of total carbohydrate intake *per se* with CVD or diabetes risk. Evidence that low-carbohydrate diets appear to be protective when consumed in association with plant-based foods, but are detrimental in animal-based diets, are consistent with the notion that effects of carbohydrates, and their restriction, on cardiometabolic risk are to some extent modulated by the nutrients and foods that replace them and the overall dietary context in which carbohydrates are consumed.

In the absence of randomized controlled trials of low-carbohydrate diets on clinical outcomes, we rely on trials with surrogate measures of CVD and diabetes risk. Such studies show benefits of restricting total carbohydrate intake, manifest most notably as ameliorations in features of atherogenic dyslipidemia, namely, plasma TG, HDL-C, and small dense LDL particles, along with improvement in glycemic control and glycated hemoglobin in individuals with T2DM.

GLYCEMIC INDEX

As mentioned earlier, the glycemic index (GI) is a measure of carbohydrate quality and represents the postprandial blood glucose response to 50 g of carbohydrates from a test food, expressed as a percentage of the blood glucose response to the same amount of carbohydrate from a reference food, namely, glucose or white bread (Wolever et al. 1991). It is used to categorize foods on the basis of their rate of digestion and absorption, with high-GI foods having a GI ≥ 70, whereas low-GI foods have a GI ≤ 55 (Augustin et al. 2015). Also as noted earlier, the concept of GL has been developed to take into consideration both carbohydrate quality and quantity, and is the product of a foods' GI and the amount of carbohydrate in a typical serving of that food. Hence, foods with a higher GL generally elicit more rapid and larger blood glucose and insulin responses.

Lipid and Lipoprotein Risk Factors

The effects of GI and GL on plasma lipids and lipoproteins are inconsistent. Several cross-sectional studies (Levitan et al. 2008, Liu et al. 2001, McKeown et al. 2009, Shikany et al. 2010) have shown reduced plasma TG and increased HDL-C levels with lower GL or GI diets and have suggested that the differential lipid effects may be more pronounced with increasing BMI (Liu et al. 2001, Shikany et al. 2010). Notably, the positive association with TG and inverse association with HDL-C appeared to be stronger for GL than GI (Liu et al. 2001). In the earlier studies, lowest vs. highest quartiles/quintiles ranged from 68 to 81 for GI (Levitan et al. 2008, Liu et al. 2001, McKeown et al. 2009, Shikany et al. 2010) and from 50 to 180 for GL (Levitan et al. 2008, Liu et al. 2001, McKeown et al. 2009, Shikany et al. 2010). Evidence from dietary intervention studies, however, is mixed. A recent meta-analysis of 28 randomized controlled feeding trials ≥4 weeks (N = 1272) reported no effect of GI on plasma TG and HDL-C, but reduced LDL-C (−6.2 mg/dL, 95% CI −9.3 to −3.1) with low-GI diets. Notably, subgroup analysis revealed that improvements in LDL-C occurred only when low-GI diets were also high in fiber, but not when fiber was matched across diets (Goff et al. 2013). The observation that low- vs. high-GI diets did not differentially affect plasma TG and HDL-C in this meta-analysis (Goff et al. 2013) suggests that GL, which captures both carbohydrate quality and quantity, and/or carbohydrate quantity as such, may be more important determinants of these biomarkers of CVD risk than GI, in agreement with an earlier meta-analysis that reported lowering of plasma TG with low-GL diets (Livesey et al. 2008). Alternatively, it is possible that benefits of low-GI diets on plasma TG and HDL-C may be attenuated if the diet has an abundance of low-GI foods that are high in fructose, a simple sugar shown to promote atherogenic dyslipidemia (Chapters 14 and 15).

The OmniCarb study is the most rigorous clinical trial to date to evaluate the effect of GI on CVD risk factors. It compared high-GI (65) vs. low-GI (40) diets in the context of DASH-like dietary patterns with high (58%E) or moderate (40%E) carbohydrate intake (Sacks et al. 2014) in 163 overweight and obese adults. In this 5-week intervention study, carbohydrate amount influenced lipid risk factors to a greater extent than GI. Low vs. high GI levels had no effect on HDL-C and apoB in the context of either moderate or high carbohydrate intake but resulted in a modest reduction in TG (5 mg/dL) on the moderate-carbohydrate diet. In keeping with the documented effect of carbohydrates on atherogenic dyslipidemia, the high- vs. moderate-carbohydrate diet increased plasma TG (18%–20%) at both high and low GI levels and reduced HDL-C (4%) at the high GI level. The authors concluded that in an otherwise healthy dietary setting, lowering the GI may not improve cardiovascular risk factors. The RISCK study tested the effects of higher GI (GI, 64) vs. lower GI (GI, 51–53) in the context of either high monounsaturated fat diets or low-fat diets, in comparison to a high-GI high saturated fat control diet, in a 24-week intervention in 548 men and women at high risk of metabolic syndrome (Jebb et al. 2010). Replacing saturated fat with either carbohydrate or monounsaturated fat reduced total cholesterol and LDL-C, but the most significant reductions were achieved for diets with low-GI carbohydrates. No other differences in plasma lipids were noted between low- and high-GI diets, in overall agreement with the Diogenes study in 932 overweight adults (Gogebakan et al. 2011), and a meta-analysis of 14 longer-term randomized controlled trials (≥6 months) that reported no differential effect of GI or GL on plasma lipids (Schwingshackl and Hoffmann 2013). Discrepancies in findings between cross-sectional studies and randomized controlled trials may reflect differences in populations studied, duration of interventions, inherent limitations associated with the variability of GI measurements (Matthan et al. 2016), and the potential for misclassification of low- vs. high-GI foods in food frequency questionnaires. It is also possible that in cross-sectional studies, GI/GL may be a reflection of dietary patterns including other bioactive components that favorably affect biomarkers of CVD risk.

Inflammation

The modest effects of GI/GL on plasma lipids as noted earlier suggest that other pathways, such as those impacting inflammation, may be implicated in the association of low-GI/low-GL diets with reduced CVD risk, as reviewed in the following text. A recent systematic review suggests that the anti-inflammatory benefits of low-GI diets documented in epidemiological studies are supported by several dietary intervention studies (Buyken et al. 2014). In cross-sectional analyses among healthy middle-aged women (WHS, N = 18,137) (Levitan et al. 2008), middle-aged women with T2DM (NHS, N = 891) (Qi et al. 2006), and smaller cohorts at high risk for CVD (PREDIMED, N = 511) (Bulló et al. 2013), or with generally impaired glucose tolerance (Dutch cohort, N = 786) (Du et al. 2008), a high dietary GI was associated with increases in two biomarkers of inflammation that are strongly associated with CVD risk (Ridker et al. 2000): CRP (Du et al. 2008, Levitan et al. 2008, Qi et al. 2006) and IL-6 (Bulló et al. 2013). The associations of dietary GL with inflammatory markers in observational studies are less consistent (Buyken et al. 2014).

The Diogenes study, involving 932 overweight adults from eight European countries, is the largest clinical trial to date to evaluate the effect of GI on inflammatory markers. After 26 weeks of weight maintenance, the low-GI diet (GI, ~56) led to a significantly greater reduction in CRP (−0.46 mg/L; 95% CI 0.79–0.13) than the high-GI diet (GI, ~61) (Gogebakan et al. 2011), in agreement with results from a 1-year Canadian study in 162 individuals with T2DM where CRP levels were 30% lower with the low-GI diet (GI, 55) than the high-GI diet (GI, 63) (CRP 1.95 vs. 2.75 mg/L, respectively; P = 0.0078) (Wolever et al. 2008). While smaller dietary trials have failed to reproduce these findings (Buyken et al. 2014), results from larger intervention studies suggest that low-GI diets may reduce low-grade inflammation in higher-risk individuals.

CVD Outcomes

There is evidence that chronically elevated fasting and postprandial glycemia and insulinemia, by promoting insulin resistance and oxidative stress as well as inflammation, are implicated in the development of both T2DM and CVD (Blaak et al. 2012). Numerous epidemiological studies have investigated the relationship of GI/GL to chronic disease risk among different cohorts and populations. In the NHS including 75,521 women and 761 cases of CHD during a 10-year follow-up, high GL and, to a lesser degree, high GI were associated with an increased risk of CHD (Liu et al. 2000b). When stratified by BMI, the increased risk of CHD with GL was most pronounced among women with BMI > 23, consistent with a recent meta-analysis in which GL was associated with increased CHD risk among men and women with a higher BMI (RR 1.49, 95% CI 1.27–1.76) but not among those with lower BMI (RR 1.03, 95% CI 0.86–1.23) (Fan et al. 2012). In a large Italian cohort of the EPICOR trial (N = 47, 749 men and women; 7.9 years follow-up and 463 CHD cases), a significant increase in the risk of CHD was observed across categories of GL (RR 2.24, 95% CI 1.26–3.98) and carbohydrates from high-GI foods (RR 1.68, 95% CI 1.01–2.75) in women, but not in men. High carbohydrate intake from low-GI foods, starch, or sugar was not associated with CHD risk in either gender (Sieri et al. 2010). Similar associations of high GL with increased CHD risk were recently reported in the EPIC Greek cohort study (20,275 men and women; 10.4 years follow-up) (Turati et al. 2015). Notably, in this cohort, high adherence to a Mediterranean diet with low/moderate GL (tertiles I and II of GL) was associated with a 40% lower risk of CHD compared with a high GL/high adherence to a Mediterranean diet, suggesting a benefit to reducing GL even in an otherwise healthy dietary pattern.

Several meta-analyses of prospective cohort studies examining the relation between GI/GL and CVD were published in 2012, with generally comparable conclusions. A meta-analysis of eight prospective cohort studies (N = 220,050 participants; 4,826 incident cases) (Dong et al. 2012), and another based on 10 cohort studies (eight overlapping with the Dong meta-analysis; N = 240,936 participants; 6,940 incident cases) (Mirrahimi et al. 2012) showed significant associations of GL and GI with CHD risk among women, but not men. Notably, GL was more strongly associated with CHD risk (55%–69% increase) than GI (26% increase). Results of another meta-analysis of 14 cohorts (90% overlap with the Mirrahimi meta-analysis, with an additional five cohorts, and extending CHD outcomes to stroke and heart failure) (N = 229,213 participants; 11,363 cases) indicated an 18% increase in risk for cardiac events per 50-unit increment of GL among Caucasians (Ma et al. 2012). Yet another meta-analysis (12 cohorts, 438,073 participants [100% overlap with Mirrahimi meta-analysis, with two additional cohorts], and 9,424 incident CHD cases and 2,123 stroke cases) (Fan et al. 2012) concluded that high GL, but not GI, was associated with an increased risk for stroke as well as CHD. In a dose–response analysis, there were 5% and 3% increases in risk of CHD and stroke, respectively, per 50-unit increment in GL level (Fan et al. 2012). A subsequent meta-analysis showing a significant association of high GL, but not of GI or total carbohydrate, to increased risk of stroke suggests that this relationship is independent of total carbohydrate intake (Cai et al. 2015).

Glucose Homeostasis and Glycemic Control

In the context of cardiometabolic health, low-GI diets are most studied for their effects on measures of glycemic control for the management of diabetes. In a meta-analysis of 14 controlled trials lasting 12 days to 12 months (N = 356 individuals with type 1 and type 2 diabetes), low-GI diets (average GI = 65) reduced HbA1c by 0.34% points and plasma fructosamine (a measure of glycosylated blood proteins that reflects glycemic control over the preceding 2–3 weeks) by 0.2 mmol/L more than that achieved with high-GI diets (average GI = 83) (Brand-Miller et al. 2003). When data from HbA1c and fructosamine were combined and the difference between the low- and high-GI diets was expressed in percentage terms, the low-GI diet reduced values by 7.4%, an effect estimated by the authors to translate into clinically meaningful reductions in diabetes-related endpoints based on data from the UKPDS trial (UKPDS 1998). In a later meta-analysis of 45 controlled diet intervention trials (N = 972/treatment arm) ≥1 week duration and including individuals who were healthy, had type 1 or type 2 diabetes, or were at risk of CHD, low-GI diets reduced fasting glucose and glycated proteins and improved measures of insulin sensitivity assessed by clamp, frequently sampled IV glucose tolerance test, or insulin tolerance test (Livesey et al. 2008). These effects were of greater magnitude in individuals with blood glucose levels >5 mmol/L (90 mg/dL) and, notably, were independent of unavailable carbohydrate (i.e., indigestible oligosaccharides and fiber) intake. In individuals with type 1 and type 2 diabetes (N = 612), the improvement in glycemic control manifest as reductions in HbA1c (0.4%) or fructosamine (0.23 mmol/L) with low- vs. high-GI diets was confirmed in a meta-analysis of 12 randomized controlled trials of ≥4 weeks duration (Thomas and Elliott 2010). A recent meta-analysis of longer-term studies (≥6 months, 16 trials, N = 3073) compared the effectiveness of popular dietary approaches (i.e., low-carbohydrate, low-GI, vegetarian, vegan, Mediterranean, and high-protein) vs. control diets on measures of glycemic control and confirmed that low-GI vs. control diets (3 trials, N = 357) improved HbA1c. However, the magnitude of the effect was small (−0.14%) and of questionable clinical relevance. Low-carbohydrate, Mediterranean, and high-protein diets were also effective at reducing HbA1c, with the greatest effect attributed to Mediterranean diets (−0.47%) (Ajala et al. 2013). The smaller effect sizes of low-GI diets in these longer-term studies, as compared to those reported in earlier meta-analyses (Brand-Miller et al. 2003, Livesey et al. 2008), raise the possibility of metabolic adaptation or reduced compliance over time with such restrictive regimens.

While clinical data generally suggest benefits of low-GI/low-GL diets for glycemic control in diabetes, the effectiveness of this approach in nondiabetics is questionable. In the 5-week OmniCarb trial in 163 overweight and obese adults discussed earlier, DASH-like low-GI diets did not improve glycemic control compared to high-GI diets and, in the context of high carbohydrate intake, actually reduced insulin sensitivity determined as areas under the curve (AUC) for glucose and insulin after a glucose tolerance test (Sacks et al. 2014). It was speculated that the low-GI diet may have promoted morning insulin resistance as a means of maintaining adequate blood glucose levels. Similar observations were reported in a controlled 28-day feeding study involving 89 healthy adults who were either normal weight or overweight/obese, and where low- and high-GL diets resulted in comparable measures of insulin sensitivity (estimated as HOMA-IR) (Runchey et al. 2012). Acutely, high-GL meals induced higher postprandial insulin and glucose responses, but the ratio of iAUC insulin/iAUC glucose was comparable for both high- and low-GL test meals, suggesting no detrimental effect of GL on ß-cell function.

Diabetes Risk

While a mechanistic relationship between GI and risk of T2DM remains uncertain, it is suggested that the increase in postprandial glucose resulting from high-GI diets raises insulin demand which, over time, may compromise ß-cell function and eventually lead to higher diabetes risk (Ludwig 2002). As is the case for CVD risk, numerous longitudinal studies have also investigated the relationship of GI/GL to risk of T2DM among different cohorts. This was first reported in the NHS in 65,173 women (40–65 years old) (Salmerón et al. 1997b) and HPFS in 42,759 men (40–75 years old) (Salmerón et al. 1997a) and later among younger women in NHSII (N = 91,249; 24–44 years old) (Schulze et al. 2004) without NIDDM or CVD at onset. At 6–8 years of follow-up, the relative risk of diabetes was increased 37%–59% in the highest vs. lowest quintile of GI (Salmerón et al. 1997a,b, Schulze et al. 2004), and 25%–47% in the highest vs. lowest quintile of GL, in models adjusted for cereal fiber intake (Salmerón et al. 1997a,b). When the effects of GL and cereal fiber were examined jointly, the risk for diabetes was even higher for the combination of high GL (>165) and low cereal fiber (<3.2 g/day) vs. low GL (<143) and higher cereal fiber intake (>5.8 g/day) (RR = 2.17–2.5) (Salmerón et al. 1997a,b). In an updated analysis of the combined NHS, NHSII, and HPFS cohorts (N = 205,157; follow-up 3,800,618 person-years), individuals in the highest vs. lowest quintiles of energy-adjusted GI and GL had a 33% and 10% higher risk of T2DM, respectively, suggesting that GI is more strongly associated with diabetes risk than GL (Bhupathiraju et al. 2014). When high-GI or high-GL diets were combined with low cereal fiber intake, the risks of T2DM were respectively 59% and 47% higher compared to low-GI/low-GL high-fiber diets, underscoring the importance of highly processed carbohydrate-containing foods in this relationship (Bhupathiraju et al. 2014, Salmerón et al. 1997a,b). The possible association between processed carbohydrates and diabetes risk was also highlighted in a subsequent analysis of NHSII (AlEssa et al. 2015) in which the starch-to-cereal fiber ratio was found to have the strongest association with diabetes risk (RR = 1.39; CI 1.27, 1.53; P-trend < 0.0001) vs. RRs of 1.28 (CI 1.17, 1.39; P-trend < 0.0001), 1.12 (CI 1.02, 1.23; P-trend = 0.03), and 1.09 (CI 1.00, 1.20; P-trend = 0.04) for carbohydrate-to-cereal fiber, starch to total fiber, and carbohydrate-to-total fiber ratios, respectively.

In addition to the findings from the NHS and HPFS cohorts, a relationship of GI and/or GL to diabetes risk has been corroborated in the Dutch EPIC cohort (Sluijs et al. 2010), the Black Women's Health Study (N = 59,000) (Krishnan et al. 2007), and in a cohort of Chinese women (N = 64,227) (Villegas et al. 2007), but not in the Women's Health Study (Meyer et al. 2000) or other prospective studies (Mosdol et al. 2007, Sahyoun et al. 2008, Simila et al. 2011). These inconsistences may reflect population/ethnic differences, the subjectivity of assigning GI values to mixed meals and local foods leading to possible misclassification, and the fact that in some studies assessment of dietary intake occurred only at baseline rather than at regular intervals during follow-up, thus failing to account for changes in dietary intake over time.

Despite inconsistencies across prospective cohort studies, several meta-analyses conducted since 2008 report a positive relationship between high-GI or high-GL diets and diabetes risk (Barclay et al. 2008, Dong et al. 2011, Greenwood et al. 2013, Livesey et al. 2013). In a meta-analysis of nine prospective cohort studies (N = 422,224) investigating the relationship of GL/GL to the risk of T2DM among mostly female participants (Barclay et al. 2008), comparison between the highest and lowest quintiles of GI/GL showed GI to be more strongly associated with diabetes risk (40% increase) than GL (27% increase), independent of dietary fiber intake. Positive associations between GI/GL and risk of T2DM were confirmed in a subsequent meta-analysis of 13 prospective cohort studies (75% overlap with cohorts from the Barclay meta-analysis, with an additional seven cohorts) conducted between 1997 and 2010 (N = 530,875; 4–14 years follow-up) (Dong et al. 2011). In the most recent dose–response meta-analysis reporting on 24 studies (N = 757,984; 7.5 million person-years follow-up), there was a 45% increase in diabetes risk per 100 g increment in GL in the fully adjusted model (Livesey et al. 2013). The relationship between GL and diabetes risk was found to be stronger among females than males, in European Americans vs. other ethnic groups (albeit the latter were not well represented), and in studies using dietary instruments of greater validity. Whereas the association of GL with diabetes risk was observed over a wide range of GL values (62–279 g/2000 kcal), it was significant only at GL > 95 g/2000 kcal, leading the authors to recommend a daily target of less than 100 g GL. In Americans consuming 48%–51% daily energy from carbohydrates (DGAC 2015), this GL would correspond to ~250 g carbohydrates with a GI = 40, but may more practically be achieved by reducing carbohydrate intake to 180 g (≅35% daily kcal) and selecting foods in the upper range of what are considered low-GI foods (<55) (Augustin et al. 2015).

WHOLE GRAINS

In the United States, an emphasis on consumption of grain products dates back to the 1992 USDA food pyramid, which advocated consumption of 6–11 servings each day of bread, cereal, rice, and pasta, with only slight consideration for the quality of foods that constituted these grain servings. In its most recent iteration, the Dietary Guidelines for Americans 2015–2020 recommends the selection of whole grains as staple items of healthy food patterns. Yet, it is estimated that the majority of the U.S. population does not meet recommendations for 3–4 oz/day whole grains and >70% of Americans exceed recommended intakes for refined grains (DGAC 2015). The absence of a universally accepted definition for what constitutes a whole grain product (Ferruzzi et al. 2014) makes identification of such foods challenging. Designations range from ≥25% to ≥51% whole grain or bran by weight. A ratio of total carbohydrate to fiber (in g/serving) ≤10:1 has also been proposed as a means of identifying whole grain foods (Lloyd-Jones et al. 2010). It is important to recognize that even if a standard definition for whole grain foods were in place, characteristics such as the structure and degree of processing of grains (e.g., the extent to which they are milled vs. cracked vs. intact) will modulate physiological responses. Yet such characteristics are rarely described or reported in observational and randomized controlled trials (Ross et al. 2015), making it difficult to evaluate the association of "whole grains" to cardiometabolic health.

Lipid and Lipoprotein Risk Factors

The cholesterol-lowering properties of whole grains have, in part, been ascribed to their content of soluble fibers, which can reduce bile acid reabsorption and favor their fecal excretion. The ensuing hepatic conversion of cholesterol to bile acids promotes LDL-receptor upregulation and increased hepatic uptake of LDL particles (Surampudi et al. 2016). In a recent meta-analysis of 24 randomized controlled trials in which effects of whole grains on plasma lipids were evaluated by type of whole grain product, total whole grain intake reduced LDL-cholesterol vs. control (−0.09 mmol/L, 95% CI −0.03, −0.15), but the magnitude of effect was greatest with whole grain oat (−0.17 mmol/L, 95% CI −0.10, −0.25) (Hollaender et al. 2015). In contrast, whole grain wheat or mixed whole grains derived mostly from wheat products showed no effect on plasma lipids, likely because wheat contains mostly insoluble fiber. The number of trials in which rye, barley, or rice were compared to control foods were too few to arrive at meaningful conclusions regarding their cholesterol-lowering potential. Notably, in a meta-regression to test whether dose could predict changes in plasma lipids, there was a negative association between whole grains and total cholesterol and LDL-C for studies in which intake was <100 g/day, but the association was positive when the entire range of intakes (28–213 g/day) was included (Hollaender et al. 2015). Together, these findings suggest possibly undesirable plasma lipid effects at higher levels of whole grain intake, possibly reflecting an effect of total carbohydrate load. This observation is consistent with results from our own study in which provision of diets high in resistant starch, a form of dietary starch which undergoes limited digestion by α-amylases in the small intestine, did not lower plasma and LDL-C compared to low-resistant-starch diets (Bergeron et al. 2016). Notably, we found that independent of the resistant starch content of the diet, high vs. low carbohydrate intake increased plasma TG and large VLDL particles, in keeping with the notion that total carbohydrate load may be an important determinant of atherogenic dyslipidemia.

To date, evidence from randomized controlled trials fails to support the notion that the protective effect of whole grains on CVD risk is due to anti-inflammatory effects (Buyken et al. 2014).

CVD Risk

Studies consistently report inverse associations between whole grain intake and the risks of CVD (Jensen et al. 2004, Mellen et al. 2008, Wu et al. 2015a, Ye et al. 2012). However, and as referred to earlier, interpretation of such studies has been complicated by the lack of a universal definition of what constitutes a whole grain food (Cho et al. 2013). In addition, most whole grain products contain dietary fiber that may or may not account for their health benefits. For example, the HPFS (Jensen et al. 2004) reported that the significant inverse association between whole grain intake and CVD risk (6% reduction in CVD risk for each 20 g increment in whole grain intake) was eliminated after adjustment for dietary fiber and other diet factors, suggesting that dietary fiber accounts, at least in part, for the protective effects of whole grain products. An earlier meta-analysis of 10 prospective cohort studies found that the highest category of whole grain intake (48–80 g/day, ≅3–5 servings) was associated with a 21% reduction in CVD risk when compared to rare or no intake, but it is unclear whether the multivariable adjustment model accounted for dietary fiber (Ye et al. 2012). An updated analysis that combined the NHS and the HPFS showed a 9% reduction in total mortality and 15% reduction in CVD mortality for the highest (33 g/day) vs. lowest quintiles (4.2 g/day) of whole grain intake when adjusted for the "healthy eating index," but adjustment was not made for dietary fiber *per se*. It was estimated that every serving of whole grain (28 g) was associated with a 9% lower CVD mortality (Wu et al. 2015a). These findings concur with an updated meta-analysis of 14 cohort studies (N = 786,076; 23,957 CVD deaths) in which the highest vs. lowest categories of whole grain intake were associated with an 18% reduction in CVD mortality; in a dose–response analysis, each 16 g increase in whole grain intake (~1 serving/day) was associated with a 9% lower risk of CVD mortality (RR 0.91, 95% CI 0.90–0.93) (Zong et al. 2016). Hence, consuming ~3–4 servings/day whole grain products (50–70 g/day, equivalent to 3–4 slices of whole grain bread), as recommended in the Dietary Guidelines for Americans, was associated with 19%–23% reduction in CVD mortality, compared with no whole grain consumption (Zong et al. 2016). Collectively, the earlier studies suggest a cardioprotective role of whole grains, likely mediated in part by the fiber (Wu et al. 2015b) and phytonutrients inherent in these products (Ras et al. 2014). In contrast, no association with CVD or CHD has been reported for total refined grain, white bread, refined breakfast cereal, or total rice intake (Aune et al. 2016, Mellen et al. 2008).

Glycemic Control

Soluble fibers in whole grain products have been proposed to improve glycemic control by delaying gastric emptying and slowing the rate of glucose absorption, thereby attenuating the postprandial excursion of blood glucose after carbohydrate-containing meals (Kaline et al. 2007). In a meta-analysis of 14 observational studies (~48,000 individuals of European descent), each serving of whole grain foods (assessed by food frequency questionnaires, 24 h recalls and food diaries) reduced fasting glucose by −0.019 mmol/L and fasting insulin by −0.021 pmol/L (Nettleton et al. 2010). While relatively few randomized controlled dietary intervention trials have examined the association of whole grains to glycemic control, the meta-analysis of Ye et al. (2012, 11 studies) showed that increased intake of whole grains vs. a control diet was associated with a reduction in fasting glucose (95% CI −1.65, −0.21), whereas reduction in plasma insulin levels was not significant (Ye et al. 2012). These findings should be interpreted with caution given the substantial heterogeneity noted across trials, likely reflecting differences in type of whole grains tested, method of estimating whole grain intake, nature of the control interventions, study duration, and health status of study participants. Importantly, in randomized controlled trials, few studies have directly compared whole vs. refined grains in otherwise comparable diets, making it difficult to determine whether improvements in cardiometabolic parameters are the result of whole grains *per se*, or of other bioactive components that typify the healthy dietary patterns in which whole grains are often incorporated.

Diabetes Risk

The relationship of whole grain intake to diabetes risk was initially reported in the Women's Health Study (with similar findings in the NHS cohort [Liu et al. 2000a]), where the relative risk of diabetes in the highest (median 20.5 servings/week) vs. lowest quintile (median 1 serving/week) of whole grain intake was 0.79 (95% CI 0.65–0.96). Whereas refined grains, soluble fiber, and fiber from fruits and vegetables were unrelated to risk, intake of cereal fiber and magnesium were associated with reduced diabetes risk (RR 0.64, 95% CI 0.53–0.79 and RR 0.67, 95% CI 0.55–0.82, respectively) suggesting that these constituents of whole grains confer protection from T2DM (Meyer et al. 2000).

In an earlier meta-analysis of six cohort studies (N = 286,125; 10,944 incident cases T2DM), it was estimated that a 2 serving/day increment in whole grain intake would reduce the risk of T2DM by 21% (95% CI 13%–28%) (de Munter et al. 2007). A subsequent dose–response meta-regression analysis (with some overlapping studies and three additional cohorts) covering a broad range of whole grain intake (2–154 g/day, the latter equivalent to ~5 servings/day) showed an absolute reduction of 0.3% in incidence of T2DM for each additional 10 g (~0.3 servings) of whole grains consumed. Based on population prevalence of T2DM, it was estimated that increasing whole grain intake from 7.5 to 45 g/day would lead to a 20% relative reduction in diabetes risk (Chanson-Rolle et al. 2015), consistent with findings of de Munter et al. (2007). Total fiber intake has also been found to be protective for diabetes risk (RR 0.81, 95% CI 0.73–0.90) in a meta-analysis of 17 studies involving 488,293 participants (19,033 cases) (Yao et al. 2014). From this pooled analysis, it is estimated that a daily intake of 30 g of dietary fiber (i.e., twofold more than what is currently consumed by U.S. adults (McGill et al. 2015)) would be required to achieve comparable reductions in diabetes risk than what is achieved with three servings of whole grain foods.

CONCLUSION

Dietary starches and grains are staple components of diets consumed worldwide. In assessing their effects on cardiometabolic health, one must consider the quantity of carbohydrates consumed and, importantly, the degree of processing of carbohydrate-containing foods. In randomized controlled trials, higher-carbohydrate (≥45%E) diets are generally associated with increased plasma TG, low HDL-C, increased abundance of small dense LDL particles, and worsened glycemic control manifest as increased fasting glucose and hemoglobin A1C levels. While observational studies indicate that total carbohydrate intake is marginally associated with the risk of cardiometabolic disease, the importance of carbohydrate quality is emphasized by the stronger associations of GI and GL (the product of GI and carbohydrate amount) with risk of T2DM and CVD, respectively. Overall, the evidence to date suggests that the risk for these diseases is benefited by dietary patterns that limit the intake of total carbohydrates and glycemic starches and include ~3 daily servings of minimally or unprocessed whole grains.

REFERENCES

Ajala, O., P. English, and J. Pinkney. 2013. Systematic review and meta-analysis of different dietary approaches to the management of type 2 diabetes. *Am J Clin Nutr* 97(3): 505–516. doi: 10.3945/ajcn.112.042457.

AlEssa, H. B., S. N. Bhupathiraju, V. S. Malik, N. M. Wedick, H. Campos, B. Rosner, W. C. Willett, and F. B. Hu. 2015. Carbohydrate quality and quantity and risk of type 2 diabetes in US women. *Am J Clin Nutr* 102(6): 1543–1553. doi: 10.3945/ajcn.115.116558.

Alhazmi, A., E. Stojanovski, M. McEvoy, and M. L. Garg. 2012. Macronutrient intakes and development of type 2 diabetes: A systematic review and meta-analysis of cohort studies. *J Am Coll Nutr* 31(4): 243–258.

Augustin, L. S. A., C. W. C. Kendall, D. J. A. Jenkins, W. C. Willett, A. Astrup, A. W. Barclay, I. Björck et al. 2015. Glycemic index, glycemic load and glycemic response: An International Scientific Consensus Summit from the International Carbohydrate Quality Consortium (ICQC). *Nutr Metab Cardiovasc Dis* 25(9): 795–815. doi: 10.1016/j.numecd.2015.05.005.

Aune, D., N. Keum, E. Giovannucci, L. T. Fadnes, P. Boffetta, D. C. Greenwood, S. Tonstad, L. J. Vatten, E. Riboli, and T. Norat. 2016. Whole grain consumption and risk of cardiovascular disease, cancer, and all cause and cause specific mortality: Systematic review and dose-response meta-analysis of prospective studies. *BMJ* 353: i2716. doi: 10.1136/bmj.i2716.

Barclay, A. W., P. Petocz, J. McMillan-Price, V. M. Flood, T. Prvan, P. Mitchell, and J. C. Brand-Miller. 2008. Glycemic index, glycemic load, and chronic disease risk—A meta-analysis of observational studies. *Am J Clin Nutr* 87(3): 627–637.

Bergeron, N., P. T. Williams, R. Lamendella, N. Faghihnia, A. Grube, X. Li, Z. Wang et al. 2016. Diets high in resistant starch increase plasma levels of trimethylamine-N-oxide, a gut microbiome metabolite associated with CVD risk. *Br J Nutr* 116(12): 2020–2029. doi: 10.1017/S0007114516004165.

Bhupathiraju, S. N., D. K. Tobias, V. S. Malik, A. Pan, A. Hruby, J. E. Manson, W. C. Willett, and F. B. Hu. 2014. Glycemic index, glycemic load, and risk of type 2 diabetes: Results from 3 large US cohorts and an updated meta-analysis. *Am J Clin Nutr* 100(1): 218–232. doi: 10.3945/ajcn.113.079533.

Blaak, E. E., J. M. Antoine, D. Benton, I. Bjorck, L. Bozzetto, F. Brouns, M. Diamant et al. 2012. Impact of postprandial glycaemia on health and prevention of disease. *Obes Rev* 13(10): 923–984. doi: 10.1111/j.1467-789X.2012.01011.x.

Brand-Miller, J., S. Hayne, P. Petocz, and S. Colagiuri. 2003. Low-glycemic index diets in the management of diabetes: A meta-analysis of randomized controlled trials. *Diabetes Care* 26(8): 2261–2267.

Bulló, M., R. Casas, M. P. Portillo, J. Basora, R. Estruch, A. García-Arellano, A. Lasa, M. Juanola-Falgarona, F. Arós, and J. Salas-Salvadó. 2013. Dietary glycemic index/load and peripheral adipokines and inflammatory markers in elderly subjects at high cardiovascular risk. *Nutr Metab Cardiovasc Dis* 23(5): 443–450. doi: 10.1016/j.numecd.2011.09.009.

Buyken, A. E., J. Goletzke, G. Joslowski, A. Felbick, G. Cheng, C. Herder, and J. C. Brand-Miller. 2014. Association between carbohydrate quality and inflammatory markers: Systematic review of observational and interventional studies. *Am J Clin Nutr* 99(4): 813–833. doi: 10.3945/ajcn.113.074252.

Cai, X., C. Wang, S. Wang, G. Cao, C. Jin, J. Yu, X. Li et al. 2015. Carbohydrate intake, glycemic index, glycemic load, and stroke: A meta-analysis of prospective cohort studies. *Asia Pac J Public Health* 27(5): 486–496. doi: 10.1177/1010539514566742.

Cao, Y., D. T. Mauger, C. L. Pelkman, G. Zhao, S. M. Townsend, and P. M. Kris-Etherton. 2009. Effects of moderate (MF) versus lower fat (LF) diets on lipids and lipoproteins: A meta-analysis of clinical trials in subjects with and without diabetes. *J Clin Lipidol* 3(1): 19–32. doi: 10.1016/j.jacl.2008.12.008.

Chanson-Rolle, A., A. Meynier, F. Aubin, J. Lappi, K. Poutanen, S. Vinoy, and V. Braesco. 2015. Systematic review and meta-analysis of human studies to support a quantitative recommendation for whole grain intake in relation to type 2 diabetes. *PLoS One* 10(6): e0131377. doi: 10.1371/journal.pone.0131377.

ChartsBin.com. 2016. Contribution of carbohydrates in total dietary consumption. Accessed Viewed October 4, 2016. http://chartsbin.com/view/1154.

Cho, S. S., L. Qi, G. C. Fahey, Jr., and D. M. Klurfeld. 2013. Consumption of cereal fiber, mixtures of whole grains and bran, and whole grains and risk reduction in type 2 diabetes, obesity, and cardiovascular disease. *Am J Clin Nutr* 98(2): 594–619. doi: 10.3945/ajcn.113.067629.

Cohen, E., M. Cragg, J. deFonseka, A. Hite, M. Rosenberg, and B. Zhou. 2015. Statistical review of US macronutrient consumption data, 1965–2011: Americans have been following dietary guidelines, coincident with the rise in obesity. *Nutrition* 31(5): 727–732. doi: 10.1016/j.nut.2015.02.007.

de Koning, L., T. T. Fung, X. Liao, S. E. Chiuve, E. B. Rimm, W. C. Willett, D. Spiegelman, and F. B. Hu. 2011. Low-carbohydrate diet scores and risk of type 2 diabetes in men. *Am J Clin Nutr* 93(4): 844–850. doi: 10.3945/ajcn.110.004333.

de Munter, J. S., F. B. Hu, D. Spiegelman, M. Franz, and R. M. van Dam. 2007. Whole grain, bran, and germ intake and risk of type 2 diabetes: A prospective cohort study and systematic review. *PLoS Med* 4(8): e261. doi: 10.1371/journal.pmed.0040261.

DGAC. 2015. U.S. Department of Agriculture and U.S. Department of Health and Human Services: Scientific Report of the 2015 Dietary Guidelines Advisory Committee.

Dong, J.-Y., L. Zhang, Y.-H. Zhang, and L.-Q. Qin. 2011. Dietary glycaemic index and glycaemic load in relation to the risk of type 2 diabetes: A meta-analysis of prospective cohort studies. *Br J Nutr* 106(11): 1649–1654. doi: 10.1017/S000711451100540X.

Dong, J. Y., Y. H. Zhang, P. Wang, and L. Q. Qin. 2012. Meta-analysis of dietary glycemic load and glycemic index in relation to risk of coronary heart disease. *Am J Cardiol* 109(11): 1608–1613. doi: 10.1016/j.amjcard.2012.01.385.

Dreon, D. M., H. A. Fernstrom, B. Miller, and R. M. Krauss. 1994. Low-density lipoprotein subclass patterns and lipoprotein response to a reduced-fat diet in men. *FASEB J* 8(1): 121–126.

Dreon, D. M., H. A. Fernstrom, P. T. Williams, and R. M. Krauss. 1997. LDL subclass patterns and lipoprotein response to a low-fat, high-carbohydrate diet in women. *Arterioscler Thromb Vasc Biol* 17(4): 707–714.

Dreon, D. M., H. A. Fernstrom, P. T. Williams, and R. M. Krauss. 1999. A very low-fat diet is not associated with improved lipoprotein profiles in men with a predominance of large, low-density lipoproteins. *Am J Clin Nutr* 69(3): 411–418.

Du, H., A. Dl van der, M. M. van Bakel, C. J. H. van der Kallen, E. E. Blaak, M. M. J. van Greevenbroek, E. H. J. M. Jansen et al. 2008. Glycemic index and glycemic load in relation to food and nutrient intake and metabolic risk factors in a Dutch population. *Am J Clin Nutr* 87(3): 655–661.

Fan, J., Y. Song, Y. Wang, R. Hui, and W. Zhang. 2012. Dietary glycemic index, glycemic load, and risk of coronary heart disease, stroke, and stroke mortality: A systematic review with meta-analysis. *PLoS One* 7(12): e52182. doi: 10.1371/journal.pone.0052182.

Ferruzzi, M. G., S. S. Jonnalagadda, S. Liu, L. Marquart, N. McKeown, M. Reicks, G. Riccardi et al. 2014. Developing a standard definition of whole-grain foods for dietary recommendations: Summary report of a multidisciplinary expert roundtable discussion. *Adv Nutr* 5(2): 164–176. doi: 10.3945/an.113.005223.

Fung, T. T., R. M. van Dam, S. E. Hankinson, M. Stampfer, W. C. Willett, and F. B. Hu. 2010. Low-carbohydrate diets and all-cause and cause-specific mortality: Two cohort studies. *Ann Intern Med* 153(5): 289–298. doi: 10.1059/0003-4819-153-5-201009070-00003.

Furtado, J. D., H. Campos, L. J. Appel, E. R. Miller, N. Laranjo, V. J. Carey, and F. M. Sacks. 2008. Effect of protein, unsaturated fat, and carbohydrate intakes on plasma apolipoprotein B and VLDL and LDL containing apolipoprotein C-III: Results from the OmniHeart Trial. *Am J Clin Nutr* 87(6): 1623–1630.

Gannon, M. C., H. Hoover, and F. Q. Nuttall. 2010. Further decrease in glycated hemoglobin following ingestion of a LoBAG30 diet for 10 weeks compared to 5 weeks in people with untreated type 2 diabetes. *Nutr Metab* 7(1): 64. doi: 10.1186/1743-7075-7-64.

Goff, L. M., D. E. Cowland, L. Hooper, and G. S. Frost. 2013. Low glycaemic index diets and blood lipids: A systematic review and meta-analysis of randomised controlled trials. *Nutr Metab Cardiovasc Dis* 23(1): 1–10. doi: 10.1016/j.numecd.2012.06.002.

Gogebakan, O., A. Kohl, M. A. Osterhoff, M. A. van Baak, S. A. Jebb, A. Papadaki, J. A. Martinez et al. 2011. Effects of weight loss and long-term weight maintenance with diets varying in protein and glycemic index on cardiovascular risk factors: The diet, obesity, and genes (DiOGenes) study: A randomized, controlled trial. *Circulation* 124(25): 2829–2838. doi: 10.1161/CIRCULATIONAHA.111.033274.

Greenwood, D. C., D. E. Threapleton, C. E. Evans, C. L. Cleghorn, C. Nykjaer, C. Woodhead, and V. J. Burley. 2013. Glycemic index, glycemic load, carbohydrates, and type 2 diabetes: Systematic review and dose-response meta-analysis of prospective studies. *Diabetes Care* 36(12): 4166–4171. doi: 10.2337/dc13-0325.

Halton, T. L., S. Liu, J. E. Manson, and F. B. Hu. 2008. Low-carbohydrate-diet score and risk of type 2 diabetes in women. *Am J Clin Nutr* 87(2): 339–346.

Halton, T. L., W. C. Willett, S. Liu, J. E. Manson, C. M. Albert, K. Rexrode, and F. B. Hu. 2006. Low-carbohydrate-diet score and the risk of coronary heart disease in women. *N Engl J Med* 355(19): 1991–2002. doi: 10.1056/NEJMoa055317.

Hollaender, P. L., A. B. Ross, and M. Kristensen. 2015. Whole-grain and blood lipid changes in apparently healthy adults: A systematic review and meta-analysis of randomized controlled studies. *Am J Clin Nutr* 102(3): 556–572. doi: 10.3945/ajcn.115.109165.

Hu, F. B., R. M. van Dam, and S. Liu. 2001. Diet and risk of Type II diabetes: The role of types of fat and carbohydrate. *Diabetologia* 44(7): 805–817. doi: 10.1007/s001250100547.

Hu, T., K. T. Mills, L. Yao, K. Demanelis, M. Eloustaz, W. S. Yancy, Jr., T. N. Kelly, J. He, and L. A. Bazzano. 2012. Effects of low-carbohydrate diets versus low-fat diets on metabolic risk factors: A meta-analysis of randomized controlled clinical trials. *Am J Epidemiol* 176(Suppl 7): S44–S54. doi: 10.1093/aje/kws264.

Jebb, S. A., J. A. Lovegrove, B. A. Griffin, G. S. Frost, C. S. Moore, M. D. Chatfield, L. J. Bluck, C. M. Williams, T. A. Sanders, and Risck Study Group. 2010. Effect of changing the amount and type of fat and carbohydrate on insulin sensitivity and cardiovascular risk: The RISCK (Reading, Imperial, Surrey, Cambridge, and Kings) trial. *Am J Clin Nutr* 92(4): 748–758. doi: 10.3945/ajcn.2009.29096.

Jenkins, D. J., T. M. Wolever, R. H. Taylor, H. Barker, H. Fielden, J. M. Baldwin, A. C. Bowling, H. C. Newman, A. L. Jenkins, and D. V. Goff. 1981. Glycemic index of foods: A physiological basis for carbohydrate exchange. *Am J Clin Nutr* 34(3): 362–366.

Jensen, M. K., P. Koh-Banerjee, F. B. Hu, M. Franz, L. Sampson, M. Gronbaek, and E. B. Rimm. 2004. Intakes of whole grains, bran, and germ and the risk of coronary heart disease in men. *Am J Clin Nutr* 80(6): 1492–1499.

Kaline, K., S. R. Bornstein, A. Bergmann, H. Hauner, and P. E. Schwarz. 2007. The importance and effect of dietary fiber in diabetes prevention with particular consideration of whole grain products. *Horm Metab Res* 39(9): 687–693. doi: 10.1055/s-2007-985811.

Krauss, R. M. 2010. Lipoprotein subfractions and cardiovascular disease risk. *Curr Opin Lipidol* 21(4): 305–311. doi: 10.1097/MOL.0b013e32833b7756.

Krauss, R. M. 2014. All low-density lipoprotein particles are not created equal. *Arterioscler Thromb Vasc Biol* 34(5): 959–961. doi: 10.1161/ATVBAHA.114.303458.

Krauss, R. M., P. J. Blanche, R. S. Rawlings, H. S. Fernstrom, and P. T. Williams. 2006. Separate effects of reduced carbohydrate intake and weight loss on atherogenic dyslipidemia. *Am J Clin Nutr* 83(5): 1025–1031; quiz 1205.

Krishnan, S., L. Rosenberg, M. Singer, F. B. Hu, L. Djoussé, L. A. Cupples, and J. R. Palmer. 2007. Glycemic index, glycemic load, and cereal fiber intake and risk of type 2 diabetes in US black women. *Arch Int Med* 167(21): 2304–2309. doi: 10.1001/archinte.167.21.2304.

Lagiou, P., S. Sandin, M. Lof, D. Trichopoulos, H. O. Adami, and E. Weiderpass. 2012. Low carbohydrate-high protein diet and incidence of cardiovascular diseases in Swedish women: Prospective cohort study. *BMJ* 344: e4026. doi: 10.1136/bmj.e4026.

Lagiou, P., S. Sandin, E. Weiderpass, A. Lagiou, L. Mucci, D. Trichopoulos, and H. O. Adami. 2007. Low carbohydrate-high protein diet and mortality in a cohort of Swedish women. *J Intern Med* 261(4): 366–374. doi: 10.1111/j.1365-2796.2007.01774.x.

Levitan, E. B., N. R. Cook, M. J. Stampfer, P. M. Ridker, K. M. Rexrode, J. E. Buring, J. E. Manson, and S. Liu. 2008. Dietary glycemic index, dietary glycemic load, blood lipids, and C-reactive protein. *Metabolism* 57(3): 437–443. doi: 10.1016/j.metabol.2007.11.002.

Liu, S., J. E. Manson, M. J. Stampfer, M. D. Holmes, F. B. Hu, S. E. Hankinson, and W. C. Willett. 2001. Dietary glycemic load assessed by food-frequency questionnaire in relation to plasma high-density-lipoprotein cholesterol and fasting plasma triacylglycerols in postmenopausal women. *Am J Clin Nutr* 73(3): 560–566.

Liu, S., J. E. Manson, M. J. Stampfer, F. B. Hu, E. Giovannucci, G. A. Colditz, C. H. Hennekens, and W. C. Willett. 2000a. A prospective study of whole-grain intake and risk of type 2 diabetes mellitus in US women. *Am J Public Health* 90(9): 1409–1415.

Liu, S., W. C. Willett, M. J. Stampfer, F. B. Hu, M. Franz, L. Sampson, C. H. Hennekens, and J. E. Manson. 2000b. A prospective study of dietary glycemic load, carbohydrate intake, and risk of coronary heart disease in US women. *Am J Clin Nutr* 71(6): 1455–1461.

Livesey, G., R. Taylor, T. Hulshof, and J. Howlett. 2008. Glycemic response and health—A systematic review and meta-analysis: Relations between dietary glycemic properties and health outcomes. *Am J Clin Nutr* 87(1): 258S–268S.

Livesey, G., R. Taylor, H. Livesey, and S. Liu. 2013. Is there a dose-response relation of dietary glycemic load to risk of type 2 diabetes? Meta-analysis of prospective cohort studies. *Am J Clin Nutr* 97(3): 584–596. doi: 10.3945/ajcn.112.041467.

Lloyd-Jones, D. M., Y. Hong, D. Labarthe, D. Mozaffarian, L. J. Appel, L. Van Horn, K. Greenlund et al. 2010. Defining and setting national goals for cardiovascular health promotion and disease reduction: The American Heart Association's strategic impact goal through 2020 and beyond. *Circulation* 121(4): 586–613. doi: 10.1161/circulationaha.109.192703.

Ludwig, D. S. 2002. The glycemic index: Physiological mechanisms relating to obesity, diabetes, and cardiovascular disease. *JAMA* 287(18): 2414–2423.

Ma, X.-Y., J.-P. Liu, and Z.-Y. Song. 2012. Glycemic load, glycemic index and risk of cardiovascular diseases: Meta-analyses of prospective studies. *Atherosclerosis* 223(2): 491–496. doi: 10.1016/j.atherosclerosis.2012.05.028.

Matthan, N. R., L. M. Ausman, H. Meng, H. Tighiouart, and A. H. Lichtenstein. 2016. Estimating the reliability of glycemic index values and potential sources of methodological and biological variability. *Am J Clin Nutr* 104(4): 1004–1013. doi: 10.3945/ajcn.116.137208.

McGill, C., L. F. Victor III, and L. Devareddy. 2015. Ten-year trends in fiber and whole grain intakes and food sources for the United States population: National Health and Nutrition Examination Survey 2001–2010. *Nutrients* 7(2): 1119.

McKeown, N. M., J. B. Meigs, S. Liu, G. Rogers, M. Yoshida, E. Saltzman, and P. F. Jacques. 2009. Dietary carbohydrates and cardiovascular disease risk factors in the Framingham offspring cohort. *J Am Coll Nutr* 28(2): 150–158.

Mellen, P. B., T. F. Walsh, and D. M. Herrington. 2008. Whole grain intake and cardiovascular disease: A meta-analysis. *Nutr Metab Cardiovasc Dis* 18(4): 283–290. doi: 10.1016/j.numecd.2006.12.008.

Meyer, K. A., L. H. Kushi, D. R. Jacobs, J. Slavin, T. A. Sellers, and A. R. Folsom. 2000. Carbohydrates, dietary fiber, and incident type 2 diabetes in older women. *Am J Clin Nutr* 71(4): 921–930.

Mirrahimi, A., R. J. de Souza, L. Chiavaroli, J. L. Sievenpiper, J. Beyene, A. J. Hanley, L. S. Augustin, C. W. Kendall, and D. J. Jenkins. 2012. Associations of glycemic index and load with coronary heart disease events: A systematic review and meta-analysis of prospective cohorts. *J Am Heart Assoc* 1(5): e000752. doi: 10.1161/JAHA.112.000752.

Mosdol, A., D. R. Witte, G. Frost, M. G. Marmot, and E. J. Brunner. 2007. Dietary glycemic index and glycemic load are associated with high-density-lipoprotein cholesterol at baseline but not with increased risk of diabetes in the Whitehall II study. *Am J Clin Nutr* 86(4): 988–994.

Mozaffarian, D. 2016. Dietary and policy priorities for cardiovascular disease, diabetes, and obesity: A comprehensive review. *Circulation* 133(2): 187–225. doi: 10.1161/CIRCULATIONAHA.115.018585.

Nakamura, Y., N. Okuda, T. Okamura, A. Kadota, N. Miyagawa, T. Hayakawa, Y. Kita et al. 2014. Low-carbohydrate diets and cardiovascular and total mortality in Japanese: A 29-year follow-up of NIPPON DATA80. *Br J Nutr* 112(6): 916–924. doi: 10.1017/S0007114514001627.

Nanri, A., T. Mizoue, K. Kurotani, A. Goto, S. Oba, M. Noda, N. Sawada, S. Tsugane, and Group Japan Public Health Center-Based Prospective Study. 2015. Low-carbohydrate diet and type 2 diabetes risk in Japanese men and women: The Japan Public Health Center-Based Prospective Study. *PLoS One* 10(2): e0118377. doi: 10.1371/journal.pone.0118377.

Nettleton, J. A., N. M. McKeown, S. Kanoni, R. N. Lemaitre, M.-F. Hivert, J. Ngwa, F. J. A. van Rooij, E. Sonestedt, M. K. Wojczynski, Z. Ye, and T. Tanaka. 2010. Interactions of dietary whole-grain intake with fasting glucose– and insulin-related genetic loci in individuals of European descent: A meta-analysis of 14 cohort studies. *Diabetes Care* 33(12): 2684–2691. doi: 10.2337/dc10-1150.

Nuttall, F. Q., K. Schweim, H. Hoover, and M. C. Gannon. 2008. Effect of the LoBAG30 diet on blood glucose control in people with type 2 diabetes. *Br J Nutr* 99(3): 511–519. doi: 10.1017/S0007114507819155.

Qi, L., R. M. van Dam, S. Liu, M. Franz, C. Mantzoros, and F. B. Hu. 2006. Whole-grain, bran, and cereal fiber intakes and markers of systemic inflammation in diabetic women. *Diabetes Care* 29(2): 207–211.

Ras, R. T., J. M. Geleijnse, and E. A. Trautwein. 2014. LDL-cholesterol-lowering effect of plant sterols and stanols across different dose ranges: A meta-analysis of randomised controlled studies. *Br J Nutr* 112(2): 214–219. doi: 10.1017/S0007114514000750.

Ridker, P. M., N. Rifai, M. Pfeffer, F. Sacks, S. Lepage, and E. Braunwald. 2000. Elevation of tumor necrosis factor-alpha and increased risk of recurrent coronary events after myocardial infarction. *Circulation* 101(18): 2149–2153.

Ross, A. B., M. Kristensen, C. J. Seal, P. Jacques, and N. M. McKeown. 2015. Recommendations for reporting whole-grain intake in observational and intervention studies. *Am J Clin Nutr* 101(5): 903–907. doi: 10.3945/ajcn.114.098046.

Runchey, S. S., M. N. Pollak, L. M. Valsta, G. D. Coronado, Y. Schwarz, K. L. Breymeyer, C. Wang, C. Y. Wang, J. W. Lampe, and M. L. Neuhouser. 2012. Glycemic load effect on fasting and post-prandial serum glucose, insulin, IGF-1 and IGFBP-3 in a randomized, controlled feeding study. *Eur J Clin Nutr* 66(10): 1146–1152. doi: 10.1038/ejcn.2012.107.

Sacks, F. M. 2015. The crucial roles of apolipoproteins E and C-III in apoB lipoprotein metabolism in normolipidemia and hypertriglyceridemia. *Curr Opin Lipidol* 26(1): 56–63. doi: 10.1097/MOL.0000000000000146.

Sacks, F. M., V. J. Carey, C. A. Anderson, E. R. Miller, T. Copeland, 3rd, J. Charleston, B. J. Harshfield et al. 2014. Effects of high vs low glycemic index of dietary carbohydrate on cardiovascular disease risk factors and insulin sensitivity: The OmniCarb randomized clinical trial. *JAMA* 312(23): 2531–2541. doi: 10.1001/jama.2014.16658.

Sahyoun, N. R., A. L. Anderson, F. A. Tylavsky, J. S. Lee, D. E. Sellmeyer, T. B. Harris, and Aging Health, and Study Body Composition. 2008. Dietary glycemic index and glycemic load and the risk of type 2 diabetes in older adults. *Am J Clin Nutr* 87(1): 126–131.

Salmerón, J., A. Ascherio, E. B. Rimm, G. A. Colditz, D. Spiegelman, D. J. Jenkins, M. J. Stampfer, A. L. Wing, and W. C. Willett. 1997a. Dietary fiber, glycemic load, and risk of NIDDM in men. *Diabetes Care* 20(4): 545–550. doi: 10.2337/diacare.20.4.545.

Salmerón, J., J. E. Manson, M. J. Stampfer, G. A. Colditz, A. L. Wing, and W. C. Willett. 1997b. Dietary fiber, glycemic load, and risk of non-insulin-dependent diabetes mellitus in women. *JAMA* 277(6): 472–477.

Schulze, M. B., S. Liu, E. B. Rimm, J. E. Manson, W. C. Willett, and F. B. Hu. 2004. Glycemic index, glycemic load, and dietary fiber intake and incidence of type 2 diabetes in younger and middle-aged women. *Am J Clin Nutr* 80(2): 348–356.

Schwingshackl, L. and G. Hoffmann. 2013. Long-term effects of low glycemic index/load vs. high glycemic index/load diets on parameters of obesity and obesity-associated risks: A systematic review and meta-analysis. *Nutr Metab Cardiovasc Dis* 23(8): 699–706. doi: 10.1016/j.numecd.2013.04.008.

Select Committee on Human Nutrition and Needs (ed.). 1977. Dietary goals for the United States. United States Senate, Washington, DC.

Sharman, M. J., W. J. Kraemer, D. M. Love, N. G. Avery, A. L. Gomez, T. P. Scheett, and J. S. Volek. 2002. A ketogenic diet favorably affects serum biomarkers for cardiovascular disease in normal-weight men. *J Nutr* 132(7): 1879–1885.

Shikany, J. M., L. F. Tinker, M. L. Neuhouser, Y. Ma, R. E. Patterson, L. S. Phillips, S. Liu, and D. T. Redden. 2010. Association of glycemic load with cardiovascular disease risk factors: The Women's Health Initiative Observational Study. *Nutrition* 26(6): 641–647. doi: 10.1016/j.nut.2009.08.014.

Shin, M. J. and R. M. Krauss. 2010. Apolipoprotein CIII bound to apoB-containing lipoproteins is associated with small, dense LDL independent of plasma triglyceride levels in healthy men. *Atherosclerosis* 211(1): 337–341. doi: 10.1016/j.atherosclerosis.2010.02.025.

Sieri, S., V. Krogh, F. Berrino, A. Evangelista, C. Agnoli, F. Brighenti, N. Pellegrini et al. 2010. Dietary glycemic load and index and risk of coronary heart disease in a large Italian cohort: The EPICOR study. *Arch Int Med* 170(7): 640–647. doi: 10.1001/archinternmed.2010.15.

Simila, M. E., L. M. Valsta, J. P. Kontto, D. Albanes, and J. Virtamo. 2011. Low-, medium- and high-glycaemic index carbohydrates and risk of type 2 diabetes in men. *Br J Nutr* 105(8): 1258–1264. doi: 10.1017/S000711451000485X.

Sluijs, I., Y. T. van der Schouw, D. L. van der A, A. M. Spijkerman, F. B. Hu, D. E. Grobbee, and J. W. Beulens. 2010. Carbohydrate quantity and quality and risk of type 2 diabetes in the European Prospective Investigation into Cancer and Nutrition–Netherlands (EPIC-NL) study. *Am J Clin Nutr* 92(4): 905–911. doi: 10.3945/ajcn.2010.29620.

Stern, L., N. Iqbal, P. Seshadri, K. L. Chicano, D. A. Daily, J. McGrory, M. Williams, E. J. Gracely, and F. F. Samaha. 2004. The effects of low-carbohydrate versus conventional weight loss diets in severely obese adults: One-year follow-up of a randomized trial. *Ann Intern Med* 140(10): 778–785.

Surampudi, P., B. Enkhmaa, E. Anuurad, and L. Berglund. 2016. Lipid lowering with soluble dietary fiber. *Curr Atheroscler Rep* 18(12): 75. doi: 10.1007/s11883-016-0624-z.

Thomas, D. E. and E. J. Elliott. 2010. The use of low-glycaemic index diets in diabetes control. *Br J Nutr* 104(6): 797–802. doi: 10.1017/S0007114510001534.

Trichopoulou, A., T. Psaltopoulou, P. Orfanos, C. C. Hsieh, and D. Trichopoulos. 2007. Low-carbohydrate-high-protein diet and long-term survival in a general population cohort. *Eur J Clin Nutr* 61(5): 575–581.

Turati, F., V. Dilis, M. Rossi, P. Lagiou, V. Benetou, M. Katsoulis, A. Naska, D. Trichopoulos, C. La Vecchia, and A. Trichopoulou. 2015. Glycemic load and coronary heart disease in a Mediterranean population: The EPIC Greek cohort study. *Nutr Metab Cardiovasc Dis* 25(3): 336–342. doi: 10.1016/j.numecd.2014.12.002.

UKPDS. 1998. Effect of intensive blood-glucose control with metformin on complications in overweight patients with type 2 diabetes (UKPDS 34). UK Prospective Diabetes Study (UKPDS) Group. *Lancet* 352(9131): 854–865.

Villegas, R., S. Liu, Y. T. Gao, G. Yang, H. Li, W. Zheng, and X. O. Shu. 2007. Prospective study of dietary carbohydrates, glycemic index, glycemic load, and incidence of type 2 diabetes mellitus in middle-aged Chinese women. *Arch Int Med* 167(21): 2310–2316. doi: 10.1001/archinte.167.21.2310.

Willett, W. C. 2007. Low-carbohydrate diets: A place in health promotion? *J Intern Med* 261(4): 363–365. doi: 10.1111/j.1365-2796.2007.01804.x.

Wolever, T. M., D. J. Jenkins, A. L. Jenkins, and R. G. Josse. 1991. The glycemic index: Methodology and clinical implications. *Am J Clin Nutr* 54(5): 846–854.

Wolever, T. M. S., A. L. Gibbs, C. Mehling, J.-L. Chiasson, P. W. Connelly, R. G. Josse, L. A. Leiter et al. 2008. The Canadian Trial of Carbohydrates in Diabetes (CCD), a 1-y controlled trial of low-glycemic-index dietary carbohydrate in type 2 diabetes: No effect on glycated hemoglobin but reduction in C-reactive protein. *Am J Clin Nutr* 87(1): 114–125.

Wu, H., A. J. Flint, Q. Qi, R. M. van Dam, L. A. Sampson, E. B. Rimm, M. D. Holmes, W. C. Willett, F. B. Hu, Q. Sun 2015a. Association between dietary whole grain intake and risk of mortality: Two large prospective studies in us men and women. *JAMA Int Med* 175(3): 373–384. doi: 10.1001/jamainternmed.2014.6283.

Wu, Y., Y. Qian, Y. Pan, P. Li, J. Yang, X. Ye, and G. Xu. 2015b. Association between dietary fiber intake and risk of coronary heart disease: A meta-analysis. *Clin Nutr* 34(4): 603–611. doi: 10.1016/j.clnu.2014.05.009.

Yang, Q., Z. Zhang, E. W. Gregg, W. D. Flanders, R. Merritt, and F. B. Hu. 2014. Added sugar intake and cardiovascular diseases mortality among US adults. *JAMA Intern Med* 174(4): 516–524. doi: 10.1001/jamainternmed.2013.13563.

Yao, B., H. Fang, W. Xu, Y. Yan, H. Xu, Y. Liu, M. Mo, H. Zhang, and Y. Zhao. 2014. Dietary fiber intake and risk of type 2 diabetes: A dose-response analysis of prospective studies. *Eur J Epidemiol* 29(2): 79–88. doi: 10.1007/s10654-013-9876-x.

Ye, E. Q., S. A. Chacko, E. L. Chou, M. Kugizaki, and S. Liu. 2012. Greater whole-grain intake is associated with lower risk of type 2 diabetes, cardiovascular disease, and weight gain. *J Nutr* 142(7): 1304–1313. doi: 10.3945/jn.111.155325.

Zong, G., A. Gao, F. B. Hu, and Q. Sun. 2016. Whole grain intake and mortality from all causes, cardiovascular disease, and cancer: A meta-analysis of prospective cohort studies. *Circulation* 133(24): 2370–2380. doi: 10.1161/CIRCULATIONAHA.115.021101.

Section IV

Dietary Protein and Cardiometabolic Health

17 Interaction of Dietary Protein and Energy Balance

Eveline A. Martens, Richard D. Mattes, and
Margriet S. Westerterp-Plantenga

CONTENTS

ABSTRACT

Nutrition plays a key role in the prevention of cardiovascular disease, acting in part, on the prevention and treatment of obesity. Here the role of dietary protein in energy balance and weight regulation with consequent implications for the prevention and management of cardiovascular diseases is described. An energy-restricted high-protein diet has been shown to achieve body weight loss and subsequent weight maintenance by reducing energy intake without changing appetite, and maintaining energy expenditure by preserving FFM. Mechanisms behind protein-induced appetite control and energy expenditure are direct and indirect effects of elevated plasma amino acid and anorexigenic hormone concentrations, increased diet-induced thermogenesis (DIT), and a ketogenic state. Mechanisms behind protein-induced energy expenditure and preservation of fat-free mass are metabolic inefficiency, due to processing, protein turn-over, and possibly gluconeogenesis. In neutral energy balance, a protein diet may prevent a positive energy balance due to the higher energy expenditure. With respect to reward homeostasis, protein-induced food reward is limited, and may affect compliance to a protein-modified diet. When applied within a range of 0.66–1.66 g/kgBW/d, protein consumption has not been associated with increased health risks. Even in the elderly, beneficial health effects of higher-protein intake might outweigh possible adverse effects.

In conclusion, higher-protein diets may reduce cardiovascular disease risk by decreasing the susceptibility for the development of obesity.

INTRODUCTION

Cardiovascular diseases are important complications of obesity. The mechanism behind the development of obesity is one or more uncompensated periods of positive energy balance. The energy consumed in excess of need is stored in body reserves resulting in body weight gain (Westerterp 2013). Treatment of obesity entails loss of body weight, which requires a negative energy balance. At a negative energy balance, energy is mobilized from body reserves (Westerterp 2013). The most efficient and effective way to achieve a negative energy balance is with an energy-restricted diet (Westerterp-Plantenga et al. 2009). However, a sudden decrease in energy intake from the habitual diet results in increased feelings of hunger and desire to eat, and in a decrease of the feeling of fullness. These changes in appetite make it difficult to sustain a lower energy intake. Furthermore, body weight loss usually results in a reduction in energy expenditure, which is mainly caused by the loss of fat-free mass (FFM). These conditions counteract the negative energy balance induced by the energy-restricted diet, hampering body weight loss. Therefore, the aims of body weight loss are to reduce energy intake without changing appetite and to maintain energy expenditure by preserving FFM. Both goals can be achieved with an energy-restricted high-protein diet (Acheson 2013, Leidy et al. 2015, Westerterp-Plantenga et al. 2012, Wycherley et al. 2012) (see Protein Intake in Negative Energy Balance section).

A relevant question is whether the consumption of high-protein diets can also prevent the development of a positive energy balance, thus preventing overweight and obesity. In this regard, longer-term intervention studies assessing the effects of high-protein diets in normal-weight individuals are evaluated (Protein Intake in Neutral Energy Balance section). This chapter also deals with the mechanisms behind protein-induced appetite modulation and energy expenditure (Mechanisms behind Protein-Induced Appetite Control and Energy Expenditure section). To complete the picture of the relation between dietary protein and energy balance, the effects of high-protein diets in positive energy balance are described (Protein Intake in Positive Energy Balance section). Reward homeostasis related to dietary protein, effects of dietary protein on cardiovascular diseases independent of energy balance, and the adverse effects of protein diets are described in Reward Homeostasis Related to Dietary Protein, Protein Intake and Cardiovascular Diseases, Adverse Effects of Protein Diets sections. Throughout this chapter, a major theme is the distinction between short-term and longer-term effects of protein diets.

PROTEIN INTAKE IN NEGATIVE ENERGY BALANCE

Achieving and maintaining a negative energy balance are necessary conditions for dietary interventions to induce body weight loss. High-protein diets have the potential to maintain a negative energy balance by sustaining satiety at the level of the original diet (Weigle et al. 2005, Westerterp-Plantenga et al. 2006) and to limit the reduction of energy expenditure through sparing of FFM (Martens and Westerterp-Plantenga 2014, Soenen et al. 2013). The strongest effects are documented with diets restricted in carbohydrate and fat intake, but without restriction of protein intake. In this case, the diet is typically relatively high in protein (as % of energy), while the protein intake (in g/day) may be comparable to the original diet.

A few conditions apply for longer-term studies aimed at elucidating the effects of high-protein diets on body weight. First, it is necessary to monitor and confirm compliance with the designated protein intake preferably with a quantitative, objective biomarker, such as urinary nitrogen. Second, differences in protein intake between the experimental and control diets must be achieved and sustained to adequately test the efficacy of the high-protein diet (Soenen et al. 2013, Westerterp-Plantenga et al. 2012, Wycherley et al. 2012). The conclusions of studies comparing high-protein with normal-protein diets may differ from those testing high-protein and low-protein diets (Westerterp-Plantenga et al. 2012). During energy restriction, sustaining protein intake at the level of the minimal requirement (0.66 g/kg body weight/day) appears not to hinder body weight loss and fat loss (Krieger et al. 2006, Soenen et al. 2013, Wycherley et al. 2012). An additional increase of protein intake may not induce a larger loss of body weight, but can be effective in maintaining a larger amount of FFM (Krieger et al. 2006, Soenen et al. 2013, Wycherley et al. 2012). For example, a 6-month energy-restricted diet with a daily protein intake just above the minimal requirement (0.8 g/kg body weight) induces a comparable reduction in body weight to an energy-restricted diet with a daily protein intake well above the minimal requirement (1.2 g/kg body weight) (Soenen et al. 2013). However, a protein intake of 1.2 g/kg body weight/day results in a greater decrease in fat mass and preservation of FFM (Soenen et al. 2013). Furthermore, high-protein diets can be beneficial for weight maintenance after weight loss. Weight regain is less with energy-restricted high-protein diets compared with normal-protein diets (Larsen et al. 2010, Soenen et al. 2013). An energy-restricted high-protein diet in combination with exercise can even increase muscle mass (Josse et al. 2011). Dietary protein intake below requirements could lead to less weight loss and a higher risk for body weight regain (Acheson 2013).

Moreover, the effects described earlier may involve concurrent changes in protein, carbohydrate, and/or fat intake. Increasing the relative protein content of a diet automatically results in a decrease in the relative content of carbohydrate and/or fat. Nevertheless, a study by Soenen et al. demonstrated that the effects of a high-protein intake on body weight loss and weight maintenance were present independent of a low-carbohydrate intake (Soenen et al. 2012). Well-controlled studies comparing energy-restricted diets with a high protein content and diets with a normal protein content, within a large range of fat contents, also showed independent effects of a high-protein intake (Wycherley et al. 2012).

PROTEIN INTAKE IN NEUTRAL ENERGY BALANCE

If the protein-induced effects on appetite and energy expenditure observed during energy restriction also hold under nonrestricted conditions, then increasing protein intake with a normal diet could prevent overweight and obesity. Alternatively, the consumption of a diet with lower protein content could increase the risk for body weight gain. Recently, a 12-week intervention study was performed comparing high-protein (30% of energy from protein) and low-protein (5% of energy from protein) diets, in weight stable individuals (Martens et al. 2014a). This was a randomized parallel group study in 14 men and 18 women on diets containing 30/35/35 or 5/60/35 percentage of energy from protein/carbohydrate/fat. Participants were able to sustain the high- and low-protein diets in this field study, according to the biomarker urinary nitrogen. Nitrogen excretion increased significantly in the high-protein diet group, from 11.8 ± 3.2 g/day at baseline to 21.7 ± 5.1 g/day during the intervention, and decreased from 12.2 ± 3.4 g/day to 7.0 ± 2.4 g/day in the low-protein diet group (Martens et al. 2014a). The low-protein diet indeed facilitated the development of a positive energy balance, while the high-protein diet was beneficial to prevent this, showing a nonsignificant positive energy balance (Martens et al. 2014b). The positive protein balance was not caused by a difference in feelings of fullness or satiety yet by a difference in energy expenditure. Total energy expenditure as measured in the respiratory chamber did not change with the high-protein diet over 12 weeks but decreased with the low-protein diet (Martens et al. 2014b).

MECHANISMS BEHIND PROTEIN-INDUCED APPETITE CONTROL AND ENERGY EXPENDITURE

APPETITE

Short-term intervention studies using energy-balanced diets with large contrasts in relative protein content have shown that high-protein diets are more satiating than diets lower in protein (Bendtsen et al. 2013, Halton and Hu 2004, Leidy et al. 2010, Lejeune et al. 2006, Veldhorst et al. 2009b,d, Westerterp-Plantenga et al. 2006). Furthermore, subjects consumed less food during an ad libitum high-protein diet relative to baseline (Weigle et al. 2005). Despite this lower total energy intake, subjects were similarly satiated and satisfied during the intervention and preintervention periods (Martens et al. 2013, 2014c, Weigle et al. 2005).

Correspondingly, small increases in fullness and satiety ratings were observed as acute responses to a high-protein diet in neutral energy balance (Martens et al. 2014b). After 1 week on the high-protein diet, fullness scores were significantly increased, while on the low-protein diet, they were decreased. In this situation, translation into large changes in energy intake was not possible, because subjects had to maintain their body weight. After 12 weeks, appetite ratings were returned to the level of the original diet, which suggests that the human body habituates to the satiating effects of high-protein intake (Martens et al. 2014b). Thus, shifts in appetite may only appear as response to changes in dietary protein content in the short term.

Protein-induced satiety is likely a combined expression with direct and indirect effects of elevated plasma amino acids and anorexigenic hormone concentrations, increased diet-induced thermogenesis (DIT), and a ketogenic state.

Elevated blood concentrations of amino acids stimulate satiety signaling in the brain (Acheson et al. 2011, Fromentin et al. 2012, Hall et al. 2003, Morrison et al. 2012, Veldhorst et al. 2009a,d). According to the "aminostatic theory," serum amino acids that cannot be channeled into protein synthesis directly serve as satiety signals (Mellinkoff et al. 1956). However, the aminostatic theory failed to garner strong support because fasting circulating amino acid levels do not correlate with appetitive sensations and there are noncongruent appetitive responses to protein sources varying in the rate of amino acid appearance. Indirectly, dietary amino acids may act on satiety signaling via receptors in the duodeno-intestinal and hepatoportal regions (Niijima et al. 2005). Depending on the type of amino acid, they increase or decrease the activity of hepatic vagal afferent fibers, innervating satiety centers in the brain (Niijima et al. 2005). The branched-chain amino acids leucine, isoleucine, and valine reportedly play an important role in these mechanisms (Acheson et al. 2011, Fromentin et al. 2012, Morrison et al. 2012, Niijima et al. 2005, Veldhorst et al. 2009a,d).

Furthermore, the satiety-stimulating effect of protein is related to increases in anorexigenic gut hormones (Belza et al. 2013, Diepvens et al. 2008, Juvonen et al. 2011, Karhunen et al. 2008, Maersk et al. 2012, Veldhorst et al. 2009a). Such hormones are produced in response to peripheral and central detection of amino acids. They react to elevated protein intake from specific sources and stimulate vagal activity in brain areas involved in the control of food intake (Davidenko et al. 2013, Leidy et al. 2013, Morrison et al. 2012, Veldhorst et al. 2009a). Concentrations of glucagon-like peptide 1, cholecystokinin, and peptide YY consistently increase in response to high-protein intakes (Belza et al. 2013, Diepvens et al. 2008, Juvonen et al. 2011, Karhunen et al. 2008, Maersk et al. 2012, Veldhorst et al. 2009a). However, it should be emphasized that changes in appetite do not consistently change in line with concentrations of amino acids or appetite hormones (Veldhorst et al. 2009a,b,c).

Acute amino acid–related effects on appetite have been reported with several high-quality proteins. A high-casein breakfast was more satiating than a normal-casein breakfast, coinciding with prolonged elevated concentrations of plasma amino acids (Veldhorst et al. 2009d). Also, a high–soy protein breakfast was more satiating than a normal–soy protein breakfast, which was related to larger increases in plasma taurine concentrations (Veldhorst et al. 2009d). Taurine is synthesized endogenously from cysteine, which in turn can be synthesized from methionine. Whey could be more satiating than casein shortly after a meal as a result of fast digestion (Veldhorst et al. 2009a). Theoretically, the digestion of *fast* proteins, such as whey, results in high and early rises of plasma amino acids and appetite hormones. Casein, which is a *slower* protein, could have a more prolonged satiety effect than whey (Boirie et al. 1997, Dangin et al. 2001). The slower digestion and absorption rates of casein give more prolonged and maintained plasma amino acid and hormone concentrations (Boirie et al. 1997, Dangin et al. 2001, Hall et al. 2003). However, no clear evidence exists for differences in satiating capacity between different types of protein, at high concentrations (Acheson et al. 2011, Adechian et al. 2012, Bendtsen et al. 2013, Bowen et al. 2006, Hall et al. 2003, Juvonen et al. 2011, Lorenzen et al. 2012, Pal et al. 2014, Veldhorst et al. 2009a). Moreover, differences in satiety responses between protein sources are scarcely observed in the longer term. It is hypothesized that the concentrations of certain amino acids have to be above a particular threshold to promote a relatively stronger hunger suppression or greater fullness (Veldhorst et al. 2009a). Certain dietary proteins, mainly complete dietary proteins, reach these thresholds at lower concentrations than other sources of protein. At high concentrations of dietary proteins, it may not be possible to discriminate between complete proteins because the amino acid concentrations are above the threshold for all sources. In the longer term, the amount of dietary protein intake rather than protein source may determine the magnitude of satiety responses.

The theoretical basis of the relationship between protein-induced satiety and DIT may be that increased energy expenditure at rest implies increases in oxygen consumption and body temperature. The feeling of oxygen deprivation may be translated into satiety feelings (Westerterp-Plantenga et al. 1999a,b). The presence of a positive relationship between the increase in satiety and in 24 h DIT has been observed with an energy-balanced high-protein diet (Westerterp-Plantenga et al. 1999b). The contribution of this mechanism to possible longer-term satiety responses remains to be determined.

With respect to a ketogenic effect, fasting β-hydroxybutyrate concentrations increase in response to a ketogenic high-protein diet that is concurrently a *low-carb* diet (Coleman and Nickols-Richardson 2005, Johnston et al. 2006, Veldhorst et al. 2009c). In a 1.5-day study, Veldhorst et al. observed that on this low-carb high-protein diet, increased concentrations of β-hydroxybutyrate directly affected appetite suppression (Veldhorst et al. 2010). A hyperketogenic state will not be reached with a common high-protein diet when its carbohydrate content is high enough to prevent strong ketogenesis. Nevertheless, the suggested contribution of ketogenesis to appetite suppression warrants further study (Johnston et al. 2006, Laeger et al. 2010, Scharrer 1999, Veldhorst et al. 2010).

Energy Intake

The studies described earlier show that protein intake itself does not automatically determine the magnitude of appetitive responses. Protein-induced satiety may depend on energy balance, and may differ between the short-term and longer-term consumption of high-protein meals. At least in the short term, ad libitum high-protein diets have been observed to sustain appetite at levels comparable to the original diet, despite a lower energy intake. Energy-restricted, high-protein diets produce, under some conditions, a sustained lower energy intake than diets with a lower protein content (Gosby et al. 2011, Martens et al. 2013, 2014c). Again, this has occurred with appetite scores comparable to those elicited by the control diet (Gosby et al. 2011, Martens et al. 2013, 2014c). As a result, individuals who consume a high-protein diet in combination with energy restriction are more satiated and potentially less likely to consume additional calories from foods extraneous to dietary prescription (Halton and Hu 2004).

The protein leverage hypothesis encompasses a geometrical model suggesting that energy intake is adjusted to reach an individual-specific target protein amount (Simpson and Raubenheimer 2005). The regulation of protein intake may be stronger than the regulation of carbohydrate and fat intake, and thus than that of total energy intake. However, evidence for a target for protein intake in humans is equivocal (Gosby et al. 2011, Griffioen-Roose et al. 2012, Martens et al. 2013, 2014c). The absence of complete protein leverage suggests that humans have a wide capacity to respond and adapt to differences in protein intake. There may be stronger protein leveraging responses in various animals than in humans (Raubenheimer and Simpson 1997, Shariatmadari and Forbes 1993, Tews et al. 1992, Theall et al. 1984, Simpson and Raubenheimer 1997, Sorensen et al. 2008). Possible species differences may reflect abilities to maintain protein intake for growth and reproduction on low-protein diets and/or limitations on metabolism of excess protein from high-protein diets.

A recent intervention study demonstrated that humans are able to maintain high-protein (30% of energy from protein) and low-protein diets (5% of energy from protein) and can respond and adapt to a range of protein intakes for a period of at least 12 weeks (Martens et al. 2014b). In contrast, the consumption of a diet extremely low in indispensable amino acids suppresses energy intake in animals. The detection of reduced concentrations of indispensable amino acids in the brain affects protein synthesis, subsequently leading to behavioral responses including underconsumption of diets that lack a minimal amount of indispensable amino acids. Evidence for comparable behavioral responses in humans is scarce. Consequently, the limits of adaptation to protein challenges acutely and over the longer term remain to be clarified.

Energy Expenditure

In addition to the effects on appetite and energy intake, dietary protein may also modulate energy expenditure. Most high-protein diet studies focusing on body weight loss have applied an energy-restriction regimen to induce a negative energy balance. The decline in energy expenditure and sleeping metabolic rate (SMR) as a result of body weight loss was less on a high-protein diet than on a normal-protein diet (Whitehead et al. 1996). In addition, higher rates of energy expenditure were observed as acute responses to energy-balanced high-protein diets (Mikkelsen et al. 2000, Veldhorst et al. 2010). Longer-term studies of individuals in energy balance support a view that higher-protein intake plays a role in the prevention of obesity via energy expenditure. In one trial, energy expenditure was maintained on a high-protein diet during energy balance for 12 weeks (Martens et al. 2014b; see also Protein Intake in Neutral Energy Balance section). In contrast, the consumption of a low-protein diet resulted in a positive energy balance after 12 weeks. Thus, at a constant body weight, a high-protein diet may protect against the development of a positive energy balance. The consumption of a low-protein diet may increase the risk for the development of a positive energy balance through adaptive thermogenesis (Martens et al. 2014b). The observations on total energy expenditure were completely underscored by changes in SMR and DIT (Martens et al. 2014b). Differential effects of dietary protein content on metabolic efficiency may contribute to the explanation for changes in DIT in response to high- and low-protein diets. The metabolic efficiency (the amount of MJ to ingest to increase 1 kg of body mass) is lower for protein than for carbohydrate and fat. Increases in protein oxidation likely contribute to the small increases in DIT in response to a high-protein diet. This may be beneficial to sustain total energy expenditure in the longer term (Westerterp et al. 1999). It may be possible that a high-protein intake induces a strong acute response on DIT, followed by a smaller but sustained effect in the longer term (Luscombe et al. 2003).

Body Composition

During energy restriction, the decline in total energy expenditure and SMR as a result of body weight loss is less on a high-protein diet than on a normal-protein diet (Whitehead et al. 1996). This has been ascribed to the potential of high-protein diets to preserve FFM, the main determinant of SMR. FFM only showed small increases and decreases after a 12-week intervention with high-protein and low-protein diets in energy balance (Martens et al. 2014a). As a consequence, SMR did not significantly change. Ultimately, a high-protein intake would be a strong stimulus for preservation of FFM.

Previous studies did observe an increase in FFM during a high-protein diet in negative (Josse et al. 2011) or neutral energy balance (Soenen et al. 2010). Likely, these changes could be explained by a high-protein intake combined with physical activity.

Although changes in protein intake will not automatically result in marked changes in FFM, this should not be interpreted to mean that metabolic function remains unaffected. Visceral adipose tissue (VAT) volume has been linked to the metabolic disturbances associated with obesity, such as diminished insulin sensitivity and dyslipidemia (Despres and Lemieux 2006). However, high ectopic lipid content, especially intrahepatic triglyceride (IHTG) content, and not VAT volume, is an independent risk factor for these metabolic disturbances (Fabbrini et al. 2009, Lettner and Roden

2008, Magkos et al. 2010). In general, weight loss improves metabolic function (Acheson 2013, Wycherley et al. 2012), but a high-protein intake may modulate the IHTG content as well (Bortolotti et al. 2009, 2011, Theytaz et al. 2012). In the context of prevention of metabolic disturbances, a 12-week intervention study determined the effects of high- and low-protein diets on the IHTG content in weight-stable individuals (Martens et al. 2014a). There was a trend for lower IHTG content after the high-protein low-carbohydrate diet compared with the low-protein high-carbohydrate diet (Martens et al. 2014a). This effect was caused by the difference in protein intake between the diets, since the fat intakes were the same, and the carbohydrate intakes were within the normal ranges (Martens et al. 2014a). This suggests that high-protein low-carbohydrate diets may be favorable for the prevention of metabolic disturbances in healthy humans. High-protein intake seems to stimulate hepatic lipid oxidation because of the high energetic demand for amino acid catabolism and ketogenesis (Veldhorst et al. 2009c, Westerterp-Plantenga et al. 2012). Furthermore, hepatic lipid oxidation may be stimulated by an increased bile acid production, a process that may also inhibit lipogenesis (Watanabe et al. 2004). Protein-induced glucagon secretion inhibits de novo lipogenesis and stimulates hepatic ketogenesis (Gannon et al. 2001, Torres and Tovar 2007). Moreover, high-protein intake may blunt the increase of very-low-density lipoprotein (VLDL)-TG concentrations induced by carbohydrate intake (Hudgins et al. 1996, 2000, Schwarz et al. 1995). High VLDL-TG concentrations may increase hepatic TG, and subsequently IHTG content (Schwarz et al. 1995). Therefore, it is likely that the observed trend for a difference in the IHTG content between the diets may be the result of combined effects involving changes in protein and carbohydrate intake.

Protein Intake and Protein Turnover

Acutely, high-protein intake stimulates protein synthesis and turnover and induces a small suppression of protein breakdown (Gilbert et al. 2011, Tang and Phillips 2009, van Loon 2012). However, it could be speculated that prolonged low-protein intake leads to muscle loss due to the lack of precursor amino acid availability for de novo muscle protein synthesis (Dideriksen et al. 2013, Symons et al. 2009). Hursel et al. (2015) observed that protein turnover was also significantly higher after a 12-week high-protein vs. low-protein diet, with significant increases in protein synthesis, protein breakdown, and protein oxidation. Protein turnover was determined in the fasted state, but protein balance was noted in the fasted as well as in the fed state (Hursel et al. 2015). Taking the fed state into account, protein balance was positive with the high-protein diet, and negative with the low-protein diet (Hursel et al. 2015). Surprisingly, net protein balance was less negative after the low-protein diet compared with the high-protein diet in the fasted state. Therefore, it is important to distinguish protein turnover in the fasted state from that in the fed state.

Wolfe et al. discussed the role of protein synthesis and protein breakdown in FFM accretion (Deutz and Wolfe 2013, Symons et al. 2009). The observed maximum response of protein synthesis after a single serving of 20–30 g of dietary protein suggests that additional effects of protein intake on FFM accretion are accounted for by the inhibition of protein breakdown. However, a beneficial reduction of protein breakdown only occurs with acute ingestion of protein (Flakoll et al. 1989, Greenhaff et al. 2008, Louard et al. 1995, Symons et al. 2009). Consequently, changes were not apparent in the basal fasted state after prolonged high-protein intake (Hursel et al. 2015). The positive protein balance observed with a high-protein diet may be due to acute postprandial responses, rather than the postabsorptive state.

Consumption of a low-protein diet for 12 weeks was not detrimental to young healthy individuals who might have the ability to adapt acutely to this condition (Hursel et al. 2015). The adaptive metabolic demand model developed by Millward may provide an explanation for the observation that the human body is able to show physiological adaptations to changes in protein intake (Millward 2003). The model proposes that the metabolic demand for amino acids comprises a fixed component and a variable adaptive component (Millward 2003). Short-term changes in protein intake are likely within the adaptive range. Adaptations in protein and amino acid metabolism to changes in protein intake largely occur via changes in whole-body protein turnover and amino acid oxidation (Tome and Bos 2000). Changes in amino acid oxidation were reflected as decreased and increased nitrogen excretion in response to the low- and high-protein diets, respectively. The activity of enzymes that regulate (1) transamination, (2) the disposal of the carbon skeletons in intermediary metabolism, and (3) the disposal of nitrogen through the urea cycle increased in response to high-protein intake (Harper 1983, Harper et al. 1984). Nevertheless, a positive nitrogen balance following high-protein intake (Garlick et al. 1999, Pannemans et al. 1995, Price et al. 1994, Tome and Bos 2000) does not automatically reflect an increase in protein anabolism (Millward 2012a). The capacity of the body to increase amino acid anabolism through an increase in lean body mass is limited (Millward 2012a). Only interventions using diets high in specific indispensable amino acids, such as leucine, might be able to stimulate protein synthesis in specific target groups such as athletes or the elderly (Millward 2012b, van Loon 2012). Therefore, transient retention or loss of body nitrogen because of a labile pool of body nitrogen may contribute to adaptations in amino acid metabolism in response to changes in protein intake (Munro 1964). Transient adaptive mechanisms may be distinguished from mechanisms that maintain homeostasis in the body in the longer term.

PROTEIN INTAKE IN POSITIVE ENERGY BALANCE

To complete the picture of the relation between dietary protein and energy balance, this section elaborates on the effects of high-protein diets in positive energy balance. Research participants are able to consume a large amount of protein during overfeeding with a high-protein diet, in a controlled setting, for 8 weeks (Bray et al. 2012). Nevertheless, it is likely that free-living individuals more readily eat in excess of energy need on a low-protein diet compared with a high-protein diet due to a lower satiating capacity of a low-protein diet. Still, support for protein leverage driving energy intake on low-protein diets is scarce (Martens et al. 2013, 2014c).

It is hypothesized that the level of protein plays a major role in FFM deposition, and in the stimulation of energy expenditure during overfeeding. In a randomized controlled trial, Bray et al. investigated the effect of dietary protein content on weight gain, body composition, and energy expenditure in young men and women in positive energy balance (Bray et al. 2012). Participants were overfed with diets low in protein (5% of energy from protein), normal in protein (15% of energy from protein), or high in protein (25% of energy from protein) for 8 weeks. Overeating produced significantly less weight gain in the low-protein diet group compared with the normal-protein or the high-protein diet groups (Bray et al. 2012). Fat mass increased similarly in all three groups. With the low-protein diet, the equivalent of more than 90% of the extra energy was stored as fat. With the normal- and high-protein diets, the equivalent of only about 50% of the excess energy was stored as fat. FFM only increased with the normal- and high-protein diets, and slightly decreased with the low-protein diet (Bray et al. 2012).

The observed acute increase in total energy expenditure corresponds with data from short-term overfeeding studies (Dallosso and James 1984, Flatt 1978, Garrow 1985, Krebs 1964). Acute increases in urinary nitrogen production to remove excess protein may significantly contribute to the increase in energy expenditure during overfeeding with normal- and high-protein diets. Total energy expenditure did not differ between the high- and normal-protein diets but was higher than with the low-protein diet. Correspondingly, resting energy expenditure (REE) increased with the normal- and high-protein diets, but did not change in response to the low-protein diet (Bray et al. 2012). The accretion of FFM in the normal- and high-protein groups was the principal contributor to the increase in REE (Bray et al. 2012). Much of the increase in REE occurred within the first 2 weeks in normal- and high-protein diet groups and was sustained throughout the remaining 6 weeks. This indicates that the acute responses were the result of increased thermogenesis rather than of the increase in body weight (Bray et al. 2012, 2015).

Thus, from this study it is suggested that among persons living in a controlled setting, excess energy intake alone may account for the increase in fat mass. Moreover, increases in energy expenditure and FFM may largely be predicted by protein intake (Bray et al. 2012).

REWARD HOMEOSTASIS RELATED TO DIETARY PROTEIN

Reward-driven eating behavior may dominate energy homeostasis (Born et al. 2013, Davidenko et al. 2013, Fromentin et al. 2012, Journel et al. 2012, Lemmens et al. 2011). Several brain areas that are involved in food reward might link high-protein intake with reduced food wanting and thereby act as a mechanism involved in the reduced energy intake following high-protein intake (Born et al. 2013, Davidenko et al. 2013, Fromentin et al. 2012, Journel et al. 2012, Lemmens et al. 2011). A hypothesized mechanism by which protein might act on brain reward centers involves direct effects of certain amino acids as precursors of the neuropeptides, serotonin, and dopamine (Davidenko et al. 2013, Journel et al. 2012). A high-protein, low-carbohydrate breakfast vs. a normal-protein, high-carbohydrate breakfast led to reduced reward-related activation in the hippocampus and parahippocampus before dinner (Fromentin et al. 2012).

Furthermore, acute food-choice compensation changed the macronutrient composition of a subsequent meal to offset the protein intervention (Born et al. 2013). A compensatory increase in carbohydrate intake was related to a decrease in liking and task-related signaling in the hypothalamus after a high-protein breakfast. After a lower-protein breakfast, an increase in wanting in the hypothalamus was related to a relative increase in protein intake in a subsequent meal (Born et al. 2013). Protein intake may directly affect the rewarding value of this macronutrient (Born et al. 2013, Griffioen-Roose et al. 2012). A limited protein-induced food-reward effect may affect compliance to a protein-modified diet.

PROTEIN INTAKE AND CARDIOVASCULAR DISEASES

Although for prevention of cardiovascular diseases prevention of overweight and obesity are important, nutrition also may play a role independently. In this respect, health effects of protein intake have been studied in epidemiological studies.

One review provided evidence for an estimated average requirement of 0.66 g good quality protein/kg body weight/day based on nitrogen balance studies. Further, a relationship was proposed between increased all-cause mortality risk and long-term low-carbohydrate high-protein diets; but data were inconclusive for a relationship between all-cause mortality risk and protein intake per se. Findings were also (1) suggestive of an inverse relationship between cardiovascular mortality and vegetable protein intake; (2) inconclusive for relationships between protein intake and cancer and cancer-related mortality; (3) inconclusive for a relationship between cardiovascular diseases and total protein intake; (4) suggestive for an inverse relationship between blood pressure and vegetable protein; (5) probable to convincing for an inverse relationship between soya protein intake and LDL cholesterol; (6) inconclusive for a relationship between protein intake and bone health, renal function, and risk of kidney stones; (7) suggestive for a relationship between increased risk of type 2 diabetes and long-term low-carbohydrate high-protein high-fat diets; (8) inconclusive for an impact of physical training on protein requirement; and (9) suggestive of an effect of physical training on whole-body protein retention. The authors conclude that the evidence is inconclusive to suggestive for protein intake and mortality and morbidity. Vegetable protein intake was associated with decreased risk in many studies (Pedersen et al. 2013).

Another study reporting data on the relationship between dietary protein sources and the risk of stroke in 84,010 women and 43,150 men during 26 and 22 years of follow-up suggests that stroke risk may be reduced by replacing red meat with other dietary sources of protein. (Bernstein et al. 2012).

On the other hand, the atherosclerosis risk in communities study on dietary protein intake and coronary heart disease did not find a relationship between type of dietary protein or major dietary protein resources and risk for coronary heart disease (Haring et al. 2014).

Finally, Clifton (2011) describes, in a review paper, that meat protein is associated with an increase in risk of heart disease. In the Nurses' Health Study, diets low in red meat, containing nuts, low-fat dairy, poultry, or fish, appeared to be associated with a 13%–30% lower risk of CHD compared with diets high in meat. Low-carbohydrate diets high in animal protein were associated with a 23% higher total mortality rate, whereas low-carbohydrate diets high in vegetable protein were associated with a 20% lower total mortality rate. Recent soy interventions have been assessed by the American Heart Association and found to be associated with only small reductions in LDL cholesterol. Although dairy intake has been associated with a lower insulin resistance and metabolic syndrome, the only long-term dairy intervention performed to date has shown no effects on these outcomes (Clifton 2011).

Taken together, epidemiological studies on health effects of protein intake report inconclusive results. It seems that consumption of red meat promotes the development of cardiovascular diseases, while consumption of vegetable protein such as nuts, low-fat dairy, poultry, or fish may be protective against cardiovascular diseases.

ADVERSE EFFECTS OF PROTEIN DIETS

There is a long-held view that high-protein intake might interfere with calcium homeostasis by increasing the acid load. It is hypothesized that this could be partially buffered by bone, subsequently resulting in bone resorption and hypercalciuria (Calvez et al. 2012). In general, high-protein intake does not seem to be associated with an impaired calcium balance. Clinically, large prospective epidemiologic studies have shown positive associations of protein intake with bone mineral mass and reduced incidence of osteoporotic fracture (Bonjour 2005). Furthermore, nitrogen intake seems to have a positive effect on calcium balance and consequent preservation of bone mineral content (Westerterp 2002). With respect to renal issues, only patients with pre-existing dysfunction reportedly have an increased risk for the development of kidney stones and renal diseases (Calvez et al. 2012). In the elderly, beneficial health effects of higher-protein intake might outweigh the adverse effects possibly because of the changes in protein metabolism with aging. In contrast, persistent total protein and amino acid intake below requirements impairs bodily functions leading to higher disease and mortality risks across the lifespan (Moughan 2012, Tome 2012). Taken together, the application of relatively high-protein diets, whereby protein intake is sustained at the customary level, does not seem to have any adverse effects in healthy individuals.

Although no clear recommendation exists that defines the safe upper limit of protein intake, consumption of up to 1.66 g/kg body weight/day has not been associated with increased health risks (Millward 2012a, WHO/FAO/UNU 2007). This means that sustaining or slightly increasing protein intake during energy restriction likely poses no adverse effects in healthy individuals. However, protein intake can exceed the suggested safe upper limit. The question arises whether and how these high intakes of protein would negatively affect health. Recent studies applying medium-term, high-protein interventions in neutral or positive energy balance did not report any adverse effects (Bray et al. 2012, Martens et al. 2014a). However, the limits of adaptation to high-protein intake over the longer term remain to be investigated.

SUMMARY

In summary, the effects of diets varying in protein differ according to energy balance. During energy restriction, sustaining protein intake at the level of requirement appears to be sufficient to aid body weight loss and fat loss. An additional increase of protein intake does not induce a larger loss of body weight, but can be effective to maintain a larger amount of FFM. Protein-induced satiety is likely a combined expression with direct and indirect effects of elevated plasma amino acid and anorexigenic hormone concentrations, increased DIT, and a ketogenic state, which all feedback on the central nervous system. In general, changes in appetite may only appear as short-term response to changes in dietary protein content, because the human body may habituate to the satiating effects of protein intake in the longer term.

The decline in energy expenditure and sleeping metabolic rate as a result of body weight loss is less on a high-protein diet than on a normal-protein diet. In addition, higher rates of energy expenditure have been observed as acute responses to energy-balanced high-protein diets. In energy balance, high-protein diets may be beneficial to prevent the development of a positive energy balance, whereas low-protein diets may facilitate this. Furthermore, high-protein, low-carbohydrate diets may be favorable for the prevention of metabolic disturbances.

With respect to protein turnover, it is important to distinguish the fasted state from the fed state. In the fed state, protein balance may be positive with high-protein diets, and negative with the low-protein diets. Surprisingly, net protein balance may be less negative after low-protein diets compared with high-protein diets in the fasted state. Therefore, a positive protein balance observed at a high-protein diet may be due to acute postprandial responses. During positive energy balance, excess energy intake alone may account for the increase in fat mass. Increases in energy expenditure and FFM may largely be predicted by protein intake.

Regarding epidemiological studies on health effects of protein intake independent of energy balance and overweight, these appear to report inconclusive results. It seems that consumption of red meat promotes the development of cardiovascular diseases, while consumption of vegetable protein such as nuts, low-fat dairy, poultry, or fish may be protective against cardiovascular diseases.

In conclusion, higher-protein diets may reduce cardiovascular disease risk by decreasing the susceptibility for the development of obesity. Results of epidemiological studies on health effects of protein intake independent of energy balance and overweight appear to be inconclusive.

ACKNOWLEDGMENT

Eveline Martens has received funding for her research described in this chapter from the European Union's Seventh Framework Programme for research, technological development and demonstration under grant agreement 266408.

REFERENCES

Acheson, K. J. 2013. Diets for body weight control and health: The potential of changing the macronutrient composition. *Eur J Clin Nutr* 67:462–466.

Acheson, K. J., A. Blondel-Lubrano, S. Oguey-Araymon, M. Beaumont, S. Emady-Azar, C. Ammon-Zufferey, I. Monnard, S. Pinaud, C. Nielsen-Moennoz, and L. Bovetto. 2011. Protein choices targeting thermogenesis and metabolism. *Am J Clin Nutr* 93:525–534.

Adechian, S., M. Balage, D. Remond, C. Migne, A. Quignard-Boulange, A. Marset-Baglieri, S. Rousset et al. 2012. Protein feeding pattern, casein feeding, or milk-soluble protein feeding did not change the evolution of body composition during a short-term weight loss program. *Am J Physiol Endocrinol Metab* 303:E973–E982.

Belza, A., C. Ritz, M. Q. Sorensen, J. J. Holst, J. F. Rehfeld, and A. Astrup. 2013. Contribution of gastroenteropancreatic appetite hormones to protein-induced satiety. *Am J Clin Nutr* 97:980–989.

Bendtsen, L. Q., J. K. Lorenzen, N. T. Bendsen, C. Rasmussen, and A. Astrup. 2013. Effect of dairy proteins on appetite, energy expenditure, body weight, and composition: A review of the evidence from controlled clinical trials. *Adv Nutr* 4:418–438.

Bernstein, A. M., A. Pan, K. M. Rexrode, M. Stampfer, F. B. Hu, D. Mozaffarian, and W. C. Willett. March 2012. Dietary protein sources and the risk of stroke in men and women. *Stroke* 43(3):637–644.

Boirie, Y., M. Dangin, P. Gachon, M. P. Vasson, J. L. Maubois, and B. Beaufrere. 1997. Slow and fast dietary proteins differently modulate postprandial protein accretion. *Proc Natl Acad Sci USA* 94:14930–14935.

Bonjour, J. P. 2005. Dietary protein: An essential nutrient for bone health. *J Am Coll Nutr* 24:526S–536S.

Born, J. M., M. J. Martens, S. G. Lemmens, R. Goebel, and M. S. Westerterp-Plantenga. 2013. Protein vs. carbohydrate intake differentially affects liking- and wanting-related brain signalling. *Br J Nutr* 109:376–381.

Bortolotti, M., R. Kreis, C. Debard, B. Cariou, D. Faeh, M. Chetiveaux, M. Ith et al. 2009. High protein intake reduces intrahepatocellular lipid deposition in humans. *Am J Clin Nutr* 90:1002–1010.

Bortolotti, M., E. Maiolo, M. Corazza, E. Van Dijke, P. Schneiter, A. Boss, G. Carrel et al. 2011. Effects of a whey protein supplementation on intrahepatocellular lipids in obese female patients. *Clin Nutr* 30:494–498.

Bowen, J., M. Noakes, C. Trenerry, and P. M. Clifton. 2006. Energy intake, ghrelin, and cholecystokinin after different carbohydrate and protein preloads in overweight men. *J Clin Endocrinol Metab* 91:1477–1483.

Bray, G. A., L. M. Redman, L. de Jonge, J. Covington, J. Rood, C. Brock, S. Mancuso, C. K. Martin, and S. R. Smith. 2015. Effect of protein overfeeding on energy expenditure measured in a metabolic chamber. *Am J Clin Nutr* 101:496–505.

Bray, G. A., S. R. Smith, L. de Jonge, H. Xie, J. Rood, C. K. Martin, M. Most, C. Brock, S. Mancuso, and L. M. Redman. 2012. Effect of dietary protein content on weight gain, energy expenditure, and body composition during overeating: A randomized controlled trial. *JAMA* 307:47–55.

Calvez, J., N. Poupin, C. Chesneau, C. Lassale, and D. Tome. 2012. Protein intake, calcium balance and health consequences. *Eur J Clin Nutr* 66:281–295.

Clifton, P. M. 2011. Protein and coronary heart disease: The role of different protein sources. *Curr Atheroscler Rep* 13:493–498.

Coleman, M. D. and S. M. Nickols-Richardson. 2005. Urinary ketones reflect serum ketone concentration but do not relate to weight loss in overweight premenopausal women following a low-carbohydrate/high-protein diet. *J Am Diet Assoc* 105:608–611.

Dallosso, H. M. and W. P. James. 1984. Whole-body calorimetry studies in adult men. 2. The interaction of exercise and over-feeding on the thermic effect of a meal. *Br J Nutr* 52:65–72.

Dangin, M., Y. Boirie, C. Garcia-Rodenas, P. Gachon, J. Fauquant, P. Callier, O. Ballevre, and B. Beaufrere. 2001. The digestion rate of protein is an independent regulating factor of postprandial protein retention. *Am J Physiol Endocrinol Metab* 280:E340–E348.

Davidenko, O., N. Darcel, G. Fromentin, and D. Tome. 2013. Control of protein and energy intake—Brain mechanisms. *Eur J Clin Nutr* 67:455–461.

Despres, J. P. and I. Lemieux. 2006. Abdominal obesity and metabolic syndrome. *Nature* 444:881–887.

Deutz, N. E. and R. R. Wolfe. 2013. Is there a maximal anabolic response to protein intake with a meal? *Clin Nutr* 32:309–313.

Dideriksen, K., S. Reitelseder, and L. Holm. 2013. Influence of amino acids, dietary protein, and physical activity on muscle mass development in humans. *Nutrients* 5:852–876.

Diepvens, K., D. Haberer, and M. Westerterp-Plantenga. 2008. Different proteins and biopeptides differently affect satiety and anorexigenic/orexigenic hormones in healthy humans. *Int J Obes* 32:510–518.

Fabbrini, E., F. Magkos, B. S. Mohammed, T. Pietka, N. A. Abumrad, B. W. Patterson, A. Okunade, and S. Klein. 2009. Intrahepatic fat, not visceral fat, is linked with metabolic complications of obesity. *Proc Natl Acad Sci USA* 106:15430–15435.

Flakoll, P. J., M. Kulaylat, M. Frexes-Steed, H. Hourani, L. L. Brown, J. O. Hill, and N. N. Abumrad. 1989. Amino acids augment insulin's suppression of whole body proteolysis. *Am J Phys* 257:E839–E847.

Flatt, J. P. 1978. The biochemistry of energy expenditure. *Rec Adv Obes Res* 2:211.

Fromentin, G., N. Darcel, C. Chaumontet, A. Marsset-Baglieri, N. Nadkarni, and D. Tome. 2012. Peripheral and central mechanisms involved in the control of food intake by dietary amino acids and proteins. *Nutr Res Rev* 25:29–39.

Gannon, M. C., J. A. Nuttall, G. Damberg, V. Gupta, and F. Q. Nuttall. 2001. Effect of protein ingestion on the glucose appearance rate in people with type 2 diabetes. *J Clin Endocrinol Metab* 86:1040–1047.

Garlick, P. J., M. A. McNurlan, and C. S. Patlak. 1999. Adaptation of protein metabolism in relation to limits to high dietary protein intake. *Eur J Clin Nutr* 53(Suppl 1):S34–S43.

Garrow, J. S. 1985. The contribution of protein synthesis to thermogenesis in man. *Int J Obes* 9(Suppl 2):97–101.

Gilbert, J. A., N. T. Bendsen, A. Tremblay, and A. Astrup. 2011. Effect of proteins from different sources on body composition. *Nutr Metab Cardiovasc Dis* 21(Suppl 2):B16–B31.

Gosby, A. K., A. D. Conigrave, N. S. Lau, M. A. Iglesias, R. M. Hall, S. A. Jebb, J. Brand-Miller, I. D. Caterson, D. Raubenheimer, and S. J. Simpson. 2011. Testing protein leverage in lean humans: A randomised controlled experimental study. *PLoS One* 6:e25929.

Greenhaff, P. L., L. G. Karagounis, N. Peirce, E. J. Simpson, M. Hazell, R. Layfield, H. Wackerhage et al. 2008. Disassociation between the effects of amino acids and insulin on signaling, ubiquitin ligases, and protein turnover in human muscle. *Am J Physiol Endocrinol Metab* 295:E595–E604.

Griffioen-Roose, S., M. Mars, E. Siebelink, G. Finlayson, D. Tome, and C. de Graaf. 2012. Protein status elicits compensatory changes in food intake and food preferences. *Am J Clin Nutr* 95:32–38.

Hall, W. L., D. J. Millward, S. J. Long, and L. M. Morgan. 2003. Casein and whey exert different effects on plasma amino acid profiles, gastrointestinal hormone secretion and appetite. *Br J Nutr* 89:239–248.

Halton, T. L. and F. B. Hu. 2004. The effects of high protein diets on thermogenesis, satiety and weight loss: A critical review. *J Am Coll Nutr* 23:373–385.

Haring, B., N. Gronroos, J. A. Nettleton, M. C. Wyler von Ballmoos, E. Selvin, and A. Alonso. 2014. Dietary protein intake and coronary heart disease in a large community based cohort: Results from the Atherosclerosis Risk in Communities (ARIC) Study. *PLoS One* 9(10):e109552. doi: 10.1371/journal.pone.0109552.

Harper, A. E. 1983. Some recent developments in the study of amino acid metabolism. *Proc Nutr Soc* 42:437–449.

Harper, A. E., R. H. Miller, and K. P. Block. 1984. Branched-chain amino acid metabolism. *Annu Rev Nutr* 4:409–454.

Hudgins, L. C., M. Hellerstein, C. Seidman, R. Neese, J. Diakun, and J. Hirsch. 1996. Human fatty acid synthesis is stimulated by a eucaloric low fat, high carbohydrate diet. *J Clin Invest* 97:2081–2091.

Hudgins, L. C., M. K. Hellerstein, C. E. Seidman, R. A. Neese, J. D. Tremaroli, and J. Hirsch. 2000. Relationship between carbohydrate-induced hypertriglyceridemia and fatty acid synthesis in lean and obese subjects. *J Lipid Res* 41:595–604.

Hursel, R., E. A. Martens, H. K. Gonnissen, H. M. Hamer, J. M. Senden, L. J. van Loon, and M. Westerterp-Plantenga. 2015. Prolonged adaptation to a low or high protein diet does not modulate basal muscle protein synthesis rates—A substudy. *PLoS One* 10(9):e0137183. doi.10.1371/journal.pone.0137183.

Johnston, C. S., S. L. Tjonn, P. D. Swan, A. White, H. Hutchins, and B. Sears. 2006. Ketogenic low-carbohydrate diets have no metabolic advantage over nonketogenic low-carbohydrate diets. *Am J Clin Nutr* 83:1055–1061.

Josse, A. R., S. A. Atkinson, M. A. Tarnopolsky, and S. M. Phillips. 2011. Increased consumption of dairy foods and protein during diet- and exercise-induced weight loss promotes fat mass loss and lean mass gain in overweight and obese premenopausal women. *J Nutr* 141:1626–1634.

Journel, M., C. Chaumontet, N. Darcel, G. Fromentin, and D. Tome. 2012. Brain responses to high-protein diets. *Adv Nutr* 3:322–329.

Juvonen, K. R., L. J. Karhunen, E. Vuori, M. E. Lille, T. Karhu, A. Jurado-Acosta, D. E. Laaksonen et al. 2011. Structure modification of a milk protein-based model food affects postprandial intestinal peptide release and fullness in healthy young men. *Br J Nutr* 106:1890–1898.

Karhunen, L. J., K. R. Juvonen, A. Huotari, A. K. Purhonen, and K. H. Herzig. 2008. Effect of protein, fat, carbohydrate and fibre on gastrointestinal peptide release in humans. *Regul Pept* 149:70–78.

Krebs, H. A. 1964. The metabolic fate of amino acids. In *Mammalian Protein Metabolism*, H. N. Munro and J. B. Allison, eds. New York: Academic Press.

Krieger, J. W., H. S. Sitren, M. J. Daniels, and B. Langkamp-Henken. 2006. Effects of variation in protein and carbohydrate intake on body mass and composition during energy restriction: A meta-regression 1. *Am J Clin Nutr* 83:260–274.

Laeger, T., C. C. Metges, and B. Kuhla. 2010. Role of beta-hydroxybutyric acid in the central regulation of energy balance. *Appetite* 54:450–455.

Larsen, T. M., S. M. Dalskov, M. van Baak, S. A. Jebb, A. Papadaki, A. F. Pfeiffer, J. A. Martinez et al. 2010. Diets with high or low protein content and glycemic index for weight-loss maintenance. *N Engl J Med* 363:2102–2113.

Leidy, H. J., C. L. Armstrong, M. Tang, R. D. Mattes, and W. W. Campbell. 2010. The influence of higher protein intake and greater eating frequency on appetite control in overweight and obese men. *Obesity (Silver Spring)* 18:1725–1732.

Leidy, H. J., P. M. Clifton, A. Astrup, T. P. Wycherley, M. S. Westerterp-Plantenga, N. D. Luscombe-Marsh, S. C. Woods, and R. D. Mattes. 2015. The role of protein in weight loss and maintenance. Symposium Proceedings. Invited Review. Paper read at American Journal of Clinical Nutrition. *Am J Clin Nutr* 101:13205–13295.

Leidy, H. J., L. C. Ortinau, S. M. Douglas, and H. A. Hoertel. 2013. Beneficial effects of a higher-protein breakfast on the appetitive, hormonal, and neural signals controlling energy intake regulation in overweight/obese, "breakfast-skipping," late-adolescent girls. *Am J Clin Nutr* 97:677–688.

Lejeune, M. P., K. R. Westerterp, T. C. Adam, N. D. Luscombe-Marsh, and M. S. Westerterp-Plantenga. 2006. Ghrelin and glucagon-like peptide 1 concentrations, 24-h satiety, and energy and substrate metabolism during a high-protein diet and measured in a respiration chamber. *Am J Clin Nutr* 83:89–94.

Lemmens, S. G., E. A. Martens, J. M. Born, M. J. Martens, and M. S. Westerterp-Plantenga. 2011. Lack of effect of high-protein vs. high-carbohydrate meal intake on stress-related mood and eating behavior. *Nutr J* 10:136.

Lettner, A. and M. Roden. 2008. Ectopic fat and insulin resistance. *Curr Diab Rep* 8:185–191.

Lorenzen, J., R. Frederiksen, C. Hoppe, R. Hvid, and A. Astrup. 2012. The effect of milk proteins on appetite regulation and diet-induced thermogenesis. *Eur J Clin Nutr* 66:622–627.

Louard, R. J., E. J. Barrett, and R. A. Gelfand. 1995. Overnight branched-chain amino acid infusion causes sustained suppression of muscle proteolysis. *Metabolism* 44:424–429.

Luscombe, N. D., P. M. Clifton, M. Noakes, E. Farnsworth, and G. Wittert. 2003. Effect of a high-protein, energy-restricted diet on weight loss and energy expenditure after weight stabilization in hyperinsulinemic subjects. *Int J Obes Relat Metab Disord* 27:582–590.

Maersk, M., A. Belza, J. J. Holst, M. Fenger-Gron, S. B. Pedersen, A. Astrup, and B. Richelsen. 2012. Satiety scores and satiety hormone response after sucrose-sweetened soft drink compared with isocaloric semi-skimmed milk and with non-caloric soft drink: A controlled trial. *Eur J Clin Nutr* 66:523–529.

Magkos, F., E. Fabbrini, B. S. Mohammed, B. W. Patterson, and S. Klein. 2010. Increased whole-body adiposity without a concomitant increase in liver fat is not associated with augmented metabolic dysfunction. *Obesity (Silver Spring)* 18:1510–1515.

Martens, E. A., B. Gatta-Cherifi, H. K. Gonnissen, and M. S. Westerterp-Plantenga. October 16, 2014a. The potential of a high protein-low carbohydrate diet to preserve intrahepatic triglyceride content in healthy humans. *PLoS One* 9(10):e109617. doi: 10.1371/journal.pone.0109617.

Martens, E. A., H. K. Gonnissen, B. Gatta-Cherifi, P. L. Janssens, and M. S. Westerterp-Plantenga. November 8, 2014b. Maintenance of energy expenditure on high-protein vs. high-carbohydrate diets at a constant body weight may prevent a positive energy balance. *Clin Nutr* 34(5):968–975. doi: 10.1016/j.clnu.2014.10.007.

Martens, E. A., S. G. Lemmens, and M. S. Westerterp-Plantenga. 2013. Protein leverage affects energy intake of high-protein diets in humans. *Am J Clin Nutr* 97:86–93.

Martens, E. A., S. Y. Tan, M. V. Dunlop, R. D. Mattes, and M. S. Westerterp-Plantenga. 2014c. Protein leverage effects of beef protein on energy intake in humans. *Am J Clin Nutr* 99:1397–1406.

Martens, E. A. and M. S. Westerterp-Plantenga. 2014. Protein diets, body weight loss and weight maintenance. *Curr Opin Clin Nutr Metab Care* 17:75–79.

Mellinkoff, S. M., M. Frankland, D. Boyle, and M. Greipel. 1956. Relationship between serum amino acid concentration and fluctuations in appetite. *J Appl Physiol* 8:535–538.

Mikkelsen, P. B., S. Toubro, and A. Astrup. 2000. Effect of fat-reduced diets on 24-h energy expenditure: Comparisons between animal protein, vegetable protein, and carbohydrate. *Am J Clin Nutr* 72:1135–1141.

Millward, D. J. 2003. An adaptive metabolic demand model for protein and amino acid requirements. *Br J Nutr* 90:249–260.

Millward, D. J. 2012a. Identifying recommended dietary allowances for protein and amino acids: A critique of the 2007 WHO/FAO/UNU report. *Br J Nutr* 108(Suppl 2):S3–S21.

Millward, D. J. 2012b. Knowledge gained from studies of leucine consumption in animals and humans. *J Nutr* 142:2212S–2219S.

Morrison, C. D., S. D. Reed, and T. M. Henagan. 2012. Homeostatic regulation of protein intake: In search of a mechanism. *Am J Physiol Regul Integr Comp Physiol* 302:R917–R928.

Moughan, P. J. 2012. Dietary protein for human health. *Br J Nutr* 108(Suppl 2):S1–S2.

Munro, H. N. 1964. *General Aspects of the Regulation of Protein Metabolism by Hormones*. New York: Academic Press.

Niijima, A., K. Torii, and H. Uneyama. 2005. Role played by vagal chemical sensors in the hepato-portal region and duodeno-intestinal canal: An electrophysiological study. *Chem Senses* 30:I178–I179.

Pal, S., S. Radavelli-Bagatini, M. Hagger, and V. Ellis. 2014. Comparative effects of whey and casein proteins on satiety in overweight and obese individuals: A randomized controlled trial. *Eur J Clin Nutr* 68:980–986.

Pannemans, D. L., D. Halliday, K. R. Westerterp, and A. D. Kester. 1995. Effect of variable protein intake on whole-body protein turnover in young men and women. *Am J Clin Nutr* 61:69–74.

Pedersen, A. N., J. Kondrup, and E. Børsheim. 2013. Health effects of protein intake in healthy adults: A systematic literature review. *Food Nutr Res* 57:21245.

Price, G. M., D. Halliday, P. J. Pacy, M. R. Quevedo, and D. J. Millward. 1994. Nitrogen homeostasis in man: Influence of protein intake on the amplitude of diurnal cycling of body nitrogen. *Clin Sci (Lond)* 86:91–102.

Raubenheimer, D. and S. J. Simpson. 1997. Integrative models of nutrient balancing: Application to insects and vertebrates. *Nutr Res Rev* 10:151–179.

Scharrer, E. 1999. Control of food intake by fatty acid oxidation and ketogenesis. *Nutrition* 15:704–714.

Schwarz, J. M., R. A. Neese, S. Turner, D. Dare, and M. K. Hellerstein. 1995. Short-term alterations in carbohydrate energy intake in humans. Striking effects on hepatic glucose production, de novo lipogenesis, lipolysis, and whole-body fuel selection. *J Clin Invest* 96:2735–2743.

Shariatmadari, F. and J. M. Forbes. 1993. Growth and food intake responses to diets of different protein contents and a choice between diets containing two concentrations of protein in broiler and layer strains of chicken. *Br Poult Sci* 34:959–970.

Simpson, S. J. and D. Raubenheimer. 1997. Geometric analysis of macronutrient selection in the rat. *Appetite* 28:201–213.

Simpson, S. J. and D. Raubenheimer. 2005. Obesity: The protein leverage hypothesis. *Obes Rev* 6:133–142, Figure 5 The protein leverage effect, p. 138.

Soenen, S., A. G. Bonomi, S. G. Lemmens, J. Scholte, M. A. Thijssen, F. van Berkum, and M. S. Westerterp-Plantenga. 2012. Relatively high-protein or 'low-carb' energy-restricted diets for body weight loss and body weight maintenance? *Physiol Behav* 107:374–380.

Soenen, S., E. A. Martens, A. Hochstenbach-Waelen, S. G. Lemmens, and M. S. Westerterp-Plantenga. 2013. Normal protein intake is required for body weight loss and weight maintenance, and elevated protein intake for additional preservation of resting energy expenditure and fat free mass. *J Nutr* 143:591–596.

Soenen, S., G. Plasqui, A. J. Smeets, and M. S. Westerterp-Plantenga. 2010. Protein intake induced an increase in exercise stimulated fat oxidation during stable body weight. *Physiol Behav* 101:770–774.

Sorensen, A., D. Mayntz, D. Raubenheimer, and S. J. Simpson. 2008. Protein-leverage in mice: The geometry of macronutrient balancing and consequences for fat deposition. *Obesity (Silver Spring)* 16:566–571.

Symons, T. B., M. Sheffield-Moore, R. R. Wolfe, and D. Paddon-Jones. 2009. A moderate serving of high-quality protein maximally stimulates skeletal muscle protein synthesis in young and elderly subjects. *J Am Diet Assoc* 109:1582–1586.

Tang, J. E. and S. M. Phillips. 2009. Maximizing muscle protein anabolism: The role of protein quality. *Curr Opin Clin Nutr Metab Care* 12:66–71.

Tews, J. K., J. J. Repa, and A. E. Harper. 1992. Protein selection by rats adapted to high or moderately low levels of dietary protein. *Physiol Behav* 51:699–712.

Theall, C. L., J. J. Wurtman, and R. J. Wurtman. 1984. Self-selection and regulation of protein:carbohydrate ratio in foods adult rats eat. *J Nutr* 114:711–718.

Theytaz, F., Y. Noguchi, L. Egli, V. Campos, T. Buehler, L. Hodson, B. W. Patterson et al. 2012. Effects of supplementation with essential amino acids on intrahepatic lipid concentrations during fructose overfeeding in humans. *Am J Clin Nutr* 96:1008–1016.

Tome, D. 2012. Criteria and markers for protein quality assessment—A review. *Br J Nutr* 108(Suppl 2): S222–S229.

Tome, D. and C. Bos. 2000. Dietary protein and nitrogen utilization. *J Nutr* 130:1868S–1873S.

Torres, N. and A. R. Tovar. 2007. The role of dietary protein on lipotoxicity. *Nutr Rev* 65:S64–S68.

van Loon, L. J. 2012. Leucine as a pharmaconutrient in health and disease. *Curr Opin Clin Nutr Metab Care* 15:71–77.

Veldhorst, M. A., A. G. Nieuwenhuizen, A. Hochstenbach-Waelen, A. J. van Vught, K. R. Westerterp, M. P. Engelen, R. J. Brummer, N. E. Deutz, and M. S. Westerterp-Plantenga. 2009a. Dose-dependent satiating effect of whey relative to casein or soy. *Physiol Behav* 96:675–682.

Veldhorst, M. A., A. G. Nieuwenhuizen, A. Hochstenbach-Waelen, K. R. Westerterp, M. P. Engelen, R. J. Brummer, N. E. Deutz, and M. S. Westerterp-Plantenga. 2009b. Comparison of the effects of a high- and normal-casein breakfast on satiety, 'satiety' hormones, plasma amino acids and subsequent energy intake. *Br J Nutr* 101:295–303.

Veldhorst, M. A., K. R. Westerterp, A. J. van Vught, and M. S. Westerterp-Plantenga. 2010. Presence or absence of carbohydrates and the proportion of fat in a high-protein diet affect appetite suppression but not energy expenditure in normal-weight human subjects fed in energy balance. *Br J Nutr* 104:1395–1405.

Veldhorst, M. A., M. S. Westerterp-Plantenga, and K. R. Westerterp. 2009c. Gluconeogenesis and energy expenditure after a high-protein, carbohydrate-free diet. *Am J Clin Nutr* 90:519–526.

Veldhorst, M. A. B., A. G. Nieuwenhuizen, A. Hochstenbach-Waelen, K. R. Westerterp, M. P. K. J. Engelen, R. J. M. Brummer, N. E. P. Deutz, and M. S. Westerterp-Plantenga. 2009d. Effects of high and normal soy protein breakfasts on satiety and subsequent energy intake, including amino acid and 'satiety' hormone responses. *Eur J Nutr* 48:92–100.

Watanabe, M., S. M. Houten, L. Wang, A. Moschetta, D. J. Mangelsdorf, R. A. Heyman, D. D. Moore, and J. Auwerx. 2004. Bile acids lower triglyceride levels via a pathway involving FXR, SHP, and SREBP-1c. *J Clin Invest* 113:1408–1418.

Weigle, D. S., P. A. Breen, C. C. Matthys, H. S. Callahan, K. E. Meeuws, V. R. Burden, and J. Q. Purnell. 2005. A high-protein diet induces sustained reductions in appetite, ad libitum caloric intake, and body weight despite compensatory changes in diurnal plasma leptin and ghrelin concentrations. *Am J Clin Nutr* 82:41–48.

Westerterp, K. R. 2002. Weight loss and bone mineral content. *Obes Res* 10:559.

Westerterp, K. R. 2013. *Energy Balance in Motion.* New York: Springer.

Westerterp, K. R., S. A. Wilson, and V. Rolland. 1999. Diet induced thermogenesis measured over 24 h in a respiration chamber: Effect of diet composition. *Int J Obes Relat Metab Disord* 23:287–292.

Westerterp-Plantenga, M. S., S. G. Lemmens, and K. R. Westerterp. 2012. Dietary protein—Its role in satiety, energetics, weight loss and health. *Br J Nutr* 108(Suppl 2):S105–S112.

Westerterp-Plantenga, M. S., N. Luscombe-Marsh, M. P. G. M. Lejeune, K. Diepvens, A. Nieuwenhuizen, M. P. K. J. Engelen, N. E. P. Deutz, D. Azzout-Marniche, D. Tome, and K. R. Westerterp. 2006. Dietary protein, metabolism, and body-weight regulation: Dose–response effects. *Int J Obes* 30:S16–S23.

Westerterp-Plantenga, M. S., A. Nieuwenhuizen, D. Tome, S. Soenen, and K. R. Westerterp. 2009. Dietary protein, weight loss, and weight maintenance. *Annu Rev Nutr* 29:21–41.

Westerterp-Plantenga, M. S., V. Rolland, S. A. Wilson, and K. R. Westerterp. 1999a. Satiety related to 24 h diet-induced thermogenesis during high protein/carbohydrate vs high fat diets measured in a respiration chamber. *Eur J Clin Nutr* 53:495–502.

Westerterp-Plantenga, M. S., K. R. Westerterp, M. Rubbens, and J.-P. Richalet. 1999b. Appetite at 'high altitude' [operation Everest III (Comex-'97)]: A simulated ascent of the Mount Everest. *J Appl Physiol* 87:391–399.

Whitehead, J. M., G. McNeill, and J. S. Smith. 1996. The effect of protein intake on 24-h energy expenditure during energy restriction. *Int J Obes Relat Metab Disord* 20:727–732.

WHO/FAO/UNU. 2007. Protein and amino acid requirements in human nutrition. Report of a Joint WHO/FAO/UNU Expert Consultation. WHO Technical Report Series No 935, Geneva, Switzerland.

Wycherley, T. P., L. J. Moran, P. M. Clifton, M. Noakes, and G. D. Brinkworth. 2012. Effects of energy-restricted high-protein, low-fat compared with standard-protein, low-fat diets: A meta-analysis of randomized controlled trials. *Am J Clin Nutr* 96:1281–1298.

18 A Protein-Centric Perspective for Skeletal Muscle Metabolism and Cardiometabolic Health

Donald K. Layman

CONTENTS

ABSTRACT

High-protein diets have been shown to be beneficial for cardiometabolic health; however, the specific effects of dietary protein are often confounded by parallel changes in energy or carbohydrate intakes. In general, energy-restricted diets with higher protein and reduced carbohydrates produce a greater loss of body weight and body fat while minimizing the loss of lean tissues and lead to improvements in glycemic regulations and dyslipidemia. Specific roles of protein in cardiometabolic health may be most evident by focusing on amino acid metabolism in skeletal muscle. Research studies in areas of obesity and weight loss, aging and sarcopenia, and exercise physiology have cast new light on dietary protein needs and challenged the existing dietary guidelines as inadequate for long-term muscle health. These studies have identified a meal-based protein requirement, in large part, associated with the unique roles of the essential amino acid leucine in the regulation of skeletal muscle protein synthesis and energy metabolism. Postmeal increases in intracellular leucine concentrations initiate a signaling cascade that triggers muscle protein synthesis and increases fatty acid oxidation. These changes in muscle metabolism appear to explain the metabolic advantages of dietary protein including protecting calorie-burning muscle tissue, increasing energy expenditure characterized as diet-induced thermogenesis, and partitioning of weight loss to body fat. This review will evaluate the meal-based protein-centric needs for skeletal muscle metabolism and their relationship to cardiometabolic health.

ABBREVIATIONS

BCAA	Branched-chain amino acids
BCKAD	Branched-chain ketoacid dehydrogenase
EAA	Essential amino acids
mPS	Muscle protein synthesis
mTORC1	Mechanistic target of rapamycin complex 1
RDA	Recommended Dietary Allowance

INTRODUCTION

Cardiometabolic disorders express a cluster of metabolic and physiological risk factors including elevated body fat, abnormal blood triglycerides, and insulin resistance (Grundy et al., 2004). This cluster of factors was originally termed "syndrome X" or the "metabolic syndrome." Subsequent research questioned if the *metabolic syndrome* was fundamentally a lipid disorder, dysfunction of glycemic regulations, a consequence of obesity, or declining function of skeletal muscle (Reaven, 1996). These questions led to nutrition studies testing an array of diet combinations with higher or lower amounts of fat, carbohydrates, and protein. Diets that reduce energy intake with higher protein and lower carbohydrates have been shown to be beneficial for cardiometabolic health (Layman et al., 2008). These diets produce a greater loss of body weight and body fat while minimizing the loss of lean tissues and lead to improvements in glycemic regulations and dyslipidemia (Krieger et al., 2006; Wycherley et al., 2012). In total, higher-protein diets appear to reverse many of the risk factors associated with the *metabolic syndrome*. While the outcomes of these diets appear beneficial, defining the specific role of protein is often confounded by changes in total energy and carbohydrates.

The role of protein in cardiometabolic health can be viewed from different perspectives. Protein can be viewed simply as a macronutrient competing with carbohydrates or fats as a source of calories. Compared with carbohydrates or fats, protein provides greater satiety to reduce food intake and produces greater thermogenesis to increase energy expenditure (Westerterp-Plantenga et al., 2006). While these changes in energy balance are consistent with greater weight loss, changes in satiety and diet-induced thermogenesis do not fully explain the differences in body composition or glycemic regulations observed with higher-protein diets. Evaluating the role of protein in cardiometabolic health requires going beyond the generic role of protein as a macronutrient to considering molecular roles of individual amino acids and particularly roles in metabolic regulation within skeletal muscles.

The importance of skeletal muscle and physical activity to cardiometabolic health is well accepted. Physical activity is a standard recommendation for all cardiometabolic disorders including obesity, the *metabolic syndrome*, type 2 diabetes, and cardiovascular diseases (Klein et al., 2004; Lee et al., 2005; American Diabetes Association, 2006). Routine exercise impacts energy expenditure, glucose homeostasis, insulin sensitivity, lipid metabolism, mitochondrial function, and body composition. Exercise alters skeletal muscle metabolism by changing total energy consumption and the fuel balance of carbohydrates and fats and producing changes in both blood lipids and insulin sensitivity. Further, age-related losses of muscle mass, strength, and metabolic functions are significant risk factors for cardiometabolic disease and associated with increased morbidity and mortality (Wolfe, 2006). Much less appreciated is that changing the dietary amount of protein and the ratio of protein and carbohydrates produces similar metabolic effects on skeletal muscle as exercise. This perspective might be considered a "protein-centric" view of metabolism recognizing specific roles of dietary protein in skeletal muscle health (Layman et al., 2015).

The relationship of dietary protein to skeletal muscle mass and function is not a new concept. Athletes and trainers routinely emphasize protein for muscle performance with long-held beliefs that greater protein intake leads to greater muscle mass and performance. While many athletes overconsume protein (Phillips, 2006), there is mounting evidence that the current Recommended Dietary Allowance (RDA) of 0.8 g of protein/kg body weight/day is not adequate to optimize muscle development, repair, and remodeling (Burd et al., 2008). Likewise, there is a consensus developing that the current RDA is not adequate to maintain adult muscle health (Bauer et al., 2013). This chapter focuses on the relationships of protein and skeletal muscle to cardiometabolic health. The research will be reviewed in three areas: (1) weight management and obesity, (2) sarcopenia, and (3) amino acid regulation of muscle metabolism. These diverse areas of research are providing new perspectives about optimum daily protein needs for adult health with the focus shifting from minimum daily protein intake to the optimum amount and distribution of protein at individual meals.

PROTEIN, WEIGHT LOSS, AND MUSCLE MASS

The initial evidence linking higher-protein diets to body composition and muscle mass appeared in the 1970s with acute weight loss studies (Flatt and Blackburn, 1974; Bistrain et al., 1977). During extreme energy restrictions such as fasting or very-low-calorie diets (<900 kcal/day), the body is forced to modify the balance of metabolic fuels. In a typical American diet, carbohydrates provide ~50% of energy and >1200 kcal/day. When total energy and dietary carbohydrates are restricted, the body shifts toward the use of stored fats. In addition, lean tissues are degraded to maintain a constant supply of amino acids for hepatic gluconeogenesis to maintain blood glucose and for the synthesis of essential proteins for plasma and organs. This early research with very-low-calorie diets demonstrated that providing a diet enriched in high-quality proteins produced a "protein-sparing" effect by minimizing the degradation of lean tissues and reducing nitrogen loss. Researchers found that protein intakes of 1.5 g/kg/day could produce net protein gains even during extreme energy restriction.

During the 1990s, a carbohydrate-centric view of protein emerged with popular weight loss diets including the Atkins diet (Atkins, 1992), the Zone diet (Sears, 1999), and the *carbohydrate addict's* diet (Heller and Heller, 1993). These diets all trumpeted the dangers of excess carbohydrates and chronic hyperinsulinemia as major contributors to the onset of obesity, heart disease, and type 2 diabetes; and authors recommended replacing dietary carbohydrates with protein and/or fat. These diets were characterized as *high*-protein diets, but protein was generally only high as a percentage of calories. Dietary protein expressed as percentage of energy increases by default as carbohydrate intake is reduced. Most of these diets were moderate in the absolute amount of daily protein consumed, ranging from about 1.0 to 1.5 g/kg body weight or about 80 to 130 g/day. These diets were typically effective for short-term weight loss, but long-term efficacy was equivocal (Foster et al., 2003).

Since the late 1990s, there have been numerous well-controlled weight loss studies using higher-protein diets. Diets with protein >1.4 g/kg/day produce greater weight loss and improve body composition by protecting lean body mass and partitioning energy loss to body fat. Many of these studies have been summarized in two meta-analyses (Krieger et al., 2006; Wycherley et al., 2012). Krieger et al. (2006) evaluated 87 weight loss studies examining the substitution of protein for carbohydrates in reduced-energy diets. They found that diets with carbohydrates reduced below ~40% of energy and protein above 1.05 g/kg/day produced greater reductions of body mass, fat mass, and fat as a percentage of body weight and attenuated loss of fat-free mass. Wycherley et al. (2012) extended these findings to weight loss studies that also included measurements of blood lipids, glucose, and blood pressure. They reported that higher-protein diets increased the loss of body weight and body fat and reduced serum triglycerides and blood pressure while mitigating reductions in fat-free mass and resting energy expenditure.

While the majority of weight loss studies support the use of higher-protein diets, some randomized controlled trials report no differences in weight loss or body composition comparing diets with different macronutrient compositions (Dansigner et al., 2005; Sacks et al., 2009). These investigators concluded that the critical factor in weight loss is the caloric deficit created by the diet, and the macronutrient ratios are relatively unimportant. However, on further inspection of these studies, a confounding factor was often poor diet compliance. In large clinical trials, precise diet monitoring is impossible and producing sustained lifestyle changes is difficult. Subjects tend to relapse toward preexisting diet behaviors (Foster et al., 2003; Dansigner et al., 2005).

While diet acceptance is an important issue in evaluating diet merits, poor compliance obscures the fundamental question about the efficacy of a diet.

In total, research studies provide evidence that higher-protein diets provide metabolic advantages over high-carbohydrate diets for weight loss, but negative perceptions hinder the acceptance of these diets (St. Jeor et al., 2001). As a macronutrient, protein provides 4 kcal/g, making it equal to carbohydrates, but protein-rich foods are often energy dense, containing high amounts of cholesterol and saturated fat. Further, protein produces ammonia and urea still considered by some to be a health risk. From an energy perspective, the perceived risks of protein or protein-rich foods combined with survey data showing that Americans typically consume protein in excess of the RDA temper enthusiasm for higher-protein diets. In total, protein is often viewed as an expensive and inefficient form of calories.

Carbohydrate-centric and fat-phobic perspectives have been in*grain*ed in the U.S. Dietary Guidelines for over 50 years. Since the late 1960s, the major nutrition-related health concern for Americans has been heart disease, and U.S. nutrition policy was formulated largely around using carbohydrates to reduce the consumption of cholesterol and saturated fat (USDA, 2005). Protein was not considered to be a nutrient at risk and was downplayed in dietary guidelines. The most visual example of this policy was the iconic *food guide pyramid* emphasizing avoiding fat and specifically animal products containing cholesterol and saturated fat and increasing consumption of grains. These nutrition guidelines resulted in a reduced consumption of milk, eggs, and red meat by 31%, 30%, and 21%, respectively, from 1970 to 2000 (USDA, 2003). In place of these protein-rich foods, Americans increased consumption of grains, plant oils, and potatoes by 40%, 56%, and 62%. Coincident with these dietary changes were dramatic increases in obesity and cardiometabolic disorders. In 2010, the Dietary Guidelines Advisory Committee established by the USDA and NIH attempted to define the diet changes associated with the obesity epidemic and found that beginning in the 1980s Americans increased daily energy consumption by over 350 kcal, and the top six food categories accounting for the excess calories were grain-based desserts and snacks, yeast breads, pizza, pasta, breaded chicken products, and sugar-sweetened soda and sports drinks (USDA-HHS, 2010). Based on these findings, the USDA discontinued the use of the *food guide pyramid* and shifted nutrition policy to *MyPlate* emphasizing vegetables and protein (including dairy) as the foundation of a healthy diet.

DEVELOPING AN AMINO ACID PERSPECTIVE ABOUT CARDIOMETABOLIC HEALTH

The protein-centric perspective shifts the focus from a global view of protein as simply a macronutrient similar to carbohydrates and fat to a molecular focus that recognizes the individual roles of each of the 20 amino acids. Each amino acid has at least two important roles, one in protein synthesis as a building block for new proteins and a second in the creation of new biomolecules and/or metabolic signals (Wu, 2013). A few examples of *secondary* roles of amino acids include tryptophan for synthesis of serotonin, arginine for synthesis of creatine, cysteine for synthesis of glutathione, and lysine for synthesis of carnitine, and signal molecules include histidine for stimulation of GCN2 in the integrated stress response, arginine for nitric oxide and vascular function, and leucine for the activation of the mTORC1 signal cascade for stimulation of muscle protein synthesis (mPS). The leucine signal has received extensive attention because of its role in stimulating mPS and has become a principal factor in defining optimal dietary protein intake (Layman, 2003; Layman et al., 2015).

These diverse roles of amino acids are dependent upon intracellular concentrations and, as might be expected, are optimized at different dietary intakes. In the hierarchy of metabolic roles, the fundamental role of amino acids as building blocks for new proteins appears to be satisfied first and equates with the estimated average requirement. Additional roles of amino acids appear to be more dependent on increases in intracellular concentrations of respective amino acids. The relationship of the metabolic response to the intracellular concentration highlights the importance of the protein content of individual meals. If the intracellular concentration of a specific amino acid does not increase after a meal, the metabolic pathway or signal cascade is minimized. The protein-centric perspective emphasizes the quantity, quality, and meal distribution of protein to optimize these metabolic signals and related health outcomes.

OPTIMIZING MEAL PATTERN OF PROTEIN FOR BODY COMPOSITION AND SARCOPENIA

The fourth decade of life often marks a detectable age-related loss of muscle mass and strength known as sarcopenia (Stenholm et al., 2008). The decline in muscle mass and strength leads to the loss of mobility, increased likelihood of falls and injury, reduced glucose tolerance, and increased risk for obesity (Rosenberg, 1997). Factors contributing to sarcopenia remain to be fully elucidated. Declining physical activity certainly contributes, but there is also a progressive decline in the mPS response to dietary protein. Skeletal muscle slowly becomes more refractory to anabolic stimulus, a condition described as "anabolic resistance" (Cuthbertson et al., 2005; Rennie and Wilkes, 2005).

Maintaining muscle health requires continuous repair and remodeling of muscle structures and enzymes dependent on continuous synthesis and breakdown of muscle proteins (Burd et al., 2008). The balance between synthesis and breakdown is an oscillating pattern with anabolic periods occurring after meals and catabolic periods during postabsorptive times. The anabolic periods after meals are driven by a rapid stimulation of protein synthesis with small changes in protein breakdown. The catabolic period between meals occurs with a decline in protein synthesis, while protein breakdown is maintained at higher rates. The net balance between the anabolic and catabolic periods determines changes in muscle mass; and there is general consensus that the postmeal anabolic periods are the dominant factor. This perspective shifts the focus of dietary protein requirements from the current recommendations based on total protein per day to a focus on the meal distribution of protein.

Historically, protein requirements have been viewed as the minimum amount of dietary protein per day necessary to achieve efficient growth or prevent deficiencies. For adults, growth is not relevant and acute deficiencies are rare. Instead, adult protein requirements are based on an Estimated Average Requirement defined as the minimum amount of protein necessary to achieve nitrogen balance (Institute of Medicine, 2002). Nitrogen balance studies to determine the Estimated Average Requirement have been performed mostly in young healthy adults with short-term controlled feeding conditions. Protein intakes above that required for nitrogen balance have been viewed as unnecessary and possibly unsafe. While nitrogen balance is the conventional approach to define minimum protein requirements, it has no clear relationship to any health outcomes. Further, using the Estimated Average Requirement as the dietary guideline assumes that amino acid metabolism beyond minimum nitrogen balance provides no metabolic advantage and should be avoided. Nitrogen balance methods are widely criticized for underestimating optimal amino acid needs (Elango et al., 2008; Millward et al., 2008; Wolfe and Miller, 2008). Emphasis on adult health is shifting attention from simple nitrogen balance to functional health outcomes related to skeletal muscle mass, metabolic function, and physical performance.

Mechanisms to explain anabolic resistance and net loss of muscle mass during aging remain unclear, but likely include changes in capillary blood flow, reduced membrane transport of essential nutrients, and reduced anabolic signaling for the initiation of mPS (Cuthbertson et al., 2005; Fry et al., 2011; Wall et al., 2014). Research from Volpi et al. (1999) demonstrates that anabolic resistance originates from changes in protein synthesis (translation) versus defects in gene expression (transcription). In a series of studies, these researchers found that mPS responds similarly in older (>60 years) and younger (<25 years) adults given a large bolus of essential amino acids (EAA, 18 g). However, when subjects were given only 7 g of EAA, mPS was stimulated in the young but not in older adults. These studies demonstrated that older adults maintain similar mPS capacity if adequate amino acids are available. Subsequent studies examined the effects of individual EAA. They found that the amino acid leucine had a unique ability to overcome the anabolic resistance in older adults (Volpi et al., 2000, 2003). In a seminal study, subjects consumed a drink containing 6.7 g of EAA with leucine accounting for 26% (1.75 g) of the total EAA. The EAA and leucine contents of the test meal represent the EAA content of a 15 g whey protein meal. This EAA drink produced a normal postmeal mPS response in young adults, but no response in older adults. Then the investigators modified the drink by substituting additional leucine for equal amounts of the other EAA to enrich the formula to 41% leucine (2.75 g). The leucine-enriched formula stimulated mPS similarly in young and older subjects demonstrating that leucine was the critical EAA limiting the anabolic response in older adults (Katsanos et al., 2006).

These investigators also examined supplementing the amino acid test meal with 40 g of glucose. As expected, the glucose supplement increased plasma insulin. The glucose supplement also increased mPS in young adults but inhibited mPS in the older adults (Volpi et al., 2000). This negative effect of glucose (or insulin) was confirmed in a subsequent study (Guillet et al., 2004). Insulin is now thought to function in a permissive but not regulatory role in older adults. These findings demonstrate that high-carbohydrate diets may have differential effects on adults depending on age with insulin producing an anabolic response in young adults but contributing to anabolic resistance and reduced mPS in older adults (Volpi et al., 2000). The differential effects of glucose and/or insulin on mPS in young versus older adults have not been extensively studied. Preliminary studies indicate that older adults exhibit reduced insulin-induced blood flow reducing amino acid delivery to muscles (Rasmussen et al., 2006) and reduced signaling at mTORC1 (Cuthbertson et al., 2005) consistent with the negative effects of hyperinsulinemia (Gual et al., 2005).

Consistent with studies using free EAA, Pennings et al. (2012) reported that the mPS response for older adults was greater after a meal containing 40 g of whey protein compared with 20 or 10 g meals. In most proteins, EAA account for ~50% of total amino acid content, such that the 40 g whey meal provides ~20 g of EAA. These investigators found that the 10 g meal produced no response in mPS compared with the fasted baseline, while 20 g produced an anabolic response equal to approximately one-half of the 40 g meal. Whey protein was used in these studies because it is highly water soluble, rapidly digested, and particularly high in leucine accounting for ~11% of the total amino acids. The three whey protein meals provided approximately 4.4, 2.2, and 1.1 g of leucine, respectively.

Yang et al. (2012) extended these findings by examining the interaction of dietary protein with exercise. In a sedentary control group, they found that 40 g of whey protein increased myofibrillar protein synthesis more than 20 g, and 10 g was not different from the fasted baseline. Using the same protein meals, they found that the rate of mPS was significantly higher after each of the protein meals if subjects completed a bout of resistance exercise before the meal. The synergy of protein with exercise appeared to lower the threshold of protein required to stimulate mPS such that adults consuming 20 g of whey protein after resistance exercise produced a similar anabolic response in mPS as sedentary adults consuming the 40 g meal. These studies help define the meal threshold for protein and demonstrate that resistance exercise can reduce anabolic resistance and lower the threshold for older adults.

The meal perspective for muscle health is becoming well recognized (Paddon-Jones and Rasmussen, 2009; Layman et al., 2015). A recent international study group concluded that older adults require more protein than younger adults to maintain function and health and to offset catabolic conditions and disease risk associated with aging (Bauer et al., 2013). They recommended that daily protein should be increased at least to a range of 1.0–1.2 g/kg body weight with protein distributed in meals containing at least 30 g of protein and providing at least 2.5 g of leucine. These recommendations received additional support from a study by Mamerow et al. (2014) demonstrating that subjects consuming 90 g/day of protein had higher net daily mPS if the protein was distributed in three 30 g meals versus an unbalanced distribution with meals containing 11, 16, and 63 g, respectively.

LEUCINE DEFINING A MEAL THRESHOLD FOR DIETARY PROTEIN

Metabolic pathways for the three branched-chain amino acids (BCAA), leucine, valine, and isoleucine, have been studied extensively since the 1970s when researchers discovered that BCAA, unlike other amino acids, were not degraded in the liver, but were predominately metabolized in skeletal muscle, and that leucine had a unique role in stimulating mPS (Buse and Reid, 1975; Fulks et al., 1975; Harper et al., 1984). These discoveries served to focus attention on leucine in the relationship between dietary protein and muscle mass and led to the development of a meal threshold theory.

Equally important, the mPS response to leucine appears to contribute to the metabolic advantage of dietary protein to increase thermogenesis, increase fat utilization, and improve body composition.

The unique roles of leucine are, at least in part, associated with the absence of the branched-chain aminotransferase enzyme in liver, resulting in an enriched supply of the BCAA appearing in blood (Harper et al., 1984). Dietary BCAA reach the blood virtually unaltered from the levels in the diet, while all other dietary amino acids are extensively metabolized by the GI tract and liver with the removal of 60%–98% before reaching the blood. Further, BCAA transport is in near equilibrium balance between extracellular and intracellular concentrations, allowing leucine concentration within skeletal muscle to directly reflect dietary intake (Bergstrom et al., 1974). Muscle responds to changes in leucine concentrations through multiple pathways including mTORC1, the branched-chain ketoacid dehydrogenase (BCKAD) complex, Sirt-1, and adenosine monophosphate (AMP) kinase (AMPK) (Suryawan et al., 1998; Vary and Lynch, 2007; Sun and Zemel, 2009; Wilson et al., 2011). Collectively, these pathways connect the regulation of skeletal muscle protein turnover and energy metabolism with dietary protein intake.

mPS is cyclical with stimulation after meals and inhibition during postabsorptive periods. After a meal, the intracellular leucine concentration increases in proportion to the protein content of the meal. If the meal contains adequate protein to produce approximately a threefold increase in intracellular leucine (from fasted ~100 μmol/L to fed ~300 μmol/L), then mTORC1 is activated stimulating downstream activation of translation factors eIF4E (initiation factor 4E) and rpS6 (ribosomal protein S6). These translation factors serve to target specific mRNAs that increase the capacity for the synthesis of structural myofibrillar proteins by 30%–40% (Crozier et al., 2005; Norton et al., 2009). Meals with approximately 30 g of protein, and specifically providing more than 2.5 g of leucine, produce an anabolic response that enhances muscle protein turnover (Layman et al., 2015).

Parallel with mTORC1 activation, increased intracellular leucine stimulates BCKAD, the rate-limiting step in BCAA oxidation (Lynch et al., 2003) (Figure 18.1). BCAA (along with lysine)

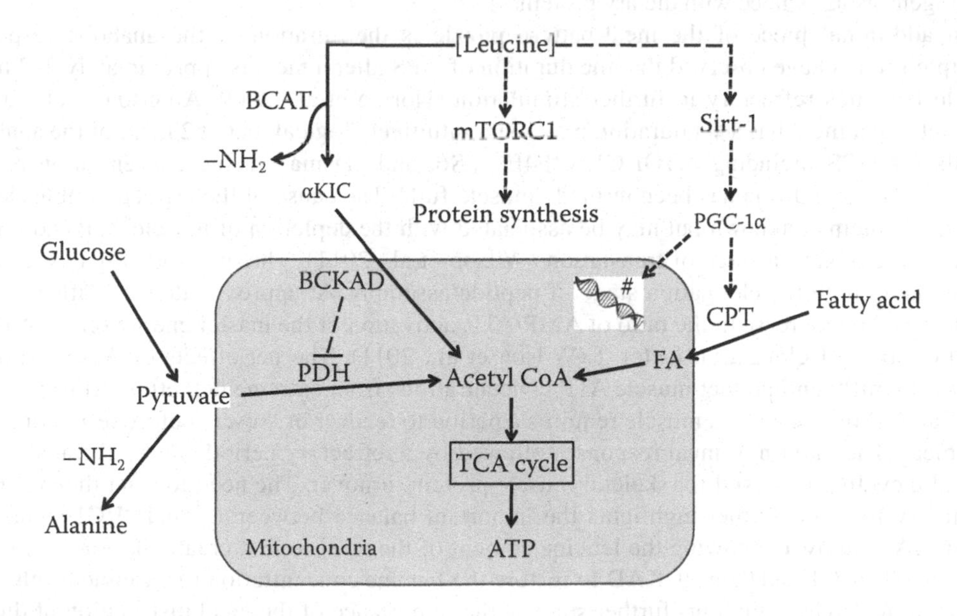

FIGURE 18.1 Roles of leucine in regulation of skeletal muscle metabolism. Increased intracellular leucine concentration stimulates mTORC1 and BCKAD and shifts the production of acetyl CoA from glucose to fatty acids. Solid lines represent metabolic pathways and dashed lines represent signaling pathways. *Abbreviations*: BCAT, branched-chain aminotransferase; BCKAD, branched-chain ketoacid dehydrogenase; αKIC, alpha-keto isocaproate; mTORC1, mechanistic target of rapamycin complex 1; Sirt-1, Sirtuin-1; PGC-1α, peroxisome proliferator-activated receptor-γ coactivator-1α; CPT, carnitine palmitoyltransferase; PDH, pyruvate dehydrogenase; #, mitochondrial biogenesis.

are the only ketogenic amino acids producing acetyl CoA similar to β-oxidation of fatty acids and providing an important fuel source for skeletal muscle. Activation of the BCKAD complex occurs through the phosphorylation of a kinase that also inhibits the pyruvate dehydrogenase complex, regulating the conversion of pyruvate to acetyl CoA for entry into the mitochondria (Chang and Goldberg, 1978). With inhibition of pyruvate dehydrogenase, pyruvate generated through glycolysis from either blood glucose or muscle glycogen is converted to alanine with the addition of a nitrogen group derived from BCAA degradation. Leucine concentration also appears to stimulate signaling through Sirt-1 and PGC-1α (peroxisome proliferator-activated receptor-γ coactivator-1α) to increase mitochondrial biogenesis and fatty acid oxidation (Sun and Zemel, 2009). The net effects of increased intracellular leucine are stimulation of mPS, increased energy expenditure, a shift of mitochondrial fuel mixture from glucose to fatty acids, and changes in glycemic regulations with increases in glucose recycling via the glucose–alanine cycle (Layman and Baum, 2004).

The magnitude of the impact of the mPS response on energy status can be appreciated by monitoring ATP depletion. After a leucine-rich protein meal, we observed a significant depletion of muscle ATP and activation of the cellular energy sensor AMPK (Wilson et al., 2011). These responses are similar to the effects of exhaustive exercise. Activating AMPK serves to protect cellular ATP levels by inhibiting mPS at the elongation stage of translation, reducing ATP expenditure, and stimulating energy production by increasing mitochondrial fatty acid oxidation and glucose uptake for glycolysis (Kahn et al., 2005). While equating a protein meal to exercise may be overextending the data, the metabolic responses are similar to changes observed with endurance training (McArdle et al., 1999) and estimates of energy costs of protein synthesis account for ~20% of total energy expenditure (Waterlow, 1995) with the response proportional to the postmeal thermogenic effects (Giordano and Castellino, 1997). Clearly, a meal pattern of dietary protein and mPS impacts daily energy expenditure. These findings suggest that mPS is likely a major component of the increased thermogenesis associated with dietary protein.

An additional piece of the meal-pattern puzzle is the duration of the anabolic response. Multiple groups have observed that the duration of mPS after a meal is approximately 2–3 h and muscle becomes refractory to further stimulation (Norton et al., 2009; Atherton et al., 2010). The fact that a meal has a set duration may seem intuitively logical, but at 2 h, all of the anabolic signals for mPS including mTORC1, eIF4E, rpS6, and plasma leucine concentration remain elevated. This condition has been termed "muscle full." The cause of the refractory, muscle full response remains unknown but may be associated with the depletion of muscle ATP and inhibition of the elongation stage of translation (Wilson et al., 2011). The major energy cost of mPS is associated with the elongation stage of peptide assembly. At approximately 2 h after a meal, we observed an increase in the ratio of AMP/ATP, activation of the master energy sensor AMPK, and inhibition of elongation factor 2 (Wilson et al., 2011). The net effects of these responses are to slow mPS and protect muscle ATP concentrations from extreme depletion. After the postprandial anabolic response, muscle requires a period to recover or "reset" before responding to a next meal. The pattern of meal response followed by a refractory period creates the anabolic to catabolic cycling observed for skeletal muscle protein turnover. The need to reset the metabolic machinery for mPS further highlights the important balance between the mTORC1 signal and the BCKAD pathway allowing the leucine content of the meal to first create the anabolic signal through mTORC1 and then BCKAD to restore the leucine concentration to baseline levels prior to a next meal. These findings further support the importance of the meal distribution of dietary protein and may ultimately determine potential metabolic advantages including diet-induced thermogenesis.

Using a criterion of a leucine threshold to define the protein quantity and quality at each meal, we designed a series of weight loss studies evaluating changes in body composition and cardiometabolic parameters. The studies were randomized controlled trials comparing a higher-protein, reduced-carbohydrate (HP/LC) diet with a high-carbohydrate, low-protein (HC/LP) diet. The HC/LP diet was designed to follow the guidelines of the Food Guide Pyramid. Both diets reduced energy intake, while the HP/LC diet provided daily protein at 1.5 g/kg body weight including a minimum of 2.5 g of leucine at each meal and carbohydrates <150 g/day; and the HC/LP diet set protein at 0.8 g/kg with carbohydrates at >200 g/day. The first study was a 10-week controlled feeding study designed to minimize behavioral aspects of diet compliance (Layman et al., 2003a,b). Participants were assigned diets with defined meal composition using a required 14-day menu rotation, and ~60% of meals prepared at our Food Research Center. Participants also completed weekly 3-day weighed food records. The HP/LC diet resulted in increased fat loss, greater improvement in body composition (greater reduction in fat mass and attenuated loss of lean body mass), reduced triglycerides, increased HDL-cholesterol, and stabilized postprandial glycemic responses including reducing postprandial insulin peak and area-under-the-curve and eliminating the 2-h postmeal drop in blood glucose. The second study was a 16-week evaluation of the same diets with or without exercise (Layman et al., 2005). Participants were required to use the same meals tested in study 1 but were allowed free choice for daily meal selection based on personal diet preferences. Participants completed weekly 3-day weighed food records, and ~20% of meals were consumed at the Food Research Center. The primary outcomes of increased fat loss, attenuated loss of lean mass, reduced triglycerides, and increased HDL-cholesterol were consistent with study 1. Exercise further increased fat loss and attenuated loss of lean mass with greater effects with the HP/LC diet. The third study was a multicenter, 12-month randomized controlled trial with free-living subjects (Layman et al., 2009). Subjects were required to attend a diet education meeting each week and complete 3-day weighed food records. The HP/LC diet resulted in more subjects losing at least 10% of initial body weight with increased fat loss while minimizing the loss of lean tissue mass compared with the HC/LP diet. In addition to improved body composition, the HP diet improved cardiometabolic parameters including reducing triglycerides and increasing HDL-cholesterol.

IMPACT OF PROTEIN VERSUS CARBOHYDRATES ON CARDIOMETABOLIC RISK FACTORS

Glycemic Regulations

Diets with increased protein and reduced carbohydrates have been shown to improve glycemic regulations and blood lipids in normal subjects, obese subjects, and people with type 2 diabetes. Improvements include reduced postprandial glucose and insulin (i.e., area-under-the-curve) and reduced triglycerides. However, the specific impact of dietary protein on cardiometabolic parameters beyond body composition and energy expenditure is difficult to differentiate from changes associated with reduced carbohydrate or energy intake.

Interactions of protein and amino acids with carbohydrate metabolism are well known. Amino acids directly contribute to de novo synthesis of glucose via gluconeogenesis and participate in the recycling of glucose carbon from skeletal muscle via the glucose–alanine cycle. Further, dietary protein and, specifically, the amino acids leucine and glycine stimulate insulin release from the pancreas, and leucine serves to modulate the intracellular insulin signal in skeletal muscle and adipose tissue. Whereas potential interactions of amino acids with glucose metabolism have been experimentally established, the physiological impact of amino acids on glucose homeostasis is dependent on the experimental or dietary conditions.

Studies by Sweeney (1927) and Himsworth (1935) reported that normal subjects fed increasing levels of carbohydrates increased their capacity for the disposal of an oral glucose load. These studies are often cited as early evidence that high-carbohydrate diets increased insulin sensitivity, and the converse, reduced-carbohydrate diets reduce the capacity for glucose disposal. Other studies reported that increasing plasma amino acid concentrations can decrease glucose disposal, induce hyperinsulinemia and hyperglycemia, and potentially lead to insulin resistance (Schwenk and Haymond, 1987; Ferrannini et al., 1988). These studies used the intravenous infusion of amino acids with euglycemic clamp techniques to measure glucose uptake and insulin resistance. Acute increases in plasma amino acids were found to increase plasma glucose concentrations, decrease glucose uptake, and increase plasma insulin levels.

Contrary to these reports, studies examining metabolic responses in normal subjects consuming meals in which protein was substituted for carbohydrates found that HP/LC meals reduced postprandial insulin response and decreased 24-h area-under-the-curve for both glucose and insulin. Floyd et al. (1966a,b) compared the intravenous infusion of amino acids with the oral consumption of a protein meal and found acute hyperinsulinemia after the intravenous infusion but minimal postprandial insulin response after oral consumption. Krezowski et al. (1986) reported similar effects on glycemic regulations for normal, weight-stable subjects. Using isoenergetic meals, they found that substituting dietary protein for carbohydrates reduced postmeal responses of both plasma glucose and insulin.

Treatment of type 2 diabetes with restriction of dietary carbohydrates produces similar improvements for glycemic regulations. HP/LC diets decrease fasting plasma glucose and reduce HbA1c when compared with responses to HC/LP diets with or without accompanying weight loss. Gannon et al. compared HP/LC and HC/LP diets in weight-stable subjects with type 2 diabetes. They found that HP/LC diets reduced fasting glucose, 24-h glucose area-under-the-curve, and HbA1c; the reduction in HbA1c was proportional to the reduction in carbohydrate consumption (Krezowski et al., 1986; Gannon et al., 1996; Gannon and Nuttall 2004). An important difference for people with type 2 diabetes is that dietary protein appears to stimulate insulin release at levels similar to dietary carbohydrates. Therefore, whereas the replacement of dietary carbohydrates with protein results in reduced postprandial glucose response, protein maintains an equivalent insulin response that is significantly higher than replacement with fat.

Blood Lipids

The most consistent effect of HP/LC diets on blood lipids is lowering serum triglycerides. Normolipidemic subjects using HP/LC diets for weight loss generally experience 30%–55% reductions in triglyceride concentrations from baseline values (Krieger et al., 2006). Other changes in blood lipids often associated with HP/LC diets include increased HDL-cholesterol concentration and larger LDL particle size, but specific responses are influenced by baseline lipoprotein patterns, fat content of the diet, total energy intake, weight loss, and insulin responsiveness of subjects (Layman et al., 2008). Specific effects of protein are often difficult to untangle from changes in energy and/or carbohydrate intakes; however, the OmniHeart Trial found the replacement of carbohydrates with protein had a greater effect on triglycerides than the replacement of carbohydrates with unsaturated fat (Appel et al., 2005).

Controlled studies for energy intake that maintained stable body weight show reduced triglyceride concentrations with HP/LC diets. Krauss et al. (2006) varied carbohydrate and protein intakes with weight-stable subjects and found reduced triglycerides and increased LDL particle size with the primary effects associated with carbohydrate restriction. Likewise, Wolfe and Giovannetti (1991) compared HP/LC and HC/LP diets that were isocaloric with weight-stable subjects. They found that HP/LC reduced triglyceride and LDL-cholesterol concentrations and increased HDL-cholesterol. Hence, both weight loss and weight-stable studies show that the isocaloric replacement of carbohydrates with protein is beneficial for blood lipoprotein patterns and particularly for triglycerides.

Investigators have long recognized the associations of glucose intolerance, insulin resistance, and increased triglycerides (Reaven, 1996). These relationships underlie the dyslipidemia of the *metabolic syndrome*. Numerous studies with nondiabetic and diabetic subjects evaluated reduced-carbohydrate diets for the treatment of dyslipidemia. Most of these studies reduced carbohydrates by replacement with fat as an energy substitute (Reaven, 1996; Schwarz et al., 2003; Volk et al., 2014). These studies consistently found that reducing dietary carbohydrates and increasing fat reduced triglycerides and increased HDL. Similar findings are observed with substituting protein for carbohydrates suggesting that the primary effects on lowering triglycerides arise from reducing dietary carbohydrates. McAuley et al. (2005) attempted to define the individual effects of protein, carbohydrates, and fats on blood lipids. In a study with insulin-resistant, overweight women, they compared changes in blood lipids using HP, high-carbohydrate (HC), or high-fat diets. After 24 weeks, the HP and high-fat groups had greater reductions in body weight and triglycerides than the HC group. LDL-cholesterol decreased for subjects in the HC and HP groups, and LDL was significantly lower in the HP compared with the high-fat group. These findings suggest that lowering carbohydrates is most important for reducing triglycerides and that replacing carbohydrates with protein may be more efficacious than using fat for improving lipoprotein patterns. Further in support of benefits with high protein intake, skeletal muscle mass appears to relate to triglyceride concentration by affecting VLDL secretion rates (Sondergaard et al., 2015).

CONCLUSIONS

Dietary protein recommendations range from minimum requirements to prevent deficiencies defined as the RDA to higher amounts established for optimal adult health. The RDA is 0.8 g/kg/day and based on maintaining nitrogen balance, while optimal health is based on protecting skeletal muscle mass and function with protein recommended at 1.2–1.5 g/kg/day (Bauer et al., 2013). Consistent with the higher-protein targets, the 2015 Dietary Guidelines Advisory Committee recommended healthy diets should provide protein at 155%–198% above the RDA (USDA, 2015). Further, optimal muscle health requires daily protein to be consumed in meals containing a minimum of 30 g of protein that also provide all of the EAA including at least 2.5 g of the EAA leucine.

Studies using energy-restricted diets for weight loss consistently find that diets with increased protein and reduced carbohydrates (HP/LC) have beneficial effects on cardiometabolic outcomes. These HP/LC diets produce a greater loss of weight and body fat while minimizing the loss of lean tissue, and have been shown to improve dyslipidemia with reduced blood triglycerides and increased HDL and to minimize postprandial swings in blood glucose and insulin. While higher-protein diets appear to be beneficial for cardiometabolic health, interpreting the specific effects of protein is difficult because of parallel changes in energy and carbohydrate intakes. Further, many long-term clinical trials are confounded by the lack of subject compliance with diet protocols.

While metabolic advantages of higher-protein diets are often intertwined with reductions in carbohydrates, evidence is accumulating that protein has unique effects on skeletal muscle including increases in protein turnover, energy expenditure, and fat oxidation. These changes are consistent with the increased fat loss and sparing of lean tissues during weight loss. Further, research studies focused on healthy aging and exercise demonstrate that protein effects arise from the meal distribution of protein and specifically the signaling effects of the EAA leucine on initiation of mPS.

Meal-based effects of dietary protein on mPS appear to be associated with the initiation phase of protein synthesis. In skeletal muscle, protein synthesis is a cyclical process stimulated during the absorptive period after a meal providing adequate protein and energy and inhibited during postabsorptive periods between meals. The signal for the postmeal stimulation of mPS is transmitted through the mTORC1 signal complex to downstream initiation factors. In adults, mTORC1 is sensitive to the amount of protein in the meal and specifically to the amount of the essential amino acid leucine. Optimum stimulation of mPS requires meals providing at least 30 g of protein containing at least 2.5 g of leucine. Studies evaluating the meal response to protein demonstrate the positive effects of protein on muscle mass and strength. Further, changes in leucine concentrations influence muscle metabolism and energy expenditure through multiple pathways including mTORC1, the BCKAD complex, Sirt-1, and AMPK. mPS is estimated to account for up to 20% of total resting energy expenditure. Together, these meal-based changes in mPS are consistent with the protection of lean tissues and the increased energy expenditure (i.e., diet-induced thermogenesis) and fatty acid oxidation observed with higher-protein diets.

The effects of HP/LC diets on glycemic regulations and blood lipoproteins appear to be largely associated with reduced-carbohydrate intake. Multiple studies have shown that reducing carbohydrate intake by energy restriction or replacing carbohydrates with protein or fats will reduce blood triglycerides, increase HDL, and reduce postmeal increases in glucose and insulin. While the primary effects appear to be associated with reducing carbohydrates, higher-protein diets may help stabilize glycemic regulations by increasing the recycling of glucose via the glucose–alanine cycle in skeletal muscle and increasing fatty acid oxidation.

REFERENCES

American Diabetes Association. 2006. Standards of medical care in diabetes—2006. *Diabetes Care* 29:S4–S42.

Appel L.J., Sacks F.M., Carey V.J., Obarzanek E., Swain J.F., Miller E.R., Conlin P.R. et al. 2005. Effects of protein, monounsaturated fat, and carbohydrate intake on blood pressure and serum lipids. Results of the OmniHeart Randomized Trial. *JAMA* 294:2455–2464.

Atherton P.J., Etheridge T., Watt P., Wilkinson D., Selby A., Rankin D., Smith K., Rennie M. 2010. Muscle full effect after oral protein: Time dependent concordance and discordance between human muscle protein synthesis and mTORC 1 signaling. *Am J Clin Nutr* 92:1080–1088.

Atkins R.C. 1992. *Dr. Atkins' New Diet Revolution*. New York: Avon Books, Inc.

Bauer J., Biolo G., Cederholm T., Cesari M., Cruz-Jentoft A.J., Morley J.E., Phillips S. et al. 2013. Evidence-based recommendations for optimal dietary protein intake in older people: A position paper from the PROT-AGE study group. *JAMDA* 14:542–559.

Bergstrom J., Furst P., Noree L.O., Vinnars E. 1974. Intracellular free amino acid concentration in human muscle tissue. *J Appl Physiol* 36:693–697.

Bistrain B.R., Winterer J., Blackburn G.L., Young V., Sherman M. 1977. Effect of a protein-sparing diet and brief fast on nitrogen metabolism in mildly obese subjects. *J Lab Clin Med* 89:1030–1035.

Burd N.A., Tang J.E., Moore D.R., Phillips S.M. 2008. Exercise training and protein metabolism: Influences of contraction, protein intake, and sex-based differences. *J Appl Physiol* 106:1692–1701.

Buse M.G., Reid S. 1975. Leucine: A possible regulator of protein turnover in muscle. *J Clin Invest* 56:1250–1261.

Chang T.W., Goldberg A.L. 1978. Leucine inhibits oxidation of glucose and pyruvate in skeletal muscle during fasting. *J Biol Chem* 253:3696–3701.

Crozier S.J., Kimball S.R., Emmert S.W., Anthony J.C., Jefferson L.S. 2005. Oral leucine administration stimulates protein synthesis in rat skeletal muscle. *J Nutr* 135:376–382.

Cuthbertson D., Smith K., Babraj J., Leese G., Waddell T., Atherton P., Wakerhage H., Taylor P., Rennie M. 2005. Anabolic signaling deficits underlie amino acid resistance of wasting, aging muscle. *FASEB J* 19:422–424.

Dansigner M.L., Gleason J.A., Griffith J.L., Selker H.P., Schaefer E.J. 2005. Comparison of the atkins, ornish, weight watchers, and zone diets for weight loss and heart disease risk reduction. *JAMA* 293:43–53.

Elango R., Ball R., Pencharz P. 2008. Indicator amino acid oxidation: Concept and application. *J Nutr* 138:243–246.

Ferrannini E., Bevilacqua S., Lanzone L., Bonadonna R., Brandi L., Oleggini M., Boni C. et al. 1988. Metabolic interactions of amino acids and glucose in healthy humans. *Diab Nutr Metab* 3:175–186.

Flatt J.P., Blackburn G.L. 1974. The metabolic fuel regulatory system: Implications for protein sparing therapies during caloric deprivation and disease. *Am J Clin Nutr* 27:175–187.

Floyd J.C., Fajans S.S., Conn J.W., Knopf R.F., Rull J. 1966a. Insulin secretion in response to protein ingestion. *J Clin Invest* 45:1479–1486.

Floyd J.C., Fajans S.S., Conn J.W., Knopf R.F., Rull J. 1966b. Stimulation of insulin secretion by amino acids. *J Clin Invest* 45:1487–1502.

Foster G.D., Wyatt H.R., Hill J.O., McGuckin B.G., Brill C., Mohammed S., Szapary P.O., Rader D.J., Edman J.S., Klein S. 2003. A randomized trial of a low-carbohydrate diet for obesity. *N Engl J Med* 348:2082–2090.

Fry C.S., Drummond M., Glynn E., Dickinson J., Gundermann D., Timmerman K., Walker D., Dhanani S., Volpi E., Rasmussen B. 2011. Aging impairs contraction-induced human skeletal muscle mTORC1 signaling and protein synthesis. *Skeletal Muscle* 1:11–21.

Fulks R.M., Li J., Goldberg A. 1975. Effects of insulin, glucose, and amino acids on protein turnover in rat diaphragm. *J Biol Chem* 250:290–298.

Gannon M.C., Nuttall F.Q. 2004. Effect of a high-protein, low-carbohydrate diet on blood glucose control in people with type 2 diabetes. *Diabetes* 53:2375–2382.

Gannon M.C., Nuttall F.Q., Lane J.T., Fang S., Gupta V., Sandhofer C. 1996. Effect of 24 hours of starvation on plasma glucose and insulin concentrations in people with untreated non-insulin-dependent diabetes mellitus. *Metabolism* 45:492–497.

Giordano M., Castellino P. 1997. Correlation between amino acid induced changes in energy expenditure and protein metabolism in humans. *Nutrition* 13:309–312.

Grundy, S.M., Brewer H.B., Cleeman J.I., Smith S.C., Lenfant C. 2004. Definition of metabolic syndrome. Report of the national heart, lung, and blood institute. *Circulation* 109:433–438.

Gual P., Marchand-Brustel Y., Tanti J.-F. 2005. Positive and negative regulation of insulin signaling through IRS-1 phosphorylation. *Biochimie* 87:99–109.

Guillet C., Prod'homme M., Balage M., Gachon P., Giraudet C., Morin L., Grizard J., Boirie Y. 2004. Impaired anabolic response of muscle protein synthesis is associated with S6K1 dysregulation in elderly humans. *FASEB J* 18:1586–1587.

Harper A.E., Miller R., Block K. 1984. Branched-chain amino acid metabolism. *Annu Rev Nutr* 4:409–454.

Heller R.F., Heller R.F. 1993. *The Carbohydrate Addict's Diet.* New York: Signet.

Himsworth H.P. 1935. The dietetic factor determining the glucose tolerance and sensitivity to insulin of healthy men. *Clin Sci* 2:67–94.

Institute of Medicine. 2002. *Food and Nutrition Board: Dietary Reference Intakes.* Washington, DC: National Academy Press.

Kahn B.B., Alquier T., Carling D., Hardie D.G. 2005. AMP-activated protein kinase: Ancient energy gauge provides clues to modern understanding of metabolism. *Cell Metab* 1:15–25.

Katsanos C.S., Kobayashi H., Sheffield-Moore M., Aarsland A., Wolfe R.R. 2006. A high proportion of leucine is required for optimal stimulation of the rate of muscle protein synthesis by essential amino acids in the elderly. *Am J Physiol Endocrinol Metab* 291:E381–E387.

Klein S., Sheard N.F., Pi-Sunyer X., Daly A., Wylie-Rosett J., Kulkarni K., Clark N.G. 2004. Weight management through lifestyle modification for the prevention and management of type 2 diabetes: Rationale and strategies. *Am J Clin Nutr* 80:257–263.

Krauss R.M., Blanche P.J., Rawlings R.S., Fernstrom H.S., Williams P.T. 2006. Separate effects of reduced carbohydrate intake and weight loss on atherogenic dyslipidemia. *Am J Clin Nutr* 83:1025–1031.

Krezowski P.A., Nuttall F.Q., Gannon M.C., Bartosh N.H. 1986. The effect of protein ingestion on the metabolic response to oral glucose in normal individuals. *Am J Clin Nutr* 44:847–856.

Krieger J.W., Sitren H.S., Daniels M.J., Langkamp-Henken B. 2006. Effects of variation in protein and carbohydrate intake on body mass and composition during energy restriction: A meta-regression. *Am J Clin Nutr* 83:260–274.

Layman D.K. 2003. The role of leucine in weight loss diets and glucose homeostasis. *J Nutr* 133:261S–267S.

Layman D.K., Anthony T.G., Rasmussen B.B., Adams S.H., Lynch C.J., Brinkworth G.D., Davis T.A. 2015. Defining meal requirements for protein to optimize metabolic roles of amino acids. *Am J Clin Nutr* 101:1330S–1338S.

Layman D.K., Baum J.I. 2004. Dietary protein impact on glycemic control during weight loss. *J Nutr* 134:968S–973S.

Layman D.K., Boileau R.A., Erickson D.J., Painter J.E., Shiue H., Sather C., Christou D.D. 2003b. A reduced ratio of dietary carbohydrate to protein improves body composition and blood lipid profiles during weight loss in adult women. *J Nutr* 133:411–417.

Layman D.K., Clifton P., Gannon M.C., Krauss R.M., Nuttall F.Q. 2008. Protein in optimal health: Heart disease and type 2 diabetes. *Am J Clin Nutr* 87:1571S–1575S.

Layman D.K., Evans E., Baum J.I., Seyler J., Erickson D.J., Boileau R.A. 2005. Dietary protein and exercise have additive effects on body composition during weight loss in adult women. *J Nutr* 135:1903–1910.

Layman D.K., Evans E.M., Erickson D., Seyler J., Weber J., Bagshaw D., Griel A., Psota T., Kris-Etherton P. 2009. A moderate-protein diet produces sustained weight loss and long-term changes in body composition and blood lipids in obese adults. *J Nutr* 139:514–521.

Layman D.K., Shiue H., Sather C., Erickson D.J., Baum J. 2003a. Increased dietary protein modifies glucose and insulin homeostasis in adult women during weight loss. *J Nutr* 133:405–410.

Lee S., Kuk J.L., Katzmarzyk P.T., Blair S.N., Church T.S., Ross R. 2005. Cardiorespiratory fitness attenuates metabolic risk independent of abdominal subcutaneous and visceral fat in men. *Diabetes Care* 28:895–901.

Lynch C.J., Halle B., Fujii H., Vary T.C., Wallin R., Damuni Z., Hutson S.M. 2003. Potential role of leucine metabolism in the leucine-signaling pathway involving mTOR. *Am J Physiol Endocrinol Metab* 285:E854–E863.

Mamerow M.M., Mettler J.A., English K.L., Casperson S.L., Arentson-Lantz E., Sheffield-Moore M., Layman D.K., Paddon-Jones D. 2014. Dietary protein distribution positively influences 24-h muscle protein synthesis in healthy adults. *J Nutr* 144:876–880.

McArdle W.D., Katch F.I., Katch V.L. 1999. *Sports & Exercise Nutrition*. Baltimore, MD: Lippincott Williams & Wilkins.

McAuley K.A., Hopkins C.M., Smith K.J., McLay R.T., Williams S.M., Taylor R.W., Mann J.I. 2005. Comparison of high-fat and high-protein diets with a high-carbohydrate diet in insulin-resistant obese women. *Diabetologia* 48:8–16.

Millward D.J., Layman D.K., Tome D., Schaafsma G. 2008. Protein quality assessment: Impact of expanding understanding of protein and amino acid needs for optimal health. *Am J Clin Nutr* 87:1576S–1581S.

Norton L.E., Layman D., Bunpo P., Anthony T., Brana D., Garlick P. 2009. The leucine content of a complete meal directs peak activation but not duration of skeletal muscle protein synthesis and mammalian target of rapamycin signaling in rats. *J Nutr* 139:1103–1109.

Paddon-Jones D., Rasmussen B. 2009. Dietary protein recommendations and the prevention of sarcopenia. *Curr Opin Clin Nutr Metab Care* 12:86–90.

Pennings B., Groen B., de Lange A., Gijsen A., Zorenc A., Senden J., van Loon L. 2012. Amino acid absorption and subsequent muscle protein accretion following graded intakes of whey protein in elderly men. *Am J Physiol Endocrinol Metab* 302:E992–E999.

Phillips S.M. 2006. Dietary protein for athletes: From requirements to metabolic advantage. *Appl Physiol Nutr Metab* 31:647–654.

Rasmussen B.B., Fujita S., Wolfe R.R., Mittendorfer B., Roy M., Rowe V.L., Volpi E. 2006. Insulin resistance of muscle protein metabolism in aging. *FASEB J* 20(6):768–769.

Reaven G.M. 1996. Pathophysiology of insulin resistance in human disease. *Physiol Rev* 76:473–486.

Rennie M., Wilkes E. 2005. Maintenance of the musculoskeletal mass by control of protein turnover: The concept of anabolic resistance and its relevance to the transplant recipient. *Ann Transplant* 10:31–34.

Rosenberg I.H. 1997 Sarcopenia: Origins and clinical relevance. *J Nutr* 127:990S–991S.

Sacks F.M., Bray G.A., Cary V.J., Smith S.R., Ryan D.H., Anton S.D., McManus K. et al. 2009. Comparison of weight-loss diets with different compositions of fat, protein, and carbohydrates. *N Engl J Med* 360:859–873.

Schwarz J.M., Linfoot P., Dare D., Aghajanian K. 2003. Hepatic de novo lipogenesis in normoinsulinemic and hyperinsulinemic subjects consuming high-fat, low-carbohydrate and low-fat, high-carbohydrate isoenergetic diets. *Am J Clin Nutr* 77:43–50.

Schwenk W.F., Haymond M.W. 1987. Decreased uptake of glucose by human forearm during infusion of leucine, isoleucine, or threonine. *Diabetes* 36:199–204.

Sears B. 1999. *The Zone Diet*. Hammersmith, London: Thorsons Publishing Group.

Sondergaard E., Nellemann B., Sorensen L.P., Christensen B., Gormsen L.C., Nielsen S. 2015. Lean body mass, not FFA, predicts VLDL-TG secretion rate in healthy men. *Obesity* 23:1379–1385.

St. Jeor S.T., Howard B.V., Prewitt E., Bovee V., Bazzarre T., Eckel R.H. 2001. Dietary protein and weight reduction. *Circulation* 104:1869–1874.

Stenholm S., Harris T.B., Rantanen T., Wisser M., Kritchevsky S.B., Ferrucci L. 2008. Sarcopenic obesity—Definition, etiology and consequences. *Curr Opin Clin Nutr Metab Care* 11(6):693–700.

Sun X., Zemel M.B. 2009. Leucine modulation of mitochondrial mass and oxygen consumption in skeletal muscle cells and adipocytes. *Nutr Metab* 6:26–34.

Suryawan A., Hawes J.W., Harris R.A., Shimomura Y., Jenkins A.E., Hutson S.M. 1998. A molecular model of human branched-chain amino acid metabolism. *Am J Clin Nutr* 68:72–81.

Sweeney J.S. 1927. Dietary factors that influence the dextrose tolerance test. *Arch Internal Med* 40:818–830.

U.S. Department of Agriculture. 2005. *Dietary Guidelines for Americans. Home and Garden Bulletin 232*, 4th edn. Washington, DC: Department of Health and Human Services.

USDA. 2003. Chapter 2: Profiling food consumption in America. In *Agriculture Fact Book 2001–2002*. Washington, DC: United States Department of Agriculture, Office of Communications. www.USDA.gov/documents/usda-factbook-2001-2002.pdf.

USDA and Department of Health and Human Services (HHS). 2010. *Dietary Guidelines for Americans 2010*, 7th edn. Washington, DC: U.S. Government Printing Office.

USDA. 2015. *Scientific Report of the 2015 Dietary Guidelines Advisory Committee*. Washington, DC: USDA Department of Health & Human Services, Table D1.33, p. 126. www.health.gov/dietaryguidelines/2015-scientific-report/.

Vary T.C., Lynch C.J. 2007. Nutrient signaling components controlling protein synthesis in striated muscle. *J Nutr* 137:1835–1843.

Volk B.M., Kunces L.J., Freidenreich D.J., Kupchak B.R., Saenz C., Artistizabal J.C., Fernandez M.L. et al. 2014. Effects of step-wise increases in dietary carbohydrate on circulating saturated fatty acids and palmitoleic acid in adults with Metabolic Syndrome. *PLoS One* 9(11):e113605. doi: 10.1371/journal.pone.0113605.

Volpi E., Kobayashi H., Sheffield-Moore M., Mittendorfer B., Wolfe R.R. 2003. Essential amino acids are primarily responsible for the amino acid stimulation of muscle protein anabolism in healthy elderly adults. *Am J Clin Nutr* 78:250–258.

Volpi E., Mittendorfer B., Rasmussen B.B., Wolfe R.R. 2000. The response of muscle protein anabolism to combined hyperaminoacidemia and glucose-induced hyperinsulinemia is impaired in the elderly. *J Clin Endocrinol Metab* 85:4481–4490.

Volpi E., Mittendorfer B., Wolf S.E., Wolfe R.R. 1999. Oral amino acids stimulate muscle protein anabolism in the elderly despite higher first-pass splanchnic extraction. *Am J Physiol* 277:E513–E520.

Wall B.T., Cermak N.M., van Loon L.J.C. 2014. Dietary protein considerations to support active aging. *Sports Med* 44:S185–S194.

Waterlow J.C. 1995. Whole-body protein turnover in humans—Past, present, and future. *Annu Rev Nutr* 15:57–92.

Westerterp-Plantenga M.A., Luscombe-March N., Lejeune M.P.G.M., Diepvens K., Nieuwenhuizen A., Engelen M.P.K.J., Deutz N.E.P., Azzout-Marniche D., Tome D., Westerterp K.R. 2006. Dietary protein, metabolism, and body-weight regulation: Dose-response effects. *Int J Obes* 30:S16–S23.

Wilson G.J., Layman D.K., Moulton C.J., Norton L.E., Anthony T.G., Proud C.G., Rupassara S.I., Garlick P.J. 2011. Leucine or carbohydrate supplementation reduces AMPK and eEF2 phosphorylation and extends postprandial muscle protein synthesis in rats. *Am J Physiol Endocrinol Metab* 301:E1236–E1242.

Wolfe B.M., Giovannetti P.M. 1991. Short-term effects of substituting protein for carbohydrate in diets of moderately hypercholesterolemic human subjects. *Metabolism* 40:338–343.

Wolfe R.R. 2006. The underappreciated role of muscle in health and disease. *Am J Clin Nutr* 84:475–482.

Wolfe R.R., Miller S. 2008. The recommended dietary allowance of protein: A misunderstood concept. *JAMA* 299:2891–2893.

Wu G. 2013. *Amino Acids*. Boca Raton, FL: Taylor & Francis.

Wycherley T.P., Moran L.J., Clifton P.M., Noakes M., Brinkworth G.D. 2012. Effects of energy-restricted high-protein, low-fat compared with standard-protein, low-fat diets: A meta-analysis of randomized controlled trials. *Am J Clin Nutr* 96:1281–1298.

Yang Y., Breen L., Burd N., Hector A.J., Churchward-Venne T.A., Josse A.R., Tarnopolsky M.A., Phillips S.M. 2012. Resistance exercise enhances myofibrillar protein synthesis with graded intakes of whey protein in older men. *Br J Nutr* 108:1780–1788.

19 Protein Sources, CVD, Type 2 Diabetes, and Total Mortality

Peter Clifton

CONTENTS

ABSTRACT

Each of the main protein sources red and processed meat, dairy, poultry, chicken, fish, egg, and soy will be discussed commencing with epidemiology relating to these foods and total mortality, CVD, CHD, and stroke events and mortality and type 2 diabetes as well as risk markers of these diseases such as weight, lipids and blood pressure. Acute and chronic interventions with these foods will then be discussed. Although there is epidemiological evidence for red and processed meat to increase the risk of CVD and type 2 diabetes, and for dairy to protect there is a complete absence of any evidence from intervention studies to support these findings, except for a high dairy diet as part of the DASH diet lowering blood pressure. Red meat in place of carbohydrate also lowers blood pressure. The epidemiological findings are very heterogeneous and only yogurt appears to be protective in the majority of studies.

ABBREVIATIONS

CARDIA	Coronary Artery Risk Development in Young Adults
CCL5	Chemokine (C-C motif) ligand 5
CHD	Coronary heart disease
CVD	Cardiovascular disease
EPIC	European Prospective Investigation into Cancer and Nutrition
IHD	Ischemic heart disease
MESA	The Multi-Ethnic Study of Atherosclerosis
PREDIMED	Prevención con Dieta Mediterránea
RANTES	Regulated on activation, normal T cell expressed and secreted

INTRODUCTION

This is a very complex area in which it is almost impossible to isolate the protein source *per se* from other macronutrients associated with that protein source in its usual food form at least in epidemiological studies. Thus, red meat is always accompanied by a varied amount of saturated fat; dairy with calcium, magnesium, and saturated fat; and fish with very widely varying amounts of long-chain omega-3 (N3) fats, and poultry may be eaten with or without fatty skin. Vegetable sources of protein except soy are always accompanied by carbohydrate and fiber and polyphenols. Only in acute studies are isolated sources of protein available, and interpretation of the physiological significance of these studies is difficult. There are many differences in the way protein sources are consumed in the United States, Europe, and Asia, so combining data from many regions may obscure any relationships. In addition, as in all epidemiological studies, the results may be confounded by unmeasured variables, for example, red meat eaters have higher mortality and fish eaters lower mortality because of other behavioral attributes inadequately captured by the data and not due to meat or fish itself.

SCOPE OF REVIEW

Sources of protein in the U.S. diet (O'Neil et al. 2012) are shown in Table 19.1. Although wheat- and corn flour–based products rank first in contribution to protein in this table, they will not be discussed in detail except for acute studies using gluten. Eggs are an important source of protein, but the accompanying cholesterol makes interpretation of the effect of protein difficult except in acute studies using egg albumin. Although soy and other legumes contribute only 1%–2% protein, they will be discussed as they are important in non-U.S. diets. Nuts and seeds will not be discussed as they are not major contributors to protein intake for most people and contribute mostly fat. This is similar for legumes, which contribute fat, carbohydrate, and fiber. Red meat epidemiology usually includes unprocessed pork as red meat, whereas in this analysis it is mixed with pork-based processed goods. Red and processed meats together are the major source of protein at 24.1%, while animal protein accounts for about 75%–78%. Meat, poultry, and fish account for about 25% of the saturated fat intake as does dairy.

TABLE 19.1
Data from NHANES 2003–2006 Was Used to Look at Protein Sources in the U.S. Diet in 9490 Individuals

Food Group	Adults 19 Years and Over (% Total)
Bread, cakes, biscuits, etc. (wheat and corn)	At least 20
Poultry	14.4
Beef	14.0
Cheese	8.5
Milk	6.9
Pork, ham, and bacon	5.7
Fish and shellfish	5.0
Frankfurters, sausages, luncheon meats	4.4
Eggs	3.2
Nuts, seeds	2.1

Source: O'Neil, C.E. et al., *Nutrients*, 4(12), 2097, 2012.

RED AND PROCESSED MEAT

Epidemiological Studies

Total Mortality/CVD Mortality/CVD Events

Total mortality is shown in Table 19.2 and CVD mortality and events in Table 19.3. The most recent meta-analysis done by Wang et al. (2015) found a 15% increase in total mortality and CVD mortality per 100 g of processed meats/day (both $p < 0.001$; five and six studies, respectively) with similar findings for total meat. There was evidence of a nonlinear relationship for CVD mortality (steeper for the first 20 g and flatter thereafter), and the effect was seen only in U.S. populations and not in European and Asian populations. An ecological study of eight Asian prospective studies found no association between red meat and all-cause or CVD mortality (Lee et al. 2013). However, in Shanghai, red meat intake (mostly pork) was associated with an 18% difference in total and IHD mortality between top and bottom quintiles in men

TABLE 19.2
Total Mortality: Increase in Risk from Highest to Lowest Intake Group or per 50–100 g

Study	Total Meat (High vs. Low)	Total Meat (per 100 g)	Processed Meat (High vs. Low)	Processed Meat (per 50 g)	Fresh Meat (High vs. Low)	Fresh Meat (per 100 g)
Wang et al. (2015) Meta-analysis		15% (n = 6)		15% (per 100 g) (n = 5)		
Larsson and Orsini (2014) Meta-analysis	29% (n = 5)		23% (n = 6)		10% (NS) Significant only in men, USA	
Abete et al. (2014) Meta-analysis			22%			
Takata et al. (2013) Shanghai study	18% (men only)					

Notes: Lowest intake varied from <1 day/week, <6 times/month, or 0.25 servings/day, 0.51 servings/day, 0.28 servings per 1000 kcal, 9.1 g/1000 kcal, 15 g/day, or 21.4 g/day (all for total meat). Highest intake was 4–7 times/week, >45 times/month, 1.2 servings/1000 kcal, 65.8–68 g/1000 kcal, 2.07–2.17 servings/day, 160 g/day. Overall 4–11 times greater than the lowest.

TABLE 19.3
CVD Mortality: Increase in Risk from Highest to Lowest Intake Group or per 50–100 g/day

Study	Total Meat (High vs. Low)	Total Meat (per 100 g)	Processed Meat (High vs. Low)	Processed Meat (per 50 g)	Fresh Meat (High vs. Low)	Fresh Meat (per 100 g)
Wang et al. (2015) Meta-analysis		15%		15% (per 100 g) (n = 6)		
Micha et al. (2010, 2012) Meta-analysis				42% (incidence) (n = 5)		
Abete et al. (2014) Meta-analysis	16%		18%			
Takata et al. (2013) Shanghai study	18% (men only)					
Kaluza et al. (2012) Meta-analysis 6 cohorts		Stroke 13% per serving		Stroke 11% per serving		Stroke 11% per serving

only (Takata et al. 2013). In Japan no effect of meat was seen on IHD, stroke, or total CVD deaths (Nagao et al. 2012). Larsson and Orsini (2014) separated out fresh red meat from total meat and found that the risk for this component for total mortality was not significant (risk ratio [RR] 1.10, six studies) but also found a higher risk for processed meat (highest vs. lowest consumption of about 50 g/day, RR 1.23, six studies) and total meat (1.29 or 100 g/day, five studies). They also found that the relationship for unprocessed meat was significant only in men and in U.S. populations, whereas processed meat and total meat were significant in both men and women and in both the United States and Europe. Some of the same authors examined six cohorts (Kaluza et al. 2012) and found a significant relationship between red meat and stroke. For each serving per day increase in fresh red meat, processed meat, and total red meat consumption, the RRs of total stroke were 1.11, 1.13, and 1.11, respectively (all $p < 0.05$), and unlike the studies on total and CVD mortality, there was no heterogeneity in the stroke studies. Only thrombotic stroke was related to meat intake (four cohorts). Abete et al. (2014) examined CVD mortality in 13 cohorts and found similar results to Wang et al. (2015) with a 22% and 18% increase in all-cause and CVD mortality in the highest category of consumption of processed meat and 16% for total red meat consumption and CVD mortality. Micha et al. (2010) found that red meat intake was not related to CHD risk (four studies) while processed meat was related to a 42% increase per 50 g (five studies, $p = 0.04$). Similar results were found in an updated analysis, and it was concluded that the 400% difference in sodium content between fresh and processed meat could explain two-thirds of the difference in risk (Micha et al. 2012). In the ARIC study, protein sources were unrelated to CHD risk (Haring et al. 2014).

Diabetes

The most recent meta-analysis was performed by Feskens et al. (2013). Per 100 g of total meat, the relative risk for type 2 diabetes was 1.15 and for unprocessed red meat 1.13, and for processed meat, the relative risk per 50 g was 1.32, and all were significant. Poultry intake was unrelated to risk. Pan et al. (2011) estimated that substitutions of one serving of nuts, low-fat dairy, and whole grains per day for one serving of red meat per day were associated with a 16%–35% lower risk of type 2 diabetes. Pan et al. (2013) also examined the effects of changes in red meat intake. Increasing red meat intake of more than 0.50 servings/day (1 serving = 13 g for bacon; 28–45 g for various processed meat items; 85 g for unprocessed red meat) was associated with a 48% ($p < 0.001$) elevated risk in the subsequent

4-year period, and the association was modestly attenuated to 30% after further adjustment for initial body mass index (BMI) and concurrent weight gain. Reducing red meat consumption by more than 0.5 servings/day from baseline to the first 4 years of follow-up was associated with a significant 14% lower risk during the subsequent entire follow-up through 2006 or 2007. In the Malmo study, there was a 16% increased risk with processed meat intake in the highest quintile (Ericson et al. 2013). In the MESA study, a higher intake of meat saturated fat was associated with greater CVD risk with an increase of 5 g/day or 5% of energy from meat increasing risk significantly by 26% and 48%, respectively, with a clear dose–response relationship. The substitution of 2% of energy from meat saturated fat with energy from dairy saturated fat was associated with a 25% lower CVD risk (de Oliveira Otto et al. 2012). A meta-analysis of seven vegetarian studies showed a 29% lower mortality from IHD and a 12% lower mortality from cerebrovascular disease (Huang et al. 2012). This result is a summation of the absence of meat plus the addition of more fruit and vegetables. In meat eaters, increasing fruit and vegetable intake from less than 3 servings/day to more than 5 servings/day reduces CHD risk by 17% suggesting that half of the protective effect seen in vegetarians may be due to the absence of meat (He et al. 2007).

Characteristics of Red Meat Eaters

In the EPIC study (N = 449,000), men and women in the top categories of processed meat intake in general consumed fewer fruits and vegetables than those with low intake. Red and processed meat consumers were more likely to be current smokers and less likely to have a university degree. Men with high red meat intake consumed more alcohol than men with a low intake, which was not seen in women. Individuals consuming more than 80 g poultry/day had a higher consumption of fruits and vegetables than those with an intake of less than 5 g/day; there was no difference in smoking habits at baseline. After adjustment for these factors, processed meat was associated with 44% higher mortality. Mutual adjustment for other meat sources did not change the processed meat association. The authors estimated that 3.3% of all deaths could be avoided if processed meat consumption was less than 20 g/day (Rohrmann et al. 2013).

In the Health Professional Follow-Up Study (HPFS), men in the top quintile of meat consumption were heavier and less active and a greater proportion of them were smokers compared with men in the bottom quintile. They also had 50% greater energy intake, consumed more alcohol, eggs, coffee, soft drinks, dairy, and trans fat and slightly less fish, poultry, and fruit and vegetables, and consumed 60% less fiber (Pan et al. 2013). Their polyunsaturated-fat-to-saturated-fat ratio was about 60% of that in the bottom quintile. Similar but less dramatic findings were seen in both Nurses' Health Study (NHS) cohorts (Pan et al. 2013), although in NHSII the high red meat consumers also ate more fish and more poultry. A diabetes score was calculated from *trans* fat and glycemic load, cereal fiber, and the ratio of polyunsaturated to saturated fat, and this score and BMI, along with alcohol, energy intake, and physical activity, were used to adjust the RRs. Using dietary variables rather than the diet score did not change the results.

Possible Mechanisms of a Harmful Effect of Red Meat

Red meat has variable amounts of saturated fat and is rich in iron, phosphatidylcholine, and carnitine, the latter two of which are sources of trimethylamine, which, as discussed in later text, has been linked to CVD and type 2 diabetes (Koeth et al. 2013, Tang et al. 2013). Processed meat is rich in fat, salt, and nitrates. Although iron intake and iron stores have been linked to CVD (Hunnicutt et al. 2014), many cuts of chicken have more myoglobin than does pork (http://ndb.nal.usda.gov/ndb/search), so the relationship of CVD with food sources of iron is not clear. Advanced glycation end products in meat is another possibility. Overall, although there are many mechanisms for effects of red meat on both CVD and diabetes (Kim et al. 2015), none stand out as obvious candidates.

Red Meat and CVD/Diabetes Risk Factors

Weight

A recent meta-analysis showed that those in the highest intake group of red and processed meat had a 37% and a 32% higher BMI, respectively. Waist circumference was increased by 2.8 cm in this group. There was, however, considerable heterogeneity in the studies (Rouhani et al. 2014). A high saturated fat intake enhances the association between obesity gene risk scores and BMI, and meat contributes about 25% of saturated fat to the diet (Casas-Agustench et al. 2014).

Saturated Fat/Cholesterol

Surprisingly, there are few epidemiological studies of meat intake and serum cholesterol. The Harbin study (Na et al. 2015) showed a relationship between a high meat dietary pattern (1 of 5 patterns) and hypertriglyceridemia (86% greater in the highest tertile), but there was no relationship with hypercholesterolemia. In South Korea, a high meat and takeaway food diet was associated with more hypercholesterolemia (Shin et al. 2014).

Blood Pressure

In the Oxford cohort of the EPIC study, male meat eaters have an incidence of hypertension of 15% compared with a rate of 5.8% in male vegans. Fish eaters and vegetarians have intermediate and similar values suggesting the replacement of meat with fish will beneficially influence blood pressure (Appleby et al. 2002). In the CARDIA study (Steffen et al. 2005), positive dose–response relations for elevated blood pressure incidence were observed across increasing quintiles of meat intake (p trend = 0.004).

Telomeres

Processed meat was associated with shorter telomeres in the MESA study (Nettleton et al. 2008), and it is known that telomeres are shorter in those with CVD (Aviv 2012).

Inflammatory Markers

Although C-reactive protein (CRP) was related to meat intake in the Nurses' Health Study, the relationship was no longer significant after adjustment for BMI (Ley et al. 2014).

Serum/Urine Trimethylamine Oxide (TMAO)

Both phosphatidylcholine and carnitine can be converted by the microbiome to trimethylamine, which is absorbed and oxidized in the liver. Omnivores have fourfold higher urinary TMAO excretion and 25%–30% higher plasma TMAO compared to vegans (Koeth et al. 2013). In addition, feeding carnitine or steak increased plasma TMAO up to 6 μM in omnivores with no change in vegans. Individuals with an enterotype characterized by enriched proportions of the genus *Prevotella* (n = 4) demonstrated higher ($p < 0.05$) plasma TMAO levels than subjects with an enterotype notable for enrichment of *Bacteroides* (n = 49) genus. There were significant differences in microbiota composition between vegans/vegetarians and omnivores. Plasma carnitine levels predicted increased risks for both prevalent CVD and incident cardiac events, but only among subjects with high TMAO levels. Three-year follow-up in 4007 patients showed that plasma TMAO levels predicted increased CVD events with a 2.5-fold increase in the highest vs. the lowest quartile (Tang et al. 2013). People with type 2 diabetes also have higher levels of TMAO (Li et al. 2015). Fish, however, has high levels of TMAO that can be converted to trimethylamine by bacteria, yet as described in the following text, fish intake is associated with a reduced risk of CVD.

Metabolomics

The EPIC study was a nested case–control study of 688 cases and 1993 controls. Total red meat intake was associated with a 26% increase in risk of type 2 diabetes per 11 g/MJ. Six biomarkers (ferritin, glycine, diacylphosphatidylcholines 36:4 and 38:4, lysophosphatidylcholine 17:0, and hydroxysphingomyelin 14:1) were associated with red meat consumption and diabetes risk and, when added to the regression model, eliminated the association of red meat to risk. Because the biomarkers accounted for 69% of the variance in outcomes, it was assumed that they were mediators of risk. However, it is plausible that ferritin, for example, may only be a marker of red meat intake (Wittenbecher et al. 2015) and would thus be expected to eliminate the association of red meat with diabetes risk. As noted previously, the relationship between iron and CVD risk is conflicted and controversial.

Dietary Interventions and Biomarkers of CVD and Diabetes Risk

Feeding hypercholesterolemic volunteers lean beef, poultry, or fish for 26 days lowered LDL cholesterol by 5%–9% compared with the usual average American high saturated fat diet, with no differences between the diets (Beauchesne-Rondeau et al. 2003). This is not a surprise given the low saturated fat of all the diets, but it does not represent usual fatty American beef and so provides no insight into the effect of this kind of palmitic acid–rich beef on CVD risk factors. A meta-analysis of eight studies confirmed that there were no lipid differences comparing beef to chicken/fish (Maki et al. 2012). Nevertheless, it is clear that in experimental studies, the major saturated fat in red meat, palmitic acid, elevates LDL cholesterol (Mensink et al. 2003).

The DASH diet emphasizes a low intake of red meat in addition to high intake of fruit, vegetables, and dairy, but in a recent DASH-like study, substitution of lean pork for fish and chicken did not affect the blood pressure–lowering ability of the diet (Sayer et al. 2015). Lean red meat lowers blood pressure by 5 mmHg systolic when 5% energy from carbohydrate is replaced with protein (Hodgson et al. 2006). Notably, markers of oxidation and inflammation were not found to be increased by red meat (Hodgson et al. 2007).

One of the few studies using red meat as normally consumed showed that substituting an oily fish for red meat four times per week for 8 weeks in young women with low iron stores lowered fasting insulin and increased HDL. Adhesion molecules, lipid peroxides, and LDL cholesterol were not different across diets (Navas-Carretero et al. 2009). Insulin increased by 20% from baseline on the red meat diet and did not change with the fish diet, although saturated fat intake was the same in both diet groups and iron stores were no different. Saturated fat intake does not appear to influence insulin sensitivity in humans (Lovejoy et al. 2002), suggesting it is not the saturated fat content of meat that accounts for the apparent increased risk of type 2 diabetes. Chiu et al. (2014) showed that increased saturated fat and protein from dairy sources had no effect on insulin sensitivity.

DAIRY

Epidemiological Studies

Although dairy fat contains about 50% saturated fat and is very similar in composition to beef fat, its association with disease is quite different from red meat with no clear association with CVD and apparent protection from type 2 diabetes, although the data are very heterogeneous and often of poor quality.

Total Mortality/CVD Mortality/CVD Events

In the most recent meta-analysis in 2015, an inverse association was found between total dairy consumption and overall risk of CVD (9 studies; RR 0.88, $p < 0.05$) and stroke (12 studies; RR 0.87, $p < 0.05$). However, no association was established between dairy consumption and CHD risk (RR 0.94; 95% CI 0.82, 1.07; 12 studies). Stroke risk was significantly reduced by consumption of low-fat dairy (six studies; RR 0.93, $p < 0.05$) and cheese (four studies; RR 0.91, $p < 0.05$), and CHD risk was significantly lowered by 16% by cheese consumption (seven studies; $p = 0.05$). Heterogeneity across studies was found for stroke and CHD analyses, and publication bias was found for stroke analysis (Qin et al. 2015). A previous meta-analysis of eight prospective studies focused particularly on milk (Soedamah-Muthu et al. 2011) also reported reduced total CVD but found no effect of dairy on stroke; of note, the number of studies was limited. Milk intake was not associated with total mortality (Soedamah-Muthu et al. 2011).

Rice (2014) reviewed papers published between 2009 and 2013 and found 18 prospective studies in this time period but did not perform a meta-analysis or add them to the meta-analysis of Soedamah-Muthu et al. (2011); rather, they only discussed the findings. Six of the cohorts had at least one positive finding of protection from dairy, three had negative findings, and nine were neutral. Full-fat cheese and fermented milk are most often associated with apparent protection. Several of these studies are not included in the 2015 meta-analysis (Qin et al. 2015).

Studies not included in the 2015 meta-analysis include the Hoorn study (van Aerde et al. 2013), which showed that overall total dairy intake was not associated with CVD mortality or all-cause mortality. Each standard deviation increase in high-fat dairy; intake was associated with a significant 32% higher risk of CVD mortality. In Costa Rican adults, dairy product intake as assessed by adipose tissue fatty acids 15:0 and 17:0 and by food frequency questionnaire (FFQ) was not associated with change in the risk of myocardial infarction (MI) (Aslibekyan et al. 2012). In a nested case–control study from Sweden, milk fat biomarkers 15:0 and 17:0 were inversely associated with the risk of first MI with a significant 26% reduction in women only. Quartiles of reported intake of cheese (men and women) and fermented milk products (men) were inversely related to a first MI (p trend < 0.05 for all) (Warensjo et al. 2010).

In elderly women, yogurt intake was inversely related to carotid intima-media thickness (IMT) baseline risk factor–adjusted standard $\beta = -0.075$, $p = 0.015$. Participants who consumed >100 g yogurt/day had a significantly lower common carotid artery IMT than did participants with lower consumption (multivariable adjustment = −0.023 mm, $p = 0.003$) (Ivey et al. 2011).

In the Dutch Epic cohort (34,409 men and women), cheese was modestly inversely associated with CVD mortality, particularly stroke mortality, with a 41% reduction in the latter (Praagman et al. 2015). In the Norwegian counties study, ruminant trans fat (from the two major protein sources—beef and dairy) was associated with a 30% increase in CVD deaths, 30% increase in heart disease deaths, and a 27% increase in sudden death in women only from highest compared to lowest intake category (Laake et al. 2012). In the Swedish mammography study, the highest vs. lowest quintile of total dairy food intake was associated with a 23% decreased incidence of MI ($P < 0.05$) and the highest vs. lowest quintile of total cheese associated with a 26% decreased incidence of MI ($p = 0.006$). No significant association between milk, cultured milk, or cream and MI was seen. In the highest vs. lowest quartile of full-fat cheese, there was a 17% decreased incidence of MI ($p = 0.035$) (Patterson et al. 2013).

In an effort to determine whether calcium was a protective nutrient linking dairy to CVD, an updated analysis of mineral intake in the Nurses' Health Study showed no association between calcium intake and stroke, although potassium and magnesium were protective. In an updated meta-analysis of all cohort studies, calcium was not protective (Adebamowo et al. 2015).

Elwood et al. (2010) performed a meta-analysis of dairy intake and total mortality in eight cohorts but omitted data from two cohorts. In the six cohorts included, there was a small but significant reduction in total mortality in the subjects with the highest dairy consumption, relative to the risk in the subjects with the lowest consumption (RR) 0.87, 95% confidence limits (0.77, 0.98). However, the two omitted cohorts could have been validly included, and their omission biases the results. One, the Adventist cohort compared 3+ glasses of milk per week to <1 glass per week and found a nonsignificant 0.98 RR (Kahn et al. 1984). The Dutch Civil Servants cohort (Vijver et al. 1992) compared the top third of calcium intake to the bottom and found no significant reduction with wide risk estimates, so the addition of these two studies to the meta- analysis would likely make the relationship nonsignificant. It is reasonable to say that dairy probably does not alter total mortality, but as noted earlier, there are some studies suggesting it may increase total mortality. Kelemen et al. (2005) found a 41% increase in CHD mortality (and a 44% increase with red meat) in the highest vs. the lowest quintile of intake substituting animal protein for an equal number of servings of carbohydrate using the Willett technique (Willett 1998). Dairy was not significantly associated with total mortality, but red meat increased mortality by 16%, which fits with other meta-analytic results as discussed earlier. The Elwood meta-analysis on total mortality was dominated by van der Pols' paper on the Boyd Orr cohort (van der Pols et al. 2009), which examined childhood family dairy intake and mortality 65 years later.

Similarly, in the meta-analysis of CHD deaths and dairy (mostly milk), Elwood used a derived figure from the Hu report of the Nurses' Health Study and ignored the significant risk estimate of 1.67 for two glasses of whole milk per day vs. less than 1 glass/week and essentially used the significant skimmed milk estimate of 0.78. In the Hu paper itself (Hu et al. 1999), the ratio of high-fat to low-fat dairy was associated with CHD risk with an increase of 27% in the highest quintile ($p < 0.0004$) after full adjustment. Given this data treatment, all estimates in the paper are suspect.

Overall, it is not clear if total dairy or any dairy form is related to the risk of CVD or CHD or mortality from these diseases.

Type 2 Diabetes

The epidemiology of dairy intake and protection from type 2 diabetes is contradictory. Many studies show protection with low-fat dairy but at the same time also show protection with a fermented food—cheese (Aune et al. 2013). Perhaps the most convincing data comes from the Harvard group as their studies have dietary assessments every 4 years and a long follow-up period of 18–20 years. They showed no link with total dairy or low-fat or high-fat dairy in a combined analysis of the NHS and NHSII and the HPFS, but 1 serving/day of yogurt (226 g) was associated with a 17% reduction in the incidence of type 2 diabetes (Chen et al. 2014). They also performed a meta-analysis with the addition of one new study and the updated Harvard information to the studies in the original Aune meta-analysis (Aune et al. 2013). No protection was shown for total dairy (11 studies), whereas 1 serving of yogurt/day was associated with an 18% reduction in risk (only 6 studies separated out yogurt).

The EPIC interact study showed that cheese intake tended to have an inverse association with diabetes (p-trend = 0.01), and a higher combined intake of fermented dairy products (cheese, yogurt, and thick fermented milk) was inversely associated with diabetes (12% reduction in highest quintile, p-trend = 0.02) in adjusted analyses (Sluijs et al. 2012). In the EPIC-Norfolk study (O'Connor et al. 2014), an inverse association was found between diabetes and low-fat fermented dairy product intake (24% reduction in highest tertile p trend = 0.049) and specifically with yogurt intake (28% reduction p trend = 0.017) in multivariable adjusted analyses. In the Malmo Diet and Cancer Study, there was a 23% reduction in risk in the highest quintile of high-fat dairy, particularly cream, high-fat fermented milk, and cheese in women. Intakes of saturated fat with 4–14 carbons were associated with a decreased risk (Ericson et al. 2015). The Malmo study stands out as providing opposite results to virtually all other studies except for the findings for cheese and fermented milk. In the PREDIMED study (Díaz-López et al. 2015), total dairy and low-fat dairy were associated with a 32%–35% reduced incidence of type 2 diabetes in the top tertile. Total yogurt reduced the incidence by 40% and increasing the consumption of low-fat dairy and total yogurt reduced the risk even further to 45%–56%. However, the total number of cases (270) was relatively small, so the estimates have wide confidence intervals.

In conclusion, yogurt seems to be convincingly associated with protection, while cheese is in doubt. Astrup (2014) discusses the findings relating to yogurt in a recent review.

Dairy and Risk Factors for Type 2 Diabetes

Weight and Metabolic Syndrome

Kratz et al. (2013) examined 16 cohorts and found that high-fat dairy was associated with decreased adiposity in 11 of them. Similarly, dairy intake was inversely associated with an incidence or prevalence of the metabolic syndrome in 7 out of 13 studies. Three studies found no association and three had mixed findings (Crichton et al. 2011). The Hoorn study (Snijder et al. 2007) found that dairy intake had no relation to current weight or metabolic syndrome components (except lower diastolic blood pressure and higher glucose) and no relation to the development of metabolic syndrome over 6.4 years. In subjects with a BMI < 25, high dairy intake was associated with weight gain (Snijder et al. 2008). A review in 2011 concludes that the data linking dairy food with protection from obesity was suggestive but not consistent with 3 out of 10 studies in children and 5 of 9 studies in adults showing protection (Louie et al. 2011). In the Stanislas cohort in men only, a higher consumption of dairy products was associated with beneficial changes in the metabolic profile (lower glucose and higher HDL cholesterol) over a 5-year period; a higher calcium consumption was associated with a lower 5-year increase of the BMI and waist circumference (Samara et al. 2013). The DESIR study showed a beneficial association between dietary calcium and arterial blood pressure, insulin, and HDL cholesterol levels in women, whereas in men there was only a beneficial association with diastolic blood pressure (Drouillet et al. 2007).

Blood pressure is the CVD risk marker most strongly associated with dairy. In a meta-analysis, Soedamah-Muthu et al. (2012) showed that total dairy, low-fat dairy, and milk were associated with protection from hypertension (6–9 cohorts). The risk reduction was small at 3%–4% per 200 g/day. High-fat dairy (six studies), total fermented dairy (four studies), yogurt (five studies), and cheese (eight studies) were not significantly associated with hypertension incidence. A second meta-analysis with five cohorts showed that the highest intake of low-fat dairy reduced hypertension by 16% (Ralston et al. 2012).

In the Luxembourg study (Crichton and Alkerwi 2014a,b), higher intakes of whole-fat milk, yogurt, and cheese were associated with better cardiovascular health as defined by the American Heart Association (smoking, BMI, physical activity, total cholesterol, blood pressure, and fasting plasma glucose). Even when controlling for demographic and dietary variables, those who consumed at least 5 servings/week of these dairy products had a significantly higher cardiovascular health score than those who consumed these products less frequently. Obesity was reduced by 55% in the highest tertile of dairy intake. Clearly, a high dairy intake is a marker of those with better lifestyle choices such as less smoking and more physical activity. In Portugal, adolescents with high milk intake were 47% less likely to have a high cardiometabolic risk score than those with low milk intake (Abreu et al. 2014). No association was found between this score and total dairy, yogurt, and cheese intake. The PREDIMED study found that a higher intake of low-fat dairy, low-fat yogurt and milk, and full-fat yogurt were associated with a significant 20%–28% reduction in the incidence of metabolic syndrome in the upper tertile (Babio et al. 2015). Interestingly, cheese was associated with a 31% increase in risk. A higher prevalence of Inuit participants with metabolic syndrome was observed in the highest tertile compared with the lowest tertile of total dairy (10.3% vs. 1.6%; $p < 0.001$) (Ferland et al. 2011).

Dietary Interventions and Biomarkers of CVD and Diabetes

Longer-Term Feeding Studies

Chen et al. (2012) analyzed 29 randomized controlled trials with 2010 participants and found that dairy had no effect on weight overall with a positive effect in studies less than 1 year in duration and a negative effect in longer-term studies. Interventions focusing on changing dairy intake without changing weight or exercise patterns are sparse. We recently reviewed the dairy intervention studies and found a very mixed picture with no clear outcomes on glucose and (Turner et al. 2015a). We performed a three-way 4-week crossover diet study in 47 overweight and obese people contrasting high-dairy diets with a high-meat diet and a control diet containing neither dairy or red meat. The high-dairy diet caused increased insulin resistance relative to both red meat and control diets (Turner et al. 2015b).

A large parallel design 4-week intervention ($n = 158$) that increased fat and protein derived mostly from dairy found no effect on insulin sensitivity as assessed by intravenous glucose tolerance tests. However, changes in plasma branched-chain amino acids (BCAAs) across all diets were negatively correlated with changes in the metabolic clearance rate of insulin ($\rho = -0.18$, $p = 0.03$) and positively correlated with changes in the acute insulin response to glucose ($\rho = 0.15$, $p = 0.05$) (Chiu et al. 2014). BCCAs are related to increases in the risk of insulin resistance and in fasting and 2 h glucose levels (Würtz et al. 2012, 2013).

In the Dairy Health study (Bohl et al. 2015), 63 healthy adults with abdominal obesity were randomly allocated to 1 of 4 diets: 60 g casein or whey plus 63 g of milk fat with either high or low medium-chain saturated fatty acids for 12 weeks. No effects on fasting lipids or glucose were seen, but whey reduced postprandial apoB48 and decreased glucagon-like peptide 1 (GLP1) compared with casein. There was no control diet. It was hypothesized that CVD risk would be lowered by whey because of its effects on apoB48.

Benatar et al. (2013) examined 20 studies with 1677 participants over a mean of 26 weeks. Dairy was increased by 3.6 servings, and there was a weight increase with low- and high-fat dairy of 0.4–0.8 kg. No other variable changed significantly.

Dairy fat increases both HDL and LDL cholesterol as expected based on their fatty acid composition compared with control diets, but no meta-analysis has been performed to look at different components of dairy or to contrast saturated fat from dairy vs. saturated fat from other food sources (Huth and Park 2012). Tholstrup et al. (2004) originally showed that cheese elevated LDL cholesterol less than expected based on its composition and less than butter for the same amount of saturated fat, and a meta-analysis of 12 studies showed a 0.22 mmol/L difference in LDL cholesterol between cheese and butter for the same amount of saturated fat (de Goede et al. 2015). Rosqvist et al. (2015) examined 40 g/day of dairy fat with and without a milk fat globule membrane (whipped cream or butter) for 8 weeks in a parallel study. LDL cholesterol increased by 0.36 mmol/L with butter and by 0.04 mmol/L with whipped cream ($p = 0.024$ for difference). Sphingolipids are important components of the milk globule membrane and have been shown to reduce cholesterol absorption (Conway et al. 2013). Butter milk also lowers blood pressure compared with a macro- and micronutrient-matched placebo (Conway et al. 2014). Metabolomic studies have been performed on dairy interventions examining either urine or postprandial plasma and have found distinctive changes, but these have not so far been related to CVD and dietary risk markers (Piccolo et al. 2015, Zheng et al. 2015)

A meta-analysis of 14 randomized placebo-controlled trials involving 702 participants showed that probiotic fermented milk produced a significant reduction of 3.10 mmHg in systolic BP and 1.09 mmHg in diastolic BP (Dong et al. 2013). A second meta-analysis of nine studies showed that probiotic consumption significantly changed systolic BP by −3.56 mmHg and diastolic BP by −2.38 mmHg compared with control groups. A greater reduction was found with multiple as compared with single species of probiotics, and interventions of <8 weeks did not result in a significant reduction in systolic or diastolic BP. A daily dose of probiotics $>10^{11}$ colony-forming units was required for a significant effect (Khalesi et al. 2014).

Probiotics compared with placebo significantly reduced fasting glucose (−0.31 mmol/L; $p = 0.02$) and fasting plasma insulin (−1.29 μU/mL; $p = 0.004$) in 17 randomized trials with 1105 participants (Ruan et al. 2015).

Acute Feeding Studies

Clemente et al. (2003) examined postprandial lipemia after milk, mozzarella cheese, and butter and found the same triglyceride peak height, but the peak occurred earlier for milk than cheese or butter. This may reflect differences between solid and liquid foods rather than anything specific to the individual whole dairy foods.

Most of the acute studies have examined isolated dairy proteins rather than intact dairy products. Four liquid test meals containing whey, tuna, turkey, and egg albumin and eaten on four separate occasions were followed 4 h later by a standard ad libitum test meal in 22 lean healthy men. The blood glucose response was significantly lower with the whey meal than with the turkey ($p < 0.023$) and egg ($p < 0.001$) meals, but it was similar to the tuna meal. The area under the curve (AUC) for blood insulin was significantly higher with the whey meal than with the tuna, turkey, and egg meals (all $p < 0.001$). The AUC for the rating of hunger was significantly lower with the whey meal than with the tuna ($p < 0.033$), turkey ($p < 0.001$), and egg ($p < 0.001$) meals. Mean energy intake for an ad libitum meal consumed 4 h after the test meal was significantly lower ($p < 0.001$) with the whey meal than with the tuna, egg, and turkey meals. There was a strong relationship between self-rated appetite, postprandial insulin response, and energy intake at lunch (Pal and Ellis 2010).

Twenty-five healthy subjects consumed 10% or 25% of meal energy either as casein, soy, or whey protein. At both levels of the protein, whey triggered the strongest responses in concentrations of active GLP1 ($p < 0.05$) and insulin ($p < 0.05$) compared with casein and/or soy. There were no differences in energy intake at a test meal 3 h later (Veldhorst et al. 2009).

Cod protein was compared with cottage cheese or soy in 17 healthy women (von Post-Skagegård et al. 2006). The blood glucose response after the cod protein meal differed from that of the soy protein meal, with a larger AUC calculated up to 120 min. The serum insulin response after the cottage cheese differed from that of the cod protein meal with a larger insulin AUC calculated up to 240 min. The insulin/C-peptide was higher after the cottage cheese meal (suggesting delayed insulin clearance) compared to the cod and soy protein meals at 120 min. The insulin/glucose ratio was lower after the cod protein meal compared to the cottage cheese and soy protein meals at 120 min. Based on these observations, it was suggested that cottage cheese may be metabolically harmful.

Protein-rich meals containing 45 g casein, whey, cod, or gluten as part of a 100 g butter meal were fed to 12 people with type 2 diabetes. The incremental area under the curve (iAUC) for triglyceride was significantly lower after the whey meal than after the other meals. Free fatty acids were most pronouncedly suppressed after the whey meal. The glucose response was lower after the whey meal than after the other meals, whereas no significant differences were found in insulin, glucagon, GLP1, and glucose-dependent insulinotropic peptide responses (Mortensen et al. 2009).

Eleven obese nondiabetic subjects were fed a fat-rich meal with either whey, casein, or gluten. Whey protein caused lower postprandial lipemia ($p < 0.05$) compared to supplementation with cod protein and gluten. This was primarily due to lower triglyceride concentrations in the chylomicron-rich fraction ($p < 0.05$) (Holmer-Jensen et al. 2013). The iAUC for CCL5/RANTES (pro-inflammatory molecules) was significantly lower after the whey meal compared with the cod and casein meals ($p = 0.0053$). The iAUC for monocyte chemoattractant protein 1 was significantly higher after the whey meal compared to the cod and gluten meals ($p = 0.04$), which would be interpreted as adverse for atherosclerosis development despite the lower postprandial lipemia. The overall effect on the risk of atherosclerosis is not clear.

An acute intervention with 45 g casein, whey, or glucose supplemented to a breakfast test meal had no differential effects over 6 h on blood pressure, vascular function, or IL-6, TNF-α, and CRP (Pal and Ellis 2011). However, there was a significant decrease in the triglyceride AUC by 21% and 27% after consuming the whey meal compared to control and casein meals, respectively (Pal et al. 2010).

Overall, whey appears to stimulate insulin and lower triglyceride and glucose responses compared with other proteins. The increased insulin may stimulate lipoprotein lipase and enhance triglyceride clearance. Although this would be perceived as beneficial, it is possible that enhanced stimulation of insulin may not be metabolically benign in those individuals predisposed to pancreatic failure. The metabolic benefit of whey has been reviewed by Sousa et al. (2012), while the use of dairy foods for the management of type 2 diabetes has also been reviewed (Astrup 2014). Whey-containing premeal drinks can dampen meal glycemic responses (Clifton et al. 2014).

POULTRY

Poultry in moderate amounts is a component of the Mediterranean diet, and it and other dietary patterns that replace red meat with white meat are associated with lower rates of CVD and type 2 diabetes (Esposito et al. 2010), but whether poultry *per se* has a protective as opposed to a neutral effect is not clear. The healthy dietary patterns reduced type 2 diabetes by 15%–83% in all 10 prospective cohorts examined. Poultry is recommended as an important component of a healthy diet (Marangoni et al. 2015).

EGGS

Because dietary cholesterol elevates LDL cholesterol to a small degree (Weggemans et al. 2001), there has been controversy about the role of whole eggs as a source of dietary protein. Two meta-analyses have been performed examining the relationship between eggs and CVD. Li et al. (2013a) examined 14 studies with 320,778 subjects. Comparing the highest to the lowest egg intake groups, CVD risk was increased significantly in the whole population by 19%. In those with diabetes, the risk was greater, with a significant 83% increase. For each 4 eggs/week increase in intake, the risk for CVD increased by 6% and the development of type 2 diabetes increased by 40% in the whole population, and both were significant. For unknown reasons, eggs appeared to be twice as harmful in non-U.S. Western countries compared with the United States (Li et al. 2013a). A second meta-analysis (Shin et al. 2013) examined 22 separate cohorts and did not find any increase in risk for CVD or its separate components for a comparison of the highest (1 egg/day or more) to the lowest (<1 egg/week) intake. However in people with type 2 diabetes, there was a significant increase in overall CVD risk of 69%. There was also a 42% increase in the risk of developing type 2 diabetes. Despite this and Weggemans meta-analysis from egg intervention studies, the 2015 Dietary Guidelines Advisory Committee removed dietary cholesterol from its nutrients of concern. Notably, eggs are rich in choline, a dietary precursor of trimethylamine, which has been associated with CVD risk (Miller et al. 2014), but the trimethylamine area is controversial.

FISH

Epidemiological Studies of Fish Consumption and CVD and Diabetes

Epidemiology relating fish to CVD has been mixed. The Physicians Health Study found no association of fish to CVD risk (Morris et al. 1995), whereas a meta-analysis of 14 cohort and 5 case–control studies found that any vs. no fish consumption was associated with 14% less total CHD and 17% less fatal CHD (Whelton et al. 2004). A second meta-analysis (He et al. 2004a) found that weekly fish intake reduced fatal CHD by 15%, with a 38% reduction when fish was consumed five or more times per week. Fish type was not assessed. A very small amount (~20 g/day) of fish could reduce fatal CHD by 7% (He et al. 2004a). Strokes were also reduced by this low level of intake (He et al. 2004b). This level of fish intake would be unlikely to change levels of N3 fatty acids in RBC membranes, and indeed lean fish is also protective (Kromhout et al. 1985), so N3 fats may not be required for protection. In PREDIMED, the Mediterranean diet, which reduced CVD rates by 13% for a two-point change in diet score, is a fish-rich diet (Martinez-Gonzalez and Bes-Rastrollo, 2014). Although measurement of N3 fats in plasma phospholipids is related to total and CHD mortality (27% reduction in the highest quintile) in older adults (Mozaffarian et al. 2013), this does not necessarily mean that the N3 fats are the cause of the reduction as they may be a marker of a healthy diet abundant in fish and with little red meat. A higher N3 fat level may also reflect individuals with superior incorporation of N3 fats into phospholipids as well as a higher intake of fish. A primary prevention intervention using 1 g/day of fish oil fatty acids in high-risk individuals had no effect on cardiovascular disease endpoints (Risk and Prevention Study Collaborative Group 2013).

In Japan a high fish intake of 180 g/day (8 times/week) was associated with reduced definite myocardial infarction by 56% compared with a low intake of 23 g/day of fish. The effect was predominantly on nonfatal events as opposed to the U.S. epidemiology. The effect appeared to be related to N3 fatty acids rather than fish protein as the highest intake of N3 fats reduced definite MI by 65% (Iso et al. 2006).

A recent meta-analysis examined 11 prospective studies and found that the highest intake of fish (>4 times/week) was associated with a 21% reduction in acute coronary syndromes. Each 100 g serving of fish per week lowered the risk by 5% (Leung Yinko et al. 2014). Heart failure was also reduced by fish consumption in five prospective studies with a 14% reduction for consumption five or more times per week. An increase of 20 g/day of fish reduced the risk by a further 6% (Li et al. 2013b).

In some studies a separation of the effect of fish *per se* and fish oil fatty acids could be seen. For instance, in the Nurses' Health Study in diabetic women, there was a 74% reduction in CHD mortality in the highest fish consumption group (5 or more times/week), while higher consumption of long-chain N3 fatty acids was associated with an insignificant 31% reduction in CHD mortality (Hu et al. 2003). This suggests that there was a benefit from fish protein (or some other components in fish) replacing other forms of protein, in particular red meat, for reducing the risk of CHD mortality. In addition, in Western populations, red meat intake may also be a significant source of long-chain N3 fatty acids (Welch et al. 2010), which will confound the relationships. This disparity between fish and N3 fats was not seen in the whole Nurses' Health Study cohort (Hu et al. 2002) for CHD, but total strokes were reduced by 52% in the highest fish intake group and by 33% in the highest quintile of fish oil intake (Iso et al. 2001).

Diabetes

Fish/seafood or DHA and EPA consumption had no overall effect on the risk of type 2 diabetes in 18 separate cohorts (Wu et al. 2012). However, in Asian cohorts, there was an 11% reduced risk in the highest intake, while there was a significant 20% increase ($p < 0.02$ for interaction) risk in diabetes in Western populations (North America and Europe). Asian subjects with type 2 diabetes also had significantly lower tissue levels of 22:6 N3 compared with those without diabetes (Zheng et al. 2012). Another meta-analysis found a significant protective effect of oily fish only, with a 20% reduced risk of type 2 diabetes per 80 g of fish/day. Ethnicity was not assessed in this study

(Zhang et al. 2013). In Japan, fish intake was associated with a significant 27%–32% reduced risk of type 2 diabetes in men, but there was no significant effect in women. The fat content of fish was unrelated to risk (Nanri et al. 2011). In the Women's Health Study, both fish and N3 intake were associated with increased risk of type 2 diabetes, but adjustment of fish for DHA content removed the risk, suggesting it was not fish *per se* but fish oil fatty acids that increased the risk (Djoussé et al. 2011). This may be due to N3 fats modulating the insulin receptor lipid microdomain.

Dietary Interventions

Most fish interventions have aimed to increase the intake of long-chain N3 fats, and there are few studies using lean fish. The WISH-CARE study examined 273 people with metabolic syndrome after 8 weeks of intervention with 100 g/day of hake, a lean fish. There was no control nonfish protein used, but participants had an 8-week fish-and-seafood-free period in a randomized crossover study. The investigators found a significant effect of the intervention with white fish on reducing waist circumference ($p < 0.001$) and diastolic blood pressure ($p = 0.014$). A significant lowering of serum LDL cholesterol concentrations ($p = 0.048$) was also seen. A significant rise in serum EPA and DHA following white fish consumption suggested that the effects may not be due only to fish protein (Vázquez et al. 2014).

Four weeks of lean fish per week (100–150 g per meal) decreased systolic and diastolic blood pressure ($p < 0.01$ and $p < 0.02$, respectively, group by time interaction) in volunteers with cardiac disease, with no effects in the fatty fish or lean meat fed control groups (Erkkilä et al. 2008).

Eight weeks of four mixed fish meals per week compared to a control group had no effect on CRP ($n = 80$), IL-1β ($n = 33$), or IL-6 ($n = 21$) concentrations, blood pressure, or lipids (Grieger et al. 2014). Daily fish diets in people with type 2 diabetes increased HbA1c by 0.5% and fasting glucose by 0.57 mmol/L (Dunstan et al. 1997).

The effects of lean white fish on plasma lipoproteins also have been investigated in pre- and postmenopausal women fed a low-fat, high-polyunsaturated/saturated-fat ratio diet (Jacques et al. 1992). In postmenopausal women, lean white fish compared with other animal protein products induced higher concentrations of plasma cholesterol, LDL-apoB and HDL cholesterol, mainly in the HDL3 fraction. In premenopausal women, lean white fish induced lower concentrations of VLDL triglycerides and higher concentrations of LDL-apoB in plasma (Gascon et al. 1996).

SOY INTAKE, HEART DISEASE, AND TYPE 2 DIABETES

The Singapore Chinese Health Study was a population-based study that recruited 63,257 Chinese adults aged 45–74 years old from 1993 to 1998. The median intake was 5.2 g/day for soy protein, 15.8 mg/day for soy isoflavones, and 87.4 g/day for soy expressed as tofu equivalents. Cardiovascular deaths ($n = 4780$) occurred until 2011. After adjustment for sociodemographic, lifestyle, and other dietary factors, soy protein intake was not significantly associated with cardiovascular disease. Similarly, no significant association was observed for soy isoflavones and total tofu equivalents when deaths from CHD ($n = 2697$) and stroke ($n = 1298$) were considered separately (Talaei et al. 2014). In the same cohort (Mueller et al. 2012), the highest quintile of unsweetened soy intake was associated with a 28% reduced risk of type 2 diabetes (p trend = 0.015), while sweetened soybean was associated with 13% more diabetes in the highest quintile of intake (p trend = 0.013).

In a case–control study in women from Fukuoka City, Japan, with 660 cases and 1277 controls, tofu consumption was inversely related to the risk of acute myocardial infarction; relative risks for eating tofu <2, 2–3, and 4 or more times per week were 1.0, 0.8, and 0.5, respectively, after adjustment for nondietary factors (p trend = 0.01). Further adjustment for the consumption of fruit and fish did not alter the findings (Sasazuki et al. 2001). In the Japan Public Health Center–based cohort of 40,462 men and women, consuming soy more than five times per week was associated with a 69% reduction in CVD mortality. Similar relationships were seen with isoflavone intake. The observation was mostly in postmenopausal women and was not seen in men (Kokubo et al. 2007).

Dietary Patterns Containing Soy

A dietary pattern rich in soy, fruits, and vegetables (Odegaard et al. 2014) was associated with a 25% reduction in all-cause mortality in the highest quintile (p trend < 0.0001), while a diet rich in dim sum and meat was associated with a 27% increase in CVD mortality in the highest quintile (p trend = 0.001). In never smokers only, type 2 diabetes was reduced by 25% (p = 0.0005) with the healthy diet and increased by 47% (p < 0.0001) with the meat diet (Odegaard et al. 2011).

In the INTERHEART China case–control study (Guo et al. 2013), the fruit and vegetables and tofu groups had a 30% reduction in risk of type 2 diabetes in the highest vs. lowest intake quartile (p = 0.0001).

Isoflavonoid Excretion

In a nested case–control study (377 cases and 753 controls) with the Shanghai cohort, urinary equol excretion (but not total isoflavonoids) showed a significant inverse association with CHD in women with a 54% reduction in the highest vs. lowest quartile (Hall et al. 2005).

Interventions with Soy on Cardiovascular and Diabetes Risk Markers

LDL Cholesterol

Soy protein has been shown in many studies to lower LDL cholesterol, and there have been several meta-analyses confirming these findings. The most recent one was performed by Anderson and Bush (2011), and 20 parallel studies and 23 crossover studies were examined. LDL cholesterol was lowered by 5.5% in parallel studies and 4.2% in crossover studies with a median dose of 30 g/day of soy protein in comparison with non-soy protein. Only in parallel studies was HDL cholesterol elevated by 3.2% and triglyceride lowered by 10.2%. Studies of soy protein with intact isoflavones (n = 23) showed very similar effects to the earlier meta-analysis (Zhan and Ho 2005) with a dose–response relationship found between isoflavone daily intake and LDL cholesterol lowering, but this was not adjusted for soy protein intake. Soy may be effective because it is displacing other protein sources that may be associated with LDL-elevating components such as saturated fat.

A meta-analysis showed no overall effect of isoflavone extracts on lipids (Taku et al. 2008), and a comparison of soy enriched or depleted in isoflavones (11 studies) showed no reduction in total cholesterol but isoflavone enrichment resulting in a small significant reduction in LDL cholesterol of 3.5% (Taku et al. 2007). Thus, it would appear that isolated soy protein lowers LDL cholesterol with some additional benefit from intrinsic isoflavones. Isolated isoflavones appear to have no effect, and there is no dose–response relationship between the amount of isoflavones and LDL cholesterol lowering (Weggemans and Trautwein 2003). A Cochrane meta-analysis found no effect of isoflavones on plasma lipids (Qin et al. 2013).

Nontraditional Risk Factors

There have been few studies on nontraditional risk markers, but 40 g of soy protein (89.3 mg of isoflavones) for 8 weeks in comparison with 40 g milk protein supplement or 40 g complex carbohydrate in a randomized crossover study lowered E-selectin (p = 0.014) and leptin (p = 0.011). However, given that 20 comparisons were made, these changes could well have occurred by chance (Rebholz et al. 2013). No effect was found on adhesion molecules in postmenopausal women (Blum et al. 2003), on adhesion molecules or other inflammatory markers in 117 postmenopausal women (Hall et al. 2005), or on CRP in a meta-analysis of 17 studies, but there was some evidence of benefit of soy in women with a high baseline CRP (Dong et al. 2011). In the Hall study (Hall et al. 2005), there was no effect of soy on lipids, glucose, and insulin.

Thirty men were fed 25 g/day of protein from soy with or without isoflavones, or milk. A high-fat test meal resulted in an increase in postprandial triglycerides after the soy alone diet and not the other two diets (Santo et al. 2010). Feeding natto (viscous fermented soybeans) and viscous vegetables as a breakfast with rice for 2 weeks compared with nonviscous soybeans, potatoes, and broccoli and rice breakfast improved glucose and insulin responses to the breakfast, while the comparator showed no improvement with time. Furthermore, the test meal of natto and viscous vegetables also lowered glucose and insulin response compared with the control meal prior to the 2-week feeding period (Taniguchi-Fukatsu et al. 2012).

Acute Studies with Soy

These have been mostly confined to muscle protein synthesis studies that find that soy is inferior to whey but is better than (Tang et al. 2009), equivalent (Luiking et al. 2011), or worse than casein (Luiking et al. 2005) at acutely stimulating protein synthesis. Soy is similar to whey and gluten at reducing appetite over 3 h and reducing food intake at a buffet meal by 10% and stimulating GLP1 and CCK (Bowen et al. 2006).

CONCLUSION

Meat is associated with worse outcomes, while dairy is probably neutral, although yogurt may protect against type 2 diabetes. Fish is mostly associated with protection from CVD but the exact mechanism is not clear. Poultry is neutral and soy may be beneficial. Most data are based on epidemiology, while the few interventions that have been performed have failed to show clear cardiometabolic benefit.

REFERENCES

Abete I, Romaguera D, Vieira AR, Lopez de Munain A, Norat T. 2014. Association between total, processed, red and white meat consumption and all-cause, CVD and IHD mortality: A meta-analysis of cohort studies. *Br J Nutr* 112(5):762–775.

Abreu S, Moreira P, Moreira C et al. 2014. Intake of milk, but not total dairy, yogurt, or cheese, is negatively associated with the clustering of cardiometabolic risk factors in adolescents. *Nutr Res* 34(1):48–57.

Adebamowo SN, Spiegelman D, Willett WC, Rexrode KM. 2015. Association between intakes of magnesium, potassium, and calcium and risk of stroke: 2 cohorts of US women and updated meta-analyses. *Am J Clin Nutr* 101(6):1269–1277.

Anderson JW, Bush HM. 2011. Soy protein effects on serum lipoproteins: A quality assessment and meta-analysis of randomized, controlled studies. *J Am Coll Nutr* 30(2):79–91.

Appleby PN, Davey GK, Key TJ. 2002. Hypertension and blood pressure among meat eaters, fish eaters, vegetarians and vegans in EPIC-Oxford. *Public Health Nutr* 5(5):645–654.

Aslibekyan S, Campos H, Baylin A. 2012. Biomarkers of dairy intake and the risk of heart disease. *Nutr Metab Cardiovasc Dis* 22:1039–1045.

Astrup A. 2014. Yogurt and dairy product consumption to prevent cardiometabolic diseases: Epidemiologic and experimental studies. *Am J Clin Nutr* 99(5 Suppl):1235S–1242S.

Aune D, Norat T, Romundstad P, Vatten LJ. 2013. Dairy products and the risk of type 2 diabetes: A systematic review and dose-response meta-analysis of cohort studies. *Am J Clin Nutr* 98(4):1066–1083.

Aviv A. 2012. Genetics of leukocyte telomere length and its role in atherosclerosis. *Mutat Res* 730(1–2):68–74.

Babio N, Becerra-Tomás N, Martínez-González MA et al.; on behalf of the PREDIMED Investigators. 2015. Consumption of yogurt, low-fat milk, and other low-fat dairy products is associated with lower risk of metabolic syndrome incidence in an elderly Mediterranean population. *J Nutr* 102(1):20–30.

Beauchesne-Rondeau E, Gascon A, Bergeron J, Jacques H. 2003. Plasma lipids and lipoproteins in hypercholesterolemic men fed a lipid-lowering diet containing lean beef, lean fish, or poultry. *Am J Clin Nutr* 77(3):587–593.

Benatar JR, Sidhu K, Stewart RA. 2013. Effects of high and low fat dairy food on cardio-metabolic risk factors: A meta-analysis of randomized studies. *PLoS One* 8(10):e76480.

Blum A, Lang N, Peleg A et al. 2003. Effects of oral soy protein on markers of inflammation in postmenopausal women with mild hypercholesterolemia. *Am Heart J* 145(2):e7.

Bohl M, Bjørnshave A, Rasmussen KV et al. 2015. Dairy proteins, dairy lipids, and postprandial lipemia in persons with abdominal obesity (DairyHealth): A 12-wk, randomized, parallel-controlled, double-blinded, diet intervention study. *Am J Clin Nutr* 101(4):870–878.

Bowen J, Noakes M, Clifton PM. 2006. Appetite regulatory hormone responses to various dietary proteins differ by body mass index status despite similar reductions in ad libitum energy intake. *J Clin Endocrinol Metab* 91(8):2913–2919.

Casas-Agustench P, Arnett DK, Smith CE et al. December 2014. Saturated fat intake modulates the association between an obesity genetic risk score and body mass index in two US populations. *J Acad Nutr Diet* 114(12):1954–1966.

Chen M, Pan A, Malik VS, Hu FB. 2012. Effects of dairy intake on body weight and fat: A meta-analysis of randomized controlled trials. *Am J Clin Nutr* 96(4):735–747.

Chen M, Sun Q, Giovannucci E et al. 2014. Dairy consumption and risk of type 2 diabetes: 3 cohorts of US adults and an updated meta-analysis. *BMC Med* 12:215.

Chiu S, Williams PT, Dawson T et al. 2014. Diets high in protein or saturated fat do not affect insulin sensitivity or plasma concentrations of lipids and lipoproteins in overweight and obese adults. *J Nutr* 144(11):1753–1759.

Clemente G, Mancini M, Nazzaro F et al. 2003. Effects of different dairy products on postprandial lipemia. *Nutr Metab Cardiovasc Dis* 13(6):377–383.

Clifton PM, Galbraith C, Coles L. 2014. Effect of a low dose whey/guar preload on glycemic control in people with type 2 diabetes—A randomised controlled trial. *Nutr J* 13:103.

Conway V, Couture P, Gauthier S, Pouliot Y, Lamarche B. 2014. Effect of buttermilk consumption on blood pressure in moderately hypercholesterolemic men and women. *Nutrition* 30(1):116–119.

Conway V, Couture P, Richard C, Gauthier SF, Pouliot Y, Lamarche B. 2013. Impact of buttermilk consumption on plasma lipids and surrogate markers of cholesterol homeostasis in men and women. *Nutr Metab Cardiovasc Dis* 23(12):1255–1262.

Crichton GE, Alkerwi A. 2014a. Whole-fat dairy food intake is inversely associated with obesity prevalence: Findings from the Observation of Cardiovascular Risk Factors in Luxembourg study. *Nutr Res* 34(11):936–943.

Crichton GE, Alkerwi A. 2014b. Dairy food intake is positively associated with cardiovascular health: Findings from Observation of Cardiovascular Risk Factors in Luxembourg study. *Nutr Res* 34(12):1036–1044.

Crichton GE, Bryan J, Buckley J, Murphy KJ. 2011. Dairy consumption and metabolic syndrome: A systematic review of findings and methodological issues. *Obes Rev* 12(5):e190–e201.

de Goede J, Geleijnse JM, Ding EL, Soedamah-Muthu SS. 2015. Effect of cheese consumption on blood lipids: A systematic review and meta-analysis of randomized controlled trials. *Nutr Rev* 73(5):259–275.

de Oliveira Otto MC, Mozaffarian D, Kromhout D et al. 2012. Dietary intake of saturated fat by food source and incident cardiovascular disease: The Multi-Ethnic Study of Atherosclerosis. *Am J Clin Nutr* 96(2):397–404.

Díaz-López A, Bulló M, Martínez-González MA et al. 2015. Dairy product consumption and risk of type 2 diabetes in an elderly Spanish Mediterranean population at high cardiovascular risk. *Eur J Nutr* 55(1):349–360. February 7. [Epub ahead of print].

Djoussé L, Gaziano JM, Buring JE, Lee IM. 2011. Dietary omega-3 fatty acids and fish consumption and risk of type 2 diabetes. *Am J Clin Nutr* 93(1):143–150.

Dong JY, Szeto IM, Makinen K et al. 2013. Effect of probiotic fermented milk on blood pressure: A meta-analysis of randomised controlled trials. *Br J Nutr* 110(7):1188–1194.

Dong JY, Wang P, He K, Qin LQ. 2011. Effect of soy isoflavones on circulating C-reactive protein in postmenopausal women: Meta-analysis of randomized controlled trials. *Menopause* 18(11):1256–1262.

Drouillet P, Balkau B, Charles MA, Vol S, Bedouet M, Ducimetière P; Desir Study Group. 2007. Calcium consumption and insulin resistance syndrome parameters. Data from the Epidemiological Study on the Insulin Resistance Syndrome (DESIR). *Nutr Metab Cardiovasc Dis* 17(7):486–492.

Dunstan DW, Mori TA, Puddey IB et al. 1997. The independent and combined effects of aerobic exercise and dietary fish intake on serum lipids and glycemic control in NIDDM. A randomized controlled study. *Diabetes Care* 20(6):913–921.

Elwood PC, Janet E, Pickering JE, Givens DI, Gallacher JE. 2010. The consumption of milk and dairy foods and the incidence of vascular disease and diabetes: An overview of the evidence. *Lipids* 45(10):925–939.

Ericson U, Hellstrand S, Brunkwall L et al. 2015. Food sources of fat may clarify the inconsistent role of dietary fat intake for incidence of type 2 diabetes. *Am J Clin Nutr* 101(5):1065–1080.

Ericson U, Sonestedt E, Gullberg B et al. 2013. High intakes of protein and processed meat associate with increased incidence of type 2 diabetes. *Br J Nutr* 109(6):1143–1153.

Erkkilä AT, Schwab US, de Mello VD et al. 2008. Effects of fatty and lean fish intake on blood pressure in subjects with coronary heart disease using multiple medications. *Eur J Nutr* 47(6):319–328.

Esposito K, Kastorini CM, Panagiotakos DB, Giugliano D. 2010. Prevention of type 2 diabetes by dietary patterns: A systematic review of prospective studies and meta-analysis. *Metab Syndr Relat Disord* 8(6):471–476.

Ferland A, Lamarche B, Chateau-Degat ML et al. 2011. Dairy product intake and its association with body weight and cardiovascular disease risk factors in a population in dietary transition. *J Am Coll Nutr* 30:92–99.

Feskens EJ, Sluik D, van Woudenbergh GJ. 2013. Meat consumption, diabetes, and its complications. *Curr Diab Rep* 13(2):298–306.

Gascon A, Jacques H, Moorjani S et al. 1996. Plasma lipoprotein profile and lipolytic activities in response to the substitution of lean white fish for other animal protein sources in premenopausal women. *Am J Clin Nutr* 63(3):315–321.

Grieger JA, Miller MD, Cobiac L. 2014. Investigation of the effects of a high fish diet on inflammatory cytokines, blood pressure, and lipids in healthy older Australians. *Food Nutr Res* 15:58.

Guo J, Li W, Wang Y et al. 2013. INTERHEART China study investigators. Influence of dietary patterns on the risk of acute myocardial infarction in China population: The INTERHEART China study. *Chin Med J (Engl)* 126(3):464–470.

Hall WL, Vafeiadou K, Hallund J et al. 2005. Soy-isoflavone-enriched foods and inflammatory biomarkers of cardiovascular disease risk in postmenopausal women: Interactions with genotype and equol production. *Am J Clin Nutr* 82(6):1260–1268.

Haring B, Gronroos N ,Nettleton JA, von Ballmoos MC, Selvin E, Alonso A. 2014. Dietary protein intake and coronary heart disease in a large community based cohort: Results from the Atherosclerosis Risk in Communities (ARIC) study [corrected]. *PLoS One* 9(10):e109552.

He FJ, Nowson CA, Lucas M, MacGregor GA. 2007. Increased consumption of fruit and vegetables is related to a reduced risk of coronary heart disease: Meta-analysis of cohort studies. *J Hum Hypertens* 21(9):717–728.

He K, Song Y, Daviglus ML et al. 2004a. Accumulated evidence on fish consumption and coronary heart disease mortality: A meta-analysis of cohort studies. *Circulation* 109(22):2705–2711.

He K, Song Y, Daviglus ML et al. 2004b. Fish consumption and incidence of stroke: A meta-analysis of cohort studies. *Stroke* 35(7):1538–1542.

Hodgson JM, Burke V, Beilin LJ, Puddey IB. 2006. Partial substitution of carbohydrate intake with protein intake from lean red meat lowers blood pressure in hypertensive persons. *Am J Clin Nutr* 83(4):780–787.

Hodgson JM, Ward NC, Burke V, Beilin LJ, Puddey IB. 2007. Increased lean red meat intake does not elevate markers of oxidative stress and inflammation in humans. *J Nutr* 137(2):363–367.

Holmer-Jensen J, Mortensen LS, Astrup A et al. 2013. Acute differential effects of dietary protein quality on postprandial lipemia in obese non-diabetic subjects. *Nutr Res* 33(1):34–40.

Hu FB, Stampfer MJ, Manson JE et al. December 1999. Dietary saturated fats and their food sources in relation to the risk of coronary heart disease in women. *Am J Clin Nutr* 70(6):1001–1008.

Hu FB, Bronner L, Willett WC et al. 2002. Fish and omega-3 fatty acid intake and risk of coronary heart disease in women. *JAMA* 287(14):1815–1821.

Hu FB, Cho E, Rexrode KM, Albert CM, Manson JE. 2003. Fish and long-chain omega-3 fatty acid intake and risk of coronary heart disease and total mortality in diabetic women. *Circulation* 107(14):1852–1857.

Huang T, Yang B, Zheng J, Li G, Wahlqvist ML, Li D. 2012. Cardiovascular disease mortality and cancer incidence in vegetarians: A meta-analysis and systematic review. *Ann Nutr Metab* 60(4):233–240.

Hunnicutt J, He K, Xun P. 2014. Dietary iron intake and body iron stores are associated with risk of coronary heart disease in a meta-analysis of prospective cohort studies. *J Nutr* 144(3):359–366.

Huth PJ, Park KM. 2012. Influence of dairy product and milk fat consumption on cardiovascular disease risk: A review of the evidence. *Adv Nutr* 3(3):266–285.

Iso H, Kobayashi M, Ishihara J et al.; JPHC Study Group. 2006. Intake of fish and n3 fatty acids and risk of coronary heart disease among Japanese: The Japan Public Health Center-Based (JPHC) Study Cohort I. *Circulation* 13(2):195–202.

Iso H, Rexrode KM, Stampfer MJ et al. 2001. Intake of fish and omega-3 fatty acids and risk of stroke in women. *JAMA* 285(3):304–312.

Ivey KL, Lewis JR, Hodgson JM et al. 2011. Association between yogurt, milk, and cheese consumption and common carotid artery intima-media thickness and cardiovascular disease risk factors in elderly women. *Am J Clin Nutr* 94:234–239.

Jacques H, Noreau L, Moorjani S. 1992. Effects on plasma lipoproteins and endogenous sex hormones of substituting lean white fish for other animal-protein sources in diets of postmenopausal women. *Am J Clin Nutr* 55(4):896–901.

Kahn HA, Phillips RL, Snowdon DA, Choi W. 1984. Association between reported diet and all-cause mortality. Twenty-one-year follow-up on 27,530 adult Seventh-Day Adventists. *Am J Epidemiol* 119:775–787.

Kaluza J, Wolk A, Larsson SC. 2012. Red meat consumption and risk of stroke: A meta-analysis of prospective studies. *Stroke* 43:2556–2560.

Kelemen LE, Kushi LH, Jacobs Jr DR, Cerhan JR. 2005. Associations of dietary protein with disease and mortality in a prospective study of postmenopausal women. *Am J Epidemiol* 161:239–249.

Khalesi S, Sun J, Buys N, Jayasinghe R. 2014 Effect of probiotics on blood pressure: A systematic review and meta-analysis of randomized, controlled trials. *Hypertension* 64(4):897–903.

Kim Y, Keogh J, Clifton P. 2015. A review of potential metabolic etiologies of the observed association between red meat consumption and development of type 2 diabetes mellitus. *Metabolism* 64(7):768–779.

Koeth RA, Wang Z, Levison BS et al. 2013. Intestinal microbiota metabolism of L-carnitine, a nutrient in red meat, promotes atherosclerosis. *Nat Med* 19(5):576–585.

Kokubo Y, Iso H, Ishihara J, Okada K, Inoue M, Tsugane S; JPHC Study Group. 2007. Association of dietary intake of soy, beans, and isoflavones with risk of cerebral and myocardial infarctions in Japanese populations: The Japan Public Health Center-based (JPHC) study cohort I. *Circulation* 116(22):2553–2562.

Kratz M, Baars T, Guyenet S. 2013. The relationship between high-fat dairy consumption and obesity, cardiovascular, and metabolic disease. *Eur J Nutr* 52(1):1–24.

Kromhout D, Bosschieter EB, de Lezenne Coulander C. 1985. The inverse relation between fish consumption and 20-year mortality from coronary heart disease. *N Engl J Med* 312:1205–1209.

Laake I, Pedersen JI, Selmer R et al. 2012. A prospective study of intake of trans-fatty acids from ruminant fat, partially hydrogenated vegetable oils, and marine oils and mortality from CVD. *Br J Nutr* 108(4):743–754.

Larsson SC, Orsini N. 2014. Red meat and processed meat consumption and all-cause mortality: A meta-analysis. *Am J Epidemiol* 179:282–289.

Lee JE, McLerran DF, Rolland B et al. 2013. Meat intake and cause-specific mortality: A pooled analysis of Asian prospective cohort studies. *Am J Clin Nutr* 98(4):1032–1041.

Leung Yinko SS, Stark KD, Thanassoulis G, Pilote L. 2014. Fish consumption and acute coronary syndrome: A meta-analysis. *Am J Med* 127(9):848–857.e2.

Ley SH, Sun Q, Willett WC et al. 2014. Associations between red meat intake and biomarkers of inflammation and glucose metabolism in women. *Am J Clin Nutr* 99(2):352–360.

Li D, Kirsop J, Tang WH. 2015. Listening to our gut: Contribution of gut microbiota and cardiovascular risk in diabetes pathogenesis. *Curr Diab Rep* 15(9):634.

Li Y, Zhou C, Zhou X, Li L. 2013a. Egg consumption and risk of cardiovascular diseases and diabetes: A meta-analysis. *Atherosclerosis* 229(2):524–530.

Li YH, Zhou CH, Pei HJ et al. 2013b. Fish consumption and incidence of heart failure: A meta-analysis of prospective cohort studies. *Chin Med J (Engl)* 126(5):942–948.

Louie JC, Flood VM, Hector DJ, Rangan AM, Gill TP. 2011. Dairy consumption and overweight and obesity: A systematic review of prospective cohort studies. *Obes Rev* 12(7):e582–e592.

Lovejoy JC, Smith SR, Champagne CM et al. 2002. Effects of diets enriched in saturated (palmitic), monounsaturated (oleic), or trans (elaidic) fatty acids on insulin sensitivity and substrate oxidation in healthy adults. *Diabetes Care* 25(8):1283–1288.

Luiking YC, Deutz NE, Jäkel M, Soeters PB. 2005. Casein and soy protein meals differentially affect whole-body and splanchnic protein metabolism in healthy humans. *J Nutr* 135(5):1080–1087.

Luiking YC, Engelen MP, Soeters PB, Boirie Y, Deutz NE. 2011. Differential metabolic effects of casein and soy protein meals on skeletal muscle in healthy volunteers. *Clin Nutr* 30(1):65–72.

Maki KC, Van Elswyk ME, Alexander DD, Rains TM, Sohn EL, McNeill S. 2012. A meta-analysis of randomized controlled trials that compare the lipid effects of beef versus poultry and/or fish consumption. *J Clin Lipidol* 6(4):352–361.

Marangoni F, Corsello G, Cricelli C et al. 2015. Role of poultry meat in a balanced diet aimed at maintaining health and wellbeing: An Italian consensus document. *Food Nutr Res* 59:27606.

Martinez-Gonzalez MA, Bes-Rastrollo M. February 2014. Dietary patterns, Mediterranean diet, and cardiovascular disease. *Curr Opin Lipidol* 25(1):20–26.

Mensink RP, Zock PL, Kester AD, Katan MB. 2003. Effects of dietary fatty acids and carbohydrates on the ratio of serum total to HDL cholesterol and on serum lipids and apolipoproteins: A meta-analysis of 60 controlled trials. *Am J Clin Nutr* 77(5):1146–1155.

Micha R, Michas G, Mozaffarian D. 2012. Unprocessed red and processed meats and risk of coronary artery disease and type 2 diabetes—An updated review of the evidence. *Curr Atheroscler Rep* 14(6):515–524.

Micha R, Wallace SK, Mozaffarian D. 2010. Red and processed meat consumption and risk of incident coronary heart disease, stroke, and diabetes mellitus: A systematic review and meta-analysis. *Circulation* 121(21):2271–2283.

Miller CA, Corbin KD, da Costa KA et al. 2014. Effect of egg ingestion on trimethylamine-N-oxide production in humans: A randomized, controlled, dose-response study. *Am J Clin Nutr* 100(3):778–786.

Morris MC, Manson JE, Rosner B, Buring JE, Willett WC, Hennekens CH. 1995. Fish consumption and cardiovascular disease in the physicians' health study: A prospective study. *Am J Epidemiol* 142(2):166–175.

Mortensen LS, Hartvigsen ML, Brader LJ et al. 2009. Differential effects of protein quality on postprandial lipemia in response to a fat-rich meal in type 2 diabetes: Comparison of whey, casein, gluten, and cod protein. *Am J Clin Nutr* 90(1):41–48.

Mozaffarian D, Lemaitre RN, King IB et al. 2013. Plasma phospholipid long-chain ω-3 fatty acids and total and cause-specific mortality in older adults: A cohort study. *Ann Intern Med* 158(7):515–525.

Mueller NT, Odegaard AO, Gross MD et al. 2012. Soy intake and risk of type 2 diabetes in Chinese Singaporeans [corrected]. *Eur J Nutr* 51(8):1033–1040.

Na L, Han T, Zhang W et al. 2015. A snack dietary pattern increases the risk of hypercholesterolemia in northern Chinese adults: A prospective cohort study. *PLoS One* 10(8):e0134294.

Nagao M, Iso H, Yamagishi K, Date C, Tamakoshi A. 2012. Meat consumption in relation to mortality from cardiovascular disease among Japanese men and women. *Eur J Clin Nutr* 66:687–693.

Nanri A, Mizoue T, Noda M et al.; Japan Public Health Center-based Prospective Study Group. 2011. Fish intake and type 2 diabetes in Japanese men and women: The Japan Public Health Center-based Prospective Study. *Am J Clin Nutr* 94(3):884–891.

Navas-Carretero S, Pérez-Granados AM, Schoppen S, Vaquero MP. 2009. An oily fish diet increases insulin sensitivity compared to a red meat diet in young iron-deficient women. *Br J Nutr* 102(4):546–553.

Nettleton JA, Diez-Roux A, Jenny NS, Fitzpatrick AL, Jacobs Jr DR. 2008 Dietary patterns, food groups, and telomere length in the Multi-Ethnic Study of Atherosclerosis (MESA). *Am J Clin Nutr* 88(5):1405–1412.

O'Connor LM, Lentjes MA, Luben RN, Khaw KT, Wareham NJ, Forouhi NG. 2014. Dietary dairy product intake and incident type 2 diabetes: A prospective study using dietary data from a 7-day food diary. *Diabetologia* 57(5):909–917.

O'Neil CE, Keast DR, Fulgoni VL, Nicklas TA. 2012. Food sources of energy and nutrients among adults in the US: NHANES 2003–2006. *Nutrients* 4(12):2097–2120.

Odegaard AO, Koh WP, Butler LM. 2011. Dietary patterns and incident type 2 diabetes in Chinese men and women: The Singapore Chinese health study. *Diabetes Care* 34(4):880–885.

Odegaard AO, Koh WP, Yuan JM, Gross MD, Pereira MA. 2014. Dietary patterns and mortality in a Chinese population. *Am J Clin Nutr* 100(3):877–883.

Pal S, Ellis V. 2010. The acute effects of four protein meals on insulin, glucose, appetite and energy intake in lean men. *Br J Nutr* 104(8):1241–1248.

Pal S, Ellis V. 2011. Acute effects of whey protein isolate on blood pressure, vascular function and inflammatory markers in overweight postmenopausal women. *Br J Nutr* 105(10):1512–1519.

Pal S, Ellis V, Ho S. 2010. Acute effects of whey protein isolate on cardiovascular risk factors in overweight, post-menopausal women. *Atherosclerosis* 212(1):339–344.

Pan A, Sun Q, Bernstein AM, Manson JE, Willett WC, Hu FB. 2013. Changes in red meat consumption and subsequent risk of type 2 diabetes mellitus: Three cohorts of US men and women. *JAMA Intern Med* 173(14):1328–1335.

Pan A, Sun Q, Bernstein AM et al. 2011. Red meat consumption and risk of type 2 diabetes: 3 cohorts of US adults and an updated meta-analysis. *Am J Clin Nutr* 94(4):1088–1096.

Patterson E, Larsson SC, Wolk A, Akesson A. 2013. Association between dairy food consumption and risk of myocardial infarction in women differs by type of dairy food. *J Nutr* 143:74–79.

Piccolo BD, Comerford KB, Karakas SE, Knotts TA, Fiehn O, Adams SH. 2015. Whey protein supplementation does not alter plasma branched-chain amino acid profiles but results in unique metabolomics patterns in obese women enrolled in an 8-week weight loss trial. *J Nutr* 145(4):691–700.

Praagman J, Dalmeijer GW, van der Schouw YT et al. 2015. The relationship between fermented food intake and mortality risk in the European Prospective Investigation into Cancer and Nutrition-Netherlands cohort. *Br J Nutr* 113(3):498–506.

Qin LQ, Xu JY, Han SF, Zhang ZL, Zhao YY, Szeto IM. 2015. Dairy consumption and risk of cardiovascular disease: An updated meta-analysis of prospective cohort studies. *Asia Pac J Clin Nutr* 24(1):90–100.

Qin Y, Niu K, Zeng Y et al. June 6, 2013. Isoflavones for hypercholesterolaemia in adults. *Cochrane Database Syst Rev* 6:CD009518.

Ralston RA, Lee JH, Truby H, Palermo CE, Walker KZ. 2012. A systematic review and meta-analysis of elevated blood pressure and consumption of dairy foods. *J Hum Hypertens* 26(1):3–13.

Rebholz CM, Reynolds K, Wofford MR et al. 2013. Effect of soybean protein on novel cardiovascular disease risk factors: A randomized controlled trial. *Eur J Clin Nutr* 67(1):58–63.

Rice BH. 2014. Dairy and cardiovascular disease: A review of recent observational research. *Curr Nutr Rep* 3(2):130–138.

Risk and Prevention Study Collaborative Group. 2013. n-3 fatty acids in patients with multiple cardiovascular risk factors. *N Engl J Med* 368(19):1800–1808.

Rohrmann S, Overvad K, Bueno-de-Mesquita HB et al. 2013. Meat consumption and mortality—Results from the European Prospective Investigation into Cancer and Nutrition. *BMC Med* 11:63.

Rosqvist F, Smedman A, Lindmark-Månsson H. 2015. Potential role of milk fat globule membrane in modulating plasma lipoproteins, gene expression, and cholesterol metabolism in humans: A randomized study. *Am J Clin Nutr* 102(1):20–30.

Rouhani MH, Salehi-Abargouei A, Surkan PJ, Azadbakht L. September 2014. Is there a relationship between red or processed meat intake and obesity? A systematic review and meta-analysis of observational studies. *Obes Rev* 15(9):740–748. doi: 10.1111/obr.12172. Epub May 12, 2014.

Ruan Y, Sun J, He J, Chen F, Chen R, Chen H. 2015. Effect of probiotics on glycemic control: A systematic review and meta-analysis of randomized, controlled trials. *PLoS One* 10(7):e0132121.

Samara A, Herbeth B, Ndiaye NC et al. 2013. Dairy product consumption, calcium intakes, and metabolic syndrome-related factors over 5 years in the STANISLAS study. *Nutrition* 29(3):519–524.

Santo AS, Santo AM, Browne RW et al. 2010. Postprandial lipemia detects the effect of soy protein on cardiovascular disease risk compared with the fasting lipid profile. *Lipids* 45(12):1127–1138.

Sasazuki S; Fukuoka Heart Study Group. 2001. Case-control study of nonfatal myocardial infarction in relation to selected foods in Japanese men and women. *Jpn Circ J* 65(3):200–206.

Sayer RD, Wright AJ, Chen N, Campbell WW. 2015. Dietary approaches to stop hypertension diet retains effectiveness to reduce blood pressure when lean pork is substituted for chicken and fish as the predominant source of protein. *Am J Clin Nutr* 102(2):302–308.

Shin HJ, Cho E, Lee HJ et al. 2014. Instant noodle intake and dietary patterns are associated with distinct cardiometabolic risk factors in Korea. *J Nutr* 144:1247–1255.

Shin JY, Xun P, Nakamura Y, He K. 2013. Egg consumption in relation to risk of cardiovascular disease and diabetes: A systematic review and meta-analysis. *Am J Clin Nutr* 98(1):146–159.

Sluijs I, Forouhi NG, Beulens JW et al.; InterAct Consortium. 2012. The amount and type of dairy product intake and incident type 2 diabetes: Results from the EPIC-InterAct Study. *Am J Clin Nutr* 96(2):382–390.

Snijder MB, van Dam RM, Stehouwer CD, Hiddink GJ, Heine RJ, Dekker JM. 2008. A prospective study of dairy consumption in relation to changes in metabolic risk factors: The Hoorn Study. *Obesity (Silver Spring)* 16(3):706–709.

Snijder MB, van der Heijden AA, van Dam RM et al. 2007. Is higher dairy consumption associated with lower body weight and fewer metabolic disturbances? The Hoorn Study. *Am J Clin Nutr* 85(4):989–995.

Soedamah-Muthu SS, Ding EL, Al-Delaimy WK et al. 2011. Milk and dairy consumption and incidence of cardiovascular diseases and all-cause mortality: Dose-response meta-analysis of prospective cohort studies. *Am J Clin Nutr* 93(1):158–171.

Soedamah-Muthu SS, Verberne LD, Ding EL, Engberink MF, Geleijnse JM. 2012. Dairy consumption and incidence of hypertension: A dose-response meta-analysis of prospective cohort studies. *Hypertension* 60(5):1131–1137.

Sousa GT, Lira FS, Rosa JC et al. 2012. Dietary whey protein lessens several risk factors for metabolic diseases: A review. *Lipids Health Dis* 11:67.

Steffen LM, Kroenke CH, Yu X et al. 2005. Associations of plant food, dairy product, and meat intakes with 15-y incidence of elevated blood pressure in young black and white adults: The Coronary Artery Risk Development in Young Adults (CARDIA) Study. *Am J Clin Nutr* 82(6):1169–1177.

Takata Y, Shu XO, Gao YT et al. 2013. Red meat and poultry intakes and risk of total and cause-specific mortality: Results from cohort studies of Chinese adults in Shanghai. *PLoS One* 8:e56963.

Taku K, Umegaki K, Ishimi Y, Watanabe S. 2008. Effects of extracted soy isoflavones alone on blood total and LDL cholesterol: Meta-analysis of randomized controlled trials. *Ther Clin Risk Manag* 4(5):1097–1103.

Taku K, Umegaki K, Sato Y, Taki Y, Endoh K, Watanabe S. 2007. Soy isoflavones lower serum total and LDL cholesterol in humans: A meta-analysis of 11 randomized controlled trials. *Am J Clin Nutr* 85(4):1148–1156.

Talaei M, Koh WP, van Dam RM, Yuan JM, Pan A. 2014. Dietary soy intake is not associated with risk of cardiovascular disease mortality in Singapore Chinese adults. *J Nutr* 144(6):921–928.

Tang JE, Moore DR, Kujbida GW, Tarnopolsky MA, Phillips SM. 2009. Ingestion of whey hydrolysate, casein, or soy protein isolate: Effects on mixed muscle protein synthesis at rest and following resistance exercise in young men. *J Appl Physiol* 107(3):987–992.

Tang WH, Wang Z, Levison BS et al. 2013. Intestinal microbial metabolism of phosphatidylcholine and cardiovascular risk. *N Engl J Med* 368(17):1575–1584.

Taniguchi-Fukatsu A, Yamanaka-Okumura H, Naniwa-Kuroki Y et al. 2012. Natto and viscous vegetables in a Japanese-style breakfast improved insulin sensitivity, lipid metabolism and oxidative stress in overweight subjects with impaired glucose tolerance. *Br J Nutr* 107(8):1184–1191.
Tholstrup T, Høy CE, Andersen LN, Christensen RD, Sandström B. 2004. Does fat in milk, butter and cheese affect blood lipids and cholesterol differently? *J Am Coll Nutr* 23(2):169–176.
Turner KM, Keogh JB, Clifton PM. 2015a. Dairy consumption and insulin sensitivity: A systematic review of short- and long-term intervention studies. *Nutr Metab Cardiovasc Dis* 25 (1):3–8.
Turner KM, Keogh JB, Clifton PM. 2015b. Red meat, dairy, and insulin sensitivity: A randomized crossover intervention study. *Am J Clin Nutr* 101(6):1173–1179.
van Aerde MA, Soedamah-Muthu SS, Geleijnse JM et al. 2013. Dairy intake in relation to cardiovascular disease mortality and all-cause mortality: The Hoorn Study. *Eur J Nutr* 52(2):609–616.
van der Pols JC, Gunnell D, Williams GM, Holly JM, Bain C, Martin RM. 2009. Childhood dairy and calcium intake and cardiovascular mortality in adulthood: 65-year follow-up of the Boyd Orr cohort. *Heart* 19:1600–1606.
Vázquez C, Botella-Carretero JI, Corella D et al.; WISH-CARE Study Investigators. 2014. White fish reduces cardiovascular risk factors in patients with metabolic syndrome: The WISH-CARE study, a multicenter randomized clinical trial. *Nutr Metab Cardiovasc Dis* 24(3):328–335.
Veldhorst MA, Nieuwenhuizen AG, Hochstenbach-Waelen A et al. 2009. Dose-dependent satiating effect of whey relative to casein or soy. *Physiol Behav* 96(4–5):675–682.
Vijver LPL, Waal MAE, Weterings KGC, Dekker JM, Schouten EG, Kok F. 1992. Calcium intake and 28-year cardiovascular and coronary heart disease mortality in Dutch civil servants. *Int J Epidemiol* 21:36–39.
von Post-Skagegård M, Vessby B, Karlström B. 2006. Glucose and insulin responses in healthy women after intake of composite meals containing cod-, milk-, and soy protein. *Eur J Clin Nutr* 60(8):949–954.
Wang X, Lin X, Ouyang YY et al. 2015. Red and processed meat consumption and mortality: Dose-response meta-analysis of prospective cohort studies. *Public Health Nutr* 19(5):1–13. July 6. [Epub ahead of print]
Warensjo E, Jansson JH, Cederholm T et al. 2010. Biomarkers of milk fat and the risk of myocardial infarction in men and women: A prospective, matched case–control study. *Am J Clin Nutr* 2:194–202.
Weggemans RM, Trautwein EA. 2003. Relation between soy-associated isoflavones and LDL and HDL cholesterol concentrations in humans: A meta-analysis. *Eur J Clin Nutr* 57(8):940–946.
Weggemans RM, Zock PL, Katan MB. 2001. Dietary cholesterol from eggs increases the ratio of total cholesterol to high-density lipoprotein cholesterol in humans: A meta-analysis. *Am J Clin Nutr* 73(5):885–891.
Welch AA, Shakya-Shrestha S, Lentjes MA, Wareham NJ, Khaw KT. 2010. Dietary intake and status of n-3 polyunsaturated fatty acids in a population of fish-eating and non-fish-eating meat-eaters, vegetarians, and vegans and the product-precursor ratio [corrected] of α-linolenic acid to long-chain n-3 polyunsaturated fatty acids: Results from the EPIC-Norfolk cohort. *Am J Clin Nutr* 92(5):1040–1051.
Whelton SP, He J, Whelton PK, Muntner P. 2004. Meta-analysis of observational studies on fish intake and coronary heart disease. *Am J Cardiol* 93(9):1119–1123.
Willett WC. 1998. *Nutritional Epidemiology*, 2nd edn. New York: Oxford University Press.
Wittenbecher C, Mühlenbruch K, Kröger J et al. 2015. Amino acids, lipid metabolites, and ferritin as potential mediators linking red meat consumption to type 2 diabetes. *Am J Clin Nutr* 101(6):1241–1250.
Wu JH, Micha R, Imamura F et al. 2012. Omega-3 fatty acids and incident type 2 diabetes: A systematic review and meta-analysis. *Br J Nutr* 107(Suppl 2):S214–S227.
Würtz P, Soininen P, Kangas AJ et al. 2013. Branched-chain and aromatic amino acids are predictors of insulin resistance in young adults. *Diabetes Care* 36(3):648–655.
Würtz P, Tiainen M, Mäkinen VP et al. 2012. Circulating metabolite predictors of glycemia in middle-aged men and women. *Diabetes Care* 35(8):1749–1756.
Zhan S, Ho SC. 2005. Meta-analysis of the effects of soy protein containing isoflavones on the lipid profile. *Am J Clin Nutr* 81(2):397–408.
Zhang M, Picard-Deland E, Marette A. 2013. Fish and marine omega-3 polyunsaturated Fatty Acid consumption and incidence of type 2 diabetes: A systematic review and meta-analysis. *Int J Endocrinol* 2013:501015.
Zheng H, Clausen MR, Dalsgaard TK, Bertram HC. 2015. Metabolomics to explore impact of dairy intake. *Nutrients* 7(6):4875–4896.
Zheng JS, Huang T, Yang J, Fu YQ, Li D. 2012. Marine N-3 polyunsaturated fatty acids are inversely associated with risk of type 2 diabetes in Asians: A systematic review and meta-analysis. *PLoS One* 7(9):e44525.

Section V

Dietary Food Groups, Patterns, and Cardiometabolic Health

20 Consumption of Foods, Food Groups, and Cardiometabolic Risk

Edward Yu and Frank B. Hu

CONTENTS

ABSTRACT

Knowledge about the effect of regular intake of specific food groups on cardiometabolic health is primarily derived from large prospective cohort studies. With careful study design and analysis, results from observational data offer opportunities for causal inference. Sugar-sweetened beverage intake is consistently associated with increased risk of obesity, cardiovascular disease (CVD), and type 2 diabetes owing to the excess amounts of added sugar, as well as mediation by increased weight gain. Coffee consumption is associated with lower incidence of CVD, with the largest benefit observed around 3–5 cups/day. Higher consumption of fruits and vegetables is associated with lower risk of heart disease, although data on type 2 diabetes is conflicted. Dairy consumption has mixed associations with cardiometabolic diseases, depending on the types of dairy products. Red meat, especially processed red meat, is associated with increased risk of diabetes and CVD. Fish intake is inversely associated with CVD incidence, although high-dose fish oil supplementation does not appear to be beneficial. Regular consumption of whole grains and nuts is associated with lower risk of both diabetes and CVD. Future research should focus on studying food subtypes, as well as adopting a holistic view of nutrition.

INTRODUCTION

For decades, scientists have recommended the intake of specific foods in order to achieve a balanced diet. As a result, food groups have become a popular area of study in nutritional science, as they allow for easier understanding, reporting, and public health recommendations.

At present, the evidence for the effects of intake of specific foods is dominated by epidemiologic studies. Although randomized clinical trials are regarded as the gold standard for causal inference, such studies are especially difficult to carry out for foods, owing to the high attrition rate, lack of compliance, short follow-up time, and small sample sizes. Narrowness of exposure is also a problem; an investigator of a randomized trial must specify a quantity of food or drink to administer before the study commences, whereas epidemiologic studies may draw from a range of intakes provided by the participants. Finally, dietary trials are difficult to blind, and so the interventional nature of trials may affect participant expectations and results.

On the contrary, epidemiologic studies collect information from free-living participants and consist primarily of case–control and cohort studies. Case–control studies are most often conducted retrospectively, when the investigation begins after the outcome has occurred. As a result, they are prone to both recall bias and reverse causation, which prevents strong arguments for causation. Consequently, large prospective cohort studies provide the best current knowledge for the cardiometabolic effects of food groups. Cohorts such as the European Prospective Investigation into Cancer and Nutrition (EPIC), the Health Professionals' Follow-Up Study (HPFS), and the Nurses' Health Study (NHS) consist of tens of thousands of participants that periodically report their eating habits and incidence of disease. The prospective nature of cohort studies obviates the problems of reverse causation and recall bias, although residual confounding remains a major obstacle to causal inference. However, with prudent study design and statistical analysis, such studies can provide a robust case for causation. Major well-known covariates such as smoking, body mass index, and common demographic variables will almost always be accounted for in the analyses of published studies. Furthermore, once data regarding food groups from several populations have been released, a meta-analysis can be performed to quantitatively combine results in order to report a pooled effect of exposure. Meta-analyses provide much more statistical power than a single study alone, and sources of heterogeneity can also be explored. Though they are still imperfect, such results have provided the basis for many public health recommendations and policies.

Assessment of food intake has long been a source of both criticism and misunderstanding. While diet records provide the reference method for quantifying food and drink, the expense and burden of this technique has kept its widespread use in all but small randomized trials and validation studies (Bingham et al. 1994, Newby et al. 2003). Random dietary recalls, where a trained investigator interviews participants on their eating habits, have also been shown to be highly reliable and accurate (Briefel 1994, Hu 2008, Wright et al. 2007). For large prospective cohort studies, semiquantitative food frequency questionnaires (FFQs) remain the method of choice for dietary assessment. Different FFQs, such as the Block or Willett FFQ, have been validated against reference methods for both accuracy and reproducibility (Kroke et al. 1999, Subar et al. 2001). Although precise measurement of food quantity is difficult if not impossible with FFQs, investigators can gain great insight by examining the relative ranking of food intakes among participants.

The present chapter summarizes the current knowledge of nine major groups of food and drink that have been linked to cardiometabolic risk (Tables 20.1 and 20.2). Evidence originates primarily from the systematic review and meta-analyses of large prospective cohort studies. Potential mechanisms based on results from animal studies, as well as small randomized trials, will also be discussed.

BEVERAGES

SUGAR-SWEETENED BEVERAGES

Sugar-sweetened beverages (SSBs) are a class of drinks that include soft drinks, sports drinks, energy drinks, and fruit juices with added sugar. This class of beverage represents the primary source of added sugar in the U.S. diet and is composed of sweeteners such as sucrose, high-fructose corn syrup, and fruit juice concentrate (100% fruit juice with no added sugar is not considered a SSB)

TABLE 20.1
Summary of Food Group Constituents and Nutrients

Food/Beverage	Constituents of Interest	Major Nutrients/Compounds
Sugar-sweetened beverages	Soft drinks, sports drinks, energy drinks, fruit juice	Added sugar
Coffee	Caffeinated and decaffeinated, filtered and unfiltered	Caffeine, chlorogenic acid, lignans, flavonoids
Alcohol	Beer, wine, spirits	Ethanol, resveratrol (red wine)
Fruits	Tree fruits, berries, melons, citrus	Phytochemicals, flavonoids, folate, fiber
Vegetables	Green leafy, cruciferous, root	
Dairy	Milk, cheese, yogurt	Saturated fat, ruminant fat, protein, lactose, calcium, probiotics
Eggs		Cholesterol, protein, sodium
Red meats	Beef, pork, lamb, game meats	Sodium, preservatives, L-carnitine, protein, fatty acids
White meats	Chicken, turkey	
Fish	Oily (sardines, herring, anchovies, salmon, trout, tuna), whitefish (cod, kutum, whiting, haddock, hake, pollock)	Polyunsaturated fatty acids, protein
Grains	Rice, wheat, bread, corn	Starch, fiber
Nuts and legumes	Tree nuts, peanuts, peas, beans	Unsaturated fats, plant protein, minerals, vitamins, polyphenols

(Malik et al. 2010a). Data from the National Health and Nutrition Examination Survey (NHANES) from 2005 to 2008 have shown that roughly half the U.S. population consumes SSBs on any given day, that at least a quarter of the population consumes at least 200 calories from SSBs, and that 5% consume at least 567 calories (Ogden et al. 2011). Although consumption has seen a modest decline over the past decade, soft drink sales continue to rise outside the United States (Kleiman et al. 2012, Welsh et al. 2011), and such a trend poses a major public health challenge.

As also discussed in Chapters 13 and 14 of this text, ample observational evidence has strongly suggested a detrimental effect of SSB consumption in relation to obesity, type 2 diabetes mellitus (T2DM), and CVD. Most (Hu and Malik 2010, Malik et al. 2006, 2009, 2010a, Vartanian et al. 2007), but not all (Forshee et al. 2008), systematic reviews of epidemiologic studies have concluded that there is a positive relationship between SSB intake and risk of overweight/obesity in both children and adults. This association is strongest among large prospective cohort studies with long duration of follow-up and without adjustment for total energy intake (Malik et al. 2009). Findings from experimental studies also support this hypothesis. A meta-analysis of six randomized trials performed by Mattes et al. (2011) demonstrates that the addition of SSBs to the diets of participants significantly increased body weight, although in the same publication, no weight loss benefit was seen in a meta-analysis of six different trials aimed at reducing SSB intake. However, Mattes et al. (2011) note methodological limitations of these trials, including short duration, small sample sizes, poor compliance, and lack of blinding. Genetic factors may also affect the strength of association between SSB intake and weight gain. Based on a genetic predisposition score of 32 obesity genes, those who consumed >1 serving/day of SSBs showed more than twice the genetic effect on obesity risk compared to those who consumed <1 serving/month, suggesting that the benefit of healthy beverage choice is greater among individuals genetically predisposed to weight gain (Qi et al. 2012).

Systematic reviews and meta-analyses of prospective cohort studies have also clearly linked SSB consumption with risk of type 2 diabetes and metabolic syndrome (Hu and Malik 2010, Malik et al. 2010a,b, Vartanian et al. 2007). Among 310,819 individuals, those in the highest category of SSB intake (most often 1–2 servings/day) had a 26% greater incidence of T2DM compared to those in

TABLE 20.2
Summary of Relative Risks of Food Groups in Relation to CVD, T2DM, and Strength of Evidence

Food or Beverage	Pooled Risk Ratio for CVD	Overall	Level of Evidence	Pooled Risk Ratio for T2DM	Overall	Level of Evidence
SSBs	1.16 (1.10–1.23)[a] (Huang et al. 2014)	+	Strong	1.26 (1.12–1.41)[b] (Malik et al. 2010a)	+	Strong
Coffee	0.85 (0.80–0.90)[c] (Ding et al. 2014b)	U	Strong	0.91 (0.89–0.94)[a] (Ding et al. 2014a)	–	Moderate
Alcohol	0.80 (0.78–0.83)[b] (Corrao et al. 2000)	U	Strong	0.87 (0.76–1.00)[d] (Baliunas et al. 2009)	U	Weak
Fruits and Vegetables	0.96 (0.92–0.99)[a] (Wang et al. 2014)	–	Strong	0.90 (0.80–1.01)[c] (Cooper et al. 2012)	0	Moderate
Dairy	0.92 (0.80–0.99)[c] (Elwood et al. 2010)	–	Moderate	0.99 (0.98, 1.01)[a] (Chen et al. 2014)	–	Moderate
Eggs	0.96 (0.88–1.05)[c] (Shin et al. 2013)	0	Moderate	1.06 (0.86–1.30)[c] (Djoussé et al. 2016)	+	Weak
Red Meats	1.09 (1.01–1.18)[c] (Chen et al. 2013)	+	Weak	1.19 (1.04–1.37)[a] (Pan et al. 2011)	+	Moderate
Processed Meats	1.42 (1.07–1.89)[a] (Micha et al. 2010)	+	Strong	1.51 (1.25–1.83)[a] (Pan et al. 2011)	+	Strong
White Meats	1.00 (0.87–1.15)[a] (Abete et al. 2014)	0	Weak	1.04 (0.82–1.32)[a] (Feskens et al. 2013)	0	Weak
Fish	0.62 (0.46–0.82)[c] (He et al. 2004)	–	Strong	0.99 (0.85–1.16)[c] (Xun and He 2012)	0	Moderate
Whole Grains	0.79 (0.74–0.85)[c] (Ye et al. 2012)	–	Strong	0.74 (0.69–0.80)[b] (Ye et al. 2012)	–	Strong
Refined Grains	1.07 (0.94–1.22)[c] (Mellen et al. 2008)	0	Moderate	0.95 (0.88–1.04)[b] (Aune et al. 2013b)	0	Moderate
Nuts/Legumes	0.71 (0.59–0.85)[a] (Luo et al. 2014)	–	Strong	0.72 (0.64–0.81)[a] (Luo et al. 2014)	–	Strong

[a] For 1 serving/day increase.
[b] For 3–5 serving/day increase.
[c] Comparing those in highest to lowest categories of intake.
[d] U-shaped relationship where relative risk is at optimal intake.

the lowest category of intake (none or <1 serving/month) (95% CI = 1.12–1.41). For metabolic syndrome, the relative risk was 1.20 (95% CI = 1.02–1.42) (Malik et al. 2010b). SSB intake has also been shown to have a detrimental effect on cardiovascular health, leading to an increased risk of total cardiovascular disease, hypertension, and coronary heart disease (CHD), but not stroke (Huang et al. 2014, Xi et al. 2015). In particular, a pooled analysis of 173,753 participants indicated that a one serving per day increase in SSB consumption was associated with a 16% increased risk in CHD (95% CI = 1.10–1.23) and that the effect was especially prominent among men and for individuals living in the United States (Huang et al. 2014).

It is thought that SSBs lead to weight gain through their high levels of added sugar, which provide ample energy but low satiety due to the liquid calorie content, leading to additional food intake and net positive energy balance (Malik et al. 2006, 2010a). Widespread consumption of SSBs contributes to high glycemic load, which has been shown to lead to increased concentrations of inflammatory biomarkers, such as C-reactive protein (Liu et al. 2002), and insulin resistance, especially among overweight individuals (Schulze et al. 2004). The effect of SSB intake on type 2 diabetes and metabolic syndrome is thought to act in part through weight gain. However, the added sugar in SSBs may also have an independent effect in the development of these diseases. Schulze et al. (2004) estimate that roughly half the effect of SSBs on type diabetes was through obesity. SSBs have also been shown to dramatically increase postprandial blood glucose and insulin concentrations (Janssens et al. 1999). Recent experimental studies have indicated an important role of fructose, a constituent of both sucrose and high-fructose corn syrup, in inducing adverse metabolic effects. Fructose has been shown to increase hepatic lipogenesis, lower high density lipoprotein (HDL) cholesterol, and promote insulin resistance (Bray 2007). Compared to glucose-containing beverages, fructose-containing beverages may promote additional visceral adiposity (Stanhope et al. 2009).

Although the case against SSB consumption is robust, observational data continue to be criticized on the grounds that they cannot infer causality. Both Hu (2013) and Huffman (2012) have appealed to the Hill's criteria, a set of conditions to establish causality, to argue for the true effect of SSBs consumption on negative cardiometabolic outcomes. While the health consequences of SSBs have been well established, additional research into appropriate and cost–effect measures to curb SSB use is needed.

Coffee

Coffee is one of the most widely consumed beverages in the world. Historically, the link between coffee and disease had remained unclear due to strong confounding by smoking, but research on coffee consumption has seen a recent flurry of interest following the initial publication of a strong decrease in risk of type 2 diabetes with increasing coffee consumption among 17,111 Dutch adults (van Dam and Feskens 2002). In this study, those who drank at least seven cups of coffee a day were half as likely to develop type 2 diabetes compared to those who drank two cups or fewer a day. This finding was subsequently confirmed in several other large cohorts, including the NHS/HPFS (Salazar-Martinez et al. 2004), NHANES (Greenberg et al. 2005), and the Women's Health Study (Song et al. 2005). A meta-analysis of prospective cohort studies including 50,595 cases of T2DM among 1,096,647 participants reported a relative risk of 0.71 (95% CI = 0.67–0.76) for the highest level of coffee intake compared to lowest (Jiang et al. 2014).

Interestingly, caffeine content did not appear to alter the magnitude of the results, with decaffeinated coffee having a similar relative risk of 0.79 (95% CI = 0.69–0.91), as well as total caffeine content alone with a relative risk of 0.70 (95% CI = 0.65–0.75) (Jiang et al. 2014). In a dose–response analysis, Ding et al. (2014a) reported that a 1 cup/day increase was associated with a 0.91 (95% CI = 0.89–0.94) reduction in T2DM risk for regular coffee and 0.94 (95% CI = 0.91–0.98) for decaffeinated coffee. This trend appeared to be linear, with more coffee leading to a monotonically increasing benefit.

Pooled analyses by Sofi et al. (2006) and Malerba et al. (2013) show that risk of both CHD and CVD mortality are reduced when comparing heavy to light coffee drinkers. Two additional meta-analyses that are modeling nonlinear associations point to drinking 3–5 cups/day to have the optimal reduction in risk of approximately 15% (95% CI = 0.80–0.90), and heavy coffee intake having a null effect (Ding et al. 2014b, Mostofsky et al. 2012). A meta-analysis performed by Mesas et al. (2011) concluded that although administration of caffeine produces an acute increase in blood pressure, there was no evidence of an increased risk of CVD among hypertensive subjects.

The primary component responsible for the cardiometabolic benefit of coffee remains unclear, as brewed coffee contains over a thousand identified chemicals. Caffeine, once thought to be detrimental to insulin sensitivity and glucose tolerance (Cheraskin et al. 1967, Keijzers et al. 2002, Pizziol et al. 1998), appears to have little effect, since both caffeinated and decaffeinated coffee are independently associated with benefit. One hypothesis is that long-term intake of coffee causes a tolerance to develop against caffeine (van Dam et al. 2004). Another hypothesis is that other components found in coffee antagonize the adverse effects of caffeine (Natella and Scaccini 2012).

Several clinical studies have suggested important roles for polyphenols and antioxidants, similar to those found in fruits and vegetables. Findings from randomized trials indicate that improved adipocyte and hepatocyte function induced by changes in adiponectin and fetuin-A concentrations may play a role in the benefit of coffee (Wedick et al. 2011). Coffee also appears to improve markers of inflammation and endothelial dysfunction, such as TNF-α, E-selectin, C-reactive protein, and VCAM-1 (Kempf et al. 2010, Natella and Scaccini 2012). The presence of phytochemicals in coffee such as flavonoids, lignans, and chlorogenic acid has also been observed to independently increase glucose tolerance and insulin sensitivity (Natella and Scaccini 2012, van Dijk et al. 2009). Chlorogenic acid in particular has recently caught the attention of researchers, as it appears to reduce fasting glucose (Rodriguez de Sotillo et al. 2006), increase insulin sensitivity (Shearer et al. 2003), and attenuate the appearance of glucose in blood after challenging with glucose (Bassoli et al. 2008).

Method of preparation is an area deserving of future research. Although Ranheim and Halvorsen (2005) speculate that boiled coffee is particularly beneficial due to its antioxidant content, van Dam et al. (2006) reported that there was no difference in the benefit of filtered coffee (RR = 0.86, 95% CI = 0.82–0.90) or instant coffee (RR = 0.83, 95% CI = 0.74–0.93) on T2DM.

Alcohol

Alcohol intake has been studied extensively in the past several decades. Among food groups examined in epidemiologic studies of diet, modest alcohol has presented the most consistent association with lower cardiometabolic risk (Rimm et al. 1996). This is also discussed in Chapter 31 of this text. Alcohol can be classified into beers, wines, and distilled beverages (spirits), although there appears to be no difference in the type of drink on health benefit (Rimm et al. 1996), offering enticing evidence that the causal component of risk reduction is due to the ethanol itself.

Pooled analyses of alcohol intake have also repeatedly shown a U-shaped relationship with both CVD risk (Holmes et al. 2014, Ronksley et al. 2011) and T2DM risk (Baliunas et al. 2009, Carlsson et al. 2005, Schrieks et al. 2015). Reviewing 84 eligible studies, Ronksley et al. (2011) reported that the relative risks for drinkers vs. nondrinkers were 0.75 (95% CI = 0.70–0.80) for total CVD mortality, 0.71 (95% CI = 0.66–0.77) for incident CHD, 0.75 (95% CI = 0.68–0.81) for CHD-specific mortality, 0.98 (95% CI = 0.91–1.06) for incident stroke, and 1.06 (95% CI = 0.91–1.23) for stroke-specific mortality. The strongest reduction in CVD risk was seen at one to two drinks per day. Corrao et al. (2000) report similar results, with optimal intake of one to two drinks per day but a deleterious effect above six drinks per day. Evidence from experimental studies is also encouraging, as a meta-analysis of 42 trials demonstrated that moderate alcohol intake was associated with increased HDL, apolipoprotein A1, and lower fibrinogen (Rimm et al. 1999).

For T2DM, a recent meta-analysis found a similar U-shaped relationship (Baliunas et al. 2009). Incidence of T2DM was lowest among men drinking 22 g alcohol/day (about 2 drinks) with a relative risk of 0.87 (95% CI = 0.76–1.00), and increased significantly compared to nondrinkers at over 60 g/day (about 5 drinks). The effects among women are even stronger, with consumption of 24 g/day alcohol having a relative risk of 0.60 (95% CI = 0.52–0.69), and becoming deleterious at 50 g/day (about 4 drinks). A meta-analysis of 14 clinical trials indicated that moderate alcohol consumption reduced fasting insulin and improved insulin sensitivity among women but not men (Schrieks et al. 2015).

Alcohol has been shown to increase circulating HDL cholesterol, which is thought to be the most important mechanism for its cardioprotective effect (Gaziano et al. 1993). It is estimated that approximately two drinks per day increases HDL levels by 4.0 mg/dL (Rimm et al. 1999), which is greater than that produced by gemfibrozil, a drug used to raise HDL levels (Stampfer et al. 1991). However, a risk reduction is observed for CHD even when controlling for HDL cholesterol, implicating additional pathways (Criqui et al. 1987). Moreover, as discussed elsewhere in this volume (Chapter 31), there is little evidence to date that an increase in HDL cholesterol causes a reduction in CVD risk. Ethanol also modulates several biochemical pathways, including platelet aggregation and clotting, omega-3 fatty acid processing, and vascular integrity (Di Castelnuovo et al. 2009).

Moderate alcohol intake may also affect inflammation, a process associated with atherosclerosis, and lower plasma concentration of C-reactive protein, a molecule correlated with CVD risk (Albert et al. 2003). On the other hand, alcohol consumption appears to increase levels of triglyceride, which is associated with an increased incidence of CVD (Stampfer et al. 1996). However, the balance appears to be in favor of reduced risk.

While epidemiologic studies have indicated the benefits of moderate alcohol intake on health outcomes, public health experts have not endorsed alcohol consumption as a prophylactic for cardiometabolic disease, owing to the dangers of overconsumption. At higher intake, risk of death attributed to CVD has been found to be comparable or worse in relation to nondrinkers, which may due to direct myocardial toxicity or tendency of alcohol to induce arrhythmias (Moore and Pearson 1986). Researchers have pointed out the strong potential for confounding in observational studies of alcohol (Mukamal and Rimm 2001). Abstainers may not drink due to illness or have quit due to former alcohol abuse. Moderate drinkers also tend be younger, leaner, more physically active, and of higher socioeconomic status and are likelier to be married compared to nondrinkers (Mukamal and Rimm 2001). Furthermore, although randomized trials of alcohol address the question of causality, they tended to be of small sample size, short duration, and measure only intermediate outcomes (Rimm et al. 1999, Schrieks et al. 2015).

A novel way of addressing the causal role of alcohol has originated from genetic studies. Because polymorphisms in alcohol dehydrogenase and aldehyde dehydrogenase are associated with aversion to alcohol, a genetic association study of single nucleotide polymorphisms in these genes may act as a Mendelian randomized trial of alcohol consumption. Studies of alcohol dehydrogenase (Hines et al. 2001) and cholesteryl ester transfer protein (Jensen et al. 2008) indicate a benefit of moderate alcohol consumption that was modified by genotype. However, in a large pooled analysis of 261,991 individuals, Holmes et al. (2014) reported that carriers of a genetic variant in alcohol dehydrogenase 1B, which is associated with nondrinking, presented lower systolic blood pressure, interleukin-6 levels, waist circumference, body mass index, odds of CHD, and odds of ischemic stroke. The authors concluded that alcohol consumption increases cardiovascular risk among all drinkers, including those who drink moderately, contrasting with the body of epidemiologic evidence. However, the use of genetic variants as instrumental variables in dietary association analyses remains controversial, and thus additional studies are needed.

FOODS

Fruits and Vegetables

Fruits are the seed-bearing structures that develop from ovaries of flowering plants, whereas vegetables are all the other plant parts, such as leaves, roots, and stems. However, both fruits and vegetables are similar in that they are rich in folate, fiber, vitamins, minerals, and phytochemicals, including polyphenols (Dauchet et al. 2006). They have been historically recommended as part of a healthy diet since the earliest iteration of the USDA guidelines in 1980 and for good reason—evidence for fruits and vegetables overwhelmingly support their positive effects on cardiometabolic and overall health.

Among the earliest systematic reviews, examining fruits and vegetables was conducted by Ness and Powles (1997), who found a strong protective effect against stroke and weaker benefit for CHD. The earliest quantitative meta-analysis of fruits and vegetables for CHD risk was performed by Dauchet et al. (2006), who reported a relative risk of 0.96 (95% CI = 0.93–0.99) for each additional serving of fruits and vegetables. In the same year, He et al. (2006) reported a reduction of 26% in stroke incidence for those consuming 3–5 servings/d of fruits and vegetables. A later analysis performed by He et al. (2007) reached a similar conclusion for CHD: compared with those who had less than 3 servings/d of fruits and vegetables, those who consumed more than 5 servings/d had a relative risk of 0.83 (95% CI = 0.77–0.89) for CHD. The most recent meta-analysis of fruits and vegetables conducted by Wang et al. (2014) consisted of 833,234 subjects—more than triple to that of the analysis conducted by He et al. (2007). It found that a 1 serving/day increase in fruits or vegetables was associated with a risk ratio of 0.96 (95% CI = 0.92–0.99) for CVD mortality.

The findings for fruit and vegetable consumption on the risk of T2DM are less clear. A meta-analysis of four cohort studies consisting of 223,512 subjects conducted by Carter et al. (2010) reported that there was no association between vegetable, fruit, or total fruit and vegetables and T2DM incidence, although green leafy vegetables specifically were associated with a relative risk of 0.86 (95% CI = 0.77–0.97). Cooper et al. (2012) reported no association between total fruits and vegetables and T2DM, although root and green leafy vegetables specifically may reduce T2DM incidence. An updated meta-analysis of 10 cohort studies consisting of 434,342 subjects performed by Li et al. (2014) concluded that a 1 serving/day increase in total fruit intake was associated with a 7% decrease in T2DM risk (RR = 0.93, 95% CI = 0.88–0.99). No association was found for total vegetable intake (RR = 0.90, 95% CI = 0.80–1.01). Again, similar to the previous study by Carter et al. (2010) and Cooper et al. (2012), green leafy vegetables were found to be protective against T2DM, with a 0.2 serving/day increase conferring a relative risk of 0.87 (95% CI = 0.81–0.93).

A major component of the cardioprotective effect of fruits and vegetables is thought to arise from plant-derived phytochemicals, such as sulfides, carotenoids, flavonoids, phenols, lignans, and resveratrol (Van Duyn and Pivonka 2000). These biomolecules are not found in other nonplant foods and have been shown to modulate the detoxification of enzymes, stimulate the immune system, reduce inflammation, regulate cholesterol synthesis and hormone metabolism, and also demonstrate antioxidant, antibacterial, and antiviral effects (Lampe 1999). Such effects have been reported not only in animal and cell-culture models but also in numerous clinical trials (Dillard and Bruce German 2000).

One developing frontier of research has been into flavonoids, a class of polyphenols found exclusively in plant and plant products such as tea and wine. Interest in flavonoids originated from examination of the French paradox, the observation that Mediterranean populations consuming diets high in red wine and saturated fat (SFA) present low CVD mortality rate (Nijveldt et al. 2001). As isolated molecules, flavonoids have been easier to study in a clinical context than whole foods and have been shown to protect cells against oxidative damage, interfere with nitric-oxide synthase activity, scavenge free radicals, mobilize leukocytes, and interact with other enzymes to produce beneficial effects (Nijveldt et al. 2001). Among observational data, regular flavonoid intake has been shown to be associated with reduced blood pressure (Cassidy et al. 2011) and T2DM incidence (Liu et al. 2014). In a meta-analysis of 133 randomized trials of flavonoids among 6557 participants, Hooper et al. (2008) concluded that soy protein isolate, cocoa, and green tea confer the strongest effects of cardiovascular risk factors via antihypertensive and LDL-lowering actions. Additional research is required to elucidate the different mechanisms through which flavonoid subclasses operate.

There is also a growing need to study the effects of specific fruit and vegetable subtypes because the composition of micronutrients and phytochemicals differ between food classes. For example, the specific benefit of green leafy vegetables on T2DM may be attributed to its high magnesium and α-linolenic acid content compared to other types of vegetables (Carter et al. 2010). Regarding flavonoids, citrus fruits contain virtually all the flavanones consumed in the American diet, whereas berries are the richest sources of anthocyanins (Cassidy et al. 2011). Furthermore, different nutritional constituents, such as flavonoid subclasses, may have different physiological effects (Hooper et al. 2008). Muraki et al. (2013) recently published results from the NHS and HPFS and found significant heterogeneity between individual fruits. For instance, 3 servings/week of blueberries were strongly protective (RR = 0.74, 95% CI = 0.66–0.83) while 3 servings/week of cantaloupe appeared to be detrimental (RR = 1.10, 95% CI = 1.02–1.18). These results signify that future studies should not classify all fruits and vegetables into one exposure category but should differentiate between individual foods wherever possible.

Dairy (Cheese, Milk, Yogurt)

Dairy consists of milk or products derived from milk, such as cheese, butter, and yogurt. They are a major source of SFAs in the United States, accounting for about 21% of total SFA consumption (U.S. Department of Agriculture 2015). As a result, research into dairy has been closely linked to the controversy regarding SFA. Current recommendations from the World Health Organization and from federal dietary guidelines in the United States suggest consuming less than 10% of total energy from SFA in order to decrease the risk of CVD, with the American Heart Association setting a target at less than 7% of total energy. SFAs have been known to increase circulatory low-density lipoprotein (LDL) cholesterol (Mensink et al. 2003), a major risk factor of CVD risk. Furthermore, it is known that following a diet high in polyunsaturated fat compared to SFA leads to a lower risk of total CHD events (Mozaffarian et al. 2010, Skeaff and Miller 2009).

Despite the high SFA content in dairy, current findings from prospective cohort studies indicate no clear evidence of an increased risk in CVD with milk or dairy consumption. Qin et al. (2015) reported that among 22 studies, dairy intake was found to be associated with a modest reduction in overall CVD risk (RR = 0.88, 95% CI = 0.81–0.96), stroke (RR = 0.87, 95% CI = 0.77–0.99), but not CHD (RR = 0.94, 95% CI = 0.82–1.07). No link was found comparing high-fat dairy and CHD (RR = 1.04, 95% CI = 0.89–1.21) or low-fat dairy and CHD (RR = 0.93, 95% CI = 0.74–1.17) (Soedamah-Muthu et al. 2011). However, low-fat dairy may reduce the risk of stroke (RR = 0.93, 95% CI = 0.88–0.99).

Results regarding T2DM are conflicting. Two meta-analyses of 14 and 17 cohort studies, each consisting of over 400,000 subjects, have concluded that a significant inverse association exists between dairy consumption and T2DM risk (Aune et al. 2013a, Gao et al. 2013), but a more recent analysis concluded a null association (Chen et al. 2014). However, yogurt intake specifically has been shown to be predictive of reduced T2DM risk (Chen et al. 2014, Gao et al. 2013).

Several hypotheses have been proposed to explain the null or modest benefit of dairy despite its high SFA content. One explanation is that milk and dairy products are rich mixtures of macro- and micronutrients, many of which confer cardioprotective effects. For example, epidemiologic evidence has suggested an inverse association between vitamin D and calcium intake and the development of metabolic syndrome and T2DM (Tremblay and Gilbert 2009). Another explanation is that while SFAs may elevate LDL cholesterol, SFAs may also affect other lipid biomarkers in different ways depending on the macronutrient composition of the food (Micha and Mozaffarian 2010, Mozaffarian and Clarke 2009). For example, substituting carbohydrates with SFAs increase total cholesterol and LDL cholesterol, but also lowers triglycerides (TG) and increases HDL cholesterol. The overall effect is that the TG/HDL cholesterol ratio is not altered, which is arguably the best predictor of CVD risk (Micha and Mozaffarian 2010). Additionally, the possibilities of residual confounding and measurement error cannot be excluded when considering observational evidence. Finally, the type of dairy product is seldom considered in these studies. Fermented dairy like yogurt and cheese may have different effects from unfermented varieties such as milk (St-Onge et al. 2000).

Despite the need for experimental studies, well-conducted trials of dairy are extremely rare. Steinmetz et al. (1994) assessed the lipid profile of eight males consuming 2–3 cups/day of whole or skimmed milk and found that compared to whole milk, skimmed milk significantly lowered total cholesterol and LDL cholesterol, but did not alter other lipids, lipoproteins, or apolipoproteins. In a study of 49 males, Hjerpsted et al. (2011) reported that a 6-week intervention of cheese lowered serum total, LDL, and HDL cholesterol concentrations and raised glucose concentrations compared to a butter diet. There has also been interest in yogurt, owing to its probiotic potential, but evidence from randomized trials has been vitiated by various design issues such as adequate control for energy and macronutrient intake, adjustment for bacterial concentration, study duration, and prebiotic confounding (Huth and Park 2012). Nonetheless, results from a few randomized trials support the conclusion that yogurts fermented by probiotic strains may affect the lipid profile more favorably compared to conventional yogurts (Cho and Kim 2015, Ejtahed et al. 2011, Mohamadshahi et al. 2014). Future studies should incorporate dairy into long-term interventions and continue to track lipids, inflammatory markers, and gut hormones as predictors of cardiometabolic risk.

Eggs

Historically, the health benefits of regular egg consumption have been viewed with skepticism from consumers and scientists alike due to its high cholesterol content. The 1980 USDA Dietary Guidelines admonished that "[eggs] can be eaten in moderation, as long as your overall cholesterol intake is not excessive" (USDA 1980). Indeed, a single large 50 g egg contains about 186 mg of total cholesterol (USDA 2015). However, most randomized trials conclude that high doses of dietary cholesterol are not significantly associated with serum cholesterol (Bowman et al. 1988, Buzzard et al. 1982, Chenoweth et al. 1981, Kummerow et al. 1977, Vorster et al. 1992). A meta-analysis of 395 metabolic ward studies indicated that consuming 1 egg/d increased both LDL cholesterol by 4.1 mg/dL and HDL cholesterol by 0.9 mg/dL, resulting in a negligible effect on LDL/HDL ratio, a significant predictor of CHD (Clarke et al. 1997). Research by Miettinen and Kesäniemi (1989) demonstrated that endogenous cholesterol levels are highly regulated and that greater cholesterol intake is offset by higher rates of biliary secretion and fecal elimination, and lower rates of cholesterol synthesis.

With respect to cardiovascular disease, a meta-analysis of 17 total studies concluded a null relationship for each additional egg consumed per day and risk of CHD (RR = 0.99, 95% CI = 0.85–1.15) (Rong et al. 2013). Consumption of 1 egg/d was also not associated with total stroke (RR = 0.91, 95% CI = 0.81–1.02), although the authors noted a significant decrease in risk of hemorrhagic stroke (RR = 0.75, 95% CI = 0.57–0.99). Among diabetic patients, however, those in the highest category of egg consumption were found to have a 1.54-fold (95% CI = 1.14–2.09) increase in CHD risk compared to those in the lowest category, signifying possible effect modification by pre-existing illness. For total CVD risk, a later meta-analysis of 14 studies and 320,778 subjects indicated that an additional 4 eggs/week was associated with a significant increase in total CVD (RR = 1.06, 95% CI = 1.03–1.10) and that the effect is strengthened among diabetics (RR = 1.40, 95% CI = 1.25–1.57) (Li et al. 2013). However, a contemporary meta-analysis of 16 studies found that compared to an intake of <1 egg/d, intake of ≥1 egg/d was not associated with total CVD (RR = 0.96, 95% CI = 0.88–1.05), ischemic heart disease (IHD) (RR = 0.97, 95% CI = 0.86–1.09), stroke (RR = 0.93, 95% CI = 0.81–1.07), IHD mortality (RR = 0.98, 95% CI = 0.77–1.24), or stroke mortality (RR = 0.92, 95% CI = 0.56–1.50) (Shin et al. 2013). The disparity in results for total CVD may be due to differences in methodologies and included studies, although the observation that egg consumption is detrimental for heart disease in populations with T2DM is consistent. However, these findings contrast with a randomized trial of 140 T2DM patients assigned to 12 eggs/week vs. <2 eggs/week, which indicated no between-group differences for HDL, LDL, total cholesterol, triglycerides, or glycemic control after 3 months (Fuller et al. 2015).

In contrast to CVD, those consuming high amounts of eggs appear to be at heightened risk for T2DM. Every increase in consumption by 4 eggs/week was associated with a 1.29-fold (95% CI = 1.21–1.37) greater risk of T2DM (Li et al. 2013), and an alternate categorical comparison of ≥1 egg/d vs. <1 egg/d yielded similar results (RR = 1.42, 95% CI = 1.09–1.86) (Shin et al. 2013). However, a more recent meta-analysis of egg intake and T2DM considered 12 cohorts totaling 219,979 individuals and concluded a null relationship when comparing highest to lowest category of intake (RR = 1.06, 95% CI = 0.86–1.30). The authors discovered heterogeneity by country of origin, reporting that among studies conducted in the United States only, those in the highest category of consumption had a 1.39-fold (95% CI = 1.21–1.60) risk of T2DM compared to those in the lowest category (Djoussé et al. 2016). An association for T2DM comparing highest vs. lowest intake in non-U.S. countries was not observed (RR = 0.89, 95% CI = 0.79–1.02). Although several publications have suggested that high cholesterol intake alone increases chronic inflammation (Tannock et al. 2005) and risk of T2DM (Feskens and Kromhout 1990, Meyer et al. 2001, Salmerón et al. 2001), a 12-week randomized trial that assigned 31 subjects to 3 eggs/d vs. placebo (egg substitute with no cholesterol) reported no changes in fasting blood glucose or insulin sensitivity (Mutungi et al. 2008, Ratliff et al. 2009).

The relationship between eggs and cardiometabolic risk remains unsettled. The conflicting conclusions involving T2DM outcomes demonstrate the unique challenges of the study of eggs in an epidemiologic context. Likely explanations for these conflicting results include unmeasured confounding in the observational data, particularly strong measurement error, and short follow-up duration in RCTs. Future research should focus on reconciling these differences and exploring plausible biological mechanisms that may mediate an increase in T2DM incidence. Another unexplored area of interest is the method of preparation (e.g., raw, fried, scrambled, hard-boiled), since different methods can alter the nutrient content of the eggs, especially with the addition of cooking oils and salt or when used as an ingredient in baked goods.

Meats

Meats consist of a heterogeneous range of foods from white meat (e.g., turkey, chicken) to red meat (e.g., pork, beef) to seafood. The most often studied meats in observational studies are red meat and white meat. Fish is also commonly consumed, but is covered in a separate section. Meats present several nutritional benefits, as they are rich in protein, iron, zinc, and B vitamins, but they also contain high amounts of SFAs and cholesterol (Rohrmann et al. 2013).

Red meats consist of beef, lamb, pork, and game meat and exclude poultry and fish. They may come in processed or unprocessed varieties. Processed meats are defined as meats that have been preserved by smoking, curing, salting, or addition of chemical preservatives. Examples of processed meats include hamburgers, bacon, salami, sausages, hot dogs, and deli and luncheon meats. A meta-analysis of 20 prospective and case–control studies consisting of 1,218,380 individuals (Micha et al. 2010) indicated that a 100 g/day increase in red meat consumption was not associated with CHD (RR = 1.00, 95% CI = 0.81–1.23). However, the authors note the critical gaps in the literature when it comes to differentiating between processed and unprocessed meats. In the same meta-analysis, Micha et al. (2010) note that a 50 g/day increased in processed meat consumption was associated with a relative risk of 1.42 for CHD (95% CI = 1.07–1.89) and 1.19 for T2DM (95% CI = 1.11–1.27). However, it should be noted that this meta-analysis included only a small number of studies, and additional research is warranted. A later analysis of six cohort studies revealed that unprocessed red meat, processed meat, and total red meat consumption were all associated with elevated risks of total stroke (Kaluza et al. 2012). Finally, data from the EPIC cohort consisting of 448,568 individuals who were not included in the previous analyses indicated no association between red meat intake and mortality but a moderate positive association between processed meat consumption (RR = 1.30, 95% CI = 1.17–1.45 for a 50 g/day increase) and mortality (Rohrmann et al. 2013). A pooled analysis by Pan et al. (2011) addressed the issue of T2DM; they conclude that a 1 serving/day intake of unprocessed, processed, or total red meat were all associated with an increased risk of T2DM.

On the other hand, regular intake of white meats, which include chicken, turkey, and rabbit, was not found to be associated with CVD risk based on a meta-analysis of 13 cohort studies of 1,674,272 participants (Abete et al. 2014). A 100 g/day increase in white meats was associated with a relative risk for CVD mortality of 1.00 (95% CI = 0.87–1.15), and 1.10 (95% CI = 0.63–1.89) for IHD mortality. Similarly, the consumption of unprocessed poultry was not associated with T2DM risk (RR = 1.04, 95% CI = 0.82–1.32) (Feskens et al. 2013).

The subject of unprocessed red meat and CVD risk warrants further investigation. Traditionally, the high SFA content found in red meat (but not in white meat) is thought to heighten cardiovascular risk by increasing LDL cholesterol levels. However, a randomized trial of lean red meats and lean white meats showed no significant difference in serum lipid levels among hypercholesterolemic patients (Davidson et al. 1999). Heme iron has been implicated as a mediator in the relationship between red meat intake and CVD, as high concentrations have been shown to be linked with chronic inflammation and increased oxidative stress (Wagener et al. 2001). Studies in mice have also indicated that L-carnitine, a nutrient found in high levels in red meat, may be processed by intestinal microbiota to produce trimethylamine-N-oxide, which may reduce reverse cholesterol transport and precipitate atherosclerosis (Koeth et al. 2013). Yet, processed meats contain much lower levels of L-carnitine levels than red meats and are also associated with higher CVD risk. This may be explained by the addition of preservatives to processed meats. In the United States, processed meats contain on average four times the amount of sodium and 50% more nitrates than unprocessed varieties (Micha et al. 2010).

Future investigations should aim to clarify the link between fresh meats and CVD risk. Using data from the Nurses' Health Study, Bernstein et al. (2010) concluded that replacing red meats with alternative protein sources such as poultry, fish, low-fat dairy, nuts, and beans is associated with a significant reduction in CHD incidence. Cutting out meats altogether may also be a potential method of reducing cardiometabolic risk; compared to non-vegetarians, vegetarians present lower risk of IHD, CVD mortality, stroke, all-cause mortality, and cancer (Huang et al. 2012), although there is strong potential for confounding by lifestyle factors among these individuals. However, clinical trials of vegetarian diets have shown their potential for lowering blood pressure as well as improving glycemic control (Yokoyama et al. 2014a,b). Such a dietary pattern may prove meaningful as a nonpharmacologic method of improving health.

Fish

Epidemiologists have long suspected fish intake to be protective against CHD based on early studies of Alaskan and Greenland Eskimo (Bang et al. 1980, Kromann and Green 1980). This is also discussed in Chapter 19. Fish has also historically been an integral component of a Mediterranean dietary pattern, which has been shown to drastically reduce the incidence of CVD (Estruch et al. 2013). Indeed, the current body of evidence suggests that whole fish intake is inversely associated with heart disease. Two meta-analyses published concurrently in 2004 both concluded that fish intake is an important modifiable lifestyle factor for reducing CHD risk. He et al. (2004) reported that among 11 prospective cohort studies and 222,364 individuals, a higher consumption of fish was associated with a dose-dependent reduction in CHD mortality, with the highest category of intake of 2–4 times per week resulting in a risk ratio of 0.62 (95% CI = 0.46–0.82). In a meta-analysis of 228,864 subjects, comparing all fish consumers to nonconsumers, Whelton et al. (2004) reported a risk ratio of 0.83 (95% CI = 0.76–0.90) for fatal CHD and 0.86 (95% CI = 0.81–0.92) for total CHD incidence.

While fish appears to be salutary for heart health, epidemiologic data do not support the same benefit for T2DM. In a recent meta-analysis of nine cohort studies and 438,214 individuals, Xun and He (2012) reported that comparing those eating fish five or more times per week to those who did not eat or ate fish less than once per week, the risk of developing T2DM over follow-up was 0.99 (95% CI = 0.85–1.16). The authors note that significant heterogeneity existed when comparing studies in Eastern vs. Western populations, with fish intake being significantly beneficial in populations based in the East (Japan and China).

Traditionally, the cardioprotective effect of fish has been explained by the rich amounts of polyunsaturated fatty acids (PUFA) found in fish, especially omega-3 fatty acids such as eicosapentaenoic and docosahexaenoic acid. As discussed further in Chapter 10, the physiological benefits of these fatty acids are numerous and act through various molecular pathways to lower inflammation and maintain vascular function (Mozaffarian and Wu 2011). Furthermore, various studies have indicated that omega-3 fatty acids decrease the risk of cardiac arrest, reduce blood pressure, improve the lipid profile, and decrease platelet aggregation (Dyerberg et al. 1978, Kris-Etherton et al. 2002, Nestel 1990, Siscovick et al. 1995). Nonetheless, Rizos et al. (2012) concluded in a meta-analysis of 20 clinical trials of 68,680 patients that fish oil supplementation conferred no significant benefit for total CVD, CVD subtypes, or all-cause mortality. Similarly, Chowdhury et al. (2012) found a significant protective effect of fish in epidemiologic studies, but no benefit of omega-3 supplementation in randomized trials.

The discordance between the epidemiologic and experimental evidence has led scientists to believe that other nutrients in fish, such as vitamins, trace elements, and essential amino acids, may drive its effect on CVD. Others have argued that insufficient attention has been paid to confounders such as red meat intake, baseline drug use, or method of preparation (Chowdhury et al. 2012). Furthermore, FFQs typically do not specify type of fish consumed (e.g., oily fish vs. whitefish), only total intake of fish. Since different fish species contain varying amounts of omega-3 fatty acids, pooling fish intake into one exposure type may introduce measurement error. Lastly, although fish intake correlates with circulating omega-3 fatty acid concentration, only 20%–25% of this variation can be explained by fish intake alone (Welch et al. 2006).

Despite the effectiveness of high-dose fish oil supplementation being called into question, consumption of whole fish remains a wise choice for maintaining cardiovascular health. However, public health officials must also note complications arising from mercury and polychlorinated biphenyl and consider the risks vs. benefits of regularly consuming seafood (Storelli 2008). Future research should focus on elucidating the mechanism by which fish helps to lower CHD risk, as well as whether whole fish intake confers any additional benefit for T2DM and glycemic control and insulin resistance.

Grains and Fiber

Grains provide about two-thirds of the total energy and protein intake in the world, even more in developing countries, and about a quarter of total energy in the United States (Pedersen et al. 1989). Cereal grains include wheat, rice, corn, barley, sorghum, millet, oat, and rye. These grains are usually processed in order to modify flavor, color, texture, and appearance. Whereas whole grains are left with the bran, germ, and endosperm intact, refined grains undergo additional processing and retain only the endosperm in order to produce a finer texture and prolong shelf life. This refining process decreases the nutritional value of the grain because while the bran and germ are rich in dietary fiber, phytochemicals, iron, and B vitamins (such as folate), the endosperm contains mostly starch (Slavin 2000).

Regular intake of whole grains is inversely associated with all CVD events (RR = 0.79, 95% CI = 0.73–0.85) according to a meta-analysis of seven cohort studies (Mellen et al. 2008). Similar estimates were indicated for CVD subtypes, such as CHD, stroke, and CVD death. An expanded meta-analysis conducted in 2012 consisting of 66 studies arrived at a very similar estimate (RR = 0.79, 95% CI = 0.74–0.85) (Ye et al. 2012). In contrast, refined grain intake was found to have no association with all CVD events (RR = 1.07, 95% CI = 0.94–1.22) (Mellen et al. 2008). Investigators have also analyzed epidemiologic data from the perspective of dietary fiber, which is thought to be a major contributor to the cardioprotective effect of whole grains. A meta-analysis of 22 cohort studies by Threapleton et al. (2013) found that greater total dietary fiber intake was significantly associated with a lower risk of first stroke, with an additional 7 g/day conferring a relative risk of 0.93 (95% CI = 0.88–0.98). Total fiber intake was also found to be protective for CHD incidence (RR = 0.93, 95% CI = 0.91–0.96), and for CHD mortality (RR = 0.83, 95% CI = 0.76–0.91) in a meta-analysis of 18 studies involving 672,408 participants (Wu et al. 2015).

Whole grain intake also appears to be associated with a decreased risk of T2DM. A meta-analysis of six studies among 286,125 participants conducted by de Munter et al. (2007) indicates that a 2 serving/d (20 g/day) increase in whole grain intake was associated with a relative risk of 0.79 (95% CI = 0.72–0.87). Similarly, a 3–5 servings/d increase was associated with a relative risk of 0.74 (95% CI = 0.69–0.80) (Ye et al. 2012). For refined grains, Aune et al. (2013b) conclude from a pooled analysis of 16 cohort studies that a 3 serving/day increase of refined grains was not associated with T2DM (RR = 0.95, 95% CI = 0.88–1.04). There has also been recent interest in white rice, as it is one of the most commonly consumed food items in the world, especially in Asian countries. Combining data from four cohort studies consisting of 352,384 subjects, Hu et al. (2012) found that a 1 serving/day increment in white rice intake was associated with a relative risk of 1.11 (95% CI = 1.08–1.14) of T2DM. Finally, a meta-analysis of total dietary fiber and T2DM reported an inverse correlation, with a 2 g/day increment resulting in a risk ratio of 0.94 (95% CI = 0.93–0.96) (Yao et al. 2014).

Although micronutrients and phytochemicals may play a role in the differences between whole and refined grains, dietary fiber has been the most studied component. Regarding its cardioprotective effects, dietary fibers in the form of guar gum, glucan, and psyllium have been shown to lower blood pressure (Anderson et al. 2009) and decrease LDL cholesterol (Anderson et al. 2000, Brown et al. 1999, Whitehead et al. 2014). It is thought that fiber binds to bile acids in the small intestine and increases their excretion in the feces; the fermentation of fibers in the colon with production of propionate may also contribute to the hypocholesterolemic effects of fiber (Anderson et al. 2009). Dietary fiber also improves glycemic control and insulin sensitivity, although additional studies will be needed to elucidate this mechanism (Weickert and Pfeiffer 2008).

Currently, few studies have differentiated between soluble and insoluble fiber, and from what sources these fibers originate. Threapleton et al. (2013) found a null relationship between soluble fiber intake (RR = 0.94, 95% CI = 0.88–1.01) and risk of first stroke, but also remarked that more studies of fiber types needed to be performed. The differences in physiological response between soluble and insoluble fiber are well known. Insoluble fiber slows gastric emptying, reduces nutrient intake, and can blunt the rise in plasma glucose after a glucose challenge. Soluble fiber, due to its high water-retaining capacity, can be fermented by intestinal bacteria, and may increase utilization of fatty acids, thereby increasing energy absorption. Although both types appear to lead to weight loss, how insoluble and soluble fiber interacts with diet is not well understood, and more research is needed in this area (Lattimer and Haub 2010).

Nuts and Legumes

Although nuts were once considered unhealthy foods due to their high caloric and fat content, their cardioprotective effects (further discussed in Chapter 24) have been demonstrated by recent epidemiologic and clinical data. In a review of 25 observational studies and 501,791 subjects, Afshin et al. (2014) report that nut consumption was inversely associated with fatal IHD (RR = 0.76, 95% CI = 0.69–0.84), nonfatal IHD (RR = 0.78, 95% CI = 0.67–0.92), but not stroke. Similarly, legume consumption was associated with a lower risk of total IHD (RR = 0.86, 95% CI = 0.78–0.94), but not stroke. Two other concurrent meta-analyses corroborate these findings (Luo et al. 2014, Zhou et al. 2014). Luo et al. (2014) additionally reported that nut consumption also reduced the risk of all-cause mortality (RR = 0.85, 95% CI = 0.79–0.91). Zhou et al. (2014) meta-analyzed 40,102 subjects in studies of blood pressure as well and found that nut consumption was protective against hypertension (RR = 0.66, 95% CI = 0.44–1.00). In a recent cohort study of 120,852 subjects not included in previous pooled analyses, van den Brandt and Schouten (2015) indicate that total nut but not peanut butter intake was related to lower incidence of cardiovascular disease. The PREDIMED trial, an exceptional intervention study of 7,447 individuals, demonstrated that compared to a traditional low-fat diet, a Mediterranean diet supplemented with 30 g/day of nuts had a relative risk for all cardiovascular events of 0.72 (95% CI = 0.54–0.96) (Estruch et al. 2013).

All three of the previous meta-analyses concluded a null effect of nut consumption on the risk of T2DM after adjustment for BMI (Afshin et al. 2014, Luo et al. 2014, Zhou et al. 2014), although the point estimate for risk reduction remained below 1, signaling that the pooled analyses may still be underpowered. Furthermore, van den Brandt and Schouten (2015) reported an inverse association between nut intake and diabetes in the Netherlands Cohort Study. Despite a historic aversion to nuts owing to their high-energy density, nuts have not been linked to obesity (Rajaram and Sabate 2006). This may be due to both decreased fat absorption and the satiating effect of nut consumption (Ros 2009). Furthermore, nuts and legumes typically have low glycemic indices (i.e., they do not drastically increase postprandial blood glucose levels), and consumption of low glycemic index foods in place of high glycemic index foods have been linked to lower risk of T2DM (Willett et al. 2002).

One of the main explanations for the health benefits of nuts is their high unsaturated fat content. Indeed, numerous clinical studies have demonstrated that short-term nut supplementation decreases LDL cholesterol, total cholesterol, apoB, and triglycerides (Del Gobbo et al. 2015, Sabate et al. 2010). However, nuts and legumes additionally contain ample amounts of plant protein, fiber, folate, vitamins, minerals, and phytochemicals such as flavonoids. Key constituents also include L-arginine, the precursor of nitric oxide, α-linolenic acid and phenolic antioxidants (Ros 2010). All of these nutrients have been shown to boost cardiovascular health beyond their effects on blood cholesterol modulation (Mozaffarian et al. 2011). Various short-term clinical trials have shown that nut and legume consumption may improve insulin sensitivity and produce beneficial endothelial effects (Nash and Nash 2008). Nuts also decrease LDL oxidation, and favorably modulate biomarkers such as adiponectin (Ros 2009).

Future studies should focus on T2DM risk, as well as provide data on specific nut and legume subtypes. It is known that different nuts offer different nutrient profiles, for example, walnuts contain the highest concentration of PUFAs among any nut subtype (Ros 2010). Moreover, evidence from the NHS and NHSII confirm that consumption of walnuts was linearly associated with decreased risk of T2DM, with those consuming at least 2 servings/week having a relative risk of 0.67 (95% CI = 0.54–0.82) compared to nonconsumers (Pan et al. 2013). Furthermore, a meta-analysis of clinical trials revealed that walnuts significantly decrease total and LDL cholesterol (Banel and Hu 2009). A higher consumption of peanuts has also been associated with lower risk of CHD (Hu et al. 1998) and T2DM (Jiang et al. 2002). In the latter study, even peanut butter was found to lower the risk of T2DM when comparing those consuming ≥5 times a week to nonconsumers (RR = 0.79, 95% CI = 0.68–0.91).

CONCLUSION

This chapter aimed to summarize the epidemiologic and clinical evidence regarding food groups and their relationships with cardiometabolic disease. Different foods and beverages confer different health consequences depending on their macro- and micronutrient composition. However, the effects of foods appear similar for both CVD and T2DM. In other words, there does not appear to be a food item that is clearly beneficial for one condition and detrimental for the other, perhaps due to similar metabolic mechanisms underlying both conditions. Public health officials should recommend foods such as nuts, whole grains, fruits, and vegetables and discourage excessive consumption of red meats and sugar-sweetened beverages. Furthermore, processed varieties are generally unhealthier than unprocessed varieties of foods, as is the case with whole grains vs. refined grains. Coffee appears to be beneficial with moderate intake but neutral with heavy intake. Moderate alcohol consumption is also beneficial, but heavy consumption is associated with deleterious effects on both diabetes and CVD. One should exercise caution when prescribing these beverages for improving health. These recommendations are described in more detail in the 2015 Dietary Guidelines for Americans (U.S. Department of Health and Human Services and U.S. Department of Agriculture 2015).

Our present knowledge of food groups originates from data from large prospective cohort studies in conjunction with results from randomized trials. Yet, despite our gains in knowledge, questions of causation still linger for various types of foods and beverages. For these concerns, future investigators may require large randomized trials to settle issues once and for all. However, such trials, which are often infeasible due to practical and ethical considerations, present their own set of disadvantages, such as expense, high attrition rates, nonadherence, and inadequate blinding (Satija et al. 2015).

Nutrition research has also begun to see a shift in thinking from a reductionist to a holistic perspective. The traditional reductionist perspective holds that parts of the diet, such as single nutrients, are responsible for the health benefits or detriments observed in the literature (Hoffmann 2003). Following the pharmacological paradigm, classical nutritionists and clinicians have isolated hundreds of active ingredients in hopes of finding a magic bullet, but very few have been successful. Among many randomized trials, for example, there has been no significant effect of the use of multivitamins/multiminerals on death due to vascular causes or cancer (Macpherson et al. 2013), fish oil supplements on heart disease (Rizos et al. 2012), or antioxidant vitamins on heart disease (Ye et al. 2013). Furthermore, dosages administered in trials are often much greater than what one would normally consume from food sources. In one case, concentrated doses of vitamin A, as well as beta-carotene in combination with vitamin E, appeared to increase incidence of all-cause mortality (Bjelakovic et al. 2013). On the contrary, the holistic view of nutrition incorporates complex relationships between foods, as well as multicausal nonlinear associations (Fardet and Rock 2014). Such a view can facilitate the translation of scientific evidence into healthful dietary patterns for the prevention of cardiometabolic diseases.

REFERENCES

Abete, I., D. Romaguera, A. R. Vieira, A. Lopez de Munain, and T. Norat. 2014. Association between total, processed, red and white meat consumption and all-cause, CVD and IHD mortality: A meta-analysis of cohort studies. *Br J Nutr* 112 (5):762–775. doi: 10.1017/s000711451400124x.

Afshin, A., R. Micha, S. Khatibzadeh, and D. Mozaffarian. 2014. Consumption of nuts and legumes and risk of incident ischemic heart disease, stroke, and diabetes: A systematic review and meta-analysis. *Am J Clin Nutr* 100 (1):278–288. doi: 10.3945/ajcn.113.076901.

Albert, M. A., R. J. Glynn, and P. M. Ridker. 2003. Alcohol consumption and plasma concentration of C-reactive protein. *Circulation* 107 (3):443–447.

Anderson, J. W., L. D. Allgood, A. Lawrence, L. A. Altringer, G. R. Jerdack, D. A. Hengehold, and J. G. Morel. 2000. Cholesterol-lowering effects of psyllium intake adjunctive to diet therapy in men and women with hypercholesterolemia: Meta-analysis of 8 controlled trials. *Am J Clin Nutr* 71 (2):472–479.

Anderson, J. W., P. Baird, R. H. Davis, Jr., S. Ferreri, M. Knudtson, A. Koraym, V. Waters, and C. L. Williams. 2009. Health benefits of dietary fiber. *Nutr Rev* 67 (4):188–205. doi: 10.1111/j.1753-4887.2009.00189.x.

Aune, D., T. Norat, P. Romundstad, and L. J. Vatten. 2013a. Dairy products and the risk of type 2 diabetes: A systematic review and dose-response meta-analysis of cohort studies. *Am J Clin Nutr* 98 (4):1066–1083. doi: 10.3945/ajcn.113.059030.

Aune, D., T. Norat, P. Romundstad, and L. J. Vatten. 2013b. Whole grain and refined grain consumption and the risk of type 2 diabetes: A systematic review and dose–response meta-analysis of cohort studies. *Eur J Epidemiol* 28 (11):845–858. doi: 10.1007/s10654-013-9852-5.

Baliunas, D. O., B. J. Taylor, H. Irving, M. Roerecke, J. Patra, S. Mohapatra, and J. Rehm. 2009. Alcohol as a risk factor for type 2 diabetes: A systematic review and meta-analysis. *Diabetes Care* 32 (11):2123–2132. doi: 10.2337/dc09-0227.

Banel, D. K. and F. B. Hu. 2009. Effects of walnut consumption on blood lipids and other cardiovascular risk factors: A meta-analysis and systematic review. *Am J Clin Nutr* 90 (1):56–63. doi: 10.3945/ajcn.2009.27457.

Bang, H. O., J. Dyerberg, and H. M. Sinclair. 1980. The composition of the Eskimo food in north western Greenland. *Am J Clin Nutr* 33 (12):2657–2661.

Bassoli, B. K., P. Cassolla, G. R. Borba-Murad, J. Constantin, C. L. Salgueiro-Pagadigorria, R. B. Bazotte, R. S. da Silva, and H. M. de Souza. 2008. Chlorogenic acid reduces the plasma glucose peak in the oral glucose tolerance test: Effects on hepatic glucose release and glycaemia. *Cell Biochem Funct* 26 (3):320–328. doi: 10.1002/cbf.1444.

Bernstein, A. M., Q. Sun, F. B. Hu, M. J. Stampfer, J. E. Manson, and W. C. Willett. 2010. Major dietary protein sources and risk of coronary heart disease in women. *Circulation* 122 (9):876–883. doi: 10.1161/circulationaha.109.915165.

Bingham, S. A., C. Gill, A. Welch, K. Day, A. Cassidy, K. T. Khaw, M. J. Sneyd, T. J. Key, L. Roe, and N. E. Day. 1994. Comparison of dietary assessment methods in nutritional epidemiology: Weighed records v. 24 h recalls, food-frequency questionnaires and estimated-diet records. *Br J Nutr* 72 (4):619–643.

Bjelakovic, G., D. Nikolova, and C. Gluud. 2013. Meta-regression analyses, meta-analyses, and trial sequential analyses of the effects of supplementation with beta-carotene, vitamin A, and vitamin E singly or in different combinations on all-cause mortality: Do we have evidence for lack of harm? *PLoS One* 8 (9):e74558. doi: 10.1371/journal.pone.0074558.

Bowman, M. P., J. Van Doren, L. J. Taper, F. W. Thye, and S. J. Ritchey. 1988. Effect of dietary fat and cholesterol on plasma lipids and lipoprotein fractions in normolipidemic men. *J Nutr* 118 (5):555–560.

Bray, G. A. 2007. How bad is fructose? *Am J Clin Nutr* 86 (4):895–896.

Briefel, R. R. 1994. Assessment of the US diet in national nutrition surveys: National collaborative efforts and NHANES. *Am J Clin Nutr* 59 (1 Suppl):164s–167s.

Brown, L., B. Rosner, W. W. Willett, and F. M. Sacks. 1999. Cholesterol-lowering effects of dietary fiber: A meta-analysis. *Am J Clin Nutr* 69 (1):30–42.

Buzzard, I. M., M. R. McRoberts, D. L. Driscoll, and J. Bowering. 1982. Effect of dietary eggs and ascorbic acid on plasma lipid and lipoprotein cholesterol levels in healthy young men. *Am J Clin Nutr* 36 (1):94–105.

Carlsson, S., N. Hammar, and V. Grill. 2005. Alcohol consumption and type 2 diabetes meta-analysis of epidemiological studies indicates a U-shaped relationship. *Diabetologia* 48 (6):1051–1054. doi: 10.1007/s00125-005-1768-5.

Carter, P., L. J. Gray, J. Troughton, K. Khunti, and M. J. Davies. 2010. Fruit and vegetable intake and incidence of type 2 diabetes mellitus: Systematic review and meta-analysis. *BMJ* 341:c4229. doi: 10.1136/bmj.c4229.

Cassidy, A., É. J. O'Reilly, C. Kay, L. Sampson, M. Franz, J. P. Forman, G. Curhan, and E. B. Rimm. 2011. Habitual intake of flavonoid subclasses and incident hypertension in adults. *Am J Clin Nutr* 93 (2):338–347. doi: 10.3945/ajcn.110.006783.

Chen, G. C., D. B. Lv, Z. Pang, and Q. F. Liu. 2013. Red and processed meat consumption and risk of stroke: A meta-analysis of prospective cohort studies. *Eur J Clin Nutr* 67 (1):91–95. doi: 10.1038/ejcn.2012.180.

Chen, M., Q. Sun, E. Giovannucci, D. Mozaffarian, J. E. Manson, W. C. Willett, and F. B. Hu. 2014. Dairy consumption and risk of type 2 diabetes: 3 cohorts of US adults and an updated meta-analysis. *BMC Med* 12:215. doi: 10.1186/s12916-014-0215-1.

Chenoweth, W., M. Ullmann, R. Simpson, and G. Leveille. 1981. Influence of dietary cholesterol and fat on serum lipids in men. *J Nutr* 111 (12):2069–2080.

Cheraskin, E., W. M. Ringsdorf, Jr., A. T. Setyaadmadja, and R. A. Barrett. 1967. Effect of caffeine versus placebo supplementation on blood-glucose concentration. *Lancet* 1 (7503):1299–1300.

Cho, Y. A. and J. Kim. 2015. Effect of probiotics on blood lipid concentrations: A meta-analysis of randomized controlled trials. *Medicine* 94 (43):e1714. doi: 10.1097/md.0000000000001714.

Chowdhury, R., S. Stevens, D. Gorman, A. Pan, S. Warnakula, S. Chowdhury, H. Ward et al. 2012. Association between fish consumption, long chain omega 3 fatty acids, and risk of cerebrovascular disease: Systematic review and meta-analysis. *BMJ* 345:e6698. doi: 10.1136/bmj.e6698.

Clarke, R., C. Frost, R. Collins, P. Appleby, and R. Peto. 1997. Dietary lipids and blood cholesterol: Quantitative meta-analysis of metabolic ward studies. *BMJ* 314 (7074):112–117.

Cooper, A. J., N. G. Forouhi, Z. Ye, B. Buijsse, L. Arriola, B. Balkau, A. Barricarte et al. 2012. Fruit and vegetable intake and type 2 diabetes: EPIC-InterAct prospective study and meta-analysis. *Eur J Clin Nutr* 66 (10):1082–1092. doi: 10.1038/ejcn.2012.85.

Corrao, G., L. Rubbiati, V. Bagnardi, A. Zambon, and K. Poikolainen. 2000. Alcohol and coronary heart disease: A meta-analysis. *Addiction* 95 (10):1505–1523. doi: 10.1046/j.1360-0443.2000.951015056.x.

Criqui, M. H., L. D. Cowan, H. A. Tyroler, S. Bangdiwala, G. Heiss, R. B. Wallace, and R. Cohn. 1987. Lipoproteins as mediators for the effects of alcohol consumption and cigarette smoking on cardiovascular mortality: Results from the lipid research clinics follow-up study. *Am J Epidemiol* 126 (4):629–637.

Dauchet, L., P. Amouyel, S. Hercberg, and J. Dallongeville. 2006. Fruit and vegetable consumption and risk of coronary heart disease: A meta-analysis of cohort studies. *J Nutr* 136 (10):2588–2593.

Davidson, M. H., D. Hunninghake, K. C. Maki, P. O. Kwiterovich, Jr., and S. Kafonek. 1999. Comparison of the effects of lean red meat vs lean white meat on serum lipid levels among free-living persons with hypercholesterolemia: A long-term, randomized clinical trial. *Arch Intern Med* 159 (12):1331–1338.

de Munter, J. S., F. B. Hu, D. Spiegelman, M. Franz, and R. M. van Dam. 2007. Whole grain, bran, and germ intake and risk of type 2 diabetes: A prospective cohort study and systematic review. *PLoS Med* 4 (8):e261. doi: 10.1371/journal.pmed.0040261.

Del Gobbo, L. C., M. C. Falk, R. Feldman, K. Lewis, and D. Mozaffarian. 2015. Effects of tree nuts on blood lipids, apolipoproteins, and blood pressure: Systematic review, meta-analysis, and dose-response of 61 controlled intervention trials. *Am J Clin Nutr* 102 (6):1347–1356. doi: 10.3945/ajcn.115.110965.

Di Castelnuovo, A., S. Costanzo, R. di Giuseppe, G. de Gaetano, and L. Iacoviello. 2009. Alcohol consumption and cardiovascular risk: Mechanisms of action and epidemiologic perspectives. *Future Cardiol* 5 (5):467–477. doi: 10.2217/fca.09.36.

Dillard, C. J. and J. Bruce German. 2000. Phytochemicals: Nutraceuticals and human health. *J Sci Food Agric* 80 (12):1744–1756. doi: 10.1002/1097-0010(20000915)80:12<1744::AID-JSFA725>3.0.CO;2-W.

Ding, M., S. N. Bhupathiraju, M. Chen, R. M. van Dam, and F. B. Hu. 2014a. Caffeinated and decaffeinated coffee consumption and risk of type 2 diabetes: A systematic review and a dose-response meta-analysis. *Diabetes Care* 37 (2):569–586. doi: 10.2337/dc13-1203.

Ding, M., S. N. Bhupathiraju, A. Satija, R. M. van Dam, and F. B. Hu. 2014b. Long-term coffee consumption and risk of cardiovascular disease: A systematic review and a dose–response meta-analysis of prospective cohort studies. *Circulation* 129 (6):643–659. doi: 10.1161/circulationaha.113.005925.

Djoussé, L., O. A. Khawaja, and J. Michael Gaziano. 2016. Egg consumption and risk of type 2 diabetes: A meta-analysis of prospective studies. *Am J Clin Nutr* 103(2):474–480. doi: 10.3945/ajcn.115.119933.

Dyerberg, J., H. O. Bang, E. Stoffersen, S. Moncada, and J. R. Vane. 1978. Eicosapentaenoic acid and prevention of thrombosis and atherosclerosis? *Lancet* 2 (8081):117–119.

Ejtahed, H. S., J. Mohtadi-Nia, A. Homayouni-Rad, M. Niafar, M. Asghari-Jafarabadi, V. Mofid, and A. Akbarian-Moghari. 2011. Effect of probiotic yogurt containing *Lactobacillus acidophilus* and *Bifidobacterium lactis* on lipid profile in individuals with type 2 diabetes mellitus. *J Dairy Sci* 94 (7):3288–3294. doi: http://dx.doi.org/10.3168/jds.2010-4128.

Elwood, P. C., J. E. Pickering, D. I. Givens, and J. E. Gallacher. 2010. The consumption of milk and dairy foods and the incidence of vascular disease and diabetes: An overview of the evidence. *Lipids* 45 (10):925–939. doi: 10.1007/s11745-010-3412-5.

Estruch, R., E. Ros, J. Salas-Salvadó, M.-I. Covas, D. Corella, F. Arós, E. Gómez-Gracia et al. 2013. Primary prevention of cardiovascular disease with a Mediterranean diet. *N Engl J Med* 368 (14):1279–1290. doi: 10.1056/NEJMoa1200303.

Fardet, A. and E. Rock. 2014. Toward a new philosophy of preventive nutrition: From a reductionist to a holistic paradigm to improve nutritional recommendations. *Adv Nutr* 5 (4):430–446. doi: 10.3945/an.114.006122.

Feskens, E. J. and D. Kromhout. 1990. Habitual dietary intake and glucose tolerance in euglycaemic men: The Zutphen study. *Int J Epidemiol* 19 (4):953–959.

Feskens, E. J., D. Sluik, and G. J. van Woudenbergh. 2013. Meat consumption, diabetes, and its complications. *Curr Diab Rep* 13 (2):298–306. doi: 10.1007/s11892-013-0365-0.

Forshee, R. A., P. A. Anderson, and M. L. Storey. 2008. Sugar-sweetened beverages and body mass index in children and adolescents: A meta-analysis. *Am J Clin Nutr* 87 (6):1662–1671.

Fuller, N. R., I. D. Caterson, A. Sainsbury, G. Denyer, M. Fong, J. Gerofi, K. Baqleh, K. H. Williams, N. S. Lau, and T. P. Markovic. 2015. The effect of a high-egg diet on cardiovascular risk factors in people with type 2 diabetes: The Diabetes and Egg (DIABEGG) study—A 3-mo randomized controlled trial. *Am J Clin Nutr* 101(4):705–713. doi: 10.3945/ajcn.114.096925.

Gao, D., N. Ning, C. Wang, Y. Wang, Q. Li, Z. Meng, Y. Liu, and Q. Li. 2013. Dairy products consumption and risk of type 2 diabetes: Systematic review and dose-response meta-analysis. *PLoS One* 8 (9):e73965. doi: 10.1371/journal.pone.0073965.

Gaziano, J. M., J. E. Buring, J. L. Breslow, S. Z. Goldhaber, B. Rosner, M. VanDenburgh, W. Willett, and C. H. Hennekens. 1993. Moderate alcohol intake, increased levels of high-density lipoprotein and its subfractions, and decreased risk of myocardial infarction. *N Engl J Med* 329 (25):1829–1834. doi: 10.1056/NEJM199312163292501.

Greenberg, J. A., K. V. Axen, R. Schnoll, and C. N. Boozer. 2005. Coffee, tea and diabetes: The role of weight loss and caffeine. *Int J Obes Relat Metab Disord* 29 (9):1121–1129.

He, F. J., C. A. Nowson, M. Lucas, and G. A. MacGregor. 2007. Increased consumption of fruit and vegetables is related to a reduced risk of coronary heart disease: Meta-analysis of cohort studies. *J Hum Hypertens* 21 (9):717–728.

He, F. J., C. A. Nowson, and G. A. MacGregor. 2006. Fruit and vegetable consumption and stroke: Meta-analysis of cohort studies. *Lancet* 367 (9507):320–326. doi: 10.1016/S0140-6736(06)68069-0.

He, K., Y. Song, M. L. Daviglus, K. Liu, L. Van Horn, A. R. Dyer, and P. Greenland. 2004. Accumulated evidence on fish consumption and coronary heart disease mortality: A meta-analysis of cohort studies. *Circulation* 109 (22):2705–2711. doi: 10.1161/01.cir.0000132503.19410.6b.

Hines, L. M., M. J. Stampfer, J. Ma, J. M. Gaziano, P. M. Ridker, S. E. Hankinson, F. Sacks, E. B. Rimm, and D. J. Hunter. 2001. Genetic variation in alcohol dehydrogenase and the beneficial effect of moderate alcohol consumption on myocardial infarction. *N Engl J Med* 344 (8):549–555. doi: 10.1056/nejm200102223440802.

Hjerpsted, J., E. Leedo, and T. Tholstrup. 2011. Cheese intake in large amounts lowers LDL-cholesterol concentrations compared with butter intake of equal fat content. *Am J Clin Nutr* 94 (6):1479–1484. doi: 10.3945/ajcn.111.022426.

Hoffmann, I. 2003. Transcending reductionism in nutrition research. *Am J Clin Nutr* 78 (3):514S–516S.

Holmes, M. V., C. E. Dale, L. Zuccolo, R. J. Silverwood, Y. Guo, Z. Ye, D. Prieto-Merino et al. 2014. Association between alcohol and cardiovascular disease: Mendelian randomisation analysis based on individual participant data. *BMJ* 349:g4164. doi: 10.1136/bmj.g4164.

Hooper, L., P. A. Kroon, E. B. Rimm, J. S. Cohn, I. Harvey, K. A. Le Cornu, J. J. Ryder, W. L. Hall, and A. Cassidy. 2008. Flavonoids, flavonoid-rich foods, and cardiovascular risk: A meta-analysis of randomized controlled trials. *Am J Clin Nutr* 88 (1):38–50.

Hu, E. A., A. Pan, V. Malik, and Q. Sun. 2012. White rice consumption and risk of type 2 diabetes: Meta-analysis and systematic review. *BMJ* 344. doi: 10.1136/bmj.e1454.

Hu, F. 2008. *Obesity Epidemiology*. Oxford University Press, Cary, NC.

Hu, F. B. 2013. Resolved: There is sufficient scientific evidence that decreasing sugar-sweetened beverage consumption will reduce the prevalence of obesity and obesity-related diseases. *Obes Rev* 14 (8):606–619. doi: 10.1111/obr.12040.

Hu, F. B., M. J. Stampfer, J. E. Manson, E. B. Rimm, G. A. Colditz, B. A. Rosner, F. E. Speizer, C. H. Hennekens, and W. C. Willett. 1998. Frequent nut consumption and risk of coronary heart disease in women: Prospective cohort study. *BMJ* 317 (7169):1341–1345. doi: 10.1136/bmj.317.7169.1341.

Hu, F. B. and V. S. Malik. 2010. Sugar-sweetened beverages and risk of obesity and type 2 diabetes: Epidemiologic evidence. *Physiol Behav* 100 (1):47–54. doi: 10.1016/j.physbeh.2010.01.036.

Huang, C., J. Huang, Y. Tian, X. Yang, and D. Gu. 2014. Sugar sweetened beverages consumption and risk of coronary heart disease: A meta-analysis of prospective studies. *Atherosclerosis* 234 (1):11–16. doi: http://dx.doi.org/10.1016/j.atherosclerosis.2014.01.037.

Huang, T., B. Yang, J. Zheng, G. Li, M. L. Wahlqvist, and D. Li. 2012. Cardiovascular disease mortality and cancer incidence in vegetarians: A meta-analysis and systematic review. *Ann Nutr Metab* 60 (4):233–240. doi: 10.1159/000337301.

Huffman, M. D. 2012. Association or causation of sugar-sweetened beverages and coronary heart disease: Recalling Sir Austin Bradford Hill. *Circulation* 125 (14):1718–1720. doi: 10.1161/circulationaha.112.097634.

Huth, P. J. and K. M. Park. 2012. Influence of dairy product and milk fat consumption on cardiovascular disease risk: A review of the evidence. *Adv Nutr Int Rev J* 3 (3):266–285. doi: 10.3945/an.112.002030.

Janssens, J. P., N. Shapira, P. Debeuf, L. Michiels, R. Putman, L. Bruckers, D. Renard, and G. Molenberghs. 1999. Effects of soft drink and table beer consumption on insulin response in normal teenagers and carbohydrate drink in youngsters. *Eur J Cancer Prev* 8 (4):289–295.

Jensen, M. K., K. J. Mukamal, K. Overvad, and E. B. Rimm. 2008. Alcohol consumption, TaqIB polymorphism of cholesteryl ester transfer protein, high-density lipoprotein cholesterol, and risk of coronary heart disease in men and women. *Eur Heart J* 29 (1):104–112. doi: 10.1093/eurheartj/ehm517.

Jiang, R., J. E. Manson, M. J. Stampfer, S. Liu, W. C. Willett, and F. B. Hu. 2002. Nut and peanut butter consumption and risk of type 2 diabetes in women. *JAMA* 288 (20):2554–2560. doi: 10.1001/jama.288.20.2554.

Jiang, X., D. Zhang, and W. Jiang. 2014. Coffee and caffeine intake and incidence of type 2 diabetes mellitus: A meta-analysis of prospective studies. *Eur J Nutr* 53 (1):25–38. doi: 10.1007/s00394-013-0603-x.

Kaluza, J., A. Wolk, and S. C. Larsson. 2012. Red meat consumption and risk of stroke: A meta-analysis of prospective studies. *Stroke* 43:2556–2560. doi: 10.1161/strokeaha.112.663286.

Keijzers, G. B., B. E. De Galan, C. J. Tack, and P. Smits. 2002. Caffeine can decrease insulin sensitivity in humans. *Diabetes Care* 25 (2):364–369.

Kempf, K., C. Herder, I. Erlund, H. Kolb, S. Martin, M. Carstensen, W. Koenig et al. 2010. Effects of coffee consumption on subclinical inflammation and other risk factors for type 2 diabetes: A clinical trial. *Am J Clin Nutr* 91 (4):950–957. doi: 10.3945/ajcn.2009.28548.

Kleiman, S., S. W. Ng, and B. Popkin. 2012. Drinking to our health: Can beverage companies cut calories while maintaining profits? *Obes Rev* 13 (3):258–274. doi: 10.1111/j.1467-789X.2011.00949.x.

Koeth, R. A., Z. Wang, B. S. Levison, J. A. Buffa, E. Org, B. T. Sheehy, E. B. Britt et al. 2013. Intestinal microbiota metabolism of L-carnitine, a nutrient in red meat, promotes atherosclerosis. *Nat Med* 19 (5):576–585. doi: 10.1038/nm.3145. http://www.nature.com/nm/journal/v19/n5/abs/nm.3145.html#supplementary-information.

Kris-Etherton, P. M., W. S. Harris, L. J. Appel, and for the Nutrition Committee. 2002. Fish consumption, fish oil, omega-3 fatty acids, and cardiovascular disease. *Circulation* 106 (21):2747–2757. doi: 10.1161/01.cir.0000038493.65177.94.

Kroke, A., K. Klipstein-Grobusch, S. Voss, J. Möseneder, F. Thielecke, R. Noack, and H. Boeing. 1999. Validation of a self-administered food-frequency questionnaire administered in the European Prospective Investigation into Cancer and Nutrition (EPIC) Study: Comparison of energy, protein, and macronutrient intakes estimated with the doubly labeled water, urinary nitrogen, and repeated 24-h dietary recall methods. *Am J Clin Nutr* 70 (4):439–447.

Kromann, N. and A. Green. 1980. Epidemiological studies in the Upernavik district, Greenland. Incidence of some chronic diseases 1950–1974. *Acta Med Scand* 208 (5):401–406.

Kummerow, F. A., Y. Kim, J. Hull, J. Pollard, P. Ilinov, D. L. Drossiev, and J. Valek. 1977. The influence of egg consumption on the serum cholesterol level in human subjects. *Am J Clin Nutr* 30 (5):664–673.

Lampe, J. W. 1999. Health effects of vegetables and fruit: Assessing mechanisms of action in human experimental studies. *Am J Clin Nutr* 70 (3 Suppl):475s–490s.

Lattimer, J. M. and M. D. Haub. 2010. Effects of dietary fiber and its components on metabolic health. *Nutrients* 2 (12):1266–1289. doi: 10.3390/nu2121266.

Li, M., Y. Fan, X. Zhang, W. Hou, and Z. Tang. 2014. Fruit and vegetable intake and risk of type 2 diabetes mellitus: Meta-analysis of prospective cohort studies. *BMJ Open* 4 (11):e005497. doi: 10.1136/bmjopen-2014-005497.

Li, Y., C. Zhou, X. Zhou, and L. Li. 2013. Egg consumption and risk of cardiovascular diseases and diabetes: A meta-analysis. *Atherosclerosis* 229 (2):524–530. doi: 10.1016/j.atherosclerosis.2013.04.003.

Liu, S., J. E. Manson, J. E. Buring, M. J. Stampfer, W. C. Willett, and P. M. Ridker. 2002. Relation between a diet with a high glycemic load and plasma concentrations of high-sensitivity C-reactive protein in middle-aged women. *Am J Clin Nutr* 75 (3):492–498.

Liu, Y.-J., J. Zhan, X.-L. Liu, Y. Wang, J. Ji, and Q.-Q. He. 2014. Dietary flavonoids intake and risk of type 2 diabetes: A meta-analysis of prospective cohort studies. *Clin Nutr* 33 (1):59–63. doi: http://dx.doi.org/10.1016/j.clnu.2013.03.011.

Luo, C., Y. Zhang, Y. Ding, Z. Shan, S. Chen, M. Yu, F. B. Hu, and L. Liu. 2014. Nut consumption and risk of type 2 diabetes, cardiovascular disease, and all-cause mortality: A systematic review and meta-analysis. *Am J Clin Nutr* 100 (1):256–269. doi: 10.3945/ajcn.113.076109.

Macpherson, H., A. Pipingas, and M. P. Pase. 2013. Multivitamin-multimineral supplementation and mortality: A meta-analysis of randomized controlled trials. *Am J Clin Nutr* 97(2):437–444. doi: 10.3945/ajcn.112.049304.

Malerba, S., F. Turati, C. Galeone, C. Pelucchi, F. Verga, C. La Vecchia, and A. Tavani. 2013. A meta-analysis of prospective studies of coffee consumption and mortality for all causes, cancers and cardiovascular diseases. *Eur J Epidemiol* 28 (7):527–539. doi: 10.1007/s10654-013-9834-7.

Malik, V. S., B. M. Popkin, G. A. Bray, J.-P. Després, and F. B. Hu. 2010a. Sugar-sweetened beverages, obesity, type 2 diabetes mellitus, and cardiovascular disease risk. *Circulation* 121 (11):1356–1364. doi: 10.1161/circulationaha.109.876185.

Malik, V. S., B. M. Popkin, G. A. Bray, J.-P. Després, W. C. Willett, and F. B. Hu. 2010b. Sugar-sweetened beverages and risk of metabolic syndrome and rype 2 diabetes: A meta-analysis. *Diabetes Care* 33 (11):2477–2483. doi: 10.2337/dc10-1079.

Malik, V. S., M. B. Schulze, and F. B. Hu. 2006. Intake of sugar-sweetened beverages and weight gain: A systematic review. *Am J Clin Nutr* 84 (2):274–288.

Malik, V. S., W. C. Willett, and F. B. Hu. 2009. Sugar-sweetened beverages and BMI in children and adolescents: Reanalyses of a meta-analysis. *Am J Clin Nutr* 89 (1):438–439. doi: 10.3945/ajcn.2008.26980.

Mattes, R. D., J. M. Shikany, K. A. Kaiser, and D. B. Allison. 2011. Nutritively sweetened beverage consumption and body weight: A systematic review and meta-analysis of randomized experiments. *Obes Rev* 12 (5):346–365. doi: 10.1111/j.1467-789X.2010.00755.x.

Mellen, P. B., T. F. Walsh, and D. M. Herrington. 2008. Whole grain intake and cardiovascular disease: A meta-analysis. *Nutr Metab Cardiovasc Dis* 18 (4):283–390. doi: 10.1016/j.numecd.2006.12.008.

Mensink, R. P., P. L. Zock, A. D. M. Kester, and M. B. Katan. 2003. Effects of dietary fatty acids and carbohydrates on the ratio of serum total to HDL cholesterol and on serum lipids and apolipoproteins: A meta-analysis of 60 controlled trials. *Am J Clin Nutr* 77 (5):1146–1155.

Mesas, A. E., L. M. Leon-Munoz, F. Rodriguez-Artalejo, and E. Lopez-Garcia. 2011. The effect of coffee on blood pressure and cardiovascular disease in hypertensive individuals: A systematic review and meta-analysis. *Am J Clin Nutr* 94 (4):1113–1126. doi: 10.3945/ajcn.111.016667.

Meyer, K. A., L. H. Kushi, D. R. Jacobs, Jr., and A. R. Folsom. 2001. Dietary fat and incidence of type 2 diabetes in older Iowa women. *Diabetes Care* 24 (9):1528–1535.

Micha, R. and D. Mozaffarian. 2010. Saturated fat and cardiometabolic risk factors, coronary heart disease, stroke, and diabetes: A fresh look at the evidence. *Lipids* 45 (10):893–905. doi: 10.1007/s11745-010-3393-4.

Micha, R., S. K. Wallace, and D. Mozaffarian. 2010. Red and processed meat consumption and risk of incident coronary heart disease, stroke, and diabetes mellitus: A systematic review and meta-analysis. *Circulation* 121 (21):2271–2283. doi: 10.1161/circulationaha.109.924977.

Miettinen, T. A. and Y. A. Kesäniemi. 1989. Cholesterol absorption: Regulation of cholesterol synthesis and elimination and within-population variations of serum cholesterol levels. *Am J Clin Nutr* 49 (4):629–635.

Mohamadshahi, M., M. Veissi, F. Haidari, A. Z. Javid, F. Mohammadi, and E. Shirbeigi. 2014. Effects of probiotic yogurt consumption on lipid profile in type 2 diabetic patients: A randomized controlled clinical trial. *J Res Med Sci* 19 (6):531–536.

Moore, R. D. and T. A. Pearson. 1986. Moderate alcohol consumption and coronary artery disease. A review. *Medicine (Baltimore)* 65 (4):242–267.

Mostofsky, E., M. S. Rice, E. B. Levitan, and M. A. Mittleman. 2012. Habitual coffee consumption and risk of heart failure: A dose-response meta-analysis. *Circul Heart Fail* 5 (4):401–405. doi: 10.1161/circheartfailure.112.967299.

Mozaffarian, D., L. J. Appel, and L. Van Horn. 2011. Components of a cardioprotective diet: New insights. *Circulation* 123 (24):2870–2891. doi: 10.1161/circulationaha.110.968735.

Mozaffarian, D. and R. Clarke. 2009. Quantitative effects on cardiovascular risk factors and coronary heart disease risk of replacing partially hydrogenated vegetable oils with other fats and oils. *Eur J Clin Nutr* 63 (Suppl 2):S22–S33. doi: 10.1038/sj.ejcn.1602976.

Mozaffarian, D., R. Micha, and S. Wallace. 2010. Effects on coronary heart disease of increasing polyunsaturated fat in place of saturated fat: A systematic review and meta-analysis of randomized controlled trials. *PLoS Med* 7 (3):e1000252. doi: 10.1371/journal.pmed.1000252.

Mozaffarian, D. and J. H. Y. Wu. 2011. Omega-3 fatty acids and cardiovascular disease effects on risk factors, molecular pathways, and clinical events. *J Am Coll Cardiol* 58 (20):2047–2067. doi: 10.1016/j.jacc.2011.06.063.

Mukamal, K. J. and E. B. Rimm. 2001. Alcohol's effects on the risk for coronary heart disease. *Alcohol Res Health* 25 (4):255–261.

Muraki, I., F. Imamura, J. E. Manson, F. B. Hu, W. C. Willett, R. M. van Dam, and Q. Sun. 2013. Fruit consumption and risk of type 2 diabetes: Results from three prospective longitudinal cohort studies. *BMJ* 347:f5001. doi: 10.1136/bmj.f5001.

Mutungi, G., J. Ratliff, M. Puglisi, M. Torres-Gonzalez, U. Vaishnav, J. O. Leite, E. Quann, J. S. Volek, and M. L. Fernandez. 2008. Dietary cholesterol from eggs increases plasma HDL cholesterol in overweight men consuming a carbohydrate-restricted diet. *J Nutr* 138 (2):272–276.

Nash, S. D. and D. T. Nash. 2008. Nuts as part of a healthy cardiovascular diet. *Curr Atheroscler Rep* 10 (6):529–535.

Natella, F. and C. Scaccini. 2012. Role of coffee in modulation of diabetes risk. *Nutr Rev* 70 (4):207–217. doi: 10.1111/j.1753-4887.2012.00470.x.

Ness, A. R. and J. W. Powles. 1997. Fruit and vegetables, and cardiovascular disease: A review. *Int J Epidemiol* 26 (1):1–13. doi: 10.1093/ije/26.1.1.

Nestel, P. J. 1990. Effects of N-3 fatty acids on lipid metabolism. *Annu Rev Nutr* 10:149–167. doi: 10.1146/annurev.nu.10.070190.001053.

Newby, P. K., F. B. Hu, E. B. Rimm, S. A. Smith-Warner, D. Feskanich, L. Sampson, and W. C. Willett. 2003. Reproducibility and validity of the Diet Quality Index revised as assessed by use of a food-frequency questionnaire. *Am J Clin Nutr* 78 (5):941–949.

Nijveldt, R. J., E. van Nood, D. E. C. van Hoorn, P. G. Boelens, K. van Norren, and P. A. M. van Leeuwen. 2001. Flavonoids: A review of probable mechanisms of action and potential applications. *Am J Clin Nutr* 74 (4):418–425.

Ogden, C. L., B. K. Kit, M. D. Carroll, and S. Park. 2011. Consumption of sugar drinks in the United States, 2005–2008. *NCHS Data Brief* 71:1–8.

Pan, A., Q. Sun, A. M. Bernstein, M. B. Schulze, J. E. Manson, W. C. Willett, and F. B. Hu. 2011. Red meat consumption and risk of type 2 diabetes: 3 cohorts of US adults and an updated meta-analysis. *Am J Clin Nutr* 94 (4):1088–1096. doi: 10.3945/ajcn.111.018978.

Pan, A., Q. Sun, J. E. Manson, W. C. Willett, and F. B. Hu. 2013. Walnut consumption is associated with lower risk of type 2 diabetes in women. *J Nutr* 143 (4):512–518. doi: 10.3945/jn.112.172171.

Pedersen, B., K. E. Knudsen, and B. O. Eggum. 1989. Nutritive value of cereal products with emphasis on the effect of milling. *World Rev Nutr Diet* 60:1–91.

Pizziol, A., V. Tikhonoff, C. D. Paleari, E. Russo, A. Mazza, G. Ginocchio, C. Onesto, L. Pavan, E. Casiglia, and A. C. Pessina. 1998. Effects of caffeine on glucose tolerance: A placebo-controlled study. *Eur J Clin Nutr* 52 (11):846–849.

Qi, Q., A. Y. Chu, J. H. Kang, M. K. Jensen, G. C. Curhan, L. R. Pasquale, P. M. Ridker et al. 2012. Sugar-sweetened beverages and genetic risk of obesity. *N Engl J Med* 367 (15):1387–1396. doi: 10.1056/NEJMoa1203039.

Qin, L. Q., J. Y. Xu, S. F. Han, Z. L. Zhang, Y. Y. Zhao, and I. M. Szeto. 2015. Dairy consumption and risk of cardiovascular disease: An updated meta-analysis of prospective cohort studies. *Asia Pac J Clin Nutr* 24 (1):90–100. doi: 10.6133/apjcn.2015.24.1.09.

Rajaram, S. and J. Sabate. 2006. Nuts, body weight and insulin resistance. *Br J Nutr* 96 (Suppl 2):S79–S86.

Ranheim, T. and B. Halvorsen. 2005. Coffee consumption and human health—Beneficial or detrimental?—Mechanisms for effects of coffee consumption on different risk factors for cardiovascular disease and type 2 diabetes mellitus. *Mol Nutr Food Res* 49 (3):274–284. doi: 10.1002/mnfr.200400109.

Ratliff, J., G. Mutungi, M. J. Puglisi, J. S. Volek, and M. L. Fernandez. 2009. Carbohydrate restriction (with or without additional dietary cholesterol provided by eggs) reduces insulin resistance and plasma leptin without modifying appetite hormones in adult men. *Nutr Res* 29 (4):262–268. doi: 10.1016/j.nutres.2009.03.007.

Rimm, E. B., A. Klatsky, D. Grobbee, and M. J. Stampfer. 1996. Review of moderate alcohol consumption and reduced risk of coronary heart disease: Is the effect due to beer, wine, or spirits? *BMJ* 312 (7033):731–736. doi: 10.1136/bmj.312.7033.731.

Rimm, E. B., P. Williams, K. Fosher, M. Criqui, and M. J. Stampfer. 1999. Moderate alcohol intake and lower risk of coronary heart disease: Meta-analysis of effects on lipids and haemostatic factors. *BMJ* 319 (7224):1523–1528. doi: 10.1136/bmj.319.7224.1523.

Rizos, E. C., E. E. Ntzani, E. Bika, M. S. Kostapanos, and M. S. Elisaf. 2012. Association between omega-3 fatty acid supplementation and risk of major cardiovascular disease events: A systematic review and meta-analysis. *JAMA* 308 (10):1024–1033. doi: 10.1001/2012.jama.11374.

Rodriguez de Sotillo, D. V., M. Hadley, and J. E. Sotillo. 2006. Insulin receptor exon 11+/– is expressed in Zucker (fa/fa) rats, and chlorogenic acid modifies their plasma insulin and liver protein and DNA. *J Nutr Biochem* 17 (1):63–71. doi: 10.1016/j.jnutbio.2005.06.004.

Rohrmann, S., K. Overvad, H. B. Bueno-de-Mesquita, M. U. Jakobsen, R. Egeberg, A. Tjønneland, L. Nailler et al. 2013. Meat consumption and mortality—Results from the European Prospective Investigation into Cancer and Nutrition. *BMC Med* 11:63. doi: 10.1186/1741-7015-11-63.

Rong, Y., L. Chen, T. Zhu, Y. Song, M. Yu, Z. Shan, A. Sands, F. B. Hu, and L. Liu. 2013. Egg consumption and risk of coronary heart disease and stroke: Dose-response meta-analysis of prospective cohort studies. *BMJ* 346:e8539. doi: 10.1136/bmj.e8539.

Ronksley, P. E., S. E. Brien, B. J. Turner, K. J. Mukamal, and W. A. Ghali. 2011. Association of alcohol consumption with selected cardiovascular disease outcomes: A systematic review and meta-analysis. *BMJ* 342:d671. doi: 10.1136/bmj.d671.

Ros, E. 2009. Nuts and novel biomarkers of cardiovascular disease. *Am J Clin Nutr* 89 (5):1649s–1656s. doi: 10.3945/ajcn.2009.26736R.

Ros, E. 2010. Health benefits of nut consumption. *Nutrients* 2 (7):652–682. doi: 10.3390/nu2070652.

Sabate, J., K. Oda, and E. Ros. 2010. Nut consumption and blood lipid levels: A pooled analysis of 25 intervention trials. *Arch Intern Med* 170 (9):821–827. doi: 10.1001/archinternmed.2010.79.

Salazar-Martinez, E., W. C. Willett, A. Ascherio, J. E. Manson, M. F. Leitzmann, M. J. Stampfer, and F. B. Hu. 2004. Coffee consumption and risk for type 2 diabetes mellitus. *Ann Intern Med* 140 (1):1–8.

Salmerón, J., F. B. Hu, J. E. Manson, M. J. Stampfer, G. A. Colditz, E. B. Rimm, and W. C. Willett. 2001. Dietary fat intake and risk of type 2 diabetes in women. *Am J Clin Nutr* 73 (6):1019–1026.

Satija, A., E. Yu, W. C. Willett, and F. B. Hu. 2015. Understanding nutritional epidemiology and its role in policy. *Adv Nutr Int Rev J* 6 (1):5–18. doi: 10.3945/an.114.007492.

Schrieks, I. C., A. L. J. Heil, H. F. J. Hendriks, K. J. Mukamal, and J. W. J. Beulens. 2015. The effect of alcohol consumption on insulin sensitivity and glycemic status: A systematic review and meta-analysis of intervention studies. *Diabetes Care* 38 (4):723–732. doi: 10.2337/dc14-1556.

Schulze, M. B., J. E. Manson, D. S. Ludwig, G. A. Colditz, M. J. Stampfer, W. C. Willett, and F. B. Hu. 2004. Sugar-sweetened beverages, weight gain, and incidence of type 2 diabetes in young and middle-aged women. *JAMA* 292 (8):927–934. doi: 10.1001/jama.292.8.927.

Shearer, J., A. Farah, T. de Paulis, D. P. Bracy, R. R. Pencek, T. E. Graham, and D. H. Wasserman. 2003. Quinides of roasted coffee enhance insulin action in conscious rats. *J Nutr* 133 (11):3529–3532.

Shin, J. Y., P. Xun, Y. Nakamura, and K. He. 2013. Egg consumption in relation to risk of cardiovascular disease and diabetes: A systematic review and meta-analysis. *Am J Clin Nutr* 98 (1):146–159. doi: 10.3945/ajcn.112.051318.

Siscovick, D. S., T. E. Raghunathan, I. King, S. Weinmann, K. G. Wicklund, J. Albright, V. Bovbjerg et al. 1995. Dietary intake and cell membrane levels of long-chain n-3 polyunsaturated fatty acids and the risk of primary cardiac arrest. *JAMA* 274 (17):1363–1367.

Skeaff, C. M. and J. Miller. 2009. Dietary fat and coronary heart disease: Summary of evidence from prospective cohort and randomised controlled trials. *Ann Nutr Metab* 55 (1–3):173–201. doi: 10.1159/000229002.

Slavin, J. L. 2000. Whole grains, refined grains and fortified refined grains: What's the difference? *Asia Pac J Clin Nutr* 9 (S1):S23–S27. doi: 10.1046/j.1440-6047.2000.00171.x.

Soedamah-Muthu, S. S., E. L. Ding, W. K. Al-Delaimy, F. B. Hu, M. F. Engberink, W. C. Willett, and J. M. Geleijnse. 2011. Milk and dairy consumption and incidence of cardiovascular diseases and all-cause mortality: Dose-response meta-analysis of prospective cohort studies. *Am J Clin Nutr* 93 (1):158–171. doi: 10.3945/ajcn.2010.29866.

Sofi, F., A. A. Conti, A. M. Gori, M. L. E. Luisi, A. Casini, R. Abbate, and G. F. Gensini. 2006. Coffee consumption and risk of coronary heart disease: A meta-analysis. *Nutr Metab Cardiovasc Dis* 17 (3):209–223. doi: 10.1016/j.numecd.2006.07.013.

Song, Y., J. E. Manson, J. E. Buring, H. D. Sesso, and S. Liu. 2005. Associations of dietary flavonoids with risk of type 2 diabetes, and markers of insulin resistance and systemic inflammation in women: A prospective study and cross-sectional analysis. *J Am Coll Nutr* 24 (5):376–384.

St-Onge, M.-P., E. R. Farnworth, and P. J. H. Jones. 2000. Consumption of fermented and nonfermented dairy products: Effects on cholesterol concentrations and metabolism. *Am J Clin Nutr* 71 (3):674–681.

Stampfer, M. J., R. M. Krauss, J. Ma, P. J. Blanche, L. G. Holl, F. M. Sacks, and C. H. Hennekens. 1996. A prospective study of triglyceride level, low-density lipoprotein particle diameter, and risk of myocardial infarction. *JAMA* 276 (11):882–888.

Stampfer, M. J., F. M. Sacks, S. Salvini, W. C. Willett, and C. H. Hennekens. 1991. A prospective study of cholesterol, apolipoproteins, and the risk of myocardial infarction. *N Engl J Med* 325 (6):373–381. doi: 10.1056/nejm199108083250601.

Stanhope, K. L., J. M. Schwarz, N. L. Keim, S. C. Griffen, A. A. Bremer, J. L. Graham, B. Hatcher et al. 2009. Consuming fructose-sweetened, not glucose-sweetened, beverages increases visceral adiposity and lipids and decreases insulin sensitivity in overweight/obese humans. *J Clin Invest* 119 (5):1322–1334. doi: 10.1172/JCI37385.

Steinmetz, K. A., M. T. Childs, C. Stimson, L. H. Kushi, P. G. McGovern, J. D. Potter, and W. K. Yamanaka. 1994. Effect of consumption of whole milk and skim milk on blood lipid profiles in healthy men. *Am J Clin Nutr* 59 (3):612–618.

Storelli, M. M. 2008. Potential human health risks from metals (Hg, Cd, and Pb) and polychlorinated biphenyls (PCBs) via seafood consumption: Estimation of target hazard quotients (THQs) and toxic equivalents (TEQs). *Food Chem Toxicol* 46 (8):2782–2788. doi: http://dx.doi.org/10.1016/j.fct.2008.05.011.

Subar, A. F., F. E. Thompson, V. Kipnis, D. Midthune, P. Hurwitz, S. McNutt, A. McIntosh, and S. Rosenfeld. 2001. Comparative validation of the Block, Willett, and National Cancer Institute food frequency questionnaires: The Eating at America's Table Study. *Am J Epidemiol* 154 (12):1089–1099.

Tannock, L. R., K. D. O'Brien, R. H. Knopp, B. Retzlaff, B. Fish, M. H. Wener, S. E. Kahn, and A. Chait. 2005. Cholesterol feeding increases C-reactive protein and serum amyloid A levels in lean insulin-sensitive subjects. *Circulation* 111 (23):3058–3062. doi: 10.1161/circulationaha.104.506188.

Threapleton, D. E., D. C. Greenwood, C. E. Evans, C. L. Cleghorn, C. Nykjaer, C. Woodhead, J. E. Cade, C. P. Gale, and V. J. Burley. 2013. Dietary fibre intake and risk of cardiovascular disease: Systematic review and meta-analysis. *BMJ* 347:f6879. doi: 10.1136/bmj.f6879.

Tremblay, A. and J. A. Gilbert. 2009. Milk products, insulin resistance syndrome and type 2 diabetes. *J Am Coll Nutr* 28 (Suppl 1):91s–102s.

U.S. Department of Agriculture. 1980. Dietary guidelines for Americans. Accessed January 13, 2017. Available from https://health.gov/dietaryguidelines/1980thin.pdf.

U.S. Department of Agriculture. 2015. USDA National Nutrient Database for Standard Reference, Release 28. Version current: September 2015. Accessed January 13, 2016. Available from http://www.ars.usda.gov/nea/bhnrc/ndl.

U.S. Department of Health and Human Services and U.S. Department of Agriculture. 2015. 2015–2020 Dietary guidelines for Americans. (8) 2015 [cited 1/12/16 2015]. Accessed 13 Jan 2016. Available from http://health.gov/dietaryguidelines/2015/guidelines/.

van Dam, R. M. and E. J. Feskens. 2002. Coffee consumption and risk of type 2 diabetes mellitus. *Lancet* 360 (9344):1477–1478. doi: 10.1016/s0140-6736(02)11436-x.

van Dam, R. M., W. J. Pasman, and P. Verhoef. 2004. Effects of coffee consumption on fasting blood glucose and insulin concentrations: Randomized controlled trials in healthy volunteers. *Diabetes Care* 27 (12):2990–2992.

van Dam, R. M., W. C. Willett, J. E. Manson, and F. B. Hu. 2006. Coffee, caffeine, and risk of type 2 diabetes: A prospective cohort study in younger and middle-aged U.S. women. *Diabetes Care* 29 (2):398–403. doi: 10.2337/diacare.29.02.06.dc05-1512.

van den Brandt, P. A. and L. J. Schouten. 2015. Relationship of tree nut, peanut and peanut butter intake with total and cause-specific mortality: A cohort study and meta-analysis. *Int J Epidemiol* 44(3):1038–1049. doi: 10.1093/ije/dyv039.

van Dijk, A. E., M. R. Olthof, J. C. Meeuse, E. Seebus, R. J. Heine, and R. M. van Dam. 2009. Acute effects of decaffeinated coffee and the major coffee components chlorogenic acid and rrigonelline on glucose tolerance. *Diabetes Care* 32 (6):1023–1025. doi: 10.2337/dc09-0207.

Van Duyn, M. A. and E. Pivonka. 2000. Overview of the health benefits of fruit and vegetable consumption for the dietetics professional: Selected literature. *J Am Diet Assoc* 100 (12):1511–1521. doi: 10.1016/s0002-8223(00)00420-x.

Vartanian, L. R., M. B. Schwartz, and K. D. Brownell. 2007. Effects of soft drink consumption on nutrition and health: A systematic review and meta-analysis. *Am J Public Health* 97 (4):667–675. doi: 10.2105/ajph.2005.083782.

Vorster, H. H., A. J. Benade, H. C. Barnard, M. M. Locke, N. Silvis, C. S. Venter, C. M. Smuts, G. P. Engelbrecht, and M. P. Marais. 1992. Egg intake does not change plasma lipoprotein and coagulation profiles. *Am J Clin Nutr* 55 (2):400–410.

Wagener, F. A., A. Eggert, O. C. Boerman, W. J. Oyen, A. Verhofstad, N. G. Abraham, G. Adema, Y. van Kooyk, T. de Witte, and C. G. Figdor. 2001. Heme is a potent inducer of inflammation in mice and is counteracted by heme oxygenase. *Blood* 98 (6):1802–1811. doi: 10.1182/blood.V98.6.1802.

Wang, X., Y. Ouyang, J. Liu, M. Zhu, G. Zhao, W. Bao, and F. B. Hu. 2014. Fruit and vegetable consumption and mortality from all causes, cardiovascular disease, and cancer: Systematic review and dose-response meta-analysis of prospective cohort studies. *BMJ* 349:g4490. doi: 10.1136/bmj.g4490.

Wedick, N. M., A. M. Brennan, Q. Sun, F. B. Hu, C. S. Mantzoros, and R. M. van Dam. 2011. Effects of caffeinated and decaffeinated coffee on biological risk factors for type 2 diabetes: A randomized controlled trial. *Nutr J* 10 (1):1–9. doi: 10.1186/1475-2891-10-93.

Weickert, M. O. and A. F. H. Pfeiffer. 2008. Metabolic effects of dietary fiber consumption and prevention of diabetes. *J Nutr* 138 (3):439–442.

Welch, A. A., S. A. Bingham, J. Ive, M. D. Friesen, N. J. Wareham, E. Riboli, and K. T. Khaw. 2006. Dietary fish intake and plasma phospholipid n–3 polyunsaturated fatty acid concentrations in men and women in the European Prospective Investigation into Cancer–Norfolk United Kingdom cohort. *Am J Clin Nutr* 84 (6):1330–1339.

Welsh, J. A., A. J. Sharma, L. Grellinger, and M. B. Vos. 2011. Consumption of added sugars is decreasing in the United States. *Am J Clin Nutr* 94 (3):726–734. doi: 10.3945/ajcn.111.018366.

Whelton, S. P., J. He, P. K. Whelton, and P. Muntner. 2004. Meta-analysis of observational studies on fish intake and coronary heart disease. *Am J Cardiol* 93 (9):1119–1123. doi: 10.1016/j.amjcard.2004.01.038.

Whitehead, A., E. J. Beck, S. Tosh, and T. M. Wolever. 2014. Cholesterol-lowering effects of oat beta-glucan: A meta-analysis of randomized controlled trials. *Am J Clin Nutr* 100 (6):1413–1421. doi: 10.3945/ajcn.114.086108.

Willett, W., J. Manson, and S. Liu. 2002. Glycemic index, glycemic load, and risk of type 2 diabetes. *Am J Clin Nutr* 76 (1):274S–280S.

Wright, J. D., L. G. Borrud, M. A. McDowell, C. Y. Wang, K. Radimer, and C. L. Johnson. 2007. Nutrition assessment in the National Health and Nutrition Examination Survey 1999–2002. *J Am Diet Assoc* 107 (5):822–829. doi: 10.1016/j.jada.2007.02.017.

Wu, Y., Y. Qian, Y. Pan, P. Li, J. Yang, X. Ye, and G. Xu. 2015. Association between dietary fiber intake and risk of coronary heart disease: A meta-analysis. *Clin Nutr* 34 (4):603–611.

Xi, B., Y. Huang, K. H. Reilly, S. Li, R. Zheng, M. T. Barrio-Lopez, M. A. Martinez-Gonzalez, and D. Zhou. 2015. Sugar-sweetened beverages and risk of hypertension and CVD: A dose-response meta-analysis. *Br J Nutr* 113 (5):709–717. doi: 10.1017/s0007114514004383.

Xun, P. and K. He. 2012. Fish consumption and incidence of diabetes: Meta-analysis of data from 438,000 individuals in 12 independent prospective cohorts with an average 11-year follow-up. *Diabetes Care* 35 (4):930–938. doi: 10.2337/dc11-1869.

Yao, B., H. Fang, W. Xu, Y. Yan, H. Xu, Y. Liu, M. Mo, H. Zhang, and Y. Zhao. 2014. Dietary fiber intake and risk of type 2 diabetes: A dose-response analysis of prospective studies. *Eur J Epidemiol* 29 (2):79–88. doi: 10.1007/s10654-013-9876-x.

Ye, E. Q., S. A. Chacko, E. L. Chou, M. Kugizaki, and S. Liu. 2012. Greater whole-grain intake is associated with lower risk of type 2 diabetes, cardiovascular disease, and weight gain. *J Nutr* 142 (7):1304–1313. doi: 10.3945/jn.111.155325.

Ye, Y., J. Li, and Z. Yuan. 2013. Effect of antioxidant vitamin supplementation on cardiovascular outcomes: A meta-analysis of randomized controlled trials. *PLoS One* 8 (2):e56803. doi: 10.1371/journal.pone.0056803.

Yokoyama, Y., N. D. Barnard, S. M. Levin, and M. Watanabe. 2014a. Vegetarian diets and glycemic control in diabetes: A systematic review and meta-analysis. *Cardiovasc Diagn Ther* 4 (5):373–382.

Yokoyama, Y., K. Nishimura, N. D. Barnard, M. Takegami, M. Watanabe, A. Sekikawa, T. Okamura et al. 2014b. Vegetarian diets and blood pressure: A meta-analysis. *JAMA Intern Med* 174 (4):577–587. doi: 10.1001/jamainternmed.2013.14547.

Zhou, D., H. Yu, F. He, K. H. Reilly, J. Zhang, S. Li, T. Zhang, B. Wang, Y. Ding, and B. Xi. 2014. Nut consumption in relation to cardiovascular disease risk and type 2 diabetes: A systematic review and meta-analysis of prospective studies. *Am J Clin Nutr* 100 (1):270–277. doi: 10.3945/ajcn.113.079152.

21 Dietary Patterns and Cardiometabolic Disease

Elizabeth M. Cespedes Feliciano and Frank B. Hu

CONTENTS

ABSTRACT

Appropriate dietary recommendations are essential to the prevention and management of cardiovascular disease. Dietary patterns attempt to encompass the synergistic and cumulative effects of the whole diet and, as such, may be more easily translated into guidelines for healthful nutrition than knowledge of the disease associations of single foods or nutrients. In this chapter, we describe the methodology used to study dietary patterns, synthesize the evidence for the most commonly studied dietary patterns and cardiovascular health, and describe the emerging role of dietary patterns in national nutrition policy. The benefits of a Mediterranean dietary pattern characterized by the abundant consumption of olive oil, fruits, and vegetables and moderate consumption of fish, dairy, and alcohol and low intake of red and processed meats are among the best studied, strongest, and the most consistent. While the Mediterranean diet is the only dietary pattern to have been tested in a large, randomized controlled trial for the primary prevention of cardiovascular endpoints, there are other patterns, such as the Dietary Approaches to Stop Hypertension (DASH), whose effects on cardiovascular disease risk factors such as blood pressure, blood lipids, and glycemic control have been rigorously tested and show compelling benefits. Across healthful dietary patterns, there are common elements that likely drive their protective associations with cardiovascular disease, including an emphasis on plant foods including fruits, vegetables, and whole grains. Often, fish is a signature component, while red and processed meat and added sugar are limited and nuts, legumes, and moderate alcohol consumption are considered beneficial. In sum, the study of dietary patterns provides a complementary evidence base to the study of individual foods and nutrients and has great potential for informing nutrition policy to reduce cardiovascular disease risk.

INTRODUCTION

Identifying the optimal diet (or diets) for the prevention of cardiometabolic diseases is a public health priority. While traditional nutrition research in cardiovascular health has focused on single nutrients or specific foods as exposures, there are limitations to this classical approach to nutritional epidemiology: foods and nutrients are often highly correlated and may have cumulative, synergistic, or antagonistic effects. Dietary pattern analysis offers a complementary approach by describing the overall diet: the foods, food groups, and nutrients included in the pattern; their combination and variety; and the frequency and quantity with which they are habitually consumed (Hu 2002). Further, the overall quality of the diet may have a stronger relationship with cardiovascular outcomes than do individual foods or nutrients. This makes dietary pattern analysis a potentially useful tool to detect effects in the context of measurement error and misclassification, which reduce a study's statistical power (Willett 2012). Dietary pattern analysis can also provide a summary measure of diet quality with which to control for potential confounding by diet when studying the relationship of other exposures (e.g., physical activity or individual dietary components) to cardiovascular risk. From the perspective of national guidelines, recommendations based on a composite measure of diet quality may be most applicable: individuals consume foods in combination, and when intake is manipulated, there are important substitution effects best captured by examining the entirety of the diet. As methods have been refined and standardized, recent dietary guidelines in the United States (United States Department of Agriculture 2015a) and other countries (United Kingdom Department of Health 1994) have shifted toward advice based on dietary patterns.

This chapter describes prominent methods for assessing dietary patterns, current evidence on the role of major dietary patterns for the primary prevention and management of cardiometabolic diseases and major cardiovascular risk factors in adult populations, implications, and future directions for research.

DIETARY PATTERNS METHODOLOGY

The most prominent statistical methods to assess dietary patterns can be divided into *a posteriori* and *a priori* approaches, as shown in Figure 21.1.

A posteriori methods take nutritional data (typically semiquantitative food frequency questionnaires or diet records) and apply multivariable statistical techniques to empirically identify correlated groups of foods. Principal components analysis identifies nonexclusive *factors* to explain variation among food items based on intercorrelations, whereas cluster analysis groups individuals into mutually

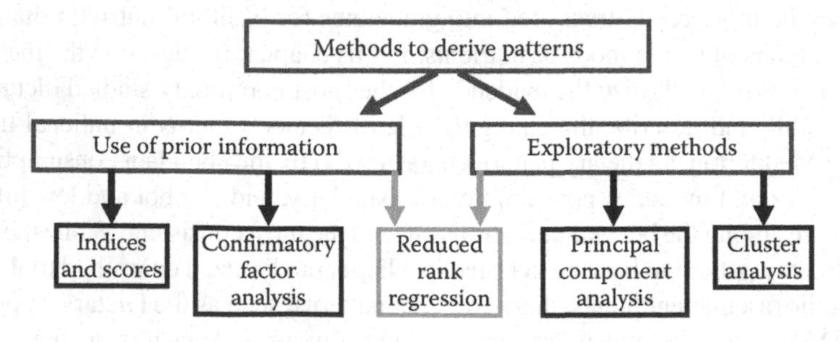

FIGURE 21.1 Major approaches to dietary patterns analysis (Jackson and Hu 2014, Horton 2005). (Adapted from Schulze, M.B. and Hoffmann, K., *Br. J. Nutr.*, 95(5), 860, 2006; Hu, F., *Obesity Epidemiology*, New York, Oxford University Press, 2008.)

exclusive *clusters* based on differences in mean intakes (Newby and Tucker 2004). In both of these *outcome-independent* techniques, foods and nutrients are typically grouped into a smaller number of input variables (e.g., food groups, quantified by frequency of consumption, weight, or contribution to daily energy) before patterns are derived. Reduced rank regression is another type of *a posteriori* technique but is *outcome dependent*: it incorporates scientific knowledge by deriving patterns that explain the largest variation in intermediate outcomes such as biomarkers or nutrients previously known to be associated with disease (Hoffmann et al. 2004). Often, patterns derived via reduced rank regression are more strongly associated with cardiovascular disease (CVD) endpoints than those obtained from *outcome-independent* techniques. Regardless of the method of derivation, *a posteriori* patterns are often grouped into two broad categories: *healthy/prudent* and *unhealthy/Western*. The most common characteristics of these two categories of empirical dietary patterns are described in Table 21.1.

Importantly, dietary patterns defined using *a posteriori* techniques are empirically derived and thus may not represent optimal diets based on scientific evidence for chronic disease prevention. One alternative to describe a dietary pattern consistent with the current knowledge on dietary risk factors and/or on current dietary recommendations is to use an *a priori* approach such as numerical indices, which measure adherence to predefined diets. As is the case for *a posteriori* methods, the dietary input variables for *a priori* methods are typically assessed through self-reported intake on a food frequency questionnaire, diet record, or 24-hour recall. Food and nutrient intakes recorded through these instruments are then used to characterize the overall diet. One approach to quantifying dietary patterns is to define the pattern based on individual preference or behavior or on excluded foods; lacto-ovo-vegetarianism is a prominent example. However, the most common *a priori* approach is to create numerical indices that describe the degree to which an individual's habitual intake represents the predefined dietary pattern in question. Table 21.2 lists the most

TABLE 21.1
Major *A Posteriori* Dietary Patterns: Constituents and Scoring Criteria

Dietary Pattern	Constituents Emphasized	Scoring Criteria[a]
A posteriori	*A posteriori* patterns describe clusters of foods and nutrients commonly eaten together identified through statistical methods (factor analysis, utilizing intercorrelations between dietary items, or cluster analysis that is based on individual differences in mean intakes).	For factor analysis, input variables are typically entered into principal components analysis using varimax (orthogonal) rotation and eigenvalues (which indicate that the factor explains more of the variance in the correlations than is explained by a single variable). Often, factor scores are categorized for further analysis. The number of factors that are derived ranges substantially depending on the analysis from just a few to dozens. The percent variance explained by the factors may also range.
Prudent	• Fruit • Vegetables • Legumes • Fish • Whole grains • Poultry	A pattern with high-factor loadings for several healthy foods, including fruit, vegetables, legumes, and fish, is typically called *prudent*. Individuals receive a score that defines the position of each individual along a gradient for each derived pattern.
Western	• Red and processed meats • Eggs • Refined grains • Sweets/sweetened beverages • Fried foods	Pattern with high-factor loadings for red and processed meats, eggs, refined grains, and sugar is typically called *Western*.

[a] For both *a posteriori* and *a priori* methods, the primary dietary assessment method may be a 24-hour recall or diet record, though food frequency questionnaires are used most often in prospective cohort studies. In both cases, different dietary input variables may be quantified differently, for example, by frequency (servings), weight (grams), or daily percent energy contribution and are at times adjusted for total energy intake.

TABLE 21.2
Scoring Criteria for Major Diet Quality Indices with Sample Population Intakes[a]

	HEI-2010 (Guenther et al. 2013) 0–100 Points 12 Components, Each 5–20 Points				AHEI-2010 (Chiuve et al. 2012) 0–110 Points 11 Components, Each 10 Points				DASH (Fung et al. 2008) 8–40 Points 8 Components, Each 5 Points				aMED (Fung et al. 2009) 0–9 Points 9 Components, Each 1 Point			
Criteria and Score	Min		Max		Min		Max		Min		Max		Min		Max	
Fruit	0 cups	0	≥0.8 cup total fruit; ≥0.4 cup whole fruit/1000 kcal	5	0 cups	0	≥4 servings/day excluding juices	10	Low quintile 0.46 cups	1	High quintile 3 cups	5	<Median	0	>Median	1
Vegetables	0 cups	0	≥1.1 cup total; ≥0.2 cup greens/beans	5	0 cups	0	≥5 servings/day	10	Low quintile 0.44 cups	1	High quintile 2 cups	5	<Median	0	>Median 1 cup/day	1
Dairy	0 cups	0	≥1.3 cup/1000 kcal, includes high fat	10		0		10	Low quintile 0.09 cups	1	High quintile 3 cups	5				
Nuts and legumes			Allocated to total or plant proteins or vegetables		0 serving/day	0	≥1 servings/day	10	High quintile 0.09 oz	1	Low quintile 2 oz	5	<Median	0	>Median 0.25 cups/day legumes, 0.15 oz/day nuts	1
Fish	0 oz	0	≥0.8 oz/1000 kcal (seafood/plant proteins)										<Median	0	>Median 0.45 oz/day	1
Oils/fats			Ratio (PUFA + MUFA):SFA		>4% trans; 0 mg EPA + DHA; <2% PUFA	0	≤0.5% trans; 250 mg EPA + DHA; ≥10% PUFA	10					<Median	0	>Median ratio MUFA:SFA 1.14	1
Total protein foods	0 oz	0	>2.5 oz/1000 kcal	10												
Whole grains	0 oz	0	>1.5 oz/1000 kcal	10	0 g/day	0	75 (women) or 90 (men) g/day	10	Low quintile 0.22 oz	1	High quintile 3 oz	5	<Median	0	>Median 1 oz/day	1

(Continued)

TABLE 21.2 (*Continued*)
Scoring Criteria for Major Diet Quality Indices with Sample Population Intakes[a]

	HEI-2010 (Guenther et al. 2013) 0–100 Points 12 Components, Each 5–20 Points				AHEI-2010 (Chiuve et al. 2012) 0–110 Points 11 Components, Each 10 Points				DASH (Fung et al. 2008) 8–40 Points 8 Components, Each 5 Points				aMED (Fung et al. 2009) 0–9 Points 9 Components, Each 1 Point			
Criteria and Score	**Min**		**Max**		**Min**		**Max**		**Min**		**Max**		**Min**		**Max**	
Refined grains	≥4.3 oz	0	≤1.8 oz/1000 kcal	10												
Sugar-sweetened beverages					>1 servings including juice	0	0 serving	10	High quintile 1 serving/day	1	Low quintile 0 serving/day	5				
Red and processed meats					≥1.5 serving/day	0	0 oz	10	High quintile 0.34 oz	1	Low quintile 4 oz	5	>Median	0	<Median 1 oz/day	1
Sodium	≥2.0 g	0	≤1.1 g per 1000 kcal	10	High decile mg/day	0	Low decile mg/day	10	High quintile 1382 mg	1	Low quintile 4314 mg	5				
Empty calories	≥50% kcal	0	≤19% kcal from solid fat, added sugars, alcohol													
Alcohol			>2 drinks/day toward empty kcal		≥2.5 (women) or ≥3.5 (men) drinks/day; nondrinker 2.5 pts	0	0.5–1.5 (women) or 2 (men) drinks/day	10					<5 or >15 g	0	5–15 g	1

[a] Adapted from Cespedes et al. (2016) and George et al. (2014), with sample intakes from Cespedes et al. (2016) analysis of multiple dietary patterns and diabetes risk in the Women's Health Initiative.

common components and scoring criteria for the major numerical indices. Adherence to the dietary pattern is represented in a summary score based on assigning points for the consumption of component foods and nutrients in predefined relative or absolute quantities. Often, multiple indices describe variations of the same dietary pattern, for example, multiple indices describe adherence to a Mediterranean-style dietary pattern, with two of the most prominent being the Mediterranean Diet Score (MDS) (Trichopoulou et al. 2003) and the Alternate Mediterranean Diet Score (aMED) (Fung et al. 2009). Different numerical indices also use different scoring and weighting schemes. For example, some use population-specific intakes (e.g., Dietary Approaches to Stop Hypertension [DASH] (Fung et al. 2008) scores individuals based on quintiles of intake for the population studied) versus fixed cutoffs for recommended intakes (e.g., Alternate Healthy Eating Index [AHEI] (Chiuve et al. 2012) scores individuals primarily on the servings/day of particular foods or nutrient groups). These differences in scoring criteria make synthesizing evidence across studies a challenge. Dietary patterns methodology continues to evolve to address these limitations, with recent efforts to standardize numerical dietary quality indices across various population-based cohorts (Liese et al. 2015).

MAJOR STUDY DESIGNS

In addition to multiple approaches to quantifying dietary patterns, there are multiple study designs, from the ecologic to the prospective cohort to the randomized controlled trial, for testing their associations with disease. While observational studies of dietary patterns and health outcomes are often cost effective and allow for wider exposure ranges and longer follow-up in which clinical endpoints can be observed, testing the efficacy of dietary patterns through randomized controlled trials of intermediate endpoints provides a complementary evidence base. One such approach is controlled feeding trials, in which all food is provided to participants over the course of weeks or months. These studies allow the researcher to precisely define the dietary exposures tested. Prominent examples include the evaluation of the effects of the DASH diet with and without sodium reduction on blood pressure lowering (Appel et al. 1997, Sacks et al. 2001); the benefits of DASH for CVD outcomes were later affirmed in large cohort studies showing that adherence to the DASH-style diet decreased the risk of CVD, coronary heart disease, stroke, and heart failure by 20%, 21%, 19%, and 29%, respectively (Salehi-Abargouei et al. 2013). Long-term randomized trials of dietary pattern interventions on hard endpoints are rare due to prohibitive cost and lack of dietary compliance in the long run, though there are important exceptions (e.g., the Prevención con Dieta Mediterránea [PREDIMED] trial) (Estruch et al. 2013).

Table 21.3 presents pooled relative risk (RR) estimates drawn from meta-analyses comparing the highest to lowest categories of adherence to major *a priori* and *a posteriori* dietary patterns. In the case of Mediterranean-style diets, the evidence base is particularly strong: meta-analyses of prospective cohort studies are accompanied with published results of a randomized controlled trial of clinical endpoints. For the *a posteriori* patterns, not only are there no interventions testing the influence of these diets on clinical outcomes, findings from prospective cohort studies have yielded inconsistent or null results, and, as indicated by the blanks in the table, there are some clinical outcomes for which no existing meta-analysis of the dietary pattern could be found. The subsequent section of the chapter describes in greater detail the current state of knowledge for each of the dietary patterns.

MEDITERRANEAN DIET

Research on the role of the Mediterranean diet for the primary prevention of CVD began to take off after the Seven Countries Study in the 1960s (Keys 1970), which observed exceptional longevity among populations living along the shores of the Mediterranean. The lower incidence of CVD was hypothesized to be due in part to the traditional dietary pattern characterized by olive oil as a primary culinary fat; abundant plant-based foods; moderate consumption of fish, dairy, and alcohol with

TABLE 21.3
Relationship of Major Dietary Patterns to Cardiovascular Disease and Cardiovascular Risk Factors

	Relative Risk (95% Confidence Interval)			
Dietary Pattern	**CVD**	**CHD**	**Stroke**	**T2D**
A posteriori				
Prudent	0.69 (0.60–0.78)[a]	0.83 (0.75–0.92)[a]	0.86 (0.74–1.01)[a]	0.85 (0.80–0.91)[b]
Western	1.14 (0.92–1.42)[a]	1.03 (0.90–1.17)[a]	1.05 (0.91–2.22)[a]	1.41 (1.32–1.52)[b]
A priori				
Mediterranean	0.90 (0.87–0.92)[c]	0.63 (0.53–0.72)[e]	0.71 (0.57–0.89)[f]	0.77 (0.66–0.89)[g]
	0.87 (0.87–0.90)[d]			
DASH	0.80 (0.74–0.86)[h]	0.79 (0.71–0.88)[h]	0.81 (0.72–0.92)[h]	0.79 (0.66–0.95)[i]
	0.80 (0.76–0.85)[h]			
AHEI-2010	0.74 (0.72–0.77)[i]			0.77 (0.68–0.86)[i]
HEI-2010	0.82 (0.79–0.85)[i]			0.82 (0.76–0.88)[i]

[a] Rodriguez-Monforte, Flores-Mateo, and Sanchez (2015).
[b] McEvoy et al. (2014).
[c] Includes CHD and stroke in composite "CVD" endpoint and reports result per 2-point increase in a Mediterranean diet adherence scores Sofi et al. (2014).
[d] Martinez-Gonzalez and Bes-Rastrollo (2014).
[e] Mente et al. (2009).
[f] Psaltopoulou et al. (2013).
[g] Koloverou et al. (2014).
[h] Salehi-Abargouei et al. (2013).
[i] Schwingshackl and Hoffmann (2015).

meals; and a comparatively low intake of red meat. Contemporary prospective cohort studies provide consistent evidence regarding the benefits of adherence to a Mediterranean-style diet for CVD prevention (notably, the findings for CVD prevention are more consistent than the results observed for CHD or for cerebrovascular disease individually) (D'Alessandro and De Pergola 2015). Of all of the dietary patterns described in this chapter, the Mediterranean diet has arguably the strongest evidence of causality since this dietary pattern has been tested in a large, randomized controlled trial for the primary prevention of CVD. Testing a dietary pattern through a randomized controlled trial is very rare due to the expense, difficulty, and length of follow-up required; thus, the PREDIMED trial (Estruch et al. 2013) represents a key advance that warrants description here.

Conducted in Spain among 7447 participants with CVD risk factors, PREDIMED compared advice to follow a low-fat diet (control) with advice to follow a Mediterranean-style diet (high in vegetables, fruits, legumes, fish, and poultry but low in red meats, sweets, and whole-fat dairy) along with the provision of either extra virgin olive oil (~1 L per week) or nuts (30 g/day; half walnuts and one-quarter each hazelnuts and almonds). It bears mention that a major criticism of the trial was the lack of a comparably intense intervention in the low-fat group, which did not achieve radical reductions in fat intake. Indeed, one reason that low-fat diets have not been effective for long-term CVD risk reduction may be the substitution of fat by refined carbohydrate, as well as the difficulty of adhering to such a diet in the long term without continued reinforcement (Howard et al. 2006). Despite these limitations, compared to the low-fat control group, both PREDIMED intervention groups experienced ~30% reductions in CVD events after a median 4.8 years of follow-up, and the data safety monitoring board stopped the trial early. While subgroup analyses of randomized trials must be interpreted with caution, those within the PREDIMED trial suggested a beneficial effect of the Mediterranean diet on multiple CVD endpoints and intermediate markers of risk. For example, there was a clear protective effect of a Mediterranean diet supplemented with olive oil on stroke compared to the low-fat control, but the protective effects for myocardial infarction (MI) and CVD death did not achieve statistical significance (Estruch et al. 2013). Building on this success, the PREDIMED research group has launched the "PREDIMED-Plus" trial, which will test the efficacy for the primary prevention of adding calorie restriction, an intensive lifestyle program with physical activity and behavioral therapy to achieve weight loss goals to the original PREDIMED diet (Corella et al. 2013). The results from the landmark PREDIMED trial, together with consistent observational evidence from prospective cohort studies (Martinez-Gonzalez and Bes-Rastrollo 2014) indicating that greater adherence to a Mediterranean-style diet (see Figure 21.2) is strongly associated with lower incidence of CVD, provide convincing evidence to support the health benefits of the Mediterranean diet for the primary prevention of CVD.

As mentioned earlier, in addition to robust evidence from randomized controlled trials, a large body of observational evidence has examined adherence to a Mediterranean diet with results that are generally consistent with findings from short- and long-term randomized trials (Estruch et al. 2013; Martinez-Gonzalez and Bes-Rastrollo 2014). One challenge in summarizing this evidence, however, is that more than a dozen scores describe adherence to a "Mediterranean-style diet" (D'Alessandro and De Pergola 2015). One of the most popular is an adaptation of the MDS (Trichopoulou et al. 2003) known as the aMED (Fung et al. 2009), which ranges from 0 (minimal adherence to the Mediterranean diet) to 9 (maximal adherence). Table 21.2 shows the components and scoring criteria for aMED in comparison with other major dietary pattern indices. For each of nine foods or

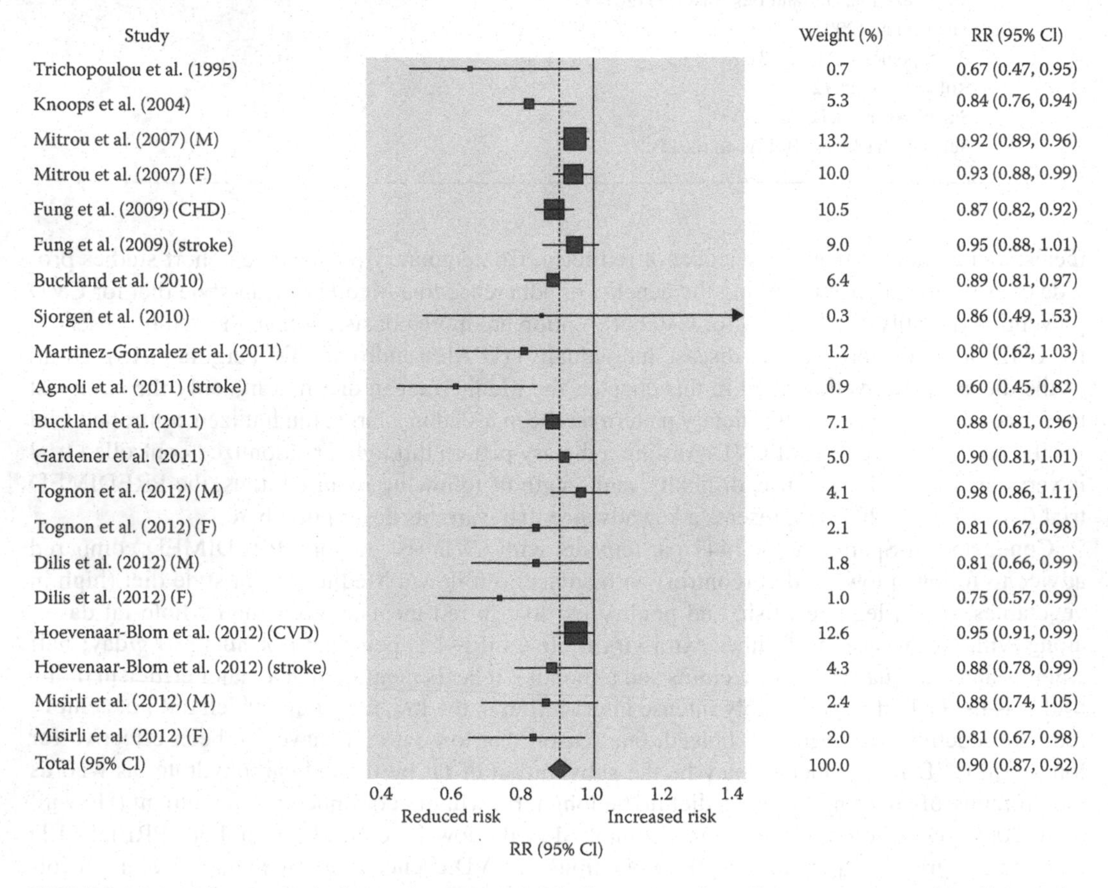

FIGURE 21.2 Meta-analysis forest plot of greater Mediterranean diet adherence scores and cardiovascular incidence and/or mortality risk. (From Sofi, F. et al., *Public Health Nutr.*, 17(12), 2769, December 2014.)

nutrients, the score assigns a value of 1 to beneficial components for which the individual studied consumes *above* the sex-specific median intake (vegetables, legumes, fruits and nuts, cereal, fish, ratio of monounsaturated to saturated fat) as well as detrimental components for which the individual consumption is *below* the sex-specific median (meat, poultry, and dairy products). The aMED is scored identically to the original MDS but includes dietary patterns and eating behaviors consistently associated with lower risks of chronic disease, for example, excluding potato products from the vegetable group, including only whole-grain products in the cereal category, and assigning a lower (15 g instead of 25 g) value to moderate alcohol intake. In the following summary of the Mediterranean diet's influence on major cardiometabolic risk factors, we summarize evidence from randomized controlled trials where available (primarily subgroup analyses of the PREDIMED trial) and rely on observational research utilizing *a priori* scores such as the aMED otherwise.

In addition to CVD endpoints, adherence to a Mediterranean-style dietary pattern has also been associated with a lower risk of metabolic syndrome and beneficial effects on components including waist circumference, high-density lipoprotein (HDL) cholesterol, triglycerides (TG), systolic and diastolic blood pressure, and blood glucose (Kastorini et al. 2011), as well as lower annual weight gain and lower risk of obesity, which have been reported in some but not all studies (Beunza et al. 2010, Romaguera et al. 2010). Importantly, though trials show benefits of a Mediterranean dietary pattern on both blood pressure and lipids as summarized earlier, there is very limited observational research examining benefits of Mediterranean-style diets on blood pressure (Nunez-Cordoba et al. 2009) and results for lipids have been inconsistent (Tortosa et al. 2007, Rumawas et al. 2009) suggesting that the level of adherence achieved through an intensive dietary intervention may be critical to achieving maximum CVD protection.

With regard to risk of type 2 diabetes (T2D), the trials leading up to PREDIMED as well as post hoc analyses of PREDIMED suggest a protective effect of Mediterranean diets supplemented with olive oil on the incidence of T2D (Salas-Salvadó et al. 2011, 2014) and glycemic control: compared to control (advice to follow a low-fat diet), the Mediterranean diet supplemented with extra virgin olive oil (RR 0.60, 95% confidence interval [CI] 0.43–0.85) and the Mediterranean diet supplemented with nuts (RR 0.82, 95% CI 0.61–1.10) reduced the risk for T2D (Salas-Salvadó et al. 2014). In observational research, most scores measuring a greater adherence to a Mediterranean-style diet have a protective association with T2D overall (Schwingshackl et al. 2015). However, in research examining multiethnic populations in the United States, results have been mixed, with some studies finding no association or disparate associations according to race/ethnicity (Abiemo et al. 2013, Jacobs et al. 2014, Cespedes et al. 2016). One potential reason for the weaker and at times null associations in diverse U.S. populations is that a major source of monounsaturated fat (a signature component of the Mediterranean diet) is meat, which also contains a large amount of saturated fat, possibly confounding the benefits of plant-source monounsaturated fats. To know whether translating the Mediterranean diet to additional cultural contexts or substituting key ingredients will provide the same benefit observed in the primarily European and European-descended populations examined to date will require randomized trials of CVD outcomes in diverse regions of the world.

With respect to maintaining a healthy body weight, a meta-analysis of Mediterranean diet trials found that while the dietary pattern was associated with lower weight overall (mean difference between Mediterranean diet and control diet, −1.75 kg [95% CI −2.86 to −0.64 kg]), this difference was stronger when combined with energy restriction or physical activity (Esposito et al. 2011). Notably, the Mediterranean diet was not significantly associated with weight gain in any of the studies examined despite the high-fat content of the diet: in PREDIMED the intervention resulted in a change in the type of fat rather than the quantity of fat consumed, as % energy from fat was >40% in both intervention arms at follow-up due to the supplementation with olive oil and mixed nuts. There are various suggested reasons for the lack of weight gain, including increased satiety (e.g., increased protein and dietary fiber in the case of nuts) and possibly reduced energy storage (e.g., unsaturated fats may increase oxidation) (Jackson and Hu 2014).

The PREDIMED trial reported clear benefits of the intervention on blood pressure (Estruch et al. 2006) and on HDL cholesterol (HDL-C), total-C/HDL-C ratio, and TG (Estruch et al. 2013). Similarly, a Cochrane meta-analysis of randomized trials of dietary interventions consistent with a Mediterranean dietary pattern noted overall reductions in total and low-density lipoprotein (LDL) cholesterol as well as blood pressure (Rees et al. 2013). With regard to inflammation, subanalyses of the PREDIMED trial (Urpi-Sarda et al. 2012) and further research from the same group (Esposito et al. 2004) suggest that a Mediterranean diet reduces circulating inflammatory markers such as high-sensitivity C-reactive protein (hs-CRP) and interleukin (IL)-6, which have been implicated in endothelial dysfunction and atherosclerosis.

Intervention trials of secondary prevention among participants with existing CVD are few; prominent examples include the Lyon Diet Heart Study (de Lorgeril et al. 1999) and the Indo-Mediterranean Diet Heart Study (Singh et al. 2002). Both compared a Mediterranean-style diet to a low-fat dietary pattern and reported benefits for CVD mortality but have been criticized: important concerns about data reliability were raised after the publication of the Indo-Mediterranean Diet Heart Study (Horton 2005), while the Lyon Diet Heart Study and PREDIMED were both stopped due to significant beneficial effects in interim analyses, which can exaggerate the magnitude of intervention effect, particularly in small trials (Guyatt et al. 2012).

It bears mention that the Women's Health Initiative observational study, an epidemiologic cohort, has examined additional CVD outcomes not investigated in trial settings (e.g., heart failure and sudden cardiac death). For example, in the Women's Health Initiative observational study, DASH scores were not associated with sudden cardiac death, while higher Mediterranean diet scores predicted lower sudden cardiac death risk (comparing highest to lowest quintile RR 0.64 [95% CI 0.43–0.94]) (Bertoia et al. 2014). For heart failure, results from Women's Health Initiative showed a (nonsignificant) trend toward a protective association with greater adherence to a Mediterranean-style diet (Levitan et al. 2013).

OTHER COMMONLY USED *A PRIORI* DIETARY PATTERNS

Often, major indices of diet quality are calculated and compared in the same study; for example, Fung et al. examined the association between change in diet quality indices and concurrent weight change in a large sample of male health professionals and female nurses and found that a one standard deviation increase in the aMed, AHEI-2010, and DASH adherence scores was associated with significantly less weight gain over 4-year periods in both men and women (Fung et al. 2015). Similarly, a recent meta-analysis found that diets of the highest quality, as assessed by the HEI, AHEI, and DASH score, reduced by 22% the risk of T2D (RR 0.78, 95% CI 0.72–0.85) and CVD incidence/mortality (RR 0.78, 95% CI 0.75–0.81) (Schwingshackl and Hoffmann 2015). These findings are consistent with the standardized analyses conducted by the Dietary Patterns Methods Project; while the highest scores (signifying higher diet quality) on each of the indices examined (aMed, HEI-2010, AHEI-2010, and DASH) were associated with marked reductions in mortality, the benefits were already evident at relatively lower levels of diet quality (Liese et al. 2015). This suggests that even incremental improvements in overall diet quality—achievable through a variety of dietary modifications—could lead to clinically relevant reductions in risk. The flexibility offered by a variety of healthful dietary patterns with a variety of components is an advantage in the sense that healthful eating may be tailored to individual preferences and culture; for example, an increase in the AHEI-2010 could be accomplished by eliminating sugar-sweetened beverages or by reducing the intake of red and processed meats to <2.5 oz/day. However, a limitation of these methods is the implication that an incremental improvement in diet quality, for example, ten points on the AHEI-2010, is associated with a similar reduction in CVD risk regardless of how it is accomplished. Thus, there is an inherent tension between describing the relationship of the entirety of the diet and disease and the individual relationships of specific food groups that make up the dietary pattern.

DASH DIET

As mentioned in the Introduction of this chapter, the DASH feeding trials (Sacks et al. 1995, Appel et al. 1997, Sacks et al. 2001) and the variations of DASH with different macronutrient compositions tested in the OmniHeart trial (Miller, Erlinger, and Appel 2006) are signature examples of randomized interventions testing the efficacy of a dietary pattern on CVD risk factors. The primary endpoint in these trials was blood pressure, though benefits were also observed for blood lipids. The original DASH intervention trials[12] provided all food to 459 participants with mild hypertension for 8 weeks. The diet provided was high in vegetables, fruits, low-fat dairy products, whole grains, poultry, fish, and nuts; low in sweets and sugar-sweetened beverages; and lower in red and processed meats. Further, the DASH dietary pattern is high in fiber, potassium, magnesium, calcium, and protein and low in sodium, saturated fat, total fat, and cholesterol. When compared to a dietary pattern high in saturated fat and sodium and low in vegetables and fruits, the DASH-style dietary pattern reduced blood pressure by approximately 6/3 mmHg (systolic blood pressure/diastolic blood pressure) across diverse age, sex, and race subgroups. Variations on the DASH diet also had marked benefits for key CVD risk factors: the DASH sodium trials observed a greater benefit with the combined intervention of sodium reduction plus the DASH diet than with either alone (Sacks et al. 2001). With respect to the variations of the DASH dietary pattern, the OmniCarb trial found no difference in CVD risk factors or insulin resistance comparing DASH diets with low and high glycemic index, suggesting that carbohydrate intake and not glycemic index was the primary drive of lipid profiles (Sacks et al. 2014). The OmniHeart trial (Miller, Erlinger, and Appel 2006) found favorable effects of the DASH diet on LDL-C and total-C, and total-C/HDL-C ratio regardless of macronutrient composition, with no appreciable effect on TG. Notably, the OmniHeart trial (Miller, Erlinger, and Appel 2006) found the greatest improvements in CVD risk factors when carbohydrate was partially replaced with monounsaturated fat or protein (Molitor et al. 2014). Overall, the DASH diet showed marked benefits for blood pressure and blood lipids across populations defined by sex, race/ethnicity, and hypertension status, with additional benefits when sodium was reduced or carbohydrate replaced with high-quality fat or protein. Most recently, replacement of low-fat with high-fat dairy was tested within the context of a DASH-like diet; the resulting higher intake of saturated fat and lower intake of sugar achieved equivalent reductions in blood pressure as the original DASH, and even greater reductions in plasma triglyceride and VLDL concentrations (Chiu et al. 2016).

While the DASH feeding trials provide robust evidence of the diet's benefit on CVD risk factors, these trials were short in follow-up and never intended to evaluate clinical endpoints such as CVD, CHD, stroke, and T2D; for this, we turn to prospective cohort studies that quantify adherence to a DASH-style diet in a score or index. While multiple scores exist to quantify adherence to a DASH-style dietary pattern, the most frequently used is the DASH score by Fung et al. (2008). The summary DASH score ranges from 8 (nonadherence) to 40 points (perfect adherence). Based on population-specific quintiles, individual DASH components are scored between 1 (worst) and 5 (best) with points awarded for higher intakes of eight food groups related to a lower risk of hypertension (one point per higher quintile of fruits, vegetables, dairy, nuts and legumes, and whole grains) and lower intakes of harmful foods (one point per lower quintile of sodium, red/processed meats, and sweetened beverages).

Overall, the observational evidence is consistent with the CVD protection expected based on the interventions' impact on key CVD risk factors. For example, a recent meta-analysis of prospective cohort studies observed a dose–response association between DASH-style diet adherence and overall CVD protection (Salehi-Abargouei et al. 2013). However, this is not without exception: despite the consistent benefits on blood pressure in feeding trials, when long-term benefits were examined in observational studies of community-dwelling populations, associations with higher scores on a DASH-style dietary pattern and reduced blood pressure were small in magnitude and no association was seen with incident hypertension, suggesting that consistent and strong adherence is a key factor (Folsom, Parker, and Harnack 2007, Camoes et al. 2010).

Cohort studies have also been useful in evaluating additional CVD endpoints and risk factors not examined in the DASH trials. For example, in the Swedish Mammography Cohort, a greater adherence to a DASH-style diet was associated with a lower risk of heart failure (Levitan, Wolk, and Mittleman 2009). Meanwhile, in the Cardiovascular Health Study, none of the dietary patterns examined (AHEI, DASH, and an American Heart Association 2020 dietary goals score) were associated with incident heart failure (Del Gobbo et al. 2015). Fung et al. found that, independent of CVD factors including body mass index, adherence to the DASH-style diet was associated with reduced CHD and stroke among middle-aged women during 24 years of follow-up, and in cross-sectional analysis in a subgroup of women, the DASH score was inversely associated with lower plasma levels of hs-CRP and IL-6, suggesting inflammation as a potential mechanism (Fung et al. 2008). A greater adherence to a DASH-style diet has also been associated with lower levels of inflammatory markers in other studies (Nowlin, Hammer, and D'Eramo Melkus 2012).

With respect to body fatness, a recent meta-analysis of four prospective studies estimated that the pooled RR comparing the highest DASH category to the lowest was 0.79 (95% CI 0.66–0.95) (Schwingshackl and Hoffmann 2015). Not all studies have found this association; for example, in the Multi-Ethnic Study of Atherosclerosis, higher DASH scores were associated with lesser gain in waist circumference but not with reduced risk of T2D (de Oliveira Otto et al. 2015). A recent meta-analysis of randomized controlled trials suggests that the DASH diet can significantly reduce fasting insulin (mean difference −0.15 (95% CI −0.22 to −0.08) but not fasting blood glucose or the homeostatic model assessment of insulin resistance (HOMA-IR) (Shirani, Salehi-Abargouei, and Azadbakht 2013). This echoes the conclusion of another systematic review that concluded that significant improvements in insulin sensitivity are observed only when adherence to a DASH-style dietary pattern is part of lifestyle modification including exercise and weight loss (Hinderliter et al. 2011).

HEALTHY EATING INDEX

The HEI was first developed to measure adherence to federal dietary guidelines in 1995 and later adapted to reflect the revisions to the guidelines every 5 years. Contemporary studies use the latest update and validation that reflects the 2010 Dietary Guidelines for Americans (Guenther et al. 2013, 2014), though the HEI will likely be updated to reflect the recently released 2015 Guidelines. The HEI-2010 has 12 components expressed in terms of nutrient density (with the idea of uncoupling nutrient quality from quantity), most weighted equally at 10 points. There are nine adequacy components (all receive a score of zero for zero intake, other than fatty acids, for which the 15th percentile of the 2001–2002 population distribution of one-day's intake is set as the minimum) and three moderation components (empty calories, sodium, and refined grains). For moderation components, intakes at the level of the standard or lower receive maximum points (for sodium, the maximum score is assigned to <1100 mg of sodium per 1000 calories). This score also includes beans and peas under protein foods when protein requirements are not otherwise met to enable healthy vegetarian dietary patterns to receive a perfect score. For additional components and scoring criteria, consult Table 21.2.

Few prospective studies have evaluated the relationship of HEI-2010 to CVD, CHD, stroke, diabetes, or CVD risk factors. The meta-analysis cited in Table 21.3 combined estimates from eight studies for the highest versus lowest categories of HEI scores from various years and reported a pooled RR of 0.82 (95% CI 0.76–0.89) for CVD incidence and mortality (Schwingshackl and Hoffmann 2015). While no other review or meta-analysis provided information on subtypes of CVD, a well-known prospective study by Chiuve et al. assessed associations among 71,495 female nurses and 41,029 male health professionals during ≥24 years of follow-up and reported RRs comparing the highest to lowest categories of HEI-2005 of 0.79 (95% CI 0.71–0.88) for CVD, 0.76 (95% CI 0.68–0.84) for CHD, and 0.82 (95% CI 0.72–0.93) for stroke (Chiuve et al. 2012). Notably, this study also updated the AHEI to its present form, the AHEI-2010, with additional chronic disease risk factors and found similar associations as with HEI-2005 with stroke, but stronger association of the AHEI-2010 than of the HEI-2005 with CHD and T2D.

Few prospective studies have evaluated the relationship of HEI-2010 to T2D or other CVD risk factors. No meta-analysis has presented a pooled estimate of this relationship; thus, the best existing evidence is from the study described earlier in which Chiuve et al. report a RR of 0.82 (95% CI 0.76–0.89) for T2D comparing the highest to lowest categories of HEI-2005 (Chiuve et al. 2012). Analyses with the updated HEI-2010 in the more racially and ethnically diverse populations in the Women's Health Initiative[39] found similar results overall, while there was no association of HEI-2010 with T2D in the Multiethnic Cohort.[37] A potential reason for these disparate findings could be culturally specific foods not captured through dietary assessment methods, such as the FFQ, leading to misclassification of diet quality, or differences in the consumption of specific food groups, leading to the same index score, but potentially with differing strengths of association with disease.

In the Multi-Ethnic Study of Atherosclerosis, higher HEI-2010 scores had a small but significant inverse association with incident obesity, BMI, and waist circumference overall, with stronger associations in non-Hispanic whites than in other racial/ethnic groups (Gao et al. 2008). Cross-sectionally, higher HEI-2010 scores are also associated with lower odds of abdominal obesity in the National Health and Nutrition Survey (NHANES) (Tande, Magel, and Strand 2010). Together, these results provide weak but suggestive evidence that the long-term maintenance of a healthful diet as characterized by the HEI-2010 could be protective against excessive weight gain.

Also in cross-sectional analyses in the NHANES, the total HEI-2005 score was not associated with any CVD risk factors (blood pressure, fasting glucose and insulin, HOMA-IR, HDL-C, LDL-C, TG, and hs-CRP) after adjustment for body mass index. The few studies that have examined HEI-2010 scores have not observed significant benefits on blood lipid levels with greater adherence to the 2010 Dietary Guidelines for Americans (Mertens et al. 2015). With regard to inflammation, Fung et al. found no association of higher HEI-2010 scores with hs-CRP, IL-6, E-selectin, soluble intercellular adhesion molecule 1, or soluble vascular cell adhesion molecule 1 (sVCAM-1), whereas in the same study AHEI-2010 was inversely associated with all of these other than sVCAM-1 (Fung et al. 2005).

ALTERNATE HEALTHY EATING INDEX

The AHEI is originally based on features of the HEI but adapted to incorporate scientific knowledge of foods and nutrients predictive of chronic disease risk, such as the specific type of fat, carbohydrate, or protein consumed. By contrast to the HEI, which uses nutrient densities to express foods and nutrients, the AHEI uses primarily absolute intakes. The most recent update is the AHEI-2010 by Chiuve et al. (2012), which ranges from 0 (nonadherence) to 110 (perfect adherence) with the ten food components scored from 0 (worst) to 10 (best), and points awarded proportionally for intermediate intakes. Points are allocated for higher intakes for healthful food groups (fruits, vegetables, nuts and legumes, whole grains, long-chain n-3 fats, polyunsaturated fats), moderate consumption of alcohol, lower intakes for unhealthy foods (red/processed meats and sweetened beverages), and the lowest population-specific decile for sodium. While the contemporary AHEI-2010 and HEI-2010 scores emphasize many of the same components (e.g., awarding points for greater consumption of fruits and vegetables, consideration of fatty acid quality), these indices also differ not only in the methods of scoring but also with respect to key components (e.g., alcohol, see Table 21.2). These differences likely explain to some degree the differences in findings.

CARDIOVASCULAR DISEASE

In addition to strong observational evidence that higher-quality diets as measured via the AHEI reduce the incidence of CVD, CHD, and stroke (Chiuve et al. 2012, Reedy et al. 2014, Liese et al. 2015, Wu et al. 2016), the dietary pattern also appears to have favorable effects on inflammation and other intermediate markers of cardiovascular risk such as T2D (Fung et al. 2007, de Koning et al. 2011, Chiuve et al. 2012, Jacobs et al. 2014, Cespedes et al. 2016, Wu et al. 2016).

With respect to secondary prevention, among participants in the Nurses' Health Study and Health Professionals Follow-Up Study, greater increases in AHEI-2010 scores from pre- to post-myocardial infarction were significantly associated with lower all-cause and cardiovascular mortality (Li et al. 2013).

CVD Risk Factors

Type 2 Diabetes

In the meta-analysis cited in Table 21.3, the pooled RR estimate across six studies comparing the highest to lowest categories of the AHEI was 0.77 (95% CI 0.68–0.86) (Schwingshackl and Hoffmann 2015). Two studies not included in this meta-analysis also found the AHEI-2010 to be protective against T2D, though the strength of association was inconsistent across racial and ethnic groups (Jacobs et al. 2014, Cespedes et al. 2016).

Body Fatness and Body Mass Index

As is the case for the HEI, evidence for an association of AHEI-2010 with the prevention of excessive weight gain is suggestive but extremely limited. Aside from the Fung et al. study described earlier that showed that adherence as measured by a variety of dietary scores (including AHEI-2010) was associated with significantly less weight gain (Fung et al. 2015), few studies have examined the association of AHEI-2010 scores with body fatness. One longitudinal analysis in the Whitehall II study found long-term adherence to a healthful diet as measured by AHEI-2010 was associated with reversal of the metabolic syndrome, driven by the association of AHEI-2010 among participants with elevated TG and central obesity (waist circumference >102 cm in men or >88 cm in women) rather than those with other metabolic derangements (Akbaraly et al. 2010).

Blood Pressure, Blood Lipids, and Inflammation

Similarly, very little research has examined AHEI-2010 in relation to biomarkers of CVD risk, and most available studies examining the benefits of greater AHEI-2010 adherence with blood pressure and blood lipids have focused on diabetic patients (Huffman et al. 2011, Wu et al. 2016). With regard to inflammation, in the Whitehall II study in England, participants who maintained a high AHEI-2010 score or who improved their score over time showed significantly lower mean levels of IL-6 (1.84 pg/mL [95% CI 1.71–1.98] and 1.84 pg/mL [95% CI 1.70–1.99], respectively) than those who had a low AHEI score over the 6-year exposure period (2.01 pg/mL [95% CI 1.87–2.17]) (Akbaraly et al. 2015).

Taken together, these results suggest that additional prospective research characterizing the relationship of various *a priori* dietary indices to intermediate biomarkers of CVD risk such as blood lipids and blood pressure would further our understanding of the mechanisms underlying the associations of each of these individual dietary patterns to CVD incidence and mortality.

OTHER POPULAR DIETS

In addition to the dietary patterns discussed here, there are many other *a priori* patterns that are commonly consumed or commercially available, including vegetarian and vegan diets, defined by the exclusion of select animal products, and the Atkins and Paleolithic diets, defined by the near-elimination of carbohydrates and of processed foods, respectively. Vegetarian dietary patterns appear cardioprotective, with a meta-analysis showing lower mortality from ischemic heart disease (29%) and cerebrovascular (16%) and circulatory (12%) diseases compared to nonvegetarians (Huang et al. 2012). Importantly, some authors argue that the protective association is driven primarily by studies of Seventh Day Adventists (a Protestant sect that consumes a vegetarian diet rich in legumes, whole grains, nuts, fruits, and vegetables), with less robust evidence of CVD reduction in other populations (Kwok et al. 2014). Others argue that the benefits of a vegetarian diet are not unique, but rather attributable to having a plant-based diet that limits (but does not necessarily eliminate) red and processed meats, as this is associated with a reduced risk of coronary heart disease and T2D (McEvoy, Temple, and Woodside 2012). A meta-analysis of prospective studies comparing an omnivorous diet to loosely defined vegetarian diets found reductions in blood pressure also (Yokoyama et al. 2014), but the evidence on vegetarian diets and other CVD risk factors has not been rigorously reviewed.

The Paleolithic diet takes its name from the nutritional habits of our pre-agricultural ancestors of the Paleolithic era, whose diets likely varied substantially in the quantity of animal versus plant foods depending on climate and latitude, but would have had in common heat as the main form of food processing, very limited carbohydrate and a complete lack of dairy outside infancy (Cordain et al. 2005). A recent meta-analysis including four randomized controlled trials testing the efficacy of the Paleolithic diet compared to control diets based on dietary guidelines concluded that there was moderate evidence that the Paleolithic diet resulted in greater short-term improvements in metabolic syndrome components (i.e., significant reductions in waist circumference, TG, and blood pressure, and nonsignificant reductions in fasting glucose and improvements in HDL-C) (Manheimer et al. 2015). Importantly, these endpoints were all assessed at <6 months after intervention began. The restrictiveness of the Paleolithic diet (complete lack of dairy, very limited food processing) could pose a challenge to long-term adherence, but to date this is unknown; there is no evidence regarding the long-term maintenance or efficacy of these diets compared to guidelines-based dietary patterns.

Unlike the Paleolithic diet, Atkins does not emphasize the consumption of unprocessed foods. Atkins is a four-phase diet plan based on very-low-carbohydrate intake (it is a ketogenic diet, with <20% of energy from carbohydrates) and unlimited fat and protein, which has only been assessed in short-term interventions on intermediate endpoints (Atallah et al. 2014). With respect to weight loss, while initially Atkins resulted in superior weight loss compared to low-fat controls, it had inconsistent efficacy at 12–24 months. With regard to lipids, Akins had a suggestively beneficial effect in short-term trials on HDL-C and TG. There was no effect on LDL-C at 12–24 months, despite the early suggestion of an adverse influence. Effects on blood pressure were inconsistent compared to control diets, and there was no evidence of a benefit for glycemic control (Atallah et al. 2014).

In sum, despite the scale of the weight loss industry in the United States, there is insufficient evidence to compare the long-term maintenance or benefits of various popular commercial diets for the prevention of CVD in the long term.

A POSTERIORI PATTERNS

Cardiovascular Disease

As described earlier, empirically derived *a posteriori* dietary patterns typically identify two broad categories that explain the most variation in study participants' consumption: *healthy/prudent* and *unhealthy/Western*. While it strengthens the case for causality when similar dietary patterns show consistent benefits in populations with different confounding structures and health behaviors, it also complicates the task of summarizing a heterogeneous body of evidence. For example, diets designated as *healthy/prudent* or *unhealthy/Western* using principal components analysis may have different components or different factor loadings for individual components depending on the study population. The meta-analysis cited in Table 21.3 illustrates the advantages and complications of pooling results across studies (Rodriguez-Monforte, Flores-Mateo, and Sanchez 2015). The authors evaluated results from cohort and case–control studies investigating the association between *a posteriori* dietary patterns and CVD. Patterns designated as *healthy/prudent* had high-factor loadings for vegetables, fruit, legumes, whole grains, fish, and poultry, and those designated as *unhealthy/Western* had high-factor loadings for red and processed meat, refined grains, French fries, sweets, desserts, high-fat dairy products, and alcohol. The authors found a lower risk of all CVD endpoints with greater adherence to a *healthy/prudent* pattern, with the exception of stroke. Meanwhile, for the *unhealthy/Western*, despite highly significant results in some individual studies, the overall pooled estimate did not achieve statistical significance. As an explanation for why *healthy/prudent* dietary patterns might be more consistently associated with (decreased) CVD risk than *unhealthy/Western* patterns with (increased) CVD risk, the authors proposed, first, that dietary patterns are socially and culturally mediated and, second, that the foods that explain the greatest variation in a dietary pattern labeled as *unhealthy* may in fact have inverse relationships with select chronic disease outcomes, even if they increased the risk of others. For example, a *dairy product* dietary pattern examined among Japanese adults was associated with a reduced risk of stroke; despite including butter, the pattern also included other types of dairy, fruits, and other items typically in the *healthy* patterns (Maruyama et al. 2013). In another study focused on black Americans, a pattern defined by a high intake of sweets and saturated fats was associated with a reduction in stroke risk, and the authors hypothesized that perhaps adherence to the dietary pattern could be associated with a higher risk of cancer or some kinds of CHD that might lead to death before a stroke could occur (Judd et al. 2013). Meanwhile, other studies characterizing *a posteriori* dietary patterns did find a protective association of *healthy/prudent* dietary patterns with stroke: a meta-analysis assessing the influence of food patterns identified via principal component analysis, cluster analysis, and/or factor analysis concluded that the highest compared with the lowest categories of *healthy/prudent* dietary patterns were associated with a decreased risk of stroke (summary RR 0.77 [95% CI 0.63–0.93]), whereas *unhealthy/Western* dietary patterns were not associated with stroke (Zhang et al. 2015).

Often, dietary patterns derived via a hybrid method called reduced rank regression, which identifies food patterns that explain maximal variation in intermediate disease risk factors, are more strongly associated with CVD risk than purely empirical patterns derived without regard to outcome. For example, a recent study using data from nearly 35,000 participants in the European Prospective Investigation into Cancer–Netherlands identified seven dietary patterns using reduced rank regression and principal components analysis that could be grouped into three broad categories: a *Western*, *prudent*, and *traditional* pattern (Biesbroek et al. 2015). Despite deriving similar dietary patterns, the reduced rank regression approach, which derived a pattern to explain maximal variation in body mass index, total-C/HDL-C ratio, and systolic blood pressure, resulted in small differences in food items that contributed to a stronger association with coronary artery disease than patterns derived from principal components analysis: the reduced rank regression *Western* pattern included a fewer number of important foods (high consumption of French fries, fast food, sausages, and soft drinks) and was significantly associated to coronary artery disease, whereas the *Western* pattern derived through principal components analysis (without the use of intermediate risk factors) was not associated with coronary artery disease despite having a larger number of components with higher-factor loadings (e.g., alcohol, bread, sweets, and low-fiber cereal were included in the principal components pattern) (Biesbroek et al. 2015). Similarly, in the Whitehall II study, researchers used reduced rank regression to derive a dietary pattern associated with serum total-C and HDL-C and TG levels as dependent variables. Among 7314 participants, researchers derived a diet characterized by "high consumption of white bread, fried potatoes, sugar in tea and coffee, burgers and sausages, soft drinks, and low consumption of French dressing and vegetables" that was associated with >50% increased risk of CHD, even after an adjustment for the intermediates blood pressure and BMI (RR for top versus bottom quartile, 1.57 [95% CI 1.08–2.27]) (McNaughton, Mishra, and Brunner 2009).

CVD Risk Factors

Type 2 Diabetes

Many empirically derived dietary patterns are associated with T2D risk (Alhazmi et al. 2014, Maghsoudi, Ghiasvand, and Salehi-Abargouei 2015). A recent review meta-analysis of nine prospective cohort studies (totaling 309,430 participants and 16,644 incident cases) found a 15% lower T2D risk for those in the highest category of *healthy/prudent* pattern compared with those in the lowest category (RR 0.85, 95% CI 0.80–0.91) (McEvoy et al. 2014). Compared with the lowest category of *unhealthy/Western* pattern, those in the highest category had a 41% increased risk of T2D (RR 1.41, 95% CI 1.32–1.52) (McEvoy et al. 2014). Another meta-analysis of cohort studies found a protective RR of 0.79 (95% CI 0.74–0.86) for T2D comparing the highest to the lowest adherence to empirically derived *healthy/prudent* dietary patterns, which emphasized whole grain products, fruits, and vegetables (Alhazmi et al. 2014). By contrast, when comparing the highest to lowest adherence to *unhealthy/Western* dietary patterns, which emphasized red or processed meats, high-fat dairy, refined grains, and sweets, an adverse RR of 1.44 was observed (95% CI 1.33–1.57) (Alhazmi et al. 2014).

Body Fatness and Body Mass Index

Empirically derived *healthy/prudent* dietary patterns characterized by the presence of vegetables, fruit, whole grains, and reduced-fat dairy are also associated with a lower risk of obesity, healthier weight or BMI, and lower weight and waist gain, whereas *unhealthy/Western* associated with a higher risk of obesity were characterized by the presence of red meat and processed meats, sugar-sweetened foods and drinks, and refined grains (Quatromoni et al. 2002, Newby et al. 2003, 2004a, Newby, Muller, and Tucker 2004b, Schulze et al. 2006, McNaughton et al. 2007, Boggs et al. 2011, Hosseini-Esfahani et al. 2012). However, the methods employed and study populations examined were heterogeneous, and not all studies found significant associations.

Blood Pressure, Blood Lipids, and Inflammation

Very few prospective studies have examined blood pressure, blood lipids, or inflammation in relation to *a posteriori* dietary patterns (Jiang et al. 2015). With regard to inflammation, most available studies have been relatively small and cross-sectional and show inconsistent results (Barbaresko et al. 2013). For example, research conducted in the Nurses' Health Study's female participants found an inverse association of a *healthy/prudent* diet with the markers of inflammation and endothelial dysfunction such as hs-CRP and E-selectin (Lopez-Garcia et al. 2004); while among men in the Health Professionals Follow-up Study, there was no association (Fung et al. 2001). While results have not been wholly consistent, another recent narrative review concluded that studies have shown an overall adverse association of *unhealthy/Western* dietary patterns with markers of inflammation and endothelial dysfunction (Barbaresko et al. 2013).

Similarly, little research has addressed the association of *a posteriori* dietary patterns with blood lipids and the available findings are inconsistent. For example, a study in the Cardiovascular Risk in Young Finns Study suggesting that adherence to a *health-conscious* pattern (similar to the *healthy/prudent* pattern and rich in fruit and vegetables, fish, legumes and nuts, tea, rye, cheese and other dairy products, and alcoholic beverages) was associated with lower LDL-C and insulin in women but not in men. Meanwhile, adherence to a *traditional* pattern (high consumption of potatoes, sausages, milk, coffee, rye, and butter) was associated with higher LDL-C, apolipoprotein B, and CRP concentrations in both men and women (Mikkila et al. 2007).

IMPLICATIONS AND DIRECTIONS FOR FUTURE RESEARCH

The overall body of evidence suggests that a healthful dietary pattern is strongly associated with a decreased risk of CVD and associated risk factors, while unhealthy dietary patterns are associated with an increased risk of CVD and associated risk factors. For example, meta-analyses indicate that diets of the highest quality, as assessed by the HEI, AHEI, and DASH scores, reduce the risk of CVD (incidence or mortality) by 22% (Schwingshackl and Hoffmann 2015). Variations in the strength of associations between dietary patterns with disease outcomes may be due to small differences in how dietary patterns characterize an optimally healthy diet. For example, alcohol in moderation was included as a positive component (e.g., Mediterranean style or AHEI-2010) and consumption of red and processed meats as a negative component in some (e.g., Mediterranean or DASH) but not all patterns. How dairy, poultry, or added sugars were treated also varied. While examining the associations of these individual components with cardiometabolic disease may help in identifying the most *active ingredients* in a healthful dietary pattern, isolating these foods and nutrients may not provide a realistic picture of what people eat in combination and its health impact; it is likely the cumulative and interactive effects of multiple components of diet that predict disease, and when one component of the diet changes, it is typically substituted by another. This is where dietary pattern analyses become particularly useful: not only do dietary patterns encompass the totality of diet but also they allow for multiple ways to achieve a healthy diet. Thus, public health guidelines and recommendations may be most easily translated into eating behaviors when described by the composite measure of diet quality encompassed in dietary patterns. Increasingly, this is recognized; for example, the 2015 Dietary Guidelines Advisory Committee (DGAC) focused its evidence review and recommendations on healthful dietary patterns instead of individual nutrients or foods in its recently released scientific report. The DGAC noted remarkable consistency in the findings over a wide range of disease outcomes, including cardiometabolic diseases, and across different dietary pattern assessment methods (United States Department of Agriculture 2015b). This suggests that dietary modifications to improve CVD risk may also benefit other chronic disease outcomes. Remarkably, despite different approaches to deriving dietary patterns, common elements—nutrients and foods—emerge over and over and are likely to be drivers of the observed effects. In essence, dietary patterns associated with decreased risk of CVD feature fruits, vegetables, whole grains, low-fat dairy, and fish as signature components. In these dietary patterns, red and processed meat and added sugar were limited, while nuts and legumes and moderate consumption of alcohol were often beneficial. Further, where specific nutrients are included in the dietary patterns, those low in saturated fat and sodium but rich in fiber and potassium showed the greatest potential for reducing CVD risk (United States Department of Agriculture National Evidence Library 2014, United States Department of Agriculture 2015b).

Despite the consistency of the characteristics of a healthful dietary pattern across studies, there remain significant gaps in the research literature and an urgent need to develop effective strategies to improve diet quality at the population level. First, the vast majority of studies examined European or European-descent populations. With this in mind, one consideration when developing guidelines on the basis of dietary patterns research is that many signature foods vary by region or are culturally specific. Already, there have been efforts to tackle this translational challenge; for example, a recent report from a 3-day consensus workshop convened by the World Heart Federation argued that the essence of the Mediterranean diet could be translated to regions and cultures and concretized this by suggesting replacement with specific foods that represent staples of particular regions, for example, "whole grains" might be sorghum or millet in East Asia, but brown or rye bread in Europe or North America (Anand et al. 2015). Nevertheless, prospective research and large-scale trials of healthful dietary patterns in diverse regions and populations of the globe would strengthen the evidence base for relevant dietary guidelines at the country level.

Recently, there has been interest in testing the efficacy of national dietary guidelines on intermediate biomarkers of cardiovascular risk through short-term randomized controlled trials; this represents a promising approach to evaluating the efficacy of national dietary guidance. For example, a recent trial of 165 adults found that the current UK dietary guidelines had favorable effects on blood pressure and lipids compared to a traditional British diet (Reidlinger et al. 2015). In addition to randomized controlled trials, continued analysis of adherence to healthful dietary patterns in the general population through the nationally representative studies with repeated cross-sectional measures of diet (such as NHANES) will be critical. One reason is that recent improvements in diet quality, while estimated to account for substantial reduction in disease burden (13% fewer T2D cases and 9% fewer CVD cases [Wang et al. 2015]), have not been shared equally; despite steady improvement in AHEI-2010 scores in the U.S. population overall from the 1999 to 2010 surveys by NHANES, absolute scores remain low and the gap between low and high socioeconomic status widened over time (Wang et al. 2014). Monitoring changes in diet quality in the population overall and among subgroups can inform public health and policy interventions to address these nutritional disparities and therefore mitigate disparities in cardiometabolic diseases. Further, the use of diet quality indices provides a surveillance tool to evaluate the efficacy of dietary guidelines for the prevention of cardiometabolic disease at the population level.

REFERENCES

Abiemo, E. E., A. Alonso, J. A. Nettleton, L. M. Steffen, A. G. Bertoni, A. Jain, and P. L. Lutsey. 2013. Relationships of the Mediterranean dietary pattern with insulin resistance and diabetes incidence in the Multi-Ethnic Study of Atherosclerosis (MESA). *Br J Nutr* 109(08):1490–1497.

Akbaraly, T. N., M. J. Shipley, J. E. Ferrie, M. Virtanen, G. Lowe, M. Hamer, and M. Kivimaki. 2015. Long-term adherence to healthy dietary guidelines and chronic inflammation in the prospective Whitehall II study. *Am J Med* 128(2):152–160.e4.

Akbaraly, T. N., A. Singh-Manoux, A. G. Tabak, M. Jokela, M. Virtanen, J. E. Ferrie, M. G. Marmot, M. J. Shipley, and M. Kivimaki. 2010. Overall diet history and reversibility of the metabolic syndrome over 5 years the Whitehall II Prospective Cohort Study. *Diabetes Care* 33(11):2339–2341.

Alhazmi, A., E. Stojanovski, M. McEvoy, and M. L. Garg. 2014. The association between dietary patterns and type 2 diabetes: A systematic review and meta-analysis of cohort studies. *J Hum Nutr Diet* 27(3):251–260. doi: 10.1111/jhn.12139.

Anand, S. S., C. Hawkes, R. J. De Souza, A. Mente, M. Dehghan, R. Nugent, M. A. Zulyniak, T. Weis, A. M. Bernstein, and R. M. Krauss. 2015. Food consumption and its impact on cardiovascular disease: Importance of solutions focused on the globalized food system: A report from the workshop convened by the World Heart Federation. *J Am Coll Cardiol* 66(14):1590–1614.

Appel, L. J., T. J. Moore, E. Obarzanek, W. M. Vollmer, L. P. Svetkey, F. M. Sacks, G. A. Bray et al. 1997. A clinical trial of the effects of dietary patterns on blood pressure. DASH Collaborative Research Group. *N Engl J Med* 336(16):1117–1124. doi: 10.1056/nejm199704173361601.

Atallah, R., K. B. Filion, S. M. Wakil, J. Genest, L. Joseph, P. Poirier, S. Rinfret, E. L. Schiffrin, and M. J. Eisenberg. 2014. Long-term effects of 4 popular diets on weight loss and cardiovascular risk factors: A systematic review of randomized controlled trials. *Circ Cardiovasc Qual Outcomes* 7(6):815–827.

Barbaresko, J., M. Koch, M. B. Schulze, and U. Nöthlings. 2013. Dietary pattern analysis and biomarkers of low-grade inflammation: A systematic literature review. *Nutr Rev* 71(8):511–527.

Bertoia, M. L., E. W. Triche, D. S. Michaud, A. Baylin, J. W. Hogan, M. L. Neuhouser, L. F. Tinker et al. 2014. Mediterranean and dietary approaches to stop hypertension dietary patterns and risk of sudden cardiac death in postmenopausal women. *Am J Clin Nutr* 99(2):344–351. doi: 10.3945/ajcn.112.056135.

Beunza, J. J., E. Toledo, F. B. Hu, M. Bes-Rastrollo, M. Serrano-Martinez, A. Sanchez-Villegas, J. A. Martinez, and M. A. Martinez-Gonzalez. 2010. Adherence to the Mediterranean diet, long-term weight change, and incident overweight or obesity: The Seguimiento Universidad de Navarra (SUN) cohort. *Am J Clin Nutr* 92(6):1484–1493. doi: 10.3945/ajcn.2010.29764.

Biesbroek, S., A. Dl van der, M. C. Brosens, J. W. Beulens, W. M. Verschuren, Y. T. van der Schouw, and J. M. Boer. 2015. Identifying cardiovascular risk factor-related dietary patterns with reduced rank regression and random forest in the EPIC-NL cohort. *Am J Clin Nutr* 102(1):146–154. doi: 10.3945/ajcn.114.092288.

Boggs, D. A., J. R. Palmer, D. Spiegelman, M. J. Stampfer, L. L. Adams-Campbell, and L. Rosenberg. 2011. Dietary patterns and 14-y weight gain in African American women. *Am J Clin Nutr* 94(1):86–94. doi: 10.3945/ajcn.111.013482.

Camoes, M., A. Oliveira, M. Pereira, M. Severo, and C. Lopes. 2010. Role of physical activity and diet in incidence of hypertension: A population-based study in Portuguese adults. *Eur J Clin Nutr* 64(12): 1441–1449. doi: 10.1038/ejcn.2010.170.

Cespedes, E. M., F. B. Hu, L. Tinker, B. Rosner, S. Redline, L. Garcia, M. Hingle, L. Van Horn, B. V. Howard, and E. B. Levitan. 2016. Multiple healthful dietary patterns and type 2 diabetes in the women's health initiative. *Am J Epidemiol* 183(7):622–633.

Chiu, S., N. Bergeron, P. T. Williams, G. A. Bray, B. Sutherland, and R. M. Krauss. 2016. Comparison of the DASH (Dietary Approaches to Stop Hypertension) diet and a higher-fat DASH diet on blood pressure and lipids and lipoproteins: A randomized controlled trial. *Am J Clin Nutr* 103(2):341–347.

Chiuve, S. E., T. T. Fung, E. B. Rimm, F. B. Hu, M. L. McCullough, M. Wang, M. J. Stampfer, and W. C. Willett. 2012. Alternative dietary indices both strongly predict risk of chronic disease. *J Nutr* 142(6):1009–1018. doi: 10.3945/jn.111.157222.

Cordain, L., S. Boyd Eaton, A. Sebastian, N. Mann, S. Lindeberg, B. A. Watkins, J. H. O'Keefe, and J. Brand-Miller. 2005. Origins and evolution of the Western diet: Health implications for the 21st century. *Am J Clin Nutr* 81(2):341–354.

Corella, D., R. Estruch, M. Fitó, M. Á. Martínez-Gonzíalez, E. Ros, and J. Salas-Salvadó. 2013. Effect of an intensive lifestyle intervention with an energy-restricted Mediterranean diet, increased physical activity, and behavioural treatment on the primary prevention of cardiovascular diseases: The PREDIMED-PLUS randomized clinical trial 2013 [cited January 2, 2016]. Available from http://predimedplus.com/uk/public/abstract.html.

D'Alessandro, A. and G. De Pergola. 2015. Mediterranean diet and cardiovascular disease: A critical evaluation of a priori dietary indexes. *Nutrients* 7(9):7863–7888.

de Koning, L., S. E. Chiuve, T. T. Fung, W. C. Willett, E. B. Rimm, and F. B. Hu. 2011. Diet-quality scores and the risk of type 2 diabetes in men. *Diabetes Care* 34(5):1150–1156. doi: 10.2337/dc10-2352.

de Lorgeril, M., P. Salen, J. L. Martin, I. Monjaud, J. Delaye, and N. Mamelle. 1999. Mediterranean diet, traditional risk factors, and the rate of cardiovascular complications after myocardial infarction: Final report of the Lyon Diet Heart Study. *Circulation* 99(6):779–785.

de Oliveira Otto, M. C., N. S. Padhye, A. G. Bertoni, D. R. Jacobs Jr, and D. Mozaffarian. 2015. Everything in moderation-dietary diversity and quality, central obesity and risk of diabetes. *PLoS One* 10(10):e0141341.

Del Gobbo, L. C., S. Kalantarian, F. Imamura, R. Lemaitre, D. S. Siscovick, B. M. Psaty, and D. Mozaffarian. 2015. Contribution of major lifestyle risk factors for incident heart failure in older adults: The Cardiovascular Health Study. *JACC Heart Fail* 3(7):520–528. doi: 10.1016/j.jchf.2015.02.009.

Esposito, K., C. M. Kastorini, D. B. Panagiotakos, and D. Giugliano. 2011. Mediterranean diet and weight loss: Meta-analysis of randomized controlled trials. *Metab Syndr Relat Disord* 9(1):1–12. doi: 10.1089/met.2010.0031.

Esposito, K., R. Marfella, M. Ciotola, C. Di Palo, F. Giugliano, G. Giugliano, M. D'Armiento, F. D'Andrea, and D. Giugliano. 2004. Effect of a Mediterranean-style diet on endothelial dysfunction and markers of vascular inflammation in the metabolic syndrome: A randomized trial. *JAMA* 292(12):1440–1446. doi: 10.1001/jama.292.12.1440.

Estruch, R., M. A. Martinez-Gonzalez, D. Corella, J. Salas-Salvadó, V. Ruiz-Gutierrez, M. I. Covas, M. Fiol et al. 2006. Effects of a Mediterranean-style diet on cardiovascular risk factors: A randomized trial. *Ann Intern Med* 145(1):1–11.

Estruch, R., E. Ros, J. Salas-Salvadó, M. I. Covas, D. Corella, F. Aros, E. Gomez-Gracia et al. 2013. Primary prevention of cardiovascular disease with a Mediterranean diet. *N Engl J Med* 368(14):1279–1290. doi: 10.1056/NEJMoa1200303.

Folsom, A. R., E. D. Parker, and L. J. Harnack. 2007. Degree of concordance with DASH diet guidelines and incidence of hypertension and fatal cardiovascular disease. *Am J Hypertens* 20(3):225–232. doi: 10.1016/j.amjhyper.2006.09.003.

Fung, T. T., S. E. Chiuve, M. L. McCullough, K. M. Rexrode, G. Logroscino, and F. B. Hu. 2008. Adherence to a DASH-style diet and risk of coronary heart disease and stroke in women. *Arch Intern Med* 168(7):713–720. doi: 10.1001/archinte.168.7.713.

Fung, T. T., M. McCullough, R. M. van Dam, and F. B. Hu. 2007. A prospective study of overall diet quality and risk of type 2 diabetes in women. *Diabetes Care* 30(7):1753–1757. doi: 10.2337/dc06-2581.

Fung, T. T., M. L. McCullough, P. K. Newby, J. E. Manson, J. B. Meigs, N. Rifai, W. C. Willett, and F. B. Hu. 2005. Diet-quality scores and plasma concentrations of markers of inflammation and endothelial dysfunction. *Am J Clin Nutr* 82(1):163–173.

Fung, T. T., A. Pan, T. Hou, S. E. Chiuve, D. K. Tobias, D. Mozaffarian, W. C. Willett, and F. B. Hu. 2015. Long-term change in diet quality is associated with body weight change in men and women. *J Nutr* 145(8):1850–1856.

Fung, T. T., K. M. Rexrode, C. S. Mantzoros, J. E. Manson, W. C. Willett, and F. B. Hu. 2009. Mediterranean diet and incidence of and mortality from coronary heart disease and stroke in women. *Circulation* 119(8):1093–1100. doi: 10.1161/circulationaha.108.816736.

Fung, T. T., E. B. Rimm, D. Spiegelman, N. Rifai, G. H. Tofler, W. C. Willett, and F. B. Hu. 2001. Association between dietary patterns and plasma biomarkers of obesity and cardiovascular disease risk. *Am J Clin Nutr* 73(1):61–67.

Gao, S. K., S. A. A. Beresford, L. L. Frank, P. J. Schreiner, G. L. Burke, and A. L. Fitzpatrick. 2008. Modifications to the Healthy Eating Index and its ability to predict obesity: The Multi-Ethnic Study of Atherosclerosis. *Am J Clin Nutr* 88(1):64–69.

George, S. M., R. Ballard-Barbash, J. E. Manson, J. Reedy, J. M. Shikany, A. F. Subar, L. F. Tinker, M. Vitolins, and M. L. Neuhouser. 2014. Comparing indices of diet quality with chronic disease mortality risk in postmenopausal women in the Women's Health Initiative Observational Study: Evidence to inform national dietary guidance. *Am J Epidemiol* 180(6):616–625.

Guenther, P. M., K. O. Casavale, J. Reedy, S. I. Kirkpatrick, H. A. B. Hiza, K. J. Kuczynski, L. L. Kahle, and S. M. Krebs-Smith. 2013. Update of the healthy eating index: HEI-2010. *J Acad Nutr Diet* 113(4):569–580.

Guenther, P. M., S. I. Kirkpatrick, J. Reedy, S. M. Krebs-Smith, D. W. Buckman, K. W. Dodd, K. O. Casavale, and R. J. Carroll. 2014. The Healthy Eating Index-2010 is a valid and reliable measure of diet quality according to the 2010 Dietary Guidelines for Americans. *J Nutr* 144(3):399–407.

Guyatt, G. H., M. Briel, P. Glasziou, D. Bassler, and V. M. Montori. 2012. Problems of stopping trials early. *BMJ* 344:e3863.

Hinderliter, A. L., M. A. Babyak, A. Sherwood, and J. A. Blumenthal. 2011. The DASH diet and insulin sensitivity. *Curr Hypertens Rep* 13(1):67–73.

Hoffmann, K., M. B. Schulze, A. Schienkiewitz, U. Nothlings, and H. Boeing. 2004. Application of a new statistical method to derive dietary patterns in nutritional epidemiology. *Am J Epidemiol* 159(10):935–944.

Horton, R. 2005. Expression of concern: Indo-Mediterranean diet heart study. *Lancet* 366(9483):354–356.

Hosseini-Esfahani, F., S. A. Djazaieri, P. Mirmiran, Y. Mehrabi, and F. Azizi. 2012. Which food patterns are predictors of obesity in Tehranian adults? *J Nutr Educ Behav* 44(6):564–573. doi: 10.1016/j.jneb.2010.08.004.

Howard, B. V., L. Van Horn, J. Hsia, J. E. Manson, M. L. Stefanick, S. Wassertheil-Smoller, L. H. Kuller, A. Z. LaCroix, R. D. Langer, and N. L. Lasser. 2006. Low-fat dietary pattern and risk of cardiovascular disease: The Women's Health Initiative Randomized Controlled Dietary Modification Trial. *JAMA* 295(6):655–666.

Hu, F. 2008. *Obesity Epidemiology*. Oxford University Press, New York.

Hu, F. B. 2002. Dietary pattern analysis: A new direction in nutritional epidemiology. *Curr Opin Lipidol* 13(1):3–9.

Huang, T., B. Yang, J. Zheng, G. Li, M. L. Wahlqvist, and D. Li. 2012. Cardiovascular disease mortality and cancer incidence in vegetarians: A meta-analysis and systematic review. *Ann Nutr Metab* 60(4):233–240. doi: 10.1159/000337301.

Huffman, F. G., G. G. Zarini, E. Mcnamara, and A. Nagarajan. 2011. The Healthy Eating Index and the Alternate Healthy Eating Index as predictors of 10-year CHD risk in Cuban Americans with and without type 2 diabetes. *Public Health Nutr* 14(11):2006–2014.

Jackson, C. L. and F. B. Hu. 2014. Long-term associations of nut consumption with body weight and obesity. *Am J Clin Nutr* 100(Suppl 1):408S–411S.

Jacobs, S., B. E. Harmon, C. J. Boushey, Y. Morimoto, L. R. Wilkens, L. Le Marchand, J. Kroger, M. B. Schulze, L. N. Kolonel, and G. Maskarinec. 2014. A priori-defined diet quality indexes and risk of type 2 diabetes: The Multiethnic Cohort. *Diabetologia* 58(1):98–112. doi: 10.1007/s00125-014-3404-8.

Jiang, J., M. Liu, F. Parvez, B. Wang, F. Wu, M. Eunus, S. Bangalore et al. 2015. Association of major dietary patterns and blood pressure longitudinal change in Bangladesh. *J Hypertens* 33(6):1193–1200. doi: 10.1097/hjh.0000000000000534.

Judd, S. E., O. M. Gutiérrez, P. K. Newby, G. Howard, V. J. Howard, J. L. Locher, B. M. Kissela, and J. M. Shikany. 2013. Dietary patterns are associated with incident stroke and contribute to excess risk of stroke in black Americans. *Stroke* 44(12):3305–3311.

Kastorini, C. M., H. J. Milionis, K. Esposito, D. Giugliano, J. A. Goudevenos, and D. B. Panagiotakos. 2011. The effect of Mediterranean diet on metabolic syndrome and its components: A meta-analysis of 50 studies and 534,906 individuals. *J Am Coll Cardiol* 57(11):1299–1313. doi: 10.1016/j.jacc.2010.09.073.

Keys, A. 1970. Coronary heart disease in seven countries. *Circulation* 41(1):186–195.

Koloverou, E., K. Esposito, D. Giugliano, and D. Panagiotakos. 2014. The effect of Mediterranean diet on the development of type 2 diabetes mellitus: A meta-analysis of 10 prospective studies and 136,846 participants. *Metabolism* 63(7):903–911.

Kwok, C. S., S. Umar, P. K. Myint, M. A. Mamas, and Y. K. Loke. 2014. Vegetarian diet, Seventh Day Adventists and risk of cardiovascular mortality: A systematic review and meta-analysis. *Int J Cardiol* 176(3):680–686. doi: 10.1016/j.ijcard.2014.07.080.

Levitan, E. B., C. E. Lewis, L. F. Tinker, C. B. Eaton, A. Ahmed, J. E. Manson, L. G. Snetselaar, L. W. Martin, M. Trevisan, and B. V. Howard. 2013. Mediterranean and DASH diet scores and mortality in women with heart failure: The Women's Health Initiative. *Circ Heart Fail* 6(6):1116–1123.

Levitan, E. B., A. Wolk, and M. A. Mittleman. 2009. Consistency with the DASH diet and incidence of heart failure. *Arch Intern Med* 169(9):851–857.

Li, S., S. E. Chiuve, A. Flint, J. K. Pai, J. P. Forman, F. B. Hu, W. C. Willett, K. J. Mukamal, and E. B. Rimm. 2013. Better diet quality and decreased mortality among myocardial infarction survivors. *JAMA Intern Med* 173(19):1808–1819.

Liese, A. D., S. M. Krebs-Smith, A. F. Subar, S. M. George, B. E. Harmon, M. L. Neuhouser, C. J. Boushey, T. E. Schap, and J. Reedy. 2015. The dietary patterns methods project: Synthesis of findings across cohorts and relevance to dietary guidance. *J Nutr* 145(3):393–402. doi: 10.3945/jn.114.205336.

Lopez-Garcia, E., M. B. Schulze, T. T. Fung, J. B. Meigs, N. Rifai, J. E. Manson, and F. B. Hu. 2004. Major dietary patterns are related to plasma concentrations of markers of inflammation and endothelial dysfunction. *Am J Clin Nutr* 80(4):1029–1035.

Maghsoudi, Z., R. Ghiasvand, and A. Salehi-Abargouei. 2015. Empirically derived dietary patterns and incident type 2 diabetes mellitus: A systematic review and meta-analysis on prospective observational studies. *Public Health Nutr* 1(2):1–12. doi: 10.1017/s1368980015001251.

Manheimer, E. W., E. J. van Zuuren, Z. Fedorowicz, and H. Pijl. 2015. Paleolithic nutrition for metabolic syndrome: Systematic review and meta-analysis. *Am J Clin Nutr* 102(4):922–932.

Martinez-Gonzalez, M. A. and M. Bes-Rastrollo. 2014. Dietary patterns, Mediterranean diet, and cardiovascular disease. *Curr Opin Lipidol* 25(1):20–26. doi: 10.1097/mol.0000000000000044.

Maruyama, K., H. Iso, C. Date, S. Kikuchi, Y. Watanabe, Y. Wada, Y. Inaba, A. Tamakoshi, and JACC Study Group. 2013. Dietary patterns and risk of cardiovascular deaths among middle-aged Japanese: JACC Study. *Nutr Metabol Cardiovasc Dis* 23(6):519–527.

McEvoy, C. T., C. R. Cardwell, J. V. Woodside, I. S. Young, S. J. Hunter, and M. C. McKinley. 2014. A posteriori dietary patterns are related to risk of type 2 diabetes: Findings from a systematic review and meta-analysis. *J Acad Nutr Diet* 114(11):1759–1775.e4. doi: 10.1016/j.jand.2014.05.001.

McEvoy, C. T., N. Temple, and J. V. Woodside. 2012. Vegetarian diets, low-meat diets and health: A review. *Public Health Nutr* 15(12):2287–2294.

McNaughton, S. A., G. D. Mishra, and E. J. Brunner. 2009. Food patterns associated with blood lipids are predictive of coronary heart disease: The Whitehall II study. *Br J Nutr* 102(4):619–624. doi: 10.1017/s0007114509243030.

McNaughton, S. A., G. D. Mishra, A. M. Stephen, and M. E. Wadsworth. 2007. Dietary patterns throughout adult life are associated with body mass index, waist circumference, blood pressure, and red cell folate. *J Nutr* 137(1):99–105.

Mente, A., L. de Koning, H. S. Shannon, and S. S. Anand. 2009. A systematic review of the evidence supporting a causal link between dietary factors and coronary heart disease. *Arch Intern Med* 169(7):659–669.

Mertens, E., B. Deforche, P. Mullie, J. Lefevre, R. Charlier, S. Knaeps, I. Huybrechts, and P. Clarys. 2015. Longitudinal study on the association between three dietary indices, anthropometric parameters and blood lipids. *Nutr Metabol* 12(1):1.

Mikkila, V., L. Rasanen, O. T. Raitakari, J. Marniemi, P. Pietinen, T. Ronnemaa, and J. Viikari. 2007. Major dietary patterns and cardiovascular risk factors from childhood to adulthood. The Cardiovascular Risk in Young Finns Study. *Br J Nutr* 98(1):218–225.

Miller III, E. R., T. P. Erlinger, and L. J. Appel. 2006. The effects of macronutrients on blood pressure and lipids: An overview of the DASH and OmniHeart trials. *Curr Atheroscler Rep* 8(6):460–465.

Molitor, J., I. J. Brown, Q. Chan, M. Papathomas, S. Liverani, N. Molitor, S. Richardson et al. 2014. Blood pressure differences associated with Optimal Macronutrient Intake Trial for Heart Health (OMNIHEART)-like diet compared with a typical American Diet. *Hypertension* 64(6):1198–1204. doi: 10.1161/hypertensionaha.114.03799.

Newby, P. K., D. Muller, J. Hallfrisch, R. Andres, and K. L. Tucker. 2004a. Food patterns measured by factor analysis and anthropometric changes in adults. *Am J Clin Nutr* 80(2):504–513.

Newby, P. K., D. Muller, J. Hallfrisch, N. Qiao, R. Andres, and K. L. Tucker. 2003. Dietary patterns and changes in body mass index and waist circumference in adults. *Am J Clin Nutr* 77(6):1417–1425.

Newby, P. K., D. Muller, and K. L. Tucker. 2004b. Associations of empirically derived eating patterns with plasma lipid biomarkers: A comparison of factor and cluster analysis methods. *Am J Clin Nutr* 80(3):759–767.

Newby, P. K. and K. L. Tucker. 2004. Empirically derived eating patterns using factor or cluster analysis: A review. *Nutr Rev* 62(5):177–203.

Nowlin, S. Y., M. J. Hammer, and G. D'Eramo Melkus. 2012. Diet, inflammation, and glycemic control in type 2 diabetes: An integrative review of the literature. *J Nutr Metabol* 2012, Article ID 542698, 21 pages. doi: 10.1155/2012/542698.

Nunez-Cordoba, J. M., F. Valencia-Serrano, E. Toledo, A. Alonso, and M. A. Martinez-Gonzalez. 2009. The Mediterranean diet and incidence of hypertension: The Seguimiento Universidad de Navarra (SUN) Study. *Am J Epidemiol* 169(3):339–346. doi: 10.1093/aje/kwn335.

Psaltopoulou, T., T. N. Sergentanis, D. B. Panagiotakos, I. N. Sergentanis, R. Kosti, and N. Scarmeas. 2013. Mediterranean diet, stroke, cognitive impairment, and depression: A meta-analysis. *Ann Neurol* 74(4):580–591.

Quatromoni, P. A., D. L. Copenhafer, R. B. D'Agostino, and B. E. Millen. 2002. Dietary patterns predict the development of overweight in women: The Framingham Nutrition Studies. *J Am Diet Assoc* 102(9):1239–1246.

Reedy, J., S. M. Krebs-Smith, P. E. Miller, A. D. Liese, L. L. Kahle, Y. Park, and A. F. Subar. 2014. Higher diet quality is associated with decreased risk of all-cause, cardiovascular disease, and cancer mortality among older adults. *J Nutr* 144(6):881–889. doi: 10.3945/jn.113.189407.

Rees, K., L. Hartley, N. Flowers, A. Clarke, L. Hooper, M. Thorogood, and S. Stranges. 2013. 'Mediterranean' dietary pattern for the primary prevention of cardiovascular disease. *Cochrane Database Syst Rev* 8:Cd009825. doi: 10.1002/14651858.CD009825.pub2.

Reidlinger, D. P., J. Darzi, W. L. Hall, P. T. Seed, P. J. Chowienczyk, and T. A. Sanders. 2015. How effective are current dietary guidelines for cardiovascular disease prevention in healthy middle-aged and older men and women? A randomized controlled trial. *Am J Clin Nutr* 101(5):922–930. doi: 10.3945/ajcn.114.097352.

Rodriguez-Monforte, M., G. Flores-Mateo, and E. Sanchez. 2015. Dietary patterns and CVD: A systematic review and meta-analysis of observational studies. *Br J Nutr* 114(9):1341–1359. doi: 10.1017/s0007114515003177.

Romaguera, D., T. Norat, A. C. Vergnaud, T. Mouw, A. M. May, A. Agudo, G. Buckland et al. 2010. Mediterranean dietary patterns and prospective weight change in participants of the EPIC-PANACEA project. *Am J Clin Nutr* 92(4):912–921. doi: 10.3945/ajcn.2010.29482.

Rumawas, M. E., J. B. Meigs, J. T. Dwyer, N. M. McKeown, and P. F. Jacques. 2009. Mediterranean-style dietary pattern, reduced risk of metabolic syndrome traits, and incidence in the Framingham Offspring Cohort. *Am J Clin Nutr* 90(6):1608–1614. doi: 10.3945/ajcn.2009.27908.

Sacks, F. M., V. J. Carey, C. A. M. Anderson, E. R. Miller, T. Copeland, J. Charleston, B. J. Harshfield, N. Laranjo, P. McCarron, and J. Swain. 2014. Effects of high vs low glycemic index of dietary carbohydrate on cardiovascular disease risk factors and insulin sensitivity: The OmniCarb randomized clinical trial. *JAMA* 312(23):2531–2541.

Sacks, F. M., E. Obarzanek, M. M. Windhauser, L. P. Svetkey, W. M. Vollmer, M. McCullough, N. Karanja et al. 1995. Rationale and design of the Dietary Approaches to Stop Hypertension trial (DASH). A multicenter controlled-feeding study of dietary patterns to lower blood pressure. *Ann Epidemiol* 5(2):108–118.

Sacks, F. M., L. P. Svetkey, W. M. Vollmer, L. J. Appel, G. A. Bray, D. Harsha, E. Obarzanek et al. 2001. Effects on blood pressure of reduced dietary sodium and the Dietary Approaches to Stop Hypertension (DASH) diet. DASH-Sodium Collaborative Research Group. *N Engl J Med* 344(1):3–10. doi: 10.1056/nejm200101043440101.

Salas-Salvadó, J., M. Bullo, N. Babio, M. A. Martinez-Gonzalez, N. Ibarrola-Jurado, J. Basora, R. Estruch et al. 2011. Reduction in the incidence of type 2 diabetes with the Mediterranean diet: Results of the PREDIMED-Reus nutrition intervention randomized trial. *Diabetes Care* 34(1):14–19. doi: 10.2337/dc10-1288.

Salas-Salvadó, J., M. Bullo, R. Estruch, E. Ros, M. I. Covas, N. Ibarrola-Jurado, D. Corella et al. 2014. Prevention of diabetes with Mediterranean diets: A subgroup analysis of a randomized trial. *Ann Intern Med* 160(1):1–10. doi: 10.7326/m13-1725.

Salehi-Abargouei, A., Z. Maghsoudi, F. Shirani, and L. Azadbakht. 2013. Effects of Dietary Approaches to Stop Hypertension (DASH)-style diet on fatal or nonfatal cardiovascular diseases—Incidence: A systematic review and meta-analysis on observational prospective studies. *Nutrition* 29(4):611–618. doi: 10.1016/j.nut.2012.12.018.

Schulze, M. B., T. T. Fung, J. E. Manson, W. C. Willett, and F. B. Hu. 2006. Dietary patterns and changes in body weight in women. *Obesity (Silver Spring)* 14(8):1444–1453. doi: 10.1038/oby.2006.164.

Schulze, M. B. and K. Hoffmann. 2006. Methodological approaches to study dietary patterns in relation to risk of coronary heart disease and stroke. *Br J Nutr* 95(5):860–869.

Schwingshackl, L. and G. Hoffmann. 2015. Diet quality as assessed by the Healthy Eating Index, the Alternate Healthy Eating Index, the Dietary Approaches to Stop Hypertension score, and health outcomes: A systematic review and meta-analysis of cohort studies. *J Acad Nutr Diet* 115(5):780–800.e5. doi: 10.1016/j.jand.2014.12.009.

Schwingshackl, L., B. Missbach, J. Konig, and G. Hoffmann. 2015. Adherence to a Mediterranean diet and risk of diabetes: A systematic review and meta-analysis. *Public Health Nutr* 18(7):1292–1299. doi: 10.1017/s1368980014001542.

Shirani, F., A. Salehi-Abargouei, and L. Azadbakht. 2013. Effects of Dietary Approaches to Stop Hypertension (DASH) diet on some risk for developing type 2 diabetes: A systematic review and meta-analysis on controlled clinical trials. *Nutrition* 29(7–8):939–947. doi: 10.1016/j.nut.2012.12.021.

Singh, R. B., G. Dubnov, M. A. Niaz, S. Ghosh, R. Singh, S. S. Rastogi, O. Manor, D. Pella, and E. M. Berry. 2002. Effect of an Indo-Mediterranean diet on progression of coronary artery disease in high risk patients (Indo-Mediterranean Diet Heart Study): A randomised single-blind trial. *Lancet* 360(9344):1455–1461. doi: 10.1016/s0140-6736(02)11472-3.

Sofi, F., C. Macchi, R. Abbate, G. F. Gensini, and A. Casini. 2014. Mediterranean diet and health status: An updated meta-analysis and a proposal for a literature-based adherence score. *Public Health Nutr* 17(12):2769–2782. doi: 10.1017/s1368980013003169.

Tande, D. L., R. Magel, and B. N. Strand. 2010. Healthy Eating Index and abdominal obesity. *Public Health Nutr* 13(2):208–214. doi: 10.1017/s1368980009990723.

Tortosa, A., M. Bes-Rastrollo, A. Sanchez-Villegas, F. J. Basterra-Gortari, J. M. Nunez-Cordoba, and M. A. Martinez-Gonzalez. 2007. Mediterranean diet inversely associated with the incidence of metabolic syndrome: The SUN prospective cohort. *Diabetes Care* 30(11):2957–2959. doi: 10.2337/dc07-1231.

Trichopoulou, A., T. Costacou, C. Bamia, and D. Trichopoulos. 2003. Adherence to a Mediterranean diet and survival in a Greek population. *N Engl J Med* 348(26):2599–2608. doi: 10.1056/NEJMoa025039.

United Kingdom Department of Health. 1994. Nutritional aspects of cardiovascular disease. Committee on Medical Aspects of Food Policy. Report on Health and Social Subjects No 46. HMSO, London, U.K.

United States Department of Agriculture. February 2015a. Scientific report of the 2015 Dietary Guidelines Advisory Committee: Advisory to the Secretary of Health and Human Services and the Secretary of Agriculture. Accessed March 1 2015. Available from http://www.health.gov/dietaryguidelines/2015-scientific-report/PDFs/Scientific-Report-of-the-2015-Dietary-Guidelines-Advisory-Committee.pdf.

United States Department of Agriculture. February 2015b. Scientific report of the 2015 Dietary Guidelines Advisory Committee: Advisory to the Secretary of Health and Human Services and the Secretary of Agriculture; Part B. Chapter 2: 2015 DGAC themes and recommendations: Integrating the evidence, p. 2. Accessed March 1, 2015. Available from http://www.health.gov/dietaryguidelines/2015-scientific-report/PDFs/Scientific-Report-of-the-2015-Dietary-Guidelines-Advisory-Committee.pdf.

United States Department of Agriculture National Evidence Library. 2014. A series of systematic reviews on the relationship between dietary patterns and health outcomes. United States Department of Agriculture, 2014 [cited November 5, 2014]. Available from http://www.nel.gov/vault/2440/web/files/DietaryPatterns/DPRptFullFinal.pdf.

Urpi-Sarda, M., R. Casas, G. Chiva-Blanch, E. S. Romero-Mamani, P. Valderas-Martinez, S. Arranz, C. Andres-Lacueva et al. 2012. Virgin olive oil and nuts as key foods of the Mediterranean diet effects on inflammatory biomakers related to atherosclerosis. *Pharmacol Res* 65(6):577–583. doi: 10.1016/j.phrs.2012.03.006.

Wang, D. D., C. W. Leung, Y. Li, E. L. Ding, S. E. Chiuve, F. B. Hu, and W. C. Willett. 2014. Trends in dietary quality among adults in the United States, 1999 through 2010. *JAMA Intern Med* 174(10):1587–1595.

Wang, D. D., Y. Li, S. E. Chiuve, F. B. Hu, and W. C. Willett. 2015. Improvements in US diet helped reduce disease burden and lower premature deaths, 1999–2012; But overall diet remains poor. *Health Aff* 34(11):1916–1922.

Willett, W. 2012. *Nutritional Epidemiology*. Oxford University Press, New York.

Wu, P. Y., C. L. Huang, W. S. Lei, and S. H. Yang. 2016. Alternative health eating index and the Dietary Guidelines from American Diabetes Association both may reduce the risk of cardiovascular disease in type 2 diabetes patients. *J Hum Nutr Diet* 29(3):363–373.

Yokoyama, Y., K. Nishimura, N. D. Barnard, M. Takegami, M. Watanabe, A. Sekikawa, T. Okamura, and Y. Miyamoto. 2014. Vegetarian diets and blood pressure: A meta-analysis. *JAMA Intern Med* 174(4):577–587. doi: 10.1001/jamainternmed.2013.14547.

Zhang, X., L. Shu, C. Si, X. Yu, W. Gao, D. Liao, L. Zhang, X. Liu, and P. Zheng. 2015. Dietary patterns and risk of stroke in adults: A systematic review and meta-analysis of prospective cohort studies. *J Stroke Cerebrovasc Dis* 24(10):2173–2182.

22 The Mediterranean Diet to Prevent Type 2 Diabetes and Cardiovascular Disease

Michel de Lorgeril

CONTENTS

ABSTRACT

The traditional Mediterranean diet (MD) was shown to be associated with a lower incidence of cardiovascular disease (CVD) in the 1950s. Randomized controlled trials and epidemiological studies have subsequently reported lower CVD rates in people following a traditional or a "modernized" form of MD. In 1994 and 1999, the reports of the intermediate and final analyses of the trial *Lyon Diet Heart Study* showed a striking protection of the MD against CVD complications. In 2003, a major epidemiological study in Greece showed a strong inverse association between a "*Mediterranean diet score*" and the risk of cardiovascular complications. In 2011–2012, several reports showed that even non-Mediterranean populations can gain benefits from long-term adherence to the MD. In 2013, the PREDIMED trial demonstrated a significant risk reduction of CVD complications with MD in a lower risk population than that of the Lyon trial. Contrary to the pharmacological approach, the adoption of MD is also associated with a significant reduction in new cancers and overall mortality. Thus, in terms of evidence-based medicine, the full adoption of a modern version of the MD pattern should be considered as one of the most effective approaches for the prevention of CVD complications. On the other hand, there is a worldwide type 2 diabetes epidemic with no clear biological explanation. Lifestyle factors are probably important and lifestyle interventions, including physical exercise and healthy nutrition, have been proposed to prevent type 2 diabetes and its complications. The optimal dietary pattern seems to be again the MD model that appears to also be the most appropriate to maintain the pleasure of eating—and therefore the long-term adherence to the MD pattern—and thus protect against the main complications of type 2 diabetes, that is, cardiovascular diseases and cancers, and to prolong survival with a good quality of life.

INTRODUCTION

A number of diets have received attention for their potential health effect. One of them, the Mediterranean diet (MD), has been evaluated in many clinical and epidemiological studies. Before examining these studies, we must define what the MD is.

The definition varies with experts and geography. The traditional dietary habits of the Italians are not those of the Spaniards, and those of the Greeks are not those of the Moroccans, to make the story short. All of them, however, live close to the Mediterranean Sea. An acceptable definition of the MD could be that it is a modern nutritional pattern inspired by the traditional dietary habits of Greece and southern Italy. The principal components include consumption of olive oil, legumes, unrefined cereals, nuts, and vegetables; moderate consumption of fish and wine; and low consumption of animal products except fermented dairy products made from sheep and goat's milk (see Box 22.1 for additional comments).

Each aspect deserves comment, although a full description of that complex dietary pattern is not possible here. We can take the *dietary fat issue* as an example of its complexity.

The Mediterranean dietary fat issue cannot be summarized—qualitatively and quantitatively—with a single statement about olive oil. We must indicate the approximate amounts of each type of fat provided by the (traditional or modernized) MD in comparison with the typical Western diet. It is important to differentiate the monounsaturated fatty acid oleic acid provided by olive oil (or other vegetable oils) and the oleic acid provided by animal fat, although it is the same chemical. Also, it is important to separate the different categories of *essential* polyunsaturated fatty acids (omega-6 vs. omega-3) and to differentiate the sources of omega-3 (plant vs. marine) and of omega-6 (plant vs. meat). Finally, it is critical to separate industrial and natural (ruminant) *trans* fatty acids. All these items are critical to understand the "modern" concept of MD. They are probably more important than, for instance, the "total fat intake" when analyzing the MD concept compared to the Western diet. Conventional issues such as "low fat" versus "high fat" are not relevant when comparing the Western diet and the MD. In other words, it is quite clear that both "high fat" and "low fat" MD are similarly protective against CVD complications.

Type 2 diabetes (T2D) is a devastating disease with rapidly increasing prevalence worldwide; a similar evolution is seen with the metabolic syndromes [1,2]. They are characterized by insulin resistance, defined as a decreased ability of insulin to exert its metabolic effects in key target tissues, despite an elevation of insulin blood levels [3,4]. Besides cardiovascular, infectious, eye and kidney diseases, other critical complications of T2D and insulin resistance are cancers [5–8]. The prevention of T2D and metabolic syndromes is therefore critical to protect health in general. The biological explanations of the worldwide T2D epidemic are unknown. However, it is usually accepted that lifestyle factors are probably key to this issue. In contrast, it is important to recall that most of the drugs prescribed to supposedly prevent CVD by reducing cholesterol levels (and blood pressure) increase insulin resistance and the risk of T2D [9–23]. These major toxic side effects, in particular those of statins, are usually underestimated by scientists working with the pharmaceutical industry [9–14]. In fact, most trial data (and meta-analyses) are derived from commercial studies entailing major conflicts of interest [19–21]. In contrast, studies independent from the industry clearly show that statins greatly increase insulin resistance and the risk of T2D [15,16]. Biological mechanisms of statin toxicity have been partly identified [9,17]. At the same time, the protective effects of statins against CVD complications in diabetics remain debatable [18–22]. For instance, the main meta-analysis pooling the results of studies examining the effects of statins in diabetics [22] was obviously flawed [18].

Finally, as T2D and insulin resistance increase the risk of many diseases, including cancer [5], the claims that the protective effects of statins against CVD complications in T2D patients outweigh their toxic effects appear terribly naive [11–14]. Finally, most drugs used to control blood glucose levels and to prevent T2D, and the risk of CVD complications, may be considerably less effective—probably not effective at all—than previously suspected [23–26]. Thus, it is critical to define nondrug treatments to prevent T2D, insulin resistance, and their various—not only CVD—complications. Lifestyle interventions, including physical exercise and healthy nutrition, have been proposed [27–30]. Nutrition is critical in preventing T2D, managing existing T2D, and preventing—or slowing—the development of T2D complications [31]. According to the American Diabetic Association (ADA), the main goals of nutrition in individuals with T2D are to maintain blood glucose levels in the "normal" range, achieve a lipoprotein profile that reduces CVD risk (in accordance with the so-called "conventional" targets), maintain blood pressure levels within the normal range, prevent (or slow) the development of the various complications of T2D, address individual nutrition needs, and maintain the pleasure of eating by only limiting food choices when indicated by scientific evidence [31].

The next question is: what is the best nutritional approach to achieve these goals?

There are still controversies regarding the importance of reducing total energy intake, total fat intake, specific fat intake, carbohydrate intake, and/or the benefits of foods with a low glycemic index [32–34].

So far, the optimal dietary pattern to meet the ADA goals [31] seems to be the MD model, which is, on the other hand, the most appropriate to maintain the (gastronomic) pleasure of eating and thus actually protect against the main complications of T2D—CVD and cancers—and to prolong survival with a good quality of life [35–38]. What is the scientific evidence for this claim?

THE MEDITERRANEAN DIET PATTERN: HISTORY, EPIDEMIOLOGY, AND RANDOMIZED TRIALS

The term MD was first coined by a nonphysician American scientist (Ancel Keys) who observed a lower mortality rate from CVD among people living in Greece—as well as certain parts of Italy and the former Yugoslavia—than in Western cohorts (United States and the Netherlands, for instance), while conducting large multinational studies in the 1950s through 1980s [39–41], in particular the *Seven Countries Study*. As this study was observational and failed to demonstrate a cause–effect relationship, the concept of MD was not widely recognized until the 1990s.

It was in 1994, when the preliminary results of the *Lyon Diet Heart Study*, a randomized controlled trial testing a modern version of the MD in survivors of a prior acute myocardial infarction, were reported [35] that the MD began to be accepted as a major scientific concept to prevent CVD complications. The *Lyon trial* data were published in two steps. The first, in 1994, was the report of intermediate results after an average follow-up of 27 months [35], upon the request of the Scientific Committee whose members intended to stimulate the replication of the trial results in different conditions (and countries). The second step was the final report, which was published in 1999 [36] after a follow-up of about 4 years and 275 CVD endpoints. The delay—from 27 months to 4 years—was due to the time needed to recontact and determine the health status of all the patients. Thus, the total duration of the trial was ultimately close to the follow-up initially calculated to test the primary hypothesis. Contrary to the claims of certain scientists, the *Lyon trial* was not prematurely terminated. Not only was an impressive 50%–70% reduction in the risk of new heart attack or CVD complication demonstrated among patients in the MD group, but fewer cancers were also observed, as well as a significant reduction of all-cause mortality [36,37]. Because of these impressive data, experts of the French National Institute for Health Research (INSERM) were commissioned to thoroughly review the individual raw data, the whole dataset, and the analyses in the *Lyon trial*, but failed to identify significant bias [42], which confirmed the validity of the trial results.

Curiously, there have been misunderstandings about the MD tested in the *Lyon trial*, the main one related to the omega-3-rich rapeseed oil margarine that was used to replace butter and cream in the MD group. Butter and cream were still intensively used at that time in the area around the city of Lyon, where the patients were recruited. It was therefore essential to obtain good compliance of the patients with the experimental MD by offering them an acceptable substitute, the rapeseed oil margarine. There have been claims that the *Lyon trial* was in fact testing the effects of omega-3 fatty acids. This is wrong. As shown in the *Seven Countries Study* when comparing the blood fatty acid patterns of the Greek and Dutch cohorts [43], it was clear that the Greek diet was traditionally rich in the plant omega-3 alpha-linolenic acid (ALA). At the time of the *Lyon trial*, however, the exact dietary sources of ALA in the Greek diet were not known. Since then, Simopoulos and others have identified some of the ALA-rich plants consumed in the Mediterranean areas [44,45], explaining the high blood ALA levels observed in the Greek cohort, along with the low blood levels of omega-6 fatty acid linoleic acid [43]. Thus, to best mimic the traditional MD, the patients of the *Lyon trial* were advised to eat some ALA-rich foods. Olive oil being poor in ALA, rapeseed oil—with a saturated/monounsaturated fatty acid composition close to that of olive oil—was chosen as a source of dietary ALA [35–37]. Efforts were made to avoid increasing omega-6 intakes, as plasma omega-6 levels were lowest in the blood of the Greeks with the lowest mortality rate from CVD in the *Seven Countries Study* [43]. Thus, rapeseed oil was identified as the adequate edible oil, in association with olive oil, in the experimental group of the *Lyon trial* [35–37].

In summary, the *Lyon Trial* was the first trial to report health benefits of a "modernized" MD, even though some confusion remained about the true characteristics of that dietary pattern [46–50].

About 10 years after the first results of the *Lyon trial* were published [35], a new wave of scientific data about the health benefits of the MD appeared. In 2003, Trichopoulos published the first modern epidemiological study examining the health effects of the MD [51]. In a large prospective investigation, involving 22,043 adults in Greece, adherence to a MD pattern was measured through the use of a MD score: the higher the score, the lower the mortality from CVD [51]. Both death due to coronary heart disease and death due to cancer were inversely associated with greater compliance with the MD, after adjustment for many confounders including physical activity and some socioeconomic factors [51]. The Greek study thus confirmed the results of the *Lyon trial* [35–37]. Lower all-cause mortality also observed by Trichopoulos—including reduction of cancer mortality—suggested that the MD is not associated with any major adverse effect. This is a critical issue in view of the many side effects of drug-based CVD prevention [9–23]. Following the Greek study, and using similar approaches with a MD score, several groups analyzed datasets from various populations [52–54] and reported similar lower CVD and overall mortality. In brief, higher MD score was associated with lower CVD complication rates and increased life expectancy, including after adjustment for confounders such as physical activity and socioeconomic factors [52–54].

Despite these strong data, international organizations—such as the European Society of Cardiology and the American Heart Association—still did not recommend at that time the MD for CVD prevention. That "intellectual" resistance might have resulted from two factors: (1) the lack of a large randomized trial clearly confirming the findings of the *Lyon Diet Heart Study*, and (2) the use of the MD score in epidemiological studies that may have contributed to oversimplifying (and confusing) the notion of MD—modernized versus traditional—in both theory and practice. It was in that context that the *PREDIMED study* investigators reported the main results of their trial in February 2013 [55].

The Spanish investigators of the *PREDIMED study* reported that adopting a MD reduced the risk of CVD complications by 30%, and specifically the risk of stroke by 40%, over a follow-up of about 5 years [55]. In this multicenter trial involving 7500 persons, three randomized groups were compared: a control group advised to follow a low-fat diet and two experimental groups advised to follow a MD supplemented with either extra-virgin olive oil or mixed nuts. While the sample size was large, the total numbers of CVD complications were small in the three groups. This indicated that the recruited population was at very low risk. Observing a significant protective effect in this context suggests that the two dietary interventions tested were clearly effective. The analysis of the dietary habits in these three Spanish groups is likely to explain the low rate of CVD complications in the entire study: in fact, the average diet in the three groups, including the "low-fat" control group, was a Mediterranean-type of diet known to be cardioprotective. As a consequence, the differences between the three groups for most of the Mediterranean diet items were small; for certain items, such as the use of olive oil as main culinary fat, wine drinking, the consumption of commercial wheat baked products, and others, the differences were small and even not statistically significant [55]. Observing a significant protection in this context suggests that the whole Mediterranean dietary pattern—and the interactions between various nutrients—was the real biological source of protection, rather than any small difference in specific nutrients. The *PREDIMED study* is thus a confirmation of the *Lyon trial* and of the Trichopoulos study data.

In terms of specific foods, the main differences explaining the different complication rates in the three groups were essentially the wide use of extra-virgin olive oil in one experimental group and the consumption of mixed nuts in the other one. Biomarkers of the consumption of these foods were measured and higher levels of the plant omega-3 ALA in the mixed nuts group and a higher urinary excretion of the olive polyphenol hydroxytyrosol in the extra-virgin olive oil group were found. This is not unexpected as many studies have shown the protective effects of both omega-3 fatty acids and polyphenols (see also the Box 22.1). Further studies are required to confirm that Mediterranean polyphenols and plant omega-3 fatty acids are major factors of the health benefits of the MD pattern and also, importantly, to determine whether the modern foods consumed by the Mediterranean (and other) populations are still rich in these critical ingredients.

Thus, the *PREDIMED study* confirmed the findings of the *Lyon Diet Heart Study* [35–37] in a primary prevention setting, as well as those of the many epidemiological studies [52–54] published since Trichopoulos' 2003 report [51]. However, many questions have been raised. For instance, experts stated that "*The PREDIMED trial is neither a pure test of a Mediterranean-style diet ... Interpretation of the PREDIMED trial is similar in complexity to that of the Lyon Diet Heart Study, which tested provision of a margarine rich in alpha-linolenic acid, coupled with brief advice to consume a Mediterranean diet*" [56]. Clarification about the use of rapeseed oil in the *Lyon trial* is given in the previous section of this article. It is also noteworthy that the dietary intervention in the *Lyon trial* was not "brief advice" [35–37]. In contrast, in the same issue of the *New England Journal of Medicine*, an editorial stated that "*the Mediterranean diet has become the standard for healthy eating*" and that "*the PREDIMED results reinforce the Mediterranean diet's value for health internationally, suggesting a dietary template that may be of particular value as chronic disease becomes a global issue*" [57].

THE MEDITERRANEAN DIET IN THE PREVENTION OF TYPE 2 DIABETES

It may be clinically important to differentiate the prevention of T2D itself, on one hand, and the management of diabetic patients to prevent or delay the various complications resulting from T2D, in particular CVD complications, on the other hand. However, this may be a very theoretical distinction as careful analysis of the international literature clearly indicates that the MD prevents both the occurrence of T2D and the complications of T2D in various populations [58–65]. Not only does the MD actually reduce the risk of T2D, but this dietary pattern also reduces the rate of complications, in particular CVD

BOX 22.1 MEDITERRANEAN DIET AND POLYPHENOLS

Generally speaking, both the traditional and "modernized" Mediterranean diets are rich in cereals (especially wheat), legumes, vegetables and fruits and quite poor in animal foods.

The consumption of seafood is variable, and the main everyday beverages (other than water) are extremely rich in **polyphenols**, that is, wine on the Christian North bank of the sea, tea on the Muslim South bank. This is an important aspect as plant polyphenols, especially those found in typical Mediterranean foods such as olive products, may be useful for the prevention of insulin resistance and T2D [1,2]. Other polyphenols—such as the anthocyanins found in grapes and wine—have been shown to increase the endogenous synthesis (from the plant precursor alpha-linolenic acid) of the marine very long-chain omega-3 fatty acids [3,4]. It is noteworthy that both plant and marine omega-3—which are major substances in the traditional Mediterranean diet—were shown to be inversely associated with the risk of T2D, in particular alpha-linolenic acid found in plants [5]. As discussed in this chapter, alpha-linolenic acid is a major component of the Mediterranean diet.

REFERENCES

1. de Bock M, Derraik JG, Brennan CM, Biggs JB, Morgan PE, Hodgkinson SC, Hofman PL, Cutfield WS. Olive (*Olea europaea* L.) leaf polyphenols improve insulin sensitivity in middle-aged overweight men: A randomized, placebo-controlled, crossover trial. *PLoS One*. 2013;8(3):e57622.
2. Wainstein J, Ganz T, Boaz M, Bar Dayan Y, Dolev E, Kerem Z, Madar Z. Olive leaf extract as a hypoglycemic agent in both human diabetic subjects and in rats. *J Med Food*. July 2012;15(7):605–610.
3. de Lorgeril M, Salen P, Martin JL. Interactions of wine drinking with omega-3 fatty acids in patients with coronary heart disease: A fish-like effect of moderate wine drinking. *Am Heart J*. 2008;155:175–181.
4. Toufektsian MC, Salen P, Laporte F, Tonelli C, de Lorgeril M. Dietary flavonoids increase plasma very long-chain (n-3) fatty acids in rats. *J Nutr*. 2011;141:37–41.
5. Feskens EJ. The prevention of type 2 diabetes: Should we recommend vegetable oils instead of fatty fish? *Am J Clin Nutr*. August 2011;94(2):369–370.

complications, associated with T2D. This is not very surprising, since the major foods that characterize the MD are each individually linked with the risks of T2D and its complications [66–68].

One major issue that remains to be studied is whether typical Mediterranean foods with prebiotic properties play a role in the modulation of the T2D risks. Actually, data in animals, but also observational studies in patients, have suggested that the composition of gut microbiota differs in patients with diabetes versus patients without diabetes [69].

Finally, in addition to adhering to a MD, it is critical for the prevention of T2D in our societies to stop taking (and prescribing) drugs with prodiabetic effects with the aim of reducing cholesterol, blood glucose, or blood pressure [9–17].

CONCLUSIONS

Observational studies and randomized trials indicate that the MD may be considered as an effective nutritional approach to CVD reduction in particular in patients at high risk for diabetes. Recommendations should be adapted depending on geographic location, the cultural or religious background, and the available foods in each geographical area, in order to obtain long-term compliance. This is what we call the "modernized" Mediterranean diet.

One difficulty is the fact that many foods offered to consumers at the present time do not contain the nutrients expected to be present in those traditionally consumed by Mediterranean populations because of the modern practices of crop farming and modern techniques of the food industry.

Some of our foods are not those that could be found in grocery shops and open-air markets in the 1950s through 1970s. For example, the bread consumed today differs from the bread consumed by our grandparents, because the wheat varieties that are grown and harvested today are genetically and biologically very different from the wheat of the 1950s through 1970s [70,71].

Although this dietary pattern has been proposed as yielding long life expectancy, recent research has found that certain Mediterranean populations are giving up their traditional dietary habits and associated healthy lifestyles to adopt unhealthy Westernized food patterns instead. Recent studies have shown that people with little education, overweight, or diabetes and those who were less physically active, single, divorced or separated, or smokers, were less likely to comply with the MD [72]. These groups will require special educational efforts.

REFERENCES

1. Lam DW, LeRoith D. The worldwide diabetes epidemic. *Curr Opin Endocrinol Diabetes Obes*. 2012;19:93–96.
2. Seidell JC. Obesity, insulin resistance and diabetes—A worldwide epidemic. *Br J Nutr*. 2000;83(Suppl 1):S5–S8.
3. Haffner SM. The insulin resistance syndrome revisited. *Diabetes Care*. 1996;19:275–277.
4. Hanley AJ, Williams K, Stern MP, Haffner SM. Homeostasis model assessment of insulin resistance in relation to the incidence of cardiovascular disease: The San Antonio Heart Study. *Diabetes Care*. 2002;25:1177–1184.
5. Emerging Risk Factors Collaboration, Seshasai SR, Kaptoge S, Thompson A et al. Diabetes mellitus, fasting glucose, and risk of cause-specific death. *N Engl J Med*. 2011;364:829–841; Erratum, *N Engl J Med*. 2011;364:1281.
6. Smith U, Gale EA. Cancer and diabetes: Are we ready for prime time? *Diabetologia*. 2010;53:1541–1544.
7. Pollak M. Insulin and insulin-like growth factor signalling in neoplasia. *Nat Rev Cancer*. 2008;8:915–928; Erratum, *Nat Rev Cancer*. 2009;9:224.
8. Hirakawa Y, Ninomiya T, Mukai N et al. Association between glucose tolerance level and cancer death in a general Japanese population: The Hisayama Study. *Am J Epidemiol*. November 15, 2012;176(10):856–864.
9. Goldstein MR, Mascitelli L. Do statins cause diabetes? *Curr Diab Rep*. 2013;13:381–390.
10. Danaei G, Rodríguez LA, Cantero OF, Hernán MA. Statins and risk of diabetes: An analysis of electronic medical records to evaluate possible bias due to differential survival. *Diabetes Care* 2013;36:1236–1240.

11. Sattar N, Preiss D, Murray HM et al. Statins and risk of incident diabetes: A collaborative meta-analysis of randomised statin trials. *Lancet*. February 27, 2010;375(9716):735–742.
12. Preiss D, Seshasai SR, Welsh P et al. Risk of incident diabetes with intensive-dose compared with moderate-dose statin therapy: A meta-analysis. *JAMA*. June 22, 2011;305(24):2556–2564.
13. Izzo R, de Simone G, Trimarco V et al. Primary prevention with statins and incident diabetes in hypertensive patients at high cardiovascular risk. *Nutr Metab Cardiovasc Dis*. 2013;23:1101–1106.
14. Axsom K, Berger JS, Schwartzbard AZ. Statins and diabetes: The good, the bad, and the unknown. *Curr Atheroscler Rep*. February 2013;15(2):299.
15. Culver AL, Ockene IS, Balasubramanian R et al. Statin use and risk of diabetes mellitus in postmenopausal women in the Women's Health Initiative. *Arch Intern Med*. 2012;172:144–152.
16. Koh KK, Quon MJ, Han SH, Lee Y, Kim SJ, Shin EK. Atorvastatin causes insulin resistance and increases ambient glycemia in hypercholesterolemic patients. *J Am Coll Cardiol*. 2010;55:1209–1216.
17. de Lorgeril M, Salen P, Defaye P, Rabaeus M. Recent findings on the health effects of omega-3 fatty acids and statins, and their interactions: Do statins inhibit omega-3? *BMC Med*. January 4, 2013;11:5.
18. de Lorgeril M, Hamazaki T, Kostucki W et al. Is the use of cholesterol-lowering drugs for the prevention of cardiovascular complications in type 2 diabetics evidence-based? A systematic review. *Rev Recent Clin Trials*. 2012;7:150–157.
19. Colhoun HM, Betteridge DJ, Durrington PN et al. CARDS Investigators. Primary prevention of cardiovascular disease with atorvastatin in type 2 diabetes in the Collaborative Atorvastatin Diabetes Study (CARDS): Multicentre randomised placebo-controlled trial. *Lancet*. 2004;364:685–696.
20. Knopp RH, d'Emden M, Smilde JG, Pocock SJ. Efficacy and safety of atorvastatin in the prevention of cardiovascular end points in subjects with type 2 diabetes: The Atorvastatin Study for Prevention of Coronary Heart Disease Endpoints in non-insulin-dependent diabetes mellitus (ASPEN). *Diabetes Care*. 2006;29:1478–1485.
21. Wanner C, Krane V, März W et al. German Diabetes and Dialysis Study Investigators. Atorvastatin in patients with type 2 diabetes mellitus undergoing hemodialysis. *N Engl J Med*. 2005;353:238–248.
22. Cholesterol Treatment Trialists' Collaborators, Kearney PM, Blackwell L, Collins R et al. Efficacy of cholesterol-lowering therapy in 18,686 people with diabetes in 14 randomised trials of statins. *Lancet*. 2008;371:117–125.
23. Boussageon R, Supper I, Bejan-Angoulvant T et al. Reappraisal of metformin efficacy in the treatment of type 2 diabetes: A meta-analysis of randomised controlled trials. *PLoS Med*. 2012;9(4):e1001204.
24. Hemmingsen B, Lund SS, Gluud C et al. Intensive glycaemic control for patients with type 2 diabetes: Systematic review with meta-analysis and trial sequential analysis of randomised clinical trials. *BMJ*. November 24, 2011;343:d6898.
25. Ray KK, Seshasai SR, Wijesuriya S et al. Effect of intensive control of glucose on cardiovascular outcomes and death in patients with diabetes mellitus: A meta-analysis of randomised controlled trials. *Lancet*. May 23, 2009;373(9677):1765–1772.
26. Boussageon R, Bejan-Angoulvant T, Saadatian-Elahi M et al. Effect of intensive glucose lowering treatment on all-cause mortality, cardiovascular death, and microvascular events in type 2 diabetes: Meta-analysis of randomised controlled trials. *BMJ*. July 26, 2011;343:d4169.
27. Knowler WC, Barrett-Connor E, Fowler SE et al. Diabetes Prevention Program Research Group. Reduction in the incidence of type 2 diabetes with lifestyle intervention or metformin. *N Engl J Med*. 2002;346:393–403.
28. Lindström J, Peltonen M, Eriksson JG et al. Finnish Diabetes Prevention Study (DPS). Improved lifestyle and decreased diabetes risk over 13 years: Long-term follow-up of the randomised Finnish Diabetes Prevention Study (DPS). *Diabetologia*. February 2013;56(2):284–293.
29. Uusitupa M, Peltonen M, Lindström J et al. Finnish Diabetes Prevention Study Group. Ten-year mortality and cardiovascular morbidity in the Finnish Diabetes Prevention Study—Secondary analysis of the randomized trial. *PLoS One*. May 21, 2009;4(5):e5656.
30. Li G, Zhang P, Wang J et al. The long-term effect of lifestyle interventions to prevent diabetes in the China Da Qing Diabetes Prevention Study: A 20-year follow-up study. *Lancet*. May 24, 2008;371(9626):1783–1789.
31. American Diabetes Association, Evert AB, Boucher JL Cypress M et al. Nutrition therapy recommendations for the management of adults with diabetes. *Diabetes Care*. 2013;36(11):3821–3842.
32. Ajala O, English P, Pinkney J. Systematic review and meta-analysis of different dietary approaches to the management of type 2 diabetes. *Am J Clin Nutr*. March 2013;97(3):505–516.
33. Nield L, Summerbell CD, Hooper L, Whittaker V, Moore H. Dietary advice for the prevention of type 2 diabetes mellitus in adults. *Cochrane Database Syst Rev*. July 16 2008;(3):CD005102. doi: 10.1002/14651858.CD005102.pub2.

34. Franz MJ. Diabetes mellitus nutrition therapy: Beyond the glycemic index. *Arch Intern Med*. November 26, 2012;172(21):1660–1661.
35. de Lorgeril M, Renaud S, Mamelle N. Mediterranean alpha-linolenic acid-rich diet in secondary prevention of coronary heart disease. *Lancet*. 1994;343:1454–1459.
36. de Lorgeril M, Salen P, Martin JL. Mediterranean diet, traditional risk factors and the rate of cardiovascular complications after myocardial infarction. Final report of the Lyon Diet Heart Study. *Circulation*. 1999;99:779–785.
37. de Lorgeril M, Salen P, Martin JL et al. Mediterranean dietary pattern in a randomized trial: Prolonged survival and possible reduced cancer rate. *Arch Intern Med*. 1998;158:1181–1187.
38. de Lorgeril M, Salen P. The Mediterranean diet: Rationale and evidence for its benefit. *Curr Atheroscler Rep*. 2008;10:518–522.
39. Keys A. *Seven Countries: A Multivariate Analysis of Death and Coronary Heart Disease*. Boston, MA, Harvard University Press, 1980.
40. Keys A, Menotti A, Karvonen MJ et al. The diet and 15-year death rate in the seven countries study. *Am J Epidemiol*. 1986;124(6):903–915.
41. Keys A. Mediterranean diet and public health: Personal reflections. *Am J Clin Nutr*. 1995;61 (6 Suppl):1321S–1323S.
42. de Lorgeril M, Salen P, Caillat-Vallet E et al. Control of bias in dietary trial to prevent coronary recurrences: The Lyon Diet Heart Study. *Eur J Clin Nutr*. 1997;51(2):116–122.
43. Sandker GW, Kromhout D, Aravanis C et al. Serum cholesteryl ester fatty acids and their relation with serum lipids in elderly men in Crete and The Netherlands. *Eur J Clin Nutr*. 1993;47(3):201–208.
44. Simopoulos AP. Omega-3 fatty acids and antioxidants in edible wild plants. *Biol Res*. 2004;37(2):263–277.
45. Zeghichi S, Kallithraka S, Simopoulos AP, Kypriotakis Z. Nutritional composition of selected wild plants in the diet of Crete. *World Rev Nutr Diet*. 2003;91:22–40.
46. Willett WC. The Mediterranean diet: Science and practice. *Public Health Nutr*. 2006;9(1A):105–110.
47. Willett WC. *Eat, Drink, and Be Healthy: The Harvard Medical School Guide to Healthy Eating*. Boston, MA, Free Press, 2005.
48. Ascherio A, Willett WC. New directions in dietary studies of coronary heart disease. *J Nutr*. 1995;125 (3 Suppl):647S–655S.
49. Trichopoulos D. In defense of the Mediterranean diet. *Eur J Clin Nutr*. 2002;56(9):928–929.
50. Ferro-Luzzi A, James WP, Kafatos A. The high-fat Greek diet: A recipe for all? *Eur J Clin Nutr*. 2002;56(9):796–809.
51. Trichopoulos A, Costacou T, Bamia C, Trichopoulos D. Adherence to a Mediterranean diet and survival in a Greek population. *N Engl J Med*. 2003;348(26):2599–2608.
52. Knoops KT, de Groot LC, Kromhout D et al. Mediterranean diet, lifestyle factors, and 10-year mortality in elderly European men and women. *JAMA*. 2004;292:1433–1439.
53. Mitrou PN, Kipnis V, Thiébaut AC et al. Mediterranean dietary pattern and prediction of all-cause mortality in a US population. *Arch Intern Med*. 2007;167:2461–2468.
54. Fung TT, Rexrode KM, Mantzoros CS, Manson JE, Willett WC, Hu FB. Mediterranean diet and incidence of and mortality from coronary heart disease and stroke in women. *Circulation*. 2009;119:1093–1100.
55. Estruch R, Ros E, Salas-Salvadó J et al. PREDIMED Study Investigators. Primary prevention of cardiovascular disease with a Mediterranean diet. *N Engl J Med*. 2013;368(14):1279–1290.
56. Appel LJ, Van Horn L. Did the PREDIMED trial test a Mediterranean diet? *N Engl J Med*. 2013;368(14):1353–1354.
57. Tracy SW. Something new under the sun? The Mediterranean diet and cardiovascular health. *N Engl J Med*. 2013;368(14):1274–1276.
58. Domínguez LJ, Bes-Rastrollo M, de la Fuente-Arrillaga C, Toledo E, Beunza JJ, Barbagallo M, Martínez-González MA. Similar prediction of decreased total mortality, diabetes incidence or cardiovascular events using relative- and absolute-component Mediterranean diet score: The SUN cohort. *Nutr Metab Cardiovasc Dis* 2013;23:451–458.
59. Esposito K, Maiorino MI, Ciotola M, Di Palo C, Scognamiglio P, Gicchino M, Petrizzo M et al. Effects of a Mediterranean-style diet on the need for antihyperglycemic drug therapy in patients with newly diagnosed type 2 diabetes: A randomized trial. *Ann Intern Med*. September 1, 2009;151(5):306–314.
60. Hodge AM, English DR, Itsiopoulos C, O'Dea K, Giles GG. Does a Mediterranean diet reduce the mortality risk associated with diabetes: Evidence from the Melbourne Collaborative Cohort Study. *Nutr Metab Cardiovasc Dis*. September 2011;21(9):733–739.
61. Sjögren P, Becker W, Warensjö E, Olsson E, Byberg L, Gustafsson IB, Karlström B, Cederholm T. Mediterranean and carbohydrate-restricted diets and mortality among elderly men: A cohort study in Sweden. *Am J Clin Nutr*. October 2010;92(4):967–974.

62. Abiemo EE, Alonso A, Nettleton JA, Steffen LM, Bertoni AG, Jain A, Lutsey PL. Relationships of the Mediterranean dietary pattern with insulin resistance and diabetes incidence in the Multi-Ethnic Study of Atherosclerosis (MESA). *Br J Nutr*. 2013;109:1490–1497.
63. Salas-Salvadó J, Bulló M, Babio N et al. PREDIMED Study Investigators. Reduction in the incidence of type 2 diabetes with the Mediterranean diet: Results of the PREDIMED-Reus nutrition intervention randomized trial. *Diabetes Care*. January 2011;34(1):14–19.
64. InterAct Consortium, Romaguera D, Guevara M, Norat T et al. Mediterranean diet and type 2 diabetes risk in the European Prospective Investigation into Cancer and Nutrition (EPIC) study: The InterAct project. *Diabetes Care*. September 2011;34(9):1913–1918.
65. Itsiopoulos C, Brazionis L, Kaimakamis M, Cameron M, Best JD, O'Dea K, Rowley K. Can the Mediterranean diet lower HbA1c in type 2 diabetes? Results from a randomized cross-over study. *Nutr Metab Cardiovasc Dis*. September 2011;21(9):740–777.
66. Feskens EJ, Sluik D, van Woudenbergh GJ. Meat consumption, diabetes, and its complications. *Curr Diab Rep*. April 2013;13(2):298–306.
67. Beulens JW, van der Schouw YT, Bergmann MM et al. InterAct Consortium. Alcohol consumption and risk of type 2 diabetes in European men and women: Influence of beverage type and body size The EPIC-InterAct study. *J Intern Med*. October 2012;272(4):358–370.
68. de Lorgeril M. PREDIMED trial: Mediterranean diet may reduce the risk of type 2 diabetes. *Evid Based Med*. October 2011;16(5):152–153.
69. Delzenne NM, Neyrinck AM, Cani PD. Gut microbiota and metabolic disorders: How prebiotic can work? *Br J Nutr*. January 2013;109(Suppl 2):S81–S85.
70. Hedden P. The genes of the Green Revolution. *Trends Genet*. January 2003;19(1):5–9.
71. Song X, Ni Z, Yao Y et al. Wheat (*Triticum aestivum* L.) root proteome and differentially expressed root proteins between hybrid and parents. *Proteomics*. 2007;7(19):3538–3557.
72. Hu EA, Toledo E, Diez-Espino J et al. Lifestyles and risk factors associated with adherence to the Mediterranean diet: A baseline assessment of the PREDIMED trial. *PLoS One*. 2013;8(4):e60166.

23 The DASH Diet

Catherine M. Champagne

CONTENTS

ABSTRACT

This chapter describes the Dietary Approaches to Stop Hypertension (DASH) feeding trials and subsequent studies undertaken in free-living individuals that evolved from DASH: the PREMIER and Weight Loss Maintenance intervention trials. The DASH trials demonstrated efficacy of an intervention that emphasized the intake of fruits, vegetables, and low-fat dairy products with higher protein and lower dietary fat intake, in lowering blood pressure. This was followed by the PREMIER and Weight Loss Maintenance trials that showed the effectiveness of the DASH diet in a more realistic clinical setting. While the results were less robust, participants were able to lower their blood pressure in a free-living environment. The DASH diet has been used in many other studies with modifications that show that other sources of protein can be used and that full-fat dairy products are as effective as low-fat dairy products. These primarily address cardiometabolic health and include improvements in lipid profiles and cardiovascular biomarkers, kidney disease, heart failure and stroke, all-cause mortality, and some cancers. The DASH diet is effective in all age groups and in different ethnicities. A number of health organizations have endorsed the DASH diet including it as a recommended dietary pattern in the Dietary Guidelines. It has been selected as the best overall diet in the United States by U.S. News and World Report.

DEVELOPMENT OF THE DASH DIET AND VALIDATION IN THE DASH-SODIUM STUDY

THE DASH (DIETARY APPROACHES TO STOP HYPERTENSION) TRIAL (APPEL ET AL. 1997)

Hypertension is a major public health problem with significant cardiovascular risk. At the time the DASH trial began, efforts to reduce the prevalence of hypertension had focused primarily on nonpharmacologic approaches that lower blood pressure. Among these recommendations were weight control, reduced intake of sodium chloride primarily as salt, reduced alcohol consumption, and possibly increased dietary potassium and calcium.

Observational studies showed significant inverse associations of blood pressure with intake of magnesium, potassium, calcium, fiber, and protein. However, in trials that tested these nutrients, often as dietary supplements, the reduction in blood pressure has typically been small and inconsistent. To test the concept that combining these nutrients through dietary patterns would be more effective, the National Heart Lung and Blood Institute initiated a call for proposals to test the effect of dietary patterns on change in blood pressure. Four institutions, including Harvard School of Public Health, Johns Hopkins School of Public Health, Duke University, and the Pennington Biomedical Research Center of Louisiana State University, were selected to develop and test different dietary patterns and the coordinating center was located at the Kaiser Permanente Center for Health Research in Portland, Oregon. The DASH (Dietary Approaches to Stop Hypertension) diet was the result of this multicenter trial. Planning for this trial began in early 1994.

Prior observational and intervention studies had revealed that vegetarians had lower blood pressures than their meat-eating counterparts (Sacks et al. 1974). Similarly, higher dietary potassium, magnesium, calcium, and fiber were associated with lower blood pressure, although trials of these agents individually had provided inconsistent results except for potassium (Vogt et al. 1999). Dietary protein and polyunsaturated fat also affected blood pressure; and where excessive amounts of protein were consumed, dietary cholesterol and saturated fat were associated with higher blood pressure (Vogt et al. 1999). Prior to the DASH study, trials of dietary protein and fat showed inconsistent results on blood pressure (Vogt et al. 1999).

The goal of the DASH trial was to identify a dietary pattern that lowered blood pressure, yet was palatable and acceptable to the general population. In the DASH trial, the nutrient targets for potassium, magnesium, and calcium were set at the 25th percentile of average consumption for the control diet and at the 75th percentile of average consumption as targets for the two "test" diets. No micronutrient supplements were used to increase micronutrient targets—as the mandate was that the difference in micronutrients was to come from natural food products. There was a 3-week run-in period, after which the participants were randomized to one of three diets for a period of 8 weeks. The first diet was a "standard American diet" with micronutrient levels for potassium, magnesium, and calcium at the 25th percentile. The second diet was the fruits and vegetables diet that contained fruits and vegetables in amounts sufficient to raise the potassium and magnesium intake to the 75th percentile of average intake; the third diet, known as the DASH, was designed with higher fruits and vegetables and low-fat dairy products to raise potassium, magnesium, and calcium to the 75th percentile of average intake. This diet also had 18% protein and 27% total fat. Sodium intake was constant across the three diets. Participants were recruited from the respective communities and randomized to one of the three diets. Food was provided, with 1 or 2 meals eaten on-site and the other as a takeout meal. Weekend food was also taken home on Friday.

The composition of the three diets is shown in the following:

1. The control diet was an average American diet, high in fat, with the following targets:
    a. Total fat at 37% of energy, and high in saturated fat (16% of energy)
    b. Moderate in protein at 15% of energy, with 48% of energy from carbohydrate and low in fiber at about 9 g/2000 kcal
    c. Fairly low in potassium—1700 mg/2000 kcal
    d. Low in magnesium—165 mg/2000 kcal
    e. Low in calcium—450 mg/2000 kcal
2. The fruit and vegetable diet (sometimes referred to as the intermediate diet) contained the same macronutrient targets as the control diet, with the difference being that the micronutrient targets were obtained by the addition of fruits and vegetables:
    a. Fiber was increased to about 31 g/2000 kcal.
    b. Potassium and magnesium were almost three times that of the control diet:
        i. Potassium was 4700 mg/2000 kcal
        ii. Magnesium was 500 mg/2000 kcal

3. The DASH diet (sometimes referred to as the combination diet) was designed to be lower in fat and saturated fat, with the same fiber, potassium, and magnesium targets as the fruit and vegetable diet, but with the addition of a calcium target at the 25th percentile of average intake through the use of low-fat dairy products. The major differences between this diet and the other two include the following:
   - Total fat at 27% of energy, predominantly through the reduction of saturated fat to a level of 6% of energy.
   - Protein was higher, at 18% of energy, predominantly from low-fat and nonfat dairy products.
   - Carbohydrate was higher at 55% of energy.
   - Calcium was increased to three times that of the control and fruit and vegetable diets, containing approximately 1240 mg/2000 kcal, brought about primarily by dairy products.

DASH Nutrient Targets at the 2100 kcal Level

	Control	F/V	Combination
Fat (% kcal)	37	37	**27**
Sat fat (% kcal)	16	16	**6**
CHO (% kcal)	48	48	**55**
Protein (% kcal)	15	15	**18**
Fiber (g/day)	9	**31**	**31**
Potassium (mg/day)	1700	**4700**	**4700**
Magnesium (mg/day)	165	**500**	**500**
Calcium (mg/day)	450	450	**1240**
Sodium (g/day)	3–3.5	3–3.5	3–3.5

The main differences are shown in **bold** font.

Four hundred and fifty-nine (459) participants were randomized and 49% were women. Minorities represented 66% of the sample. The mean age was 45 years. Most subjects were overweight (mean BMI for women was 28.7 kg/m^2; for men was 27.7 kg/m^2). Mean blood pressure was 132/85 mmHg, with approximately 29% of the population being hypertensive.

Both systolic and diastolic blood pressures were significantly lowered in those individuals consuming both test diets, with the DASH diet (mean systolic −5.5 mmHg, mean diastolic −3.0 mmHg; compared to control, $P < 0.001$) also producing a significantly greater reduction of blood pressure than the fruits and vegetables diet. The blood pressure responses to the DASH diet are shown in Table 23.1.

The DASH diet lowered systolic and diastolic blood pressures significantly for both men and women. Minorities consuming the DASH diet had a much greater drop in both systolic and diastolic blood pressure than the nonminority groups.

The drop in blood pressure produced by the DASH diet in the hypertensive population was comparable to drug therapy. Both hypertensive and nonhypertensive individuals had blood pressure reductions that were significant with the DASH diet compared to the control diet. One important message from the DASH trial and a basis for its popularity was the suggestion that if one eats according to the DASH dietary pattern, blood pressure medications may be decreased or discontinued.

The DASH diet affected serum lipids (Obarzanek et al. 2001). Although baseline lipid values did not differ among the three treatment arms, individuals consuming the DASH diet had a reduction of 13.7 mg/dL in total cholesterol, a decrease in low-density lipoprotein cholesterol (LDL-C) of 10.7 mg/dL, and a decrease in high-density lipoprotein cholesterol (HDL-C) of 3.7 mg/dL relative to the control diet ($P < 0.001$ for each of the lipid values). This was probably due to the reduced saturated fat intake in the DASH diet. For those individuals consuming the fruit and vegetable diet, there was no change

TABLE 23.1
Blood Pressure Changes in the Dietary Approaches to Stop Hypertension (DASH) Trial and in the Dietary Approaches to Stop Hypertension (DASH)-Sodium Trial

	Blood Pressure Mean mmHg (95% CI)	
Overall (Change with Control Group Subtracted Out)	**Systolic**	**Diastolic**
DASH Trial		
DASH diet	−5.5 (−7.4 to −3.7)***	−3.0 (−4.3 to −1.6)***
Fruit and vegetable diet	−2.8 (−4.7 to −0.9)***	−1.1 (−2.4 to 0.3)
Gender effects of DASH diet		
Males	−4.9 (−7.3 to −2.5)***	−3.3 (−5.1 to −1.5)***
Females	−6.2 (−9.2 to −3.3)***	−2.7 (−4.8 to −0.7)**
Ethnicity responses to the DASH diet		
Minority population	−6.8 (−9.2 to −4.4)***	−3.5 (−5.2 to −1.8)***
Nonminority population	−3.0 (−5.9 to −0.1)*	−2.0 (−4.2 to 0.2)*
Hypertensive status and the DASH diet		
Hypertensives	−11.4 (−15.9 to −6.9)***	−5.5 (−8.2 to −2.7)***
Nonhypertensives	−3.5 (−5.3 to −1.6)***	−2.1 (−3.6 to −0.5)**
DASH-Sodium Trial		
DASH vs. Average American Diet (Comparison Diet)		
High sodium level	−5.9 (−8.0 to −3.7)***	−2.9 (−4.3 to −1.5)***
Intermediate sodium level	−5.0 (−7.6 to −2.5)***	−2.5 (−4.1 to −0.8)**
Low sodium level	−2.2 (−4.4 to −0.1)*	−1.0 (−2.5 to 0.4)
DASH Diet		
Change from high to intermediate sodium	−1.3 (−2.6 to 0.0)*	−0.6 (−1.5 to 0.2)
Change from intermediate to low sodium	−1.7 (−3.0 to −0.4)**	−1.0 (−1.9 to −0.1)**
Average American diet at high sodium (comparison diet)		
Change from high to intermediate sodium	−2.1 (−3.4 to −0.8)***	−1.1 (−1.9 to −0.2)**
Change from intermediate to low sodium	−4.6 (−5.9 to −3.2)***	−2.4 (−3.3 to −1.5)***

Source: Adapted from Champagne, C.M., *Nutr. Rev.*, 64(2 Pt 2), S53, 2006.
* $P < 0.05$, ** $P < 0.01$, *** $P < 0.001$.

in total cholesterol, LDL-C, or HDL-C. Women had smaller reductions in total cholesterol and LDL-C than men (10.3 mg/dL; $P = 0.052$; 11.2 mg/dL; $P < 0.02$, respectively). African Americans and non-African Americans had similar lipid responses to the DASH diet. Individuals with a higher baseline plasma HDL responded to the DASH diet with greater reductions in HDL at a level of 3.7 mg/dL ($P < 0.05$). The investigators concluded that the DASH diet is likely to reduce coronary heart disease risk by decreasing both total cholesterol and LDL-C in addition to lowering blood pressure. The implications of the DASH results are significant since a 5 mmHg reduction in systolic blood pressure is associated with 15% lower coronary heart disease risk and 27% lower risk of stroke (Obarzanek et al. 2001).

The DASH-Sodium Trial (Sacks et al. 2001)

Sodium intake was held constant in the DASH diet, raising the question of whether dietary sodium would affect the response to the DASH diet. The DASH-Sodium trial was conducted by the same four centers that did the original DASH trial and was designed to test the effect of three levels of dietary sodium on the response to the DASH dietary pattern or the average American diet on changes in blood pressure.

The primary aim was to determine the effect on blood pressure of three levels of dietary sodium set at 50, 100, and 150 mmol/day, in individuals consuming the average American diet (the control diet) or the DASH diet.

Since this was an "efficacy" study, participants received their meals from the clinical centers 5 days a week with takeout food on the weekends. A total of 412 individuals were recruited. Women comprised 56% of the participants versus 49% in the DASH trial and 56% of the subjects were African Americans. The mean age was 49 years and the mean BMI was 29 kg/m^2, which was slightly higher than in the first DASH trial. The mean blood pressure was similar to the first DASH trial (135/86 mmHg), but there was a higher proportion of people who were hypertensive (41% vs. 29%). After a run-in period of 11–14 days on a control diet, participants were randomized to three periods on either the control or DASH diet with the three levels of sodium presented in random order for 30 consecutive days each in a crossover design with a 7-day washout between each sodium level.

The effect of sodium intake on both systolic and diastolic blood pressure was fairly linear, but the DASH diet, especially at the high and intermediate sodium levels, reduced blood pressure more than the standard American diet. The difference between the low sodium levels on systolic blood pressure with the average American (control) diet was less compared with the DASH diet at the lower sodium level; diastolic blood pressure did not show a difference in response. This trial showed that the DASH diet appears to be superior to the average American diet in lowering blood pressure at each sodium level.

In contrast to the original DASH study, the DASH-Sodium interventions did not affect total cholesterol, LDL-C, HDL-C, or triglyceride concentrations (Harsha et al. 2004). Although there was no dose response based on sodium intakes, at each level of sodium the levels of serum total cholesterol, LDL-C, and HDL-C were lower on the DASH diet compared with the average American diet.

In summary, the DASH-Sodium trial showed that sodium reduction lowered blood pressure in persons eating the DASH diet as well as those eating the average American diet. Blood pressure was significantly higher with higher versus lower sodium intakes, and this response for the three levels was linear. The DASH diet was associated with lower blood pressure at higher, intermediate, and lower sodium intakes than the average American diet, but the combination of the DASH diet and the lowest sodium level tested was superior in lowering blood pressure to the comparison diet. The blood pressure results from the DASH-Sodium trial are displayed in Table 23.1.

SUBSEQUENT STUDIES WITH THE DASH DIET CONCEPT: PREMIER AND WEIGHT LOSS MAINTENANCE

PREMIER Clinical Trial

The efficacy of the DASH diet in reducing blood pressure led to the question of whether this diet could be translated into everyday practice. Over the long haul, people need to learn to prepare the DASH diet on their own since they will not have their meals prepared for them on a daily basis with strict attention to detail unless they are institutionalized. To test the effectiveness, as opposed to the efficacy of the DASH diet, NHLBI funded the PREMIER study, which was designed to test the effectiveness of the DASH diet in free-living populations.

A total of 810 individuals were randomized in the PREMIER study to one of the three conditions: (1) advice only, (2) established strategies to lower blood pressure (EST), or (3) the established procedures plus the DASH diet (EST + DASH). The primary outcome measures were assessed at 6 months (Appel et al. 2003), with end of intervention at 18 months (Elmer et al. 2006).

The PREMIER study suggested that individuals with suboptimal blood pressure and stage 1 hypertension can make multiple lifestyle changes when motivated to do so. These lifestyle changes may lower their blood pressure and reduce cardiovascular disease risk, provided the changes are sustained, but the DASH diet did not add to this effect.

Other Trials Using the DASH-Type Diet

DASH Diet Compared to a High-Fat DASH Diet

The DASH dietary pattern is high in fruits, vegetables, and low-fat dairy foods. Although it significantly lowers blood pressure as well as low-density lipoprotein (LDL), it also lowers high-density lipoprotein (HDL) cholesterol, which may be undesirable. This raises the question of whether the low-fat dairy provides any advantage over regular dairy products. This study was designed to test the effects of substituting regular (full-fat) dairy products for low-fat dairy products in the DASH diet (Chiu et al. 2015). The increased fat content was achieved by reducing sugar intake. The trial was a three-period randomized crossover design in free-living healthy individuals who consumed in random order a control diet, a standard DASH diet, and a higher-fat, lower-carbohydrate modification of the DASH diet (HF-DASH diet) for 3 weeks each, separated by a 2-week washout period. Lipoprotein particle concentrations were determined at the end of each experimental diet by ion mobility. Thirty-six participants completed all three dietary periods. Blood pressure was reduced similarly with the DASH and HF-DASH diets when compared with the control diet. The HF-DASH diet significantly reduced triglycerides and large and medium very-low-density lipoprotein (VLDL) particle concentrations and increased LDL peak particle diameter compared with the DASH diet. The DASH diet, but not the HF-DASH diet, significantly reduced LDL cholesterol, HDL cholesterol, apolipoprotein A-I, intermediate density lipoprotein and large LDL particles, and LDL peak diameter compared with the control diet. This study suggests that the improvements in blood pressure are comparable with the DASH diet and the HF-DASH diet. The HF-DASH diet has the additional advantage of reducing plasma triglycerides and plasma VLDL concentrations without significantly increasing LDL cholesterol (Chiu et al. 2015).

DASH-Type Diet with Alternative Protein Sources

The protein sources in a DASH-type can be substituted without altering the effect on blood pressure. In a study by Roussell et al. (2012), 36 hypercholesterolemic participants (with LDL-cholesterol concentrations >2.8 mmol/L) were randomly assigned to consume each of the four diets, HAD (33% total fat, 12% SFA, 17% protein, and 20 g beef/day), DASH (27% total fat, 6% SFA, 18% protein, and 28 g beef/day), BOLD (28% total fat, 6% SFA, 19% protein, and 113 g beef/day), and BOLD+ (28% total fat, 6% SFA, 27% protein, and 153 g beef/day), for 5 weeks. Blood pressure was reduced with the higher quantities of beef. LDL cholesterol and TC decreased after consumption of the DASH, BOLD, and BOLD+ diets when the baseline C-reactive protein (CRP) concentration was <1 mg/L; LDL cholesterol and TC decreased when baseline CRP concentration was >1 mg/L with the BOLD and BOLD+ diets. Thus, lean beef appears to improve the lipid response to the DASH diet without impairing the reduction in blood pressure.

In a second study, Sayer et al. substituted pork for chicken and fish in a two-arm parallel study in a randomized crossover study of 13 women and 6 men (mean age of 61 years; BMI of 31.2 and elevated BP [130/85 mmHg]). Both pork and chicken plus fish reduced blood pressure to a similar degree.

The Omni-Heart (Optimal Macronutrient Intake Trial to Prevent Heart Disease) Study

This three-period study examined the effect of replacing saturated fat with protein (25% vs. 15%) or carbohydrate (58% vs. 48%) or unsaturated fat (predominantly monounsaturated fat 37%) in a three-period crossover with the DASH diet as basic component of the dietary structure. The carbohydrate diet used in this trial is similar to the DASH diet, except that the carbohydrate intake of the DASH diet was 55% of kcal, versus 58% of kcal in the carbohydrate diet, and the protein intake of the DASH diet was 18% of kcal, versus 15% of kcal in the carbohydrate diet. The protein intake was reduced to 15% of kcal to achieve a 10% of kcal contrast with the protein diet. Approximately two-thirds of the increase in protein from the carbohydrate to the protein diets came from plants (legumes, grains, nuts, and seed). However, sources of protein were varied and also included meat, poultry, egg product substitutes, and dairy products. The protein diet included some soy products, but the amount was low, on average just 7.3 g/day. The unsaturated fat diet emphasized monounsaturated fat. This diet included olive, canola, and safflower oils, as well as a variety of nuts and seeds, to meet its target fatty acid distributions. The type of carbohydrate in each diet was similar, as indicated by the total dietary glycemic index (68 in carbohydrate diet, 71 in the protein diet, and 75 in unsaturated fat diet, relative to the white bread index). Blood pressure, low-density lipoprotein cholesterol, and estimated coronary heart disease risk were lower on each diet compared with baseline. The protein diet further decreased mean systolic blood pressure by 1.4 mmHg (P = 0.002) and by 3.5 mmHg (P = 0.006) among those with hypertension and decreased low-density lipoprotein cholesterol by 3.3 mg/dL (0.09 mmol/L; P = 0.01), high-density lipoprotein cholesterol by 1.3 mg/dL (0.03 mmol/L; P = 0.02), and triglycerides by 15.7 mg/dL (0.18 mmol/L; P = 0.001) compared to the carbohydrate diet. A comparison of the carbohydrate diet showed that the unsaturated fat diet decreased systolic blood pressure by 1.3 mmHg (P = 0.005) and by 2.9 mmHg among those with hypertension (P = 0.02), increased high-density lipoprotein cholesterol by 1.1 mg/dL (0.03 mmol/L; P = 0.03), and lowered triglycerides by 9.6 mg/dL (0.11 mmol/L; P = 0.02) but had no significant effect on low-density lipoprotein cholesterol. Compared with the carbohydrate diet, estimated 10-year coronary heart disease risk was lower and similar on the protein and unsaturated fat diets. In the setting of a healthful diet, partial substitution of carbohydrate with either protein or monounsaturated fat can further lower blood pressure, improve lipid levels, and reduce estimated cardiovascular risk.

EFFECT OF THE DASH DIET ON CARDIOMETABOLIC HEALTH

A total of 466 publications were found when the term "DASH diet" was searched in PubMed, 214 of which were published in the last 5 years. Overviews of selected studies are presented in the following table, which compares the (1) study objectives, (2) design, (3) study population, (4) outcome measures, and (5) results (Table 23.2).

A systematic review and meta-analysis of the DASH diet on cardiovascular endpoints was published in 2015 by Siervo et al. (2015). In their meta-regression analyses, they examined the association between effect sizes, baseline values of the risk factors, BMI, age, quality of trials, salt intake, and study duration. A total of 20 articles reporting data for 1917 participants were included in the meta-analysis. The duration of interventions ranged from 2 to 24 weeks. The DASH diet was found to result in significant decreases in systolic BP (−5.2 mmHg, 95% CI −7.0, −3.4; P < 0.001) and diastolic BP (−2.6 mmHg, 95% CI −3.5, −1.7; P < 0.001) and in the concentrations of total cholesterol (−0.20 mmol/L, 95% CI −0.31, −0.10; P < 0.001) and LDL (−0.10 mmol/L, 95% CI −0.20, −0.01; P = 0.03). Changes in both systolic and diastolic BP were greater in participants with higher baseline BP or BMI. These changes predicted a reduction of approximately 13% in the 10-year Framingham risk score for CVD. The DASH diet improved cardiovascular risk factors and appeared to have greater beneficial effects in subjects with an increased cardiometabolic risk. The DASH diet is an effective nutritional strategy to prevent CVD.

If the DASH diet, which is recommended by several U.S. health organizations as a strategy for preventing and managing blood pressure, were generally adopted, it would result in a reduction of 13% in the 10-year Framingham risk score for cardiovascular events based on the results of their review and meta-analysis. These findings reinforce the evidence that adherence to the DASH dietary pattern could make a significant contribution to the prevention of cardiovascular disease, above and beyond lowering of blood pressure.

The original DASH diet lowered red meat consumption and raised protein intake to 18% with chicken and fish. As described earlier, whether other meats would improve or impair the response

TABLE 23.2
Selected Studies That Have Utilized the DASH Diet as a Main or Comparative Focus

Article	Objective	Design	Subjects (n)	Outcome Measure(s)	Results	Conclusions
Asemi Z et al. "Effects of DASH diet on lipid profiles and biomarkers of oxidative stress in overweight and obese women with polycystic ovary syndrome: A randomized clinical trial." *Nutrition* 2014 November–December; 30(11–12): 1287–1293.	To assess the effects of the Dietary Approaches to Stop Hypertension (DASH) diet on lipid profiles and biomarkers of oxidative stress in overweight and obese women with polycystic ovary syndrome (PCOS).	Randomized controlled clinical trial • Women were randomly assigned to consume either control or DASH diet for 8 weeks—both diets were calorie-restricted. • Both diets consisted of 52% carbohydrates, 18% proteins, and 30% total fats.	48 women with PCOS.	• Lipid profiles • Biomarkers of oxidative stress—plasma total antioxidant capacity (TAC) and total glutathione (GSH).	Adherence to the DASH diet resulted in a significant decrease in weight, BMI, decreased serum triglycerides and VLDL cholesterol levels compared to the control group. Increased TAC and GSH concentrations were also observed in the DASH group.	The DASH diet group resulted in a significant decrease in serum insulin, triglycerides and VLDL cholesterol and a significant increase in TAC and GSH levels. (Asemi et al. 2014)
Jacobs DR et al. "The effects of dietary patterns on urinary albumin excretion: Results of the Dietary Approaches to Stop Hypertension (DASH) Trial." *Am J Kidney Dis* 2009; 53(4): 638–646.	To evaluate albumin excretion rate (AER) while increasing protein intake in the DASH trial.	Randomized, parallel group, 8-week controlled feeding: • Followed DASH diet or control diet.	378 individuals without diabetes with prehypertension or stage 1 hypertension.	• Albumin excretion rate (AER).	The decrease in AER after 8 weeks occurred in only those with high-normal baseline AER in the FV diet, in a pattern distinct from the blood pressure decrease. The DASH diet did not increase AER despite a 3% increase in energy from protein.	The DASH diet can be especially beneficial in slowing disease progression for people with early stage (1 or 2) kidney disease. (Jacobs et al. 2009)

(*Continued*)

TABLE 23.2 (*Continued*)
Selected Studies That Have Utilized the DASH Diet as a Main or Comparative Focus

Article	Objective	Design	Subjects (n)	Outcome Measure(s)	Results	Conclusions
Sacks FM et al. "Effects of high vs low glycemic index of dietary carbohydrate on cardiovascular disease risk factors and insulin sensitivity: The OmniCarb randomized clinical trial." *JAMA* 2014 December 17; 312(23): 2531–2541.	To determine the effect of glycemic index and amount of total dietary carbohydrate on risk factors for CVD and diabetes.	Randomized crossover controlled feeding trial: • Given 4 diets based on healthful DASH-type diet, each for 5 weeks Inclusion criteria: • ≥30 years of age • Systolic BP 120–159 mmHg; Diastolic BP 70–99 mmHg • BMI ≥25 Exclusion criteria: • CV disease, DM, or CKD • Taking medication that lowers BP or lipids • FBG ≥ 125 mg/dL	163 overweight adults: • 85 (52%) females. • 78 (51%) males. Race/ethnicity: • Black 83 (51%). • Non-Hispanic white 66 (40%). • Asian 4 (2%). • Other 5 (3%).	• Insulin sensitivity. • LDL cholesterol. • HDL cholesterol. • Triglycerides. • Systolic blood pressure.	Diets with low glycemic index of dietary carbohydrate, compared with high glycemic index of dietary carbohydrate, did not result in improvements in insulin sensitivity, lipid levels, or systolic blood pressure.	Low glycemic index foods not needed for full cardiovascular benefits with DASH diet. DASH again proven to lower blood pressure and cholesterol, benefits independent of glycemic index of foods in diet. (Sacks et al. 2014)
Appel LJ et al. "Effects of protein, monounsaturated fat, and carbohydrate intake on blood pressure and serum lipids: Results of the OmniHeart randomized trial." *JAMA* 2005 November 16; 294(19): 2455–2464.	To compare the effects of 3 healthful diets, each with reduced saturated fat intake, on blood pressure and serum lipids.	Randomized, 3-period, crossover feeding study conducted in Baltimore, Maryland and Boston, Massachusetts. • Each feeding period was 6 weeks and body weight kept constant. • Diets: Diet rich in carbs, diet rich in protein (half from plant sources), diet rich in unsaturated fat.	164 adults with prehypertension or stage 1 hypertension.	• Systolic blood pressure. • LDL cholesterol.	In the setting of a healthful diet, partial substitution of carbohydrate with either protein or monounsaturated fat can further lower blood pressure, improve lipid levels, and reduce estimated cardiovascular risk.	Replacing added-sugars and refined starchy foods with either lean protein-rich foods and/or foods rich in monounsaturated fats improved blood pressure and blood lipid results in a DASH eating pattern. (Appel et al. 2005)

(*Continued*)

TABLE 23.2 (*Continued*)
Selected Studies That Have Utilized the DASH Diet as a Main or Comparative Focus

Article	Objective	Design	Subjects (n)	Outcome Measure(s)	Results	Conclusions
Couch SC et al. "The efficacy of a clinic-based behavioral nutrition intervention emphasizing a DASH-type diet for adolescents with elevated blood pressure." *J Pediatr* 2008 April; 152(4): 494–501.	To examine the efficacy of a 3-month clinic-based behavioral nutrition intervention (the DASH diet) vs. routine outpatient hospital-based nutrition care (RC) on diet and blood pressure in adolescents with elevated BP.	57 adolescents with a clinical diagnosis of prehypertension or hypertension were randomly assigned to DASH or RC. SBP, DBP, 3-day diet recall, weight, and height were assessed at pretreatment, posttreatment, and 3 months later (follow-up).	57 adolescents with prehypertension or hypertension.	• Blood pressure.	DASH had a greater decrease in systolic BP and a trend for a greater decrease in SBP over the study period. Additionally, DASH had a greater increase in the intake of fruits, potassium, and magnesium, and a greater decrease in total fat, compared to RC.	Teens that followed the DASH diet, consuming more fruits, vegetables, low-fat dairy, and nuts, were more effectively able to lower their blood pressure and improve their diets than those who followed the RC diet. (Couch et al. 2008)
Blumenthal JA et al. "Effects of the DASH diet alone and in combination with exercise and weight loss on blood pressure and cardiovascular biomarkers in men and women with high blood pressure: The ENCORE study." *Arch Intern Med* 2010 January; 170(2): 126–135.	To compare the DASH diet alone or combined with a weight management program with usual diet controls among participants with prehypertension or stage 1 hypertension.	Randomized controlled trial • Assessments at baseline and 4 months, with each patient assigned one of the following diets: Usual diet controls, DASH diet alone, and DASH diet plus weight management.	144 overweight or obese, unmedicated outpatients with high BP.	• Main outcome measure: BP. • Secondary outcome measures: Pulse wave velocity, flow-mediated dilation of the brachial artery, baroreflex sensitivity, and left ventricular mass.	For overweight or obese persons with above-normal BP, the addition of exercise and weight loss to the DASH diet resulted in even larger BP reductions, greater improvements in vascular and autonomic function, and reduced left ventricular mass, as compared to the DASH diet alone.	Adding weight loss and exercise to the DASH diet improves blood pressure regulation and showed improvements in other measures of cardiovascular health. (Blumenthal et al. 2010)

(*Continued*)

TABLE 23.2 (*Continued*)
Selected Studies That Have Utilized the DASH Diet as a Main or Comparative Focus

Article	Objective	Design	Subjects (n)	Outcome Measure(s)	Results	Conclusions
Levitan EB et al. "Relation of consistency with the dietary approaches to stop hypertension diet and incidence of heart failure in men aged 45 to 79 years." *Am J Cardiol* 2009b; 104(10): 1416–1420.	To examine if the DASH diet is associated with lower rates of heart failure in men, as it has been shown in women.	Followed participants over 7 years to examine consistency with the DASH diet (using DASH scores) and rates of heart failure hospitalization or mortality.	38,987 Swedish men aged 45–79.	• Heart failure (HF).	Men in the greatest quartile of the DASH component score had a 22% lower rate of HF events than those in the lowest quartile.	Greater consistency with the DASH diet was associated with lower rates of HF events in men aged 45–79 years. (Levitan et al. 2009b)
Levitan EB et al. "Consistency with the DASH diet and incidence of heart failure." *Arch Intern Med* 2009a 169(9): 851–857.	To test the hypothesis that diets consistent with the DASH diet would be associated with a lower incidence of heart failure.	Observational study conducted in the Swedish mammography cohort • Diet measured using FFQs and used DASH score to assess consistency with DASH diet; also recorded rates of HF-associated hospitalization or death.	36,019 women aged 48–83.	• Heart failure (HF).	Women in the top quartile of the DASH diet score based on ranking DASH diet components had a 37% lower rate of HF.	Women who followed the DASH diet were associated with lower incidence of heart failure. (Levitan et al. 2009a)

(*Continued*)

TABLE 23.2 (*Continued*)
Selected Studies That Have Utilized the DASH Diet as a Main or Comparative Focus

Article	Objective	Design	Subjects (n)	Outcome Measure(s)	Results	Conclusions
Fung TT et al. "Adherence to a DASH-style diet and risk of coronary heart disease and stroke in women." *Arch Intern Med* 2008 April 14; 168(7): 713–720.	To assess the association between a DASH-style diet score and risk of coronary heart disease (CHD) and stroke in women.	Diet assessed seven times during 24 years of follow-up with FFQs; given DASH score; recorded numbers of confirmed incident cases of nonfatal myocardial infarction, CHD death, and stroke.	88,517 women aged 34 to 59 years with no history of CVD or diabetes before 1980.	• Nonfatal myocardial infarction. • CHD death. • Stroke.	Higher DASH scores were associated with lower risks of CHD, nonfatal myocardial infarction, fatal CHD, stroke, and lower plasma levels of C-reactive protein and interleukin.	Adherence to the DASH-style diet is associated with a lower risk of CHD and stroke among middle-aged women during 24 years of follow-up. (Fung et al. 2008)
Harmon BE et al. "Associations of key diet-quality indexes with mortality in the Multiethnic Cohort: The Dietary Patterns Methods Project." *Am J Clin Nutr* 2015 March; 101(3): 587–597.	To assess the ability of 4 diet-quality Indexes: Healthy Eating Index-2010 (HEI-2010), Alternative HEI-2010 (AHEI-2010), alternate Mediterranean diet score (aMED), and the Dietary Approaches to Stop Hypertension (DASH) to predict the reduction in risk of mortality from all causes, cardiovascular disease (CVD), and cancer.	Prospective cohort: • Subjects completed a quantitative FFQ. • Scores for each dietary index were computed. • Mortality was documented over 13–18 years of follow-up.	156,804 adults 70,170 men: • White (17,330). • African American (9,014). • Native Hawaiian (4,992). • Japanese American (21,239). • Latino (17,595). 86,634 women: • White (20,653). • African American (16,072). • Native Hawaiian (6,368). • Japanese American (24,785). • Latina (18,756).	• All-cause mortality. • CVD mortality. • Cancer mortality.	High DASH scores were inversely associated with the risk of mortality from all causes, CVD, and cancer in both men and women.	Consuming a dietary pattern that has a high diet-quality index score is associated with lower risk of mortality from all causes, CVD, and cancer in men and women. (Harmon et al. 2015)

(*Continued*)

TABLE 23.2 (*Continued*)
Selected Studies That Have Utilized the DASH Diet as a Main or Comparative Focus

Article	Objective	Design	Subjects (n)	Outcome Measure(s)	Results	Conclusions
Taylor EN et al. "DASH-style diet associates with reduced risk for kidney stones." *J Am Soc Nephrol* October; 20(10): 2253–2259.	To examine the impact of the DASH diet on kidney stone formation.	Used 14–18 years of follow-up; constructed a DASH score and recorded incidents of kidney stones.	45,821 men. 94,108 older women. 101,337 younger women.	• Impact on kidney stone formation.	For participants in the highest compared with the lowest quintile of DASH score, the multivariate relative risks for kidney stones were 0.55 (95% CI, 0.46–0.65) for men, 0.58 (95% CI, 0.49–0.68) for older women, and 0.60 (95% CI, 0.52–0.70) for younger women.	There was a 45% reduction in the risk of kidney stones in men and 52% reduction in women who were consistent with the DASH diet. (Taylor et al. 2009)
Shenoy SF et al. "Weight loss in individuals with metabolic syndrome given DASH diet counseling when provided a low sodium vegetable juice: A randomized controlled trial." *J. Nutr* 2010 February 23; 9: 8.	To evaluate the effects of a ready-to-serve vegetable juice as part of a calorie-appropriate Dietary Approaches to Stop Hypertension (DASH) diet in an ethnically diverse population of people with metabolic syndrome on weight loss and their ability to meet vegetable intake recommendations, and on their clinical characteristics of metabolic syndrome.	Prospective 12-week, 3-group parallel-arm randomized controlled trial • Participants assigned to one of three groups—0, 8, or 16 fl oz of low sodium vegetable juice; educated on the DASH diet and limited calorie intake.	81 participants with metabolic syndrome: 22 men. 59 women.	• Weight loss in individuals with metabolic syndrome.	Those consuming juice lost more weight, consumed more vitamin C, potassium, and dietary vegetables than individuals who were in the group that only received diet counseling ($p < 0.05$).	Participants in a program to promote weight loss in people with metabolic syndrome lost more weight by adding low-sodium vegetable juice, as a component of the DASH diet. (Shenoy et al. 2010)

(*Continued*)

TABLE 23.2 (*Continued*)
Selected Studies That Have Utilized the DASH Diet as a Main or Comparative Focus

Article	Objective	Design	Subjects (n)	Outcome Measure(s)	Results	Conclusions
Fung TT et al. "Low-carbohydrate diets, dietary approaches to stop hypertension-style diets, and the risk of postmenopausal breast cancer." *Am J Epidemiol* 2011 September 15; 174(6): 652–660.	To examine the association between the DASH diet score, overall, animal-based, and vegetable-based low-carbohydrate-diet scores, and major plant food groups and the risk of postmenopausal breast cancer.	• Obtained number of incidences of breast cancer, DASH diet score, FFQs.	86,621 women.		A diet high in fruits and vegetables, such as one represented by the Dietary Approaches to Stop Hypertension diet score, was associated with a lower risk of ER-breast cancer. In addition, a diet high in plant protein and fat and moderate in carbohydrate content was associated with a lower risk of ER-cancer.	DASH diet is associated with a lower risk of developing Estrogen Receptor negative breast cancer. In particular, the increased intake of fruits and vegetables associated with the DASH diet appeared to be beneficial. (Fung et al. 2011)
Fung TT et al. "The Mediterranean and Dietary Approaches to Stop Hypertension (DASH) diets and colorectal cancer." *Am J Clin Nutr* 2010 December; 92(6): 1429–1435.	To prospectively assess the association between the alternate Mediterranean diet (aMed) and the DASH-style diet scores and risk of colorectal cancer in middle-aged men and women.	• Followed participants for up to 26 years, calculated aMed, DASH scores, and colorectal cancer relative risks for each participant that was assessed up to 7 times during follow-up.	87,256 women and 45,490 men without a history of cancer.			People following the DASH diet were less likely to develop colorectal cancer. Following the Mediterranean diet did not show similar benefits. (Fung et al. 2010)

has been tested by Roussell et al. (2012). They studied the effects on lipids, lipoproteins, and apolipoproteins in a heart-healthy diet that contained lean beef compared to a DASH dietary pattern. While this study investigated lipids and not blood pressure, the result was that incorporation of lean beef in a low-saturated-fat, heart-healthy dietary pattern that mimicked the DASH macronutrient targets elicited favorable cardiovascular effects comparable to DASH.

Other researchers studied a modification of the DASH diet when they substituted lean pork for the poultry and fish recommendations of the DASH diet (Sayer et al. 2015). In assessing blood pressure responses, DASH diets containing pork compared to those containing chicken and fish equally reduced all measures of blood pressures. Their results suggest that lean pork within the DASH-style diet is effective for blood pressure reduction.

CONCLUSIONS

From the material presented in this chapter, it is clear that a lifestyle that includes the DASH eating plan is a good one. The DASH eating plan, developed from the findings of the DASH feeding trials, is based on solid scientific evidence and has documented health benefits. The Dietary Guidelines for Americans 2010 endorsed the DASH eating plan in the development of a healthy eating pattern, indicating that "the USDA Food Patterns and the DASH Eating Plan apply these Dietary Guidelines recommendations and provide flexible templates for making healthy choices within and among various food groups." The 2015 Dietary Guidelines have also described the DASH dietary pattern as having many of the same characteristics as the Healthy U.S.-Style Eating Pattern (USDA Dietary Guidelines 2015).

In January 2011, U.S. News and World Report began a column in their Health Section on the U.S. News Best Diets. By convening a panel of diet and nutrition experts, this media entity unveils rankings of many eating plans and/or diets. Since the launch in 2011, the DASH diet has now been ranked Number 1 as the best overall diet every year this column has been published. Of the 38 diets evaluated in 2016, the DASH diet maintains the Number 1 position for the sixth consecutive year, truly an example of science that has health benefits for Americans and perhaps other population groups.

ACKNOWLEDGMENTS

George Bray and the DASH, DASH-Sodium, PREMIER, and Weight Loss Maintenance Investigative Teams.

CONFLICTS OF INTEREST

No conflicts of interest to report.

REFERENCES

Appel, L. J., C. M. Champagne, D. W. Harsha, L. S. Cooper, E. Obarzanek, P. J. Elmer, V. J. Stevens et al. 2003. Effects of comprehensive lifestyle modification on blood pressure control: Main results of the PREMIER clinical trial. *JAMA* 289(16): 2083–2093. doi: 10.1001/jama.289.16.2083.

Appel, L. J., T. J. Moore, E. Obarzanek, W. M. Vollmer, L. P. Svetkey, F. M. Sacks, G. A. Bray et al. 1997. A clinical trial of the effects of dietary patterns on blood pressure. DASH Collaborative Research Group. *N Engl J Med* 336(16): 1117–1124. doi: 10.1056/nejm199704173361601.

Appel, L. J., F. M. Sacks, V. J. Carey, E. Obarzanek, J. F. Swain, E. R. Miller, P. R. Conlin, 3rd et al. 2005. Effects of protein, monounsaturated fat, and carbohydrate intake on blood pressure and serum lipids: Results of the OmniHeart randomized trial. *JAMA* 294(19): 2455–2464. doi: 10.1001/jama.294.19.2455.

Asemi, Z., M. Samimi, Z. Tabassi, H. Shakeri, S. S. Sabihi, and A. Esmaillzadeh. 2014. Effects of DASH diet on lipid profiles and biomarkers of oxidative stress in overweight and obese women with polycystic ovary syndrome: A randomized clinical trial. *Nutrition* 30(11–12): 1287–1293. doi: 10.1016/j.nut.2014.03.008.

Blumenthal, J. A., M. A. Babyak, A. Hinderliter, L. L. Watkins, L. Craighead, P. H. Lin, C. Caccia, J. Johnson, R. Waugh, and A. Sherwood. 2010. Effects of the DASH diet alone and in combination with exercise and weight loss on blood pressure and cardiovascular biomarkers in men and women with high blood pressure: The ENCORE study. *Arch Intern Med* 170(2): 126–135. doi: 10.1001/archinternmed.2009.470.

Champagne, C. M. 2006. Dietary interventions on blood pressure: The Dietary Approaches to Stop Hypertension (DASH) trials. *Nutr Rev* 64(2 Pt 2): S53–S56.

Chiu, S., N. Bergeron, P. T. Williams, G. A. Bray, B. Sutherland, and R. M. Krauss. December 30, 2015. Comparison of the DASH (Dietary Approaches to Stop Hypertension) diet and a higher-fat DASH diet on blood pressure and lipids and lipoproteins: A randomized controlled trial. *Am J Clin Nutr* 103(2): 341–347.

Couch, S. C., B. E. Saelens, L. Levin, K. Dart, G. Falciglia, and S. R. Daniels. 2008. The efficacy of a clinic-based behavioral nutrition intervention emphasizing a DASH-type diet for adolescents with elevated blood pressure. *J Pediatr* 152(4): 494–501. doi: 10.1016/j.jpeds.2007.09.022.

Elmer, P. J., E. Obarzanek, W. M. Vollmer, D. Simons-Morton, V. J. Stevens, D. R. Young, P. H. Lin et al. 2006. Effects of comprehensive lifestyle modification on diet, weight, physical fitness, and blood pressure control: 18-month results of a randomized trial. *Ann Intern Med* 144(7): 485–495.

Fung, T. T., S. E. Chiuve, M. L. McCullough, K. M. Rexrode, G. Logroscino, and F. B. Hu. 2008. Adherence to a DASH-style diet and risk of coronary heart disease and stroke in women. *Arch Intern Med* 168(7): 713–720. doi: 10.1001/archinte.168.7.713.

Fung, T. T., F. B. Hu, S. E. Hankinson, W. C. Willett, and M. D. Holmes. 2011. Low-carbohydrate diets, dietary approaches to stop hypertension-style diets, and the risk of postmenopausal breast cancer. *Am J Epidemiol* 174(6): 652–660. doi: 10.1093/aje/kwr148.

Fung, T. T., F. B. Hu, K. Wu, S. E. Chiuve, C. S. Fuchs, and E. Giovannucci. 2010. The Mediterranean and Dietary Approaches to Stop Hypertension (DASH) diets and colorectal cancer. *Am J Clin Nutr* 92(6): 1429–1435. doi: 10.3945/ajcn.2010.29242.

Harmon, B. E., C. J. Boushey, Y. B. Shvetsov, R. Ettienne, J. Reedy, L. R. Wilkens, L. Le Marchand, B. E. Henderson, and L. N. Kolonel. 2015. Associations of key diet-quality indexes with mortality in the Multiethnic Cohort: The Dietary Patterns Methods Project. *Am J Clin Nutr* 101(3): 587–597. doi: 10.3945/ajcn.114.090688.

Harsha, D. W., F. M. Sacks, E. Obarzanek, L. P. Svetkey, P. H. Lin, G. A. Bray, M. Aickin, P. R. Conlin, E. R. Miller, 3rd, and L. J. Appel. 2004. Effect of dietary sodium intake on blood lipids: Results from the DASH-sodium trial. *Hypertension* 43(2): 393–398. doi: 10.1161/01.HYP.0000113046.83819.a2.

Jacobs, D. R., Jr., M. D. Gross, L. Steffen, M. W. Steffes, X. Yu, L. P. Svetkey, L. J. Appel et al. 2009. The effects of dietary patterns on urinary albumin excretion: Results of the Dietary Approaches to Stop Hypertension (DASH) Trial. *Am J Kidney Dis* 53(4): 638–646. doi: 10.1053/j.ajkd.2008.10.048.

Levitan, E. B., A. Wolk, and M. A. Mittleman. 2009a. Consistency with the DASH diet and incidence of heart failure. *Arch Intern Med* 169(9): 851–857. doi: 10.1001/archinternmed.2009.56.

Levitan, E. B., A. Wolk, and M. A. Mittleman. 2009b. Relation of consistency with the dietary approaches to stop hypertension diet and incidence of heart failure in men aged 45 to 79 years. *Am J Cardiol* 104(10): 1416–1420. doi: 10.1016/j.amjcard.2009.06.061.

Obarzanek, E., F. M. Sacks, W. M. Vollmer, G. A. Bray, E. R. Miller, 3rd, P. H. Lin, N. M. Karanja et al. 2001. Effects on blood lipids of a blood pressure-lowering diet: The Dietary Approaches to Stop Hypertension (DASH) Trial. *Am J Clin Nutr* 74(1): 80–89.

Roussell, M. A., A. M. Hill, T. L. Gaugler, S. G. West, J. P. Heuvel, P. Alaupovic, P. J. Gillies, and P. M. Kris-Etherton. January 2012. Beef in an optimal lean diet study: Effects on lipids, lipoproteins, and apolipoproteins. *Am J Clin Nutr* 95(1): 9–16. doi: 10.3945/ajcn.111.016261. Epub December 14, 2011.

Sacks, F. M., V. J. Carey, C. A. Anderson, E. R. Miller, T. Copeland, 3rd, J. Charleston, B. J. Harshfield et al. 2014. Effects of high vs low glycemic index of dietary carbohydrate on cardiovascular disease risk factors and insulin sensitivity: The OmniCarb randomized clinical trial. *JAMA* 312(23): 2531–2541. doi: 10.1001/jama.2014.16658.

Sacks, F. M., B. Rosner, and E. H. Kass. 1974. Blood pressure in vegetarians. *Am J Epidemiol* 100(5): 390–398.

Sacks, F. M., L. P. Svetkey, W. M. Vollmer, L. J. Appel, G. A. Bray, D. Harsha, E. Obarzanek et al. 2001. Effects on blood pressure of reduced dietary sodium and the Dietary Approaches to Stop Hypertension (DASH) diet. DASH-Sodium Collaborative Research Group. *N Engl J Med* 344(1): 3–10. doi: 10.1056/nejm200101043440101.

Sayer, R. D., A. J. Wright, N. Chen, and W. W. Campbell. August 2015. Dietary Approaches to Stop Hypertension diet retains effectiveness to reduce blood pressure when lean pork is substituted for chicken and fish as the predominant source of protein. *Am J Clin Nutr* 102(2): 302–308. doi: 10.3945/ajcn.115.111757. Epub June 10, 2015.

Shenoy, S. F., W. S. Poston, R. S. Reeves, A. G. Kazaks, R. R. Holt, C. L. Keen, H. J. Chen et al. 2010. Weight loss in individuals with metabolic syndrome given DASH diet counseling when provided a low sodium vegetable juice: A randomized controlled trial. *Nutr J* 9: 8. doi: 10.1186/1475-2891-9-8.

Siervo, M., J. Lara, S. Chowdhury, A. Ashor, C. Oggioni, and J. C. Mathers. 2015. Effects of the Dietary Approach to Stop Hypertension (DASH) diet on cardiovascular risk factors: A systematic review and meta-analysis. *Br J Nutr* 113(1): 1–15. doi: 10.1017/S0007114514003341.

Taylor, E. N., T. T. Fung, and G. C. Curhan. 2009. DASH-style diet associates with reduced risk for kidney stones. *J Am Soc Nephrol* 20(10): 2253–2259. doi: 10.1681/asn.2009030276.

USDA Dietary Guidelines. 2015. USDA Dietary Guidelines. http://health.gov/dietaryguidelines/.

Vogt, T. M., L. J. Appel, E. Obarzanek, T. J. Moore, W. M. Vollmer, L. P. Svetkey, F. M. Sacks et al. 1999. Dietary approaches to stop hypertension: Rationale, design, and methods. DASH Collaborative Research Group. *J Am Diet Assoc* 99(8 Suppl): S12–S18.

24 Nut Consumption and Coronary Heart Disease (CHD) Risk and Mortality

Christina Link, Alyssa Tindall, Jordi Salas-Salvadó, Caitlin Lynch, and Penny Kris-Etherton

CONTENTS

ABSTRACT

The purpose of this chapter is to review the evidence about the role of nuts in cardiovascular disease (CVD) risk reduction. CVD risk reduction has been the target of dietary intervention for decades as a result of the disease burden. Approximately 25% of all deaths in the United States are from heart disease (CHD) each year, ranking CVD the number one cause of death, both in the United States and worldwide. Epidemiological and clinical studies have been conducted that demonstrate the benefits of nuts on CVD morbidity and mortality. In addition, there is impressive evidence demonstrating beneficial effects of nuts on CVD risk factors.

Several landmark epidemiological studies, including the Adventist Study and The Nurse's Health Study, have reported beneficial associations between nut consumption and CVD risk, incidence, and mortality with different populations. One seminal randomized, controlled trial (RCT), PREDIMED, has also shown benefits of nut consumption on CVD risk, events, and mortality. This study, along with many others, has reported favorable changes in blood lipids, inflammation, and other markers of CVD with nut consumption.

The studies discussed in this chapter have added to the evidence base that informs Dietary Guidelines. The 2015–2020 Dietary Guidelines recommend a healthful dietary pattern that includes nuts, for health promotion, as well as the prevention of chronic diseases, including CVD.

INTRODUCTION

Cardiovascular disease (CVD) is the leading cause of death in both the United States and worldwide. Approximately one in four Americans die from coronary heart disease (CHD) every year (CDC, 2015). Moreover, a systematic analysis of descriptive epidemiology of 291 diseases in the United States reported that ischemic heart disease (IHD) was one of the most prevalent diseases with the largest number of years of life lost due to premature mortality (U.S. Burden of Disease Collaborators, 2013). This report also found that dietary risks are the leading cause of preventable mortality (U.S. Burden of Disease Collaborators, 2013). Authors of the 2010 Global Burden of Disease Study used meta-regression to estimate the pooled effect of fruits, vegetables, nuts and seeds, whole grains, fish, and dietary fiber on systolic blood pressure and LDL cholesterol, based on controlled feeding studies (six treatment groups from three studies for blood pressure and six treatment groups from two studies for cholesterol), and reported low nut and seed consumption was the leading dietary risk factor attributable to IHD (Lim et al., 2012).

A healthy diet is the primary strategy for the prevention and treatment of CVD. The 2015–2020 Dietary Guidelines for Americans recommend a healthy dietary pattern that includes a variety of vegetables from all of the subgroups—dark green, red and orange, legumes (beans and peas), starchy, and others; fruits, especially whole fruits; grains, at least half of which are whole grains; fat-free or low-fat dairy, including milk, yogurt, cheese, and/or fortified soy beverages; a variety of protein foods, including seafood, lean meats and poultry, eggs, legumes, and nuts, seeds, and soy products; and liquid vegetable oils (http://health.gov/dietaryguidelines/2015/guidelines/). In addition, a healthy eating pattern limits saturated fats, trans fats, added sugars, and sodium. The recommendation for nuts in the Healthy U.S. Eating Pattern is 5 oz/week for a 2000-calorie diet. Other organizations also have issued dietary recommendations for nuts (Lloyd-Jones et al., 2010; Sacco, 2011; Vannice and Rasmussen, 2014). The purpose of this chapter is, thus, to review the evidence base in support of dietary recommendations for nuts and the benefits they have on cardiometabolic health.

EARLY EPIDEMIOLOGICAL ASSOCIATIONS

Epidemiological evidence has demonstrated a consistent beneficial association between the consumption of nuts and CHD risk and mortality (Albert et al., 2002; Fraser et al., 1992, 1995; Hu et al., 1998). The Adventist Health Study, a landmark study, was the first to investigate nut consumption and CHD risk in 31,208 healthy individuals (Fraser et al., 1992). In this study, there were fewer fatal CHD events [relative risk (RR) = 0.52 (95% confidence interval [CI]: 0.36–0.76; $P < 0.0001$)] and fewer nonfatal myocardial infarctions [RR = 0.49 (95% CI: 0.28–0.85; $P < 0.005$)] in individuals who consumed nuts (type of nut undefined) ≥5 times/week (categories ranged from "never consume" to "consume more than 1 oz/day") compared to those who consumed nuts <1 time/week. Data from this study were used to assess lifetime risk of developing CHD and a first coronary event in response to nut consumption. Individuals who ate nuts ≥5 servings/week had a 12% lifetime reduction in risk of developing CHD ($P = 0.05$) compared to those who rarely consumed nuts (Fraser et al., 1995). In addition, men who developed the disease had a prolonged onset of CHD, approximately 5–6 years later, in comparison to men who rarely consumed nuts (Fraser et al., 1995). The Adventist Health Study subgroups, oldest-old adults (≥84 years; n = 603) and blacks (n = 3229), were also evaluated and similar reductions in the risk for CHD mortality and all-cause mortality were reported (Fraser et al., 1997; Fraser and Shavlikm, 1997). Oldest-old adults who consumed nuts ≥5 times/week had a RR of 0.82 (95% CI: 0.70–0.96; $P < 0.01$) for death and RR of 0.61 (95% CI: 0.45–0.83; $P < 0.001$) for death from CHD compared with those consuming nuts <1 time/week (Fraser and Shavlikm, 1997). Similarly, a decreased hazard ratio (HR) for death among black participants consuming nuts ≥5 times/week versus <1 time/week [HR = 0.6 (95% CI: 0.3–1.0)] has been observed (Fraser et al., 1997). The Iowa Women's Health Study examined the frequency of nut intake (type of nut undefined) and CHD death in a population of healthy postmenopausal women (n = 34,486) over a

7-year period. Women in the highest nut consumption quartile (>4 servings/week, serving size undefined) had a 40% reduction in risk of fatal CHD [RR = 0.60 (95% CI: 0.36–1.01; P = 0.016)] compared to those who did not consume nuts (Kushi et al., 1996). The Nurses' Health Study (NHS) was another large, prospective study (n = 86,016) that evaluated the relationship between nut consumption and CHD in middle-aged women (Hu et al., 1998). After a 14-year follow-up, a 39% decrease in the risk of fatal CHD [RR = 0.61 (95% CI: 0.35–1.05; P = 0.007)] was observed in women consuming ≥5 servings nuts/week (1 serving = 1 oz nuts) compared to those consuming <1 serving nuts/month (type of nut not defined) (Hu et al., 1998). In 2002, Albert and colleagues evaluated nut consumption and the risk of CHD in 22,071 males enrolled in the Physicians' Health Study (PHS) (Albert et al., 2002). After a 17-year follow-up, men who consumed nuts (type of nut undefined) ≥2 times/week (1 serving = 1 oz nuts) had a reduced risk of total CHD death [RR = 0.53 (95% CI: 0.30–0.92; P = 0.01)] compared to men who rarely or never consumed nuts. The reduction in CHD observed in this study was primarily attributable to a reduction in sudden cardiac death. Relative risk of sudden cardiac death was 47% lower in men who consumed nuts ≥2 times/week [RR = 0.53 (95% CI: 0.30–0.92; P = 0.01]) (Albert et al., 2002). Furthermore, the reduced risk of CHD was independent of age, body mass index, alcohol use, or presence of other CVD risk factors.

A pooled analysis of these four large U.S. studies demonstrated a 35% reduced risk of CHD incidence for the group with the highest nut intake of ≥5 times/week [RR = 0.65 (95% CI: 0.47–0.89)] (Kris-Etherton et al., 2008). The nonfatal CHD RR for persons consuming nuts ≥5 times/week was 0.68 (95% CI: 0.47–1.00). These studies demonstrate a beneficial relationship between frequency of nut consumption and CHD risk, resulting in an 8.3% reduction in risk of CHD for each serving weekly of nuts consumed (Kelly and Sabate, 2006). Collectively, the results from these studies consistently demonstrate beneficial associations between nut consumption on CHD (Table 24.1 presents an overview of the studies discussed).

MORE RECENT EPIDEMIOLOGICAL STUDIES

The association between nut consumption and the risk of CVD and all-cause mortality remains an active area of research. A study published in 2015 assessed the association between nut consumption and risk of 15-year total and CVD mortality in 2893 adults (Gopinath et al., 2015). Participants in the second tertile for nut consumption (0.9–4.55 g nuts/day) versus those in the first tertile (0.00–0.5 g nuts/day) had a 24% reduced risk of total mortality (P-trend = 0.81), with reduced risk of CVD [HR = 0.76 (95% CI: 0.61–0.94); P-trend = 0.43], and IHD mortality [HR = 0.77 (95% CI: 0.60–0.98); P-trend = 0.76] (Gopinath et al., 2015). Eslamparast et al. (2017) evaluated nut consumption and all-cause and cause-specific mortality in 50,045 adults enrolled in the Golestan cohort. The majority of prospective cohort studies have been conducted predominantly in Western countries, making this particular cohort unique because of the geographic location in northeastern Iran. Researchers observed similar results in the Golestan cohort as those seen in Western cohorts. After a 7-year period, the pooled multivariate-adjusted HRs for death among those who ate nuts, compared to those who did not, were 0.89 (95% CI: 0.82–0.95) for consumption of <1 serving/week (1 serving = 28 g), 0.75 (95% CI: 0.67–0.85) for 1 to <3 servings/week, and 0.71 (95% CI: 0.58–0.86) for ≥3 servings/week. This study provides further evidence of benefits of nut consumption and mortality in a cohort that differs from others previously studied (Eslamparast et al., 2017).

Several recent epidemiological studies have explored nut consumption and CVD risk in populations that vary in socioeconomic status (SES). In a secondary analysis using data from the NHS (a more affluent cohort), researchers assessed nut consumption and incidence of CVD in 6309 women with type 2 diabetes (Li et al., 2009). The authors reported that women who consumed 5 servings/week of tree nuts or peanut butter [serving size = 28 g (1 oz) for nuts and 16 g (1 tablespoon) for peanut butter] had a 44% lower risk [RR = 0.56 (95% CI: 0.36–0.89; P = 0.44)] compared to women who rarely or never consumed tree nuts or peanut butter. In that study, a strong inverse association with CVD in women who consumed ≥5 servings/week of nuts and peanut butter

TABLE 24.1
A Review of Observational Studies on Nut Consumption and Risk of Cardiometabolic Diseases

Author/Year	Study	Population	Nut Type	Follow-Up (Years)	Main Results
Fraser et al. (1992)	The Adventist Health Study	31,208 healthy men and women	Nuts (undefined)	6	RR = 0.52 (95% CI: 0.37–0.76; P < 0.05) for nonfatal and 0.49 (95% CI: 0.28–0.85; P = 0.005) *Comparison*: >5 times/week compared to <1 time/week
Fraser et al. (1995)	The Adventist Health Study	27,321 healthy men and women	Nut (undefined)	6	12% lifetime reduction in developing CHD (P = 0.05) *Comparison*: >5 servings/week compared to rare consumption
Kushi et al. (1996)	Iowa Women's Health Study	34,486 healthy postmenopausal woman	Nuts (undefined)	7	RR = 0.60 (95% CI: 0.36–1.01; P = 0.016) of fatal CHD *Comparison*: >4 times/week compared to 0 times/week
Fraser et al. (1997)	The Adventist Health Study	3,229 black California adults	Nuts (undefined)	7–11	HR = 0.6 (95% CI: 0.3–1.0) for nut consumption for death *Comparison*: >5 times/week compared to <1 time/week
Fraser and Shavlikm (1997)	The Adventist Health Study	603 adults ≥84 years	Nuts (undefined)	12	RR = 0.82 (95% CI, 0.70-0.96; P < 0.01) for death and RR = 0.61 (95% CI, 0.45–0.83; P < 0.001) for death from CHD
Hu et al. (1998)	Nurses' Health Study	86,016 healthy middle-aged women	1. Nuts (undefined) 2. Peanuts	14	RR = 0.61 (95% CI: 0.35–1.05; P = 0.007) for CVD risk *Comparison*: ≥5 servings/week of compared to <1 serving RR = 0.92 (95% CI: 0.74–1.15; P = 0.094) for CHD risk RR = 0.76 (95% CI: 0.51–1.15; P = 0.09) for fatal CHD *Comparison*: ≥5 times/week compared to almost never
Jiang et al. (2002)	Nurses' Health Study	83,818 women with type 2 diabetes	Nuts (undefined) Peanut butter	16	Nuts: RR = 0.73 (95% CI: 0.60–0.89; P = 0.001) for if type 2 diabetes *Comparison*: ≥5 servings/week compared to never/almost never Peanut butter: RR = 0.79 (95% CI: 0.68–0.91; P < 0.001) for risk of diabetes *Comparison*: ≥5 servings/week compared to never
Albert et al. (2002)	Physicians' Health Study	22,071 healthy men	Nuts (undefined)	17	RR = 0.53 (95% CI: 0.30–0.92; P = 0.01) for fatal *and* 47% decrease in sudden death *Comparison*: ≥2 servings/week compared to never or <1 time/month

(*Continued*)

TABLE 24.1 (*Continued*)

A Review of Observational Studies on Nut Consumption and Risk of Cardiometabolic Diseases

Author/Year	Study	Population	Nut Type	Follow-Up (Years)	Main Results
Kochar et al. (2010)	Physicians' Health Study	20,224 healthy men	Nuts (undefined)	1	No association for risk of diabetes. HR = 0.87 (95% CI: 0.61–1.24; P = 0.99)
Lutsey et al. (2008)	Atherosclerotic Risk in Community Study	9,514 white and black men and women	Nuts (undefined)	9	No association for nut consumption and MetS RR = 0.99 (95% CI: 0.91–1.08; P = 0.52) *Comparison*: Highest to lowest quintile
Li et al. (2009)	Nurses' Health Study II	6,309 women with type 2 diabetes	Tree nuts (undefined) Peanuts Peanut butter	22	RR = 0.56 (95% CI: 0.36–0.89; P = 0.44) for CVD risk *Comparison*: ≥5 servings/week compared to rarely or never consumed
O'Neil et al. (2011)	NHANES data 1999–2004	13,292	Nuts: peanuts, peanut butter, tree nuts (i.e., almonds, Brazil nuts, cashews, hazelnuts, macadamia nut, pecans, pistachios, walnuts, and pine nuts), and tree nut butters	6	Percentage of prevalence in MetS: (21.2% ± 2.1% vs. 26.6% ± 0.7%; P < 0.05) *Comparison*: Consumers (≥1/4 oz/day compared to <1/4 oz/day
Bao et al. (2013)	Nurses' Health Study Health Professionals Follow-Up Study	76,464 healthy women 42,498 male professionals	Tree Nuts (undefined) peanuts	30	HR = 0.86 (95% CI: 0.82–0.89) for total nuts for cause death HR = 0.88 (95% CI: 0.84–0.93) for peanuts for all-cause death HR = 0.83 (95% CI: 0.79–0.88) for tree nuts for all-cause death *Comparison*: ≥7 servings/week compared to never consumed
Fernández-Montero et al. (2013)	Seguimiento Universidad de Navarra (the SUN study)	9,887 young men and women	Nuts (undefined)	6	32% lower risk of MetS *Comparison*: ≥2 servings/week compared to those who never/rarely consumed
Ibarrola-Jurado et al. (2013)	PREDIMED (cross-sectional)	7,210 men and women at high CVD risk	Nuts (undefined)	N/A	OR = 0.75 (95%CI: 0.65–0.85; P < 0.001) for prevalence of MetS *Comparison*: >3 servings/week compared to <1 serving/week
Pan et al. (2013)	Nurses' Health Study Nurses' Health Study II	58,063 healthy women 79,893 healthy women	Walnuts	10	HR = 0.76 (0.62–0.94; P = 0.002) for risk of type 2 diabetes *Comparison*: ≥2 servings/week compared to reference (HR = 1.00) never/rarely consumed

(*Continued*)

TABLE 24.1 (*Continued*)
A Review of Observational Studies on Nut Consumption and Risk of Cardiometabolic Diseases

Author/Year	Study	Population	Nut Type	Follow-Up (Years)	Main Results
Jaceldo-Siegl et al. (2014)	Adventist Health Study-2 (cross-sectional)	803 adults	Total nuts, tree nuts, and peanuts	N/A	OR = (95% CI) were 0.77 (0.47, 1.28) for low tree nut/high peanut, 0.65 (0.42, 1.00) for high tree nut/high peanut and 0.68 (0.43, 1.07) for high tree nut/low peanut consumers, compared to tree nut/low peanut consumers (P for trend = 0.056)
O'Neil et al. (2015)	NHANES Data (2005–2010)	14,386 adults ≥19 years	Tree nuts (i.e., almonds, Brazil nuts, cashews, hazelnuts, macadamia nuts, pecans, pine nuts, pistachios, and walnuts)	6	Associated with lower BMI, waist circumference, systolic blood pressure, HOMA-IR, and higher HDL *Comparison*: Nut consumers (≥1/4 oz/day) and nonconsumers (<1/4 oz/day)
Gopinath et al. (2015)	The Blue Mountains Eye Study (BMES)	2,893 participants ≥49 years	Nuts (undefined)	15	HR = 0.76 (95%CI: 0.65–0.89) for nut consumption for total mortality *Comparison*: Second tertile and first tertile of nut intake
Luu et al. (2015)	Southern Community Cohort Study Shanghai Women's Health Study and Shanghai Men's Health Study	71,764 U.S. individuals with African and European descent, low SES 134,265 men and women of Asian descent	Peanuts and other nuts (undefined)	5.4 6.5 12.2	HR = 0.62 (95% CI: 0.45–0.85; P = 0.01) in African descent for ischemic heart disease HR = 0.60 (95% CI: 0.39–0.92; P = 0.007) in European descent for ischemic heart disease HR = 0.70 (95% CI: 0.54–0.89; P = 0.001) in Asian descent for ischemic heart disease *Comparison*: Highest and lowest quartile of nut intake
Eslamparast et al. (2017)	Golestan cohort study	50,045 participants ≥40 years	Nuts (undefined)	7	HR = 0.89 (95% CI: 0.82–0.95) for nut consumption for death *Comparison*: Did not consume nuts and <1 serving/week HR = 0.75 (95% CI: 0.67–0.85) for nut consumption for death *Comparison*: Did not consume nuts and 1 to <3 servings/week HR = 0.71 (95% CI: 0.58–0.86) for nut consumption for death *Comparison*: Did not consume nuts and ≥3 servings/week

compared to women who consumed less was observed. The multivariate-adjusted analysis for an incremental increase of 1 serving/day for nuts and peanut butter was associated with a significantly lower CVD risk. Authors reported improvements in LDL-C (−6.56 mg/dL, P = 0.008), non-HDL-C (−6.95 mg/dL, P = 0.014), TC (−7.34 mg/dL, P = 0.007), and ApoB (b coefficients) (−4 mg/dL, P = 0.016) (Li et al., 2009).

Bao et al. (2013) investigated the relationship between nut consumption and total and cause-specific mortality using data from the NHS (76,464 women) and the Health Professionals Follow-up Study (HPFS) (42,498 men) (another more affluent cohort). Results demonstrated that participants who consumed ≥7 servings/week of nuts (peanuts and tree nuts) had a 20% lower rate of mortality compared to those who did not consume nuts (Bao et al., 2013). The pooled multivariate-adjusted HRs for death from all causes were 0.86 (95% CI: 0.82–0.89) for total nuts, 0.88 (95% CI: 0.84–0.93) for peanuts, and 0.83 (95% CI: 0.79 to 0.88) for tree nuts (Bao et al., 2013).

Recent studies targeted populations of lower SES, since most epidemiological studies on nut consumption and CHD risk have been conducted primarily with U.S. populations of European ancestry with a higher SES. Luu et al. (2015) examined nut consumption in Americans of African and European descent that were predominantly of low SES and in Chinese individuals in Shanghai, China. The study showed an inverse association between nut intake and CVD mortality for all three ethnic groups (all P < 0.001). The HRs for IHD were 0.62 (95% CI: 0.045–0.85; P = 0.01) in those of African descent; 0.60 (95% CI: 0.39–0.92; P = 0.007) in those of European descent; and 0.70 (95% CI: 0.54–0.89; P = 0.001) in those of Asian descent for the highest versus lowest quintile of intake, respectively. The associations for ischemic stroke (HR = 0.77; 95% CI: 0.60–1.00 for the highest vs. lowest quintile of nut intake) and hemorrhagic stroke (HR = 0.77; 95% CI: 0.60–0.99 for the highest vs. lowest quintile of nut intake) were significant only in Asians (P = 0.003 for both). The association between the frequency of nut consumption and all-cause mortality and CVD mortality has also recently been observed in the Netherlands Cohort Study, analyzing 120,852 men and women aged 55–69 years (van den Brant and Schouten, 2015). In this study, peanuts and tree nuts were inversely related to mortality, whereas peanut butter was not.

Finally, a recent systematic review and meta-analysis including 20 prospective cohort studies and 467,389 participants has demonstrated that the frequency of nut consumption was significantly associated with a lower risk of all-cause mortality (10 studies; Risk Ratio [RR] = 0.81; 95% CI: 0.77–0.85 for highest vs. lower quintile of intake), CVD mortality (5 studies; RR 0.73; 95% CI: 0.68–0.78), all CHD (3 studies; RR 0.66; 95% CI: 0.48–0.91) and CHD mortality (7 studies; RR 0.70; 95% CI: 0.64–0.76), as well as a statistically nonsignificant reduction in the risk of nonfatal CHD (3 studies; RR 0.71; 95% CI: 0.49–1.03) and stroke mortality (3 studies; RR 0.83; 95% CI: 0.69–1.00) (Mayhew et al., 2016). However, no evidence of association was found for total stroke. These findings demonstrate that nut consumption is consistently associated with a decrease in all-cause mortality, total CVD and CVD mortality, CHD and CHD mortality and sudden cardiac death in different ethnic groups, as well as ischemic stroke in a Chinese cohort. Collectively, recent as well as earlier epidemiological studies demonstrate that frequent nut consumption is associated with lower CVD risk on a population-wide basis. It is important to note that epidemiological studies, and all studies to some extent, have limitations. Several of the studies reviewed report associations between the frequency of nut consumption, rather than the quantity of nuts consumed. However, the associations reported between frequent nut consumption and reduced CVD risk have provided support for the clinical studies that have been conducted to better understand cause-and-effect relationships (Covered in the next section).

NUT CONSUMPTION AND RISK OF TYPE 2 DIABETES

Jiang et al. (2002) analyzed data from the NHS to evaluate the relationship between tree nut and peanut consumption on risk of type 2 diabetes. The RR ratios across the categories of nut consumption (never/almost never, <once/week, 1–4 times/week, ≥5 times/week) were 1.0 (reference), 0.92

(95% CI: 0.85–1.00), 0.84 (95% CI: 0.76–0.93), and 0.73 (95% CI: 0.60–0.89) ($P < 0.001$), respectively (Jiang et al., 2002). The authors also examined the relationship between peanut butter consumption and diabetes risk. When comparing women who consumed peanut butter at least 5 times/week in a multivariate analysis, the RR for diabetes for a 28 g serving was 0.79 (95% CI: 0.68–0.91 [$P < 0.001$]) compared to those who did not eat peanut butter (Jiang et al., 2002). However, subsequent studies have reported conflicting results. For example, results from the Iowa Women's Health Study indicated that postmenopausal women who consumed nuts often (≥5 times/week) did not have a reduced risk of diabetes compared to those who consumed nuts occasionally (never/almost never), after adjusting for multiple confounding factors. Results, however, indicated an 18% reduction in RR between highest and lowest categories of peanut butter consumption (Parker et al., 2003; Parker and Folsom, 2003). By contrast, in the Shanghai Women's Health Study, an inverse association was demonstrated between the frequency of peanut consumption and type 2 diabetes risk incidence. The PHS did not find a significant relationship between nut consumption and incidence of type 2 diabetes (Kochar et al., 2010). The multivariable adjusted HRs were 1.0 (reference), 1.06 (95% CI: 0.93–1.20), 1.10 (95% CI: 0.95–1.26), 0.97 (95% CI: 0.82–1.14), 0.99 (95% CI: 0.76–1.30), and 0.87 (95% CI: 0.61–1.24) from the lowest to the highest category of nut consumption, respectively (P-trend = 0.99) (Kochar et al., 2010). Pan et al. (2013) studied the relationship of walnut intake and risk of type 2 diabetes using the original NHS I & II database. Walnut consumption lowered the risk of type 2 diabetes (Pan et al., 2013). Specifically, the HRs for individuals consuming 1–3 servings/month (1 serving = 28 g), 1 serving/week, and ≥2 servings/week of walnuts were 0.93 (95% CI: 0.88–0.99), 0.81 (95% CI: 0.70–0.94), and 0.67 (95% CI: 0.54–0.82) compared with women who never/rarely consumed walnuts (P-trend < 0.001).

In a report published using data from the PREDIMED cohort (n = 3541 participants without diabetes at baseline), 273 cases of new-onset diabetes occurred after 4.1 years follow-up: 80 in the Mediterranean diet supplemented with extra virgin olive oil (MeDiet + EVOO) group, 92 in the Mediterranean diet supplemented with nuts (MeDiet + nuts) group, and 101 in the control group. After multivariable adjustment, hazard ratios for diabetes were 0.60 (95% CI: 0.43, 0.85) for MeDiet + EVOO and 0.82 (95% CI: 0.61, 1.10) for MeDiet + nuts compared with the control group (Martinez-Gonzalez et al., 2015).

Collectively, these studies suggest that consumption of nuts may elicit benefits on risk of diabetes. The discrepancies among the studies conducted to date warrant further investigation (Table 24.1 summarizes the epidemiological studies reviewed).

NUT CONSUMPTION AND METABOLIC SYNDROME RISK

Few studies have evaluated tree nut and peanut consumption and the risk of Metabolic Syndrome (MetS). The Atherosclerosis Risk in Community Study prospectively analyzed data from over 9500 healthy participants aged 45–64 years of white and black race (Lutsey et al., 2008) and reported no association between nut intake and risk of MetS (RR = 0.99; 95% CI: 0.91–1.08; P = 0.52) (Lutsey et al., 2008). Other studies have observed different outcomes when using individual diagnostic criteria for MetS. O'Neil et al. (2011) evaluated the association of risk factors of MetS with consumption of all types of nuts. Nuts were defined as peanuts, peanut butter, tree nuts (i.e., almonds, Brazil nuts, cashews, hazelnuts, macadamias, pecans, pistachios, walnuts, and pine nuts), or tree nut butters. Nut consumption was defined as intakes of at least ¼ oz (7.09 g) of nuts/day, while nonconsumers were defined by an intake of <¼ oz/day (O'Neil et al., 2011). Nut consumption was associated with benefits for the following MetS criteria: lower prevalence of abdominal obesity (43.6% ± 1.6% vs. 49.5% ± 0.8%; $P \leq 0.01$), hypertension (31.4% ± 1.2% vs. 33.9% ± 0.8%; $P \leq 0.05$), low HDL-C (27.9% ± 1.7% vs. 34.5% ± 0.8%; $P < 0.01$), elevated fasting blood glucose (11.5% ± 1.4% vs. 15.0% ± 0.7%; $P \leq 0.05$), and MetS (21.2% ± 2.1% vs. 26.6% ± 0.7%; $P < 0.05$) (O'Neil et al., 2011). In the context of the Adventist Health Study, the frequency of tree nut consumption was also inversely associated with metabolic syndrome prevalence (Jaceldo-Siegl et al., 2014).

The Seguimiento Universidad de Navarra (SUN) cohort study investigated nut consumption in a Mediterranean population of university graduates (n = 9887) (Fernandez-Montero et al., 2013). After a 6-year follow-up, researchers observed a 32% reduction in MetS risk with nut consumption of >2 servings/week compared with those who never/almost never consumed nuts (adjusted OR = 0.68, 95% CI: 0.50–0.92; P = 0.075) (Fernandez-Montero et al., 2013). This inverse association was stronger in women (RR = 0.29; 95% CI: 0.15–0.56; P < 0.001) and was not significant among men (RR = 0.90; 95% CI: 0.63 = 1.29; P = 0.91), indicating that the association differed by sex. Ibarrola-Jurado et al. (2013) reported a lower adjusted odds ratio (OR = 0.74, 0.65–0.85; P = 0.001) in individuals consuming >3 servings/week of nuts compared to individuals consuming <1 serving/week. Interestingly, the higher nut intake also was associated with a lower risk of abdominal obesity (OR = 0.68, 95% CI: 0.60–0.79; P < 0.001) with no significant associations for hypertension, dyslipidemia, or elevated fasting glucose (Ibarrola-Jurado et al., 2013). O'Neil et al. (2015) used the National Health and Nutrition Examination Survey (NHANES) to investigate tree nut consumption, and adiposity measures, CVD, and MetS diagnostics. The authors categorized participants as nonconsumers (<¼ oz/day tree nuts) or consumers (>¼ oz/day tree nuts). Results showed tree nut consumers had significantly lower BMI (27.9 ± 0.3 vs. 28.7 ± 0.1 kg/m^2; P = 0.004) and waist circumference (WC) (95.8 ± 0.7 vs. 98.1 ± 0.3 cm; P = 0.008) than nonconsumers. Systolic blood pressure (SBP) was also lower in tree nut consumers (119.5 ± 0.8 vs. 122.1 ± 0.2 mmHg; P = 0.001). This study demonstrates an association between tree nut consumption and better weight status in addition to improvements in CVD and MetS risk factors (O'Neil et al., 2015). This epidemiological study, in conjunction with others, provides further affirmation that consumption of tree nuts and peanuts is associated with decreased risk of CVD, diabetes, and MetS. A dose–response relationship has also been observed between nut consumption and improved diagnostic criteria for MetS.

A beneficial effect of nut supplementation on MetS status was also observed in the PREDIMED trial (described in detail in the next section). In comparison with the control group, participants randomized to either MeDiet were more likely to show reversal of MetS, with HR 1.35 (CI: 1.15–1.58) for the MeDiet + EVOO, and HR 1.28 (CI: 1.08–1.51) for the MeDiet + nuts (Babio et al., 2014; Salas-Salvadó et al., 2008). Of note, participants in the group supplemented with nuts showed a significant decrease in central obesity.

The epidemiological evidence has continued to show a strong beneficial relationship between nut intake and CVD risk in a diverse sample that is representative of the general public. However, randomized controlled trials (RCTs) are needed to establish cause-and-effect relationships and identify the nutrients and/or bioactive compounds responsible for the beneficial associations reported for tree nuts and peanuts and reduced risk of CVD, diabetes, and MetS.

CLINICAL TRIALS ON NUT CONSUMPTION AND CORONARY HEART DISEASE

CVD Events

The Prevención con Dieta Mediterránea (PREDIMED) trial was a major clinical nutritional intervention designed to assess the efficacy of the Mediterranean diet in the primary prevention of CVD. Participants (n = 7447) were 55–80 years of age with type 2 diabetes or with three or more major CVD risk factors (hypertension, hypercholesterolemia, family history of heart disease, tobacco use, or overweight/obesity) and were randomized to (1) a Mediterranean diet supplemented with extra-virgin olive oil (1 L/week/family; 50 g/day per participant; 41.2% total fat, 9.4% SFA), (2) a Mediterranean diet supplemented with nuts (30 g/day: 15 g walnuts, 7.5 g hazelnuts, 7.5 g almonds; 41.5% total fat; 9.3% SFA), or (3) a control diet (37.0% total fat; 9.1% SFA). The primary endpoint was rate of major CVD events (myocardial infarction, stroke, or death from cardiovascular causes), which occurred in 288 participants. The HRs were 0.70 (95% CI: 0.54–0.92) and 0.72 (95% CI: 0.54–0.96) for the group supplemented with extra-virgin olive oil group (96 events) and the group supplemented with nuts (83 events), respectively, versus the control group (109 events) (Estruch et al., 2013). Thus, a

Mediterranean diet supplemented with extra-virgin olive oil or nuts reduced the rate of major CVD events compared with a lower-fat diet among individuals at high CVD risk.

Major CVD Risk Factors

The strong epidemiological evidence for benefits of nut consumption and chronic disease risk reduction has been the impetus for many clinical trials that have been conducted to evaluate the effects of nuts on CHD risk factors and their underlying mechanism(s) of action. These studies have shown beneficial effects on lipids and lipoproteins (Casas-Agustench et al., 2011a,b; Griel et al., 2007; Nouran et al., 2010; Sheridan et al., 2007; Tey et al., 2011) and numerous other risk factors for cardiometabolic diseases (Blanco Mejia et al., 2014; Viguiliouk et al., 2014). The first clinical trial evaluating the effect of nut consumption on CVD risk factors was the Loma Linda University walnut study (Sabate et al., 1993). In this study, healthy men were randomized to one of two cholesterol-lowering diets: a diet providing 20% of energy from walnuts [total fat was 31% of energy, 6% from saturated fatty acids (SFA), and 16% from polyunsaturated fatty acids (PUFA)] versus a Step-1 diet (total fat was 30% of energy, 10% SFA, and 10% PUFA). Total cholesterol (TC) and LDL-C significantly decreased by 12% ($P < 0.0001$) and 16% ($P < 0.001$), respectively, from the walnut diet versus the Step-1 diet.

Studies evaluating walnuts (Rajaram et al., 2009; Torabian et al., 2010), almonds (Berryman et al., 2013; Jenkins et al., 2002), pistachios (Sauder et al., 2013; Sheridan et al., 2007), hazelnuts (Mercanligil et al., 2007), peanuts (Lokko et al., 2007), and macadamia nuts (Griel et al., 2008) have reported decreases in LDL-C ranging from 9% to 16%. A pooled analysis of 25 nut intervention studies conducted in 7 countries with 583 men and women (normolipidemic and hypercholesterolemic) reported a dose–response improvement in lipids/lipoproteins with nut consumption (Sabaté et al., 2010). The mean daily intake was 67 g of nuts (walnuts, almonds, pistachios, pecan, macadamia nut, and peanuts) with the following reductions achieved: TC (10.9 mg/dL [5.1% change]), LDL-C (10.2 mg/dL [7.4% change]), LDL: HDL-C ratio (0.22 [8.3% change]), and TC: HDL-C ratio (0.24 [5.6% change]) ($P < 0.001$ for all). No significant effect was reported for HDL-C or triglycerides (TG), except in individuals with TG > 150 mg/dL, in whom there was a 20.6 mg/dL (10.2%) decrease in TG. The effects of nut consumption were dose-related and different nuts had similar effects on lipids/lipoproteins. The effects were greatest in those with higher LDL-C values (≥160 vs. <130 mg/dL), with a lower body mass (<25 vs. ≥25 BMI). Benefits were also greater when nuts were part of a Western diet or lower-fat diet compared to a Mediterranean diet (Sabaté et al., 2010).

A meta-analysis of 13 clinical trials with 365 participants (healthy individuals and individuals at high CVD risk) evaluated the effects of walnut consumption on lipids/lipoproteins and CVD risk factors (Banel and Hu, 2009). The diets were consumed for 4–24 weeks; walnuts provided 10%–24% of total energy. Compared to the control diets, the walnut diets significantly decreased TC (−10.3 mg/dL, $P < 0.001$) and LDL-C (−9.2 mg/dL, $P = 0.001$). There was no significant effect of walnuts on HDL-C or TG. This decrease in LDL-C (6.7%) is consistent with findings from a pooled analysis of 25 intervention trials (Sabaté et al., 2010) in which a 7.4% decrease in LDL-C was reported with consumption of different nuts (Sabaté et al., 2010). A recent systematic review and meta-analysis was conducted to evaluate the dose–response effects of different nuts on lipids, lipoproteins, and apolipoprotein B. Del Gobbo et al. (2015) evaluated 61 RCTs with 2582 participants (healthy individuals and individuals with comorbidities) who consumed different types and amounts of nuts for 3–26 weeks. Compared with control diets (habitual, American Heart Association, low-fat, high-fat, and Mediterranean-type diets), consumption of tree nuts significantly decreased TC (weight mean difference per 28 g/day: −4.7; 95% CI: −5.3, −4.0), LDL-C (−4.8%; 95% CI: −5.5, −4.2), ApoB (−3.7; 95% CI: −5.2, −2.3), and TGs (−2.2; 95% CI: −3.8, −0.5). TC and LDL-C decreased in a nonlinear fashion ($P < 0.001$); stronger effects were reported when consumption was ≥60 g/day. Linear dose–response relationships were reported between nut intake and ApoB ($r = -0.12$) and TG ($r = -0.16$). There were no significant differences among type of tree nuts. Stronger effects were observed for ApoB in participants with type 2 diabetes (−11.5 mg/dL; 95% CI: −16.2, −6.8 mg/dL) than in healthy individuals (−2.5 mg/dL; 95% CI: −4.7, −0.3 mg/dL) (P-heterogeneity = 0.015). These findings demonstrate that the quantity of nuts consumed is a major determinant of the lipid/lipoprotein effects rather than the type of nut.

A recent systematic review and meta-analysis of 12 RCTs lasting ≥3 weeks with 450 individuals with type 2 diabetes evaluated the effect of diets that included tree nuts (average amount was 56 g/day) compared to isocaloric control diets without nuts (i.e., high-fat, low-fat, ad libitum diet, NCEP Step-2 diet) on HbA1c, fasting glucose, fasting insulin, and HOMA-IR (Viguiliouk et al., 2014). The tree nut diets significantly lowered HbA1c (−0.07%; 95% CI: −0.10 to −0.03%; P = 0.0003) and fasting glucose (−1.44 mg/dL; 95% CI: −4.86 to 0.36 mg/dL; P = 0.03) compared to the control diets. No significant treatment effects were reported for fasting insulin and HOMA-IR levels. Beyond this meta-analysis that evaluated the effects of nuts on endpoints related to diabetes control, there have been few trials conducted that have reported beneficial effects of nuts on lipids and lipoproteins in individuals with type 2 diabetes (Lovejoy et al., 2002; Sauder et al., 2015; Tapsell et al., 2004). Of the three studies conducted, two reported decreases in TC (−6 to −9 mg/dL) after consumption of almonds (10% of total fat or 2 oz/day) (Lovejoy et al., 2002) or pistachios (20% of total energy) (Sauder et al., 2015). Tapsell et al. (2004) reported a 10% decrease in LDL-C (P = 0.032) after consumption of 30 g walnuts/day incorporated into a lower-fat diet (<30% fat).

A systematic review and meta-analysis (Blanco Mejia et al., 2014) of 49 RCTs with 2226 participants (healthy individuals or individuals diagnosed with dyslipidemia, MetS or type 2 diabetes) assessed the effects of nut consumption on MetS criteria. A median intake of 50 g/day of nuts (almonds, hazelnuts, cashews, walnuts, pistachio, macadamia, and mixed nuts) with a median follow-up of 8 weeks improved MetS criteria with decreases in TG [(−5.30 mg/dL; 95% CI: −7.96 to −2.56 mg/dL) with evidence of moderate heterogeneity ($I^2 = 34\%$, P = 0.02)], and fasting blood glucose [(−7.08 mg/dL; 95% CI: −14.16 to −0.88) with evidence of moderate heterogeneity ($I^2 = 41\%$, P < 0.05)] compared with the control intervention (i.e., usual, Step-1, average American diet, low-fat diets). There was no effect on waist circumference, HDL-C, or blood pressure. In a review of six nut intervention trials focusing on individuals with MetS (Salas-Salvado et al., 2014a,b), the authors reported a 25.8% reduction in fasting insulin and 27.6% reduction in HOMA-IR in individuals who received 30 g of nuts/day and advice on health compared to the control group. Wu et al. (2010) conducted a study in which 283 Asian individuals with MetS were randomly assigned to one of three treatments: (1) lifestyle counseling (LC) on the AHA guidelines, (2) LC + 30 g flaxseed/day, or (3) LC + 30 g walnuts/day. After the 12-week intervention, prevalence of MetS decreased significantly in all groups: −16.9% (LC only), −20.2% (LC + flaxseed), and −16.0% (LC + walnuts) (P < 0.05). In addition, there was a greater decrease in central obesity in the LC + flaxseed group (19.2%; P = 0.008) and LC + walnuts (16.0%; P = 0.04) than in the LC-only group (6.3%) (Wu et al., 2010). These findings suggest that nut supplementation decreases risk of MetS criteria and prevalence in healthy individuals and individuals with MetS (Table 24.2 summarizes the studies discussed).

Other CVD Risk Factors

Lipoprotein Particles

Lipoprotein subfractions that are differentiated by particle diameter, density, and composition differentially affect CVD risk (Carmena et al., 2004). While all LDL particles increase risk of CVD events, there is evidence that small LDL particles are particularly atherogenic. The Quebec Heart Study (Lamarche et al., 1995), Veterans Administration HDL Intervention Trial (VA-HIT) (Otvos et al., 2006), Cardiovascular Health Study (Kuller et al., 2002), Women's Health Study (Blake et al., 2002), Atherosclerosis in Communities (ARIC) (Hallman et al., 2004), and Framingham Offspring Study (Cromwell et al., 2007) have shown that higher concentrations of small, dense LDL (between 18.0 and 27.8 nmol/L) increase CVD risk. Some studies (e.g., the Strong Heart Study [Howard et al., 2000] and Cholesterol and Recurrent Events (CARE) study [Campos et al., 2001]), however, do not agree

TABLE 24.2
A Review of Clinical Trials on Nut Consumption and Risk Factors for Cardiometabolic Diseases

Authors	Study Design	Participants	Diet Design	Endpoints	Results
Fraser et al. (2002)	Crossover	Male and female participants (n = 81)	Supplemented 320 kcal almonds or 0 kcal almonds for 6 months	Weight	Weight increased 0.40 kg (P approximately 0.09)
Lovejoy et al. (2002)	RCT, controlled feeding	30 individuals with type 2 diabetes	Diets: 1. High-fat, high-almond (HFA; 37% total fat, 10% from almonds) 2. Low-fat, high-almond (LFA; 25% total fat, 10% from almonds) 3. High-fat control (HFC; 37% total fat, 10% from olive or canola oil) 4. Low-fat control (LFC; 25% total fat, 10% from olive or canola oil) for 4 weeks	Lipids/lipoproteins	TC lowest in HFA diet (172.5 ± 0.14, 174.8 ± 0.14, 179 ± 0.14, and 179 ± 0.14 mg/dL) compared with HFA, HFC, LFA and LDC (P = 0.0004)
Tapsell et al. (2004)	RCT, given dietary advice	58 individuals with type 2 diabetes	Diets: Low fat (control) Low fat/modified fat Walnut (low fat/modified fat including 30 g/day of walnuts) for 4 weeks	Lipids/lipoproteins	TC: HDL-C ratio (+0.33 + 0.10 vs. 0.29 + 0.07 and 0.26 + 0.06; P = 0.049) compared to the modified fat and control group, respectively. LDL—10% reduction (P = 0.032)
Banel and Hu (2009)	Meta-analysis	365 participants (healthy individuals and individuals at high CVD risk)	10%–24% energy of walnuts/day; diets lasting 4–24 weeks	Lipids/lipoproteins	TC (–10.3 mg/dL, P < 0.001) and LDL-C (–9.2 mg/dL, P = 0.001)
Sabaté et al. (2010)	Pooled analysis	583 men and women (normolipidemic and hypercholesterolemic)	67 g/day of nuts (walnuts, almonds, pistachios, pecans, macadamia nut, and peanuts, with durations of 3–6 weeks	Lipids/lipoproteins	TC (–10.9 mg/dL [5.1% change]) LDL-C (–10.2 mg/dL [7.4% change]) LDL: HDL-C ratio (0.22 [8.3% change]) TC: HDL-C ratio (0.24 [5.6% change]) (P < 0.001 for all)

(*Continued*)

TABLE 24.2 (*Continued*)
A Review of Clinical Trials on Nut Consumption and Risk Factors for Cardiometabolic Diseases

Authors	Study Design	Participants	Diet Design	Endpoints	Results
Wu et al. (2010)	RCT	283 Asian individuals with MetS	One of three treatments: 1. Lifestyle counseling (LC) on the AHA guidelines 2. LC + 30 g flaxseed/day 3. LC + 30 g walnuts/day for 12 weeks	Prevalence of MetS and MetS components	Prevalence of MetS decreased significantly in all groups: −16.9% (LC only), −20.2% (LC + flaxseed), and −16.0% (LC + walnuts) ($P < 0.05$) Reversion rate of central obesity was higher in the LC + flaxseed group (19.2%; $P = 0.008$) and LC + walnuts (16.0%; $P = 0.04$) than in the LC-only group (6.3%)
Baer et al. (2012)	Randomized, crossover, controlled feeding	Healthy adults (n = 16)	Three test diets that included 0 g/day pistachios, 42 g/day pistachios, or 84 g/day pistachios for 3 weeks	Measured energy (ME) value	Pistachios ME in the diet: (5.4 kcal/g); 5% less than the calculated Atwater factors (5.7 kcal/g)
Foster et al. (2012)	RCT	Overweight and obese individuals (n = 123)	Supplemented two 28 g packages of almonds per day for 18 months or nut-free diet	Weight	NFD lost more weight than AED (−7.4 compared with −5.5 kg; $P = 0.04$); No significant differences at 18 months
				Lipids and lipoproteins	Significantly greater reductions in triglycerides and TC in AED versus NFD group at 6 months but not at 18 months
Novotny et al. (2012)	Randomized, crossover, controlled feeding	Healthy adults (n = 18)	Three diets that included 0 g/day whole almonds, 42 g/day almonds, or 84 g/day almonds for 18 days	Measured energy (ME) value	Almonds ME in the diet: 4.6 ± 0.8 kcal/g (equivalent to 129 kcal/28 g serving); significantly less than 6.0–6.1 kcal/g (168–170 kcal/serving), the energy density determined by Atwater factors ($P < 0.001$)

(*Continued*)

TABLE 24.2 (*Continued*)
A Review of Clinical Trials on Nut Consumption and Risk Factors for Cardiometabolic Diseases

Authors	Study Design	Participants	Diet Design	Endpoints	Results
Zhang et al. (2012)	Randomized, controlled, postprandial feeding study	Healthy overweight participants (n = 15)	Four test diets: 85 g of ground whole walnuts, 34 g of ground de-fatted walnut meat, 51 g of walnut oil or 5.6 g of ground defatted walnut skins	Lipoprotein function	85 g of whole increased cholesterol efflux by 3.3% (P = 0.02) compared to the baseline
Damasceno et al. (2013)	RCT	PREDIMED cohort (n = 169) with type 2 diabetes or with 3 or more major CVD risk factors (hypertension, hypercholesterolemia, family history of heart disease, tobacco use, or overweight/obesity)	1. Mediterranean diet supplemented with extra-virgin olive oil (1 L/week/family; 50 g/day per participant; 39.1% total fat, 10.2% SFA) 2. A Mediterranean diet supplemented with nuts (30 g/day: 15 g walnuts, 7.5 g hazelnuts, 7.5 g almonds; 37.4% total fat; 9.8% SFA) 3. A control diet (39.8% total fat; 10.6% SFA) for 1 year	Lipoprotein subparticles	Traditional Mediterranean diet w/nuts increased large LDL (54 nmol/L; 95% CI: 18–90) and decreased very small, dense LDL (−111 nmol/L: 95% CI: −180 to −42; P = 0.017 for both values) No significant differences in total LDL-C among groups (P = 0.942)
Estruch et al. (2013)	Randomized trial	PREDIMED cohort (n = 7447) with type 2 diabetes or with 3 or more major CVD risk factors (hypertension, hypercholesterolemia, family history of heart disease, tobacco use, or overweight/obesity)	1. Mediterranean diet supplemented with extra-virgin olive oil (1 L/week/family; 50 g/day per participant; 41.2% total fat, 9.4% SFA) 2. A Mediterranean diet supplemented with nuts (30 g/day: 15 g walnuts, 7.5 g hazelnuts, 7.5 g almonds; 41.5% total fat; 9.3% SFA) 3. A control diet (37.0% total fat; 9.1% SFA) for 1 year	Rate of major CVD events (MI, stroke, or death from CVD causes)	HR = 0.70 (95% CI: 0.54–0.92) for extra-virgin olive oil group (96 events) and 0.72 (95% CI: 0.54–0.96) for nut group (83 events) versus the control group (109 events)

(*Continued*)

TABLE 24.2 (*Continued*)
A Review of Clinical Trials on Nut Consumption and Risk Factors for Cardiometabolic Diseases

Authors	Study Design	Participants	Diet Design	Endpoints	Results
Babio et al. (2014)	Randomized trial	PREDIMED cohort	1. Mediterranean diet supplemented with extra-virgin olive oil (50 g/day) 2. A Mediterranean diet supplemented with nuts (30 g/day) 3. A control diet for 4.8-year follow-up	Incidence and reversion of metabolic syndrome	Incidence: HR = 1.10 (95% CI: 0.94–1.30, p = 0.231) for control versus extra-virgin olive oil; HR = 1.08 (95% CI: 0.92–1.27, P = 0.3) for control versus nuts Reversion: HR = 1.35 (95% CI: 1.15–1.58, P < 0.001) for control versus extra-virgin olive oil; HR = 1.28 (95% CI: 1.08–1.51, P < 0.001) for control versus nuts
Blanco Mejia et al. (2014)	Review and meta-analysis	2226 participants (healthy individuals or individuals diagnosed with dyslipidemia, MetS or type 2 diabetes)	Median nut (almonds, hazelnuts, cashews, walnuts, pistachio, macadamia, and mixed nuts) dose was 49.3 g/day (42–70.5 g/day). Median follow-up was 8 weeks (4–12 weeks) compared to control diets (usual, Step-1, average American diet, low-fat diets)	MetS criteria	TG (–0.06 mmol; 95% CI: –0.09 to –0.03 mmol/L) Fasting blood glucose (–0.08 mmol; 95% CI: –0.16 to –0.01)
Holligan et al. (2014)	RCT	Individuals (n = 28) with elevated LDL-C levels	One of three diets: a lower-fat control diet (control; 25% total fat and 8% SFA); a diet that provided 10% of energy from pistachios (32–65 g/day [1PD]; 30% total fat and 8% SFA); a diet that provided 20% of energy from pistachios (63–126 g/day [2PD]; 34% total fat and 8% SFA) for 4 weeks	Lipoprotein subclasses Cholesterol efflux	10% and 20% pistachio diets reduced sdLDL levels (least square means [LSM] = 1.00 mmol/L [SE 0.03], P = 0.001) and (LSM = 0.86 [SE 0.03], P = 0·03) compared to the control average American diet (LSM = 1.07 [SE] 0.03) No effect except in individuals with baseline CRP values < 0.2 mg/dL had significant increases in ABCA1-mediated efflux and global efflux following the 2 servings of pistachios compared to 1 serving of pistachios (9.89% [SE 0.74] vs. 7.35% [SE 0.74], P = 0.016)

(*Continued*)

TABLE 24.2 (*Continued*)
A Review of Clinical Trials on Nut Consumption and Risk Factors for Cardiometabolic Diseases

Authors	Study Design	Participants	Diet Design	Endpoints	Results
Salas-Salvado et al. (2014b)	Review of RCTs	6 RCTs with 1,746 total individuals	30 g of nuts/day compared to advice on health compared to the control group 8 weeks to 1 year	Fasting insulin HOMAR-IR	25.8% reduction in fasting insulin 27.6% reduction in HOMAR-IR
Salas-Salvadó et al. (2014a)	Randomized trial	PREDIMED cohort	1. Mediterranean diet supplemented with extra-virgin olive oil 2. A Mediterranean diet supplemented with nuts 3. A control diet for 4.1-year follow-up	Diabetes incidence	HRs = 0.60 (95% CI, 0.43–0.85) for the Mediterranean diet supplemented with extra-virgin olive oil and 0.82 (CI, 0.61–1.10) for the Mediterranean diet supplemented with nuts versus control
Viguiliouk et al. (2014)	Systematic review	450 individuals with type 2 diabetes	56 g/day of tree nuts for 4–24 weeks	HbA1c, fasting glucose, fasting insulin, HOMA-IR	HbA1c (–0.07%; 95% CI: –0.10% to –0.03%; P = 0.0003) fasting glucose (–1.44 mg/dL; 95% CI: –4.86 to 0.36 mg/dL; P = 0.03)
Berryman et al. (2015)	RCT	Individuals (n = 48) with elevated LDL-C	Cholesterol-lowering moderate-fat diet (26% calories from fat) with almonds (1.5 oz/day) was compared with an isocaloric lower-fat (32%) diet with 106 g banana muffin + 2.7 g butter for 6 weeks	Lipoprotein subparticles	No effects for LDL_1, LDL_2, LDL_3 or LDL_4; Higher-fat almond diet decreased IDL1 (–0.06 ± 0.33 vs. 0.76 ± 0.33 mg/dL; P = 0.01), total VLDL (0.15 ± 0.91 vs. 2.46 ± 0.91 mg/dL; P = 0.02), VLDL3 (0.01 ± 0.49 vs. 1.18 ± 0.49 mg/dL; P = 0.02), and apoB (–9.7 ± 1.8 vs. –5.5 ± 1.8 mg/dL; P = 0.01)
Del Gobbo et al. (2015)	Systematic review and meta-analysis	2,582 (healthy individuals and individuals with comorbidity)	28 g/day of nuts for 3–26 weeks	Lipids/lipoproteins	TC (–4.7; 95% CI: –5.3, –4.0) LDL-C (–4.8%; 95% CI: –5.5, –4.2) ApoB (–3.7: 95% CI: –5.2, –2.3) TGs (–2.2; 95% CI: –3.8, –0.5)

(*Continued*)

TABLE 24.2 (*Continued*)
A Review of Clinical Trials on Nut Consumption and Risk Factors for Cardiometabolic Diseases

Authors	Study Design	Participants	Diet Design	Endpoints	Results
Hernandez-Alonso et al. (2015)	RCT	Individuals (n = 54) with prediabetes	Pistachio diet (PD, 50% carbohydrates, 33% fat, including 57 g/day of pistachios) or a control diet (55% carbohydrates, 30% fat) for 4 months	Lipoprotein subclasses	Greater decrease in small, dense LDL from the higher-fat pistachio diet compared to the lower-fat control diet (−28.07 nM [95%CI: −60.43, 4.29] versus −16.49 nM [95% CI: −14.19, 47.18] P = 0.023)
Sauder et al. (2015)	RCT, controlled feeding	30 individuals with type 2 diabetes	Matched diets with either incorporations of 20% pistachios into the diet or no pistachios for 4 weeks	Lipids/lipoproteins	TC (−5.8 mg) TC: HDL ratio (−0.31) (P < 0.05)
Baer et al. (2016)	Randomized, crossover, controlled feeding	Healthy adults (n = 18)	Two test diets that included: 0 g/day walnuts or 42 g/day walnuts	Measured energy (ME) value	Walnuts ME in the diet: 5.22 ± 0.16 kcal/g (146 kcal/28 g serving); significantly lower than calculated Atwater factors (6.61 kcal/g; 185 g/serving); overestimating by 21%
Estruch et al. (2016)	Randomized trial	PREDIMED cohort	1. Mediterranean diet supplemented with extra virgin olive oil 2. A Mediterranean diet supplemented with nuts 3. A control diet for 4.8-year follow-up	Bodyweight and waist circumference	Mediterranean diet with extra-virgin olive oil group was −0.43 kg (95% CI −0.86 to −0.01; P = 0.044) and in the nut group was −0.08 kg (−0.50 to 0.35; P = 0.730) versus control group Changes in waist circumference were −0.55 cm (−1.16 to −0.06; P = 0.048) in the Mediterranean diet with extra-virgin olive oil group and −0.94 cm (−1.60 to −0.27; P = 0.006) in the nut group versus control group

with these results. This discrepancy may be due to differences in study populations and different methods used to quantify lipoprotein particle size. The Strong Heart Study included individuals with type 2 diabetes and the CARE study included individuals with history of myocardial infarctions, while the previous studies were conducted in persons with no history of CVD. In addition to the predictive value of LDL size, HDL subpopulations have also been shown to predict CHD risk. The Framingham Offspring Study reported that every 1 mg/dL increase in apoA-I in very large α-1 HDL was associated with a 26% ($P < 0.0001$) decrease in CHD risk (Asztalos et al., 2004). In the VA-HIT trial, logistic regression indicated each 1 mg/dL decrease in α-1 increased the odds of CHD 13% ($P < 0.0001$) in participants with low HDL-C, after adjustment for lipid and nonlipid CHD risk factors (Asztalos et al., 2005). Thus, evaluation of lipoprotein particles may provide further insight into CVD risk.

In a subset of the PREDIMED study cohort (n = 169), consumption of a traditional Mediterranean diet with nuts increased large LDL (54 nmol/L; 95% CI: 18–90) and decreased very small, dense LDL (−111 nmol/L; 95% CI: −180 to −42; P = 0.017 for both values) (Damasceno et al., 2013). There were no significant differences in total LDL-C among groups (P = 0.942). In a study conducted by Berryman et al., the effects of a cholesterol-lowering moderate-fat diet (32% calories from fat) with almonds (1.5 oz/day) were compared with an isocaloric lower-fat (26%) diet with 106 g banana muffin + 2.7 g butter for 6 weeks (Berryman et al., 2015), in individuals (n = 48) with elevated LDL-C (149 ± 3 mg/dL). There were no treatment effects for LDL_1, LDL_2, LDL_3, or LDL_4; however, the higher-fat almond diet significantly decreased IDL_1 (−0.06 ± 0.33 vs. 0.7 6 ± 0.33 mg/dL; P = 0.01), total VLDL (0.15 ± 0.91 vs. 2.46 ± 0.91 mg/dL; P = 0.02), VLDL3 (0.01 ± 0.49 vs. 1.18 ± 0.49 mg/dL; P = 0.02), and apoB (−9.7 ± 1.8 vs. −5.5 ± 1.8 mg/dL; P = 0.01) compared with the lower-fat diet. Pistachios also have been studied for their effects on lipoprotein subclasses. One randomized, crossover controlled-feeding study was designed to evaluate the effects of pistachio consumption on lipoprotein subclasses in individuals (n = 28) with elevated LDL-C levels (≥110.6 mg/dL) (Holligan et al., 2014). There were three experimental diets: a lower-fat control diet (control; 25% total fat and 8% SFA); a diet that provided 10% of energy from pistachios (32–65 g/day (1PD); 30% total fat and 8% SFA); and a diet that provided 20% of energy from pistachios (63–126 g/day (2PD); 34% total fat and 8% SFA). Both the 10% and 20% pistachio diets significantly reduced small, dense LDL levels [least square means [LSM] = 1.00 mmol/L (SE 0.03), P = 0.001 and LSM = 0.86 (SE 0.03), P = 0.03, respectively], compared to the lower-fat control diet [LSM = 1.07 (SE) 0.03]. A similar effect also has been reported in individuals at risk for diabetes. In a study of 54 adults with prediabetes, subjects were randomized to a diet with pistachios (PD, 50% carbohydrates, 33% fat, including 57 g/day of pistachios) or a control diet (55% carbohydrates, 30% fat) for 4 months. There was a significantly greater decrease in small, dense LDL from the higher fat pistachio diet compared to the lower-fat control diet [−28.07 nM (95% CI: −60.43, 4.29) vs. −16.49 nM (95% CI: −14.19, 47.18); P = 0.023, respectively] (Hernandez-Alonso et al., 2015). Collectively, these studies demonstrate a beneficial relationship between nut consumption and reduced CVD risk in relation to lipoprotein subclass distribution within the context of a moderate-fat diet compared with a lower-fat control diet without nuts.

Lipoprotein Function

Reverse cholesterol transport (measured as cholesterol efflux) is the process by which cholesterol is removed from macrophages. In a U.S. cohort study of 2924 healthy individuals, there was a 67% reduction in cardiovascular risk in the highest quartile of cholesterol efflux capacity versus the lowest quartile [HR = 0.33; (95% CI: 0.19–0.55)]. Efflux capacity was measured using fluorescence-labeled cholesterol and assayed, evaluating cholesterol efflux as mediated by ATP-binding cassette transporter A1 (ABCA1) (Rohatgi et al., 2014). Studies have shown that dietary intervention can impact cholesterol efflux. Walnuts, walnut oil, and alpha-linolenic acid (ALA), a component of walnuts, have been shown to increase cholesterol efflux (Berryman et al., 2013; Zhang et al., 2011, 2012). Zhang et al. (2011) demonstrated that consumption of 51 g walnut oil incorporated in diet Jell-O™ increased cholesterol efflux from macrophage-derived foam cells by 17% in participants with low C-reactive protein (CRP, a marker of systemic inflammation) levels (<2 mg/L), but not in those with higher CRP (≥2 mg/L) compared to baseline. In addition, consumption of 85 g of whole walnuts incorporated into diet Jell-O increased cholesterol efflux by 3.3% (P = 0.02) compared to the baseline (fasted state) (Berryman et al., 2013). In the study by Holligan et al. (2014), consumption of one serving of pistachios (10% energy from pistachios) or two servings of pistachios (20% energy from pistachios) did not affect ABCA1-mediated cholesterol efflux or global serum efflux. However, individuals with baseline CRP values <0.2 mg/dL had significant increases in ABCA1-mediated efflux and global efflux following the two servings of pistachios compared to one serving of pistachios treatment [9.89% (SE 0.74) vs. 7.35% (SE 0.74), P = 0.016]. Thus, the effects of diet on efflux capacity may be blunted in persons with chronic inflammation. These studies suggest that one cardioprotective benefit of nuts may be due to an increase in cholesterol efflux capacity in the absence of low-grade inflammation.

Oxidation and Inflammation

Nuts are a rich source of bioactive compounds that contain antioxidants including tocopherols, phenolic compounds, phytosterols, melatonin, and selenium that may contribute to improved oxidative status (Ros, 2009). Early in vitro studies using nut extracts demonstrated reductions in lipid peroxidation and oxidative DNA damage (Anderson et al., 2001; Chen et al., 2005, 2007; Gentile et al., 2007). Acute and long-term animal studies reported improved oxidative biomarkers and beneficial effects on lipid peroxidation, antioxidant enzymatic activity, and cholesterol oxidation products (Aksoy et al., 2007; Davis et al., 2006; Hatipoglu et al., 2004; Iwamoto et al., 2002; Reiter et al., 2005). RCTs conducted in humans consuming various tree nuts (i.e., almonds, walnuts, pistachios, cashews, pecans, and Brazil nuts) and peanuts, with intakes ranging from 17 to 168 g/day for 3–12 weeks, reported an improvement in oxidative stress markers (i.e., antioxidant capacity, serum oxidized LDL, urinary isoprostanes, malondialdehyde concentration, DNA damage) (Lopez-Uriarte et al., 2009). In a postprandial study conducted by Berryman et al. (2013), the ferric-reducing antioxidant potential was significantly greater (P < 0.01) after consumption of walnut oil (51 g) and walnuts skins (56 g) compared to the nutmeat group. In addition, nuts have also been shown to decrease oxidized LDL. In the PREDIMED trial, a subsection of individuals (n = 372) was evaluated at 3 months to measure the effects of the dietary interventions on lipid oxidative damage. There were significant decreases in oxidized LDL after consumption of the Mediterranean diet with extra-virgin olive oil (−10.6 U/L; 95% CI: −14.2 to −6.1; P = 0.02) and nonsignificant decreases following the Mediterranean diet with nuts (−7.3 U/L; 95% CI: −11.2 to −3.3), compared to a lower-fat diet (−2.9 U/L; −7.3 to 1.5) (Fito et al., 2007). The Mediterranean diet with nuts also significantly decreased adhesion molecules IL-6 by 97 μg/L (P < 0.018), sICAM-1 by 167 μg/L (P < 0.003), and sVCAM by 167 μg/L compared to the lower-fat diet (P < 0.003) (Estruch et al., 2006).

In the pistachio study described earlier, pistachio intake of 1 and 2 servings/day reduced oxidized LDL compared to a lower-fat control diet (1 serving/day pistachio diet = 46.57 ± 3.03 U/L; 2 servings/day pistachio diet = 43.43 ± 3.02 U/L; vs. control = 48.57 ± 3.02 U/L, P < 0.05) (Kay et al., 2010). This study also reported greater serum antioxidant levels following the 2PD (421.89 ± 21.89 nmol/L) and 1PD (337.77 ± 22.03 nmol/L) compared to the lower-fat diet (239.37 ± 21.89 nmol/L), with greater increases following the 2PD indicating a dose effect (P < 0.001). After controlling for the change in LDL-C, increases in serum lutein and γ-tocopherol following the 2PD period were modestly associated with decreases in oxidized LDL (r = −0.36, P = 0.06 and r = −0.35, P = 0.08, respectively). This beneficial effect has also been shown in individuals with MetS. In a study conducted in 50 individuals with MetS (Lopez-Uriarte et al., 2010), 30 g mixed nuts (15, 7.5, and 7.5 g/day of walnuts, almonds, and hazelnuts, respectively) incorporated into a healthy dietary pattern (defined by meeting both nutrient and food-based dietary recommendations) had no effect on oxidized LDL (Lopez-Uriarte et al., 2010), but DNA damage evaluated by 8-oxo-7,8-dihydro-2'-deoxyguanosine was reduced significantly in the nut group (−6.35 nmol/mmol creatine; 95% CI: −7.20 to −5.51; P < 0.001). These findings suggest that nut consumption decreases both oxidative stress and markers of inflammation, which may contribute to their CVD protective effects.

Inflammation plays a key role in the progression of CHD from the initial lesion to the later-stage thrombotic complications (Libby, 2006). Studies evaluating nut consumption on inflammation have reported favorable effects on inflammatory markers and mediators (Estruch et al., 2006; Ros et al., 2004). Zhao et al. (2007) reported a decrease in CRP in participants who consumed 37 g of walnuts + 15 g walnut oil/day for 6 weeks (<0.08). Furthermore, the study diet decreased adhesion molecules ICAM-1 by 18% ($P < 0.05$) and E-selectin by 6% ($P < 0.05\%$). In healthy individuals ($n = 25$), after 4 weeks of consuming almonds corresponding to 10% or 20% of total energy, serum CRP levels were significantly lower both in the low-almond group (1.40 mg/dL) and high-almond group (1.47 mg/dL) compared to control (1.54 mg/dL) ($P < 0.05$). Walnuts incorporated into a meal also have been shown to reduce post-prandial mRNA expression of Il-6 in circulating blood mononuclear cells (Cortes et al., 2006) and consumption of a breakfast meal with walnuts reduced monocyte expression of pro-inflammatory ligands (Jimenez-Gomez et al., 2009) compared to a breakfast meal containing butter. The consumption of tree nuts and peanuts and the resulting decreases in oxidative and inflammatory markers suggest this may be an important mechanism by which tree nuts and peanuts provide CHD protection.

Vascular Health

The effect of nut consumption on blood pressure has been evaluated as a secondary outcome measure (Casas-Agustench et al., 2011a,b; Chisholm et al., 2005; Edwards et al., 1999; Estruch et al., 2006; Fito et al., 2007; Iwamoto et al., 2002; Jenkins et al., 2002; Llorente-Cortes et al., 2010; Mukuddem-Petersen et al., 2007; Olmedilla-Alonso et al., 2008; Ros et al., 2004; Sabate et al., 1993; Sari et al., 2010; Schutte et al., 2006; Sheridan et al., 2007; Spaccarotella et al., 2008; Wien et al., 2003, 2010; Wu et al., 2010). These trials have been conducted with healthy participants and individuals at risk of CVD. Daily intakes ranged from 30 to 108 g/day of different types of nuts (almonds, walnuts, hazelnuts, pistachios, cashews, and mixed nuts). Of these studies, four reported a decrease in SBP and diastolic blood pressure (DBP) in the nut consumption group compared to control (Estruch et al., 2006; Fito et al., 2007; Llorente-Cortes et al., 2010; Wien et al., 2003), and the remaining studies found no effect on resting blood pressure (Casas-Agustench et al., 2011a,b; Chisholm et al., 2005; Edwards et al., 1999; Iwamoto et al., 2002; Jenkins et al., 2002; Mukuddem-Petersen et al., 2007; Olmedilla-Alonso et al., 2008; Ros et al., 2004; Sabate et al., 1993; Sari et al., 2010; Schutte et al., 2006; Sheridan et al., 2007; Spaccarotella et al., 2008; Wien et al., 2010; Wu et al., 2010). A recent systematic review and meta-analysis of 21 clinical trials with 1652 adults found that nut consumption (i.e., walnuts, almonds, pistachios, cashews, hazelnuts, macadamia nuts, pecans, peanuts, and soy nuts) resulted in a significant reduction in SBP (−1.29 mmHg; 95% CI: −2.35–0.22; $P = 0.02$) in individuals not diagnosed with type 2 diabetes, but not in the total population (Mohammadifard et al., 2015). A subgroup analysis of different types of nuts suggests that pistachios, but not other nuts, significantly decrease SBP (−1.82 mmHg; 95% CI: −2.97, −0.67; $P = 0.002$), while both pistachios and mixed nuts significantly reduce DBP (−0.80 mmHg, $P = 0.01$; −1.19 mmHg, $P = 0.04$), respectively.

Other techniques that have been used to measure vascular health include ambulatory blood pressure, central blood pressure, and flow-mediated dilation (FMD). Ambulatory blood pressure is a technique used to measure blood pressure at regular intervals over 24 hours. This method avoids the effect of "white coat hypertension" which is the increase in blood pressure due to anxiety caused by the examination process (Jhalani et al., 2005; Ogedegbe et al., 2008). Ambulatory blood pressure monitoring over a 24-hour period also assesses nocturnal blood pressure with a dip in blood pressure during the night being considered normal and desirable (Pickering et al., 2005). Absence of this dip is associated with poorer health outcomes, including increased mortality (Minutolo et al., 2011). In a randomized, crossover controlled-feeding study, individuals with type 2 diabetes consumed either a low-fat diet (27% fat) containing a low-fat/fat-free carbohydrate snack (i.e., pretzels, string cheese, etc.) or a moderate-fat diet containing pistachios (33% total fat; 20% of energy from pistachios) for 4 weeks (Sauder et al., 2014). The pistachio diet resulted in no significant changes in resting SBP ($P = 0.76$) or DBP ($P = 0.28$). However, systolic ambulatory blood pressure was significantly decreased (−3.5 mmHg, $P = 0.046$), with the greatest reduction observed during sleep (−5.7 mmHg, $P = 0.052$). Similarly, in the PREDIMED study, consuming a Mediterranean-style diet supplemented with 30 g/day of mixed nuts (15 g walnuts, 7.5 g hazelnuts, and 7.5 g almonds) for 1 year decreased ambulatory SBP (−2.6 mmHg; 95% CI: −4.3 to −0.9; P < 0.001) and DBP (−1.2 mmHg; 95% CI: −2.2 to −0.2; P = 0.017) compared with a lower-fat diet (Domenech et al., 2014). These results provide further evidence for multiple mechanisms by which nut consumption decreases CVD risk.

Arterial stiffness is a consequence of biological processes such as aging and atherosclerosis. It is often measured by pulse wave velocity (PWV), the rate at which pressure waves move down the vessel and reflect back (Hansen et al., 2006). To date, only one study has evaluated nut consumption on arterial stiffness. The study was designed to assess measures of arterial stiffness after a 30-month intervention of a lifestyle modification (physical activity and adherence to the "therapeutic lifestyle change" diet) with or without the addition of 80 g/day of pistachios in adults with mild dyslipidemia (Kasliwal et al., 2015). The lifestyle modification with pistachios lowered carotid PWV (770.9 ± 96.5 vs. 846.4 ± 162.0 cm/s; P = 0.08), left brachial-ankle (baPWV) (1192.4 ± 152.5 vs. 1326.3 ± 253.7 cm/s; P = 0.05), and average baPWV (1208.2 ± 118.4 vs. 1295.8 ± 194.1 cm/s; P = 0.08) compared with the lifestyle modification group without nuts. Because arterial stiffening typically precedes atherosclerosis, these findings are important as they suggest a protective role of tree nuts in the prevention of CVD.

Endothelial dysfunction is a pathological state that represents an imbalance between vasodilation and vasoconstriction (Deanfield et al., 2005), which also can precede the onset of atherosclerosis (Aoki et al., 2006). FMD is a noninvasive method to measure endothelial function quantified by brachial artery ultrasound imaging (Peretz et al., 2007). This technique works by inducing reactive hyperemia via temporary arterial occlusion and measuring the relative increase in blood vessel diameter through ultrasound (Quinaglia et al., 2015). A growing number of clinical trials have demonstrated that nuts favorably affect endothelial function (Cortes et al., 2006; Ma et al., 2010; Ros et al., 2004; West et al., 2010). In hypercholesterolemic men and women (n = 18), consumption of a walnut-rich diet (i.e., 18% of energy) for 4 weeks compared with a Mediterranean diet without walnuts significantly improved endothelial-dependent vasodilation from 3.6% to 5.9% (P = 0.043) (Ros et al., 2004). This effect was also observed when pistachios were included in a Mediterranean diet (~20% energy) for 4 weeks. The pistachio diet increased FMD compared with the traditional Mediterranean diet without pistachios (10.29% ± 2.76% vs. 7.86% ± 2.28%; P = 0.002) in healthy participants (Sari et al., 2010). This effect was also reported when hypercholesterolemic subjects consumed a step-2 diet that replaced 18%–21% of energy with hazelnuts daily for 4 weeks; there was a significant increase in FMD (56.6%; P < 0.001) compared to a control diet (step-2 diet without hazelnuts) (Orem et al., 2013). Other studies have also reported this effect in individuals diagnosed with type 2 diabetes. When individuals with type 2 diabetes consumed an ad libitum diet with walnuts (56 g/day) FMD significantly increased compared to an ad libitum diet without walnuts (2.2% ± 1.7% vs. 1.2% ± 1.6%; P = 0.04) (Ma et al., 2010).

The benefits reported in long-term nut interventions (treatment periods lasting 4 weeks to 3 months) have also been reported in postprandial studies. Researchers have demonstrated acute improvement in dilation after consumption of nuts, particularly walnuts (Berryman et al., 2015; Cortes et al., 2006). In a study by Cortes et al. (2006), healthy individuals (n = 12) and hypercholesterolemic individuals (n = 12) consumed two high-fat meals (80 g of fat; 35% saturated fat) to which either walnuts (40 g) or olive oil (25 mL) was added. Postprandial FMD was reduced after the olive oil meal in both healthy (−17%) and hypercholesterolemic subjects (−36%) compared to the control group. However, after the walnut-enriched meal, FMD was unchanged in the healthy subjects and increased by 24% in the hypercholesterolemic subjects (P < 0.006). In order to understand the contribution of individual components of walnuts, Berryman et al. (2013) studied the effects of acute consumption of walnut skin, defatted walnut meat and walnut oil compared with whole walnuts on reactive hyperemia (measured by pulse amplitude tonometry). Walnut oil (51 g) improved reactive hyperemia index (RHI) compared to walnut skins (5.6 g) (P = 0.01). The authors explained this finding as being due to a greater bioavailability of bioactives in walnut oil compared with the nutmeat and skins.

The beneficial effects of nut consumption have also been reported at the microvascular level, although the number of studies is limited (Holt et al., 2015; Huguenin et al., 2015; Maranhao et al., 2011).

Microvascular reactivity is associated with CVD risk factors (Baumbach et al., 1991). In a parallel design study with 38 hypercholesterolemic, postmenopausal women, consumption of 40 versus 5 g/day of walnuts significantly increased the fasting reactive hyperemia index (RHI) (2.63 ± 0.10 vs. 2.23 ± 0.13, respectively, P = 0.025). However, two studies assessing Brazil nuts (13–25 g/day) with treatment durations between 3 and 4 months reported no effect on microvascular parameters (i.e., capillary diameter) (Huguenin et al., 2015; Maranhao et al., 2011). The conflicting results and limited number of studies highlight the need for additional research of nuts on microvascular function.

Insulin Resistance and Glycemic Response

Decreasing postprandial glycemia lowers the risk of developing hypertension, diabetes, and CHD in high-risk individuals (Chiasson et al., 2002, 2003). Post-meal hyperglycemia is also an independent risk factor for CVD (Levitan et al., 2004). There is no postprandial glycemic response when nuts are consumed alone, likely due to their very low carbohydrate content. When consumed with carbohydrate-rich foods, nuts have shown to blunt postprandial glycemia (Jenkins et al., 2006; Josse et al., 2007; Kendall et al., 2011a,b). In a postprandial study of 15 healthy subjects, glycemic indices were measured after consumption of three test meals: almond meal, 60 g almonds + 97 g of bread; parboiled rice meal, 68 g cheese + 14 g butter + 60 g parboiled rice; and mashed potato meal, 62 g cheese and 16 g butter and 68 g mashed potatoes (Jenkins et al., 2006). Glycemic indices for the rice (38 ± 6) and almond meals (55 ± 7) were less than for the potato meal (94 ± 11) (P < 0.003), as were the postprandial areas under the insulin concentration time curve (P < 0.001). A subsequent study with nine healthy participants evaluated the effects of varying amounts of almonds on the postprandial blood glucose response to a carbohydrate meal. Each test meal contained bread as the source of carbohydrate (50 g) to be eaten alone or with 30, 60, and 90 g of almonds. The addition of almonds to white bread resulted in a dose-dependent reduction in the glycemic index for the 30 g (105.8 ± 23.3), 60 g (63.0 ± 9.0), and 90 g (45.2 ± 5.8) doses of almonds (r = −0.524, P = 0.001) (Josse et al., 2007). Pistachio nuts also have a beneficial effect on postprandial glycemia. In 10 healthy volunteers, the consumption of 28 g of pistachios with white bread (50 g) resulted in reduced relative glycemic response (89.1 ± 6.0; P = 0.100), with a greater reduction achieved when 84 g of pistachios were added (51.5 ± 7.5; P < 0.001) compared to the white bread control (100 g) (Kendall et al., 2011a,b). An expansion of this study conducted with subjects with the MetS found 50 g of white bread +85 g of pistachios significantly blunted the postprandial glucose response compared to consuming white bread alone (Kendall et al., 2014), but no differences were observed for postprandial insulin levels. In a study by Kendall et al. (2011a,b), the effects of 30, 60, and 90 g of mixed nuts (almonds, macadamias, walnuts, pistachios, hazelnuts, and pecans in equal portions by weight) alone and in combination with white bread on postprandial glycemia were examined in 14 healthy subjects and 10 subjects with type 2 diabetes. The relative glycemic response was significantly lower with the three doses of mixed nuts compared to the white bread control in both normoglycemic subjects (2%–6% of control; P < 0.001) and in subjects with type 2 diabetes (4%–8% of control, P < 0.001). In normoglycemic subjects, the addition of 30, 60, and 90 g of nuts to the bread reduced the glycemic response by 11.2% ± 11.6%, 29.7% ± 12.2%, and 53.5% ± 8.5% (P = 0.35, P = 0.031, and P < 0.001, respectively). However, in subjects with type 2 diabetes, the reduction in glycemic response of 30, 60, and 90 g nuts was half that observed for the normoglycemic subjects (6.6% ± 8.8%, 16.6% ± 9.3%, 30.8% ± 7.6%; P = 0.474, P = 0.113, and P = 0.015, respectively). Interestingly, a study by Casas-Agustench et al. (2011a,b) found that subjects with the MetS were less responsive to the cholesterol-lowering effect of mixed nuts compared to previous reports with healthy individuals. Collectively, these studies demonstrate that individuals with metabolic conditions are less responsive to the cardioprotective benefits of nuts on some CVD risk factors.

Body Weight

Cross-sectional studies have reported an inverse association between nut consumption and BMI (Almario et al., 2001; Alper and Mattes, 2002; Fraser et al., 1992; Hu et al., 1998; Jackson and Hu,

2014; Kris-Etherton et al., 1999; Martinez-Gonzalez and Bes-Rastrollo, 2011; O'Byrne et al., 1997). Studies also have reported reduced waist circumference with increased nut consumption (Casas-Agustench et al., 2011a; Martinez-Gonzalez et al., 2012; O'Neil et al., 2011). Smith et al. (2015) reported results from a prospective investigation involving three cohorts that included 120,877 healthy U.S. women and men from the NHS I (n = 50,422 women) NHS II (n = 47,898 women) and the HPFS (n = 22,557 men). After 4 years, weight change was inversely associated with the intake of nuts (−0.57 lb; 95% CI: −0.97 to −0.17; P = 0.005).

A meta-analysis of 33 clinical trials (n = 1888 participants) evaluated the effects of tree nut (almonds, walnuts, pistachios, hazelnuts) and peanut consumption on body weight in diets that include nuts versus controlled diets (i.e., habitual, lower-fat, American Diabetes Association, Step-2, low-calorie diets) (Flores-Mateo et al., 2013). Pooled results indicated a nonsignificant effect on body weight (−0.47 kg; 95% CI: −1.17, 0.22 kg; I^2 = 7%), BMI (−0.40 kg/m^2; 95% CI: −0.97, 0.17 kg/m^2; I^2 = 49%), and waist circumference (−1.25 cm; 95% CI: −2.82, 0.31 cm; I^2 = 28%) of diets including nuts compared with control diets. These epidemiological and clinical trial findings indicate no increase and perhaps a decrease in body weight following nut consumption.

The mechanism is unclear for the association between nuts and body weight (Almario et al., 2001; Alper and Mattes, 2002; Flores-Mateo et al., 2013; Fraser et al., 1992; Hu et al., 1998; Kris-Etherton et al., 1999; Martinez-Gonzalez and Bes-Rastrollo, 2011; O'Byrne et al., 1997). One possible explanation is the recent discovery related to the discrepancy between the Atwater energy factor predicted for almonds, pistachios, and walnuts and the empirically measured energy value when the nuts are consumed (Baer et al., 2012, 2016; Novotny et al., 2012). Atwater-specific factors are a series of energy values for macronutrients that take digestibility and heat of combustion into account. Three studies were conducted to measure the available energy in almonds, pistachios, and walnuts compared to the corresponding calculated Atwater factor value. Each of the studies used a controlled diet, crossover design with one or two treatment diets and a control diet. Almonds were studied in 18 healthy adults fed three different diets for 18 days each, including 0, 42, and 84 g almonds/day. The authors reported the energy content of almonds in the diet as 4.6 ± 0.8 kcal/g (equivalent to 129 kcal/28 g-serving), which is significantly less than 6.0–6.1 kcal/g (168–170 kcal/serving), the energy density determined by the Atwater factors (P < 0.001). This study concluded that the Atwater factors overestimate the measured energy content of almonds by 32% (Novotny et al., 2012). Similarly, in a study examining the energy value of pistachios, 16 healthy adults consumed 0 g/day pistachios, 42 and 84 g/day for 3 weeks. Baer et al. (2012) reported a measured energy value for pistachios (5.4 kcal/g) that was 5% less than the calculated Atwater factors (5.7 kcal/g). The researchers found similar results for walnuts in 18 healthy adults. The measured energy value of walnuts [42 or 0 g/day was 5.22 ± 0.16 kcal/g (146 kcal/28 g-serving)] was significantly lower than the calculated Atwater factors (6.61 kcal/g; 185 g/serving), resulting in a 21% overestimation of energy content (Baer et al., 2016).

The measured versus absorbed energy content of almonds and walnuts may be a mechanism, in part, to explain the relationship between nut consumption and reduced body weight. However, some studies (Foster et al., 2012; Fraser et al., 2002) have shown weight gain (albeit very small) with nut consumption. Using a crossover study design, Fraser et al. (2002) tested the effects of providing a free daily supplement (averaging 320 kcal) of almonds or no supplement to 81 male and female participants for six months. After the almond feeding period, average body weight increased only 0.40 kg (P ~ 0.09), suggesting there was not significant weight change after almonds were incorporated isocalorically in the diet for other foods. Weight change was dependent on baseline BMI (P = 0.05). Only those who were initially in the lower BMI tertiles experienced a small weight gain (0.40 kg) with the almonds. Foster et al. (2012) reported similar results in 123 overweight and obese individuals who were randomly assigned to consume an almond-enriched diet (AED) or nut-free diet (NFD) for 18 months and instructed in traditional behavioral methods of weight control, such as self-monitoring and stimulus control. Participants in the AED group lost slightly, but significantly, less weight than did those in the NFD group at 6 months (−5.5 compared with −7.4 kg; P = 0.04), but there were no differences at 18 months.

No significant differences in body composition were found between the groups at 6 or 18 months. It is important to address the difference between the addition of nuts to the diet compared to the isocaloric substitution of nuts in the diet for other foods.

In a recent analysis of the PREDIMED trial, the long-term effects of an ad libitum, lower-fat control diet, a Mediterranean diet supplemented with extra-virgin olive oil, and a Mediterranean diet supplemented with mixed nuts on body weight and waist circumference were assessed in older people at risk of cardiovascular disease, most of whom were overweight or obese. After a median 4.8 years of follow-up, participants in all three groups had a marginally reduced body weight and increased waist circumference (Estruch et al., 2016). The adjusted difference in 5-year changes in body weight in the Mediterranean diet supplemented with extra-virgin olive oil group was –0.43 kg (95% CI 0.86, –0.01; P = 0.044) and in the nut group was –0.08 kg (–0.50, 0.35; P = 0.730), compared with the control group. The adjusted difference in 5-year changes in waist circumference was –0.55 cm (–1.16, –0.06; P = 0.048) in the Mediterranean diet supplemented with extra-virgin olive oil group and –0.94 cm (–1.60, –0.27; P = 0.006) in the nut supplemented group, compared with the control group. This study suggests that a long-term intervention with a Mediterranean diet that includes extra-virgin olive oil or nuts was associated with decreases in body weight and less gain in central adiposity compared with a control diet.

Collectively, the majority of research conducted to date demonstrates benefits of nut consumption on body weight, as well as measures of visceral adiposity. These findings provide further support for including nuts in a healthy eating pattern that meets energy needs for body weight control.

SUMMARY

Many health benefits of nut consumption have been reported in both epidemiological and clinical studies. Landmark population studies, such as the Adventist Health Study, the Iowa Women's Health Study, the NHS, and the PHS have demonstrated that the consumption of nuts was associated with decreased risk for CHD. A pooled analysis of these four large U.S. studies demonstrated a 35% reduced risk of CHD incidence for the highest nut intake of >5 times/week (Kris-Etherton et al., 2008). Studies in populations of different geographical regions and socioeconomic status have also reported similar benefits (Eslamparast et al., 2017; Gopinath et al., 2015; Luu et al., 2015). In addition, a beneficial relationship has been reported for nut consumption and risk reduction of type 2 diabetes and the MetS (O'Neil et al., 2011; Pan et al., 2013).

In the groundbreaking PREDIMED trial, a Mediterranean dietary pattern with nuts (30 g/day), or extra-virgin olive oil, decreased cardiovascular events by approximately 30% and decreased risk of stroke by almost 50% in men and women at high risk for CVD. Many clinical trials have reported benefits of nut consumption on numerous CVD risk factors including blood lipids/lipoproteins, inflammation, oxidation, vascular function, insulin resistance, and glycemic response. Studies evaluating walnuts (Rajaram et al., 2009; Torabian et al., 2010), almonds (Berryman et al., 2013; Jenkins et al., 2002), pistachios (Sauder et al., 2013; Sheridan et al., 2007), hazelnuts (Mercanligil et al., 2007), peanuts (Lokko et al., 2007), and macadamia nuts (Griel et al., 2008) have reported decreases in LDL-C ranging from 9% to 16%. Additionally, a pooled analysis of 25 nut intervention studies conducted in 7 countries with 583 men and women reported a dose–response improvement in lipids/lipoproteins with nut consumption (Sabaté and Wien, 2010). In summary, the clinical studies demonstrate multiple cardiovascular benefits of nut and peanut consumption when they are isocalorically substituted for other foods. In addition, recent evidence from PREDIMED and other studies supports no restriction on intake of healthy fats (such as those provided by nuts) as appropriate for body weight maintenance and overall cardiometabolic health, as recently acknowledged by the Dietary Guidelines Advisory Committee (2015).

The 2015–2020 Dietary Guidelines recommend specific food substitutions for a healthy diet. The guidelines state: "choose nutrient-dense foods and beverages across and within all food groups in place of less healthy choices" (U.S. Department of Health and Human Services and

U.S. Department of Agriculture, 2015). The 2015–2020 Dietary Guidelines further recommend "use oils rather than solid fats … when cooking, increasing the intake of foods that naturally contain oils, such as seafood and nuts, in place of some meat and poultry, and choosing other foods, such as salad dressings and spreads, made with oils instead of solid fats".

Three healthy food-based dietary patterns are recommended to implement the 2015–2020 Dietary Guidelines (U.S. Department of Health and Human Services and U.S. Department of Agriculture, 2015). Two of the USDA Food Patterns (Healthy U.S.-Style Pattern and Healthy Mediterranean-Style Pattern) recommend 5 oz equivalents/week of nuts/seeds and the third (Healthy Vegetarian Pattern) recommends 14 oz equivalents/week. The U.S. diet falls short of meeting all food-based dietary recommendations, including those made for nuts/seeds. Achieving these recommendations on a population-wide basis is expected to confer many health benefits. In addition, based on the evidence summarized herein, adoption of just the recommendations for nuts/seeds by the U.S. population would confer marked benefits on cardiometabolic risk. At this juncture, it is important to increase consumer and health care professional awareness of the many health benefits of nuts/seeds, and teach implementation strategies for incorporating them in a healthy dietary pattern. Future research on nuts will advance our understanding of their mechanisms of action as well as provide better behavior change strategies for incorporating nuts into a heart-healthy diet.

REFERENCES

Aksoy, N., Aksoy, M., Bagci, C. et al. (2007). Pistachio intake increases high density lipoprotein levels and inhibits low-density lipoprotein oxidation in rats. *Tohoku J Exp Med*, *212*(1), 43–48.

Albert, C. M., Gaziano, J. M., Willett, W. C., and Manson, J. E. (2002). Nut consumption and decreased risk of sudden cardiac death in the Physicians' Health Study. *Arch Intern Med*, *162*(12), 1382–1387.

Almario, R. U., Vonghavaravat, V., Wong, R., and Kasim-Karakas, S. E. (2001). Effects of walnut consumption on plasma fatty acids and lipoproteins in combined hyperlipidemia. *Am J Clin Nutr*, *74*(1), 72–79.

Alper, C. M. and Mattes, R. D. (2002). Effects of chronic peanut consumption on energy balance and hedonics. *Int J Obes*, *26*(8), 1129–1137.

Anderson, K. J., Teuber, S. S., Gobeille, A., Cremin, P., Waterhouse, A. L., and Steinberg, F. M. (2001). Walnut polyphenolics inhibit in vitro human plasma and LDL oxidation. *J Nutr*, *131*(11), 2837–2842.

Aoki, R., Ikarugi, H., Naemura, A., Ijiri, Y., Yamashita, T., and Yamamoto, J. (2006). Endothelial dysfunction precedes atherosclerotic lesions and platelet activation in high fat diet-induced prothrombotic state. *Thromb Res*, *117*(5), 529–535.

Asztalos, B. F., Collins, D., Cupples, L. A., Demissie, S., Horvath, K. V., Bloomfield, H. E., Robins, S. J., and Schaefer, E. J. (2005). Value of high-density lipoprotein (HDL) subpopulations in predicting recurrent cardiovascular events in the veterans affairs HDL intervention trial. *Arterioscler Thromb Vasc Biol*, *25*(10), 2185–2191.

Asztalos, B. F., Cupples, L. A., Demissie, S., Horvath, K. V., Cox, C. E., Batista, M. C., and Schaefer, E. J. (2004). High-density lipoprotein subpopulation profile and coronary heart disease prevalence in male participants of the Framingham Offspring Study. *Arterioscler Thromb Vasc Biol*, *24*(11), 2181–2187.

Babio, N., Toledo, E., Estruch, R. et al. (2014). Mediterranean diets and metabolic syndrome status in the PREDIMED randomized trial. *CMAJ*, *186*(17), 649–657.

Baer, D. J., Gebauer, S. K., and Novotny, J. A. (2012). Measured energy value of pistachios in the human diet. *Br J Nutr*, *107*(1), 120–125.

Baer, D. J., Gebauer, S. K., and Novotny, J. A. (2016). Walnuts consumed by healthy adults provide less available energy than predicted by the atwater factors. *J Nutr*, *146*(1), 9–13.

Banel, D. K. and Hu, F. B. (2009). Effects of walnut consumption on blood lipids and other cardiovascular risk factors: A meta-analysis and systematic review. *Am J Clin Nutr*, *90*(1), 56–63.

Bao, Y., Han, J., Hu, F. B., Giovannucci, E. L., Stampfer, M. J., Willett, W. C., and Fuchs, C. S. (2013). Association of nut consumption with total and cause-specific mortality. *N Engl J Med*, *369*(21), 2001–2011.

Baumbach, G. L., Siems, J. E., and Heistad, D. D. (1991). Effects of local reduction in pressure on distensibility and composition of cerebral arterioles. *Circ Res*, *68*(2), 338–351.

Berryman, C. E., Grieger, J. A., West, S. G., Chen, C. Y., Blumberg, J. B., Rothblat, G. H., Sankaranarayanan, S., and Kris-Etherton, P. M. (2013). Acute consumption of walnuts and walnut components differentially affect postprandial lipemia, endothelial function, oxidative stress, and cholesterol efflux in humans with mild hypercholesterolemia. *J Nutr*, *143*(6), 788–794.

Berryman, C. E., West, S. G., Fleming, J. A., Bordi, P. L., and Kris-Etherton, P. M. (2015). Effects of daily almond consumption on cardiometabolic risk and abdominal adiposity in healthy adults with elevated LDL-cholesterol: A randomized controlled trial. *J Am Heart Assoc*, *4*(1), e000993.

Blake, G. J., Otvos, J. D., Rifai, N., and Ridker, P. M. (2002). Low-density lipoprotein particle concentration and size as determined by nuclear magnetic resonance spectroscopy as predictors of cardiovascular disease in women. *Circulation*, *106*(15), 1930–1937.

Blanco Mejia, S., Kendall, C. W., Viguiliouk, E. et al. (2014). Effect of tree nuts on metabolic syndrome criteria: A systematic review and meta-analysis of randomised controlled trials. *BMJ Open*, *4*(7), e004660.

Campos, H., Moye, L. A., Glasser, S. P., Stampfer, M. J., and Sacks, F. M. (2001). Low-density lipoprotein size, pravastatin treatment, and coronary events. *JAMA*, *286*(12), 1468–1474.

Carmena, R., Duriez, P., and Fruchart, J. C. (2004). Atherogenic lipoprotein particles in atherosclerosis. *Circulation*, *109*(23), 2–7.

Casas-Agustench, P., Bullo, M., Ros, E., Basora, J., Salas-Salvado, J., and Nureta-PREDIMED Investigators. (2011a). Cross-sectional association of nut intake with adiposity in a Mediterranean population. *Nutr Metab Cardiovasc Dis*, *21*(7), 518–525.

Casas-Agustench, P., Lopez-Uriarte, P., Bullo, M., Ros, E., Cabre-Vila, J. J., and Salas-Salvado, J. (2011b). Effects of one serving of mixed nuts on serum lipids, insulin resistance and inflammatory markers in patients with the metabolic syndrome. *Nutr Metab Cardiovasc Dis*, *21*(2), 126–135.

CDC. (2015). NCHS. Underlying Cause of Death 1999–2013 on CDC WONDER Online Database, released 2015. Data are from the Multiple Cause of Death Files, 1999–2013, as compiled from data provided by the 57 vital statistics jurisdictions through the Vital Statistics Cooperative Program (accessed February 3, 2015). https://www.cdc.gov/heartdisease/facts.htm.

Chen, C. Y., Milbury, P. E., Chung, S. K., and Blumberg, J. (2007). Effect of almond skin polyphenolics and quercetin on human LDL and apolipoprotein B-100 oxidation and conformation. *J Nutr Biochem*, *18*(12), 785–794.

Chen, C. Y., Milbury, P. E., Lapsley, K., and Blumberg, J. B. (2005). Flavonoids from almond skins are bioavailable and act synergistically with vitamins C and E to enhance hamster and human LDL resistance to oxidation. *J Nutr*, *135*(6), 1366–1373.

Chiasson, J. L., Josse, R. G., Gomis, R., Hanefeld, M., Karasik, A., Laakso, M., and STOP-NIDDM Trail Research Group. (2002). Acarbose for prevention of type 2 diabetes mellitus: The STOP-NIDDM randomised trial. *Lancet*, *359*(9323), 2072–2077.

Chiasson, J. L., Josse, R. G., Gomis, R., Hanefeld, M., Karasik, A., Laakso, M., and STOP-NIDDM Trail Research Group. (2003). Acarbose for patients with hypertension and impaired glucose tolerance—Reply. *JAMA*, *290*(23), 3067–3069.

Chisholm, A., Mc Auley, K., Mann, J., Williams, S., and Skeaff, M. (2005). Cholesterol lowering effects of nuts compared with a Canola oil enriched cereal of similar fat composition. *Nutr Metab Cardiovasc Dis*, *15*(4), 284–292.

Cortes, B., Nunez, I., Cofan, M., Gilabert, R., Perez-Heras, A., Casals, E., Deulofeu, R., and Ros, E. (2006). Acute effects of high-fat meals enriched with walnuts or olive oil on postprandial endothelial function. *J Am Coll Cardiol*, *48*(8), 1666–1671.

Cromwell, W. C., Otvos, J. D., Keyes, M. J., Pencina, M. J., Sullivan, L., Vasan, R. S., Wilson, P. W. F., and D'Agostino, R. B. (2007). LDL particle number and risk of future cardiovascular disease in the framingham offspring study—Implications for LDL management. *J Clin Lipidol*, *1*(6), 583–592.

Damasceno, N. R. T., Sala-Vila, A., Cofan, M. et al. (2013). Mediterranean diet supplemented with nuts reduces waist circumference and shifts lipoprotein subfractions to a less atherogenic pattern in subjects at high cardiovascular risk. *Atherosclerosis*, *230*(2), 347–353.

Davis, P., Valacchi, G., Pagnin, E., Shao, Q., Gross, H. B., Calo, L., and Yokoyama, W. (2006). Walnuts reduce aortic ET-1 mRNA levels in hamsters fed a high-fat, atherogenic diet. *J Nutr*, *136*(2), 428–432.

Deanfield, J., Donald, A., Ferri, C. et al. (2005). Endothelial function and dysfunction. Part I: Methodological issues for assessment in the different vascular beds: A statement by the Working Group on Endothelin and Endothelial Factors of the European Society of Hypertension. *J Hypertens*, *23*(1), 7–17.

Del Gobbo, L. C., Falk, M. C., Feldman, R., Lewis, K., and Mozaffarian, D. (2015). Effects of tree nuts on blood lipids, apolipoproteins, and blood pressure: Systematic review, meta-analysis, and dose-response of 61 controlled intervention trials. *Am J Clin Nutr*, *102*(6), 1347–1356.

Dietary Guidelines Advisory Committee. (2015). Scientific report, Part D, Chapter 3: Individual diet and physical activity behavior change. www.health.gov/dietaryguidelines/2015-scientific-report/ (accessed April 14, 2016).

Domenech, M., Roman, P., Lapetra, J. et al. (2014). Mediterranean diet reduces 24-hour ambulatory blood pressure, blood glucose, and lipids one-year randomized, clinical trial. *Hypertension*, *64*(1), 69–76.

Edwards, K., Kwaw, I., Matud, J., and Kurtz, I. (1999). Effect of pistachio nuts on serum lipid levels in patients with moderate hypercholesterolemia. *J Am Coll Nutr, 18*(3), 229–232.

Eslamparast, T., Sharafkhah, M., Poustchi, H. et al. (2017). Nut consumption and total and cause-specific mortality: Results from the Golestan Cohort Study. *Int J Epidemiol, 46*(1), 75–85.

Estruch, R., Martinez-Gonzalez, M. A., Corella, D. et al. (2006). Effects of a Mediterranean-style diet on cardiovascular risk factors—A randomized trial. *Ann Int Med, 145*(1), 1–11.

Estruch, R., Martínez-González, M. A., Corella, D. et al. (2016). Effect of a high-fat Mediterranean diet on bodyweight and waist circumference: A prespecified secondary outcomes analysis of the PREDIMED randomised controlled trial. *Lancet Diabetes Endocrinol, 4*(8), 666–676.

Estruch, R., Ros, E., Salas-Salvadó, J. et al. (2013). Primary prevention of cardiovascular disease with a Mediterranean diet. *N Engl J Med, 368*(14), 1279–1290.

Fernandez-Montero, A., Bes-Rastrollo, M., Beunza, J. J., Barrio-Lopez, M. T., de la Fuente-Arrillaga, C., Moreno-Galarraga, L., and Martinez-Gonzalez, M. A. (2013). Nut consumption and incidence of metabolic syndrome after 6-year follow-up: The SUN (Seguimiento Universidad de Navarra, University of Navarra Follow-up) cohort. *Public Health Nutr, 16*(11), 2064–2072.

Fito, M., Guxens, M., Corella, D. et al. (2007). Effect of a traditional mediterranean diet on lipoprotein oxidation—A randomized controlled trial. *Arch Intern Med, 167*(11), 1195–1203.

Flores-Mateo, G., Rojas-Rueda, D., Basora, J., Ros, E., and Salas-Salvado, J. (2013). Nut intake and adiposity: Meta-analysis of clinical trials. *Am J Clin Nutr, 97*(6), 1346–1355.

Foster, G. D., Shantz, K. L., Vander Veur, S. S., Oliver, T. L., Lent, M. R., Virus, A., Szapary, P. O., Rader, D. J., Zemel, B. S., and Gilden-Tsai, A. (2012). A randomized trial of the effects of an almond-enriched, hypocaloric diet in the treatment of obesity. *Am J Clin Nutr, 96*(2), 249–254.

Fraser, G. E., Bennett, H. W., Jaceldo, K. B., and Sabaté, J. (2002). Effect on body weight of a free 76 Kilojoule (320 calorie) daily supplement of almonds for six months. *J Am Coll Nutr, 21*(3), 275–283.

Fraser, G. E., Lindsted, K. D., and Beeson, W. L. (1995). Effect of risk factor values on lifetime risk of and age at first coronary event. The Adventist Health Study. *Am J Epidemiol, 142*(7), 746–758.

Fraser, G. E., Sabate, J., Beeson, W. L., and Strahan, T. M. (1992). A possible protective effect of nut consumption on risk of coronary heart-disease—The adventist health study. *Arch Intern Med, 152*(7), 1416–1424.

Fraser, G. E. and Shavlikm, D. J. (1997). Risk factors for all-cause and coronary heart disease mortality in the oldest-old: The adventist health study. *Arch Intern Med, 157*(19), 2249–2258

Fraser, G. E., Sumbureru, D., Pribis, P., Neil, R. L., and Frankson, M. A. (1997). Association among health habits, risk factors, and all-cause mortality in a black California population. *Epidemiology, 8*(2), 168–174.

Gentile, C., Tesoriere, L., Butera, D., Fazzari, M., Monastero, M., Allegra, M., and Livrea, M. A. (2007). Antioxidant activity of *Sicilian pistachio* (*Pistacia vera* L. var. Bronte) nut extract and its bioactive components. *J Agric Food Chem, 55*(3), 643–648.

Gopinath, B., Flood, V. M., Burlutksy, G., and Mitchell, P. (2015). Consumption of nuts and risk of total and cause-specific mortality over 15 years. *Nutr Metab Cardiovasc Dis, 25*(12), 1125–1131.

Griel, A. E., Bagshaw, D. M., Cifelli, A. M., Cao, Y. M., and Kris-Etherton, P. M. (2007). A macadamia nut-rich diet reduces levels of total and LDL-cholesterol in mildly hypercholesterolemic individuals. *FASEB J, 21*(5), A696.

Griel, A. E., Cao, Y. M., Bagshaw, D. D., Cifelli, A. M., Holub, B., and Kris-Etherton, P. M. (2008). A macadamia nut-rich diet reduces total and LDL-Cholesterol in mildly hypercholesterolemic men and women. *J Nutr, 138*(4), 761–767.

Hallman, D. M., Brown, S. A., Ballantyne, C. M., Sharrett, A. R., and Boerwinkle, E. (2004). Relationship between low-density lipoprotein subclasses and asymptomatic atherosclerosis in subjects from the Atherosclerosis Risk in Communities (ARIC) Study. *Biomarkers, 9*(2), 190–202.

Hansen, T. W., Staessen, J. A., Torp-Pedersen, C., Rasmussen, S., Thijs, L., Ibsen, H., and Jeppesen, J. (2006). Prognostic value of aortic pulse wave velocity as index of arterial stiffness in the general population. *Circulation, 113*(5), 664–670.

Hatipoglu, A., Kanbagli, O., Balkan, J., Kucuk, M., Cevikbas, U., Aykac-Toker, G., Berkkan, H., and Uysal, M. (2004). Hazelnut oil administration reduces aortic cholesterol accumulation and lipid peroxides in the plasma, liver, and aorta of rabbits fed a high-cholesterol diet. *Biosci Biotechnol Biochem, 68*(10), 2050–2057.

Hernandez-Alonso, P., Salas-Salvado, J., Baldrich-Mora, M., Mallol, R., Correig, X., and Bullo, M. (2015). Effect of pistachio consumption on plasma lipoprotein subclasses in pre-diabetic subjects. *Nutr Metab Cardiovasc Dis, 25*(4), 396–402.

Holligan, S. D., West, S. G., Gebauer, S. K., Kay, C. D., and Kris-Etherton, P. M. (2014). A moderate-fat diet containing pistachios improves emerging markers of cardiometabolic syndrome in healthy adults with elevated LDL levels. *Br J Nutr, 112*(5), 744–752.

Holt, R. R., Yim, S. J., Shearer, G. C., Hackman, R. M., Djurica, D., Newman, J. W., Shindel, A. W., and Keen, C. L. (2015). Effects of short-term walnut consumption on human microvascular function and its relationship to plasma epoxide conten. *J Nutr Biochem 26*(12), 1458–1466.

Howard, B. V., Robbins, D. C., Sievers, M. L. et al. (2000). LDL cholesterol as a strong predictor of coronary heart disease in diabetic individuals with insulin resistance and low LDL—The Strong Heart Study. *Arterioscler Thromb Vasc Biol, 20*(3), 830–835.

Hu, F. B., Stampfer, M. J., Manson, J. E., Rimm, E. B., Colditz, G. A., Rosner, B. A., Speizer, F. E., Hennekens, C. H., and Willett, W. C. (1998). Frequent nut consumption and risk of coronary heart disease in women: Prospective cohort study. *BMJ, 317*(7169), 1341–1345.

Huguenin, G. V., Moreira, A. S., Saint'pierre, T. D., Goncalves, R. A., Rosa, G., Oliveira, G. M., Luiz, R. R., and Tibirica, E. (2015). Effects of dietary supplementation with brazil nuts on microvascular endothelial function in hypertensive and dyslipidemic patients: A randomized crossover placebo-controlled trial. *Microcirculation, 22*(8), 687–699.

Ibarrola-Jurado, N., Bullo, M., Guasch-Ferre, M. et al. (2013). Cross-sectional assessment of nut consumption and obesity, metabolic syndrome and other cardiometabolic risk factors: The PREDIMED study. *PLoS One, 8*(2), e57367.

Iwamoto, M., Kono, M., Kawamoto, D., Tomoyori, H., Sato, M., and Imaizumi, K. (2002). Differential effect of walnut oil and safflower oil on the serum cholesterol level and lesion area in the aortic root of apolipoprotein E-deficient mice. *Biosci Biotechnol Biochem, 66*(1), 141–146.

Jaceldo-Siegl, K., Haddad, E., Oda, K., Fraser, G. E., and Sabaté, J. (2014). Tree nuts are inversely associated with metabolic syndrome and obesity: The Adventist health study-2. *PLoS One, 9*(1), e85133.

Jackson, C. L. and Hu, F. B. (2014). Long-term associations of nut consumption with body weight and obesity. *Am J Clin Nutr, 100*(1), 408s–411s.

Jenkins, D. J., Kendall, C. W., Josse, A. R., Salvatore, S., Brighenti, F., Augustin, L. S., Ellis, P. R., Vidgen, E., and Rao, A. V. (2006). Almonds decrease postprandial glycemia, insulinemia, and oxidative damage in healthy individuals. *J Nutr, 136*(12), 2987–2992.

Jenkins, D. J., Kendall, C. W., Marchie, A. et al. (2002). Dose response of almonds on coronary heart disease risk factors: Blood lipids, oxidized low-density lipoproteins, lipoprotein(a), homocysteine, and pulmonary nitric oxide: A randomized, controlled, crossover trial. *Circulation, 106*(11), 1327–1332.

Jhalani, J., Goyal, T., Clemow, L., Schwartz, J. E., Pickering, T. G., and Gerin, W. (2005). Anxiety and outcome expectations predict the white-coat effect. *Blood Press Monit, 10*(6), 317–319.

Jiang, R., Manson, J. E., Stampfer, M. J., Liu, S., Willett, W. C., and Hu, F. B. (2002). Nut and peanut butter consumption and risk of type 2 diabetes in women. *JAMA, 288*(20), 2554–2560.

Jimenez-Gomez, Y., Lopez-Miranda, J., Blanco-Colio, L. M., Marin, C., Perez-Martinez, P., Ruano, J., Paniagua, J. A., Rodríguez, F., Egido, J., and Perez-Jimenez, F. (2009). Olive oil and walnut breakfasts reduce the postprandial inflammatory response in mononuclear cells compared with a butter breakfast in healthy men. *Atherosclerosis, 204*(2), e70–e76.

Josse, A. R., Kendall, C. W., Augustin, L. S., Ellis, P. R., and Jenkins, D. J. (2007). Almonds and postprandial glycemia—A dose-response study. *Metabolism, 56*(3), 400–404.

Kasliwal, R. R., Bansal, M., Mehrotra, R., Yeptho, K. P., and Trehan, N. (2015). Effect of pistachio nut consumption on endothelial function and arterial stiffness. *Nutrition, 31*(5), 678–685.

Kay, C. D., Gebauer, S. K., West, S. G., and Kris-Etherton, P. M. (2010). Pistachios increase serum antioxidants and lower serum oxidized-LDL in hypercholesterolemic adults. *J Nutr, 140*(6), 1093–1098.

Kelly, J. H., Jr. and Sabate, J. (2006). Nuts and coronary heart disease: An epidemiological perspective. *Br J Nutr, 96*(Suppl 2), S61–S67.

Kendall, C. W., Esfahani, A., Josse, A. R., Augustin, L. S., Vidgen, E., and Jenkins, D. J. (2011a). The glycemic effect of nut-enriched meals in healthy and diabetic subjects. *Nutr Metab Cardiovasc Dis, 21* (Suppl 1), S34–S39.

Kendall, C. W., West, S. G., Augustin, L. S. et al. (2014). Acute effects of pistachio consumption on glucose and insulin, satiety hormones and endothelial function in the metabolic syndrome. *Eur J Clin Nutr, 68*(3), 370–375.

Kendall, C. W. C., Josse, A. R., Esfahani, A., and Jenkins, D. J. A. (2011b). The impact of pistachio intake alone or in combination with high-carbohydrate foods on post-prandial glycemia. *Eur J Clin Nutr, 65*(6), 696–702.

Kochar, J., Gaziano, J. M., and Djousse, L. (2010). Nut consumption and risk of type II diabetes in the Physicians' Health Study. *Eur J Clin Nutr, 64*(1), 75–79.

Kris-Etherton, P. M., Hu, F. B., Ros, E., and Sabate, J. (2008). The role of tree nuts and peanuts in the prevention of coronary heart disease: Multiple potential mechanisms. *J Nutr, 138*(9), 1746S–1751S.

Kris-Etherton, P. M., Yu-Poth, S., Sabate, J., Ratcliffe, H. E., Zhao, G. X., and Etherton, T. D. (1999). Nuts and their bioactive constituents: Effects on serum lipids and other factors that affect disease risk. *Am J Clin Nutr*, *70*(3), 504s–511s.

Kuller, L., Arnold, A., Tracy, R., Otvos, J., Burke, G., Psaty, B., Siscovick, D., Freedman, D. S., and Kronmal, R. (2002). Nuclear magnetic resonance spectroscopy of lipoproteins and risk of coronary heart disease in the cardiovascular health study. *Arterioscler Thromb Vasc Biol*, *22*(7), 1175–1180.

Kushi, L. H., Folsom, A. R., Prineas, R. J., Mink, P. J., Wu, Y., and Bostick, R. M. (1996). Dietary antioxidant vitamins and death from coronary heart disease in postmenopausal women. *N Engl J Med*, *334*(18), 1156–1162.

Lamarche, B., Despres, J. P., Moorjani, S., Cantin, B., Dagenais, G. R., and Lupien, P. J. (1995). Prevalence of dyslipidemic phenotypes in ischemic heart disease (prospective results from the Quebec Cardiovascular Study). *Am J Cardiol*, *75*(17), 1189–1195.

Levitan, E. B., Song, Y. Q., Ford, E. S., and Liu, S. M. (2004). Is nondiabetic hyperglycemia a risk factor for cardiovascular disease? A meta-analysis of prospective studies. *Arch Intern Med*, *164*(19), 2147–2155.

Li, T. Y., Brennan, A. M., Wedick, N. M., Mantzoros, C., Rifai, N., and Hu, F. B. (2009). Regular consumption of nuts is associated with a lower risk of cardiovascular disease in women with type 2 diabetes. *J Nutr*, *139*(7), 1333–1338.

Libby, P. (2006). Inflammation and cardiovascular disease mechanisms. *Am J Clin Nutr*, *83*(2), 456s–460s.

Lim, S. S., Vos, T., Flaxman, A. D. et al. (2012). A comparative risk assessment of burden of disease and injury attributable to 67 risk factors and risk factor clusters in 21 regions, 1990–2010: A systematic analysis for the Global Burden of Disease Study 2010. *Lancet*, *380*(9859), 2224–2260.

Llorente-Cortes, V., Estruch, R., Mena, M. P., Ros, E., Gonzalez, M. A., Fito, M., Lamuela-Raventós, R. M., and Badimon, L. (2010). Effect of Mediterranean diet on the expression of pro-atherogenic genes in a population at high cardiovascular risk. *Atherosclerosis*, *208*(2), 442–450.

Lloyd-Jones, D., Adams, R. J., Brown, T. M. et al. (2010). Heart disease and stroke statistics—2010 update: A report from the American Heart Association. *Circulation*, *121*(7):e46–e215.

Lokko, P., Lartey, A., Armar-Klemesu, M., and Mattes, R. D. (2007). Regular peanut consumption improves plasma lipid levels in healthy Ghanaians. *Int J Food Sci Nutr*, *58*(3), 190–200.

Lopez-Uriarte, P., Bullo, M., Casas-Agustench, P., Babio, N., and Salas-Salvado, J. (2009). Nuts and oxidation: A systematic review. *Nutr Rev*, *67*(9), 497–508.

Lopez-Uriarte, P., Nogues, R., Saez, G., Bullo, M., Romeu, M., Masana, L., Tormos, C., Casas-Agustench, P., and Salas-Salvado, J. (2010). Effect of nut consumption on oxidative stress and the endothelial function in metabolic syndrome. *Clin Nutr*, *29*(3), 373–380.

Lovejoy, J. C., Most, M. M., Lefevre, M., Greenway, F. L., and Rood, J. C. (2002). Effect of diets enriched in almonds on insulin action and serum lipids in adults with normal glucose tolerance or type 2 diabetes. *Am J Clin Nutr*, *76*(5), 1000–1006.

Lutsey, P. L., Steffen, L. M., and Stevens, J. (2008). Dietary intake and the development of the metabolic syndrome: The Atherosclerosis Risk in Communities study. *Circulation*, *117*(6), 754–761.

Luu, H. N., Blot, W. J., Xiang, Y. B. et al. (2015). Prospective evaluation of the association of nut/peanut consumption with total and cause-specific mortality. *JAMA Intern Med*, *175*(5), 755–766.

Ma, Y. Y., Njike, V. Y., Millet, J., Dutta, S., Doughty, K., Treu, J. A., and Katz, D. L. (2010). Effects of walnut consumption on endothelial function in type 2 diabetic subjects—A randomized controlled crossover trial. *Diabetes Care*, *33*(2), 227–232.

Maranhao, P. A., Kraemer-Aguiar, L. G., de Oliveira, C. L., Kuschnir, M. C. C., Vieira, Y. R., Souza, M. G. C., Koury, J. C., and Bouskela, E. (2011). Brazil nuts intake improves lipid profile, oxidative stress and microvascular function in obese adolescents: A randomized controlled trial. *Nutr Metab*, *8*, 32.

Martinez-Gonzalez, M. A. and Bes-Rastrollo, M. (2011). Nut consumption, weight gain and obesity: Epidemiological evidence. *Nutr Metab Cardiovasc Dis*, *21*, S40–S45.

Martinez-Gonzalez, M. A., Garcia-Arellano, A., Toledo, E. et al. (2012). A 14-item Mediterranean diet assessment tool and obesity indexes among high-risk subjects: The PREDIMED trial. *PLoS One*, *7*(8), e43134.

Martinez-Gonzalez, M. A., Salas-Salvadó, J., Estruch, R., Corella, D., Fitó, M., Ros, E., and PREDIMED Investigators. (2015). Benefits of the mediterranean diet: Insights from the PREDIMED Study. *Prog Cardiovasc Dis*, *58*(1), 50–60.

Mayhew, A. J., de Souza, R. J., Meyre, D., Anand, S. S., and Mente, A. (2016). A systematic review and meta-analysis of nut consumption and incident risk of CVD and all-cause mortality. *Br J Nutr*, *115*(2), 212–225.

Mercanligil, S. M., Arslan, P., Alasalvar, C., Okut, E., Akgul, E., Pinar, A., Geyik, P. O., Tokgözoğlu, L., and Shahidi, F. (2007). Effects of hazelnut-enriched diet on plasma cholesterol and lipoprotein profiles in hypercholesterolemic adult men. *Eur J Clin Nutr*, *61*(2), 212–220.

Minutolo, R., Agarwal, R., Borrelli, S. et al. (2011). Prognostic role of ambulatory blood pressure measurement in patients with nondialysis chronic kidney disease. *Arch Intern Med*, *171*(12), 1090–1098.

Mohammadifard, N., Salehi-Abargouei, A., Salas-Salvado, J., Guasch-Ferre, M., Humphries, K., and Sarrafzadegan, N. (2015). The effect of tree nut, peanut, and soy nut consumption on blood pressure: A systematic review and meta-analysis of randomized controlled clinical trials. *Am J Clin Nutr*, *101*(5), 966–982.

Mukuddem-Petersen, J., Stonehouse, W., Jerling, J. C., Hanekom, S. M., and White, Z. (2007). Effects of a high walnut and high cashew nut diet on selected markers of the metabolic syndrome: A controlled feeding trial. *Br J Nutr*, *97*(6), 1144–1153.

Nouran, M. G., Kimiagar, M., Abadi, A., Mirzazadeh, M., and Harrison, G. (2010). Peanut consumption and cardiovascular risk. *Public Health Nutr*, *13*(10), 1581–1586.

Novotny, J. A., Gebauer, S. K., and Baer, D. J. (2012). Discrepancy between the Atwater factor predicted and empirically measured energy values of almonds in human diets. *Am J Clin Nutr*, *96*(2), 296–301.

O'Byrne, D. J., Knauft, D. A., and Shireman, R. B. (1997). Low fat-monounsaturated rich diets containing high-oleic peanuts improve serum lipoprotein profiles. *Lipids*, *32*(7), 687–695.

Ogedegbe, G., Pickering, T. G., Clemow, L., Chaplin, W., Spruill, T. M., Albanese, G. M., Eguchi, K., Burg, M., and Gerin, W. (2008). The misdiagnosis of hypertension: The role of patient anxiety. *Arch Intern Med*, *168*(22), 2459–2465.

Olmedilla-Alonso, B., Granado-Lorencio, F., Herrero-Barbudo, C., Blanco-Navarro, I., Blazquez-Garcia, S., and Perez-Sacristan, B. (2008). Consumption of restructured meat products with added walnuts has a cholesterol-lowering effect in subjects at high cardiovascular risk: A randomised, crossover, placebo-controlled study. *J Am Coll Nutr*, *27*(2), 342–348.

O'Neil, C. E., Fulgoni, V. L., and Nicklas, T. A. (2015). Tree Nut consumption is associated with better adiposity measures and cardiovascular and metabolic syndrome health risk factors in U.S. Adults: NHANES 2005–2010. *Nutr J*, *14*, 64.

O'Neil, C. E., Keast, D. R., Nicklas, T. A., and Fulgoni, V. L. (2011). Nut consumption is associated with decreased health risk factors for cardiovascular disease and metabolic syndrome in U.S. adults: NHANES 1999–2004. *J Am Coll Nutr*, *30*(6), 502–510.

Orem, A., Yucesan, F. B., Orem, C., Akcan, B., Kural, B. V., Alasalvar, C., and Shahidi, F. (2013). Hazelnut-enriched diet improves cardiovascular risk biomarkers beyond a lipid-lowering effect in hypercholesterolemic subjects. *J Clin Lipidol*, *7*(2), 123–131.

Otvos, J. D., Collins, D., Freedman, D. S., Shalaurova, I., Schaefer, E. J., McNamara, J. R., Bloomfield, H. E., and Robins, S. J. (2006). Low-density lipoprotein and high-density lipoprotein particle subclasses predict coronary events and are favorably changed by gemfibrozil therapy in the Veterans Affairs High-Density Lipoprotein Intervention Trial. *Circulation*, *113*(12), 1556–1563.

Pan, A., Sun, Q., Manson, J. E., Willett, W. C., and Hu, F. B. (2013). Walnut consumption is associated with lower risk of type 2 diabetes in women. *J Nutr*, *143*(4), 512–518.

Parker, E. D. and Folsom, A. R. (2003). Intentional weight loss and incidence of obesity-related cancers: The Iowa Women's Health Study. *Int J Obes Relat Metab Disord*, *27*(12), 1447–1452.

Parker, E. D., Harnack, L. J., and Folsom, A. R. (2003). Nut consumption and risk of type 2 diabetes. *JAMA*, *290*(1), 38–39; author reply 39–40.

Peretz, A., Leotta, D. F., Sullivan, J. H., Trenga, C. A., Sands, F. N., Aulet, M. R., Paun, M., Gill, E. A., and Kaufman, J. D. (2007). Flow mediated dilation of the brachial artery: An investigation of methods requiring further standardization. *BMC Cardiovasc Disord*, *7*, 11.

Pickering, T. G., Hall, J. E., Appel, L. J., Falkner, B. E., Graves, J., Hill, M. N., Jones, D. W., Kurtz, T., Sheps, S. G., Roccella, E. J., and Subcommittee of Professional and Public Education of the American Heart Association Council on High Blood Pressure Research. (2005). Recommendations for blood pressure measurement in humans and experimental animals: Part 1: Blood pressure measurement in humans: A statement for professionals from the Subcommittee of Professional and Public Education of the American Heart Association Council on High Blood Pressure Research. *Hypertension*, *45*(1), 142–161.

Quinaglia, T., Matos-Souza, J. R., Feinstein, S. B., and Sposito, A. C. (2015). Flow-mediated dilation: An evolving method. *Atherosclerosis*, *241*(1), 143–144.

Rajaram, S., Haddad, E. H., Mejia, A., and Sabate, J. (2009). Walnuts and fatty fish influence different serum lipid fractions in normal to mildly hyperlipidemic individuals: A randomized controlled study. *Am J Clin Nutr*, *89*(5), S1657–S1663.

Reiter, R. J., Manchester, L. C., and Tan, D. X. (2005). Melatonin in walnuts: Influence on levels of melatonin and total antioxidant capacity of blood. *Nutrition*, *21*(9), 920–924.

Rohatgi, A., Khera, A., Berry, J. D. et al. (2014). HDL cholesterol efflux capacity and incident cardiovascular events. *N Engl J Med*, *371*(25), 2383–2393.

Ros, E. (2009). Nuts and novel biomarkers of cardiovascular disease. *Am J Clin Nutr*, *89*(5), 1649S–1656S.

Ros, E., Nunez, I., Perez-Heras, A., Serra, M., Gilabert, R., Casals, E., and Deulofeu, R. (2004). A walnut diet improves endothelial function in hypercholesterolemic subjects—A randomized crossover trial. *Circulation*, *109*(13), 1609–1614.

Sabate, J., Fraser, G. E., Burke, K., Knutsen, S. F., Bennett, H., and Lindsted, K. D. (1993). Effects of walnuts on serum-lipid levels and blood-pressure in normal men. *N Engl J Med*, *328*(9), 603–607.

Sabaté, J. and Wein, M. (2010). Nuts, blood lipids and cardiovascular disease. *Asia Pac J Clin Nutr*, *19*, 131–136.

Sabaté, J., Oda, K., and Ros, E. (2010). Nut consumption and blood lipid levels: A pooled analysis of 25 intervention trials. *Arch Intern Med*, *170*(9), 821–827.

Sacco, R. L. (2011). The new American Heart Association 2020 goal: Achieving ideal cardiovascular health. *J Cardiovasc Med (Hagerstown)*, *12*(4), 255–257.

Salas-Salvadó, J., Bulló, M., Estruch, R. et al. (2014a). Prevention of diabetes with Mediterranean diets: A subgroup analysis of a randomized trial. *Ann Intern Med*, *160*, 1–10.

Salas-Salvadó, J., Fernández-Ballart, J., Ros, E. et al. (2008). Effect of a Mediterranean diet supplemented with nuts on metabolic syndrome status: One-year results of the PREDIMED randomized trial. *Arch Intern Med*, *168*(22), 2449–2458.

Salas-Salvado, J., Guasch-Ferre, M., Bullo, M., and Sabate, J. (2014b). Nuts in the prevention and treatment of metabolic syndrome. *Am J Clin Nutr*, *100*(1), 399s–407s.

Sari, I., Baltaci, Y., Bagci, C., Davutoglu, V., Erel, O., Celik, H., Ozer, O., Aksoy, N., and Aksoy, M. (2010). Effect of pistachio diet on lipid parameters, endothelial function, inflammation, and oxidative status: A prospective study. *Nutrition*, *26*(4), 399–404.

Sauder, K. A., McCrea, C. E., Kris-Etherton, P. M., Ulbrecht, J. S., and West, S. G. (2013). Effect of pistachios on lipids, lipoproteins, glucose metabolism, and insulin sensitivity in type 2 diabetes. *FASEB J*, *27*.

Sauder, K. A., McCrea, C. E., Ulbrecht, J. S., Kris-Etherton, P. M., and West, S. G. (2014). Pistachio nut consumption modifies systemic hemodynamics, increases heart rate variability, and reduces ambulatory blood pressure in well-controlled type 2 diabetes: A randomized trial. *J Am Heart Assoc*, *3*(4), e000873.

Sauder, K. A., McCrea, C. E., Ulbrecht, J. S., Kris-Etherton, P. M., and West, S. G. (2015). Effects of pistachios on the lipid/lipoprotein profile, glycemic control, inflammation, and endothelial function in type 2 diabetes: A randomized trial. *Metabolism*, *64*(11), 1521–1529.

Schutte, A. E., Van Rooyen, J. M., Huisman, H. W., Mukuddem-Petersen, J., Oosthuizen, W., Hanekom, S. M., and Jerling, J. C. (2006). Modulation of baroreflex sensitivity by walnuts versus cashew nuts in subjects with metabolic syndrome. *Am J Hypertens*, *19*(6), 629–636.

Sheridan, M. J., Cooper, J. N., Erario, M., and Cheifetz, C. E. (2007). Pistachio nut consumption and serum lipid levels. *J Am Coll Nutr*, *26*(2), 141–148.

Smith, J. D., Hou, T., Hu, F. B., Rimm, E. B., Spiegelman, D., Willett, W. C., and Mozaffarian, D. (2015). A comparison of different methods for evaluating diet, physical activity, and long-term weight gain in 3 prospective cohort studies. *J Nutr*, *145*(11), 2527–2534.

Spaccarotella, K. J., Kris-Etherton, P. M., Stone, W. L., Bagshaw, D. M., Fishell, V. K., West, S. G., Lawrence, F. R., and Hartman, T. J. (2008). The effect of walnut intake on factors related to prostate and vascular health in older men. *Nutr J*, *7*, 13.

Tapsell, L. C., Gillen, L. J., Patch, C. S., Batterham, M., Owen, A., Bare, M., and Kennedy, M. (2004). Including walnuts in a low-fat/modified-fat diet improves HDL cholesterol-to-total cholesterol ratios in patients with type 2 diabetes. *Diabetes Care*, *27*(12), 2777–2783.

Tey, S. L., Brown, R. C., Chisholm, A. W., Delahunty, C. M., Gray, A. R., and Williams, S. M. (2011). Effects of different forms of hazelnuts on blood lipids and alpha-tocopherol concentrations in mildly hypercholesterolemic individuals. *Eur J Clin Nutr*, *65*(1), 117–124.

Torabian, S., Haddad, E., Cordero-MacIntyre, Z., Tanzman, J., Fernandez, M. L., and Sabate, J. (2010). Long-term walnut supplementation without dietary advice induces favorable serum lipid changes in free-living individuals. *Eur J Clin Nutr*, *64*(3), 274–279.

U.S. Burden of Disease Collaborators. (2013). The state of US health, 1990–2010: Burden of diseases, injuries, and risk factors. *JAMA*, *310*(6), 591–608.

U.S. Department of Health and Human Services and U.S. Department of Agriculture. (December 2015). *2015–2020 Dietary Guidelines for Americans*. 8th Edition. http://health.gov/dietaryguidelines/2015/guidelines/.

van den Brandt, P. A. and Schouten, L. J. (2015). Relationship of tree nut, peanut and peanut butter intake with total and cause-specific mortality: A cohort study and meta-analysis. *Int J Epidemiol*, *44*(3), 1038–1049.

Vannice, G. and Rasmussen, H. (2014). Position of the academy of nutrition and dietetics: Dietary fatty acids for healthy adults. *J Acad Nutr Diet*, *114*(1), 136–153.

Viguiliouk, E., Kendall, C. W., Blanco Mejia, S. et al. (2014). Effect of tree nuts on glycemic control in diabetes: A systematic review and meta-analysis of randomized controlled dietary trials. *PLoS One*, *9*(7), e103376.

West, S. G., Krick, A. L., Klein, L. C. et al. (2010). Effects of diets high in walnuts and flax oil on hemodynamic responses to stress and vascular endothelial function. *J Am Coll Nutr*, *29*(6), 595–603.

Wien, M., Bleich, D., Raghuwanshi, M., Gould-Forgerite, S., Gomes, J., Monahan-Couch, L., and Oda, K. (2010). Almond consumption and cardiovascular risk factors in adults with prediabetes. *J Am College Nutr*, *29*(3), 189–197.

Wien, M. A., Sabate, J. M., Ikle, D. N., Cole, S. E., and Kandeel, F. R. (2003). Almonds vs complex carbohydrates in a weight reduction program. *Int J Obes Relat Metab Disord*, *27*(11), 1365–1372.

Wu, H., Pan, A., Yu, Z. et al. (2010). Lifestyle counseling and supplementation with flaxseed or walnuts influence the management of metabolic syndrome. *J Nutr*, *140*(11), 1937–1942.

Zhang, J., Grieger, J. A., Kris-Etherton, P. M., Thompson, J. T., Gillies, P. J., Fleming, J. A., and Vanden Heuvel, J. P. (2011).Walnut oil increases cholesterol efflux through inhibition of stearoyl CoA desaturase 1 in THP-1 macrophage-derived foam cells. *Nutr Metab (Lond)*, *8*, 61.

Zhang, J., Kris-Etherton, P. M., Thompson, J. T., Hannon, D. B., Gillies, P. J., and Vanden Heuvel, J. P. (2012). Alpha-linolenic acid increases cholesterol efflux in macrophage-derived foam cells by decreasing stearoyl CoA desaturase 1 expression: Evidence for a farnesoid-X-receptor mechanism of action. *J Nutr Biochem*, *23*(4), 400–409.

Zhao, G. X., Etherton, T. D., Martin, K. R., Gillies, P. J., West, S. G., and Kris-Etherton, P. M. (2007). Dietary alpha-linolenic acid inhibits proinflammatory cytokine production by peripheral blood mononuclear cells in hypercholesterolemic subjects. *Am J Clin Nutr*, *85*(2), 385–391.

25 Dairy Product Consumption, Dairy Fat, and Cardiometabolic Health*

Benoît Lamarche

CONTENTS

ABSTRACT

Because regular-fat dairy products contribute significantly to dietary intake of saturated fatty acid (SFA), and because of the well-known cholesterol-raising effects of SFA, most dietary guidelines advocate consumption of low-fat dairy products as opposed to regular/high-fat dairy foods. Yet, results from numerous randomized controlled trials (RCTs) have reported inconsistent effects of dairy consumption, including regular/whole-fat dairy, on blood lipid levels and on many other cardiometabolic risk factors, such as blood pressure and inflammatory biomarkers. Thus, the recommendation to have low-fat dairy integrated as part of healthy eating guidelines in 2015 needs to be revisited. This review suggests that consumption of dairy foods and dairy fat appears to have a null effect on a large spectrum of cardiometabolic risk factors. Data also suggest that the purported detrimental effects of SFA on cardiometabolic health may be attenuated when provided in complex food matrices such as cheese. Despite the fact that there are still numerous research gaps to be addressed, available data suggest no potential harmful effects of dairy consumption, irrespective of dairy fat, on cardiometabolic risk. Thus, the focus on low-fat dairy products in current guidelines may need to be revisited in light of the current evidence.

* Disclosures
The author is Chair of Nutrition at Laval University. This Chair is supported by unrestricted endowments from Royal Bank of Canada, Pfizer, and Provigo/Loblaws. The author has received funding in the last 5 years for his research from the Canadian Institutes for Health Research (CIHR), Natural Sciences and Engineering Research Council of Canada (NSERC), Agriculture and Agrifood Canada, the Canola Council of Canada, Dairy Farmers of Canada (DFC), Dairy Research Institute (DRI), Atrium Innovations, the Danone Institute, Merck Frosst. The author has received speaker honoraria over the last 5 years from DFC, DRI, the Dairy Council of Northern Ireland, and the International Chair on Cardiometabolic Risk. The author is Chair of the Expert Scientific Advisory Panel of DFC, and of the ad hoc committee on saturated fat of Heart and Stroke Foundation of Canada.

ABBREVIATIONS

AIx	Augmentation index
BP	Blood pressure
CHD	Coronary heart disease
CLA	Conjugated linoleic acid
CRP	C-reactive protein
FMD	Flow-mediated dilation
HDL-C	High-density lipoprotein cholesterol
HOMA	Homeostatic model assessment
IL	Interleukin
LDL-C	Low-density lipoprotein cholesterol
MCP-1	Monocyte chemoattractant protein 1
MetS	Metabolic syndrome
MUFA	Monounsaturated fatty acids
NCEP	National Cholesterol Education Program
PUFA	Polyunsaturated fatty acids
RCT	Randomized controlled trial
SFA	Saturated fatty acids
sICAM-1	Soluble intercellular adhesion molecule-1
SSB	Sugar-sweetened beverage
sVCAM	Soluble vascular cell adhesion molecule-1
T2D	Type 2 diabetes
TFA	*trans* fatty acids
TG	triglycerides
TNF-α	Tumor necrosis factor-α

INTRODUCTION

Dairy product consumption is recommended in most dietary guidelines around the world. This is in large part justified by the contribution of dairy foods to the intake of key nutrients for health, primarily high-quality protein and calcium, but also magnesium, potassium, phosphorus, vitamin B_{12}, riboflavin, vitamin A, and vitamin D in countries where dairy is fortified (Huth et al. 2013). In general, dietary guidelines recommend consuming low-fat/reduced-fat dairy products to limit the intake of saturated fat (SFA), to which dairy foods contribute significantly. Indeed, dietary SFA increases plasma LDL-cholesterol (LDL-C), a key risk factor for coronary heart disease (CHD), compared with dietary carbohydrates, monounsaturated fat (MUFA), and polyunsaturated fat (PUFA) (Mensink et al. 2003).

However, fairly recent meta-analyses of observational cohort studies have failed to show a significant association between dietary SFA and CHD risk (Siri-Tarino et al. 2010; Chowdhury et al. 2014), thus igniting a new controversy in the area of nutrition and health. While the recommendation to limit the intake of dietary SFA remains relevant until the debate is put to rest, this whole controversy also raises the pertinence of focusing on whole foods rather than on single nutrients when crafting dietary guidelines for health. This may particularly be the case for dairy products.

We have recently performed a systematic review to ascertain the association between dairy product consumption and the risk of clinical outcomes, including cardiovascular disease, type 2 diabetes (T2D), and metabolic syndrome (Drouin-Chartier et al. 2016). The review was based on the highest level of evidence from meta-analyses of prospective cohort studies as well as on more recent cohort studies not included in these meta-analyses. This extensive review revealed no evidence of unfavorable associations between dairy intake, irrespective of product type and fat content, and the risk of CHD-related clinical outcomes. For some outcomes, dairy product intake showed no association with risk, while for others the associations were favorable. For example, total dairy, low-fat dairy, and milk intakes were each associated with reduced risk for hypertension, while total dairy, low-fat dairy, yogurt, and cheese intakes were associated with a reduced risk for T2D. Total dairy and milk consumption was inversely associated with metabolic syndrome (MetS).

Although reducing LDL-C concentrations along with proper management of high blood pressure are considered key targets for prevention and treatment of CHD (Weintraub et al. 2011), considering the impact of diet on a larger spectrum of risk factors may provide additional insight on how diet modification is likely to affect risk of clinical outcomes in the future. This is important because a large RCT on dairy with hard endpoints is highly implausible in the future. This chapter is a narrative review of the data from clinical trials in humans that have documented the impact of dairy intake, with particular focus on dairy fat, on several cardiometabolic risk factors that are involved in the etiology of atherosclerosis and CHD.

CARDIOMETABOLIC RISK

Raised LDL-C concentrations represent only one of several risk factors to consider in the etiology of atherosclerosis leading to clinical outcomes such as CHD. There are indeed a plethora of other cardiometabolic risk factors that contribute to modulating CHD risk, including vascular dysfunction with high blood pressure, plasma lipid risk factors other than elevated LDL-C such as high triglycerides and low HDL-C concentrations, increased LDL particle number and small dense LDL particles, systemic inflammation, and insulin resistance (Despres et al. 2008). While documenting the impact of dairy intake and dairy fat on LDL-C is of great interest from a CHD prevention perspective, appreciating the changes in other cardiometabolic risk factors also is of key importance.

DAIRY AND PLASMA LIPID LEVELS

Data from a meta-analysis of RCTs conducted among healthy individuals have shown that intakes of total dairy and low- and whole-fat dairy products had no significant impact on plasma LDL-C or HDL-C concentrations (Benatar et al. 2013). Results from recent studies by our group are consistent with these observations. In a crossover RCT, postmenopausal women with abdominal obesity were fed two National Cholesterol Education Program (NCEP) diets for 6 weeks each, one including 3.2 servings/day of 2% fat milk per 2000 kcal and one without milk or any other dairy products. Diets were matched for calories as well as most nutrients, with the exception of calcium and vitamin D. There was no significant difference in plasma LDL-C, HDL-C and TG levels, the total cholesterol/HDL-C ratio, and LDL particle size between the milk diet and the milk-free diet (Drouin-Chartier et al. 2015). In a larger crossover RCT, 101 men and women with hs-CRP values >1 mg/L consumed 3 servings/day of dairy (375 mL low-fat milk, 175 g low-fat yogurt, and 30 g regular-fat cheddar cheese) versus energy-matched control products (fruit juice, vegetable juice, cashews, and 1 cookie) as part of prudent diets (Abdullah et al. 2016). A slight but significant increase in plasma LDL-C was observed after the dairy diet (+3.3%, $P = 0.02$ vs. the control dairy-free diet), with no difference, however, in plasma HDL-C, TG and apoB concentrations, or in LDL particle size between the two diets (Abdullah et al. 2016). Interestingly, DNA sequence variants in two genes (ABCG5 and CYP7A1) identified among a list of 13 genes known to regulate cholesterol metabolism were found to significantly modulate the LDL-C response to dairy (Abdullah et al. 2016). This is a good example of the heterogeneous response to dietary changes among individuals, hence explaining to some extent the inconsistencies often seen in the literature regarding the impact of diet on cardiometabolic risk features.

There is increasing evidence that the food matrix influences the cardiometabolic response to various nutrients, including SFA (Siri-Tarino et al. 2015). In that respect, the LDL-C raising effect of dietary SFA may vary depending on its food of origin and background diet. For example, consumption of a Gouda-type 27% fat cheese (Norvegia® 80 g/day) for 8 weeks did not significantly increase plasma LDL-C levels compared with baseline values (Nilsen et al. 2015). In a meta-analysis of 4 RCTs combining data from a total of 100 individuals, intake of SFA from cheese reduced plasma LDL-C and HDL-C levels compared with similar amounts of SFA from butter, while effects on plasma TG concentrations were similar between cheese and butter (de Goede et al. 2015). The calcium content of cheese as well as the phospholipids present in the milk fat globule membranes of cheese fat have been evoked as potential mechanisms explaining the difference between cheese and butter in modulating plasma lipid levels, despite similar SFA content (de Goede et al. 2015). Chiu et al. (2016) have recently compared the impact of DASH diets that comprised either full-fat or low-fat dairy products on plasma lipids and other cardiometabolic outcomes. The high-fat DASH diet (14% of calories as SFA) resulted in significantly lower plasma triglycerides, large and medium VLDL concentrations, and significantly higher LDL particle size compared with the low-fat DASH diet (8% of calories as SFA). There were no differences between diets in LDL-C, apoB, and HDL-C concentrations.

The lower plasma HDL-C concentrations with SFA from cheese versus butter is puzzling from a CHD health perspective, considering that SFA intake is generally associated with increased HDL-C compared with carbohydrates and other dietary fats (Mensink et al. 2003). While increased plasma HDL-C concentrations are generally associated with a reduced risk of CHD (Gordon et al. 1977; Austin 1991), recent data from large clinical trials have challenged the importance of this risk factor in the broader scheme of CHD prevention (Barter et al. 2007; Briel et al. 2009; Schwartz et al. 2012). An emerging concept suggests that HDL structure and functionality, beyond simple "static" cholesterol measures, need to be considered when assessing the HDL-related risk of CHD (Asztalos et al. 2011). For example, cholesterol efflux capacity—a key step in reverse cholesterol transport measured *ex vivo* in cultured macrophages—has been inversely correlated with carotid intima-media thickness and with coronary disease status even after adjustment for HDL-C concentrations (Khera et al. 2011). This is a good example of how a metric of enhanced HDL function may better predict the risk of vascular disease than variations in plasma HDL-C concentrations (Khera et al. 2011). Very little is known regarding the impact of dairy and dairy fat on various metrics of HDL function and structure; this represents an exciting and novel area of research.

Finally, the impact of consuming fermented dairy products on plasma lipid levels has been of interest for more than 30 years. Agerholm-Larsen et al. (2000a) published a meta-analysis of six RCTs on Gaio®, a commercially available yogurt fermented with one strain of *Enterococcus faecium* and two strains of *Streptococcus thermophiles.* Data indicated that consumption of the fermented yogurt significantly reduced plasma LDL-C compared with consumption of control yogurts, which were of identical composition to the test yogurt, but chemically fermented with an organic acid instead of a live bacterial culture. Such data have been reproduced in some (Anderson and Gilliland 1999; Andrade and Borges 2009) but not all (de Roos et al. 1999; Sadrzadeh-Yeganeh et al. 2010) of the more recent studies of fermented dairy intake. Finally, consumption of fermented dairy of any form seems to have very little impact on plasma TG (Schaafsma et al. 1998; Bertolami et al. 1999; St-Onge et al. 2002; Hansel et al. 2007), while the effects on HDL-C concentrations have not been investigated thoroughly. In a small parallel RTC, we have shown that 4-week consumption of yogurt products containing different doses of *Bifidobacterium animalis* subsp. *lactis* (*BB-12*) and *Lactobacillus acidophilus* (*LA-5*) had no significant impact on plasma LDL-C, TG, and HDL-C concentrations compared with a control yogurt (Savard et al. 2011). This is an area that certainly deserves intensified research.

In summary, fairly robust data from meta-analyses as well as from additional RCTs suggest relatively neutral effects of dairy intake and of dairy fat at least when consumed as part of a dairy food such as cheese on plasma lipid levels, including LDL-C. The effect of dairy in general and of dairy fat more specifically on other lipid risk factors such as apoB also appears to be relatively neutral (Drouin-Chartier et al. 2015; Chiu et al. 2016), while the impact on LDL particle size is mixed, with studies showing neutral effects (Drouin-Chartier et al. 2015) and others showing increase in LDL size with dairy fat (Chiu et al. 2016). Most of the existing studies on this topic have been conducted among healthy individuals and therefore such evidence needs to be further substantiated among patients with CHD or T2D, who may show different responses to dietary changes. Data pertaining to the effect of fermented dairy on plasma lipid risk factors are mixed and additional studies in this area are also warranted.

Dairy and Low-Grade Systemic Inflammation

Low-grade systemic inflammation plays a key role in the etiology of atherosclerosis and related clinical outcomes (Libby 2002, 2006). Investigating the impact of diet on systemic inflammation is challenging. Indeed, a wide array of surrogate markers have been used to reflect different aspects of pro- and anti-inflammatory processes, and this creates a lot of heterogeneity among studies. Nevertheless, some of these markers like C-reactive protein (CRP) and serum amyloid A are considered good surrogates of low-grade systemic inflammation, while others like interleukin(IL)-6, TNF-alpha, and adiponectin may reflect localized inflammation (Libby 2007).

We have recently reviewed RCTs that have assessed the impact of dairy consumption on markers of low-grade systemic inflammation (Labonte et al. 2013). Four of the eight retrieved RCTs pointed toward a null impact of dairy consumption on inflammation, while the other four studies suggested favorable effects. However, we have stressed in our review that only one of the retrieved RCTs was designed primarily to investigate the impact of dairy intake on inflammation as a primary outcome, while all other reports are based on secondary analyses, which is a significant shortcoming. The study in which change in inflammation markers was the main outcome showed a significant favorable effect of dairy consumption on plasma levels of CRP, TNF-α, and MCP-1. In most of the available studies, dairy included a combination of different types of products, thereby limiting our ability to distinguish the effects of isolated dairy products. It must also be stressed that results in some of these studies may have been confounded by weight loss, which was part of the intervention in addition to the dairy component of the study (Labonte et al. 2013).

Partly consistent with our findings, Benatar et al. (2013) in their meta-analysis of data from seven RCTs have reported no significant impact of low- or full-fat dairy intake on plasma CRP levels. This is also consistent with recent data from a large crossover RCT by our group, in which 112 men and women with subclinical inflammation (CRP > 1 mg/L) consumed 3 servings/day of dairy products (low-fat milk, low-fat yogurt, and regular cheddar cheese) or energy-matched control products (fruit juice, vegetable juice, cashews, and 1 cookie) as part of prudent 4-week diets (Labonte et al. 2014). The study was specifically designed to assess change in biomarkers of inflammation as the primary outcome. Consumption of dairy had no significant impact on serum CRP or adiponectin concentrations but significantly reduced IL-6 concentrations compared with baseline values. The reduction in serum CRP versus baseline values with the dairy-free control diet was greater than with the dairy diet, while the reductions in serum IL-6 concentrations were similar between the two diets. These variations in surrogates of systemic inflammation were not correlated to variations in the expression level of key inflammatory genes and transcription factors in whole blood cells (Labonte et al. 2014).

In summary, evidence available to date suggests a relatively neutral effect of consuming low- or full-fat dairy products on inflammatory biomarkers. As already emphasized, most of this evidence is based on studies that were not specifically designed to investigate inflammation as a primary outcome, with sample sizes that were more appropriate to examine changes in plasma lipid levels or weight loss. Thus, more studies are warranted to characterize better the impact of dairy consumption (any form and any fat content) on low-grade, systemic inflammation.

Dairy and Glucose–Insulin Homeostasis

Insulin resistance is one of several key cardiometabolic features associated with abdominal obesity and MetS (Despres and Lemieux 2006). Elevated plasma insulin levels, which reflect to some extent a higher degree of insulin resistance, have been associated with an increased risk of hypertension and CHD (Xun et al. 2013). It remains unclear if insulin is involved etiologically or is simply a partner in crime in processes leading to atherosclerosis.

Turner et al. (2015) have systematically reviewed RCTs having assessed the effects of dairy intake on various measures of glucose–insulin homeostasis. The literature search focused on trials with minimal dietary change other than the dairy component, as well as weight stable conditions. Only 10 RCTs were retrieved. Four of the dairy interventions showed a positive effect on insulin sensitivity as assessed by HOMA, one was negative, and five had no effect. Study duration appeared to be an important confounding factor. Indeed, trials of less than 8 weeks' duration saw no significant changes in insulin sensitivity, while those between 12 and 24 weeks showed a beneficial effect of higher dairy consumption. Results from the 6-month interventions were mixed, dairy intake leading to improvement in HOMA values in one study but to no change in two other studies (Turner et al. 2015). The authors concluded their review by emphasizing the importance of relying on more and larger studies on this topic to better assess the impact of dairy on insulin and glucose metabolism.

We have recently shown in an RCT among postmenopausal women that milk consumption (3.2 servings/day, 2% fat) for 6 weeks had no impact on fasting glucose and insulin levels and on Cederholm and Matsuda insulin sensitivity indices compared with a macronutrient-matched, milk-free control diet (Drouin-Chartier et al. 2015). The Cederholm index represents mainly peripheral insulin sensitivity and muscle glucose uptake, while the Matsuda index is a composite of both hepatic and peripheral tissue insulin sensitivity. Finally, in a small RCT among 14 overweight postmenopausal women, cheese consumption (96–120 g/day) for 3 weeks compared with a macronutrient-matched nondairy, high-meat control diet and a nondairy, low-fat, high-carbohydrate control diet had no effect on the HOMA-insulin resistance index and on fasting and postprandial insulin and glucose levels (Thorning et al. 2015).

While results from prospective cohort studies suggest that dairy intake, particularly cheese and yogurt intake, may be associated with a reduced risk of T2D (Drouin-Chartier et al. 2016), RCTs provide limited and mixed results regarding the impact of dairy consumption on insulin resistance. As emphasized in the systematic review by Turner et al. (2015), additional high-quality studies with insulin resistance as primary outcome are needed in this area. Longer-term interventions may be considered, while the confounding effects of weight loss in many of the individual studies so far need to be addressed in future research efforts. Finally, the extent to which population characteristics (men vs. women, healthy vs. diabetic, lean vs. obese) influence the impact of dairy intake on insulin sensitivity also needs to be considered in future studies.

Dairy, Blood Pressure, and Vascular Function

The impact of dairy consumption on blood pressure (BP) regulation has been extensively studied. Data from epidemiological studies suggest favorable associations between total dairy and milk intake and the risk of hypertension (Drouin-Chartier et al. 2016). Surprisingly, data from shorter-term RCTs are not entirely supportive of data from observational studies. In the meta-analysis of existing RCTs by Benatar et al. (2013), total dairy intake had no significant impact on systolic and/or diastolic BP. This was true for both low-fat as well as whole-fat dairy. These data have been corroborated by additional RCTs of various dairy products, including low-fat and nonfat milk, yogurt, and full-fat cheese (Agerholm-Larsen et al. 2000b; Hilpert et al. 2009; Hjerpsted et al. 2011; Maki et al. 2013; Rideout et al. 2013; Schlienger et al. 2014; Ivey et al. 2015). We have recently examined the impact of dairy intake (low-fat milk, low-fat yogurt, and full-fat cheese, for a total of 3 servings/day) versus no dairy on ambulatory BP change in 76 mildly to moderately hypertensive patients. Dairy intake significantly reduced mean daytime systolic BP in men but not in women in comparison to the dairy-free control diet (Drouin-Chartier et al. 2014). Interestingly, Chiu et al. (2016) have shown that the BP-lowering effects associated with the DASH diet were preserved even when low-fat dairy products were replaced by high-fat dairy. Finally, the original DASH study has shown that consumption of low-fat dairy products as part of a healthy diet rich in fruits and vegetable and low in SFA led to further reduction in systolic and diastolic BP compared with the dairy-free healthy diet (Appel et al. 1997).

RCTs assessing the impact of fermented dairy on BP have recently been meta-analyzed by Dong et al. (2013). Pooled data from 13 RCTs indicated that consumption of fermented milk (100–450 g/day) compared with a milk-based placebo significantly reduced systolic and diastolic BP. Hypertensive patients appeared to be more responsive to the BP-lowering effect of fermented milk than normotensive individuals. The analysis was based on a total of 702 normo- and hypertensive subjects aged 35–75 years, using antihypertensive drugs or not. These results have been partly reproduced in the Cochrane meta-analysis by Usinger et al. (2012), according to which consumption of fermented milk was found to significantly reduce systolic BP but not diastolic BP. However, authors have emphasized that effect sizes were small and heterogeneous among individual RCTs, thus limiting the generalizability of the results.

Thus, there are apparent discrepancies between results from RCTs and from prospective cohort studies regarding the impact of dairy intake on BP regulation. This can, of course, be attributed to a number of factors. In epidemiological studies, residual confounding (i.e., unmeasured confounding factors associated with both dairy intake and BP variations) can influence the observed associations. Limitations inherent to estimation of self-reported dietary intake from FFQ and 24 h recalls should also be pointed out. Such confounding is less likely to occur in well-controlled RCTs. One the other hand, it is possible that dairy consumption *per se* may attenuate the deterioration in BP generally seen with aging and with weight gain, thereby being associated with more favorable BP outcomes in the longer term. This hypothesis needs to be pursued and validated in future studies.

Measures of vascular function such as flow-mediated dilation (FMD) as well as augmentation index (AIx) and pulse wave velocity, which both reflect arterial stiffness, have been proposed to be more holistic markers of vascular health and predictor of cardiovascular events and mortality than BP *per se* (Vlachopoulos et al. 2010; Ras et al. 2013). Vascular function can also be assessed using surrogate markers in the blood such as the soluble adhesion molecules (e.g., intercellular adhesion molecule-1 [sICAM-1], vascular cell adhesion molecule-1 [sVCAM-1], and E-selectin). However, the extent to which these adhesion molecules predict the risk of CHD independent of other known risk factors is unclear (Page and Liles 2013).

In the Caerphilly prospective cohort study of 2512 men, aged 45–59 years, who were followed up at 5-year intervals for a mean of 22.8 years, dairy intake in quartiles was inversely related to AIx (Livingstone et al. 2013), suggesting favorable impact from a cardiovascular health perspective. However, other measures of arterial stiffness such as pulse wave velocity showed no association with dairy intake. Thus, the significance of these results from a cardiovascular health perspective therefore remains unclear. Such epidemiological data are not entirely supported by data from RCTs. On the one hand, intake of 4 servings/day of nonfat dairy for 4 weeks has been shown to reduce carotid–femoral pulse wave velocity with a concomitant increase in brachial FMD and cardiovagal baroreflex sensitivity compared with baseline values among patients with elevated BP (mean BP 134 ± 1/81 ± 1 mm Hg) (Machin et al. 2015). The control, dairy-free diet (4 servings/day of fruits products) had no such effects on these measures of vascular function. On the other hand, consumption of low-fat dairy products (500 mL low-fat milk and 150 g low-fat yogurt) daily for 8 weeks had no impact on plasma levels of sICAM-1 and sVCAM-1 compared with a control dairy-free diet (600 mL fruit juice and three fruit biscuits), suggesting no effect of low-fat dairy on endothelial function (van Meijl and Mensink 2010). In an RCT from our group, consumption of 3 servings of milk, yogurt, and cheese for 4 weeks versus a dairy-free control diet had no significant impact on reactive hyperemia index in a sample of 76 men and women with stage 1 hypertension (Drouin-Chartier et al. 2014).

In general, acute and short-term (≤2 weeks) effects of dairy intake in RCTs have been associated with favorable changes in various measures of vascular function, even in the absence of concomitant changes in BP (Ballard and Bruno 2015). Longer-term interventions have provided less consistent results (Ballard and Bruno 2015). From a mechanistic perspective, the vasoprotective properties of dairy and its constituents have been suggested to be mediated through improvements in nitric oxide bioavailability as well as to potential changes in oxidative stress, inflammation, and insulin resistance (Ballard and Bruno 2015). However, the extent to which dairy foods *per se* versus the foods they replace in the diet are responsible for the beneficial changes in vascular function seen in some studies needs further investigation.

DAIRY FAT AND CARDIOMETABOLIC RISK

Dairy foods, particularly whole-fat dairy, contribute significantly to the dietary intake of SFA (Huth et al. 2013) and this has prompted most health organizations to promote consumption of low-fat dairy in place of regular fat dairy for optimal cardiovascular prevention. However, as already indicated, the impact of SFA on plasma lipids, including LDL-C, may be influenced and partly mitigated by the food matrix through which it is consumed (Siri-Tarino et al. 2015). This might explain to some extent why several epidemiological studies have failed to observe a significant association between SFA intake and CVD or CHD risk (Siri-Tarino et al. 2010; Chowdhury et al. 2014).

As reviewed in Chapter 12 of this book, dairy fats also contribute to the dietary intake of naturally occurring *trans* fatty acids (TFA). Indeed, the production of milk fat by ruminants involves bacteria that hydrogenate polyunsaturated *cis* fatty acids into TFA in the rumen of these animals, mostly in the form of vaccenic acid, but also conjugated linoleic acid (CLA). Evidence from studies in animal models has suggested potential benefits of vaccenic acid and CLA on cardiometabolic risk (Blewett et al. 2009; Gebauer et al. 2011; Jacome-Sosa et al. 2014). While epidemiological studies have reported unequivocal positive associations between intake of industrially produced hydrogenated TFA and CHD risk (Ascherio et al. 1999), neutral associations have been reported regarding naturally occurring TFA (Gebauer et al. 2011). It has been argued that the lack of a significant association between intake of naturally occurring TFA and CHD risk may be due, among others, to the very low intake of such fat in the human diet. Indeed, TFA represents only 3%–8% of total milk fat (Stender and Dyerberg 2003). In that context, very high intakes of naturally occurring TFA are virtually unattainable in the current dietary scheme of Western countries, even those with high intake of dairy foods (Stender et al. 2008). Nevertheless, we have quantified the dose–response relationship between intake of naturally occurring TFA and changes in plasma lipid levels based on data from 13 RCTs (Gayet-Boyer et al. 2014). Consistent with data from epidemiological studies, we found no relationship between intake of naturally occurring TFA of up to 4% of daily energy and changes in cardiovascular risk factors such as the total cholesterol/HDL-C and LDL-C/HDL-C ratios. On the other hand, Gebauer et al. have recently investigated in a double-blind, crossover feeding RCT involving 106 healthy adults the impact of high intakes of vaccenic acid (corresponding to 3.9% of daily energy) on blood lipids. They have shown that such high intakes of vaccenic acid significantly increased LDL-C, apoB, HDL-C, apoAI, and Lp(a) concentrations compared with a low vaccenic acid control diet (Gebauer et al. 2015). Once again, such high intakes of vaccenic acid are improbable as current estimates are well below 1% of daily energy in most countries (Gebauer et al. 2011). It has been proposed that TFA from dairy is unlikely to have adverse effects on key lipid CHD risk markers in healthy individuals at current dietary intake levels (Gayet-Boyer et al. 2014), but this is not a view shared by all (Brouwer et al. 2013).

CONCLUSIONS

This chapter has highlighted a number of key points related to intake of dairy foods and cardiometabolic health. Firstly, consumption of dairy products, even in their whole-fat versions, appears to have a neutral effect on plasma LDL-C concentrations. This is consistent with data from several epidemiological studies having failed to report significant associations between SFA intake and risk of CHD. More research is warranted to better characterize the impact of dairy consumption on other cardiometabolic risk factors such as elevated plasma apoB levels, small dense LDL particles, HDL function, markers of systemic inflammation, and glucose–insulin homeostasis. The impact of dairy intake *per se* on BP based on data from RCTs is mixed and this topic needs further research as well, with emphasis on longer-term studies.

Secondly, research pertaining to the impact of dairy fat *per se* on cardiometabolic health needs to be undertaken with caution. Indeed, dairy fat with the exception of butter is not consumed in isolation. Dairy fat is consumed as part of complex matrices that may modulate its impact on health. Research should really focus on documenting the impact of whole foods rather than individual nutrients on health. In that regard, research comparing the impact of low-fat and whole-fat versions of different dairy products on cardiometabolic health will be extremely insightful to better inform future dietary guidelines.

Thirdly, one aspect that contributes to confusion in the literature pertains to the fact that dairy intake can hardly be studied in isolation. Integrating dairy foods in the diet inevitably displaces other foods that may have more or less favorable effects on health. For example, studies have shown that isocaloric replacement of milk by sugar-sweetened beverages (SSB) leads to increased visceral adiposity and hepatic fat deposition (Maersk et al. 2012). Dairy foods in published RTCs have been replaced by a wide variety of nondairy foods, which may have intrinsic beneficial or adverse health effects of their own. Future research should be designed to compare dairy foods with other foods that they are most likely to replace in the diet, such as milk versus juice or SSBs, or cheese versus other types of snacks.

In sum, the data available to date support the inclusion of dairy as part of a healthy diet, with virtually no evidence of potential harmful effects. The extent to which dairy intake is healthy *per se* remains unclear, as dairy intake may simply be a marker of good quality diets. Further research is needed to better define optimal dietary recommendations regarding dairy intake in terms of servings per day, and whether there is a difference between low-fat and whole-fat dairy in terms of health outcomes.

REFERENCES

Abdullah, M.M., Cyr, A., Lepine, M.C., Eck, P.K., Couture, P., Lamarche, B. et al. 2016. Common variants in cholesterol synthesis- and transport-related genes associate with circulating cholesterol responses to intakes of conventional dairy products in healthy individuals. *J Nutr* **146**(5): 1008–1016.

Agerholm-Larsen, L., Bell, M.L., Grunwald, G.K., and Astrup, A. 2000a. The effect of a probiotic milk product on plasma cholesterol: A meta-analysis of short-term intervention studies. *Eur J Clin Nutr* **54**: 856–860.

Agerholm Larsen, L., Raben, A., Haulrik, N., Hansen, A.S., Manders, M., and Astrup, A. 2000b. Effect of 8 week intake of probiotic milk products on risk factors for cardiovascular diseases. *Eur J Clin Nutr* **54**: 288–297.

Anderson, J.W. and Gilliland, S.E. 1999. Effect of fermented milk (yogurt) containing *Lactobacillus acidophilus* L1 on serum cholesterol in hypercholesterolemic humans. *J Am Coll Nutr* **18**: 43–50.

Andrade, S. and Borges, N. 2009. Effect of fermented milk containing *Lactobacillus acidophilus* and *Bifidobacterium longum* on plasma lipids of women with normal or moderately elevated cholesterol. *J Dairy Res* **76**: 469–474.

Appel, L.J., Moore, T.J., Obarzanek, E., Vollmer, W.M., Svetkey, L.P., Sacks, F.M. et al. 1997. A clinical trial of the effects of dietary patterns on blood pressure. *N Engl J Med* **336**: 1117–1124.

Ascherio, A., Katan, M.B., Zock, P.L., Stampfer, M.J., and Willett, W.C. 1999. Trans fatty acids and coronary heart disease. *N Engl J Med* **340**: 1994–1998.

Asztalos, B.F., Tani, M., and Schaefer, E.J. 2011. Metabolic and functional relevance of HDL subspecies. *Curr Opin Lipidol* **22**: 176–185.

Austin, M.A. 1991. Plasma triglyceride and coronary heart disease. *Atheroscler Thromb Vasc Biol* **11**: 2–14.

Ballard, K.D. and Bruno, R.S. 2015. Protective role of dairy and its constituents on vascular function independent of blood pressure-lowering activities. *Nutr Rev* **73**: 36–50.

Barter, P.J., Caulfield, M., Eriksson, M., Grundy, S.M., Kastelein, J.J., Komajda, M. et al. 2007. Effects of torcetrapib in patients at high risk for coronary events. *N Engl J Med* **357**: 2109–2122.

Benatar, J.R., Sidhu, K., and Stewart, R.A. 2013. Effects of high and low fat dairy food on cardio-metabolic risk factors: A meta-analysis of randomized studies. *PLoS One* **8**: e76480.

Bertolami, M.C., Faludi, A.A., and Batlouni, M. 1999. Evaluation of the effects of a new fermented milk product (Gaio) on primary hypercholesterolemia. *Eur J Clin Nutr* **53**: 97–101.

Blewett, H.J., Gerdung, C.A., Ruth, M.R., Proctor, S.D., and Field, C.J. 2009. Vaccenic acid favourably alters immune function in obese JCR:LA-cp rats. *Br J Nutr* **102**: 526–536.

Briel, M., Ferreira-Gonzalez, I., You, J.J., Karanicolas, P.J., Akl, E.A., Wu, P. et al. 2009. Association between change in high density lipoprotein cholesterol and cardiovascular disease morbidity and mortality: Systematic review and meta-regression analysis. *Br Med J* **338**: b92.

Brouwer, I.A., Wanders, A.J., and Katan, M.B. 2013. Trans fatty acids and cardiovascular health: Research completed? *Eur J Clin Nutr* **67**: 541–547.

Chiu, S., Bergeron, N., Williams, P.T., Bray, G.A., Sutherland, B., and Krauss, R.M. 2016. Comparison of the DASH (Dietary Approaches to Stop Hypertension) diet and a higher-fat DASH diet on blood pressure and lipids and lipoproteins: A randomized controlled trial. *Am J Clin Nutr* **103**: 341–347.

Chowdhury, R., Warnakula, S., Kunutsor, S., Crowe, F., Ward, H.A., Johnson, L. et al. 2014. Association of dietary, circulating, and supplement fatty acids with coronary risk: A systematic review and meta-analysis. *Ann Intern Med* **160**: 398–406.

de Goede, J., Geleijnse, J.M., Ding, E.L., and Soedamah-Muthu, S.S. 2015. Effect of cheese consumption on blood lipids: A systematic review and meta-analysis of randomized controlled trials. *Nutr Rev* **73**: 259–275.

de Roos, N.M., Schouten, G., and Katan, M.B. 1999. Yoghurt enriched with *Lactobacillus acidophilus* does not lower blood lipids in healthy men and women with normal to borderline high serum cholesterol levels. *Eur J Clin Nutr* **53**: 277–280.

Despres, J.P., Cartier, A., Cote, M., and Arsenault, B.J. 2008. The concept of cardiometabolic risk: Bridging the fields of diabetology and cardiology. *Ann Med* **40**(7): 514–523.

Despres, J.P. and Lemieux, I. 2006. Abdominal obesity and metabolic syndrome. *Nature* **444**: 881–887.

Dong, J.Y., Szeto, I.M., Makinen, K., Gao, Q., Wang, J., Qin, L.Q. et al. 2013. Effect of probiotic fermented milk on blood pressure: A meta-analysis of randomised controlled trials. *Br J Nutr* **110**: 1188–1194.

Drouin-Chartier, J.P., Brassard, D., Tessier-Grenier, M., Côté, J.A., Labonte, M.E., Desroches, S. et al. 2016. Systematic review of the association between dairy product consumption and risk of cardiovascular-related clinical outcomes. *Adv Nutr* **7**(6): 1026–1040.

Drouin-Chartier, J.P., Gagnon, J., Labonte, M.E., Desroches, S., Charest, A., Grenier, G. et al. 2015. Impact of milk consumption on cardiometabolic risk in postmenopausal women with abdominal obesity. *Nutr J* **14**: 12.

Drouin-Chartier, J.P., Gigleux, I., Tremblay, A.J., Poirier, L., Lamarche, B., and Couture, P. 2014. Impact of dairy consumption on essential hypertension: A clinical study. *Nutr J* **13**: 83.

Gayet-Boyer, C., Tenenhaus-Aziza, F., Prunet, C., Marmonier, C., Malpuech-Brugere, C., Lamarche, B. et al. 2014. Is there a linear relationship between the dose of ruminant trans-fatty acids and cardiovascular risk markers in healthy subjects: Results from a systematic review and meta-regression of randomised clinical trials. *Br J Nutr* **112**: 1914–1922.

Gebauer, S.K., Chardigny, J.M., Jakobsen, M.U., Lamarche, B., Lock, A.L., Proctor, S.D. et al. 2011. Effects of ruminant trans fatty acids on cardiovascular disease and cancer: A comprehensive review of epidemiological, clinical, and mechanistic studies. *Adv Nutr* **2**: 332–354.

Gebauer, S.K., Destaillats, F., Dionisi, F., Krauss, R.M., and Baer, D.J. 2015. Vaccenic acid and trans fatty acid isomers from partially hydrogenated oil both adversely affect LDL cholesterol: A double-blind, randomized controlled trial. *Am J Clin Nutr* **102**: 1339–1346.

Gordon, T., Castelli, W.P., Hjortland, M.C., Kannel, W.B., and Dawber, T.R. 1977. High density lipoprotein as a protective factor against coronary heart disease: The Framingham study. *Am J Med* **62**: 707–714.

Hansel, B., Nicolle, C., Lalanne, F., Tondu, F., Lassel, T., Donazzolo, Y. et al. 2007. Effect of low-fat, fermented milk enriched with plant sterols on serum lipid profile and oxidative stress in moderate hypercholesterolemia. *Am J Clin Nutr* **86**: 790–796.

Hilpert, K.F., West, S.G., Bagshaw, D.M., Fishell, V., Barnhart, L., Lefevre, M. et al. 2009. Effects of dairy products on intracellular calcium and blood pressure in adults with essential hypertension. *J Am Coll Nutr* **28**: 142–149.

Hjerpsted, J., Leedo, E., and Tholstrup, T. 2011. Cheese intake in large amounts lowers LDL-cholesterol concentrations compared with butter intake of equal fat content. *Am J Clin Nutr* **94**: 1479–1484.

Huth, P.J., Fulgoni, V.L., Keast, D.R., Park, K., and Auestad, N. 2013. Major food sources of calories, added sugars, and saturated fat and their contribution to essential nutrient intakes in the U.S. diet: Data from the National Health and Nutrition Examination Survey (2003–2006). *Nutr J* **12**: 116.

Ivey, K.L., Hodgson, J.M., Kerr, D.A., Thompson, P.L., Stojceski, B., and Prince, R.L. 2015. The effect of yoghurt and its probiotics on blood pressure and serum lipid profile; a randomised controlled trial. *Nutr Metab Cardiovasc Dis* **25**: 46–51.

Jacome-Sosa, M.M., Borthwick, F., Mangat, R., Uwiera, R., Reaney, M.J., Shen, J. et al. 2014. Diets enriched in trans-11 vaccenic acid alleviate ectopic lipid accumulation in a rat model of NAFLD and metabolic syndrome. *J Nutr Biochem* **25**: 692–701.

Khera, A.V., Cuchel, M., de la Llera-Moya, M., Rodrigues, A., Burke, M.F., Jafri, K. et al. 2011. Cholesterol efflux capacity, high-density lipoprotein function, and atherosclerosis. *N Engl J Med* **364**: 127–135.

Labonte, M.E., Couture, P., Richard, C., Desroches, S., and Lamarche, B. 2013. Impact of dairy products on biomarkers of inflammation: A systematic review of randomized controlled nutritional intervention studies in overweight and obese adults. *Am J Clin Nutr* **97**: 706–717.

Labonte, M.E., Cyr, A., Abdullah, M.M., Lepine, M.C., Vohl, M.C., Jones, P. et al. 2014. Dairy product consumption has no impact on biomarkers of inflammation among men and women with low-grade systemic inflammation. *J Nutr* **144**: 1760–1767.

Libby, P. 2002. Inflammation in atherosclerosis. *Nature* **420**: 868–874.

Libby, P. 2006. Inflammation and cardiovascular disease mechanisms. *Am J Clin Nutr* **83**: 456S–460S.

Libby, P. 2007. Inflammatory mechanisms: The molecular basis of inflammation and disease. *Nutr Rev* **65**: S140–S146.

Livingstone, K.M., Lovegrove, J.A., Cockcroft, J.R., Elwood, P.C., Pickering, J.E., and Givens, D.I. 2013. Does dairy food intake predict arterial stiffness and blood pressure in men?: Evidence from the Caerphilly Prospective Study. *Hypertension* **61**: 42–47.

Machin, D.R., Park, W., Alkatan, M., Mouton, M., and Tanaka, H. 2015. Effects of non-fat dairy products added to the routine diet on vascular function: A randomized controlled crossover trial. *Nutr Metab Cardiovasc Dis* **25**: 364–369.

Maersk, M., Belza, A., Stodkilde-Jorgensen, H., Ringgaard, S., Chabanova, E., Thomsen, H. et al. 2012. Sucrose-sweetened beverages increase fat storage in the liver, muscle, and visceral fat depot: A 6-mo randomized intervention study. *Am J Clin Nutr* **95**: 283–289.

Maki, K.C., Rains, T.M., Schild, A.L., Dicklin, M.R., Park, K.M., Lawless, A.L. et al. 2013. Effects of low-fat dairy intake on blood pressure, endothelial function, and lipoprotein lipids in subjects with prehypertension or stage 1 hypertension. *Vasc Health Risk Manag* **9**: 369–379.

Mensink, R.P., Zock, P.L., Kester, A.D.M., and Katan, M.B. 2003. Effects of dietary fatty acids and carbohydrates on the ratio of serum total to HDL cholesterol and on serum lipids and apolipoproteins: A meta-analysis of 60 controlled trials. *Am J Clin Nutr* **77**: 1146–1155.

Nilsen, R., Hostmark, A.T., Haug, A., and Skeie, S. 2015. Effect of a high intake of cheese on cholesterol and metabolic syndrome: Results of a randomized trial. *Food Nutr Res* **59**: 27651.

Page, A.V. and Liles, W.C. 2013. Biomarkers of endothelial activation/dysfunction in infectious diseases. *Virulence* **4**: 507–516.

Ras, R.T., Streppel, M.T., Draijer, R., and Zock, P.L. 2013. Flow-mediated dilation and cardiovascular risk prediction: A systematic review with meta-analysis. *Int J Cardiol* **168**: 344–351.

Rideout, T.C., Marinangeli, C.P., Martin, H., Browne, R.W., and Rempel, C.B. 2013. Consumption of low-fat dairy foods for 6 months improves insulin resistance without adversely affecting lipids or bodyweight in healthy adults: A randomized free-living cross-over study. *Nutr J* **12**: 56.

Sadrzadeh-Yeganeh, H., Elmadfa, I., Djazayery, A., Jalali, M., Heshmat, R., and Chamary, M. 2010. The effects of probiotic and conventional yoghurt on lipid profile in women. *Br J Nutr* **103**: 1778–1783.

Savard, P., Lamarche, B., Paradis, M.E., Thiboutot, H., Laurin, E., and Roy, D. 2011. Impact of Bifidobacterium animalis subsp. lactis BB-12 and, Lactobacillus acidophilus LA-5-containing yoghurt, on fecal bacterial counts of healthy adults. *Int J Food Microbiol* **149**: 50–57.

Schaafsma, G., Meuling, W.J., van Dokkum, W., and Bouley, C. 1998. Effects of a milk product, fermented by *Lactobacillus acidophilus* and with fructo-oligosaccharides added, on blood lipids in male volunteers. *Eur J Clin Nutr* **52**: 436–440.

Schlienger, J.L., Paillard, F., Lecerf, J.M., Romon, M., Bonhomme, C., Schmitt, B. et al. 2014. Effect on blood lipids of two daily servings of Camembert cheese. An intervention trial in mildly hypercholesterolemic subjects. *Int J Food Sci Nutr* **65**: 1013–1018.

Schwartz, G.G., Olsson, A.G., Abt, M., Ballantyne, C.M., Barter, P.J., Brumm, J. et al. 2012. Effects of dalcetrapib in patients with a recent acute coronary syndrome. *N Engl J Med* **367**: 2089–2099.

Siri-Tarino, P.W., Chiu, S., Bergeron, N., and Krauss, R.M. 2015. Saturated fats versus polyunsaturated fats versus carbohydrates for cardiovascular disease prevention and treatment. *Annu Rev Nutr* **35**: 517–543.

Siri-Tarino, P.W., Sun, Q., Hu, F.B., and Krauss, R.M. 2010. Meta-analysis of prospective cohort studies evaluating the association of saturated fat with cardiovascular disease. *Am J Clin Nutr* **91**: 535–546.

Stender, S., Astrup, A., and Dyerberg, J. 2008. Ruminant and industrially produced trans fatty acids: Health aspects. *Food Nutr Res* **52**: 1–8.

Stender, S. and Dyerberg, J. 2003. *The Influence of Trans Fatty Acids on Health. A Report from the Danish Nutrition Council*, 4th edn. Copenhagen, Publication no. 34. The Danish Nutrition Council.

St-Onge, M.P., Farnworth, E.R., Savard, T., Chabot, D., Mafu, A., and Jones, P.J. 2002. Kefir consumption does not alter plasma lipid levels or cholesterol fractional synthesis rates relative to milk in hyperlipidemic men: A randomized controlled trial. *BMC Complement Altern Med* **2**: 1.

Thorning, T.K., Raziani, F., Bendsen, N.T., Astrup, A., Tholstrup, T., and Raben, A. 2015. Diets with high-fat cheese, high-fat meat, or carbohydrate on cardiovascular risk markers in overweight postmenopausal women: A randomized crossover trial. *Am J Clin Nutr* **102**: 573–581.

Turner, K.M., Keogh, J.B., and Clifton, P.M. 2015. Dairy consumption and insulin sensitivity: A systematic review of short- and long-term intervention studies. *Nutr Metab Cardiovasc Dis* **25**: 3–8.

Usinger, L., Reimer, C., and Ibsen, H. 2012. Fermented milk for hypertension. *Cochrane Database Syst Rev* **4**: CD008118.

van Meijl, L.E. and Mensink, R.P. 2010. Effects of low-fat dairy consumption on markers of low-grade systemic inflammation and endothelial function in overweight and obese subjects: An intervention study. *Br J Nutr* **104**: 1523–1527.

Vlachopoulos, C., Aznaouridis, K., and Stefanadis, C. 2010. Prediction of cardiovascular events and all-cause mortality with arterial stiffness: A systematic review and meta-analysis. *J Am Coll Cardiol* **55**: 1318–1327.

Weintraub, W.S., Daniels, S.R., Burke, L.E., Franklin, B.A., Goff, D.C., Jr., Hayman, L.L. et al. 2011. Value of primordial and primary prevention for cardiovascular disease: A policy statement from the American Heart Association. *Circulation* **124**: 967–990.

Xun, P., Wu, Y., He, Q., and He, K. 2013. Fasting insulin concentrations and incidence of hypertension, stroke, and coronary heart disease: A meta-analysis of prospective cohort studies. *Am J Clin Nutr* **98**: 1543–1554.

26 Paleolithic Diets

Staffan Lindeberg, Maelán Fontes Villalba, Pedro Carrera-Bastos, and Lynda Frassetto

CONTENTS

ABSTRACT

If, as indicated by some studies, prudent diets such as the Mediterranean or DASH diets can be further improved, an evolutionary approach may be helpful. Paleolithic diets represent the food habits during more than two million years of hominid and human evolution before the development of agriculture. Fruits, tubers, nuts, lean meat, larvae, insects, fish, shellfish, eggs, honey, and a large variety of vegetables have been staple foods. Contemporary non-Western populations with similar lifestyles have shown exceptionally low rates of cardiovascular disease, obesity, insulin resistance, type 2 diabetes mellitus, and hypertension.

Available evidence lends some support in favor, and less against, the notion that Paleolithic diets are an appropriate template in the dietary prevention and treatment of cardiometabolic diseases.

In Memoriam

Staffan Lindeberg, MD, PhD

The authors of this chapter will always be grateful for Dr. Lindeberg’s invaluable contributions to the clinical science behind the chapter we wrote. Dr. Lindeberg died shortly after we submitted it. May he rest in peace.

Maelán Fontes Villalba, Pedro Carrera-Bastos, and Lynda Frassetto

INTRODUCTION

Paleolithic* diets are sometimes seen as templates for healthy diets, based on the following arguments:

1. very low age-adjusted rates of cardiovascular disease and other nutrition-related disorders among contemporary hunter–gatherers and other populations minimally affected by modern habits have been reported (Eaton and Konner 1985; Lindeberg 2010).
2. hunter–gatherers and traditional horticulturalists exhibit better body composition, physical fitness, and health biomarkers, when compared to Westernized populations and even modern rural populations (Lindeberg 2010; Carrera-Bastos 2011).
3. the majority of Westerners are affected by atherosclerosis and associated metabolic abnormalities, and our understanding of the main underlying causes is very limited (Lindeberg 2005, 2010).
4. among the several lifestyle factors that are very different from those of modern urban and rural populations, diet appears to stand out (Eaton and Konner 1985; Cordain et al. 2005; Lindeberg 2010; Carrera-Bastos 2011).
5. intervention studies with Paleolithic-type diets in patients with the metabolic syndrome and/or glucose intolerance (Lindeberg et al. 2007; Jönsson et al. 2009; Manheimer et al. 2015) show superiority in various cardiometabolic biomarkers when compared to prudent diets.
6. the main characteristics of human physiology are essentially the same in all human populations and are obviously the result of a long evolution in Africa. Therefore, if there is a healthier diet for humans in general, irrespective of ethnicity, it makes sense to consider evolution and to focus on the time period up to the emergence of fully modern humans around 200,000 years ago, well before some of them left Africa some 60,000 years ago and different ethnic groups emerged (Campbell and Tishkoff 2010).

Accordingly, this review relates recent evidence of Western diseases, as well as common concepts of healthy nutrition, to probable food patterns of our Paleolithic ancestors before they left Africa. In the blogosphere and popular press, Paleolithic diets are often described as low-carbohydrate diets with lots of meat. In the scientific discourse, Paleolithic diets represent much more. They can even be high in carbohydrate and low in meat (Lindeberg 2010).

NUTRITION DURING HUMAN EVOLUTION

It could be argued that the Miocene vegetarian-like habitats, between 23 and 5 million years ago, provide a proper reference for human nutrition and that we have not changed much since then (Jenkins and Kendall 2006). In contrast, others argue that later habitats exerted strong selection pressures and that humans became adapted to a high intake of meat (Brand Miller and Colagiuri 1994; Finch and Stanford 2004; Zink and Lieberman 2016). However, neither position excludes the other since we may be adapted to a food item and thrive on it without necessarily being dependent on it for high reproductive success.

It is often impossible to determine, for any particular habitat and certainly over longer time periods, the percentage of food that came from each of the available foodstuffs. The staple food items typically consumed by our bipedal ancestors in Africa is a matter of debate, but the principal foods available included sweet and ripe fruits and berries, shoots, flowers, buds and young leaves, muscle meat, bone marrow, organ meats, fish, shellfish, insects, larvae, eggs, roots, bulbs, nuts, and non-grass seeds (Gräslund 2005; Ungar 2007). In principle, these were the only types of foods that

* The Paleolithic (or Palaeolithic) is the time period of roughly 2.5 million years when hominids and humans were using stone tools and until the development of agriculture. The first part, until around 200,000 years ago, is sometimes called the Lower Paleolithic. Thereafter, the evolution of different ethnic groups started.

were available during human evolution, which now only provide about one quarter of the caloric intake for the typical Westerner (Cordain et al. 2005). Most of us now get the greater part of our energy from grains (grass seeds), dairy products, refined fat and sugar, and legumes (Cordain et al. 2005; Statens Livsmedelsverk 2012; U.S. Department of Agriculture). In addition, we have very little variation among plant foods today.

CARBOHYDRATE-RICH FOODS

Our primate ancestors may have consumed fruits more or less regularly during the 50 million years until they became bipedal around 6 million years ago (Bloch and Boyer 2002; Gräslund 2005; Ungar 2007). For chimpanzees, bonobos, and orangutans, fruit makes up more than 75% by weight of the diet. Fruit was also the most common plant food among twentieth-century hunter–gatherers, as described in the Ethnographic Atlas (n = 229) (Cordain et al. 2000a). Fruits differ from other edible plants in that they contain appreciable amounts of fructose, a monosaccharide that typically constitutes 20%–40% of available carbohydrates in wild fruits (Ko et al. 1998; Milton 1999; Dzhangaliev et al. 2003) and 10%–30% in cultivated fruits (National Food Administration 1986). Honey, where 50% of the carbohydrate is fructose, may have been consumed in considerable amounts in some habitats, at least for a few months per year (Allsop and Miller 1996; Marlowe et al. 2014).

A high intake of fructose, in particular from sodas and processed foods, has been proposed to cause abdominal obesity and associated metabolic disturbances, including diabetes type 2, high blood pressure, blood lipid disorders (high triglycerides and low HDL cholesterol), hyperuricemia, and fatty liver (Johnson et al. 2009; Park and Yetley 1993; Sanchez-Lozada et al. 2008). However, strictly controlled experiments suggest that the amounts of fructose that may be harmful are considerably higher than what is possible to get from whole fruit (Sievenpiper et al. 2009, 2012; Cozma et al. 2012; Kuzma et al. 2015). There is much evidence suggesting that any concerns with fructose are outweighed by beneficial attributes of whole fruit, such as high nutrient density, fiber content, low glycemic index, and high water content lending volume. Notably, fruit has been an essential part of dietary patterns for which there are data for cardiovascular benefit. For comprehensive reviews of dietary fructose, see Chapters 13 through 15.

Starchy underground storage organs (roots, tubers, bulbs, corms) may have become staple foods during periods of repeatedly dry and cool climates perhaps around one million years ago (Luca et al. 2010) or even before that (Laden and Wrangham 2005). Humans have a relatively high activity of salivary amylase in comparison with other primates (Samuelson et al. 1990; Perry et al. 2007) and our tooth morphology, including incisal orientation, seems well adapted to chewing tubers (Lucas et al. 2006). In order to increase the caloric yield per workload, roots and tubers may often have been an adequate choice (O'Connell et al. 1983), especially after cooking (Wrangham and Conklin-Brittain 2003). It has been suggested that the multiplication of the salivary amylase gene became selectively advantageous in terms of evolutionary fitness only when cooking became widespread (Hardy et al. 2015). The period for this change in human subsistence with regular use of fire and habitual cooking is a matter of speculation, but it might have been more than 300,000 years before the present or possibly long before that (Hardy et al. 2015).

The excellent health status among starch-eating ethnic groups (Sinnett 1977; Lindeberg 2010), including the Kitavans described subsequently, contradicts the notion that a high intake of starch would be associated with obesity and type 2 diabetes (Spreadbury 2012; Mann et al. 2014; Naude et al. 2014). Although a high starch load undoubtedly raises blood sugar after a meal, the main causes of an individual's inability to limit blood sugar rise after eating carbohydrates (i.e., glucose intolerance) remain obscure, and it is questionable whether dietary starch plays a causative role (Reaven 2005; Due et al. 2008; Brinkworth et al. 2009). Low-carbohydrate diets can sometimes decrease fasting glucose more than low-fat diets (Samaha et al. 2003; Krebs et al. 2013; de Luis et al. 2015), but it is uncertain if this is due to the reduction of carbohydrate per se or some associated dietary changes (Gannon and Nuttal 2006; Lindeberg 2010).

In addition to the questionable effect on glucose tolerance, the proportion of carbohydrate in the diet has not been proven to materially affect body weight (Clifton et al. 2014). The marginally greater weight loss with carbohydrate restriction in obesity, as opposed to restriction of fat or protein, does not suggest that dietary starch is a major cause of obesity (Clifton et al. 2014).

OTHER PLANT FOODS OF THE PALEOLITHIC DIET

Tree nuts provide a high amount of energy even when they must be collected and cracked one by one for consumption, and were probably an essential part of the diet in some of the occupied habitats. Tree nuts are typically rich in unsaturated fat, protein, soluble fiber, and various micronutrients, while low in saturated fat (Lindeberg 2010). Despite their high energy density, in Western populations the effect of tree nuts on caloric intake and adiposity appears to be neutral (Flores-Mateo et al. 2013) and their effect on cardiovascular risk factors appears to be beneficial (Del Gobbo et al. 2015). Nuts have also been an important component of the DASH diet (Appel et al. 1997), Mediterranean diets (Estruch et al. 2013), and the Portfolio diet (Jenkins et al. 2003), all of which have shown beneficial effects in randomized controlled trials. Observational studies also suggest that increased intake of tree nuts is inversely associated with ischemic heart disease and type 2 diabetes (Afshin et al. 2014).

A large quantity of nonstarchy vegetables (leafy vegetables, flowers, buds) from many different plant species were also staple items of hunter–gatherer diets with a small contribution to caloric intake (Isaacs 1987; Kuhn and Stiner 2001; Terashima and Ichikawa 2003; Termote and van Damme 2010).

MEAT

Another food that could provide a high-energy yield for preagricultural humans is *meat*, which is even consumed in considerable amounts by the chimpanzee (Stanford 1999; Pruetz et al. 2015). In one observational study, adult chimpanzees consumed an average of 65 g meat per day in the dry season (Stanford 1999). For humans, available paleontologic evidence is consistent with, but does not prove, regular high meat intake in the last 2 million years (Finch and Stanford 2004; Ungar 2007). Contemporary hunter–gatherers have generally been able to eat large amounts of meat or fish, although the figures are based on rather imprecise ethnographic data (Cordain et al. 2000a; Panter-Brick et al. 2001). Of the 229 hunter–gatherer populations studied during the twentieth century, the majority (73%) were estimated to get more than half their caloric intake from meat, fish, and shellfish (Cordain et al. 2000a). Among five African populations, for which more exact quantitative data were available, meat and/or fish constituted on average 26%, 33%, 44%, 48%, and 68% of the food (Cordain 2006).

Contemporary hunter–gatherers have had exceptionally favorable levels of serum cholesterol, blood pressure, and other cardiovascular risk factors, even with very high meat consumption (Lindeberg 2010). For instance, Truswell found no evidence of sudden, spontaneous death when interviewing 96 adults among the San tribe, hunter–gatherers with a high meat intake in the Kalahari desert, Botswana, South Africa (Truswell and Hansen 1976). However, wild game meat has a lower fat content, a higher percentage of omega-3 fatty acids and a lower omega-6/omega-3 ratio than domestic meat (Naughton et al. 1986; Mann 2000; Cordain et al. 2002).

Observational studies among Western populations have found that a high intake of red meat, and in particular processed meats, is associated with an increased risk of cardiovascular disease and diabetes type 2 (Chen et al. 2013; Mozaffarian 2016). There is substantial controversy and uncertainty as to whether unprocessed red meats increase cardiometabolic risk and the extent to which residual confounding explains any increase (Micha et al. 2010; Mozaffarian 2016). Randomized controlled trials have shown that, within the pattern of a healthy diet, there is no difference between red and white meat effects on LDL-cholesterol (Davidson et al. 1999; Maki et al. 2012; Roussell et al. 2012). Moreover, animal experiments do not suggest that meat causes atherosclerosis and the notion that "animal protein" causes atherosclerosis is based on studies with milk proteins, typically casein (Foo et al. 2009; Lindeberg 2010). For instance, one study in hamsters found that meat protein (from bison and beef, respectively) resulted in less pronounced atherosclerosis than soy protein and casein (Wilson et al. 2000).

Furthermore, red meat is a rich source of high-quality protein and high content of bioavailable essential nutrients, many of which are lacking in the diets of some population groups (Wyness 2016). Therefore, lean nonprocessed red meat can hypothetically be a healthy option in the context of a Paleolithic diet. In addition, Paleolithic diets are not necessarily high in meat. In fact, due to its high bioavailable essential nutrients, a moderate intake (70 g/day) can be sufficient to meet nutritional requirements (Wyness et al. 2011; Wyness 2016).

FISH AND SHELLFISH

Paleolithic African humans appear to have lived at times by the shores of lakes, rivers, and, presumably, the sea, where they could catch *fish and shellfish*, although their dependence on marine food has not been proven (Richards 2002; Kuipers et al. 2010). Omega-3 fatty acids from fish have been suggested to prevent coronary heart disease, although randomized controlled trials suggest that the effect is limited (Hooper et al. 2004, 2006). Observational studies have found an approximately 20% lower cardiovascular risk among Westerners who eat fatty fish at least twice a week, compared with those who do not (Schmidt et al. 2000; Hu et al. 2001). Possibly, this only applies to high-risk populations (Marckmann and Gronbaek 1999). The notion that fish is protective originally emerged from an observed very low incidence of myocardial infarction and sudden cardiac death among the Inuits of Greenland and Canada (Schaefer 1971; Bang and Dyerberg 1972). Of all the characteristics of Inuit dietary habits that could possibly explain these findings, virtually all focus has been on omega-3 fatty acids, while the absence of common Western foods has rarely been considered. For comprehensive reviews of omega-3 fatty acids and cardiovascular prevention and treatment, see Chapter 10.

INSECTS AND LARVAE

The consumption of *insects and larvae* is thought to have been substantial in most African habitats during the Paleolithic period, and they may have provided an important source of protein and fat (DeFoliart 1999; Ungar 2007; Raubenheimer et al. 2014). Nonhuman primates regularly consume them (Basabose 2002; Raubenheimer et al. 2014; Rothman et al. 2014). Yet, our knowledge of their possible health effects is extremely limited.

ALCOHOL

The extent to which *alcohol* could have been a regular part of human's original environment is unknown (Kiple and Ornelas 2000). If storage vessels for alcohol were made of leather or plants in earlier prehistoric times, they have long since disappeared without a trace. Even without deliberate production of alcoholic beverages, a low-level dietary exposure to ethanol via ingestion of fermented fruit may have characterized our lineage of humans and human-like ancestors for about 40 million years (Smith 1999; Dudley 2002). For a comprehensive review of alcohol and cardiovascular disease, see Chapter 31.

FOODS WITH NO OR MINIMAL CONTRIBUTION IN PALEOLITHIC DIETS

In the context of public health, it may hypothetically be more crucial to focus on foods that were not staple items during human evolution, instead of trying to estimate accurately intake of foods that were. On average, roughly 75% of the calories in Western countries are today provided by foods that were practically unavailable during human evolution: wheat and other cereal grains, dairy foods, refined fats and sugar (Cordain et al. 2005). In addition, the intake of sodium and chloride is now considerably higher (Cordain et al. 2005).

PALEOLITHIC DIETS AND ABSENCE OF GRAINS

During our evolution, wild *seeds* were available from various plants, but not from the grass family (Poaceae), which includes today's wheat, rice, maize, and so on, and rarely or never from one plant species every day. There is evidence for sporadic consumption of legume seeds during the latter part of the Paleolithic period (Jones 2009). Nevertheless, seeds from *legumes* apparently became staple foods only during the emergence of agriculture, as evidenced by gradual changes in their form and quality as a consequence of domestication (Zohary and Hopf 1973; Berger et al. 2003). Contemporary hunter–gatherers, in particular those living in arid, hot, marginal environments (Australian Aborigines, Kalahari Bushmen), often include large, fatty seeds in their diet, but these provide a relatively small amount of energy on an annual basis, and much less than is now provided by wheat, rice, or maize (Lee 1968; O'Connell et al. 1983; Cordain et al. 2005).

When seeds from any one particular plant species are consumed in large quantities on a regular basis, an interesting situation arises. The plant kingdom contains thousands of bioactive substances and other natural chemicals, called phytochemicals, many of which are thought to be part of the defense system against herbivores (Wynne-Edwards 2001; Herrera and Pellmyr 2002). The highest concentrations of phytochemicals are generally found in the most vital parts of the plant, namely sprouts, seeds, and beans and can make up 5%–10% of the plant's dry weight (Perantoni 1998). Prehistoric foragers were able to limit the intake of each of them by having access to a large number of various plant species, by consciously avoiding the most poisonous ones (Ulijaszek and Strickland 1993), and by cooking, which destroys some of these plant chemicals (Wrangham and Conklin-Brittain 2003). Most phytochemicals have not been properly studied with regard to their effects on human health and only a few examples will be mentioned here.

One example is plant lectins, which are glycated sugar-binding proteins (Chrispeels and Raikhel 1991; Van Damme et al. 1998), and which are found in the highest concentration in cereal grains, beans, potatoes, and peanuts. Notably, unrefined grain products have a higher lectin content than refined seed products (van Damme et al. 1998). Lectins in wheat, rye, rice, and potatoes bind to GlcNAc-domains (GlcNAc = N-acetylglucosamine) on receptors in the "host organism," receptors of crucial importance in metabolic programming mainly through the hexosamine biosynthetic pathway (Hardivillé and Hart 2014). Lectins are not completely destroyed during normal cooking (Freed 1999), although hydrating beans and then cooking them to 100°C for a minimum of 10 min significantly decreases its lectin content (Grant et al. 1982). Nevertheless, these types of procedures are not normally applied to cereal grains, so it is expected that these type of foods present a significant lectin content even after cooking (Cordain 1999; Freed 1999). This may be clinically relevant since lectins are also relatively resistant to enzymatic breakdown in the gastrointestinal tract, are thought to penetrate the intestinal mucous membrane (Liener 1986; Pusztai et al. 1993), and thereby enter the bloodstream (Pusztai et al. 1989; Wang et al. 1998; Cordain 1999). One of the most studied lectins in *in vitro* experiments and animal models is the wheat lectin (wheat germ agglutinin, WGA). WGA may contribute to atherosclerosis since it can bind to macrophages and smooth muscle cells of the vessel wall (Davis and Glagov 1986; Kagami et al. 1991), activate the epidermal growth factor receptor (Wang et al. 2001) and the toll-like receptor-2 (Unitt and Hornigold 2011), and increase the synthesis of IL-12, IL-2, INFγ, TNFI, and IL-1 (Muraille et al. 1999; Sodhi and Kesherwani 2007). Activation of the epidermal growth factor receptor and the toll-like receptor-2, hypothetically, can cause dysfunction of the glycocalyx, the protective barrier covering the endothelium of blood vessels, thereby allowing atherosclerosis to progress (Henry and Duling 2000; Drake-Holland and Noble 2009; Becker et al. 2010; Liu et al. 2011; Reitsma et al. 2011; Pahwa et al. 2016). Another lectin of potential relevance is peanut lectin, which has been shown to enter the systemic circulation in humans (Wang et al. 1998) and to produce atherosclerosis in rabbits (Kritchevsky et al. 1981, 1998). This may offer an explanation for the unexpected atherogenic effect of peanut oil in various animal models (monkeys, rabbits, and rats) (Cordain 1998).

Wheat is also rich in gliadins, which are usually designated as prolamins with lectin-like properties. Prolamins (together with glutelins that compose gluten) are present in the wheat endosperm, while

WGA is more abundant in the germ. There is *ex vivo* human evidence that gliadins can increase intestinal permeability not only in individuals with celiac disease, but also in wheat-sensitive and normal individuals (Hollon et al. 2015), although *in vivo* human studies are necessary before we can reach a definitive conclusion. There is also *in vitro* and animal evidence that WGA may increase intestinal permeability (Cordain et al. 2000b; Dalla Pellegrina et al. 2009). Increased intestinal permeability may lead to endotoxemia, which may cause low-grade chronic inflammation (Carrera-Bastos 2011). Chronic inflammation has been proposed as an important component in the pathogenesis of atherosclerosis and insulin resistance (Frostegård 2013; Straub 2014). We need better data from randomized controlled trials before we can draw any conclusions regarding cereal grains.

The leptin receptor, which is activated by the satiety hormone leptin, is glycosylated (Haniu et al. 1998) and, as such, is expected to bind lectins and lectin-like molecules like gliadin. *In vitro*, WGA has been shown to bind to the leptin receptor (Kamikubo et al. 2007), whereas peptides derived from wheat gluten digestion inhibited the ability of leptin to bind to its receptor (Jönsson et al. 2015). Reduced leptin action and/or leptin resistance appears to be an early step in ectopic lipid deposition, lipotoxicity, and the metabolic syndrome (Unger and Scherer 2010). Highly relevant in this context are findings in C57BL/6 mice fed *ad libitum* isocaloric diets matched for macronutrient composition, where gluten intake promoted weight gain and increased plasma levels of leptin, IL-6, and other pro-inflammatory cytokines and adipokines independent of energy intake and diet macronutrient composition (Soares et al. 2013; Freire et al. 2016). In one of these studies, radiolabeled gluten was detected both in the circulation and in peripheral organs including visceral adipose tissue, showing once again that this protein is not fully degraded into amino acids before absorption, and that direct action of gluten on these tissues may be possible (Freire et al. 2016). In fact, nondegraded gliadin has been found in the breast milk of healthy mothers (Chirdo et al. 1998). Another pertinent finding is cytotoxicity and accumulation of intracellular lipid droplets in cell cultures exposed to gliadins (Dolfini et al. 2003). Together, these findings, if replicated in humans, may be relevant to the lipid-laden foam cells of early atherosclerosis (Beltowski 2006) as well as progressive beta cell failure and other aspects of the metabolic syndrome and type 2 diabetes (Jönsson et al. 2005; Unger and Scherer 2010).

Cereals may also negatively affect glucose metabolism by means of their glycated proteins. Again, the best studied and perhaps more relevant example considering the current dietary and cooking patterns is the wheat germ agglutinin, which has been found to bind to several hormone receptors including insulin receptors and other tyrosine kinase receptors (namely IGF-1 and EGF receptors) (Cuatrecasas and Tell 1973; Shechter 1983; Wang et al. 2001). The binding of WGA to the insulin receptor is strong and long-lasting with high molecular efficiency, suggesting that it may hinder insulin effects for many hours (Cuatrecasas and Tell 1973; Shechter 1983, #5701; Lindeberg 2010). Hence, it is theoretically capable of causing insulin resistance. Furthermore, WGA increases glycolysis (Yevdokimova and Yefimov 2001) as well as fat storage (Freed 1991). In contrast to insulin, which has the same effects, WGA does not seem to stimulate protein synthesis (Pusztai et al. 1993), which is relevant since loss of muscle mass (sarcopenia) has been suggested to impair insulin sensitivity (Cleasby 2016). Nevertheless, at this point, it remains a theory and data from randomized controlled trials are necessary.

Another example of phytochemicals in legumes and seeds are the *protease inhibitors*, which inhibit protein-degrading enzymes in the digestive tract such as trypsin, chymotrypsin, and amylase. This very ancient defense mechanism of plants allows their seeds to pass through the gastrointestinal system undamaged. The concentration of protease inhibitors in legumes and cereals is so high that the digestion of dietary proteins other than those in the seed can be substantially reduced (Cordain 1999). This increases the risk of undigested (and potentially bioactive) proteins and peptides entering the circulation in susceptible individuals with increased intestinal permeability. Interestingly, an *in vivo* study demonstrated that wheat alpha-amylase/trypsin inhibitors, which appear to resist proteolytic digestion (Schuppan and Zevallos 2015), can activate the innate immune system both in individuals with and without celiac disease, and therefore upregulate inflammation (Junker et al. 2012).

Our knowledge of the health effects of the many bioactive substances in grains and legumes remains fragmentary. Nevertheless, one of the few controlled dietary intervention trials with hard endpoints, DART (Diet And Reinfarction Trial), reported a tendency toward increased cardiovascular mortality in the group advised to eat more fiber, the majority of which was derived from cereal grains (Burr et al. 1989). This nonsignificant effect became statistically significant after adjustment for possible confounding factors, such as medication use and health status (Ness et al. 2002). Furthermore, Cochrane systematic reviews concluded that the quality of evidence is poor and that there is not enough evidence to recommend whole grain cereals for coronary heart disease (Kelly et al. 2007) and type 2 diabetes (Priebe et al. 2008).

Thus, although whole grains are increasingly recommended to increase fiber intake, it might be prudent for patients at high cardiovascular disease risk to obtain most of their dietary fiber from nuts, tubers, fruit and vegetables, until better and more definitive data from randomized controlled trials in cardiovascular disease patients testing whole grains against other plant foods (as opposed to refined grains as is often the case) are available.

PALEOLITHIC DIETS AND ABSENCE OF DAIRY

The impact of *dairy foods* on cardiovascular health has been debated for decades. A human autopsy study in 1960 found myocardial infarction to be more common among patients who had undergone the milk-based Sippy diet, than among those treated at hospitals where the Sippy diet had not been prescribed (Briggs et al. 1960). Internationally, cardiovascular mortality has been positively associated with the intake of dairy products (Segall 1994), and secular trends in milk consumption have correlated positively with changes in mortality rates of coronary heart disease in Europe (Moss and Freed 2003). However, prospective cohort studies within Western populations have shown a slightly lower risk with higher intake of dairy, or no association, suggesting that lifestyle factors other than dairy foods are more important to explain the variation of coronary heart disease and stroke in such populations (Elwood et al. 2005; Soedamah-Muthu et al. 2011; Rice 2014; Praagman et al. 2015).

Dairy may also improve cardiometabolic health, due to some of its numerous bioactive peptides, which have been proposed to exert various beneficial effects, namely inducing satiety and hence contributing to weight management, increasing insulin secretion, and decreasing blood pressure (Nongonierma and FitzGerald 2015). Regarding the latter effect, there is evidence from randomized controlled trials that milk-derived peptides present in both the whey and casein fractions of milk modestly decrease blood pressure (Xu et al. 2008; Nongonierma and FitzGerald 2015). In accordance with this, following the DASH diet, which includes dairy products, has been shown to lead to a reduction in blood pressure (Appel et al. 1997; Chiu et al. 2015). However, the specific effect of dairy (as opposed to isolated dairy-derived proteins or peptides) have not been properly investigated in randomized controlled trials against the DASH diet, which minimize confounders by choosing adequate control foods and matching each group for protein and calcium intake. Indeed, protein, and especially calcium intakes are normally high in the dairy groups and low in the nondairy ones (Machin et al. 2014).

It has been known for decades that milk, despite presenting a low glycemic index, elicits a high insulin response (Nilsson et al. 2004; Melnik 2015a). Theoretically, this could be beneficial for glucose control in type 2 diabetic patients, but because milk has the ability to overactivate the mechanistic target of rapamycin complex 1 (mTORC1), a high milk diet could increase insulin resistance (Melnik 2015a,b). Indeed, randomized controlled trials in Danish boys have found that high intake of cow's milk, but not meat, markedly increased plasma levels of insulin, IGF-1, and IGF-1/IGFBP-3 (Hoppe et al. 2004), and induced insulin resistance, assessed by calculation with the homeostasis model assessment (HOMA) from fasting concentrations of glucose and insulin (Hoppe et al. 2005). Moreover, animal studies have found that casein, the dominant milk protein, promotes atherosclerosis (Wilson et al. 2000; Foo et al. 2009) as well as insulin resistance (Lavigne et al. 2001) apparently by inducing lipotoxicity (Ascencio et al. 2004; Tovar et al. 2005; Tovar and Torres 2010). In addition, in obese men whey protein increases glucagon (Hutchison et al. 2015), a hormone increasingly suspected of playing a central role in the metabolic syndrome and type 2 diabetes (Unger and Scherer 2010; Lee et al. 2014).

Of interest, Allen and Cheer found a striking inverse association between diabetes and lactase persistence rates with the latter explaining almost half of the worldwide variation in diabetes prevalence, indicating cow's milk as a potential contributing factor behind type 2 diabetes (Allen and Cheer 1996).

The uncertainty of the results of a recent systematic review of randomized controlled trials analyzing the effect of dairy upon insulin sensitivity (Turner et al. 2015a) led the authors to themselves conduct a trial in overweight and obese subjects, demonstrating that a diet high in primarily low-fat dairy (from milk, yogurt, or custard) with no red meat reduced insulin sensitivity more than a diet high in lean red meat with minimal dairy, and a control diet that contained neither red meat nor dairy (Turner et al. 2015b).

Given the conflicting studies mentioned, it might be prudent not to increase dairy intake in patients with cardiometabolic diseases until more definitive data from randomized controlled trials with adequate control meals and matched nutrient intakes between groups are available.

NUTRITIONAL CHARACTERISTICS OF PALEOLITHIC DIETS

In addition to being more or less devoid of grains and dairy, *refined fats and sugar* were obviously not included in Paleolithic diets. Hence, total intake of fiber and most micronutrients was generally higher (Cordain et al. 2005; Lindeberg 2010). There are no known nutrients in grains, milk, or refined fats required by humans that are not provided by a mixture of meat, fish, shellfish, vegetables, fruit, nuts, and eggs (Lindeberg 2010). One exception is calcium intake, which may not always have achieved current recommendations, especially when the intake of green leafy vegetables was low (Cordain et al. 2005; Lindeberg 2010).

However, Paleolithic-type diets, low in salt and high in fruits, vegetables, and tuber, are net base-yielding diets, which can decrease calcium excretion and hence calcium requirements (Frassetto et al. 2001, 2007, 2008). This is because diets with high contents of fruits and vegetables are high in the proportion of base-containing precursors to acid-containing precursors derived from biochemical breakdown of amino acids, fats, and organic anions in food (Lennon and Lemann 1968). While all foods contain acid precursors, only fruits and vegetables contain base precursors (Frassetto 2008). Sebastian et al., taking into account various geographies and climates, came up with acid-base estimates of potential Paleolithic-type diets with varying food compositions, and found that the vast majority of them were net base-producing (Sebastian et al. 2002). Diets low in acid precursors lower calcium excretion, while diets high in acid precursors increase calcium excretion (Lemann et al. 1967).

As an example, a study in individuals with the metabolic syndrome showed that a Paleolithic diet led to lower calcium and magnesium excretion compared to the control diet (an isoenergetic healthy reference diet, based on the guidelines of the Dutch Health Council), which together with higher magnesium intake would not compromise calcium homeostasis (Boers et al. 2014).

Another potential nutrient possibly consumed in insufficient amounts with a Paleolithic-type diet is iodine. Since iodized salt and dairy products were not available, only those ancestors with high regular access to fish or shellfish would be expected to have reached the currently recommended intake of iodine (unless they were regularly consuming animal thyroids) (Lindeberg 2009). This suggests that including moderate amounts of fish, shellfish, and minor amounts of algae in "modern" Paleolithic-type diets might be needed to prevent possible iodine insufficiency.

Regarding macronutrients, Paleolithic diets were often high in protein, typically 15%–35% of energy (E%), but not always low in carbohydrate (Cordain et al. 2000a; Kuipers et al. 2010).

Most available foods during the Paleolithic era were voluminous, with a high water and fiber content, and therefore had a low energy density. This is possibly one of the more important characteristics of Paleolithic diets, since it may prevent excessive energy consumption, perhaps by increasing satiety (Rolls et al. 2005; Jebb 2007). In animal experiments, restriction of dietary energy has been found to increase life span in dogs, rats, mice, fish, worms, yeast, and fruit flies, but not in primates (Heilbronn and Ravussin 2003; Fontana and Klein 2007; Colman et al. 2009). Although calorie restriction has not been shown to retard atherosclerosis or prolong life, markedly beneficial effects have been noted on cardiovascular risk factors in controlled trials in nonhuman primates (Bodkin et al. 2003; Colman et al. 2009). Nevertheless, in humans, the effect of caloric restriction on hard endpoints, such as premature death, has not been investigated systematically (Zhao et al. 2014).

CONTEMPORARY HUNTER–GATHERERS AND OTHER NON-WESTERN GROUPS

The rarity of ischemic heart disease has been noted in a number of clinical investigations and autopsy studies in Melanesia, Malaysia, Africa, South America, and the Arctic. A British autopsy study in Uganda, East Africa, at the beginning of the 1950s revealed only 1 in 1427 people (0.7%) above the age of 40 years with histologic signs of previous myocardial infarction (Thomas et al. 1960). Among age-matched subjects in the United States, a high occurrence of a previous myocardial infarction was noted (Table 26.1).

Roughly, two dozen studies from Papua New Guinea paint the same clear picture; prior to urbanization, myocardial infarctions were unknown among the local population. These studies include two systematic reviews of 2000 and 3999 hospital case records, respectively, completed during the first half of the twentieth century (Campbell and Arthur 1964; Dewdney 1965).

Additional support comes from three systematic interviews in the original home environment (Truswell and Hansen 1976; Sinnett 1977; Lindeberg 1994). Truswell found no evidence of sudden, spontaneous death when interviewing 96 adults among the San tribe, hunter–gatherers in the Kalahari desert, Botswana, South Africa (Truswell and Hansen 1976). Sinnett noted no occurrence of retrosternal chest pains matching angina pectoris among the Murapin in the highlands of Papua New Guinea (Sinnett 1977). However, it is difficult to distinguish these pains from musculoskeletal pain in the rib cage during an interview.

In addition to the rarity of ischemic heart disease, the medical records from Kenya and Uganda, which became British protectorates in 1920, strongly indicate the absence of noninfectious stroke in these countries before 1940 (Trowell and Burkitt 1981; Lindeberg 2010). British doctors in the 1920s, who worked in East Africa after receiving their training in Great Britain, have documented this very convincingly. At the medical clinic in Kampala, Uganda, there was no case of noninfectious stroke among 269 consecutive patients with neurological diseases (Muwazi 1944). Furthermore, in an overview of 3000 careful autopsies in Uganda during the 1930s and 1940s, 4 cases of cerebral hemorrhaging, but no cases of ischemic stroke were uncovered (Davies 1948). Hugh Trowell, in his meticulous accounts of noninfectious diseases of East Africa, did not record any cases of ischemic stroke among the aboriginal population, despite his almost 30 years as a doctor and researcher in Uganda (Trowell 1960). The medical literature also highlights the absence of stroke in Papua New Guinea before 1970 (for review, see Lindeberg 2010).

The prevalence of diabetes among hunter–gatherers has not been studied using current methods, but indirect studies of glucose tolerance, blood sugar, serum insulin, waist circumference, and other

TABLE 26.1
Percentage of Deceased Men in the United States and Uganda 1951–1956 with Signs of Previous Myocardial Infarction at Autopsy

Age, Years	United States	Uganda
40–49	31 of 178 (17%)	0 of 178
50–59	51 of 199 (26%)	1 of 199
60–69	32 of 98 (33%)	0 of 98
70–79	8 of 24 (33%)	0 of 33
≥80	2 of 9 (22%)	0 of 9

Source: Thomas, W. et al., *Am. J. Cardiol.*, 5, 41, 1960.

TABLE 26.2
Blood Pressure at Age 40–60 Years among Hunter–Gatherers, in Kitava and in Sweden (mm Hg, Mean ± Standard Deviation)

Population	Men	Women	Reference
Kung San	108/63 ± 11/7	118/71 ± 13/6	Kaminer and Lutz (1960)
Yanomamo	104/65 ± 8/8	102/63 ± 14/12	Oliver et al. (1975)
Xingu	107/68 ± 20/11	102/66 ± 23/11	Baruzzi and Franco (1981)
Kitava	113/71 ± 13/7	121/71 ± 16/8	Lindeberg (1994)
Sweden	134/92 ± 15/10	126/86 ± 16/11	Lindeberg (1994)

related variables provide evidence of a markedly low prevalence of type 2 diabetes and the metabolic syndrome (Joffe et al. 1971; Merimee et al. 1972; Spielman et al. 1982; Lindeberg 2010).

Many studies have shown that being overweight is extremely rare among hunter–gatherers and other traditional cultures (for review, see Lindeberg 2010). This simple fact is quickly apparent to all foreign visitors. The average BMI at 40 years of age is typically around 20 kg/m² for men and 19 kg/m² for women. After the age of 40, BMI for both sexes drops, because both muscle mass and water content decrease with age and because fat is not increasingly accumulated (Gallagher et al. 2000).

Regarding hypertension, multiple studies have convincingly shown that it is very rare among hunter–gatherer populations, and that the average blood pressure is low compared to the Western world (for review, see Lindeberg 2010). Table 26.2 shows the average blood pressure in middle-aged hunter–gatherers, traditional horticulturalists in Kitava, Trobriand Islands, and in Sweden. Blood pressures increase with increasing BMI, which may be one reason why hunter–gatherers have lower blood pressures (Droyvold et al. 2005).

THE KITAVA STUDY

Around 1990, our research group performed a survey in the island of Kitava, Trobriand Islands, Papua New Guinea, where we noted an apparent absence of cardiovascular disease and associated risk factors among Kitava's 2,300 inhabitants (6% of which were 60–95 years old), as well as among the remaining 23,000 people in the Trobriand Islands (Lindeberg and Lundh 1993; Lindeberg 1994, 2010; Lindeberg et al. 1997). The Kitavans are not hunter–gatherers but their staple foods resemble what could have been available to preagricultural humans in Africa. Yam, sweet potato, taro, and fruit were staple foods in Kitava, while grains, dairy, and refined fats and sugar were absent from the diet.

In our systematic surveys, we noted a lack of sudden cardiac death, exertion-related chest pain suggestive of angina pectoris, nor any cases of hemiplegia, aphasia, or sudden imbalance (Lindeberg and Lundh 1993). The survey responses covered at least two past generations, probably more, due to detailed knowledge of living and dead fellow residents. Clinical examinations did not reveal any manifestations of stroke. The results were confirmed by physicians and medical scientists with extensive knowledge of the Trobriand Islands and other parts of Melanesia. Child mortality from malaria and other infections was relatively high, and the estimated average life span was around 45 years. The remaining life expectancy at 45 years of age is more difficult to determine, but may be similar to Swedish figures. Our age estimates were based on known historical events. The main causes of death after age 45 were infections, accidents, and senescence.

In Kitava, diabetes, being overweight, and hypertension were absent, and the average fasting serum glucose and insulin levels were markedly lower than in Sweden (Lindeberg et al. 1999). The average BMI at 40 years of age was approximately 20 kg/m² for men and 19 kg/m² for women (Lindeberg 1994). No Kitavan person was larger around their waist than around their hips.

Blood pressure was measured in 272 Kitavans, aged 4–86. Compared to Westerners, the most marked difference was seen for diastolic blood pressure, which was low in all age groups, with an average of 70.4 ± 6.7 mm Hg (range 51–89). Among adults, diastolic blood pressure did not increase with age. In a European population, half of those over age 40 would fall above the highest measured value in Kitavans (Lindeberg 1994). The extent to which blood pressure rises after middle age in traditional populations is not clear. In Kitava, after the age of 40, there was a significant increase of systolic blood pressure among men ($r = 0.12$, $p = 0.0005$, $n = 92$) and women ($r = 0.12$, $p = 0.01$, $n = 46$). On average, the systolic pressure among the 15 men over the age of 75 was 133 mm Hg (range 100–162). This was significantly ($p = 0.002$) higher than among the 31 men who were between the ages of 60 and 74, whose average blood pressure was 115 mm Hg (range 84–166). No other previous study of traditional populations had included so many different age groups as the Kitava study. In addition, the accuracy of our age estimates was unusually high.

While the metabolic syndrome was apparently absent, serum lipids showed more of an overlap with Western populations. Total and LDL cholesterol levels among Kitavan men were somewhat lower than among Swedish men, and close to today's Japanese, while Kitavan women had levels comparable with Swedish women, especially for women below 60 years of age (Lindeberg 1994). A possible contributing factor is a high intake of saturated fat from coconut, approximately the same as in Sweden (Lindeberg and Vessby 1995). In fact, one could expect an even higher level of serum cholesterol from high intake of saturated fat, and since the two major fatty acids in coconut, 12:0 lauric acid and 14:0 myristic acid, are considered to have a stronger cholesterol-raising effect than 16:0 palmitic acid, which is the dominant fatty acid in Western countries (Becker and Pearson 2002). Lauric and myristic acid raise LDL and HDL, thereby contributing to a lower Total:HDL cholesterol ratio than palmitic acid (which raises Total:HDL ratio) (Mensink et al. 2003).

In other surveys among aboriginal populations, the picture in terms of blood lipids is not as consistent as it is in terms of their lack of being overweight, or having abdominal obesity and high blood pressure. There are examples of populations with a very low prevalence of ischemic heart disease despite blood lipid levels that would be considered high risk among Westerners. The Kitava study adds to the notion that some of our most common diseases are fully preventable (Lindeberg 2010).

EFFECTS OF URBANIZATION

The emergence of ischemic heart disease has been well documented in a number of populations after adopting Western dietary habits and lower levels of physical activity (for review, see Lindeberg 2010). The first case of a myocardial infarction in New Guineans, which was verified with an autopsy, was reported in 1955 and individual cases were seen during the 1960s and 1970s (Conyers 1971; Somers 1974). After the 1970s, the number gradually increased (Kevau 1990). Among blacks in Africa, the first case of classic angina pectoris was recorded in 1958 in an overweight housewife with free access to Western food (Gelfand and Kaplan 1958). Later autopsy studies appeared to indicate that myocardial infarctions were more common among those people with a higher income (el Hassan and Wasfi 1972).

Table 26.3 shows the almost explosive growth of stroke, a previously unknown illness, among the native population of Uganda. By 1955, stroke already made up 11% of the neurological cases (Hutton 1956), and by 1968, it became the most prevalent neurological diagnosis (Billinghurst 1970). At the same time, hypertension, another previously unknown phenomenon, began to spread—a curious development that was the topic of lively debates among British doctors in Uganda and Kenya at the time (Trowell and Burkitt 1981). Parallel with the changes in the landscape of diseases, these countries also underwent rapid social change from original traditional societies to Western-style colonial societies.

The East African pattern is now being repeated in Papua New Guinea (Lindeberg 2003). The first known case of stroke at Port Moresby General Hospital was seen in 1975 (Kevau I., personal communication), a few years after the first documented case in Lae (Mathews 1974). Since then, cases

TABLE 26.3
The Proportion of Stroke among Patients with Acute Neurological Disease in Kampala, Uganda, in Three Consecutive Series

Year	N	%	Reference
1942	0	0	Muwazi (1944)
1954	11/100	11	Hutton (1956)
1968	17/50	34	Billinghurst (1970)

have become increasingly more common, and in 1998 there were almost two stroke cases per week at the Port Moresby General Hospital.

As discussed earlier, many surveys among hunter–gatherers or similar non-Western populations have found a striking absence of ischemic heart disease, stroke, diabetes, hypertension, and abdominal overweight. Not only did dietary habits differ in these populations compared to Western countries, but daily physical activity was more intense.

It has been argued that traditional populations may have been genetically protected against the chronic degenerative diseases that occur in industrialized countries, yet when non-Westernized individuals adopt a more contemporary lifestyle, their risk for chronic degenerative diseases is similar or even increased compared with modern populations (Yusuf et al. 2001; Lindeberg 2010; Carrera-Bastos 2011).

Another common counterargument is the short average life expectancy at birth of hunter–gatherers and other traditional populations. The problem with this marker is that it is influenced by childhood mortality and fatal events (e.g., accidents, warfare, infections, exposure to "outdoor dangers") (Carrera-Bastos 2011). Today, average life expectancy is higher not because of a healthier diet or lifestyle but because of less physical trauma, and improved sanitation, vaccination, medical care, and social stability (Carrera-Bastos 2011). Although it is not possible to get a fair estimate of life expectancy for Paleolithic cultures due to methodological limitations in osteology (Hoppa and Vaupel 2002), among contemporary hunter–gatherers, the frequency distribution of ages at death peaks around 70 years (Gurven and Kaplan 2007). Despite data that prehistoric hunter–gatherers had a relatively high risk of death at young age, available evidence suggests that there were elderly people and that they were important enough for the survival of grandchildren for age-related diseases to be relevant in terms of nutritional adaptation (Henke and Tattersall 2007). Of more importance, these individuals reach age 60 years or beyond without the signs and symptoms of chronic degenerative diseases that afflict the majority of the elderly in industrialized countries (Carrera-Bastos 2011). Furthermore, in Western countries, various chronic degenerative diseases, including cardiometabolic diseases, which are rare or virtually absent in hunter–gatherers, horticulturalists, and traditional pastoralists, are now increasing in younger age groups (Carrera-Bastos 2011).

Nevertheless, it should be mentioned that while it is appropriate to provide information regarding health status of hunter–gatherers and the effects of urbanization, the limitations of observational studies, in particular effects due to residual confounding, preclude the inference that dietary practices are sufficient to account for differences in disease patterns.

CONTROLLED TRIALS OF "PALEOLITHIC DIETS"

There is a paucity of randomized controlled trials of "Paleolithic diets." A systematic review using the GRADE approach (Guyatt et al. 2008), as recommended by major Health Technology Assessment organizations worldwide, found four randomized controlled trials of sufficient quality where a Paleolithic diet was compared with another prudent diet in the treatment of the five components of the metabolic syndrome (Manheimer et al. 2015). In total, 159 participants were included in the meta-analysis. The control diets were based on distinct national nutrition guidelines but were broadly similar. Food intake was *ad libitum* except for one trial where detailed menus were provided. Adherence to the diets was assessed with food records. Paleolithic nutrition resulted in greater short-term improvements (from 2 weeks to 6 months) than did the control diets (random-effects model) for waist circumference (mean difference: −2.38 cm; 95% CI: −4.73, −0.04 cm), triglycerides (−0.40 mmol/L; 95% CI: −0.76, −0.04 mmol/L), systolic blood pressure (−3.64 mm Hg; 95% CI: −7.36, 0.08 mm Hg), diastolic blood pressure (−2.48 mm Hg; 95% CI: −4.98, 0.02 mm Hg), HDL cholesterol (0.12 mmol/L; 95% CI: −0.03, 0.28 mmol/L), and fasting blood glucose (−0.16 mmol/L; 95% CI: −0.44, 0.11 mmol/L). The quality of the evidence for each of the five metabolic components was moderate.

Two of these clinical trials were performed by our group (Lindeberg et al. 2007; Jönsson et al. 2009). In the studies, we noted beneficial effects of advice to eat a "Paleolithic" diet with regard to waist circumference, glucose tolerance, blood sugar, blood pressure, and blood lipids (Lindeberg et al. 2007; Jönsson et al. 2009). In both studies, we found evidence that the "Paleolithic" diet was more satiating, such that the meals gave the same feeling of fullness at a lower level of energy intake (Jönsson et al. 2010, 2013). In the first trial (Lindeberg et al. 2007), we randomly assigned 29 subjects with type 2 diabetes or glucose intolerance to one of two prudent diets, with or without grains and dairy products, a Mediterranean or Paleolithic diet, respectively. After 3 months, the Paleolithic diet improved glucose tolerance more than the Mediterranean diet, independently of weight loss. Also, after 3 months, all 14 subjects on the Paleolithic diet had normal plasma 2 h glucose compared with 7 out of 15 in the Mediterranean group ($p = 0.0007$ for group difference). Regarding the second study, a crossover study involving 13 patients, after 3 months, the Paleolithic diet improved glycated hemoglobin, blood lipids, and blood pressure more than the recommended official diet for type 2 diabetes in Sweden (Jönsson et al. 2009). Another trial included in the foregoing meta-analysis tested the long-term effects of a Paleolithic diet in 70 obese postmenopausal women (Mellberg et al. 2014). The participants were randomized to either a Paleolithic diet or Nordic Nutrition Recommendations (NNR) (Becker et al. 2004) for 2 years. Compared to the NNR, the Paleolithic diet resulted in greater decreases in total fat loss, waist circumference, and abdominal sagittal diameter at 6 but not 24 months. The effects were not maintained at 24 months, probably due to poor compliance with protein intake in the Paleolithic diet. However, triglycerides levels were reduced more in the Paleolithic than the NNR after 6 and 24 months. Liver fat also decreased more on the Paleolithic than the NRR after 6 but not 24 months (Otten et al. 2016). The fourth study included in the meta-analysis involved 32 subjects, with at least two components of the metabolic syndrome, who were randomized to follow a 2-week Paleolithic or an isoenergetic healthy reference diet according to the Dutch Health Council (Boers et al. 2014). The Paleolithic diet improved blood pressure, blood lipids, and the number of characteristics of the metabolic syndrome (1.07) more than the reference diet.

Although the control groups in these four trials were advised to follow a prudent diet and were told that it was unknown if one diet was inferior to the other, it cannot be excluded that differences in outcomes were due to the effect of residual confounding.

In a recent short-term (21 days) study in patients with type 2 diabetes, a Paleolithic diet induced a significant reduction in HbA1c, fasting glucose, fructosamine, total and LDL cholesterol, triglycerides and increased insulin sensitivity (as measured by euglycemic hyperinsulinemic clamp), and increased HDL cholesterol (Masharani et al. 2015). However, the control diet based on recommendations by the American Diabetes Association (Bantle et al. 2008), containing moderate salt intake, low-fat dairy, whole grains and legumes, also improved HbA1c and worsened HDL cholesterol compared to the baseline diets in both groups. No differences were observed between the control and Paleolithic diets.

In a nonrandomized controlled study, after 4 months, a Paleolithic diet improved plasma lipids more than the American Heart Association heart-healthy dietary recommendation (Eckel et al. 2014), in patients with hypercholesterolemia (Pastore et al. 2015). The macronutrient composition of the AHA diet was 56%, 21%, and 23%, for carbohydrate, protein, and fat, respectively in men, and 60%, 17%, and 23% in women. The macronutrient composition of the Paleolithic diet was 23%, 37%, and 40% for carbohydrate, protein, and fat, respectively in men and women. The lack of randomization of this study represents a serious limitation.

In a metabolically controlled study, nine nonobese sedentary healthy volunteers consumed a Paleolithic diet ensuring no weight loss (Frassetto et al. 2009). The participants consumed their habitual diet for 3 days, then ate 7 days "ramp-up" diets to increase potassium and fiber intake, and finally a Paleolithic diet for 10 days. All meals were prepared by the clinical research center kitchen and provided to the participants to guarantee compliance with the dietary recommendations. Frassetto et al. found improved levels of plasma insulin in the fasting state (by 68%) as well as after a glucose load (by 39%), blood lipids, and blood pressure after the Paleolithic diet compared to their usual diet. Similarly, marked improvements in body weight, blood glucose, blood lipids, and blood pressure were noted in urbanized Aborigines with type 2 diabetes when they returned to a hunter–gatherer lifestyle for 7 weeks (O'Dea 1984). Physical activity was also increased in that study.

There are few obvious risks associated with the consumption of a Paleolithic diet. The effect of a high protein intake on kidney function is debatable in subjects with healthy kidneys and would be expected to be outweighed by any beneficial effects on abdominal obesity and other health-related variables (Lindeberg 2010). Even in patients with type 2 diabetes, but without chronic kidney disease, a low-carbohydrate diet (14% of total energy intake) high in fat and protein does not impair renal function (Tay et al. 2015). Nevertheless, a Paleolithic type diet is not always high in protein. People with genetic hemochromatosis, a hereditary disease that results in enhanced iron absorption, need to limit their intake of meat (especially red meat) and fish but should otherwise do well on a Paleolithic diet. Heterozygous carriers are advised to monitor their iron status regularly after middle age. Individuals treated with ACE-inhibitors, angiotensin II receptor blockers, or diuretics should convert slowly to a salt-free Paleolithic diet in order to avoid a sharp drop in blood pressure (Milan et al. 2002). Subjects with kidney failure cannot eat a high potassium diet, and should not attempt a Paleolithic diet, unless under the care of a kidney specialist. Patients with type 2 diabetes who are on sulfonylurea preparations (glipizid, glibenklamid, glimepirid) are at risk for hypoglycemia when making a radical switch to a Paleolithic diet. People with a history of intestinal obstruction, intestinal dysmotility, or multiple intestinal surgeries can be at risk of recurrent obstruction when eating a very high fiber diet, especially if not accompanied by an increase in fluid intake. Converting to a Paleolithic diet during ongoing warfarin treatment should be done in consultation with a physician or nurse.

CONCLUSION

A Paleolithic diet may serve as a model for healthy foods, in particular in clinical trials in comparison with other prudent diets. Hypothetically, food choice is more important than counting calories or macronutrients in order to avoid common health problems in the Western world. Diets providing wild meat, fish, shellfish, vegetables, tubers, fruit, berries, nuts, and eggs can be tested in the prevention and treatment of disease. Hypothetically, dairy products, margarine, oils, and refined sugar and cereal grains, which provide 70% or more of the dietary intake for modern humans, are not optimal food choices for long-term health. However, much more research is needed to confirm the benefits of Paleolithic diets for cardiometabolic health. Although this review has focused on what most humans would have in common, studies on possible ethnic differences in susceptibility to diet-induced disease are also needed.

REFERENCES

Afshin, A., R. Micha, S. Khatibzadeh, and D. Mozaffarian. 2014. Consumption of nuts and legumes and risk of incident ischemic heart disease, stroke, and diabetes: A systematic review and meta-analysis. *Am J Clin Nutr* 100:278–288.

Allen, J. S. and S. M. Cheer. 1996. The non-thrifty genotype. *Curr Anthropol* 37:831–842.

Allsop, K. A. and J. B. Miller. 1996. Honey revisited: A reappraisal of honey in pre-industrial diets. *Br J Nutr* 75:513–520.

Appel, L. J., T. J. Moore, E. Obarzanek et al. 1997. A clinical trial of the effects of dietary patterns on blood pressure. DASH Collaborative Research Group. *N Engl J Med* 17:1117–1124.

Ascencio, C., N. Torres, F. Isoard-Acosta et al. 2004. Soy protein affects serum insulin and hepatic SREBP-1 mRNA and reduces fatty liver in rats. *J Nutr* 134:522–529.

Bang, H. O. and J. Dyerberg. 1972. Plasma lipids and lipoproteins in Greenlandic west coast Eskimos. *Acta Med Scand* 192:85–94.

Bantle, J. P., J. Wylie-Rosett, A. L. Albright et al. 2008. Nutrition recommendations and interventions for diabetes: A position statement of the American Diabetes Association. *Diabetes Care* 31:S61–S78.

Baruzzi, R. and L. Franco. 1981. Amerindians of Brazil. In *Western Diseases: Their Emergence and Prevention*, eds. H. C. Trowel and D. P. Burkitt, pp. 138–153. London, U.K.: Edward Arnold.

Basabose, A. K. 2002. Diet composition of chimpanzees inhabiting the montane forest of Kahuzi, Democratic Republic of Congo. *Am J Primatol* 58:1–21.

Becker, B. F., D. Chappell, and M. Jacob. 2010. Endothelial glycocalyx and coronary vascular permeability: The fringe benefit. *Basic Res Cardiol* 105:687–701.

Becker, W., N. Lyhne, A. N. Pedersen et al. 2004. Nordic nutrition recommendations 2004. Integrating nutrition and physical activity. *Scand J Nutr* 48:178–187.

Becker, W. and M. Pearson. 2002. Dietary habits and nutrient intake in Sweden 1997–1998: The Second National Food Consumption Survey (in Swedish). Uppsala, Sweden: Swedish National Food Administration.

Beltowski, J. 2006. Leptin and atherosclerosis. *Atherosclerosis* 189:47–60.

Berger, J. D., L. D. Robertson, and P. S. Cocks. 2003. Agricultural potential of Mediterranean grain and forage legumes: 2. Anti-nutritional factor concentrations in the genus Vicia. *Genet Resour Crop Evol* 50:201–212.

Billinghurst, J. R. 1970. The pattern of adult neurological admissions to Mulago hospital, Kampala. *East Afr Med J* 47:653–663.

Bloch, J. I. and D. M. Boyer. 2002. Grasping primate origins. *Science* 298:1606–1610.

Bodkin, N. L., T. M. Alexander, H. K. Ortmeyer, E. Johnson, and B. C. Hansen. 2003. Mortality and morbidity in laboratory-maintained Rhesus monkeys and effects of longterm dietary restriction. *J Gerontol A Biol Sci Med Sci* 58:212–219.

Boers, I., F. A. J. Muskiet, E. Berkelaar et al. 2014. Favourable effects of consuming a Palaeolithic- type diet on characteristics of the metabolic syndrome: A randomized controlled pilot-study. *Lipids Health Dis* 13:160.

Brand Miller, J. C. and S. Colagiuri. 1994. The carnivore connection: Dietary carbohydrate in the evolution of NIDDM. *Diabetologia* 37:1280–1286.

Briggs, R. D., M. L. Rubenberg, R. M. O'Neal, W. A. Thomas, and W. S. Hartroft. April 1960. Myocardial infarction in patients treated with Sippy and other high-milk diets: An autopsy study of 15 hospitals in the U.S.A. and Great Britain. *Circulation* 21:538–542.

Brinkworth, G. D., M. Noakes, J. D. Buckley, J. B. Keogh, and P. M. Clifton. 2009. Long-term effects of a very-low-carbohydrate weight loss diet compared with an isocaloric low-fat diet after 12 mo. *Am J Clin Nutr* 90:23–32.

Burr, M. L., A. M. Fehily, J. F. Gilbert et al. 1989. Effects of changes in fat, fish, and fibre intakes on death and myocardial reinfarction: Diet and Reinfarction Trial (DART). *Lancet* 2:757–761.

Campbell, C. and R. Arthur. 1964. A study of 2000 admissions to the medical ward of Port Moresby General Hospital. *Med J Aust* 1:989–992.

Campbell, M. C. and S. A. Tishkoff. 2010. The evolution of human genetic and phenotypic variation in Africa. *Curr Biol* 20:R166–R173.

Carrera-Bastos, P., M. Fontes-Villalba, J. H. O'Keefe, S. Lindeberg, and L. Cordain. 2011. The western diet and lifestyle and diseases of civilization. *Res Rep Clin Cardiol* 2:15–35.

Chen, G. C., D. B. Lv, Z. Pang, and Q.-F. Liu. 2013. Red and processed meat consumption and risk of stroke: A meta-analysis of prospective cohort studies. *Eur J Clin Nutr* 67:91–95.

Chirdo, F. G., M. Rumbo, M. C. Anon, and C. A. Fossati. 1998. Presence of high levels of non-degraded gliadin in breast milk from healthy mothers. *Scand J Gastroenterol* 33:1186–1192.

Chiu, S., N. Bergeron, P. T. Williams, G. A. Bray, B. Sutherland, and R. M. Krauss. 2015. Comparison of the DASH (Dietary Approaches to Stop Hypertension) diet and a higher-fat DASH diet on blood pressure and lipids and lipoproteins: A randomized controlled trial. *Am J Clin Nutr* 103(2):341–347.

Chrispeels, M. J. and N. V. Raikhel. 1991. Lectins, lectin genes, and their role in plant defense. *Plant Cell* 3:1–9.

Cleasby, M. E., P. M. Jamieson, and P. J. Atherton. May 2016. Insulin resistance and sarcopenia: Mechanistic links between common co-morbidities. *J Endocrinol BioScientifica* 229(2):R67–R81.

Clifton, P. M., D. Condo, and J. B. Keogh. 2014. Long term weight maintenance after advice to consume low carbohydrate, higher protein diets—A systematic review and meta analysis. *Nutr Metab Cardiovasc Dis* 24:224–235.

Colman, R. J., R. M. Anderson, S. C. Johnson et al. 2009. Caloric restriction delays disease onset and mortality in rhesus monkeys. *Science* 325:201–204.

Conyers, R. A. 1971. Myocardial infarction in a New Guinean. *Med J Aust* 2:412–417.

Cordain, L. 1998. Atherogenic potential of peanut oil-based monounsaturated fatty acids diets. *Lipids* 33(2):229–230.

Cordain, L. 1999. Cereal grains: Humanity's double-edged sword. *World Rev Nutr Diet* 84:19–73.

Cordain, L. 2006. Saturated fat consumption in ancestral human diets: Implications for contemporary intakes. In *Phytochemicals: Nutrient-Gene Interactions*, eds. M. S. Meskin, W. R. Bidlack, and R. K. Randolph, pp. 115–126. London, U.K.: Taylor & Francis.

Cordain, L., J. Brand Miller, S. B. Eaton, N. Mann, S. H. Holt, and J. D. Speth. 2000a. Plant-animal subsistence ratios and macronutrient energy estimations in worldwide hunter-gatherer diets. *Am J Clin Nutr* 71:682–692.

Cordain, L., S. B. Eaton, A. Sebastian et al. 2005. Origins and evolution of the Western diet: Health implications for the 21st century. *Am J Clin Nutr* 81:341–354.

Cordain, L., L. Toohey, M. J. Smith, and M. S. Hickey. 2000b. Modulation of immune function by dietary lectins in rheumatoid arthritis. *Br J Nutr* 83:207–217.

Cordain, L., B. A. Watkins, G. L. Florant, M. Kelher, L. Rogers, and Y. Li. 2002. Fatty acid analysis of wild ruminant tissues: Evolutionary implications for reducing diet-related chronic disease. *Eur J Clin Nutr* 56:181–191.

Cozma, A. I., J. L. Sievenpiper, R. J. de Souza et al. 2012. Effect of fructose on glycemic control in diabetes: A systematic review and meta-analysis of controlled feeding trials. *Diabetes Care* 35:1611–1620.

Cuatrecasas, P. and G. P. Tell. 1973. Insulin-like activity of concanavalin A and wheat germ agglutinin—Direct interactions with insulin receptors. *PNAS* 70:485–489.

Dalla Pellegrina, C., O. Perbellini, M. T. Scupoli et al. 2009. Effects of wheat germ agglutinin on human gastrointestinal epithelium: Insights from an experimental model of immune/epithelial cell interaction. *Toxicol Appl Pharmacol* 237(2):146–153.

Davidson, M. H., D. Hunninghake, K. C. Maki, P. O. Kwiterovich, and S. Kafonek. 1999. Comparison of the effects of lean red meat vs lean white meat on serum lipid levels among free-living persons with hypercholesterolemia: A long-term, randomized clinical trial. *Arch Intern Med* 159:1331–1338.

Davies, J. 1948. Pathology of central African natives. IX. Cardiovascular diseases. *East Afr Med J* 25:454–467.

Davis, H. R. and S. Glagov. 1986. Lectin binding to distinguish cell types in fixed atherosclerotic arteries. *Atherosclerosis* 61:193–203.

de Luis, D. A., R. Aller, O. Izaola, and E. Romero. 2015. Effects of a high-protein/low-carbohydrate versus a standard hypocaloric diet on adipocytokine levels and cardiovascular risk factors during 9 months, role of rs6923761 gene variant of glucagon-like peptide 1 receptor. *J Endocrinol Invest* 38:1183–1189.

DeFoliart, G. R. 1999. Insects as food: Why the western attitude is important. *Annu Rev Entomol* 44:21–50.

Del Gobbo, L. C., M. C. Falk, R. Feldman, K. Lewis, and D. Mozaffarian. 2015. Effects of tree nuts on blood lipids, apolipoproteins, and blood pressure: Systematic review, meta-analysis, and dose-response of 61 controlled intervention trials. *Am J Clin Nutr* 102:1347–1356.

Dewdney, J. C. H. 1965. Maprik Hospital—A review of 3888 consecutive admissions, February 1963 to July 1964. *P N G Med J* 8:89–96.

Dolfini, E., L. Elli, S. Ferrero et al. 2003. Bread wheat gliadin cytotoxicity: A new three-dimensional cell model. *Scand J Clin Lab Invest* 63:135–141.

Drake-Holland, A. J. and M. I. Noble. 2009. The important new drug target in cardiovascular medicine—The vascular glycocalyx. *Cardiovasc Hematol Disord Drug Targets* 9:118–123.

Droyvold, W. B., K. Midthjell, T. H. Neisen, and J. Holmen. 2005. Change in body mass index and its impact on blood pressure: A prospective population study. *Int J Obes* 29:650–655.

Dudley, R. 2002. Fermenting fruit and the historical ecology of ethanol ingestion: Is alcoholism in modern humans an evolutionary hangover? *Addiction* 97:381–388.

Due, A., T. M. Larsen, K. Hermansen et al. April 2008. Comparison of the effects on insulin resistance and glucose tolerance of 6-mo high-monounsaturated-fat, low-fat, and control diets. *Am J Clin Nutr* 87(4):855–862.

Dzhangaliev, A. D., T. N. Salova, and P. M. Turekhanova. 2003. The wild fruit and nut plants of Kazakhstan. In *Horticultural Reviews: Wild Apple and Fruit Trees of Central Asia*, Ed. J. Janick, Vol. 29, pp. 305–371. Hoboken, NJ: John Wiley & Sons, Inc.

Eaton, S. and M. Konner. 1985. Paleolithic nutrition. A consideration of its nature and current implications. *N Engl J Med* 312:283–289.

Eckel, R. H., J. M. Jakicic, J. D. Ard et al. 2014. 2013 AHA/ACC guideline on lifestyle management to reduce cardiovascular risk: A report of the American College of Cardiology/American Heart Association Task Force on Practice Guidelines. *J Am Coll Cardiol* 63(25_PA):2960–2984.

el Hassan, A. M. and A. Wasfi. 1972. Cardiovascular disease in Khartoum. Post-mortem and clinical evidence. *Trop Geogr Med* 24:118–123.

Elwood, P. C., J. J. Strain, P. J. Robson et al. 2005. Milk consumption, stroke, and heart attack risk: Evidence from the Caerphilly cohort of older men. *J Epidemiol Community Health* 59:502–505.

Estruch, R., E. Ros, J. Salas-Salvadó et al. 2013. Primary prevention of cardiovascular disease with a mediterranean diet. *N Engl J Med* 368:1279–1290.

Finch, C. E. and C. B. Stanford. 2004. Meat-adaptive genes and the evolution of slower aging in humans. *Q Rev Biol* 79:3–50.

Flores-Mateo, G., D. Rojas-Rueda, J. Basora, E. Ros, and J. Salas-Salvadó. 2013. Nut intake and adiposity: Meta-analysis of clinical trials. *Am J Clin Nutr* 97:1346–1355.

Fontana, L. and S. Klein. 2007. Aging, adiposity, and calorie restriction. *JAMA* 297:986–994.

Foo, S. Y., E. R. Heller, and J. Wykrzykowska. 2009. Vascular effects of a low-carbohydrate high-protein diet. *PNAS* 106:15418–15423.

Frassetto, L., R. C. Morris Jr., D. E. Sellmeyer, K. Todd, and A. Sebastian. October 2001. Diet, evolution and aging—The pathophysiologic effects of the post-agricultural inversion of the potassium-to-sodium and base-to-chloride ratios in the human diet. *Eur J Nutr* 40(5):200–213.

Frassetto, L. A. 2008. Fruits and vegetables as a marker for dietary alkali intake. *IFAVA* 21:4.

Frassetto, L. A., R. C. Morris Jr., and A. Sebastian. August 2007. Dietary sodium chloride intake independently predicts the degree of hyperchloremic metabolic acidosis in healthy humans consuming a net acid-producing diet. *Am J Physiol Renal Physiol* 293(2):F521–F525.

Frassetto, L. A., R. C. Morris Jr., D. E. Sellmeyer, and A. Sebastian. February 2008. Adverse effects of sodium chloride on bone in the aging human population resulting from habitual consumption of typical American diets. *J Nutr* 138(2):419S–422S.

Frassetto, L. A., M. Schloetter, M. Mietus-Synder, R. C. Morris Jr., and A. Sebastian. 2009. Metabolic and physiologic improvements from consuming a paleolithic, hunter-gatherer type diet. *Eur J Clin Nutr* 63:947–955.

Freed, D. L. 1991. Lectins in food: Their importance in health and disease. *J Nutr Med* 2:45–64.

Freed, D. L. 1999. Do dietary lectins cause disease? *BMJ* 318:1023–1024.

Freire, R. H., L. R. Fernandes, R. B. Silva et al. 2016. Wheat gluten intake increases weight gain and adiposity associated with reduced thermogenesis and energy expenditure in an animal model of obesity. *Int J Obes* 40(3):479–486.

Frostegård, J. 2013. Immune mechanisms in atherosclerosis, especially in diabetes type 2. *Front Endocrinol (Lausanne)* 4:162.

Gallagher, D., E. Ruts, M. Visser et al. 2000. Weight stability masks sarcopenia in elderly men and women. *Am J Physiol Endocrinol Metab* 279:E366–E375.

Gannon, M. C. and F. Q. Nuttall. 2006. Control of blood glucose in type 2 diabetes without weight loss by modification of diet composition. *Nutr Metab (Lond)* 3:16.

Gelfand, M. and M. Kaplan. 1958. Bantu coronary insufficiency. Report of a possible case. *Central Afr J Med* 4:157–159.

Grant, G., L. J. More, N. H. McKenzie, and A. Pusztai. December 1982. The effect of heating on the haemagglutinating activity and nutritional properties of bean (*Phaseolus vulgaris*) seeds. *J Sci Food Agric* 33(12):1324–1326.

Gräslund, B. 2005. *Early Humans and Their World*. London, U.K.: Routledge.

Gurven, M. and H. Kaplan. 2007. Longevity among hunter-gatherers: A cross-cultural examination. *Popul Dev Rev* 33:321–365.

Guyatt, G. H., A. D. Oxman, G. E. Vist et al. 2008. GRADE: An emerging consensus on rating quality of evidence and strength of recommendation. *BMJ* 336:924–926.

Haniu, M., T. Arakawa, E. J. Bures et al. 1998. Human leptin receptor. Determination of disulfide structure and N-glycosylation sites of the extracellular domain. *J Biol Chem* 273:28691–28699.

Hardivillé, S. and G. W. Hart. 2014. Nutrient regulation of signaling, transcription and cell physiology by O-GlcNAcylation. *Cell Metab* 20:208–213.

Hardy, K., J. Brand-Miller, K. D. Brown, M. G. Thomas, and L. Copeland. 2015. The importance of dietary carbohydrate in human evolution. *Quart Rev Biol* 90:251–268.

Heilbronn, L. K. and E. Ravussin. 2003. Calorie restriction and aging: Review of the literature and implications for studies in humans. *Am J Clin Nutr* 78:361–369.

Henke, W. and I. Tattersall (Eds.). 2007. *Handbook of Paleoanthropology*. Berlin, Germany: Springer.

Henry, C. B. and B. R. Duling. 2000. TNF-alpha increases entry of macromolecules into luminal endothelial cell glycocalyx. *Am J Physiol Heart Circ Physiol* 279:H2815–H2823.

Herrera, C. M. and O. Pellmyr (Eds.). 2002. *Plant-Animal Interactions. An Evolutionary Approach*. Oxford, U.K.: Blackwell.

Hollon, J., E. L. Puppa, B. Greenwald, E. Goldberg, A. Guerrerio, and A. Fasano. 2015. Effect of gliadin on permeability of intestinal biopsy explants from celiac disease patients and patients with non-celiac gluten sensitivity. *Nutrients* 7(3):1565–1576.

Hooper, L., R. L. Thompson, R. A. Harrison et al. 2004. Omega 3 fatty acids for prevention and treatment of cardiovascular disease. *Cochrane Database Syst Rev* 4:CD003177.

Hooper, L., R. L. Thompson, R. A. Harrison et al. 2006. Risks and benefits of omega 3 fats for mortality, cardiovascular disease, and cancer: Systematic review. *BMJ* 332:752–760.

Hoppa, R. D. and J. W. Vaupel (Eds.). 2002. *Paleodemography: Age Distributions from Skeletal Samples*. Cambridge, U.K.: Cambridge University Press.

Hoppe, C., C. Molgaard, A. Juul, and K. F. Michaelsen. 2004. High intakes of skimmed milk, but not meat, increase serum IGF-I and IGFBP-3 in eight-year-old boys. *Eur J Clin Nutr* 58:1211–1216.

Hoppe, C., C. Molgaard, A. Vaag, V. Barkholt, and K. F. Michaelsen. 2005. High intakes of milk, but not meat, increase s-insulin and insulin resistance in 8-year-old boys. *Eur J Clin Nutr* 59:393–398.

Hu, F. B., J. E. Manson, and W. C. Willett. 2001. Types of dietary fat and risk of coronary heart disease: A critical review. *J Am Coll Nutr* 20:5–19.

Hutchison, A. T., C. Feinle-Bisset, P. C. Fitzgerald et al. 2015. Comparative effects of intraduodenal whey protein hydrolysate on antropyloroduodenal motility, gut hormones, glycemia, appetite, and energy intake in lean and obese men. *Am J Clin Nutr* 102:1323–1331.

Hutton, P. W. 1956. Neurological disease in Uganda. *East Afr Med J* 33:209–223.

Isaacs, J. 1987. *Bush Food*. The Rocks, New South Wales, Australia: Lansdowne.

Jebb, S. A. 2007. Dietary determinants of obesity. *Obes Rev* 8:93–97.

Jenkins, D. J. A. and C. W. C. Kendall. 2006. The Garden of Eden. Plant-based diets, the genetic drive to store fat and conserve cholesterol, and implications for epidemiology in the 21st century. *Epidemiology* 17:128–130.

Jenkins, D. J. A., C. W. C. Kendall, A. Marchie et al. 2003. Effects of a dietary portfolio of cholesterol-lowering foods vs lovastatin on serum lipids and C-reactive protein. *JAMA* 290:502–510.

Joffe, B. I., W. P. Jackson, M. E. Thomas et al. 1971. Metabolic responses to oral glucose in the Kalahari Bushmen. *BMJ* 4:206–208.

Jones, M. 2009. Moving North: Archaeobotanical evidence for plant diet in middle and upper paleolithic Europe. In *The Evolution of Hominin Diets: Integrating Approaches to the Study of Palaeolithic Subsistence*, Eds. J.-J. Hublin and M. P. Richards, pp. 171–180. Springer, Dordrecht, the Netherlands.

Johnson, R. J., S. E. Perez-Pozo, Y. Y. Sautin et al. February 2009. Hypothesis: Could excessive fructose intake and uric acid cause type 2 diabetes? *Endocr Rev* 30(1):96–116.

Jönsson, T., Y. Granfeldt, B. Ahren et al. 2009. Beneficial effects of a Paleolithic diet on cardiovascular risk factors in type 2 diabetes: A randomized cross-over pilot study. *Cardiovasc Diabetol* 8:35.

Jönsson, T., Y. Granfeldt, C. Erlanson-Albertsson, B. Ahrén, and S. Lindeberg. 2010. A paleolithic diet is more satiating per calorie than a mediterranean-like diet in individuals with ischemic heart disease. *Nutr Metab (Lond)* 7:85.

Jönsson, T., Y. Granfeldt, S. Lindeberg, and A. C. Hallberg. 2013. Subjective satiety and other experiences of a Paleolithic diet compared to a diabetes diet in patients with type 2 diabetes. *Nutr J* 12:105. doi: 10.1186/1475-2891-12-105.

Jönsson, T., A. A. Memon, K. Sundquist et al. 2015. Digested wheat gluten inhibits binding between leptin and its receptor. *BMC Biochem* 16:3. doi: 10.1186/s12858-015-0032-y.

Jönsson, T., S. Olsson, B. Ahren, T. C. Bog-Hansen, A. Dole, and S. Lindeberg. 2005. Agrarian diet and diseases of affluence—Do evolutionary novel dietary lectins cause leptin resistance? *BMC Endocr Disord* 5:10.

Junker, Y., S. Zeissig, S. J. Kim et al. 2012. Wheat amylase trypsin inhibitors drive intestinal inflammation via activation of toll-like receptor 4. *J Exp Med* 209:2395–2408.

Kagami, H., K. Uryu, K. Okamoto, H. Sakai, T. Kaneda, and M. Sakanaka. 1991. Differential lectin binding on walls of thoraco-cervical blood vessels and lymphatics in rats. *Okajimas Folia Anat Jpn* 68:161–170.

Kamikubo, Y., C. Dellas, D. J. Loskutoff, J. P. Quigley, and Z. M. Ruggeri. 2007. Contribution of leptin receptor N-linked glycans to leptin binding. *Biochem J* 410:595–604.

Kaminer, B. and W. P. W. Lutz. 1960. Blood pressure in Bushmen of the Kalahari desert. *Circulation* 22:289–295.

Kelly, S. A. M., C. D. Summerbell, A. Brynes, V. Whittaker, and G. Frost. 2007. Wholegrain cereals for coronary heart disease. *Cochrane Database Syst Rev* 18(2):CD005051.

Kevau, I. H. 1990. Clinical documentation of twenty cases of acute myocardial infarction in Papua New Guineans. *P N G Med J* 33:275–280.

Kiple, K. F. and K. C. Ornelas. 2000. *The Cambridge World History of Food*. Cambridge, U.K.: Cambridge University Press.

Krebs, J. D., D. Bell, R. Hall et al. 2013. Improvements in glucose metabolism and insulin sensitivity with a low-carbohydrate diet in obese patients with type 2 diabetes. *J Am Coll Nutr* 32:11–17.

Kritchevsky, D., S. A. Tepper, S. K. Czarnecki, D. M. Klurfeld, and J. A. Story. 1981. Experimental atherosclerosis in rabbits fed cholesterol-free diets. Part 9. Beef protein and textured vegetable protein. *Atherosclerosis* 39:169–175.

Kritchevsky, D., S. A. Tepper, and D. M. Klurfeld. 1998. Lectin may contribute to the atherogenicity of peanut oil. *Lipids* 33:821–823.

Ko, I., R. T. Corlett, and R. J. Xu. 1998. Sugar composition of wild fruits in Hong Kong, China. *J Tropic Ecol* 14(3):381–387.

Kuhn, S. L. and M. C. Stiner. 2001. The antiquity of hunter-gatherers. In *Hunter-Gatherers: An Interdisciplinary Perspective*, Eds. C. Panter-Brick, R. H. Layton, and P. Rowley-Conwy, pp. 99–142. Cambridge, U.K.: Cambridge University Press.

Kuipers, R. S., M. F. Luxwolda, D. A. Dijck-Brouwer et al. 2010. Estimated macronutrient and fatty acid intakes from an East African Paleolithic diet. *Br J Nutr* 104:1666–1687.

Kuzma, J. N., G. Cromer, D. K. Hagman et al. 2015. No difference in ad libitum energy intake in healthy men and women consuming beverages sweetened with fructose, glucose, or high-fructose corn syrup: A randomized trial. *Am J Clin Nutr* 102:1373–1380.

Laden, G. and R. Wrangham. 2005. The rise of the hominids as an adaptive shift in fallback foods: Plant underground storage organs (USOs) and australopith origins. *J Hum Evol* 49:482–498.

Lavigne, C., F. Tremblay, G. Asselin, H. Jacques, and A. Marette. 2001. Prevention of skeletal muscle insulin resistance by dietary cod protein in high fat-fed rats. *Am J Physiol Endocrinol Metab* 281:E62–E71.

Lee, R. B. 1968. What hunters do for a living, or, how to make out on scarce resources. In *Man the Hunter*, Eds. R. B. Lee and I. DeVore, pp. 30–48. Chicago, IL: Aldine.

Lee, Y., E. D. Berglund, X. Yu et al. 2014. Hyperglycemia in rodent models of type 2 diabetes requires insulin-resistant alpha cells. *PNAS* 111:13217–13222.

Lemann, J. Jr., J. R. LItzgow, and E. J. Lennon. 1967. Studies of the mechanism by which chronic metabolic acidosis augments urinary calcium excretion in man. *J Clin Invest* 46:1318–1328.

Lennon, E. J. and J. Lemann, Jr. 1968. Influence of diet composition on endogenous fixed acid production. *Am J Clin Nutr* 21:451–456.

Liener, I. E. 1986. Nutritional significance of lectins in the diet. In *The Lectins: Properties, Functions and Applications in Biology and Medicine*, Eds. I. E. Liener, N. Sharon, and I. J. Goldstein, pp. 527–552. New York: Academic Press.

Lindeberg, S. 1994. Apparent absence of cerebrocardiovascular disease in Melanesians. Risk factors and nutritional considerations—The Kitava Study thesis. Lund, Sweden: Lund University.

Lindeberg, S. 2003. Stroke in Papua New Guinea. *Lancet Neurol* 2:273.

Lindeberg, S. 2005. Who wants to be normal? *Eur Heart J* 26:2605–2606.

Lindeberg, S. 2009. Modern human physiology with respect to evolutionary adaptations that relate to diet in the past. In *The Evolution of Hominin Diets: Integrating Approaches to the Study of Palaeolithic Subsistence*, Eds. M. P. Richards and J. J. Hublin, pp. 43–57. Berlin, Germany: Elsevier.

Lindeberg, S. 2010. *Food and Western Disease: Health and Nutrition from an Evolutionary Perspective*. Oxford, U.K.: Wiley-Blackwell.

Lindeberg, S., E. Berntorp, P. Nilsson-Ehle, A. Terent, and Vessby. 1997. Age relations of cardiovascular risk factors in a traditional Melanesian society: The Kitava Study. *Am J Clin Nutr* 66:845–852.

Lindeberg, S., M. Eliasson, B. Lindahl, and B. Ahrén. October 1999. Low serum insulin in traditional Pacific Islanders—The Kitava Study. *Metab Clin Exp* 48(10):1216–1219.

Lindeberg, S., T. Jönsson, Y. Granfeldt, E. Borgstrand, J. Soffman, K. Sjöström, and B. Ahren. 2007. A Palaeolithic diet improves glucose tolerance more than a Mediterranean-like diet in individuals with ischaemic heart disease. *Diabetologia* 50:1795–1807.

Lindeberg, S. and B. Lundh. 1993. Apparent absence of stroke and ischaemic heart disease in a traditional Melanesian island: A clinical study in Kitava. *J Intern Med* 233:269–275.

Lindeberg, S. and B. Vessby. 1995. Fatty acid composition of cholesterol esters and serum tocopherols in Melanesians apparently free from cardiovascular disease—The Kitava study. *Nutr Metab Cardiovasc Dis* 5:45–53.

Liu, X., Y. Fan, and X. Deng. 2011. Effect of the endothelial glycocalyx layer on arterial LDL transport under normal and high pressure. *J Theor Biol* 21:71–81.

Luca, F. G., H. Perry, and A. Di Rienzo. 2010. Evolutionary adaptations to dietary changes. *Annu Rev Nutr* 30: 291–314.

Lucas, P. W., K. Y. Ang, Z. Sui, K. R. Agrawal, J. F. Prinz, and N. J. Dominy. 2006. A brief review of the recent evolution of the human mouth in physiological and nutritional contexts. *Physiol Behav* 89:36–38.

Machin, D. R., W. Park, M. Alkatan, M. Mouton, and H. Tanaka. June 20, 2014. Hypotensive effects of solitary addition of conventional nonfat dairy products to the routine diet: A randomized controlled trial. *Am J Clin Nutr* 100(1):80–87.

Maki, K. C., M. E. Van Elswyk, D. D. Alexander, T. M. Rains, E. L. Sohn, and S. McNeill. 2012. A meta-analysis of randomized controlled trials that compare the lipid effects of beef versus poultry and/or fish consumption. *J Clin Lipidol* 6:352–361.

Manheimer, E. W., E. J. van Zuuren, Z. Fedorowicz, and H. Pijl. 2015. Paleolithic nutrition for metabolic syndrome: Systematic review and meta-analysis. *Am J Clin Nutr* 102:922–932.

Mann, J., R. McLean, M. Skeaff, and L. T. Morenga. 2014. Low carbohydrate diets: Going against the grain. *Lancet* 384:1479–1480.

Mann, N. 2000. Dietary lean red meat and human evolution. *Eur J Nutr* 39:71–79.

Marckmann, P. and M. Gronbaek. 1999. Fish consumption and coronary heart disease mortality. A systematic review of prospective cohort studies. *Eur J Clin Nutr* 53:585–590.

Marlowe, F. W., J. C. Berbesque, B. Wood, A. Crittenden, C. Porter, and A. M. Honey. 2014. Hadza, hunter-gatherers, and human evolution. *J Hum Evol* 71:119–128.

Masharani, U., P. Sherchan, M. Schloetter et al. 2015. Metabolic and physiologic effects from consuming a hunter-gatherer (Paleolithic)-type diet in type 2 diabetes. *Eur J Clin Nutr* 69:944–948.

Mathews, C. L. 1974. Cardiovascular disease in Lac—A five year review. *P N G Med J* 17:251–262.

Mellberg, C., S. Sandberg, M. Ryberg et al. March 2014. Long-term effects of a Palaeolithic-type diet in obese postmenopausal women: A 2-year randomized trial. *Eur J Clin Nutr.* 68(3):350–357.

Melnik, B. C. 2015a. The pathogenic role of persistent milk signaling in mTORC1- and milk-microRNA-driven type 2 diabetes mellitus. *Curr Diabetes Rev* 11:46–62.

Melnik, B. C. 2015b. Milk—A nutrient system of mammalian evolution promoting mTORC1-dependent translation. *Int J Mol Sci* 27:17048–17087.

Mensink, R. P., P. L. Zock, A. D. Kester, and M. B. Katan. 2003. Effects of dietary fatty acids and carbohydrates on the ratio of serum total to HDL cholesterol and on serum lipids and apolipoproteins: A meta-analysis of 60 controlled trials. *Am J Clin Nutr* 77:1146–1155.

Merimee, T. J., D. L. Rimoin, and S. L. Cavalli. 1972. Metabolic studies in the African pygmy. *J Clin Invest* 51:395–401.

Micha, R., S. K. Wallace, and D. Mozaffarian. 2010. Red and processed meat consumption and risk of incident coronary heart disease, stroke, and diabetes mellitus: A systematic review and meta-analysis. *Circulation* 121:2271–2283.

Milan, A., P. Mulatero, F. Rabbia, and F. Veglio. 2002. Salt intake and hypertension therapy. *J Nephrol* 15:1–6.

Milton, K. June 1999. Nutritional characteristics of wild primate foods: Do the diets of our closest living relatives have lessons for us? *Nutrition* 15(6):488–498.

Moss, M. and D. Freed. 2003. The cow and the coronary: Epidemiology, biochemistry and immunology. *Int J Cardiol* 87:203–216.

Mozaffarian, D. 2016. Dietary and policy priorities for cardiovascular disease, diabetes, and obesity. A comprehensive review. *Circulation* 133:187–225.

Muraille, E., B. Pajak, J. Urbain, and O. Leo. 1999. Carbohydrate-bearing cell surface receptors involved in innate immunity: Interleukin-12 induction by mitogenic and nonmitogenic lectins. *Cell Immunol* 10:1–9.

Muwazi, E. 1944. Neurological disease among African natives of Uganda: A review of 269 cases. *East Afr Med J* 21:2–19.

National Food Administration. 1986. *Food Composition Tables*. Uppsala, Sweden: National Food Administration.

Naude, C. E., A. Schoonees, M. Senekal, T. Young, P. Garner, and J. Volmink. 2014. Low carbohydrate versus isoenergetic balanced diets for reducing weight and cardiovascular risk: A systematic review and meta-analysis. *PLoS One* 9:e100652.

Naughton, J. M., K. O'Dea, and A. J. Sinclair. November 1986. Animal foods in traditional Australian aboriginal diets: Polyunsaturated and low in fat. *Lipids* 21(11):684–690.

Ness, A. R., J. Hughes, P. C. Elwood et al. 2002. The long-term effect of dietary advice in men with coronary disease: Follow-up of the Diet And Reinfarction Trial (DART). *Eur J Clin Nutr* 56:512–518.

Nilsson, M., M. Stenberg, A. H. Frid, J. J. Holst, and I. M. Björck. 2004. Glycemia and insulinemia in healthy subjects after lactose-equivalent meals of milk and other food proteins: The role of plasma amino acids and incretins. *Am J Clin Nutr* 80:1246–1253.

Nongonierma, A. B. and R. J. FitzGerald. November 2015. Bioactive properties of milk proteins in humans: A review. *Peptides* 73:20–34.

O'Connell, J. F., P. K. Latz, and P. Barnett. 1983. Traditional and modern plant use among the Alyawara of central Australia. *Econ Bot* 37:80–109.

O'Dea, K. 1984. Marked improvement in carbohydrate and lipid metabolism in diabetic Australian aborigines after temporary reversion to traditional lifestyle. *Diabetes* 33:596–603.

Oliver, W. J., E. L. Cohen, and J. V. Neel. 1975. Blood pressure, sodium intake, and sodium related hormones in the Yanomamo Indians, a "no-salt" culture. *Circulation* 52:146–151.

Otten, J., C. Mellberg, M. Ryberg et al. 2016. Strong and persistent effect on liver fat with a Paleolithic diet during a two-year intervention. *Int J Obes (Lond)* 40:747–753.

Pahwa, R., P. Nallasamy, and I. Jialal. 2016. Toll-like receptors 2 and 4 mediate hyperglycemia induced macrovascular aortic endothelial cell inflammation and perturbation of the endothelial glycocalyx. *J Diab Compl* 30(4):563–572.

Panter-Brick, C., R. H. Layton, and P. Rowley-Conwy. 2001. *Hunter-Gatherers: An Interdisciplinary Perspective*. Cambridge, U.K.: Cambridge University Press.

Park, Y. K. and E. A. Yetley. 1993. Intakes and food sources of fructose in the United States. *Am J Clin Nutr* 58:737S–747S.

Pastore, R. L., J. T. Brooks, and J. W. Carbone. 2015. Paleolithic nutrition improves plasma lipid concentrations of hypercholesterolemic adults to a greater extent than traditional heart-healthy dietary recommendations. *Nutr Res* 35:474–479.

Perantoni, A. O. 1998. Carcinogenesis. In *The Biological Basis of Cancer*, Eds. R. G. McKinnell, R. E. Parchment, A. O. Perantoni, and G. B. Pierce, pp. 79–114. Cambridge, U.K.: Cambridge University Press.

Perry, G. H., N. J. Dominy, K. G. Claw et al. 2007. Diet and the evolution of human amylase gene copy number variation. *Nat Genet* 39:1256–1260.

Praagman, J., O. H. Franco, M. A. Ikram et al. 2015. Dairy products and the risk of stroke and coronary heart disease: The Rotterdam Study. *Eur J Nutr* 54(6):981–990.

Priebe, M. G., J. J. van Binsbergen, R. de Vos, and R. J. Vonk. 2008. Whole grain foods for the prevention of type 2 diabetes mellitus. *Cochrane Database Syst Rev* 23(1):CD006061.

Pruetz, J. D., P. Bertolani, K. Boyer Ontl, S. Lindshield, M. Shelley, and E. G. Wessling. 2015. New evidence on the tool-assisted hunting exhibited by chimpanzees (*Pan troglodytes verus*) in a savannah habitat at Fongoli, Sénégal. *R Soc Open Sci* 2:140507. http://dx.doi.org/10.1098/rsos.140507.

Pusztai, A., S. W. Ewen, G. Grant et al. 1993. Antinutritive effects of wheat-germ agglutinin and other N-acetylglucosamine-specific lectins. *Br J Nutr* 70:313–321.

Pusztai, A., F. Greer, and G. Grant. 1989. Specific uptake of dietary lectins into the systemic circulation of rats. *Biochem Soc Trans* 17:481–482.

Raubenheimer, D., J. M. Rothman, H. Pontzer, and S. J. Simpson. 2014. Macronutrient contributions of insects to the diets of hunteregatherers: A geometric analysis. *J Hum Evol* 71:70–76.

Reaven, G. M. 2005. The insulin resistance syndrome: Definition and dietary approaches to treatment. *Annu Rev Nutr* 25:391–406.

Reitsma, S., M. G. Oude Egbrink, V. V. Heijnen et al. 2011. Endothelial glycocalyx thickness and platelet-vessel wall interactions during atherogenesis. *Thromb Haemost* 106:939–946.

Rice, B. H. 2014. Dairy and cardiovascular disease: A review of recent observational research. *Curr Nutr Rep* 3:130–138.

Richards, M. P. 2002. A brief review of the archaeological evidence for Palaeolithic and Neolithic subsistence. *Eur J Clin Nutr* 56:1270–1279.

Rolls, B. J., A. Drewnowski, and J. H. Ledikwe. 2005. Changing the energy density of the diet as a strategy for weight management. *J Am Diet Assoc* 105:S98–S103.

Rothman, J. M., D. Raubenheimer, M. A. H. Bryer, M. Takahashi, and C. C. Gilbert. June 2014. Nutritional contributions of insects to primate diets: Implications for primate evolution. *J Hum Evol* 71:59–69.

Roussell, M. A., A. M. Hill, T. L. Gaugler et al. 2012. Beef in an optimal lean diet study: Effects on lipids, lipoproteins, and apolipoproteins. *Am J Clin Nutr* 95(1):9–16.

Samaha, F. F., N. Iqbal, P. Seshadri et al. 2003. A low-carbohydrate as compared with a low-fat diet in severe obesity. *N Engl J Med* 348:2074–2081.

Samuelson, L. C., K. Wiebauer, C. M. Snow, and M. H. Meisler. 1990. Retroviral and pseudogene insertion sites reveal the lineage of human salivary and pancreatic amylase genes from a single gene during primate evolution. *Mol Cell Biol* 10:2513–2520.

Sanchez-Lozada, L. G., M. Le, M. Segal, and R. J. Johnson. 2008. How safe is fructose for persons with or without diabetes? *Am J Clin Nutr* 88:1189–1190.

Schaefer, O. 1971. When the Eskimo comes to town. *Nutr Today* 6:8–16.

Schmidt, E. B., H. A. Skou, J. H. Christensen, and J. Dyerberg. 2000. N-3 fatty acids from fish and coronary artery disease: Implications for public health. *Public Health Nutr* 3:91–98.

Schuppan, D. and V. Zevallos. 2015. Wheat amylase trypsin inhibitors as nutritional activators of innate immunity. *Dig Dis* 33:260–263.

Sebastian, A., L. A. Frassetto, D. E. Sellmeyer, R. L. Merriam, and R. C. Morris, Jr. 2002. Estimation of the net acid load of the diet of ancestral preagricultural *Homo sapiens* and their hominid ancestors. *Am J Clin Nutr* 76:1308–1316.

Segall, J. J. 1994. Dietary lactose as a possible risk factor for ischaemic heart disease: Review of epidemiology. *Int J Cardiol* 46:197–207.

Shechter, Y. 1983. Bound lectins that mimic insulin produce persistent insulin-like activities. *Endocrinology* 113:1921–1926.

Sievenpiper, J. L., A. J. Carleton, S. Chatha et al. 2009. Heterogeneous effects of fructose on blood lipids in individuals with type 2 diabetes: Systematic review and meta-analysis of experimental trials in humans. *Diab Care* 32:1930–1937.

Sievenpiper, J. L., R. J. de Souza, A. Mirrahimi et al. 2012. Effect of fructose on body weight in controlled feeding trials: A systematic review and meta-analysis. *Ann Inter Med* 156: 291–304.

Sinnett, P. F. 1977. *The People of Murapin*. Institute of Papua New Guinea Monographs. Oxford, U.K.: EW Classey.

Smith, E. O. 1999. Evolution, substance abuse, and addiction. In *Evolutionary Medicine*, Eds. W. R. Trevathan, E. O. Smith, and J. J. McKenna, pp. 375–405. Oxford, U.K.: Oxford University Press.

Soares, F. L. P., R. de Oliveira Matoso, L. G. Teixeira et al. 2013. Gluten-free diet reduces adiposity, inflammation and insulin resistance associated with the induction of PPAR-alpha and PPAR-gamma expression. *J Nutr Biochem* 24:1105–1111.

Sodhi, A. and V. Kesherwani. 2007. Production of TNF-alpha, IL-1beta, IL-12 and IFN-gamma in murine peritoneal macrophages on treatment with wheat germ agglutinin in vitro: Involvement of tyrosine kinase pathways. *Glycoconj J* 24:573–582.

Soedamah-Muthu, S. S., E. L. Ding, W. K. Al-Delaimy et al. January 2011. Milk and dairy consumption and incidence of cardiovascular diseases and all-cause mortality: Dose-response meta-analysis of prospective cohort studies. *Am J Clin Nutr* 93(1):158–171.

Somers, K. 1974. Cardiology in Papua New Guinea. *P N G Med J* 17:235–241.

Spielman, R. S., S. S. Fajans, J. V. Neel et al. 1982. Glucose tolerance in two unacculturated Indian tribes of Brazil. *Diabetologia* 23:90–93.

Spreadbury, I. 2012. Comparison with ancestral diets suggests dense acellular carbohydrates promote an in ammatory microbiota, and may be the primary dietary cause of leptin resistance and obesity. *Diab Metabol Syndr Obes* 5:175–189.

Stanford, C. G. 1999. *The Hunting Apes. Meat Eating and the Origins of Human Behaviour*. Princeton: Princeton University Press.

Statens, L. 2012. Riksmaten—vuxna 2010–11. *Livsmedels-och näringsintag bland vuxna i Sverige [In Swedish]*. Uppsala, Sweden.

Straub, R. H. 2014. Interaction of the endocrine system with inflammation: A function of energy and volume regulation. *Arthritis Res Ther* 13:203.

Tay, J., C. H. Thompson, N. D. Luscombe-Marsh et al. 2015. Long-term effects of a very low carbohydrate compared with a high carbohydrate diet on renal function in individuals with type 2 diabetes: A randomized trial. *Medicine (Baltimore)* 94:e2181.

Terashima, H. and M. Ichikawa. 2003. A comparative ethnobotany of the Mbuti and Efe hunter-gatherers in the Ituri forest, Democratic Republic of Congo. *Afr Study Monogr* 24:1–168.

Termote, C. and P. van Damme. 2010. Eating from the wild: Turumbu indigenous knowledge on noncultivated edible plants, Tshopo District, DRCongo. *Ecol Food Nutr* 49:173–207.

Thomas, W., J. Davies, I. R. O'Nea, and A. Dimakulangan. 1960. Incidence of myocardial infarction correlated with venous and pulmonary thrombosis and embolism. A geographic study based on autopsies in Uganda, East Africa and St Louis, USA. *Am J Cardiol* 5:41–47.

Tovar, A. R. and N. Torres. 2010. The role of dietary protein on lipotoxicity. *Biochim Biophys Acta* 1801:367–371.

Tovar, A. R., I. Torre-Villalvazo, M. Ochoa et al. 2005. Soy protein reduces hepatic lipotoxicity in hyperinsulinemic obese Zucker fa/fa rats. *J Lipid Res* 46:1823–1832.

Trowell, H. C. 1960. *Non-Infective Diseases in Africa*. London, U.K.: Edward Arnold.

Trowell, H. C. and D. P. Burkitt (Eds.). 1981. *Western Diseases: Their Emergence and Prevention*. Cambridge, MA: Harvard University Press.

Truswell, A. S. and J. D. L. Hansen. 1976. Medical research among the !Kung. In *Kalahari Hunter-Gatherers*, Eds. R. B. Lee and I. DeVore, pp. 166–195. Cambridge, MA: Harvard University Press.

Turner, K. M., J. B. Keogh, and P. M. Clifton. January 2015a. Dairy consumption and insulin sensitivity: A systematic review of short- and long-term intervention studies. *Nutr Metab Cardiovasc Dis* 25(1):3–8.

Turner, K. M., J. B. Keogh, and P. M. Clifton. June 2015b. Red meat, dairy, and insulin sensitivity: A randomized crossover intervention study. *Am J Clin Nutr* 101(6):1173–1179.

Ulijaszek, S. J. and S. S. Strickland. 1993. *Nutritional Anthropology: Prospects and Perspectives*. London, U.K.: Smith-Gordon.

Ungar, P. S. (Ed.) 2007. *Evolution of the Human Diet: The Known, the Unknown, and the Unknowable*. New York: Oxford University Press.

Unger, R. H. and P. E. Scherer. 2010. Gluttony, sloth and the metabolic syndrome: A roadmap to lipotoxicity. *Trends Endocrinol Metab* 21:345–352.

Unitt, J. and D. Hornigold. 2011. Plant lectins are novel Toll-like receptor agonists. *Biochem Pharmacol* 81:1324–1328.

U.S. Department of Agriculture, Agricultural Research Service, Beltsville Human Nutrition Research Center, Food Surveys Research Group. Beltsville, Maryland, Food Patterns Equivalents Databases and Datasets. Available at: http://www.ars.usda.gov/nea/bhnrc/fsrg. Accessed July 21, 2017.

Van Damme, E. J. M., W. J. Peumans, A. Pusztai, and S. Bardocz (Eds.). 1998. *Handbook of Plant Lectins: Properties and Biomedical Applications*. New York: John Wiley.

Wang, Q., L. G. Yu, B. J. Campbell, J. D. Milton, and J. M. Rhodes. 1998. Identification of intact peanut lectin in peripheral venous blood. *Lancet* 352:1831–1832.

Wang, X. Y., K. Bergdahl, A. Heijbel, C. Liljebris, and J. E. Bleasdale. 2001. Analysis of in vitro interactions of protein tyrosine phosphatase 1B with insulin receptors. *Mol Cell Endocrinol* 173:109–120.

Wilson, T. A., R. J. Nicolosi, M. J. Marchello, and D. Kritchevsky. 2000. Consumption of ground bison does not increase early atherosclerosis development in hypercholesterolemic hamsters. *Nutr Res* 20:707–719.

Wrangham, R. and N. Conklin-Brittain. 2003. Cooking as a biological trait. *Comp Biochem Physiol A Mol Integr Physiol* 136:35–46.

Wyness, L. 2016. The role of red meat in the diet: Nutrition and health benefits *Proceedings of the Nutrition Society* 75(3):227–232.

Wyness, L., E. Weichselbaum, A. O'Connor et al. 2011. Red meat in the diet: An update. *Nutr Bull* 16:34–77.

Wynne-Edwards, K. E. 2001. Evolutionary biology of plant defenses against herbivory and their predictive implications for endocrine disruptor susceptibility in vertebrates. *Environ Health Perspect* 109:443–448.

Xu, J.-Y., L.-Q. Qin, P.-Y. Wang, W. Li, and C. Chang. October 2008. Effect of milk tripeptides on blood pressure: A meta-analysis of randomized controlled trials. *Nutrition* 24(10):933–940.

Yevdokimova, N. Y. and A. S. Yefimov. 2001. Effects of wheat germ agglutinin and con- canavalin A on the accumulation of glycosaminoglycans in pericellular matrix of human dermal fibroblasts. A comparison with insulin. *Acta Biochim Pol* 48:563–572.

Yusuf, S., S. Reddy, S. Ôunpuu, and S. Anand 2001. Global burden of cardiovascular diseases part II: Variations in cardiovascular disease by specific ethnic groups and geographic regions and prevention strategies. *Circulation* 104:2855–2864.

Zhao, G., S. Guo, M. Somel, and P. Khaitovich. 2014. Evolution of human longevity uncoupled from caloric restriction mechanisms. *PLoS One* 9(1):e84117.

Zink, K. D. and D. E. Lieberman. 2016. Impact of meat and Lower Palaeolithic food processing techniques on chewing in humans. *Nature* 531(7595):500–503.

Zohary, D. and M. Hopf. 1973. Domestication of pulses in the Old World: Legumes were companions of wheat and barley when agriculture began in the Near East. *Science* 182:887–894.

27 Fasting Intermittently or Altering Meal Frequency

Effects on Plasma Lipids

John F. Trepanowski and Krista A. Varady

CONTENTS

ABSTRACT

In this systematic review, we examined whether plasma lipids are improved by intermittent fasting (5:2 diet, modified alternate day fasting) or high meal frequency dietary patterns. We found that intermittent fasting is effective at reducing plasma triglycerides and that this effect may be secondary to weight loss. Intermittent fasting is not effective for modulating LDL-cholesterol or HDL-cholesterol. High meal frequency (at a minimum of 9 meals/day) decreases LDL-cholesterol, but plasma triglycerides and HDL-cholesterol are unaffected by this type of dietary pattern.

INTRODUCTION

A high LDL-cholesterol concentration is known to increase the risk of coronary heart disease (Lewington et al. 2007). More controversially, a high triacylglycerol concentration is believed by some scientists and clinicians to do the same (Nordestgaard and Varbo 2014). Treating these lipid abnormalities with statins and fibrates has been shown to reduce coronary heart disease risk (Jun et al. 2010, Mihaylova et al. 2012).

Intermittent fasting (IF) and high meal frequency (HMF) have recently emerged as two novel dietary patterns for improving plasma lipids (Table 27.1). Intermittent fasting alternates between a period of unrestricted food intake and a period of either substantial energy restriction (e.g., energy intake at 25% of energy needs) or no food intake at all. For example, "strict" alternate day fasting (ADSF) alternates between a "feast day" of unrestricted intake and a "fast day" in which no food is consumed (Heilbronn et al. 2005b). Modified ADF (ADMF) which allows for the consumption of one small meal equivalent to 25% of energy needs on the fast day, is an alternative to strict ADF (Varady et al. 2011a). To date, plasma lipids have been measured in studies of ADMF but not in studies of strict ADF. Another example of IF is the 5:2 diet, which consists of 5 consecutive days of

TABLE 27.1
Intermittent Fasting and High Meal Frequency Dietary Patterns

Dietary Pattern	Description
Intermittent fasting (IF)	Alternates between unrestricted food intake and substantial energy restriction or no food intake
Intermittent fasting 2 out of 7 days (IF2-5)	Alternates between 5 consecutive days of unrestricted intake and 2 consecutive days consuming 25% of energy needs
Modified alternate day fasting (ADMF)	Alternates between a day of unrestricted intake, and consumption of one small meal (25% of energy needs) on the fast day
Strict alternate day fasting (ADSF)	Alternates between a day of unrestricted intake and a day in which no food is consumed
High meal frequency	5 or 6 times/day
Very high meal frequency	>10 times/day

unrestricted intake alternated with 2 consecutive days of consuming 25% of energy needs (Harvie et al. 2011). With one exception (Soeters et al. 2009), each of the IF studies reviewed in this chapter aimed for weight loss. The putative mechanisms by which IF may improve cardiometabolic health have been reviewed recently (Horne et al. 2015). These include increased fat utilization for energy (Duan et al. 2003), a hormetic response to the stress imposed by fasting (Anson et al. 2003), and improved glucose homeostasis via activation of Forkhead Box A genes (Panowski et al. 2007).

While no universally agreed-upon definition of HMF currently exists, studies often have examined increasing meal frequency to 5 or 6 eating episodes per day although some investigations have studied 12 or even 17 eating episodes per day (Jenkins et al. 1989, Murphy et al. 1996). Studies of HMF have most commonly had a short duration, lasting anywhere between 12 hours and 4 weeks. Each of these studies prescribed energy intake for weight maintenance. In contrast, a study lasting 24 weeks and another lasting 52 weeks prescribed energy intake for weight loss (Poston et al. 2005, Bertéus et al. 2008). The main mechanism by which HMF may improve cardiometabolic health is through decreased insulin secretion, both in response to each meal and overall (Heden et al. 2013). However, HMF combined with positive energy balance has been shown to increase abdominal fat and intrahepatic triglyceride content, and to impair insulin-mediated suppression of endogenous glucose production and free fatty acids from adipose tissue (Koopman et al. 2014).

The purpose of this chapter is to review the effects of IF and HMF on plasma lipids. Additionally, this chapter reviews the putative lipid-lowering mechanisms that have been examined in trials of IF or HMF. These include weight loss, augmented insulin sensitivity, augmented fat oxidation, and delayed gastric emptying.

METHODS

For a study to have been included in this review, it must have been a randomized controlled trial enrolling human participants that measured at least one of the following as a primary outcome: body weight, plasma lipids, energy intake, energy expenditure, appetitive hormones, glucose or insulin, macronutrient oxidation, gastric emptying, or lipogenesis. These outcomes were chosen because they all relate to body weight or plasma lipids. Investigations that enrolled participants with diabetes were excluded, because diabetics experience unique plasma lipid responses when compared to nondiabetics (Rivellese et al. 2004). For the studies of IF, prescribed energy intake during the feast period must have been ≥100% of needs, and prescribed energy intake during the fast period must have been ≤25% of needs. For the studies of HMF, the difference in meal frequency between the intervention group and the control group must have been ≥2. No restrictions were placed on study duration or date of publication.

On March 5, 2015, a Pubmed search was conducted. The following input was used for the studies of IF: "alternate day fasting" or "caloric restriction" or "calorie restriction" or "intermittent calorie restriction" or "intermittent fasting." Limitations were set to include only randomized controlled trials published in the English language that enrolled adults. There were 470 potentially relevant publications identified through this search. Six publications were included after applying the inclusion and exclusion criteria mentioned earlier. An additional seven publications were identified using the references listed in these manuscripts. For the studies of HMF, the following input was used: "eating frequency" or "eating pattern" or "feeding frequency" or "feeding pattern" or "gorging" or "grazing" or "meal frequency" or "meal pattern" or "nibbling" or "snack." The same limitations as listed earlier were applied in this search. There were 365 potentially relevant publications discovered through this search. Nine publications were included after applying the inclusion and exclusion criteria. An additional eight publications were identified using the references listed in these manuscripts.

RESULTS

Effects of Intermittent Fasting on Plasma Lipids

Consistent across studies, HDL-cholesterol did not change in response to IF (Table 27.2). The findings regarding the effects of IF on other plasma lipids were heterogeneous. With the exception of one study that found a reduction in LDL-cholesterol (Varady et al. 2011a), the studies that compared IF to a negative control group that did not receive any intervention (dietary or otherwise) reported no change in any plasma lipid (Varady et al. 2011a, 2013, Bhutani et al. 2013, Hoddy et al. 2014). In contrast, the studies that did not include a negative control group found reductions in LDL-cholesterol and/or plasma triglycerides, compared to baseline plasma lipids (Harvie et al. 2011, 2013, Klempel et al. 2013b). Only one study to date has compared ADMF regimens with different macronutrient compositions. This study found that a low-fat (25% of energy) and a high-fat (45% of energy) ADMF regimen reduced LDL-cholesterol (25% and 15%, respectively) and plasma triglycerides (14% in both groups) similarly (Klempel et al. 2013b). In the absence of weight loss, fasting increases LDL-cholesterol and HDL-cholesterol, and decreases plasma triglycerides (Sävendahl and Underwood 1999, Horne et al. 2013, 2014). Studies have consistently found that ADMF improves LDL particle size (Varady et al. 2011a,b, 2013, Klempel et al. 2013a, Hoddy et al. 2014).

Mechanisms for Modulation of Plasma Lipids due to Intermittent Fasting

Weight loss is known to lower plasma triglycerides and LDL-cholesterol while increasing HDL-cholesterol (Dattilo and Kris-Etherton 1992). As shown in Table 27.2, IF consistently reduces body weight in individuals seeking weight loss. It appears that individuals do not "binge" on feast days to compensate for the large energy deficit incurred on the fast days, at least in the short term (Johnstone et al. 2002, Klempel et al. 2010, Levitsky and DeRosimo 2010), and this may partially explain why IF is successful at reducing body weight. Levels of the orexigenic hormone ghrelin do not change in response to IF (Heilbronn et al. 2005a, Harvie et al. 2011), and no other appetite hormone has been measured in IF studies to date.

Improved insulin sensitivity during weight loss is associated with improvement in plasma triglycerides (McLaughlin et al. 2001), but recent evidence suggests that alterations in nutrient flux to the liver play a more important role than alterations in insulin signaling (Otero et al. 2014) in mediating this effect. The effectiveness of IF for improving insulin sensitivity remains an open question. Only one randomized controlled trial has investigated the effect of IF on insulin sensitivity under a condition of weight maintenance (Soeters et al. 2009). This trial compared consuming 3 meals/day to an IF regimen in which participants abstained from energy intake every second day for 20 hours.

TABLE 27.2
Intermittent Fasting: Effects on Body Weight and Plasma Lipids

Reference	Subjects	Trial Length (Weeks)	Dietary Regimen	Selection of Meals	Comparison Group	Body Weight Change (%)	Total Chol. Change (%)	LDL-Chol. Change (%)	HDL-Chol. Change (%)	Triglyceride Change (%)
Bhutani et al. (2013)	n = 16, MF Age 42 ± 2 BMI 35 ± 1	12	ADMF: lunch	Fast-day meal prepared	No-intervention control	↓6	0	0	0	0
Harvie et al. (2011)	n = 42, F Age 40 ± 4 BMI 31 ± 5	24	5:2 diet	Self-selected	CR (isocaloric comparison)	↓7	↓6	↓10	0	↓17
Harvie et al. (2013)	n = 75, F Age 47 ± 1 BMI 30 ± 1	12	5:2 diet 5:2 + PF	Self-selected	CR (isocaloric comparison)	↓6 ↓6	↓5 ↓4	↓4 ↓3	0 0	↓14 ↓12
Hoddy et al. (2014)	n = 74, MF Age 45 ± 3 BMI 34 ± 1	8	ADMF: lunch ADMF: dinner ADMF: small meals	Fast-day meal prepared	Each other ADF group (isocaloric comparisons)	↓4 ↓4 ↓5	0 0 0	0 0 0	0 0 0	0 0 0
Klempel et al. (2013b)	n = 32, F Age 43 ± 3 BMI 35 ± 1	8	ADMF: high fat ADMF: low fat	All meals prepared	The other ADF group (isocaloric comparison)	↓5 ↓4	↓13 ↓16	↓18 ↓25	0 0	↓14 ↓14
Varady et al. (2011a)	n = 13, MF Age 47 ± 2 BMI 32 ± 2	12	ADMF: lunch	Fast-day meal prepared	No-intervention control	↓5	0	↓10	0	↓17
Varady et al. (2013)	n = 15, MF Age 47 ± 3 BMI 26 ± 1	12	ADMF: lunch	Fast-day meal prepared	No-intervention control	↓7	0	0	0	↓20
					Mean change:	↓6	↓4	↓6	0	↓12

Notes: ADMF, modified alternate day fasting; BMI, body mass index (kg/m^2); CR, daily calorie restriction (25%); F, female; M, male; PF, *ad libitum* protein and fat intake. Within-group differences are reported so that across-study comparisons can be made.

Energy intake, macronutrient intake, and types of food consumed were matched between conditions, and participants were provided amounts of food that were titrated to prevent weight change. Each dietary assignment lasted 2 weeks in a crossover design. Glucose uptake as measured by the euglycemic hyperinsulinemic clamp was not different between the dietary groups (Soeters et al. 2009). In studies that examined IF with weight loss, ADF did not reduce the homeostasis model assessment of insulin resistance (HOMA-IR) within group (Bhutani et al. 2013, Hoddy et al. 2014), while there was a within-group reduction in HOMA-IR in response to the 5:2 diet (Harvie et al. 2011, 2013). The studies of the 5:2 diet may have found a statistically significant reduction in HOMA-IR because they had approximately twice the sample size compared to the ADF studies. Insulin sensitivity measured during an oral glucose tolerance test worsened in female participants but improved in male participants in response to ADF (Heilbronn et al. 2005a). More favorable changes in insulin sensitivity in males versus females have also been observed in mice from the Balb/c, C57Bl/6J, and C3HJ strains (Arum et al. 2009). The reason for this sexual dimorphism is presently unknown but may be due to genotype-specific effects of IF (Goodrick et al. 1990).

Impaired fat oxidation is associated with an atherogenic lipoprotein phenotype (Faghihnia et al. 2011). One mediator of this association may be insulin resistance, as impaired fat oxidation may lead to increased intracellular (particularly intramyocellular) lipids that interfere with insulin signaling (Shulman 2000). Weight loss increases resting fat oxidation in some (Corpeleijn et al. 2008) but not all studies (Kelley et al. 1999, Blaak et al. 2001). The magnitude of total fat mass and visceral fat mass reduction may determine, in part, whether weight loss leads to increased fat oxidation (Siri-Tarino et al. 2011). Fat oxidation does not appear to change in response to IF without weight loss (Soeters et al. 2009), but does increase in response to IF with weight loss (Heilbronn et al. 2005b).

Effects of High Meal Frequency on Plasma Lipids

HMF has been tested both in short-term (≤3 days) controlled dietary conditions where meals were provided, as well as in longer-term (≥2 weeks) free-living conditions. The short-term studies have generally found that HMF does not favorably modulate plasma lipids compared to consuming 3 meals/day (Table 27.3). Two studies found no difference in the plasma triglyceride area under the curve between the HMF condition and the control condition (Schlierf and Raetzer 1972, Munsters and Saris 2012), and a third study found that the plasma triglyceride area under the curve was elevated in the HMF condition (Heden et al. 2013). Two studies found no difference in the total cholesterol area under the curve between the HMF condition and the control condition (Jones et al. 1993, Heden et al. 2013), while a third study found a lower mean level of total cholesterol in the HMF condition (Wolever 1990). The only study to measure postprandial LDL-cholesterol or HDL-cholesterol found no difference for either parameter in the incremental area under the curve between the HMF and control conditions (Heden et al. 2013). No study to our knowledge has examined the effects of HMF on LDL particle size.

The longer duration studies have generally found that HMF does not favorably affect HDL-cholesterol (Jenkins et al. 1989, Arnold et al. 1993, 1994, McGrath and Gibney 1994, Murphy et al. 1996, King and Gibney 1999, Poston et al. 2005, Bertéus et al. 2008) or plasma triglycerides in the absence of weight loss (Jenkins et al. 1989, Arnold et al. 1993, 1994, McGrath and Gibney 1994, Murphy et al. 1996, King and Gibney 1999, Poston et al. 2005) (Table 27.4). Some studies have reported reductions in total cholesterol and LDL-cholesterol (Jenkins et al. 1989, Arnold et al. 1993, McGrath and Gibney 1994, Poston et al. 2005), while other studies have reported no change in these parameters (Arnold et al. 1994, Murphy et al. 1996, King and Gibney 1999, Bertéus et al. 2008). A comparison of the studies that did or did not observe a reduction in LDL-cholesterol suggests that meal frequency may need to be changed dramatically in order for LDL-cholesterol to be reduced. Two of the studies that reported an LDL-cholesterol reduction in the absence of a change in body weight compared either a 9 meals/day diet or a 17 meals/day diet to a 3 meals/day diet

TABLE 27.3
High Meal Frequency, Short-Term Feeding: Effects on Plasma Lipids

Reference	Subjects	Trial Design	Trial Length	Dietary Regimen	Effects on Blood Lipids
Heden et al. (2013)	n = 8, F Age 39 ± 3 BMI 35 ± 1	Counterbalanced crossover	12 hours	6 meals/day	Plasma triglyceride incremental area under the curve over 12 hours was elevated in the 6 meals/day condition. The incremental areas under the curve for total cholesterol, LDL-cholesterol, and HDL-cholesterol were not different, regardless of whether energy was consumed over 3 or 6 meals.
Jones et al. (1993)	n = 6, M Age 31 ± 2 BMI 23	Parallel-arm	3 days	6 meals/day	Total cholesterol decreased similarly, regardless of whether energy was consumed over 3 or 6 meals.
Munsters and Saris (2012)	n = 12, M Age 23 ± 1 BMI 22 ± 1	Counterbalanced crossover	36 hours	14 meals/day	Plasma triglyceride area under the curve over 24 hours was similar, regardless of whether energy was consumed over 3 or 14 meals.
Schlierf and Raetzer (1972)	n = 12, MF Age 35 BMI 25	Counterbalanced crossover	24 hours	6 meals/day	In patients with normotriglyceridemia and in patients with hypertriglyceridemia, plasma triglyceride area under the curve was not different, regardless of whether energy was consumed over 3 or 6 meals.
Wolever (1990)	n = 7, M Age 23 ± 2 BMI unknown	Counterbalanced crossover	12 hours	Continuous feeding	Mean total cholesterol was lower under the continuous feeding condition relative to the 3 meals/day condition.

Notes: BMI, Body mass index (kg/m^2); F, Female; M, Male. Participants were provided all meals in each study. The control regimen was 3 meals/day in each study.

(Jenkins et al. 1989, Arnold et al. 1993). The other study that reported an LDL-cholesterol reduction in the absence of a change in body weight examined a 6 meals/day diet, but the comparison group decreased their meal frequency from a baseline of 6 to 3 meals/day during the intervention (McGrath and Gibney 1994).

Mechanisms for Modulation of Plasma Lipids due to High Meal Frequency

Observational studies have often found that HMF is associated with lower body weight (Fabry et al. 1964, Metzner et al. 1977, Ruidavets et al. 2002, Ma et al. 2003). However, a recent meta-analysis of randomized controlled trials found that meal frequency was not associated with weight loss (Schoenfeld, Aragon, and Krieger 2015). Therefore, the effects of HMF on plasma lipids are unlikely to be related to changes in body weight.

TABLE 27.4
High Meal Frequency, Longer-Term Feeding: Effects on Body Weight and Plasma Lipids

Reference	Subjects	Trial Length	Dietary Regimen (Meals/Day)	Selection of Meals	Body Weight Change (%)	Total Chol. Change (%)	LDL-Chol. Change (%)	HDL-Chol. Change (%)	Triglyceride Change (%)
Arnold et al. (1993)	n = 19, MF Age 32 ± 2 BMI 23 ± 1	2 weeks	9	Self-selected	0	↓10	↓14	↓3	0
Arnold et al. (1994)	n = 16, MF Age 50 ± 2 BMI 27 ± 1	4 weeks	9	Self-selected	0	0	0	0	0
Bertéus et al. (2008)	n = 70, MF Age 40 ± 1 BMI 38 ± 1	52 weeks	6	Self-selected	↓5	0	0	0	↓14
Jenkins et al. (1989)	n = 7, M Age 40 Bodyweight 70 ± 3	2 weeks	17	Prepared	0	↓9	↓14	0	0
King and Gibney (1999)	n = 20, M Age 48 ± 2 BMI 26 ± 1	4 weeks	6	Self-selected	0	0	0	0	0
McGrath and Gibney (1994)	n = 23, M Age 50 ± 2 BMI 24 ± 1	Not stated	6	Self-selected	0	↓8	↓12	0	0
Murphy et al. (1996)	n = 11, F Age 22 ± 1 BMI 24	2 weeks	12	Prepared	0	0	0	↓9	0
Poston et al. (2005)	n = 50, MF Age 40 ± 1 BMI 32 ± 1	24 weeks	6	Self-selected	↓5	↓4	↓5	0	0
				Mean change:	↓1	↓4	↓6	↓2	↓2

Notes: BMI, Body mass index (kg/m²); F, Female; M, Male. The control regimen was 3 meals/day in each study. The experimental and control regimens were isocaloric in each study, with one exception: Poston et al. compared 3 meal replacements/day with 3 meal replacements/day plus 3 snacks/day.

Robust measurements of insulin sensitivity in response to HMF are presently lacking. A few studies have found that fasting insulin, the major determinant of HOMA-IR (Abbasi et al. 2014), does not change in response to HMF (Finkelstein and Fryer 1971, Poston et al. 2005, Bertéus et al. 2008). On the other hand, HMF reduces the incremental area under the curve for insulin when assessed for 12 hours. This may explain why there is a decrease in cholesterol synthesis (measured by the deuterium-uptake method) under HMF (Jones, Leitch, and Pederson 1993). Indeed, insulin secretion is known to upregulate enzymes involved in cholesterol synthesis (Bhutani and Varady 2009).

Insulin also decreases the rate of fat oxidation in muscle and liver (Dimitriadis et al. 2011), and therefore HMF has been hypothesized to increase fat oxidation by reducing day-long insulin secretion (Allirot et al. 2013). However, both short-duration (≤36 hours) and long-duration (≥4 weeks) studies have found that fat oxidation does not change with HMF (Bortz et al. 1966, Verboeket-Van De Venne and Westerterp 1993, Munsters and Saris 2012, Allirot et al. 2013, 2014).

Delayed gastric emptying is known to improve plasma lipids (Meier et al. 2006). HMF has been shown to delay gastric emptying (Jackson et al. 2007), but plasma lipids were not measured in this trial.

SUMMARY AND CONCLUSION

Intermittent fasting appears to be effective at reducing plasma triglycerides, and this is likely a consequence of body weight reduction. LDL-cholesterol and HDL-cholesterol do not appear to be affected by IF. No study to date has examined the effect of IF on plasma lipids in the absence of change in body weight. This is an interesting area for future research.

Most of the studies that have examined short-duration HMF have found no favorable changes in plasma lipids. The long-duration studies suggest that LDL-cholesterol is reduced only when a dramatic change in meal frequency is made (e.g., switching from 3 to 9 meals/day). Diets with high meal frequency do not affect body weight, consistent with their lack of effect on plasma triglycerides or HDL-cholesterol.

ACKNOWLEDGMENT

Departmental grant from Kinesiology and Nutrition, University of Illinois, Chicago.

CONFLICTS OF INTEREST

The authors have no conflicts of interest to report.

REFERENCES

Abbasi, F., Q.D. Okeke, and G.M. Reaven. 2014. Evaluation of fasting plasma insulin concentration as an estimate of insulin action in nondiabetic individuals: Comparison with the homeostasis model assessment of insulin resistance (HOMA-IR). *Acta Diabetol* 51 (2):193–197.

Allirot, X., L. Saulais, K. Seyssel, J. Graeppi-Dulac, H. Roth, A. Charrié, J. Drai, J. Goudable, E. Blond, and E. Disse. 2013. An isocaloric increase of eating episodes in the morning contributes to decrease energy intake at lunch in lean men. *Physiol Behav* 110:169–178.

Allirot, X., K. Seyssel, L. Saulais, H. Roth, A. Charrié, J. Drai, J. Goudable, E. Blond, E. Disse, and M. Laville. 2014. Effects of a breakfast spread out over time on the food intake at lunch and the hormonal responses in obese men. *Physiol Behav* 127:37–44.

Anson, R.M., Z. Guo, R. de Cabo, T. Iyun, M. Rios, A. Hagepanos, D.K. Ingram, M.A. Lane, and M.P. Mattson. 2003. Intermittent fasting dissociates beneficial effects of dietary restriction on glucose metabolism and neuronal resistance to injury from calorie intake. *Proc Natl Acad Sci USA* 100 (10):6216–6220.

Arnold, L., M. Ball, and J. Mann. 1994. Metabolic effects of alterations in meal frequency in hypercholesterolaemic individuals. *Atherosclerosis* 108 (2):167–174.

Arnold, L.M., M.J. Ball, A.W. Duncan, and J. Mann. 1993. Effect of isoenergetic intake of three or nine meals on plasma lipoproteins and glucose metabolism. *Am J Clin Nutr* 57 (3):446–451.

Arum, O., M.S. Bonkowski, J.S. Rocha, and A. Bartke. 2009. The growth hormone receptor gene-disrupted mouse fails to respond to an intermittent fasting diet. *Aging Cell* 8 (6):756–760.

Bertéus, F.H., S. Klingström, H. Hagberg, M. Löndahl, J.S. Torgerson, and A.-K. Lindroos. 2008. Should snacks be recommended in obesity treatment? A 1-year randomized clinical trial. *Eur J Clin Nutr* 62 (11):1308–1317.

Bhutani, S., M.C. Klempel, C.M. Kroeger, J.F. Trepanowski, and K.A. Varady. 2013. Alternate day fasting and endurance exercise combine to reduce body weight and favorably alter plasma lipids in obese humans. *Obesity (Silver Spring)* 21 (7):1370–1379.

Bhutani, S. and K.A. Varady. 2009. Nibbling versus feasting: Which meal pattern is better for heart disease prevention? *Nutr Rev* 67 (10):591–598.

Blaak, E.E., B.H.R. Wolffenbuttel, W.H.M. Saris, M.M.A.L. Pelsers, and A.J.M. Wagenmakers. 2001. Weight reduction and the impaired plasma-derived free fatty acid oxidation in type 2 diabetic subjects 1. *J Clin Endocrinol Metab* 86 (4):1638–1644.

Bortz, W.M., A. Wroldsen, B. Issekutz, Jr, and K. Rodahl. 1966. Weight loss and frequency of feeding. *N Engl J Med* 274 (7):376–379.

Corpeleijn, E., M. Mensink, M.E. Kooi, P.M. Roekaerts, W.H. Saris, and E.E. Blaak. 2008. Impaired skeletal muscle substrate oxidation in glucose-intolerant men improves after weight loss. *Obesity (Silver Spring)* 16 (5):1025–1032.

Dattilo, A.M. and P.M. Kris-Etherton. 1992. Effects of weight reduction on blood lipids and lipoproteins: A meta-analysis. *Am J Clin Nutr* 56 (2):320–328.

Dimitriadis, G., P. Mitrou, V. Lambadiari, E. Maratou, and S.A. Raptis. 2011. Insulin effects in muscle and adipose tissue. *Diabetes Res Clin Pract* 93:S52–S59.

Duan, W., Z. Guo, H. Jiang, M. Ware, and M.P. Mattson. 2003. Reversal of behavioral and metabolic abnormalities, and insulin resistance syndrome, by dietary restriction in mice deficient in brain-derived neurotrophic factor. *Endocrinology* 144 (6):2446–2453.

Fabry, P., Z. Hejl, J. Fodor, T. Braun, and K. Zvolánková. 1964. The frequency of meals its relation to overweight, hypercholesterolaemia, and decreased glucose-tolerance. *Lancet* 284 (7360):614–615.

Faghihnia, N., P.W. Siri-Tarino, R.M. Krauss, and G.A. Brooks. 2011. Energy substrate partitioning and efficiency in individuals with atherogenic lipoprotein phenotype. *Obesity (Silver Spring)* 19 (7):1360–1365.

Finkelstein, B. and B.A. Fryer. 1971. Meal frequency and weight reduction of young women. *Am J Clin Nutr* 24 (4):465–468.

Goodrick, C.L., D.K. Ingram, M.A. Reynolds, J.R. Freeman, and N. Cider. 1990. Effects of intermittent feeding upon body weight and lifespan in inbred mice: Interaction of genotype and age. *Mech Ageing Dev* 55 (1):69–87.

Harvie, M., C. Wright, M. Pegington, D. McMullan, E. Mitchell, B. Martin, R.G. Cutler, G. Evans, S. Whiteside, and S. Maudsley. 2013. The effect of intermittent energy and carbohydrate restriction v. daily energy restriction on weight loss and metabolic disease risk markers in overweight women. *Brit J Nutr* 110 (8):1534–1547.

Harvie, M.N., M. Pegington, M.P. Mattson, J. Frystyk, B. Dillon, G. Evans, J. Cuzick et al. 2011. The effects of intermittent or continuous energy restriction on weight loss and metabolic disease risk markers: A randomized trial in young overweight women. *Int J Obes (Lond)* 35 (5):714–727.

Heden, T.D., Y. Liu, L.J. Sims, A.T. Whaley-Connell, A. Chockalingam, K.C. Dellsperger, and J.A. Kanaley. 2013. Meal frequency differentially alters postprandial triacylglycerol and insulin concentrations in obese women. *Obesity (Silver Spring)* 21 (1):123–129.

Heilbronn, L.K., A.E. Civitarese, I. Bogacka, S.R. Smith, M. Hulver, and E. Ravussin. 2005a. Glucose tolerance and skeletal muscle gene expression in response to alternate day fasting. *Obes Res* 13 (3):574–581.

Heilbronn, L.K., S.R. Smith, C.K. Martin, S.D. Anton, and E. Ravussin. 2005b. Alternate-day fasting in nonobese subjects: Effects on body weight, body composition, and energy metabolism. *Am J Clin Nutr* 81 (1):69–73.

Hoddy, K.K., C.M. Kroeger, J.F. Trepanowski, A. Barnosky, S. Bhutani, and K.A. Varady. 2014. Meal timing during alternate day fasting: Impact on body weight and cardiovascular disease risk in obese adults. *Obesity (Silver Spring)* 22 (12):2524–2531.

Horne, B.D., J.B. Muhlestein, and J.L. Anderson. 2015. Health effects of intermittent fasting: Hormesis or harm? A systematic review. *Am J Clin Nutr* 102 (2):464–470.

Horne, B.D., J.B. Muhlestein, A.R. Butler, H. Brown, and J.L. Anderson. 2014. Effects of water-only fasting among prediabetic patients. *Diabetes* 63:A590.

Horne, B.D., J.B. Muhlestein, D.L. Lappé, H.T. May, J.F. Carlquist, O. Galenko, K.D. Brunisholz, and J.L. Anderson. 2013. Randomized cross-over trial of short-term water-only fasting: Metabolic and cardiovascular consequences. *Nutr Metab Cardiovasc Dis* 23 (11):1050–1057.

Jackson, S.J., F.E. Leahy, S.A. Jebb, A.M. Prentice, W.A. Coward, and L.J.C. Bluck. 2007. Frequent feeding delays the gastric emptying of a subsequent meal. *Appetite* 48 (2):199–205.

Jenkins, D.J.A., T.M.S. Wolever, V. Vuksan, F. Brighenti, S.C. Cunnane, A. Venketeshwer Rao, A.L. Jenkins, G. Buckley, R. Patten, and W. Singer. 1989. Nibbling versus gorging: Metabolic advantages of increased meal frequency. *N Engl J Med* 321 (14):929–934.

Johnstone, A.M., P. Faber, E.R. Gibney, M. Elia, G. Horgan, B.E. Golden, and R.J. Stubbs. 2002. Effect of an acute fast on energy compensation and feeding behaviour in lean men and women. *Int J Obes Relat Metab Disord* 26:1623–1628.

Jones, P.J., C.A. Leitch, and R.A. Pederson. 1993. Meal-frequency effects on plasma hormone concentrations and cholesterol synthesis in humans. *Am J Clin Nutr* 57 (6):868–874.

Jun, M., C. Foote, J. Lv, B. Neal, A. Patel, S.J. Nicholls, D.E. Grobbee, A. Cass, J. Chalmers, and V. Perkovic. 2010. Effects of fibrates on cardiovascular outcomes: A systematic review and meta-analysis. *Lancet* 375 (9729):1875–1884.

Kelley, D.E., B. Goodpaster, R.R. Wing, and J.-A. Simoneau. 1999. Skeletal muscle fatty acid metabolism in association with insulin resistance, obesity, and weight loss. *Am J Physiol* 277 (6):E1130–E1141.

King, S. and M. Gibney. 1999. Dietary advice to reduce fat intake is more successful when it does not restrict habitual eating patterns. *J Am Diet Assoc* 99 (6):685–689.

Klempel, M.C., S. Bhutani, M. Fitzgibbon, S. Freels, and K.A. Varady. 2010. Dietary and physical activity adaptations to alternate day modified fasting: Implications for optimal weight loss. *Nutr J* 9:35.

Klempel, M.C., C.M. Kroeger, and K.A. Varady. 2013a. Alternate day fasting increases LDL particle size independently of dietary fat content in obese humans. *Eur J Clin Nutr* 67 (7):783–785.

Klempel, M.C., C.M. Kroeger, and K.A. Varady. 2013b. Alternate day fasting (ADF) with a high-fat diet produces similar weight loss and cardio-protection as ADF with a low-fat diet. *Metabolism* 62 (1):137–143.

Koopman, K.E., M.W.A. Caan, A.J. Nederveen, A. Pels, M.T. Ackermans, E. Fliers, S.E. Fleur, and M.J. Serlie. 2014. Hypercaloric diets with increased meal frequency, but not meal size, increase intrahepatic triglycerides: A randomized controlled trial. *Hepatology* 60 (2):545–553.

Levitsky, D.A. and L. DeRosimo. 2010. One day of food restriction does not result in an increase in subsequent daily food intake in humans. *Physiol Behav* 99 (4):495–499.

Lewington, S., G. Whitlock, R. Clarke, P. Sherliker, J. Emberson, J. Halsey, N. Qizilbash, R. Peto, and R. Collins. 2007. Blood cholesterol and vascular mortality by age, sex, and blood pressure: A meta-analysis of individual data from 61 prospective studies with 55 000 vascular deaths. *Lancet* 370 (9602):1829–1839.

Ma, Y., E.R. Bertone, E.J. Stanek, G.W. Reed, J.R. Hebert, N.L. Cohen, P.A. Merriam, and I.S. Ockene. 2003. Association between eating patterns and obesity in a free-living US adult population. *Am J Epidemiol* 158 (1):85–92.

McGrath, S.A. and M.J. Gibney. 1994. The effects of altered frequency of eating on plasma lipids in free-living healthy males on normal self-selected diets. *Eur J Clin Nutr* 48 (6):402–407.

McLaughlin, T., F. Abbasi, H.-S. Kim, C. Lamendola, P. Schaaf, and G. Reaven. 2001. Relationship between insulin resistance, weight loss, and coronary heart disease risk in healthy, obese women. *Metabolism* 50 (7):795–800.

Meier, J.J., A. Gethmann, O. Götze, B. Gallwitz, J.J. Holst, W.E. Schmidt, and M.A. Nauck. 2006. Glucagon-like peptide 1 abolishes the postprandial rise in triglyceride concentrations and lowers levels of non-esterified fatty acids in humans. *Diabetologia* 49 (3):452–458.

Metzner, H.L., D.E. Lamphiear, N.C. Wheeler, and F.A. Larkin. 1977. The relationship between frequency of eating and adiposity in adult men and women in the Tecumseh Community Health Study. *Am J Clin Nutr* 30 (5):712–715.

Mihaylova, B., J. Emberson, L. Blackwell, A. Keech, J. Simes, E.H. Barnes, M. Voysey, A. Gray, R. Collins, and C. Baigent. 2012. The effects of lowering LDL cholesterol with statin therapy in people at low risk of vascular disease: Meta-analysis of individual data from 27 randomised trials. *Lancet* 380 (9841):581–590.

Munsters, M.J. and W.H. Saris. 2012. Effects of meal frequency on metabolic profiles and substrate partitioning in lean healthy males. *PloS One* 7 (6):e38632.

Murphy, M.C., C. Chapman, J.A. Lovegrove, S.G. Isherwood, L.M. Morgan, J.W. Wright, and C.M. Williams. 1996. Meal frequency; does it determine postprandial lipaemia? *Eur J Clin Nutr* 50 (8):491–497.

Nordestgaard, B.G. and A. Varbo. 2014. Triglycerides and cardiovascular disease. *Lancet* 384 (9943):626–635.

Otero, Y.F., J.M. Stafford, and O.P. McGuinness. 2014. Pathway-selective insulin resistance and metabolic disease: The importance of nutrient flux. *J Biol Chem* 289 (30):20462–20469.

Panowski, S.H., S. Wolff, H. Aguilaniu, J. Durieux, and A. Dillin. 2007. PHA-4/Foxa mediates diet-restriction-induced longevity of *C. elegans*. *Nature* 447 (7144):550–555.
Poston, W.S.C., C.K. Haddock, M.M. Pinkston, P. Pace, N.D. Karakoc, R.S. Reeves, and J.P. Foreyt. 2005. Weight loss with meal replacement and meal replacement plus snacks: A randomized trial. *Int J Obes (Lond)* 29 (9):1107–1114.
Rivellese, A.A., C. De Natale, L. Di Marino, L. Patti, C. Iovine, S. Coppola, S. Del Prato, G. Riccardi, and G. Annuzzi. 2004. Exogenous and endogenous postprandial lipid abnormalities in type 2 diabetic patients with optimal blood glucose control and optimal fasting triglyceride levels. *J Clin Endocrinol Metab* 89 (5):2153–2159.
Ruidavets, J.B., V. Bongard, V. Bataille, P. Gourdy, and J. Ferrieres. 2002. Eating frequency and body fatness in middle-aged men. *Int J Obes Relat Metab Disord* 26 (11):1476–1483.
Sävendahl, L. and L.E. Underwood. 1999. Fasting increases serum total cholesterol, LDL cholesterol and apolipoprotein B in healthy, nonobese humans. *J Nutr* 129 (11):2005–2008.
Schlierf, G. and H. Raetzer. 1972. Diurnal patterns of blood sugar, plasma insulin, free fatty acid and triglyceride levels in normal subjects and in patients with type IV hyperlipoproteinemia and the effect of meal frequency. *Nutr Metab* 14 (2):113–126.
Schoenfeld, B.J., A.A. Aragon, and J.W. Krieger. 2015. Effects of meal frequency on weight loss and body composition: A meta-analysis. *Nutr Rev* 73 (2):69–82.
Shulman, G.I. 2000. Cellular mechanisms of insulin resistance. *J Clin Invest* 106 (2):171.
Siri-Tarino, P.W., A.C. Woods, G.A. Bray, and R.M. Krauss. 2011. Reversal of small, dense LDL subclass phenotype by weight loss is associated with impaired fat oxidation. *Obesity (Silver Spring)* 19 (1):61–68.
Soeters, M.R., N.M. Lammers, P.F. Dubbelhuis, M. Ackermans, C.F. Jonkers-Schuitema, E. Fliers, H.P. Sauerwein, J.M. Aerts, and M.J. Serlie. 2009. Intermittent fasting does not affect whole-body glucose, lipid, or protein metabolism. *Am J Clin Nutr* 90 (5):1244–1251.
Varady, K.A., S. Bhutani, M.C. Klempel, and C.M. Kroeger. 2011a. Comparison of effects of diet versus exercise weight loss regimens on LDL and HDL particle size in obese adults. *Lipids Health Dis* 10 (1):119.
Varady, K.A., S. Bhutani, M.C. Klempel, C.M. Kroeger, J.F. Trepanowski, J.M. Haus, K.K. Hoddy, and Y. Calvo. 2013. Alternate day fasting for weight loss in normal weight and overweight subjects: A randomized controlled trial. *Nutr J* 12 (1):146.
Varady, K.A., S. Bhutani, M.C. Klempel, and B. Lamarche. 2011b. Improvements in LDL particle size and distribution by short-term alternate day modified fasting in obese adults. *Br J Nutr* 105 (04):580–583.
Verboeket-Van De Venne, W.P. and K.R. Westerterp. 1993. Frequency of feeding, weight reduction and energy metabolism. *Int J Obes Relat Metab Disord* 17 (1):31–36.
Wolever, T.M.S. 1990. Metabolic effects of continuous feeding. *Metabolism* 39 (9):947–951.

Section VI

Other Nutritional Influences of Cardiometabolic Health

28 Early Life Nutrition, Epigenetics, and Later Cardiometabolic Health

Mark H. Vickers, Clare M. Reynolds, and Clint Gray

CONTENTS

ABSTRACT

Cardiometabolic disease arises from a complex interaction between many factors, including genetic, physiologic, behavioral, and environmental influences. The increases in rates of metabolic disorders over recent years suggest that genetics may play a relatively minor role, with increasing evidence for environmental (e.g., epigenetic) and behavioral effects, underpinning the present disease epidemic. In particular, alterations in the early-life nutritional environment (spanning the periconceptional period through to infancy) are now well established to result in a "programmed" predisposition to a range of metabolic and cardiovascular disorders in later life. In this context (preferentially termed the "developmental origins of health and disease or "DOHaD"), it has been shown in both human cohorts and experimental animal models that a range of altered early-life nutritional environments, including both under- and overnutrition, can lead to cardiometabolic disorders in offspring. Further, these effects can be amplified by the postnatal nutritional environment and also can be transmitted across generations, thus leading to cycle of disease. Although the mechanisms are not fully defined, this programming was initially considered an irreversible change in developmental trajectory. However, it has now been shown that, at least in pre-clinical models, programmed metabolic disorders are potentially reversible by nutritional or targeted therapeutic interventions during critical periods of development. Given that fixed genomic variation may only explain a small proportion of disease risk, there is an increasing interest in the role of epigenetics. As an example, epigenetic gene promoter methylation at birth has been associated with later adiposity in childhood. These findings suggest that a substantial component of disease risk may have a prenatal developmental basis and perinatal epigenetic analysis may therefore have utility in identifying individual vulnerability to later cardiometabolic disease.

BACKGROUND

Obesity and related cardiovascular and metabolic sequelae represent one of the greatest modern threats to human health and lifestyle in the developed world. The incidence of cardiometabolic disease has increased dramatically over the last two decades, driven primarily by an epidemic of obesity in Western societies. These trends are also being mirrored in those developing nations that are currently transitioning to First World lifestyles. Cardiometabolic disease arises from complex interactions between genetic, physiologic, behavioral, and environmental factors. The rise in the incidence of these metabolic disorders in recent years suggests that genetics plays a relatively minor role, with increasing evidence for environmental (e.g., epigenetically mediated) and behavioral effects, underpinning the present epidemic. Furthermore, intrauterine and early conditions are now recognized as an influential factor in the progression or susceptibility of these pathologies.

The Developmental Origins of Health and Disease, or DOHaD, hypothesis has highlighted a clear link between environmental exposures during early life development and the later risk for obesity and related cardiovascular and metabolic disorders (preferentially termed "developmental programming"). The DOHaD model speculates that during early life, adaptations occur in response to cues from the environment. These predictive (mal)adaptations can result in adjustments in the set points of homeostatic control systems in order to aid immediate survival and improve chances of survival when placed in an expected adverse postnatal environment. However, if the interpretation of prenatal cues is inappropriate or there are changes to the actual immediate environment, this can result in a "mismatch" between prenatal predictions based on early life cues and postnatal reality. As a result, these early adaptive processes, akin to the "thrifty phenotype" hypothesis developed originally by Hales and colleagues (Hales and Barker 2001) and more recently the concept of predictive adaptive response (Gluckman et al. 2008), may actually be disadvantageous to offspring in postnatal life, thus leading to an increased susceptibility for a range of diseases in adulthood and/or the transmission of risk factors leading to a "feed-forward" cycle with inheritance of disease traits across generations. Under the DOHaD framework, it is now well evidenced from epidemiological observations, clinical cohorts, and a range of experimental animal models that alterations in the nutritional environment during early development can manifest as an increased susceptibility for a range of cardiometabolic disorders in later life (Fernandez-Twinn and Ozanne 2010).

Given the role of environmental influences, the role of epigenetic contributions to disease manifestation that arise due to developmental programming has become an increasing focus of recent studies. Given the dynamic changes that occur during development, the epigenome is labile in nature, thus allowing response and adaptations to environmental stressors, including early life nutritional modifications (Jang and Serra 2014). It is understood that epigenetic switches control gene activity in a tissue-specific manner. The observation that the level of imprinting in the agouti mutant gene can be modified via changes in the maternal diet gave weight to the concept that alterations in maternal nutrition can affect the epigenetic processes in the conceptus (Wolff et al. 1998, Cooney et al. 2002). Around the time of blastocyst implantation, the majority of the genome is unmethylated and preimplantation blastocysts are likely to be sensitive to environmental cues (Watkins et al. 2008, Eckert et al. 2012). The modification of the maternal diet (i.e., supplementation or restriction) with dietary cofactors including methyl donors (folate, methionine, or choline) can affect the establishment of DNA methylation patterns in offspring (Lillycrop et al. 2005, Sinclair et al. 2007). Imprinted genes (whereby gene expression is in a parent-of-origin-specific manner) are a class of genes that are considered a potential mediator of developmental programming, because the normal expression of these genes is critically dependent upon epigenetic modifications. Further, many such imprinted genes have key roles in the regulation of fetal growth (including insulin-like growth factor-2 [IGF2]) as well as postnatal growth and metabolism. The methylation of DNA is also suggested as a mechanism underlying programming-induced changes in blood pressure and glucose tolerance (Woods 2007), and the accumulation of methionine may predispose to later development of cardiovascular disease (CVD), in both human studies and rodent models, primarily through the demethylation of methionine and resultant production of homocysteine (Sutton-Tyrrell et al. 1997, Zhou et al. 2015). Kwong et al. reported that the persistent irreversible programming of postnatal growth and physiology in rats was inducible during the preimplantation period of development using a model of maternal protein restriction. A 30% reduction in the number of cells present within preimplantation blastocysts was reported, which was associated with a reduced adult offspring kidney weight. They postulated that maternal hyperglycemia and amino acid depletion may represent early programming mechanisms that initiate "metabolic stressors," thereby restricting early embryonic cell proliferation and the subsequent generation of appropriately sized stem-cell lineages (Kwong et al. 2000). This work suggests that, in an environment that is nutrient restricted, the preimplantation embryo is able to activate physiological mechanisms during this period of developmental plasticity in order to stabilize the growth of the conceptus and enhance postnatal fitness. The activation of such acute responses, however, may also be disadvantageous in the long term and predispose to a range of cardiometabolic disorders in later life as shown in a murine model (Watkins et al. 2008).

EVIDENCE FROM EPIDEMIOLOGY AND CLINICAL COHORTS

The basic concepts that underpin environmentally induced metabolic programming, and particularly transgenerational transmission of acquired phenotypic characteristics, can be traced back to the French biologist Lamarck (1809), who developed a theory around "inheritance of acquired characteristics." Later, Kermack reported a relationship between living conditions, socioeconomic status, and subsequent death rates (Kermack et al. 1934). Forsdahl and colleagues then described a correlation between infant mortality and CVD-related deaths (Forsdahl 1977). The term "programming" was first used in scientific literature by Dörner in the early 1970s following his observation that hormone, metabolite, and neurotransmitter concentrations during sensitive periods of early development could program brain development, reproductive parameters, and metabolism in human adults (Koletzko 2005). To encompass the consequences of neonatal and early childhood nutrition, the term "nutritional programming" was later proposed by Alan Lucas, and the concept went on to gain a broad and international acceptance following the work of Hales and Barker (Hales and Barker 1992). Following these early observations, a number of epidemiological studies and clinical cohorts have now accumulated a large amount of evidence relating to the "fetal origins" or "developmental programming" of adult disease hypothesis. These studies have highlighted that disease susceptibility is more than just a consequence of adult environment and lifestyle factors and that a range of nutritional stimuli or insults during the periconceptional, gestational, or early postnatal environment can have a profound effect on developmental trajectory and propensity for metabolic disorders in later life. Mechanistically, studies in the human that link epigenetic changes to later metabolic disease risk remain largely observational in nature, although there is evidence that suggests the potential for tissue-specific inheritance of DNA methylation patterns (Silva and White 1988). There are a number of limitations to human studies, including the accuracy and availability of methods, to measure discrete nutritional components involved in the one-carbon cycle and whether disruptions to these processes exert tissue-specific effects. Different environmental exposures can lead to differential patterns of epigenetic marks in the somatic tissues of individuals with evidence for this provided in studies of twins whereby a divergence of DNA methylation and histone acetylation patterns occurs more strongly in older twin pairs that are characterized by more marked life history differences (Fraga et al. 2005). Work on human disorders, including Angelman (lack of maternally contributed region 15q11) and Prader-Willi (imprinting disorder on paternally contributed regions of chromosome 15) imprinting syndromes, further suggests that the inheritance of epigenetic marks may play a role in the development of cardiometabolic disorders in the human (Kaminsky et al. 2006).

CARDIOMETABOLIC OUTCOMES

Human data are limited, and most evidence to date on epigenetic mechanisms underpinning developmental programming has been derived from experimental animal models. Of the limited human data available, the Dutch famine cohort (1944–1945) is one of the most cited historical cohorts used to investigate early life nutritional deprivation on later health outcomes (Ravelli et al.1976, Roseboom et al. 2000, 2001). The Dutch famine was a severe famine that occurred between November 1944 and June 1945. The famine primarily affected the northwestern region of the Netherlands and resulted from a blockade imposed by the German military occupation during the Second World War. The Dutch famine cohort provides the most compelling evidence that the timing of nutritional adversity in early life appears critical for changes in the adult methylome (methylated genome). Prenatal famine exposure was linked to metabolic compromise in later life (impaired glucose handling, increased adiposity and a higher body mass index [BMI], increases in total and low-density lipoprotein cholesterol) and increased incidence of schizophrenia in later life (Lumey et al. 2011). The observations of differential DNA methylation at promoters and imprinted regions for genes involved in metabolic regulation following prenatal famine exposure indicated a role for epigenetic mechanisms in these phenotypic associations. Moreover, data derived from the Dutch famine cohort have also shown that differences in methylation after famine exposure are dependent upon the timing of exposure in addition to being sex specific (Heijmans et al. 2008, Tobi et al. 2009). As an example, a recent study in this cohort has shown that early gestation, and not mid–late gestation, is a critical period for adult DNA methylation changes, as assessed in blood, after prenatal famine exposure (Tobi et al. 2015). In the Dutch famine cohort, individuals that had been prenatally exposed to famine had, 60 years later, a reduction in the methylation of the IGF2 gene compared to same-sex siblings that were unexposed. This association was specific to the timing of periconceptional famine exposure and reinforces that very early developmental stages in mammals are crucial periods for the establishment and maintenance of epigenetic marks (Heijmans et al. 2008, Tobi et al. 2009).

Although a role for macronutrient balance is clearly implicated in developmental programming, for example, restricted or excessive protein and carbohydrate intake (McMillen et al. 2008), maternal micronutrient concentrations are of interest due to their impacts on the one-carbon metabolism involved in the regulation of DNA methylation and numerous experimental observations that an imbalance in micronutrients can influence the patterns of DNA methylation in offspring. For example, an increase in vitamin B12 concentrations during pregnancy is linked to a decrease in global DNA methylation in the human newborn, while increases in the concentration of serum B12 in newborns are associated with a reduction in IGFBP3 methylation, an IGF-binding protein involved in intrauterine growth (McKay et al. 2012). More recent work examining parental obesity has shown altered DNA methylation patterns at imprinted genes in newborns of obese parents (Soubry et al. 2015). Moreover, obesity in the father has been linked to the hypomethylation of IGF2 in newborns (Soubry et al. 2013). Of note, the observation of significant associations between paternal obesity and methylation status in offspring demonstrates that the developing sperm is susceptible to environmentally mediated insults. The acquired "imprint instability" may be transmitted across generations and increase the risk for chronic diseases in later life (Soubry et al. 2015).

EVIDENCE FROM ANIMAL MODELS

Given the short generation times and scope for transgenerational studies, tissue-specific analysis, and ability to implement intervention strategies that allow the observation of outcomes over the life course of the offspring, most data to date have been derived from a range of experimental animal models. Developmental changes to epigenetic marks may induce lifelong alterations in gene expression, leaving offspring metabolically disadvantaged and susceptible to later disease, particularly when exposed to a "secondary trigger" such as a postnatal obesogenic environment. Numerous studies in animal models, using a diverse range of nutritional challenges across different experimental species, have examined changes in DNA methylation to investigate the impact of altered early life nutrition on epigenetic regulation of both imprinted and nonimprinted genes (Gicquel et al. 2008). As described earlier, given that one-carbon metabolism is dependent upon the availability of dietary methyl donors and cofactors (including folic acid, choline, and vitamin B12), it is not unexpected that alterations in the early life nutritional environment can influence DNA methylation (MacLennan et al. 2004, Gicquel et al. 2008,

Vanhees et al. 2014). Further, maternal nutritional restriction during the periconceptional period can result in changes in the expression of microRNAs (miRNAs) in offspring that have been associated with the development of insulin resistance in later life (Lie et al. 2014). Maternal dietary manipulations including low-protein (LP) exposure can result in aberrant changes in DNA methylation in key genes, changes that can be prevented by maternal dietary supplementation with cofactors (Lillycrop et al. 2005, Cho et al. 2013). For example, in the rat, Lillycrop et al. have reported altered promoter methylation and gene expression in LP-exposed offspring for both the hepatic glucocorticoid receptor (GR) and the peroxisome proliferator–activated receptor α (PPAR-α) (Lillycrop et al. 2005, 2007), influencing carbohydrate and lipid metabolism (Burdge et al. 2007a). In this study, a maternal low-protein (MLP) diet resulted in PPAR-α and GR hypomethylation in offspring; these alterations were normalized to that of the control group when the mother was supplemented with folate (Lillycrop et al. 2005). Further, alterations in the folate content of maternal or postweaning diets in the rat can result in differential changes in phosphoenolpyruvate carboxykinase (PEPCK, an enzyme primarily involved in gluconeogenesis) gene expression and promoter methylation (Hoile et al. 2012). In addition to folate, there is emerging evidence around optimal dietary choline intake (a vitamin-like essential nutrient also involved in methylation or one-carbon transfer) for normal fetal development (Zeisel 2009). In the rat, maternal choline supply during pregnancy can impact upon fetal histone and DNA methylation, suggesting that a concerted epigenomic mechanism is in place that contributes to the long-term developmental effects evident when choline intake is varied (Davison et al. 2009). In the rat, choline is involved in the methylation of histone H3, expression of histone methyltransferases G9a (Kmt1c) and Suv39h1 (Kmt1a), and methylation of their respective genes in fetal liver and brain (Davison et al. 2009). Data on vitamin B12 and altered methylation are less clear. As with folate, B12 is a requirement for the synthesis of methionine and S-adenosyl methionine, the common methyl donor required for the maintenance of methylation patterns in DNA; thus, a deficiency in B12 can result in hypomethylation. One of the most epigenetically regulated loci that has been characterized, the paternally imprinted IGF2 gene, has a labile pattern of methylation that is dependent on the nutritional stimuli or cues that are received by the developing organism during early life (Murphy and Jirtle 2003, Waterland et al. 2006b). Of note, in postweaning animals, work by Waterland showed that the paternal allele of Igf2 differentially methylated region 2 was hypermethylated in the kidneys of mice fed a synthetic control diet. These data, if translatable, suggest that compositional differences in the diet postweaning can exert persistent effects on IGF2 expression, thus suggesting that diet in early childhood could potentially contribute to a loss of IGF2 imprinting in humans (Waterland et al. 2006b).

Cardiometabolic Outcomes

Work across a range of experimental animal models of developmental programming has provided clear evidence that a wide range of environmental challenges during the periconceptional period, pregnancy, or early neonatal life can result in changes in gene promoter methylation. These changes will subsequently either directly or indirectly affect gene expression in pathways associated with a range of cardiometabolic disorders (Pham et al. 2003, Weaver et al. 2004, Bogdarina et al. 2007, Jirtle and Skinner 2007, Dudley et al. 2011). A primary focus of work to date has been on changes in DNA methylation. However, data are emerging on histone modifications arising due to aberrant developmental programming. Alterations in histone methylation are key structural changes that can, depending on the location, impact upon gene expression, leading to either promotion or repression of gene expression. The methylation of either histone or DNA proteins requires methyl donor availability in addition to a range of methyltransferases (Wolffe 1998, Callinan and Feinberg 2006). In addition to DNA methylation and histone modifications, epigenetics also integrates small noncoding miRNAs with an emerging framework that integrates methylation, histone, and miRNAs. As described earlier, although research to date has predominantly focused on changes in DNA methylation in response to altered nutrition (Delage and Dashwood 2008), an increasing number of reports are highlighting the impact of early life nutritional challenges on miRNAs and histones. Work on miRNAs has suggested a complex network of reciprocal interconnections with miRNAs not only involved in the control of gene expression at a posttranscriptional level but also connected to methylation processes. miRNAs thus represent a new important class of regulatory molecules as via regulatory loops they are also directly connected to other components of the "epigenetic machinery" (Iorio et al. 2010). On one hand, DNA methylation and chromatin modifications can regulate the expression of certain miRNAs. Reciprocally, miRNAs can impact upon the methylation machinery and the expression of proteins involved in histone modifications (Iorio et al. 2010). As a combinatorial mechanism, this process may then ultimately determine gene expression and the ensuing offspring phenotype. Epigenetic modifications are intimately linked with embryonic development, differentiation, and stem-cell programming. These epigenetic mechanisms can be affected by environmental stimuli (e.g., pregnancy complications, maternal smoking, drug use, alcohol, and diet) and can increase predisposition to cardiometabolic disease. miRNAs lead to the posttranscriptional degradation of target gene messenger RNA and translational inhibition of protein expression. As an example of this, silencing of miRNAs targeting histone deacetylases has been linked to cancer progression, but the impact of such processes in the context of developmental programming are not well described. Currently, the epigenetic regulation of miRNA-encoding gene expression following the methylation of CpG dinucleotides within the promotor regions of these genes has not been described in the context of CVD, but proof-of-principle studies in other areas (e.g., insulin sensitivity [Flowers et al. 2015] and endothelial dysfunction [Prattichizzo et al. 2015]) suggest that miRNAs have utility as biomarkers or potential therapeutic use in the setting of programming-related disorders.

Maternal Undernutrition

The most commonly used models in rodents have utilized the models of maternal undernutrition (either global dietary restriction or isocaloric LP diets) or ligation of the uterine artery in order to induce intrauterine growth restriction (IUGR). In response to alterations in early life nutrition, gene expression can be fine-tuned by organisms to achieve environmental adaptation via epigenetic alterations of histone markers of gene accessibility (Zinkhan et al. 2012). Feeding a MLP diet or inducing uteroplacental insufficiency during pregnancy can result in altered DNA methylation, which later manifests as endothelial dysfunction, increased angiotensin II type 1 receptor expression in the kidney and adrenal gland, hypertension, and nephron deficits (Bogdarina et al. 2007, Morgado et al. 2015). In the rat adrenal gland, Bogdarina and colleagues have shown that MLP diet–induced hypertension in offspring is associated with hypomethylation and increased expression of the angiotensin type 1b (AT1b) receptor gene (Bogdarina et al. 2007). Further examples are those in the models of growth restriction whereby uteroplacental insufficiency can lead to a decrease in postnatal IGF1 mRNA variants, H3 acetylation, and the gene elongation mark histone 3 trimethylation of lysine 36 of the IGF1 gene (H3Me3K36) (Fu et al. 2004, Zinkhan et al. 2012). Tosh et al. have also shown in the rat that early patterns of body growth following early growth restriction (i.e., rapid vs. delayed catch-up growth) resulted in differential changes in hepatic IGF1 mRNA expression and histone H3K4 methylation (Tosh et al. 2010). A common molecular phenotype associated with growth-restricted rats is a decrease in the expression of pancreatic and duodenal homeobox factor-1 (PDX1). PDX1 is a key transcription factor involved in the regulation of pancreatic development, and a reduction in PDX1 activity has been associated with alterations in histone modifications (Park et al. 2008). Similar findings have also been observed in the muscle of IUGR rats for the glucose transporter GLUT4 (Raychaudhuri et al. 2008). There are also important associations between phospholipid status in the mother and the one-carbon cycle (Khot et al. 2015). The inadequacy of long-chain polyunsaturated fatty acid (LCPUFA)-containing phospholipids may cause the diversion of methyl groups toward DNA and eventually result in aberrant DNA methylation patterns (Khaire et al. 2015). Changes in these patterns of DNA methylation can lead to alterations in the expression of key genes, including angiogenesis-related genes, and may thereby contribute to aberrations in angiogenesis/vasculogenesis further affecting the development of the placenta (Khot et al. 2015).

The adipokine leptin has received significant attention in studies of developmental programming with leptin treatment to neonatal rats shown to reverse the detrimental effects of global maternal undernutrition (Vickers et al. 2005, 2008, Gluckman et al. 2007, Gibson et al. 2015) with similar effects observed in a piglet model of IUGR (Attig et al. 2008). Mechanisms underlying epigenetic modifications that result in an increased susceptibility to altered programming of leptin and insulin signaling have been discussed previously (Holness and Sugden 2006). Embedded within a CpG island, leptin has a 3kb promoter region and contains a number of putative binding sites for known transcription factors including a glucocorticoid response element. In animal models, it has been shown that the degree of variation observed in the DNA methylation of the leptin promoter varies with the degree of obesity (Shen et al. 2014, Crujeiras et al. 2015) and the epigenetic regulation of leptin signaling pathways can be modified by nutrients through altered histone modification and binding of DNA methyltransferases at the level of the leptin promoter (Haggarty 2013). In addition to leptin, a further focus regarding the potential for epigenetic regulation is that of the fat mass and obesity-associated (FTO) gene (Dina et al. 2007, Lawlor et al. 2008, Sebert et al. 2010, 2014, Mayeur et al. 2013). An overview of the potential programming effects of the FTO gene in the development of obesity has been undertaken previously by Sebert and colleagues (Sebert et al. 2014). As evidenced by experimental work in both sheep and rat models (utilizing paradigms of both undernutrition and overnutrition), the FTO gene has been identified as a potential key target for nutritional programming. As an example, leptin resistance associated with obesity in IUGR offspring and rapid postnatal catch-up growth may arise due to altered FTO methylation and gene regulation (Sebert et al. 2011). However, as is a limitation of many data around altered DNA methylation, although significant associations between FTO and BMI are consistently replicated in humans, the precise mechanisms by which FTO is involved in the regulation of weight gain remain to be defined (e.g., the impact of RNA demethylation on the control of energy balance). However, recent evidence suggests that single nucleotide polymorphisms identified within the FTO gene display a functional link to IRX3, a protein that regulates early neuronal development and is associated with obesity onset. In addition, differences in the nutritional perturbations used can lead to differential effects on the regulation of the FTO gene. For example, placental FTO expression is reduced by fetal growth restriction but not by macrosomia in rodents and humans (Mayeur et al. 2013, Smemo et al. 2014).

A range of metabolic traits that result from low birth weight can be passed to subsequent generations, thus suggesting that epigenetic changes are maintained during meiosis (see "Transgenerational Effects" section). An example of this, as noted earlier, is the variation in coat color in the agouti mouse where color variation has been correlated to epigenetic marks that are established early in development (Jirtle and Skinner 2007). This was evidenced by Dolinoy et al. using intrauterine exposure to genistein via the maternal diet to heterozygous agouti viable yellow mice (A^{vy}). This resulted in alterations in coat color toward pseudoagouti and appeared to confer protection in offspring against the development of obesity in later life, a characteristic feature of the agouti phenotype (Dolinoy et al. 2006). Utilizing mouse models, work by Waterland et al. has shown that some alleles are particularly sensitive to changes in methylation arising due to changes in maternal nutrition (Waterland et al. 2006a, Waterland and Michels 2007). This work suggested that maternal nutrition in the preconception period and during pregnancy can affect the establishment of CpG methylation patterns and the lifelong expression of metastable epialleles (epigenetically modified alleles) (Waterland et al. 2006a).

Maternal Overweight/Obesity

In addition to models of maternal dietary restriction, a number of studies have now shown that an environment of maternal excess can elicit epigenetic changes in offspring. Maternal and neonatal overnutrition can result in epigenetic modifications in key genes involved in insulin signaling in skeletal muscle and predispose to insulin resistance in later life (Liu et al. 2013). Work by Marco et al. has shown that a maternal high-fat diet (HFD) resulted in the hypermethylation of the hypothalamic pro-opiomelanocortin (POMC) promoter and postweaning obesity in the rat (Marco et al. 2013), and maternal fat intake has been associated with altered epigenetic regulation of genes related to fatty acid synthesis (Hoile et al. 2013). In a rat maternal HFD model, the inhibition of the hepatic cell cycle and associated changes in gene expression and DNA methylation has been reported in offspring, but these changes did not persist into adulthood (Dudley et al. 2011). A maternal HFD can also result in altered methylation and gene expression of dopamine- and opioid-related genes and represents a further potential mechanism for early life programming of appetite control and an increased preference for energy-dense foods postnatally (Vucetic et al. 2010).

Work in the primate has shown that, in addition to DNA methylation changes, obesity induced by a calorie-dense maternal diet can lead to alterations in fetal chromatin structure via covalent histone modifications (Aagaard-Tillery et al. 2008). Hepatic metabolism in the neonate can be altered in the setting of a maternal HFD, albeit in a sex-specific manner, and these differences, in association with histone modifications, may contribute to the known sexual dimorphism in oxidative balance (Strakovsky et al. 2014). Further work in the nonhuman primate has shown that a maternal HFD can modulate sirtuin 1 (SIRT1) histone and protein deacetylase activity in the fetus. This implicates SIRT1 as a likely mediator of the fetal epigenome and metabolome in the setting of maternal obesity (Suter et al. 2012). Via regulatory loops, miRNAs can cause histone modifications and altered DNA methylation of promoter sites, which affect the expression of target genes (Hawkins and Morris 2008, Tan et al. 2009). Further, in an ovine model of maternal obesity, miRNA expression in fetal muscle is altered and therefore may be a mechanism by which intramuscular adipogenesis is enhanced during early muscle development (Yan et al. 2013).

As described earlier, offspring of rat mothers fed a moderate HFD during pregnancy display hepatic cell cycle inhibition that is associated with short-term changes in gene expression and DNA methylation (Dudley et al. 2011). In particular, the cell cycle inhibitor cyclin-dependent kinase inhibitor (Cdkn1a, p21) is hypomethylated at specific CpG dinucleotides, and hepatic mRNA expression is increased in the liver of offspring of HFD mothers. Since the upregulation of Cdkn1a has been associated with hepatocyte growth in pathologic states, these data are suggestive of early hepatic dysfunction in neonates born to mothers consuming a HFD. Exposure to a maternal obesogenic environment therefore contributes to early perturbations in whole body and liver energy metabolism in offspring mediated in part by epigenetic effects. Early programming of mitochondrial dysfunction and a reduction in fatty acid oxidation in the liver may precede the development of obesity-associated comorbidities including insulin resistance and hepatic steatosis in later life (Brumbaugh and Friedman 2014, Kjaergaard et al. 2014, Pereira et al. 2015). Further, nutritional modulation of miRNAs may also underlie susceptibility to type 2 diabetes mellitus (T2DM) in offspring—for example, a maternal HFD has been shown to alter the levels of certain hepatic miRNAs concomitant with alterations in the expression of genes including IGF2, which is important for islet β-cell survival (Zhang et al. 2009).

Although studied less widely as an independent dietary cofactor, the effect of a high maternal salt intake, common in most Western-style dietary environments, has also been examined in relation to epigenetic changes. Work by Ding et al. examined the influence of a diet high in salt during pregnancy on the development of the heart and DNA methylation in the rat fetal heart in relation to the subtype of angiotensin receptors. A high maternal salt intake resulted in changes in a number of CpG sites in the fetal heart that were linked to the AT1b promoter. Further, cardiac AT1 receptor protein in adult offspring was also higher following exposure to a maternal high-salt diet (Ding et al. 2010).

INFLAMMATION AND PROGRAMMING

Accumulating evidence has indicated that chronic low-grade inflammation is a key factor in the progression of metabolic disease. Obesity was first linked to inflammation in 1993 when Hotamisligil et al. demonstrated an increase in the pro-inflammatory cytokine TNFα in obese, insulin-resistant mice (Hotamisligil et al. 1993). Subsequent studies have demonstrated that infiltration of innate immune cells (macrophages, dendritic cells, and T cells [Lumeng et al. 2007a,b, 2009, Reynolds et al. 2012]) and local production of pro-inflammatory mediators interrupt insulin signaling, representing an integral step in the pathogenesis of metabolic disease. While TNFα represents the first association between inflammation and obesity, there are now numerous cytokines and adipokines known to disrupt insulin responsiveness, instigating a drive toward anti-inflammatory (both pharmacological and nutritional) treatments for obesity and its comorbidities. There is increasing evidence that these inflammatory processes are governed, at least in part, by environmentally induced epigenetic changes. Peripheral blood monocytes (PBMCs) represent a useful noninvasive tool for the assessment of epigenetic alterations in the immune cells of obese subjects. A study in PBMCs from monozygotic twins indicated that obesity and metabolic dysfunction are associated with differentially methylated genes in a range of metabolically relevant targets (Ollikainen et al. 2015). Indeed, the methylation of specific inflammatory genes has been linked to metabolic dysregulation. Campion et al. determined that TNFα promoter methylation was reduced following weight loss in obese men (Campion et al. 2009). There is also evidence that obese women with calorie restriction–induced weight loss have lower adipose tissue methylation levels in both the TNFα and leptin promoter regions (Cordero et al. 2011). Finally, there is evidence from human adipocytes and THP-1 (human macrophage cell line) cells that inflammatory stimuli alter the expression of miRNA (miR-221/222, miR-155), which may be responsible for inflammation-related metabolic dysfunction (Ortega et al. 2015).

Despite the relative importance of meta-inflammation (the chronic low-grade inflammatory response to obesity) in the pathogenesis of insulin resistance and T2DM, the role of maternal programming of metabolic inflammation has not been clearly defined. However, there are indicators that give reason to speculate that epigenetic alteration of inflammatory mediators may influence metabolic disease in the offspring of mothers subjected to adverse environments during pregnancy. Evidence from human studies has indicated that the development of the immune system begins at an early embryonic stage (Naito 1993, Palmer 2011). While a rudimentary immune system is present at birth, this system does not fully mature until later in life and is therefore susceptible to programming stimuli from gestation to the postweaning period (Cedar and Bergman 2011, Palmer 2011). The immune system is highly plastic, and a series of epigenetic marks govern the differentiation of hematopoietic stem cells to functional immune mediators (Attema et al. 2007). There is significant evidence that exposure to inflammatory stimuli during pregnancy can influence the offspring's immune system in later life. Further, maternal inflammation and infection represent a major cause of preterm birth, which in itself is associated with significant effects on offspring's long-term health outcomes. This appears to be linked to epigenetic cues. Sanders et al. demonstrated that specific miRNAs present in the cervix in a cohort of 53 pregnant women were associated with several factors including inflammation and predicted gestational length (Sanders et al. 2015), while Hillman et al. indicate that distinct DNA methylation profiles associated with autophagy, oxidative stress, and hormonal regulation in preterm placentas may predispose to future disease risk (Hillman et al. 2015). Maternal infection and inflammation also represent the sources of epigenetic regulation, which may affect future disease risk in adults. Infection of pregnant mice with gram-negative bacteria (A Iwoffii F78) protected offspring from inflammatory lung disease through the alteration of histone acetylation in the promoter region of the anti-inflammatory cytokine IL-4 (Brand et al. 2011). Given that HFDs, particularly those rich in saturated fats, activate the immune system both in humans and in animal models (Fernandez-Real and Ricart 1999, Ferrante 2013), it is reasonable to speculate that this nutrient-derived inflammation may play an important role in programming immune function and indeed subsequent meta-inflammation in offspring (Li et al. 2013).

While the evidence for the role of epigenetic processes in developmentally programmed metabolic inflammatory disease is limited, there are several studies that implicate poor maternal nutrition in the development of chronic low-grade inflammation and subsequent metabolic disease. Reynolds et al. demonstrated that moderate maternal global undernutrition resulted in increased adipose tissue inflammation, which is linked to insulin resistance in Sprague-Dawley rats (Reynolds et al. 2013a). This study was followed up with evidence that bone marrow macrophages from undernourished offspring have an increased inflammatory profile upon immune stimulation and demonstrate signs of polarization from the anti-inflammatory M2 phenotype to the pro-inflammatory M1 phenotype (Reynolds et al. 2013b). Interestingly, macrophage polarization is a process that is heavily governed by epigenetics, whereby demethylases act on histones that bind to the promoters of genes that characterize the M2 phenotype. Therefore, it is plausible that the effects observed in offspring from undernourished mothers may, in part, be mediated by epigenetic alterations (Satoh et al. 2010). Indeed, inflammatory changes are also observed in relation to maternal obesity. Li et al. demonstrate that maternal obesogenic diets (rich in sugars and fat) program hepatic inflammation in rat neonates, prior to the onset on overt metabolic disease (Li et al. 2013). However, whether these effects are due to direct exposure *in utero* or via epigenetic changes remains to be examined. A recent study examining transgenerational HFD-induced programming observed progressive increases in infiltrating macrophages across generations accompanied by increased gene expression of critical innate immune mediators such as NLRP4 and TLR2/4 in adipose tissue. These findings were associated with the hypomethylation of inflammatory gene promoter regions, thus demonstrating evidence of transgenerational epigenetic transmission of meta-inflammation (Ding et al. 2014).

While direct evidence linking epigenetic changes in inflammatory genes to developmentally programmed obesity and metabolic dysfunction is limited, it is clear that epigenetics plays a key role in the pathogenesis of obesity-mediated comorbidities. There is however evidence from early life interventions with anti-inflammatory nutrients (including n-3 polyunsaturated fatty acids [PUFA] and conjugated linoleic acid [CLA]) demonstrating beneficial effects on adult onset metabolic disease. There is increasing evidence that maternal dietary supplementation with n-3 LCPUFAs ameliorates the metabolic disturbances caused by a HFD in hamsters and rats (Guermouche et al. 2004, Kasbi-Chadli et al. 2014), although the outcomes can be dependent upon the source of lipid used. Furthermore, these beneficial changes have been linked to epigenetic alterations. Casas-Agustench et al. demonstrated that pregnant rats supplemented with fish oil during early pregnancy decreased the expression of hepatic miRNAs (miR192, miR21, miR26, miR10b, and miR377) involved in glucose and insulin metabolism in offspring (Casas-Agustench et al. 2015). Supplementation with n-3 PUFA during pregnancy was also seen to alter methylation profiles in $CD4^+$ T cells derived from cord blood (Amarasekera et al. 2014). Another anti-inflammatory PUFA, CLA (found primarily in ruminant meat and dairy products), has been demonstrated to have beneficial effects in terms of developmental programming of metabolic dysfunction. The supplementation of the maternal HFD with CLA during pregnancy and lactation prevented early onset puberty and hyperlipidemia in female offspring (Reynolds et al. 2015). In normal mice, however, maternal CLA consumption induced the hypermethylation of hypothalamic POMC promoter regions in adult offspring and led to metabolic dysfunction (Zhang et al. 2014), thus providing a potential epigenetic mechanism for the differential effects of this anti-inflammatory nutrient. While there is a shortfall in the evidence regarding specific epigenetic alterations in inflammatory genes as a direct result of maternal diet–induced developmental programming, there is certainly a strong case for further investigations.

A combination of obesity-induced inflammation and adipose tissue hypertrophy promotes the release of reactive oxygen species (ROS), thus promoting a state of oxidative stress. There is evidence to suggest that this process can inhibit histone deacetylase, activating previously silenced genes (Adler et al. 1999). Increased ROS production in insulin responsive tissues has been suggested as a potential mechanism for the onset of obesity-related insulin resistance (Nishikawa et al. 2007). Indeed, oxidative stress has been observed in several models of maternal diet–induced developmental programming of metabolic dysfunction (Alfaradhi et al. 2014, Preidis et al. 2014, Rodriguez-Gonzalez et al. 2015). Furthermore, programmed oxidative stress responses have been linked to epigenetic changes in offspring. Strakovsky et al. demonstrate that a maternal HFD induces hepatic promoter histone modifications in offspring that influence oxidative balance (Strakovsky et al. 2014).

TRANSGENERATIONAL EFFECTS

Extensive evidence from experimental and human studies suggests that the process of developmental programming should be regarded as a transgenerational phenomenon with evidence for both germline and somatic inheritance of epigenetic modifications that may underlie phenotypic changes across generations. As such, programming should be viewed as a form of epigenetic inheritance, either via the maternal or paternal line (Aiken and Ozanne 2014). It has been proposed that transgenerational epigenetic transmission of phenotype allows future generations to be maximally competitive in their environment (Dunn and Bale 2011). Under this assumption, adaptations acquired during the lifespan of the parent(s) persist into the next generation, thereby enabling future generations to better survive in a potential environment of adversity. However, evidence suggests that environmental exposures including poor early life nutrition can result in maladaptive parental traits being passed to offspring. The transmission of such epigenetic traits can therefore lead to the manifestation of a phenotype at a population-wide level that occurs over several generations and can exacerbate the rapid onset of phenotypes including obesity and noncommunicable diseases (NCDs) currently observed in human populations (Dunn and Bale 2011).

A number of nutritional challenges have been reported to induce transgenerational phenotypic changes in mammals (Kaminsky et al. 2006). Following undernutrition in the F0 generation, changes in the hepatic methylation of the GR promoter are reflected in the F2 generation without any further dietary manipulation of F1 female offspring (Benyshek et al. 2006). A MLP diet during F0 pregnancy in the rat induces transgenerational changes in the hepatic transcriptome in offspring and includes altered fasting glucose homeostasis and changes in PEPCK promoter methylation and expression across three generations (Burdge et al. 2007b, Hoile et al. 2011). Using a model of a sustained environmental dietary challenge (25% increase in energy compared to control diet), the expression of DNA methyltransferase (Dnmt) 3a2, but not Dnmt1 or Dnmt3b, increased, and the methylation of its promoter decreased from F1 to F3 generations (Burdge et al. 2011). These data suggest that, within a generation, the regulation of energy balance during pregnancy and lactation can be influenced by the maternal phenotype in the preceding generation and the environment during the current pregnancy. The transgenerational effects on phenotype were associated with altered DNA methylation patterns of specific genes in a manner consistent with *de novo* induction of epigenetic marks in each generation (Burdge et al. 2011). Dietary methyl donor supplementation has been shown by Waterland et al. to prevent transgenerational amplification of obesity (Waterland et al. 2008). Although a number of studies, primarily in the rodent, have reported phenotype transmission to the F2 lineage, transmission to F3 or beyond (representing true transgenerational effects as it avoids the confounding contributions of the initial maternal environmental insult) is less clear with some studies reporting a resolution or amelioration of the programmed phenotype by the F3 generation. In a meta-analysis by Aiken and Ozanne, of nine transgenerational studies carried through to F3, five failed to show any effect at F3 (Aiken and Ozanne 2014).

Transgenerational inheritance via paternal influences has also been reported (Fullston et al. 2013), with obesity in fathers linked to metabolic disturbances across two generations of mice. Diet-induced obesity in males resulted in alterations in miRNA content in sperm and germ methylation status, thus impacting potential signals that program offspring health and initiate the transmission of obesity to future generations. Studies in sperm in the F1 generation have also suggested a potential role for alterations in IGF2 and H19 expression in the transmission of a phenotype to the F2 offspring (Ding et al. 2012). However, epigenetic alterations in the F1 sperm have not been reported in all studies reporting a paternal line transmission (Drake et al. 2011). In work by Radford et al., there was no evidence that changes in the nutritional environment altered susceptibility to epigenetic reprogramming of imprinting control regions in the germline, thus suggesting that mechanisms other than direct germline transmission may be responsible (Radford et al. 2012).

Although transgenerational transmission of phenotypic traits is often viewed as a form of epigenetic inheritance, there is also evidence for the effects of nongenomic components. This includes the interaction between the developing fetus and the intrauterine environment in the propagation of programmed phenotypes. These factors include a suboptimal reproductive tract and maternal constraint and altered maternal adaptations to pregnancy. The propagation of developmental programming effects may therefore occur *de novo* through the maternal lineage in generations beyond F2 via development in a suboptimal intrauterine tract and not necessarily directly transmitted via epigenetic mechanisms. Further, as aging can exacerbate the programmed metabolic phenotype, increases in maternal age may also be a factor in increasing the likelihood of developmental programming effects being transmitted to future generations.

PATERNAL EFFECTS

The paternal influence on epigenetic alterations in offspring cannot be neglected. As the father is the sole transmitter of genetic and epigenetic factors to the oocyte, it has been argued that the father may serve as a better model to explore epigenetic involvement in the setting of developmental programming (Vanhees et al. 2014). Ng et al. reported a chronic paternal HFD programmed β-cell dysfunction in female rat offspring paralleled by changes in DNA methylation profiles including the hypomethylation of the Il13ra2 gene. This was the first time that nongenetic, intergenerational transmission of metabolic sequelae of a HFD from father to offspring was reported in mammals (Ng et al. 2010, 2014). Offspring of male mice fed a protein-depleted diet and control-fed females display an increased expression of genes involved in fat and cholesterol biosynthesis with increases in methylation in an enhancer for PPAR-α, which could therefore regulate hepatic gene expression (Carone et al. 2010). As noted earlier, the significant association between obesity in males and methylation status in offspring suggests that the developing sperm is susceptible to environmental insults (Soubry et al. 2015). Further, studies in sperm in the F1 generation have suggested a role for altered IGF2 and H19 expression in the transmission of phenotype to the F2 offspring (Ding et al. 2012), but, as shown by Drake et al., not all studies examining paternal line transmission have reported epigenetic alterations in F1 sperm (Drake et al. 2011).

STRATEGIES FOR INTERVENTION

Animal models have provided great utility in allowing the investigation of intervention strategies aimed at ameliorating or reversing the effects of adverse early life developmental programming including those described earlier regarding neonatal leptin treatment or maternal methyl donor supplementation. Leptin was an early focus in nutritional programming studies with leptin treatment to rat neonates shown to reverse the effects of IUGR on later cardiometabolic disorders in offspring in rodents (Vickers et al. 2005, Gluckman et al. 2007) and piglets (Attig et al. 2008). The leptin gene promoter is subject to epigenetic programming, and leptin expression can be modulated by DNA methylation (Melzner et al. 2002, Stoger 2006, Iliopoulos et al. 2007). In the rat, leptin exposure during lactation confers protective effects against the development of later obesity and related metabolic disorders and may be associated with changes in promoter methylation of the hypothalamic POMC gene (Palou et al. 2011). Further, leptin receptor activation can also induce the expression of the suppressor of cytokine signaling-3 (SOCS-3) gene. SOCS-3 inhibits further leptin signaling and can also inhibit insulin signaling. Alterations in SOCS-3 methylation may therefore have persistent effects on the feedback loop that exists between leptin and insulin (the adipoinsular axis) and negatively impact on phenotype development (Holness and Sugden 2006). In 3T3-L1 cells, specific CpG site methylation and a methylation-sensitive protein may contribute to the regulation of leptin gene expression during adipocyte differentiation (Yokomori et al. 2002). During preadipocyte to adipocyte differentiation, it has also been demonstrated that both methylation of specific CpG sites and a methylation-sensitive transcription factor contribute to the regulation of the GLUT4 gene (Yokomori et al. 1999). In addition to the work on leptin and insulin signaling, differential DNA methylation has been observed in promoters of genes known to be involved in glucose metabolism including GLUT4 (Yokomori et al. 1999) and uncoupling protein 2 (UCP-2) (Carretero et al. 1998). In addition to leptin, the GLP-1 analog exendin-4 can increase histone acetylase activity and reverse epigenetic modifications that silence PDX1 in the growth-restricted rat (Pinney et al. 2011). As noted previously, hypertension in offspring of LP-fed rat mothers is associated with changes in methylation and gene expression of the AT1b receptor (Bogdarina et al. 2007)—supplementation to LP-fed mothers with metyrapone, an 11β-hydroxylase inhibitor, during the first 14 days of pregnancy, normalized blood pressure, DNA methylation, and gene expression profiles in offspring (Bogdarina et al. 2010). In a model of restricted maternal nutrition in the mouse to induce a preeclampsia-type phenotype, pulmonary vascular dysfunction is associated with alterations in DNA methylation patterns in the lungs of offspring. The administration of histone deacetylase inhibitors (butyrate and trichostatin A) to offspring of these diet-restricted mice normalized pulmonary DNA methylation and pulmonary vascular function. Further, nitroxide administration (Tempol) to the mother during dietary restriction prevented vascular dysfunction and dysmethylation in the offspring, thus further demonstrating the importance of epigenetic alterations in the programming of later vascular function (Rexhaj et al. 2011, Scherrer et al. 2015). In line with lifestyle modifications as a potential avenue for the prevention of mitochondrial dysfunction and related cardiometabolic disorders, exercise as an intervention modality has also been shown to lead to alterations in the DNA methylation of the peroxisome proliferator–activated receptor gamma coactivator 1-alpha (PGC1α) promoter that favors gene expression responsible for mitochondrial biogenesis and function (Cheng and Almeida 2014). In the MLP rat model, hypomethylation in offspring of PPAR-α and GR can be normalized following maternal supplementation with folic acid (Lillycrop et al. 2005). As shown by Hoile et al., increasing the folic acid content of either the maternal or postweaning diets in the rat leads to differential effects on PEPCK expression and promoter methylation (Hoile et al. 2012). Maternal methyl donor supplementation can reduce fatty liver and has been shown to modify the fatty acid synthase DNA methylation profile in rats fed an obesogenic diet (Cordero et al. 2013a). Similarly, hyperhomocysteinemia induced by a maternal diet high in fat and sucrose intake can be prevented via the supplementation of methyl donors during lactation, possibly via altered hepatic DNA methylation and changes in the methionine–homocysteine cycle (Cordero et al. 2013b).

Imbalances in maternal micronutrients can influence LCPUFA metabolism and global methylation in the rat placenta, mediated in part by a reduction in mRNA expression of methylene tetrahydrofolate reductase (MTHFR) and methionine synthase and increased cystathionine β-synthase (CBS) (Khot et al. 2014). Supplementation with adequate concentrations of selenium and folate in female offspring of mothers fed a HFD deficient in these factors during gestation and lactation can alter global hepatic DNA methylation (Bermingham et al. 2013). Supplementation with omega-3s can ameliorate many of these observed changes arising from maternal micronutrient imbalance through normalizing MTHFR and CBS levels. Maternal supplementation with CLA has also been shown to improve maternal and offspring outcomes, particularly as regards inflammatory profile and endothelial function in the setting of maternal obesity (Gray et al. 2015, Reynolds et al. 2015), but the experimental data on CLA are conflicting and the role of epigenetic processes is not well defined. In normal rodent pregnancies, CLA can reduce adipose tissue mass via apoptosis (Tsuboyama-Kasaoka et al. 2000), and it has also been shown that CLA supplementation can lead to the hypermethylation of the proximal specificity protein (Sp1) binding site that suppresses hypothalamic POMC in neonates and therefore may contribute to metabolic disorders in adults (Zhang et al. 2014). In addition to folic acid and B vitamins, other micronutrients including vitamins A and C, iron, chromium, zinc, taurine, and flavonoids play a role in developmental programming. A maternal diet high in zinc can attenuate intestinal inflammation by reducing DNA methylation and elevating H3K9 acetylation in the promoter of the anti-inflammatory protein A20 (Li et al. 2015a). The efficacy of the methyl donors glycine and choline and the sulfonic acid taurine in ameliorating the adverse effects of both maternal undernutrition and maternal obesity across a range of experimental animal models has also been reported (Boujendar et al. 2003, Brawley et al. 2004, Bai et al. 2012, Li et al. 2013, 2015b), although the epigenetic basis of these observations is not well defined. It is known that taurine depletion in the perinatal period can increase oxidative stress and mediate blood pressure control throughout life and that taurine depletion during early life leads to epigenetic programming that can impact on later physiological function (Lerdweeraphon et al. 2013, Roysommuti and Wyss 2014). As detailed earlier, maternal choline status modifies fetal histone and DNA methylation and is involved in histone H3 methylation, expression of histone methyltransferases, and DNA methylation of their genes in rat fetal liver and brain (Davison et al. 2009). Further, the importance of dietary methionine in the programming of hypertension in the setting of a MLP diet has been highlighted. While one MLP diet preparation containing methionine consistently produces hypertension in offspring, a further MLP diet without methionine supplementation resulted in either no change or a slight reduction in blood pressure in offspring (Langley and Jackson 1994, Langley-Evans 2000).

As regards paternal transmission, it has been shown that targeted lifestyle interventions in the obese father can normalize the transmission of disease traits to female offspring. In mice, diet or exercise interventions for 8 weeks (covering two full cycles of spermatogenesis) in obese males led to a restoration of insulin sensitivity and normalization of fat mass in female offspring (McPherson et al. 2015). The diet and/or exercise regime also normalized the abundance of X-linked sperm miRNAs that are target genes involved in cell cycle regulation and apoptosis, pathways that are central to oocyte development, and early embryogenesis. In addition, comorbidities associated with obesity, including inflammation, glucose intolerance, stress, and hypercholesterolemia, served to be good predictors for sperm miRNA abundance and offspring phenotypes.

Aims currently being pursued relate to the identification of epigenetic biomarkers in early life to assess an individual's disease susceptibility and the development of protocols for tailored dietary treatments/advice to counterbalance adverse epigenomic events. As there is no "one size fits all," such approaches will allow early diagnosis and the potential for the facilitation of targeted therapeutic strategies in a personalized "epigenomically modeled" manner to combat obesity and metabolic disorders (Martinez et al. 2012).

DISCUSSION

Developmental programming during critical windows of plasticity has shown us how later life health or an individual's susceptibility to disease may be influenced by suboptimal early life nutrition. To date, comprehensive genome-scale views of differential methylation following alterations in early life nutrition are lacking in humans. The characterization of the genomic regions and biological pathways involved are key in order to understand the environmentally induced plasticity of the epigenome and its role in disease development (Tobi et al. 2014). To date, a range of experimental models have elucidated distinct phenotypes showing marked effects of early life events on later cardiometabolic status. In addition, many studies have demonstrated how these effects are vertically passed to the offspring and increase the risk factors of cardiometabolic disorders including obesity, hypertension, and metabolic syndrome. Furthermore, continued exposure to such refined, poor-quality Western-style diets has the potential to exacerbate the effects of adverse early life programming and lead to a feed-forward cycle of adverse health outcomes through future generations. This may, in part, explain the exponential increase in NCDs observed throughout developed societies and those societies that are currently transitioning to First World economies.

Suboptimal early life nutrition can induce epigenetic alterations including altered DNA methylation, histone modifications, chromatin remodeling, and/or regulatory feedback by miRNAs, all of which can modulate gene expression and promote cardiometabolic phenotype (Desai et al. 2015). Such epigenetic mechanisms, given their importance in processes around orchestrating and stabilizing cellular differentiation, likely play a major role in controlling the physiological set points that act to promote obesity and related disorders in our current obesogenic environment (Waterland 2014). Suboptimal nutrition in the periconceptional period, pregnancy, and/or lactation can lead to a range of metabolic and cardiovascular disorders in offspring. Such programming effects are mediated in part by epigenetic processes that represent an integrated network encompassing information encrypted by DNA methylation patterns, histone modifications, and miRNAs (Martinez et al. 2012).

The extent of the windows of developmental plasticity in which epigenetic changes are induced in key physiologic systems remains to be well defined, but the period of plasticity appears to extend from the periconceptional period into early postnatal life (Weaver et al. 2004, Sinclair et al. 2007). Given the transgenerational impacts, understanding the mechanisms by which developmental programming effects can be transmitted across generations is an urgent area of research and is of particular relevance to those populations transitioning between traditional and Western lifestyles (including both changes in the types of nutritional exposures and potential for decreased physical activity). Of note, some disease traits appear to be resolved in subsequent generations where others persist suggesting that there are divergent mechanisms of transmission involved. Moreover, evidence to date suggests that those metabolic traits that do persist are capable of being transmitted via the male germline (Dunn and Bale 2011). However, human evidence remains largely unsubstantiated with most studies either observational or purely associative in nature. As such, data derived primarily from the rodent provide the strongest argument for the potential of transgenerational epigenetic inheritance in humans (Morgan and Whitelaw 2008). As most work in human cohorts to date on the epigenetic basis of disease is associative in nature, the extent to which such modifications may mediate the effects of developmental programming of cardiometabolic disorders remains to be defined. As an example, quantification of DNA methylation in blood may provide little linkage with phenotype and therefore cannot be easily justified on a functional basis (Ojha et al. 2015). However, these epigenetic markers may have utility as predictive biomarkers of later disease risk (e.g., the link between cord blood promoter methylation of retinoid X receptor alpha and adiposity and bone mineral content in childhood) (Godfrey et al. 2011, Harvey et al. 2014).

Understanding the role of the early life nutritional environment and mechanisms of epigenetic inheritance across generations is essential in order to develop and validate effective intervention strategies targeted at disease prevention to modulate not only that of the immediate adult phenotype but also that of offspring, grand-offspring, and beyond. Given that around 80% of pregnant women in the United States, for example, take supplements, the evidence surrounding maternal methyl donor and vitamin supplements, one-carbon metabolism, and altered DNA methylation patterns also raises the issue that more attention should be given to the safety and potential long-term effects of such supplements on offspring (Vanhees et al. 2014). Importantly, epigenetic modifications that occur during early development may not have any effect on phenotype development until later in life, especially if they affect genes that modulate responses to later environmental challenges or secondary triggers, such as postweaning dietary challenges with energy-dense diets (i.e., the so-called second hit). The impact of paternal effects can also not be underestimated as interventions aimed at improving paternal metabolic health during specific windows prior to conception can normalize aberrant epigenetic signals in sperm and improve the metabolic health of female offspring. In addition to parent-of-origin effects, it is also important to note that many studies to date have not considered the importance of sex-specific effects in offspring programming. Such sexually dimorphic responses to programming stimuli need to be incorporated into future experimental studies as they add translational value and aid in the mechanistic understanding of how cardiometabolic phenotypes evolve. Further, adopting a life course perspective allows earlier identification of markers of risk (Godfrey et al. 2010), with the possibility of implementing nutritional and other lifestyle interventions early in life that have obvious implications for the prevention of NCDs across generations.

REFERENCES

Aagaard-Tillery, K. M., K. Grove, J. Bishop, X. Ke, Q. Fu, R. McKnight, and R. H. Lane. 2008. Developmental origins of disease and determinants of chromatin structure: Maternal diet modifies the primate fetal epigenome. *J Mol Endocrinol* 41 (2):91–102.

Adler, V., Z. Yin, K. D. Tew, and Z. Ronai. 1999. Role of redox potential and reactive oxygen species in stress signaling. *Oncogene* 18 (45):6104–6111.

Aiken, C. E. and S. E. Ozanne. 2014. Transgenerational developmental programming. *Hum Reprod Update* 20 (1):63–75.

Alfaradhi, M. Z., D. S. Fernandez-Twinn, M. S. Martin-Gronert, B. Musial, A. Fowden, and S. E. Ozanne. 2014. Oxidative stress and altered lipid homeostasis in the programming of offspring fatty liver by maternal obesity. *Am J Physiol Regul Integr Comp Physiol* 307 (1):R26–R34.

Amarasekera, M., P. Noakes, D. Strickland, R. Saffery, D. J. Martino, and S. L. Prescott. 2014. Epigenome-wide analysis of neonatal CD4(+) T-cell DNA methylation sites potentially affected by maternal fish oil supplementation. *Epigenetics* 9 (12):1570–1576.

Attema, J. L., P. Papathanasiou, E. C. Forsberg, J. Xu, S. T. Smale, and I. L. Weissman. 2007. Epigenetic characterization of hematopoietic stem cell differentiation using miniChIP and bisulfite sequencing analysis. *Proc Natl Acad Sci USA* 104 (30):12371–12376.

Attig, L., J. Djiane, A. Gertler, O. Rampin, T. Larcher, S. Boukthir, P. M. Anton, J. Y. Madec, I. Gourdou, and L. Abdennebi-Najar. 2008. Study of hypothalamic leptin receptor expression in low-birth-weight piglets and effects of leptin supplementation on neonatal growth and development. *Am J Physiol Endocrinol Metab* 295 (5):E1117–E1125.

Bai, S., D. Briggs, and M. H. Vickers 2012. Increased systolic blood pressure in rat offspring following a maternal low-protein diet is normalized by maternal dietary choline supplementation. *J Dev Orig Hlth Dis* 3 (4):1–8.

Benyshek, D. C., C. S. Johnston, and J. F. Martin. 2006. Glucose metabolism is altered in the adequately-nourished grand-offspring (F3 generation) of rats malnourished during gestation and perinatal life. *Diabetologia* 49 (5):1117–1119.

Bermingham, E. N., S. A. Bassett, W. Young, N. C. Roy, W. C. McNabb, J. M. Cooney, D. T. Brewster, W. A. Laing, and M. P. Barnett. 2013. Post-weaning selenium and folate supplementation affects gene and protein expression and global DNA methylation in mice fed high-fat diets. *BMC Med Genet* 6:7.

Bogdarina, I., A. Haase, S. Langley-Evans, and A. J. Clark. 2010. Glucocorticoid effects on the programming of AT1b angiotensin receptor gene methylation and expression in the rat. *PLoS One* 5 (2):e9237.

Bogdarina, I., S. Welham, P. J. King, S. P. Burns, and A. J. Clark. 2007. Epigenetic modification of the renin-angiotensin system in the fetal programming of hypertension. *Circ Res* 100 (4):520–526.

Boujendar, S., E. Arany, D. Hill, C. Remacle, and B. Reusens. 2003. Taurine supplementation of a low protein diet fed to rat dams normalizes the vascularization of the fetal endocrine pancreas. *J Nutr* 133 (9):2820–2825.

Brand, S., R. Teich, T. Dicke, H. Harb, A. O. Yildirim, J. Tost, R. Schneider-Stock et al. 2011. Epigenetic regulation in murine offspring as a novel mechanism for transmaternal asthma protection induced by microbes. *J Allergy Clin Immunol* 128 (3):618–625.e1-7.

Brawley, L., C. Torrens, F. W. Anthony, S. Itoh, T. Wheeler, A. A. Jackson, G. F. Clough, L. Poston, and M. A. Hanson. 2004. Glycine rectifies vascular dysfunction induced by dietary protein imbalance during pregnancy. *J Physiol* 554 (Pt 2):497–504.

Brumbaugh, D. E. and J. E. Friedman. 2014. Developmental origins of nonalcoholic fatty liver disease. *Pediatr Res* 75 (1–2):140–147.

Burdge, G. C., S. P. Hoile, T. Uller, N. A. Thomas, P. D. Gluckman, M. A. Hanson, and K. A. Lillycrop. 2011. Progressive, transgenerational changes in offspring phenotype and epigenotype following nutritional transition. *PLoS One* 6 (11):e28282.

Burdge, G. C., K. A. Lillycrop, A. A. Jackson, P. D. Gluckman, and M. A. Hanson. 2007a. The nature of the growth pattern and of the metabolic response to fasting in the rat are dependent upon the dietary protein and folic acid intakes of their pregnant dams and post-weaning fat consumption. *Br J Nutr* 99 (3):540–549.

Burdge, G. C., J. Slater-Jefferies, C. Torrens, E. S. Phillips, M. A. Hanson, and K. A. Lillycrop. 2007b. Dietary protein restriction of pregnant rats in the F0 generation induces altered methylation of hepatic gene promoters in the adult male offspring in the F1 and F2 generations. *Br J Nutr* 97 (3):435–439.

Callinan, P. A. and A. P. Feinberg. 2006. The emerging science of epigenomics. *Hum Mol Genet* 15 (Spec No 1):R95–R101.

Campion, J., F. I. Milagro, E. Goyenechea, and J. A. Martinez. 2009. TNF-alpha promoter methylation as a predictive biomarker for weight-loss response. *Obesity (Silver Spring)* 17 (6):1293–1297.

Carone, B. R., L. Fauquier, N. Habib, J. M. Shea, C. E. Hart, R. Li, C. Bock et al. 2010. Paternally induced transgenerational environmental reprogramming of metabolic gene expression in mammals. *Cell* 143 (7):1084–1096.

Carretero, M. V., L. Torres, U. Latasa, E. R. Garcia-Trevijano, J. Prieto, J. M. Mato, and M. A. Avila. 1998. Transformed but not normal hepatocytes express UCP2. *FEBS Lett* 439 (1–2):55–58.

Casas-Agustench, P., F. S. Fernandes, M. G. Tavares do Carmo, F. Visioli, E. Herrera, and A. Davalos. 2015. Consumption of distinct dietary lipids during early pregnancy differentially modulates the expression of microRNAs in mothers and offspring. *PLoS One* 10 (2):e0117858.

Cedar, H. and Y. Bergman. 2011. Epigenetics of haematopoietic cell development. *Nat Rev Immunol* 11 (7):478–488.

Cheng, Z. and F. A. Almeida. 2014. Mitochondrial alteration in type 2 diabetes and obesity: An epigenetic link. *Cell Cycle* 13 (6):890–897.

Cho, C. E., D. Sanchez-Hernandez, S. A. Reza-Lopez, P. S. Huot, Y. I. Kim, and G. H. Anderson. 2013. High folate gestational and post-weaning diets alter hypothalamic feeding pathways by DNA methylation in Wistar rat offspring. *Epigenetics* 8 (7):710–719.

Cooney, C. A., A. A. Dave, and G. L. Wolff. 2002. Maternal methyl supplements in mice affect epigenetic variation and DNA methylation of offspring. *J Nutr* 132 (8 Suppl):2393S–2400S.

Cordero, P., J. Campion, F. I. Milagro, E. Goyenechea, T. Steemburgo, B. M. Javierre, and J. A. Martinez. 2011. Leptin and TNF-alpha promoter methylation levels measured by MSP could predict the response to a low-calorie diet. *J Physiol Biochem* 67 (3):463–470.

Cordero, P., A. M. Gomez-Uriz, J. Campion, F. I. Milagro, and J. A. Martinez. 2013a. Dietary supplementation with methyl donors reduces fatty liver and modifies the fatty acid synthase DNA methylation profile in rats fed an obesogenic diet. *Genes Nutr* 8 (1):105–113.

Cordero, P., F. I. Milagro, J. Campion, and J. A. Martinez. 2013b. Maternal methyl donors supplementation during lactation prevents the hyperhomocysteinemia induced by a high-fat-sucrose intake by dams. *Int J Mol Sci* 14 (12):24422–24437.

Crujeiras, A. B., M. C. Carreira, B. Cabia, S. Andrade, M. Amil, and F. F. Casanueva. 2015. Leptin resistance in obesity: An epigenetic landscape. *Life Sci* 140:57–63.

Davison, J. M., T. J. Mellott, V. P. Kovacheva, and J. K. Blusztajn. 2009. Gestational choline supply regulates methylation of histone H3, expression of histone methyltransferases G9a (Kmt1c) and Suv39h1 (Kmt1a), and DNA methylation of their genes in rat fetal liver and brain. *J Biol Chem* 284 (4):1982–1989.

Delage, B. and R. H. Dashwood. 2008. Dietary manipulation of histone structure and function. *Annu Rev Nutr* 28:347–366.

Desai, M., J. K. Jellyman, and M. G. Ross. 2015. Epigenomics, gestational programming and risk of metabolic syndrome. *Int J Obes* 39 (4):633–641.

Dina, C., D. Meyre, S. Gallina, E. Durand, A. Korner, P. Jacobson, L. M. Carlsson et al. 2007. Variation in FTO contributes to childhood obesity and severe adult obesity. *Nat Genet* 39 (6):724–726.

Ding, G. L., F. F. Wang, J. Shu, S. Tian, Y. Jiang, D. Zhang, N. Wang et al. 2012. Transgenerational glucose intolerance with Igf2/H19 epigenetic alterations in mouse islet induced by intrauterine hyperglycemia. *Diabetes* 61 (5):1133–1142.

Ding, Y., J. Li, S. Liu, L. Zhang, H. Xiao, J. Li, H. Chen, R. B. Petersen, K. Huang, and L. Zheng. 2014. DNA hypomethylation of inflammation-associated genes in adipose tissue of female mice after multigenerational high fat diet feeding. *Int J Obes* 38 (2):198–204.

Ding, Y., J. Lv, C. Mao, H. Zhang, A. Wang, L. Zhu, H. Zhu, and Z. Xu. 2010. High-salt diet during pregnancy and angiotensin-related cardiac changes. *J Hypertens* 28 (6):1290–1297.

Dolinoy, D. C., J. R. Weidman, R. A. Waterland, and R. L. Jirtle. 2006. Maternal genistein alters coat color and protects Avy mouse offspring from obesity by modifying the fetal epigenome. *Environ Health Perspect* 114 (4):567–572.

Drake, A. J., L. Liu, D. Kerrigan, R. R. Meehan, and J. R. Seckl. 2011. Multigenerational programming in the glucocorticoid programmed rat is associated with generation-specific and parent of origin effects. *Epigenetics* 6 (11):1334–1343.

Dudley, K. J., D. M. Sloboda, K. L. Connor, J. Beltrand, and M. H. Vickers. 2011. Offspring of mothers fed a high fat diet display hepatic cell cycle inhibition and associated changes in gene expression and DNA methylation. *PLoS One* 6 (7):e21662.

Dunn, G. A. and T. L. Bale. 2011. Maternal high-fat diet effects on third-generation female body size via the paternal lineage. *Endocrinology* 152 (6):2228–2236.

Eckert, J. J., R. Porter, A. J. Watkins, E. Burt, S. Brooks, H. J. Leese, P. G. Humpherson, I. T. Cameron, and T. P. Fleming. 2012. Metabolic induction and early responses of mouse blastocyst developmental programming following maternal low protein diet affecting life-long health. *PLoS One* 7 (12):e52791.

Fernandez-Real, J. M. and W. Ricart. 1999. Insulin resistance and inflammation in an evolutionary perspective: The contribution of cytokine genotype/phenotype to thriftiness. *Diabetologia* 42 (11):1367–1374.

Fernandez-Twinn, D. S. and S. E. Ozanne. 2010. Early life nutrition and metabolic programming. *Ann NY Acad Sci* 1212:78–96.

Ferrante, A. W., Jr. 2013. The immune cells in adipose tissue. *Diabetes Obes Metab* 15 (Suppl 3):34–38.

Flowers, E., B. E. Aouizerat, F. Abbasi, C. Lamendola, K. M. Grove, Y. Fukuoka, and G. M. Reaven. 2015. Circulating microRNA-320a and microRNA-486 predict thiazolidinedione response: Moving towards precision health for diabetes prevention. *Metabolism* 64 (9):1051–1059.

Forsdahl, A. 1977. Are poor living conditions in childhood and adolescence an important risk factor for arteriosclerotic heart disease? *Br J Prev Soc Med* 31 (2):91–95.

Fraga, M. F., E. Ballestar, M. F. Paz, S. Ropero, F. Setien, M. L. Ballestar, D. Heine-Suner et al. 2005. Epigenetic differences arise during the lifetime of monozygotic twins. *Proc Natl Acad Sci USA* 102 (30):10604–10609.

Fu, Q., R. A. McKnight, X. Yu, L. Wang, C. W. Callaway, and R. H. Lane. 2004. Uteroplacental insufficiency induces site-specific changes in histone H3 covalent modifications and affects DNA-histone H3 positioning in day 0 IUGR rat liver. *Physiol Genomics* 20 (1):108–116.

Fullston, T., E. M. Ohlsson Teague, N. O. Palmer, M. J. DeBlasio, M. Mitchell, M. Corbett, C. G. Print, J. A. Owens, and M. Lane. 2013. Paternal obesity initiates metabolic disturbances in two generations of mice with incomplete penetrance to the F2 generation and alters the transcriptional profile of testis and sperm microRNA content. *FASEB J* 27 (10):4226–4243.

Gibson, L. C., B. C. Shin, Y. Dai, W. Freije, S. Kositamongkol, J. Cho, and S. U. Devaskar. 2015. Early leptin intervention reverses perturbed energy balance regulating hypothalamic neuropeptides in the pre- and postnatal calorie-restricted female rat offspring. *J Neurosci Res* 93 (6):902–912.

Gicquel, C., A. El-Osta, and Y. Le Bouc. 2008. Epigenetic regulation and fetal programming. *Best Pract Res Clin Endocrinol Metab* 22 (1):1–16.

Gluckman, P. D., M. A. Hanson, A. S. Beedle, and H. G. Spencer. 2008. Predictive adaptive responses in perspective. *Trends Endocrinol Metab* 19 (4):109–110.

Gluckman, P. D., K. A. Lillycrop, M. H. Vickers, A. B. Pleasants, E. S. Phillips, A. S. Beedle, G. C. Burdge, and M. A. Hanson. 2007. Metabolic plasticity during mammalian development is directionally dependent on early nutritional status. *Proc Natl Acad Sci USA* 104 (31):12796–12800.

Godfrey, K. M., P. D. Gluckman, and M. A. Hanson. 2010. Developmental origins of metabolic disease: Life course and intergenerational perspectives. *Trends Endocrinol Metab* 21 (4):199–205.

Godfrey, K. M., A. Sheppard, P. D. Gluckman, K. A. Lillycrop, G. C. Burdge, C. McLean, J. Rodford et al. 2011. Epigenetic gene promoter methylation at birth is associated with child's later adiposity. *Diabetes* 60 (5):1528–1534.

Gray, C., M. H. Vickers, S. A. Segovia, X. D. Zhang, and C. M. Reynolds. 2015. A maternal high fat diet programmes endothelial function and cardiovascular status in adult male offspring independent of body weight, which is reversed by maternal conjugated linoleic acid (CLA) supplementation. *PLoS One* 10 (2):e0115994.

Guermouche, B., A. Yessoufou, N. Soulimane, H. Merzouk, K. Moutairou, A. Hichami, and N. A. Khan. 2004. n-3 fatty acids modulate T-cell calcium signaling in obese macrosomic rats. *Obes Res* 12 (11):1744–1753.

Haggarty, P. 2013. Epigenetic consequences of a changing human diet. *Proc Nutr Soc* 72 (4):363–371.

Hales, C. N. and D. J. Barker. 1992. Type 2 (non-insulin-dependent) diabetes mellitus: The thrifty phenotype hypothesis. *Diabetologia* 35 (7):595–601.

Hales, C. N. and D. J. Barker. 2001. The thrifty phenotype hypothesis. *Br Med Bull* 60:5–20.

Harvey, N. C., A. Sheppard, K. M. Godfrey, C. McLean, E. Garratt, G. Ntani, L. Davies et al. 2014. Childhood bone mineral content is associated with methylation status of the RXRA promoter at birth. *J Bone Miner Res* 29 (3):600–607.

Hawkins, P. G. and K. V. Morris. 2008. RNA and transcriptional modulation of gene expression. *Cell Cycle* 7 (5):602–607.

Heijmans, B. T., E. W. Tobi, A. D. Stein, H. Putter, G. J. Blauw, E. S. Susser, P. E. Slagboom, and L. H. Lumey. 2008. Persistent epigenetic differences associated with prenatal exposure to famine in humans. *Proc Natl Acad Sci USA* 105 (44):17046–17049.

Hillman, S. L., S. Finer, M. C. Smart, C. Mathews, R. Lowe, V. K. Rakyan, G. A. Hitman, and D. J. Williams. 2015. Novel DNA methylation profiles associated with key gene regulation and transcription pathways in blood and placenta of growth-restricted neonates. *Epigenetics* 10 (1):50–61.

Hoile, S. P., N. A. Irvine, C. J. Kelsall, C. Sibbons, A. Feunteun, A. Collister, C. Torrens et al. 2013. Maternal fat intake in rats alters 20:4n-6 and 22:6n-3 status and the epigenetic regulation of Fads2 in offspring liver. *J Nutr Biochem* 24 (7):1213–1220.

Hoile, S. P., K. A. Lillycrop, L. R. Grenfell, M. A. Hanson, and G. C. Burdge. 2012. Increasing the folic acid content of maternal or post-weaning diets induces differential changes in phosphoenolpyruvate carboxykinase mRNA expression and promoter methylation in rats. *Br J Nutr* 108 (5):852–857.

Hoile, S. P., K. A. Lillycrop, N. A. Thomas, M. A. Hanson, and G. C. Burdge. 2011. Dietary protein restriction during F0 pregnancy in rats induces transgenerational changes in the hepatic transcriptome in female offspring. *PLoS One* 6 (7):e21668.

Holness, M. J. and M. C. Sugden. 2006. Epigenetic regulation of metabolism in children born small for gestational age. *Curr Opin Clin Nutr Metab Care* 9 (4):482–488.

Hotamisligil, G. S., N. S. Shargill, and B. M. Spiegelman. 1993. Adipose expression of tumor necrosis factor-alpha: Direct role in obesity-linked insulin resistance. *Science* 259 (5091):87–91.

Iliopoulos, D., K. N. Malizos, and A. Tsezou. 2007. Epigenetic regulation of leptin affects MMP-13 expression in osteoarthritic chondrocytes: Possible molecular target for osteoarthritis therapeutic intervention. *Ann Rheum Dis* 66 (12):1616–1621.

Iorio, M. V., C. Piovan, and C. M. Croce. 2010. Interplay between microRNAs and the epigenetic machinery: An intricate network. *Biochim Biophys Acta* 1799 (10–12):694–701.

Jang, H. and C. Serra. 2014. Nutrition, epigenetics, and diseases. *Clin Nutr Res* 3 (1):1–8.

Jirtle, R. L. and M. K. Skinner. 2007. Environmental epigenomics and disease susceptibility. *Nat Rev Genet* 8 (4):253–262.

Kaminsky, Z., S. C. Wang, and A. Petronis. 2006. Complex disease, gender and epigenetics. *Ann Med* 38 (8):530–544.

Kasbi-Chadli, F., C. Y. Boquien, G. Simard, L. Ulmann, V. Mimouni, V. Leray, A. Meynier et al. 2014. Maternal supplementation with n-3 long chain polyunsaturated fatty acids during perinatal period alleviates the metabolic syndrome disturbances in adult hamster pups fed a high-fat diet after weaning. *J Nutr Biochem* 25 (7):726–733.

Kermack, W. O., A. G. McKendrick, and P. L. McKinlay. 1934. Death-rates in great Britain and Sweden: Expression of specific mortality rates as products of two factors, and some consequences thereof. *J Hyg (Lond)* 34 (4):433–457.

Khaire, A. A., A. A. Kale, and S. R. Joshi. 2015. Maternal omega-3 fatty acids and micronutrients modulate fetal lipid metabolism: A review. *Prostaglandins Leukot Essent Fatty Acids* 98:49–55.

Khot, V., P. Chavan-Gautam, and S. Joshi. 2015. Proposing interactions between maternal phospholipids and the one carbon cycle: A novel mechanism influencing the risk for cardiovascular diseases in the offspring in later life. *Life Sci* 129:16–21.

Khot, V., A. Kale, A. Joshi, P. Chavan-Gautam, and S. Joshi. 2014. Expression of genes encoding enzymes involved in the one carbon cycle in rat placenta is determined by maternal micronutrients (folic acid, vitamin B12) and omega-3 fatty acids. *Biomed Res Int* 2014:613078.

Kjaergaard, M., C. Nilsson, A. Rosendal, M. O. Nielsen, and K. Raun. 2014. Maternal chocolate and sucrose soft drink intake induces hepatic steatosis in rat offspring associated with altered lipid gene expression profile. *Acta Physiol (Oxf)* 210 (1):142–153.

Koletzko, B. 2005. Early nutrition and its later consequences: New opportunities. *Adv Exp Med Biol* 569:1–12.

Kwong, W. Y., A. E. Wild, P. Roberts, A. C. Willis, and T. P. Fleming. 2000. Maternal undernutrition during the preimplantation period of rat development causes blastocyst abnormalities and programming of postnatal hypertension. *Development* 127 (19):4195–4202.

Langley, S. C. and A. A. Jackson. 1994. Increased systolic blood pressure in adult rats induced by fetal exposure to maternal low protein diets. *Clin Sci (Lond)* 86 (2):217–222; discussion 121.

Langley-Evans, S. C. 2000. Critical differences between two low protein diet protocols in the programming of hypertension in the rat. *Int J Food Sci Nutr* 51 (1):11–17.

Lawlor, D. A., N. J. Timpson, R. M. Harbord, S. Leary, A. Ness, M. I. McCarthy, T. M. Frayling, A. T. Hattersley, and G. D. Smith. 2008. Exploring the developmental overnutrition hypothesis using parental-offspring associations and FTO as an instrumental variable. *PLoS Med* 5 (3):e33.

Lerdweeraphon, W., J. M. Wyss, T. Boonmars, and S. Roysommuti. 2013. Perinatal taurine exposure affects adult oxidative stress. *Am J Physiol Regul Integr Comp Physiol* 305 (2):R95–R97.

Li, C., S. Guo, J. Gao, Y. Guo, E. Du, Z. Lv, and B. Zhang. 2015a. Maternal high-zinc diet attenuates intestinal inflammation by reducing DNA methylation and elevating H3K9 acetylation in the A20 promoter of offspring chicks. *J Nutr Biochem* 26 (2):173–183.

Li, M., C. M. Reynolds, D. M. Sloboda, C. Gray, and M. H. Vickers. 2013. Effects of taurine supplementation on hepatic markers of inflammation and lipid metabolism in mothers and offspring in the setting of maternal obesity. *PLoS One* 8 (10):e76961.

Li, M., C. M. Reynolds, D. M. Sloboda, C. Gray, and M. H. Vickers. 2015b. Maternal taurine supplementation attenuates maternal fructose-induced metabolic and inflammatory dysregulation and partially reverses adverse metabolic programming in offspring. *J Nutr Biochem* 26 (3):267–276.

Lie, S., J. L. Morrison, O. Williams-Wyss, C. M. Suter, D. T. Humphreys, S. E. Ozanne, S. Zhang et al. 2014. Periconceptional undernutrition programs changes in insulin-signaling molecules and microRNAs in skeletal muscle in singleton and twin fetal sheep. *Biol Reprod* 90 (1):5.

Lillycrop, K. A., E. S. Phillips, A. A. Jackson, M. A. Hanson, and G. C. Burdge. 2005. Dietary protein restriction of pregnant rats induces and folic acid supplementation prevents epigenetic modification of hepatic gene expression in the offspring. *J Nutr* 135 (6):1382–1386.

Lillycrop, K. A., J. L. Slater-Jefferies, M. A. Hanson, K. M. Godfrey, A. A. Jackson, and G. C. Burdge. 2007. Induction of altered epigenetic regulation of the hepatic glucocorticoid receptor in the offspring of rats fed a protein-restricted diet during pregnancy suggests that reduced DNA methyltransferase-1 expression is involved in impaired DNA methylation and changes in histone modifications. *Br J Nutr* 97 (6):1064–1073.

Liu, H. W., S. Mahmood, M. Srinivasan, D. J. Smiraglia, and M. S. Patel. 2013. Developmental programming in skeletal muscle in response to overnourishment in the immediate postnatal life in rats. *J Nutr Biochem* 24 (11):1859–1869.

Lumeng, C. N., S. M. Deyoung, J. L. Bodzin, and A. R. Saltiel. 2007a. Increased inflammatory properties of adipose tissue macrophages recruited during diet-induced obesity. *Diabetes* 56 (1):16–23.

Lumeng, C. N., S. M. Deyoung, and A. R. Saltiel. 2007b. Macrophages block insulin action in adipocytes by altering expression of signaling and glucose transport proteins. *Am J Physiol Endocrinol Metab* 292 (1):E166–E174.

Lumeng, C. N., I. Maillard, and A. R. Saltiel. 2009. T-ing up inflammation in fat. *Nat Med* 15 (8):846–847.

Lumey, L. H., A. D. Stein, and E. Susser. 2011. Prenatal famine and adult health. *Annu Rev Public Health* 32:237–262.

MacLennan, N. K., S. J. James, S. Melnyk, A. Piroozi, S. Jernigan, J. L. Hsu, S. M. Janke, T. D. Pham, and R. H. Lane. 2004. Uteroplacental insufficiency alters DNA methylation, one-carbon metabolism, and histone acetylation in IUGR rats. *Physiol Genomics* 18 (1):43–50.

Marco, A., T. Kisliouk, A. Weller, and N. Meiri. 2013. High fat diet induces hypermethylation of the hypothalamic Pomc promoter and obesity in post-weaning rats. *Psychoneuroendocrinology* 38 (12):2844–2853.

Martinez, J. A., P. Cordero, J. Campion, and F. I. Milagro. 2012. Interplay of early-life nutritional programming on obesity, inflammation and epigenetic outcomes. *Proc Nutr Soc* 71 (2):276–283.

Mayeur, S., O. Cisse, A. Gabory, S. Barbaux, D. Vaiman, A. Vambergue, I. Fajardy et al. 2013. Placental expression of the obesity-associated gene FTO is reduced by fetal growth restriction but not by macrosomia in rats and humans. *J Dev Orig Health Dis* 4 (2):134–138.

McKay, J. A., A. Groom, C. Potter, L. J. Coneyworth, D. Ford, J. C. Mathers, and C. L. Relton. 2012. Genetic and non-genetic influences during pregnancy on infant global and site specific DNA methylation: Role for folate gene variants and vitamin B12. *PLoS One* 7 (3):e33290.

McMillen, I. C., S. M. MacLaughlin, B. S. Muhlhausler, S. Gentili, J. L. Duffield, and J. L. Morrison. 2008. Developmental origins of adult health and disease: The role of periconceptional and foetal nutrition. *Basic Clin Pharmacol Toxicol* 102 (2):82–89.

McPherson, N. O., J. A. Owens, T. Fullston, and M. Lane. 2015. Preconception diet or exercise intervention in obese fathers normalizes sperm microRNA profile and metabolic syndrome in female offspring. *Am J Physiol Endocrinol Metab* 308 (9):E805–E821.

Melzner, I., V. Scott, K. Dorsch, P. Fischer, M. Wabitsch, S. Bruderlein, C. Hasel, and P. Moller. 2002. Leptin gene expression in human preadipocytes is switched on by maturation-induced demethylation of distinct CpGs in its proximal promoter. *J Biol Chem* 277 (47):45420–45427.

Morgado, J., B. Sanches, R. Anjos, and C. Coelho. 2015. Programming of essential hypertension: What pediatric cardiologists need to know. *Pediatr Cardiol* 36(7):1327–1337.

Morgan, D. K. and E. Whitelaw. 2008. The case for transgenerational epigenetic inheritance in humans. *Mamm Genome* 19 (6):394–397.

Murphy, S. K. and R. L. Jirtle. 2003.Imprinting evolution and the price of silence. *Bioessays* 25 (6):577–588.

Naito, M. 1993. Macrophage heterogeneity in development and differentiation. *Arch Histol Cytol* 56 (4):331–351.

Ng, S. F., R. C. Lin, D. R. Laybutt, R. Barres, J. A. Owens, and M. J. Morris. 2010. Chronic high-fat diet in fathers programs beta-cell dysfunction in female rat offspring. *Nature* 467 (7318):963–966.

Ng, S. F., R. C. Lin, C. A. Maloney, N. A. Youngson, J. A. Owens, and M. J. Morris. 2014. Paternal high-fat diet consumption induces common changes in the transcriptomes of retroperitoneal adipose and pancreatic islet tissues in female rat offspring. *FASEB J* 28 (4):1830–1841.

Nishikawa, T., D. Kukidome, K. Sonoda, K. Fujisawa, T. Matsuhisa, H. Motoshima, T. Matsumura, and E. Araki. 2007. Impact of mitochondrial ROS production in the pathogenesis of insulin resistance. *Diabetes Res Clin Pract* 77 (Suppl 1):S161–S164.

Ojha, S., H. P. Fainberg, S. Sebert, H. Budge, and M. E. Symonds. 2015. Maternal health and eating habits: Metabolic consequences and impact on child health. *Trends Mol Med* 21 (2):126–133.

Ollikainen, M., K. Ismail, K. Gervin, A. Kyllonen, A. Hakkarainen, J. Lundbom, E. A. Jarvinen et al. 2015. Genome-wide blood DNA methylation alterations at regulatory elements and heterochromatic regions in monozygotic twins discordant for obesity and liver fat. *Clin Epigenetics* 7 (1):39.

Ortega, F. J., M. Moreno, J. M. Mercader, J. M. Moreno-Navarrete, N. Fuentes-Batllevell, M. Sabater, W. Ricart, and J. M. Fernandez-Real. 2015. Inflammation triggers specific microRNA profiles in human adipocytes and macrophages and in their supernatants. *Clin Epigenetics* 7 (1):49.

Palmer, A. C. 2011. Nutritionally mediated programming of the developing immune system. *Adv Nutr* 2 (5):377–395.

Palou, M., C. Pico, J. A. McKay, J. Sanchez, T. Priego, J. C. Mathers, and A. Palou. 2011. Protective effects of leptin during the suckling period against later obesity may be associated with changes in promoter methylation of the hypothalamic pro-opiomelanocortin gene. *Br J Nutr* 106 (5):769–778.

Park, J. H., D. A. Stoffers, R. D. Nicholls, and R. A. Simmons. 2008. Development of type 2 diabetes following intrauterine growth retardation in rats is associated with progressive epigenetic silencing of Pdx1. *J Clin Invest* 118 (6):2316–2324.

Pereira, T. J., M. A. Fonseca, K. E. Campbell, B. L. Moyce, L. K. Cole, G. M. Hatch, C. A. Doucette, J. Klein, M. Aliani, and V. W. Dolinsky. 2015. Maternal obesity characterized by gestational diabetes increases the susceptibility of rat offspring to hepatic steatosis via a disrupted liver metabolome. *J Physiol* 593(14):3181–3197.

Pham, T. D., N. K. MacLennan, C. T. Chiu, G. S. Laksana, J. L. Hsu, and R. H. Lane. 2003. Uteroplacental insufficiency increases apoptosis and alters p53 gene methylation in the full-term IUGR rat kidney. *Am J Physiol Regul Integr Comp Physiol* 285 (5):R962–R970.

Pinney, S. E., L. J. Jaeckle Santos, Y. Han, D. A. Stoffers, and R. A. Simmons. 2011. Exendin-4 increases histone acetylase activity and reverses epigenetic modifications that silence Pdx1 in the intrauterine growth retarded rat. *Diabetologia* 54 (10):2606–2614.

Prattichizzo, F., A. Giuliani, A. Ceka, M. R. Rippo, A. R. Bonfigli, R. Testa, A. D. Procopio, and F. Olivieri. 2015. Epigenetic mechanisms of endothelial dysfunction in type 2 diabetes. *Clin Epigenetics* 7 (1):56.

Preidis, G. A., M. A. Keaton, P. M. Campeau, B. C. Bessard, M. E. Conner, and P. J. Hotez. 2014. The undernourished neonatal mouse metabolome reveals evidence of liver and biliary dysfunction, inflammation, and oxidative stress. *J Nutr* 144 (3):273–281.

Radford, E. J., E. Isganaitis, J. Jimenez-Chillaron, J. Schroeder, M. Molla, S. Andrews, N. Didier et al. 2012. An unbiased assessment of the role of imprinted genes in an intergenerational model of developmental programming. *PLoS Genet* 8 (4):e1002605.

Ravelli, G. P., Z. A. Stein, and M. W. Susser. 1976. Obesity in young men after famine exposure *in utero* and early infancy. *N Engl J Med* 295 (7):349–353.

Raychaudhuri, N., S. Raychaudhuri, M. Thamotharan, and S. U. Devaskar. 2008. Histone code modifications repress glucose transporter 4 expression in the intrauterine growth-restricted offspring. *J Biol Chem* 283 (20):13611–13626.

Rexhaj, E., J. Bloch, P. Y. Jayet, S. F. Rimoldi, P. Dessen, C. Mathieu, J. F. Tolsa, P. Nicod, U. Scherrer, and C. Sartori. 2011. Fetal programming of pulmonary vascular dysfunction in mice: Role of epigenetic mechanisms. *Am J Physiol Heart Circ Physiol* 301 (1):H247–H252.

Reynolds, C. M., M. Li, C. Gray, and M. H. Vickers. 2013a. Pre-weaning growth hormone treatment ameliorates adipose tissue insulin resistance and inflammation in adult male offspring following maternal undernutrition. *Endocrinology* 154 (8):2676–2686.

Reynolds, C. M., M. Li, C. Gray, and M. H. Vickers. 2013b. Pre-weaning growth hormone treatment ameliorates bone marrow macrophage inflammation in adult male rat offspring following maternal undernutrition. *PLoS One* 8 (7):e68262.

Reynolds, C. M., F. C. McGillicuddy, K. A. Harford, O. M. Finucane, K. H. Mills, and H. M. Roche. 2012. Dietary saturated fatty acids prime the NLRP3 inflammasome via TLR4 in dendritic cells-implications for diet-induced insulin resistance. *Mol Nutr Food Res* 56 (8):1212–1222.

Reynolds, C. M., S. A. Segovia, X. D. Zhang, C. Gray, and M. H. Vickers. 2015. Conjugated linoleic Acid supplementation during pregnancy and lactation reduces maternal high-fat-diet-induced programming of early-onset puberty and hyperlipidemia in female rat offspring. *Biol Reprod* 92 (2):40.

Rodriguez-Gonzalez, G. L., C. C. Vega, L. Boeck, M. Vazquez, C. J. Bautista, L. A. Reyes-Castro, O. Saldana, D. Lovera, P. W. Nathanielsz, and E. Zambrano. 2015. Maternal obesity and overnutrition increase oxidative stress in male rat offspring reproductive system and decrease fertility. *Int J Obes* 39(4):549–556.

Roseboom, T. J., J. H. van der Meulen, C. Osmond, D. J. Barker, A. C. Ravelli, and O. P. Bleker. 2000. Plasma lipid profiles in adults after prenatal exposure to the Dutch famine. *Am J Clin Nutr* 72 (5):1101–1106.

Roseboom, T. J., J. H. van der Meulen, A. C. Ravelli, C. Osmond, D. J. Barker, and O. P. Bleker. 2001. Effects of prenatal exposure to the Dutch famine on adult disease in later life: An overview. *Mol Cell Endocrinol* 185 (1–2):93–98.

Roysommuti, S. and J. M. Wyss. 2014. Perinatal taurine exposure affects adult arterial pressure control. *Amino Acids* 46 (1):57–72.

Sanders, A. P., H. H. Burris, A. C. Just, V. Motta, K. Svensson, A. Mercado-Garcia, I. Pantic et al. 2015. microRNA expression in the cervix during pregnancy is associated with length of gestation. *Epigenetics* 10 (3):221–228.

Satoh, T., O. Takeuchi, A. Vandenbon, K. Yasuda, Y. Tanaka, Y. Kumagai, T. Miyake et al. 2010. The Jmjd3-Irf4 axis regulates M2 macrophage polarization and host responses against helminth infection. *Nat Immunol* 11 (10):936–944.

Scherrer, U., S. F. Rimoldi, C. Sartori, F. H. Messerli, and E. Rexhaj. 2015. Fetal programming and epigenetic mechanisms in arterial hypertension. *Curr Opin Cardiol* 30 (4):393–397.

Sebert, S., T. Salonurmi, S. Keinanen-Kiukaanniemi, M. Savolainen, K. H. Herzig, M. E. Symonds, and M. R. Jarvelin. 2014. Programming effects of FTO in the development of obesity. *Acta Physiol (Oxf)* 210 (1):58–69.

Sebert, S., D. Sharkey, H. Budge, and M. E. Symonds. 2011. The early programming of metabolic health: Is epigenetic setting the missing link? *Am J Clin Nutr* 94 (6):1953S–1958S.

Sebert, S. P., M. A. Hyatt, L. L. Chan, M. Yiallourides, H. P. Fainberg, N. Patel, D. Sharkey et al. 2010. Influence of prenatal nutrition and obesity on tissue specific fat mass and obesity-associated (FTO) gene expression. *Reproduction* 139 (1):265–274.

Shen, W., C. Wang, L. Xia, C. Fan, H. Dong, R. J. Deckelbaum, and K. Qi. 2014. Epigenetic modification of the leptin promoter in diet-induced obese mice and the effects of N-3 polyunsaturated fatty acids. *Sci Rep* 4:5282.

Silva, A. J. and R. White. 1988. Inheritance of allelic blueprints for methylation patterns. *Cell* 54 (2):145–152.

Sinclair, K. D., C. Allegrucci, R. Singh, D. S. Gardner, S. Sebastian, J. Bispham, A. Thurston et al. 2007. DNA methylation, insulin resistance, and blood pressure in offspring determined by maternal periconceptional B vitamin and methionine status. *Proc Natl Acad Sci USA* 104 (49):19351–19356.

Smemo, S., J. J. Tena, K. H. Kim, E. R. Gamazon, N. J. Sakabe, C. Gomez-Marin, I. Aneas et al. 2014. Obesity-associated variants within FTO form long-range functional connections with IRX3. *Nature* 507 (7492):371–375.

Soubry, A., S. K. Murphy, F. Wang, Z. Huang, A. C. Vidal, B. F. Fuemmeler, J. Kurtzberg et al. 2015. Newborns of obese parents have altered DNA methylation patterns at imprinted genes. *Int J Obes* 39 (4):650–657.

Soubry, A., J. M. Schildkraut, A. Murtha, F. Wang, Z. Huang, A. Bernal, J. Kurtzberg, R. L. Jirtle, S. K. Murphy, and C. Hoyo. 2013. Paternal obesity is associated with IGF2 hypomethylation in newborns: Results from a Newborn Epigenetics Study (NEST) cohort. *BMC Med* 11:29.

Stoger, R. 2006. In vivo methylation patterns of the leptin promoter in human and mouse. *Epigenetics* 1 (4):155–162.

Strakovsky, R. S., X. Zhang, D. Zhou, and Y. X. Pan. 2014. The regulation of hepatic Pon1 by a maternal high-fat diet is gender specific and may occur through promoter histone modifications in neonatal rats. *J Nutr Biochem* 25 (2):170–176.

Suter, M. A., A. Chen, M. S. Burdine, M. Choudhury, R. A. Harris, R. H. Lane, J. E. Friedman, K. L. Grove, A. J. Tackett, and K. M. Aagaard. 2012. A maternal high-fat diet modulates fetal SIRT1 histone and protein deacetylase activity in nonhuman primates. *FASEB J* 26 (12):5106–5114.

Sutton-Tyrrell, K., A. Bostom, J. Selhub, and C. Zeigler-Johnson. 1997. High homocysteine levels are independently related to isolated systolic hypertension in older adults. *Circulation* 96 (6):1745–1749.

Tan, Y., B. Zhang, T. Wu, G. Skogerbo, X. Zhu, X. Guo, S. He, and R. Chen. 2009. Transcriptional inhibition of Hoxd4 expression by miRNA-10a in human breast cancer cells. *BMC Mol Biol* 10:12.

Tobi, E. W., J. J. Goeman, R. Monajemi, H. Gu, H. Putter, Y. Zhang, R. C. Slieker et al. 2014. DNA methylation signatures link prenatal famine exposure to growth and metabolism. *Nat Commun* 5:5592.

Tobi, E. W., L. H. Lumey, R. P. Talens, D. Kremer, H. Putter, A. D. Stein, P. E. Slagboom, and B. T. Heijmans. 2009. DNA methylation differences after exposure to prenatal famine are common and timing- and sex-specific. *Hum Mol Genet* 18 (21):4046–4053.

Tobi, E. W., R. C. Slieker, A. D. Stein, H. E. Suchiman, P. E. Slagboom, E. W. van Zwet, B. T. Heijmans, and L. H. Lumey. 2015. Early gestation as the critical time-window for changes in the prenatal environment to affect the adult human blood methylome. *Int J Epidemiol* 44(4):1211–1223.

Tosh, D. N., Q. Fu, C. W. Callaway, R. A. McKnight, I. C. McMillen, M. G. Ross, R. H. Lane, and M. Desai. 2010. Epigenetics of programmed obesity: Alteration in IUGR rat hepatic IGF1 mRNA expression and histone structure in rapid vs. delayed postnatal catch-up growth. *Am J Physiol Gastrointest Liver Physiol* 299 (5):G1023–G1029.

Tsuboyama-Kasaoka, N., M. Takahashi, K. Tanemura, H. J. Kim, T. Tange, H. Okuyama, M. Kasai, S. Ikemoto, and O. Ezaki. 2000. Conjugated linoleic acid supplementation reduces adipose tissue by apoptosis and develops lipodystrophy in mice. *Diabetes* 49 (9):1534–1542.

Vanhees, K., I. G. Vonhogen, F. J. van Schooten, and R. W. Godschalk. 2014. You are what you eat, and so are your children: The impact of micronutrients on the epigenetic programming of offspring. *Cell Mol Life Sci* 71 (2):271–285.

Vickers, M. H., P. D. Gluckman, A. H. Coveny, P. L. Hofman, W. S. Cutfield, A. Gertler, B. H. Breier, and M. Harris. 2005. Neonatal leptin treatment reverses developmental programming. *Endocrinology* 146 (10):4211–4216.

Vickers, M. H., P. D. Gluckman, A. H. Coveny, P. L. Hofman, W. S. Cutfield, A. Gertler, B. H. Breier, and M. Harris. 2008. The effect of neonatal leptin treatment on postnatal weight gain in male rats is dependent on maternal nutritional status during pregnancy. *Endocrinology* 149 (4):1906–1913.

Vucetic, Z., J. Kimmel, K. Totoki, E. Hollenbeck, and T. M. Reyes. 2010. Maternal high-fat diet alters methylation and gene expression of dopamine and opioid-related genes. *Endocrinology* 151 (10):4756–4764.

Waterland, R. A. 2014. Epigenetic mechanisms affecting regulation of energy balance: Many questions, few answers. *Annu Rev Nutr* 34:337–355.

Waterland, R. A., D. C. Dolinoy, J. R. Lin, C. A. Smith, X. Shi, and K. G. Tahiliani. 2006a. Maternal methyl supplements increase offspring DNA methylation at Axin Fused. *Genesis* 44 (9):401–406.

Waterland, R. A., J. R. Lin, C. A. Smith, and R. L. Jirtle. 2006b. Post-weaning diet affects genomic imprinting at the insulin-like growth factor 2 (Igf2) locus. *Hum Mol Genet* 15 (5):705–716.

Waterland, R. A. and K. B. Michels. 2007. Epigenetic epidemiology of the developmental origins hypothesis. *Annu Rev Nutr* 27:363–388.

Waterland, R. A., M. Travisano, K. G. Tahiliani, M. T. Rached, and S. Mirza. 2008. Methyl donor supplementation prevents transgenerational amplification of obesity. *Int J Obes* 32 (9):1373–1379.

Watkins, A. J., E. Ursell, R. Panton, T. Papenbrock, L. Hollis, C. Cunningham, A. Wilkins et al. 2008. Adaptive responses by mouse early embryos to maternal diet protect fetal growth but predispose to adult onset disease. *Biol Reprod* 78 (2):299–306.

Weaver, I. C., N. Cervoni, F. A. Champagne, A. C. D'Alessio, S. Sharma, J. R. Seckl, S. Dymov, M. Szyf, and M. J. Meaney. 2004. Epigenetic programming by maternal behavior. *Nat Neurosci* 7 (8):847–854.

Wolff, G. L., R. L. Kodell, S. R. Moore, and C. A. Cooney. 1998. Maternal epigenetics and methyl supplements affect agouti gene expression in Avy/a mice. *FASEB J* 12 (11):949–957.

Wolffe, A. P. 1998. Packaging principle: How DNA methylation and histone acetylation control the transcriptional activity of chromatin. *J Exp Zool* 282 (1–2):239–244.

Woods, L. L. 2007. Maternal nutrition and predisposition to later kidney disease. *Curr Drug Targets* 8 (8):906–913.

Yan, X., Y. Huang, J. X. Zhao, C. J. Rogers, M. J. Zhu, S. P. Ford, P. W. Nathanielsz, and M. Du. 2013. Maternal obesity downregulates microRNA let-7g expression, a possible mechanism for enhanced adipogenesis during ovine fetal skeletal muscle development. *Int J Obes* 37 (4):568–575.

Yokomori, N., M. Tawata, and T. Onaya. 1999. DNA demethylation during the differentiation of 3T3-L1 cells affects the expression of the mouse GLUT4 gene. *Diabetes* 48 (4):685–690.

Yokomori, N., M. Tawata, and T. Onaya. 2002. DNA demethylation modulates mouse leptin promoter activity during the differentiation of 3T3-L1 cells. *Diabetologia* 45 (1):140–148.

Zeisel, S. H. 2009. Importance of methyl donors during reproduction. *Am J Clin Nutr* 89 (2):673S-677S.

Zhang, J., F. Zhang, X. Didelot, K. D. Bruce, F. R. Cagampang, M. Vatish, M. Hanson, H. Lehnert, A. Ceriello, and C. D. Byrne. 2009. Maternal high fat diet during pregnancy and lactation alters hepatic expression of insulin like growth factor-2 and key microRNAs in the adult offspring. *BMC Genomics* 10:478.

Zhang, X., R. Yang, Y. Jia, D. Cai, B. Zhou, X. Qu, H. Han et al. 2014. Hypermethylation of Sp1 binding site suppresses hypothalamic POMC in neonates and may contribute to metabolic disorders in adults: Impact of maternal dietary CLAs. *Diabetes* 63 (5):1475–1487.

Zhou, Y., L. Zhao, Z. Zhang, and X. Lu. 2015. Protective effect of enalapril against methionine-enriched diet-induced hypertension: Role of endoplasmic reticulum and oxidative stress. *Biomed Res Int* 2015:724876.

Zinkhan, E. K., Q. Fu, Y. Wang, X. Yu, C. W. Callaway, J. L. Segar, T. D. Scholz, R. A. McKnight, L. Joss-Moore, and R. H. Lane. 2012. Maternal hyperglycemia disrupts histone 3 lysine 36 trimethylation of the IGF-1 gene. *J Nutr Metab* 2012:930364.

29 Gene–Diet Interactions

Silvia Berciano and Jose M. Ordovas

CONTENTS

ABSTRACT

Cardiometabolic diseases are the principal cause of death globally, and are strongly driven by both genetic and environmental factors, mainly nutritional. Nutrigenetic studies investigate the relationship between genetic variants and diet in modulating cardiometabolic risk. Numerous studies have reported statistically significant gene–diet interactions related to cardiovascular risk factors (obesity, insulin resistance, and dyslipidemias) and more recently some evidence is emerging related to cardiovascular events. However, current advances in this field are hampered by the lack of reproducibility across studies. Here, we describe the current state of the field of nutrigenetics with respect to cardiometabolic disease research using some of the best characterized loci, and outline directions for the translation of this and future findings into new preventive and therapeutic options for cardiometabolic disease.

ABBREVIATIONS

APOA1	Apolipoprotein A-1
APOA2	Apolipoprotein A-2
APOA4	Apolipoprotein A-4
APOA5	Apolipoprotein A-5
APOC3	Apolipoprotein C-3
APOE	Apolipoprotein E
ARIC	Atherosclerosis risk in communities
BDNF	Brain-derived neurotrophic factor
BMI	Body mass index
BPRHS	Boston Puerto Rican Health Study
CETP	Cholesteryl ester transfer protein
CHARGE	Cohorts for Heart and Aging Research in Genomic Epidemiology
CHO	Carbohydrate
CLOCK	Clock Circadian Regulator
CVD	Cardiovascular disease
EPIC	European Prospective Investigation into Cancer and Nutrition

FTO	Fat mass and obesity-associated
GI	Glycemic index
GIPR	Gastric inhibitory polypeptide receptor
GL	Glycemic load
GOLDN	Genetics of Lipid Lowering Drugs and Diet Network
GRS	Genetic risk score
GWAS	Genome-wide association studies
HDL	High density lipoproteins
HOMA	Homeostatic model assessment
IR	Insulin resistance
IRS1	Insulin Receptor Substrate 1
LEP	Leptin
LIPC	Hepatic lipase
LOC	Loss of control
LPL	Lipoprotein lipase
MC4R	Melanocortin 4 Receptor
MDCS	Malmö Diet and Cancer Study
MedDiet	Mediterranean diet
MESA	Multi-Ethnic Study of Atherosclerosis
miRNAs	MicroRNAs
MRE	miRNA recognition elements
MRESS	MRE seed sites
MUFA	Monounsaturated fatty acids
PCSK7	Proprotein Convertase Subtilisin/Kexin Type 7
PLIN1	Perilipin 1
PPM1K	Protein Phosphatase, Mg^{2+}/Mn^{2+} Dependent, 1K
PREDIMED	PREvención con DIeta MEDiterránea
PUFA	Polyunsaturated fatty acids
SFA	Saturated fatty acids
SNP	Single nucleotide polymorphism
T2D	Type 2 diabetes
TG	Triglycerides
TCF7L2	Transcription Factor 7-Like 2
VLDL	Very low density lipoprotein

INTRODUCTION

"*The controversy concerning heredity versus environment is largely an argument of the past. It is now generally accepted that genes act within the environments in which they find themselves, and that the genetic potentialities of an individual may or may not find full expression because of the limitations of the environment in which they exist. One aspect of the environment, which may affect the expression of genes, is nutrition.*" Whereas these statements are totally appropriate and timely, we cannot take ownership as they belong to the introduction of a review published in 1969 by Lucille S. Hurley (1969), well before the advent of contemporary genetics and the upsurge of personalized nutrition. The same author went on to emphasize this last concept: "*Individual differences in reactions to food are, it is believed by the writer, an expression, in part, of innate genetic individuality.*" However, this is not by any means the first explicit description of gene–diet interactions. We can go back more than eight decades and find a similar discourse in the work by W. Franklin Dove (1935), describing differences in bodily demands between genotypes: "*Different genotypes or phenotypes controlling form or function must be closely allied to the ability to choose food wisely. In the same way that one individual is able to alter its choice of food in accordance with the requirements of each stage of its growth or life cycle, so are individuals with differing genetic make-up able to make a selection of food in accordance with their differences in form and function.*" These nuggets are not unique in the quarry of the scientific literature. Rather, they represent a minimal sample to show the oldness of many research topics and how, sometimes, we forget their existence for decades just to bring them up again to the limelight with contemporary names such as Nutrigenetics or Nutrigenomics.

The purpose of this chapter is not to review the ancient literature but rather to bring to the reader the current status of the field in relation to gene–diet interactions and cardiometabolic health and to project a vision of the future in this most relevant health area that, if properly used, may change the future of preventive medicine and how we can achieve a healthier aging. Conscientious of this potential and armed with the new weapons of genetics and molecular biology, an increased number of basic, nutritional, and clinical scientists have launched an offensive to conquer the essential knowledge needed to materialize personalized nutrition. However, it is important to warn about the overstatements that have been made in relation to personalized nutrition. The scientific objectives are far from being accomplished and what we have in our hands is a large amount of promising and, in most cases, unconnected findings that still need to crystalize into solid knowledge before the field can move into clinical practice applications.

Beginning in the 1990s, there was an extensive and growing literature related to the contemporary approach to gene–environment and particularly gene–diet interactions concerning cardiometabolic health. Nevertheless, about one-third of the articles found in PubMed on this topic are review articles. Moreover, the quantitative richness may not be paralleled by the qualitative wealth, considering that there is an appalling lack of replication among the findings that hampers the ultimate objective of translating this knowledge into better cardiovascular prevention and therapy for every member of society. The lack of replication is partially due to the limitations associated with previous study designs:

- Mostly observational and retrospective, providing a low level of evidence
- Inadequate sample size to properly address the statistical power related with the complexity inherent to the analysis of gene–environment interactions
- Uncertainty and subjectivity associated with gathering environmental information, including diet

Progress to overcome some of these caveats, specifically regarding sample size, has been made possible, thanks to the assembly of the Cohorts for Heart and Aging Research in Genomic Epidemiology (CHARGE) consortium, created to enable meta-analyses of genome-wide association studies (GWAS) and replication among many large population-based cohort studies (Bis et al., 2009). However, improved methods that allow direct measurement of individual dietary intake are urgently needed (Tucker et al., 2013).

In order to compose a bird's-eye view of the current status of this research, we have recently cataloged the literature related to cardiometabolic gene–environment interactions (Parnell et al., 2014). From this inclusive list of 386 publications, including blood lipids, glycemic traits, anthropometrics, blood pressure, and inflammation, we concluded that the gene–environment single nucleotide polymorphisms (SNPs) listed in the catalog showed little overlap with variants identified for those same traits in GWAS. These observations highlight the incomplete description of contribution to phenotypic variance by main effect associations such as those in GWAS, and strengthen the importance of gene–environment interactions as contributors to that variance. This then implies that genetic contributors alone are insufficient diagnostic tools for assessing disease risk, and that those calculations also must include the gene–environment term. Besides, the publications were enriched with SNPs related to adaptation to environmental factors, such as climate. This may have had evolutionary implications on energy homeostasis and response to physical activity. Overall, the current body of literature suggests that SNPs involved in cardiometabolic gene–environment interactions often exhibit transcriptional effects or are under positive selection.

Withstanding the relevance of other environmental factors, our focus will be on gene–diet interactions. After all, food is an essential component of our daily lives that, in addition, we can individually modify to fit our needs and our health (Ordovas and Corella, 2004).

GENETICS OF CVD AND CVD RISK FACTORS

It has long been known that CVD has a strong genetic component, thanks to evidence gathered initially from twin studies and from inborn errors of metabolism (i.e., familial hypercholesterolemia). Moreover, the knowledge of the physiology and biochemistry associated with specific metabolic pathways involved in the development of the disease (i.e., plasma lipid metabolism) facilitated the early adoption of the "candidate gene approach," well before the advent of the GWAS, thus providing a "heads-up" to the field. However, a more precise and complete identification of the genetic factors associated with CVD and its risk factors has been hampered by the significant influence of environmental variables and the intrinsic complexity of the disease (Corella and Ordovas, 2009a).

Gene–Diet Interactions and CVD Risk

We are not aiming to provide a complete list and evaluation of the knowledge accumulated since the 1990s; rather, we will focus on some representative and more impactful loci related to gene–diet interactions and cardiometabolic traits. In some cases, the choice may be clear: fat mass and obesity-associated (FTO) and energy metabolism; TCF7L2 and dysglycemia. For other CVD risk factors, the choice may not be so evident and we will use our own discretion to bring examples that represent the progress made on the field.

Gene–Diet Interactions and Energy Balance

The initial focus of gene–diet interactions in relation to cardiometabolic health fell in the area of lipid metabolism; however, the interest has been increasingly shifting toward the pressing topic of energy balance and obesity.

Obesity has become, in the mind of many, the number one public health enemy. Its prevention and therapy have proved to be extremely difficult and the mindset has been shifting from a simple balance equation based on energy in and energy out (and a conceptually simple solution: "eat less and move more") to a much more complex formula with an ever-increasing number of variables. Some of them, like the microbiota and chronobiology, are gaining increased interest and relevance alongside the more traditional factors (i.e., diet, physical activity). Even within the diet itself, we have evolved from calorie-counting to a more elaborate scenario in which the different combinations of macro (and micro) nutrients may play a key role. Finally, the complexity increases exponentially when we add genetic individuality.

In practical terms, there are two sides to the obesity conundrum. One involves the prevention of unhealthy weight gain and the other relates to successfully losing the excess of weight. Whereas both have a significant genetic component, it is becoming evident that the overlap among the genes involved is far from complete. Attaining a healthy body mass index (BMI) becomes harder at increased adiposity levels, and this is due to both genetic and environmental factors. A recent study (Fildes et al., 2015) that analyzed data for 76,704 obese men and 99,791 obese women has shown that obese individuals have low chances (1.7% for men and 2.2% for women) of recovering a normal weight or even reducing it by a modest 5% during a maximum of 9 years' follow-up, refueling disbelief in the current obesity management strategies. Lifestyle modification is a central part of these interventions, and relies on the ability of the patient to adopt new, healthier habits. This may be notoriously difficult for some individuals, and we are currently studying how the interplay between genetics, epigenetics, and environment affects cognitive inhibition—that is, one's ability to process stimuli before eliciting a response—a key function in this process. It also needs to be noted that, while the follow-up duration is limited to a few months in most studies, successful short-term adherence may not imply long-term habit formation, and further research needs to be carried out on this subject to better understand how healthy eating behaviors can become stable habits to support weight maintenance in the long term.

Regarding weight gain, the state of the art of GWAS meta-analyses has led to the identification of over 100 loci for common, polygenic anthropometric traits (i.e., BMI; waist circumference and body fat distribution) (Locke et al., 2015; Shungin et al., 2015). These variants have modest effect and for most of them their functionality remains unknown. In fact, for the most significant of these obesity-predisposing loci, the FTO gene, the increase in BMI associated with the presence of each risk allele is ~0.40 kg/m^2. To put this in practical terms, this figure is similar to the average seasonal variability in BMI found in humans through the year (van Ooijen et al., 2004), or the variability associated with BMI changes resulting from dietary habits during certain holidays (Yanovski et al., 2000).

FTO was the first gene to be strongly associated with obesity using the GWAS approach and, unsurprisingly, it has been one of the most investigated genes in terms of obesity-related associations and interactions. Nevertheless, the mechanism by which the FTO might contribute to obesity remains unsolved. In fact, despite the metabolic phenotypes found in FTO rodent models and the location of SNPs in intron 1 of the human gene, the implication of other neighboring genes in obesity cannot be disregarded. Based on the high FTO expression levels in the hypothalamus, it has been suggested that the mechanism of action could be mediated by a potential role in food intake (Fredriksson et al., 2008), which is consistent with growing evidence since its discovery and with the role proposed for many of the other newly identified obesity-predisposing genes.

Interactions between the FTO gene and environmental factors were initially reported for physical activity and the most comprehensive of these studies (Ahmad et al., 2013) was carried out in 111,421 individuals of European ancestry, with the FTO being part of a 12-loci genetic risk score (GRS). Historically, the analysis and presentation of genetic findings has focused on individual genes; however, we have to keep in mind the polygenic nature of CVD and its risk factors, and that the practical translation of this research will not rely on individual loci but in more complex algorithms incorporated in GRS. The use of GRS for prediction of risk or dietary response has two major benefits. First, it takes into account the already mentioned complex polygenic nature of common diseases. Moreover, it partially overcomes the problem of multiple comparisons associated with the statistical analysis of many individual SNPs.

Returning to the FTO, secondary analyses of the rs1121980 SNP demonstrated a significant gene by physical activity interaction ($p = 0.003$). The results emerging from the analysis of FTO by diet interactions are more complex. Our group has found a significant interaction between saturated fat (SFA) intake and FTO on BMI, in two independent American populations, the Genetics of Lipid Lowering Drugs and Diet Network (GOLDN, n ~ 1100) and the Boston Puerto Rican Health Study (BPRHS, n ~ 1300) (Corella et al., 2011a). We examined rs9939609 (in the GOLDN) and rs1121980 (in the GOLDN and BPRHS) SNPs. Our results show that subjects homozygous for the FTO-risk alleles had a higher mean BMI than those with the other genotypes only when they had a high-SFA intake, whereas no associations with BMI were found at lower SFA intakes in models adjusted for energy intake. We also examined the potential interaction with carbohydrate (CHO) intake but our analysis did not reveal any statistically significant findings. Therefore, from these data we can conclude that SFA intake modulates the association between FTO and BMI in these two populations of White and Hispanic Americans.

A second study also based on three American populations (9,623 women from the Nurses' Health Study, 6,379 men from the Health Professionals Follow-up Study, and a replication cohort of 21,421 women from the Women's Genome Health Study) posed a different, although related, question and analyzed the interactions between genetic predisposition to obesity and consumption of fried food using a GRS based on 32 BMI-associated gene variants (Qi et al., 2014a). The data revealed a significant interaction between fried food consumption and the GRS by which the genetic association with adiposity was strengthened with higher consumption of fried foods, with the FTO locus showing the strongest result. Conversely, a meta-analysis performed based on data from 177,330 adults (154,439 Whites, 5,776 African Americans, and 17,115 Asians) from 40 studies did not find significant interactions between the FTO gene and dietary intake of total energy, protein, carbohydrate, or fat on BMI (Qi et al., 2014b).

Given the potential role of FTO in food intake, this locus has been investigated in relation to emotional eating and food consumption (Cornelis et al., 2014). For this purpose, information on eating behavior and BMI was collected by questionnaires for 1471 men and 2381 women from the two U.S. cohorts indicated earlier (Nurses and Health Professionals). The same GRS used earlier was applied to this study and it was positively associated with emotional and uncontrolled eating.

Another study (Harbron et al., 2014) investigated associations between polymorphisms including the FTO rs1421085 and rs17817449 haplotypes and dietary intake and eating behavior. The population was much smaller (n = 133) than in the previous study and consisted of overweight/obese Caucasian adults seeking treatment to lose weight. Weight and height were measured and eating behavior was assessed by the Three Factor Eating questionnaire, which measures dietary restraint, disinhibition, and hunger (Stunkard and Messick, 1985). The risk alleles of the FTO SNPs were associated with poorer eating behaviors (higher hunger, internal locus for hunger, and emotional disinhibition scores), a higher intake of high fat foods and refined starches supporting an effect of the FTO locus on eating behavior.

The topic of FTO and eating behavior has been also examined in children, specifically in relation to loss of control (LOC) eating, a behavior associated with weight gain (Tanofsky-Kraff et al., 2009). For this purpose, 289 youth aged 6–19 years were studied by genotyping the FTO-rs9939609 SNP and determining their level of LOC eating, a behavior assessed by interview and by participation in a buffet meal modeling an LOC episode. Subjects carrying the A risk allele had significantly greater BMI and fat mass. Of these, ~35% reported LOC compared with ~18% of the TT subjects (p = 0.002). Despite consuming the same amount of total energy, carriers of the A allele consumed a significantly greater percentage of energy from fat than did the TT subjects. Therefore, this study suggests that the youth carrying the FTO risk allele reported more often LOC eating and selected more often the consumption of foods higher in fat. FTO is highly expressed in regions of the hypothalamus that are considered key for appetite regulation and eating behavior. The preference for fat and energy-dense foods has been proposed as a potential mechanism to explain the association between the FTO risk allele A and obesity. Both findings (LOC eating and high-density food preference) support that hypothesis. However, the authors selected a population enriched for overweight. We know that there is an interaction between this FTO risk allele and saturated fat intake that results in effective development of obesity only when the daily saturated fat intake exceeds 22 g per day. The fact that the FTO carriers in this study had a significantly higher BMI than noncarriers could have biased the results as selecting for children that are already on the road to obesity could mean that carriers that have not displayed a preference for fat are left out. Therefore, this combination of effects may be driving the increased BMI associated with this risk allele. Additional support for the hypothesis involving FTO and eating behavior comes from the LOOK-AHEAD study, where the risk allele at the FTO rs1421085 SNP predicted more eating episodes per day even after adjustment for body weight (McCaffery et al., 2012). FTO rs1421085 was also associated with an increased percentage of energy intake from fat (p = 0.019), although this effect was relatively small (0.52% per risk allele copy).

The previous findings suggest certain consistency in terms of the association between the FTO locus and eating behavior; however, the evidence is still very limited. Moreover, this question can be addressed from a different perspective by examining macronutrient intake in relation to FTO and BMI. This was examined in the Atherosclerosis Risk in Communities (ARIC) study including 10,176 Whites and 3,641 African Americans aged 45–64 years (Hardy et al., 2014). As expected, the FTO SNPs (rs17817449, rs8050136) were significantly associated with higher BMI; and in mediation analysis, the FTO high-risk alleles were associated, in Whites, with higher BMI in part through small effects on CHO and protein intake. In another meta-analysis, the FTO BMI-increasing allele at the rs1421085 SNP was associated with higher protein intake, independent of BMI (Tanaka et al., 2013). These findings and their magnitude suggest that the relationship between FTO variants and BMI could be mediated, although moderately, through food intake. On one hand, there is an interaction between saturated fat and FTO driving the BMI up. On the other hand, people with the FTO variant eat more protein and carbohydrates, suggesting two independent mechanisms associated with this gene. One is driving food intake and the other one fat storage.

Analogous findings were reported in larger populations (n = 33,533 for discovery and n = 38,360 for replication) by Chu et al. (2013). In this study, the FTO rs10163409 was among the top associations for percent of total energy intake from protein and carbohydrate, suggesting preference for these macronutrients with this SNP. Some early studies in children also showed that the energy density of the food ingested as part of the experimental design was higher among carriers of the risk allele as compared with the control genotype, which could explain some of their predisposition to obesity (Cecil et al., 2008). Similar findings were observed in adult subjects participating in a lifestyle intervention program to prevent diabetes (Haupt et al., 2009). In this study, the FTO risk allele was significantly associated with higher energy intake even during dietary restriction, adding more evidence in support of the role of the FTO gene influencing food intake (Haupt et al., 2009). However, other earlier studies, despite showing the association between FTO and BMI, did not find any nutrient-specific food preference associated with the risk allele (Bauer et al., 2009).

Gene–diet interactions related to weight loss have also been identified and have recently been reviewed by Qi (2014). This excellent review highlights both the substantial progress made toward revealing relevant gene–diet interactions as well as the many shortcomings that still need to be addressed. In brief, the following loci were found to modulate the individual success of weight loss approaches such as energy restriction and change in dietary macronutrient distribution: IRS1, TCF7L2, FTO, GIPR, PPM1K, BDNF, and MC4R. In addition, loci including LEP, FTO, and BDNF were related also to differences in weight regain following intervention. On the positive side, the availability of randomized clinical trials is allowing the identification of loci that modulate the individual response to diet interventions aimed at weight loss, as well as weight maintenance. On the negative side, the field still needs more replication and identification of the functional variants and their mechanisms before translation of this research into personalized diet interventions can be made a common clinical practice.

Since the publication of this review, other studies have been reported, but for the most part, they focused on the interaction between obesity-related genes and weight-loss diets in relation to other CVD risk factors such as plasma lipid profiles (Qi et al., 2015; Xu et al., 2015) and glucose-related variables (Huang et al., 2015; Zheng et al., 2015). These studies support the notion that dietary fat intake modifies the association between common genetic variants and plasma lipids (LIPC, CETP) as well as insulin sensitivity (FTO); whereas dietary carbohydrate was a modulator of the association between PCSK7 and insulin sensitivity.

We analyzed the association between a weighted obesity GRS, calculated on the basis of 63 obesity-associated variants, and BMI in the GOLDN study (n = 783) (Casas-Agustench et al., 2014), focusing on gene–diet interactions with total fat and SFA intake. Moreover, we tested for replication of findings in the Multi-Ethnic Study of Atherosclerosis (MESA) (n = 2035). As expected, a higher GRS was associated with increased BMI in both populations. More importantly, we found significant interactions between total fat intake and the obesity GRS for the discovery and the replication population that reached a p-level for the interaction of 0.002 in the meta-analysis. The interaction terms became even more significant for SFA intake. Thus, a high consumption of SFA in combination with an elevated GRS magnifies the allele-raising effect as compared to those that despite having the high GRS consume a low-fat diet and more specifically a low-SFA diet. A practical translation of these findings would be the strong recommendation to reduce total fat intake, mainly by limiting SFAs, among those individuals with high obesity GRS. However, we need to keep in mind that for "the whole to be greater than the sum of its parts," these parts need to be well characterized. Therefore, a detailed knowledge of each of the SNPs and their specific modes of action is needed before their incorporation into any GRS.

We already mentioned that some of the candidate genes investigated in the past for associations with CVD risk factors and related gene–diet interactions did not materialize in the corresponding GWAS for main effects. One interpretation of this lack of concordance may be that the previous associations were not real. A more positive twist is that the expression of the phenotypes associated with those genes may be subject to strong gene–environment interactions that prevented their emergence in the traditional GWAS. This may be the case for two of our best-studied candidate genes for obesity: *PLIN1* and *APOA2*.

Perilipin proteins were identified in the adipocyte, where they regulate lipid storage and lipolysis. Perilipin 1 (PLIN1) is the most abundant of the adipocyte proteins, and over a decade ago we began to investigate associations of the *PLIN1* locus with obesity and related phenotypes focusing on six SNPs (rs2289487, rs1561726, rs2304794, rs894160, rs2304795, rs1052700) (Qi et al., 2004a,b, 2015). These studies revealed relatively consistent and gender-specific (women only) associations between the SNPs and anthropometric and metabolic traits in different ethnic groups and geographical locations.

Despite this compelling evidence, some studies failed to detect associations between PLIN1 and obesity-related phenotypes. Considering that dietary intake is one of the strongest determinants of obesity, we launched a series of studies examining gene–diet interactions. The first of them involved patients attending an obesity clinic (Corella et al., 2005). Subjects were exposed to an energy-restricted intervention, and after 1-year follow-up, carriers of the minor allele at the rs894160 SNP were much more resistant to weight loss compared with major allele homozygotes. This could be related to the macronutrient composition of the diet (~40% of total energy from fat, ~20% from protein, and ~40% from CHO). This hypothesis was tested in a subsequent study based on Puerto Ricans living in the United States. In this population, dietary CHO interacted with PLIN1 rs894160 SNP, in that carriers of the minor allele were protected from increased adiposity in the context of high complex CHO intake, but were at risk of increased adiposity when complex CHO intake was low (Smith et al., 2008). Findings from other studies can be interpreted in the same light (Smith and Ordovás, 2012). The current evidence is consistent with the hypothesis that a low-fat, high complex CHO diet may be protective against obesity for individuals with the minor allele for rs894160.

Moreover, in one energy-restricted intervention (n = 177 Koreans), Jang et al. (2006) demonstrated that carriers of the minor allele for either rs894160 or rs1052700, which are in strong linkage disequilibrium in Asians, showed greater waist circumference and fat mass reduction as well as a greater change in free fatty acids following weight loss. These two observations may be physiologically linked, since free fatty acids may reflect increased lipolysis accompanying weight loss, and rs894160 is the same SNP for which Mottagui-Tabar et al. (2003) reported greater rates of lipolysis in obese women.

The well-known connection between obesity and impaired glucose metabolism led us to investigate PLIN1 in the context of glucose- and insulin-related traits. Thus, in a cohort of Spanish women (n = 801) in whom linked *PLIN1* SNPs rs2289487 and rs894160 were protective against adiposity, an association between these SNPs and lower plasma glucose was also found, and adjustment by BMI did not eliminate statistical significance of the association (Qi et al., 2004a). Another example in support of taking the analysis beyond the traditional association studies and bringing diet into the equation can be found for PLIN1 and insulin. Thus, PLIN1 genotype was not associated with plasma insulin independently of nutritional factors in Singaporean Asian women (Malays, Indians, and Chinese; n = 2198) (Qi et al., 2005); however, in these women, we detected interactions between PLIN1 rs894160 and PLIN1 rs1052700 and saturated fat and CHO, which were strongest when considered as a ratio (Corella et al., 2006). For homozygous minor allele carriers of either SNP, the SFA:CHO ratio was associated with increased plasma insulin and HOMA-IR, and this relationship was replicated in U.S. White women. In both Asian and White populations, inclusion of a measure of adiposity (BMI or waist) did not attenuate the significance of the interaction, suggesting that obesity was not the primary mediator of the SNP-related insulin resistance.

Another example of replicated evidence without support from GWAS findings comes from the apolipoprotein A2 (*APOA2)* gene and its relation to obesity. We have identified and replicated a significant interaction between the *APOA2* gene variant [APOA2-265T > C (rs5082)] (which *in vitro* has been shown to modulate APOA2 gene expression), dietary SFAs, and BMI. We analyzed gene–diet interactions between the rs5082 SNP and SFA intake on BMI and obesity in subjects from three American populations: (1) Framingham Heart Study (1454 Whites); (2) GOLDN (1078 Whites); and (3) BPRHS (930 Hispanics of Caribbean origin). We found that the magnitude of the difference in BMI between the homozygotes for the risk allele C and carriers of the major allele was dependent on SFA intake. We observed a difference of 6.2% in BMI between the two genotype groups when SFA consumption was high (>22 g/d), but no difference when SFA consumption was low. Moreover, the CC genotype was significantly associated with higher obesity prevalence in these populations only when SFA intake was high (Corella et al., 2009b). These findings in three independent populations were further replicated in other geographical areas and ethnic groups (Corella et al., 2011b), and more recently, we replicated these interactions using specific foods (i.e., dairy) (Smith et al., 2013).

Gene–Diet Interactions and Glucose-Related Risk Factors

Similar to obesity, most of the solidly established candidate genes involved in glucose metabolism emerged from GWAS. This is the case of the Transcription Factor 7-Like 2 (TCF7L2) gene, the first one to be consistently implicated in type 2 diabetes (T2D) (Grant et al., 2006; Voight et al., 2010), especially in nonobese subjects (Bouhaha et al., 2010; Kalnina et al., 2012). Similarly to FTO and obesity, the mechanistic basis for TCF7L2 and T2D is not well understood.

Several gene–diet interactions related to the TCF7L2 locus have been reported. Some of them are related to glycemic traits; however, it is important to highlight that many genes cross the boundaries of different CVD risk factors. Thus, we have already indicated that the TCF7L2 is also involved in gene–diet interactions related to obesity (Fisher et al., 2012; Mattei et al., 2012; Roswall et al., 2014). Moreover, one of the first TCF7L2 by diet interactions was reported in relation to postprandial lipemia (Warodomwichit et al., 2009). In that study, we reported that high habitual intake (above the population median of 6.6% of total daily energy intake) of n-6 polyunsaturated fatty acids (PUFA) was associated with atherogenic dyslipidemia (fasting plasma VLDL concentrations and postprandial TG-rich lipoproteins) in carriers of the high-risk T-allele at the TCF7L2 rs7903146 SNP as compared with CC subjects or T-carriers consuming low levels (below the median) of n-6 PUFA.

In terms of glycemic traits, Fisher et al. (2009) investigated whether the protective effect of whole grains related to postprandial glucose response and insulin demand might be attenuated in the presence of the rs7903146 risk-conferring T-allele. These investigators tested their hypothesis using a case-cohort approach that included 2318 randomized individuals and 724 incident T2D cases from the European Prospective Investigation into Cancer and Nutrition (EPIC)-Potsdam cohort. As expected, whole-grain intake was protective against T2D risk among rs7903146 CC carriers, C being the low-risk allele. Conversely, carriers of the T high-risk allele did not benefit from the protective action of whole-grain intake. A similar question was posed in the context of a prospective population-based study (Wirström et al., 2013). The investigators examined the 8–10-year incidence of prediabetes and T2D in relation to the intake of whole grains in 2297 men and 3180 women. Overall, a higher intake of whole grains was protective, with the exception of men carrying the high-risk alleles at the TCF7L2 gene. Therefore, both studies support the notion that the beneficial effect of whole-grain intake on T2D risk is modified by the common TCF7L2 rs7903146 SNP. These findings are further supported by another cohort of 24,799 nondiabetic individuals from the Malmö Diet and Cancer Study (MDCS), who were followed for 12 years and in whom high dietary fiber intake was associated with protection from T2D only among carriers of the low-risk allele for rs7903146. During this time, 1649 subjects developed incident T2D

(Hindy et al., 2012). Once again, this study demonstrates that the protective effect of a dietary component—in this case, dietary fiber—may work preferably in those subjects who are nonrisk allele carriers.

The interaction between this locus and dietary carbohydrates, with modulation of the effect of the high-risk T-allele on T2D, was also investigated in the Nurses' Health Study after stratifying this population according to glycemic load and glycemic index (Cornelis et al., 2009). Using the GG genotype as a reference, the multivariate-adjusted ORs (95% CI) of T2D associated with the TT genotype were 2.71 (1.64, 4.46) and 2.69 (1.64, 4.43) in those subjects in the highest tertile of GL and GI, respectively. The ORs (95% CIs) for TT subjects in the lowest tertile of GL and GI were 1.66 (0.95, 2.88) and 1.82 (1.11, 3.01). A more recent study in an Algerian population (Ouhaibi-Djellouli et al., 2014) observed gene–diet interactions related to dessert and milk intake and T2D risk. This risk was greater in T-allele carriers with high dessert and milk intakes as compared with CC subjects or T-allele carriers with low dessert and milk consumption. Overall, similar to studies in other populations, the T-allele at the TCF7L2 rs7903146 SNP was associated with a higher risk of T2D and this association was magnified by high dessert and milk intakes; however, the specific nutrients involved in these interactions were not reported in this study.

Although the experimental designs and the questions differ considerably across these studies, there seems to be an agreement regarding the significant interaction between the TCF7L2 locus, carbohydrate intake, and T2D risk.

Perhaps the most relevant of all the gene–diet interactions described so far relates to the risk of stroke in the PREvención con DIeta MEDiterránea (PREDIMED) study (Corella et al., 2013). The PREDIMED study was a randomized dietary intervention trial (two MedDiet intervention groups and a control group) with 7018 participants. In this context, we investigated whether the associations of the TCF7L2-rs7903146 SNP with T2D, glucose, lipids, and CVD incidence were modulated by a Mediterranean diet (MedDiet). Data were analyzed at baseline and after a median follow-up of 4.8 years. Consistent with current knowledge, the TCF7L2-rs7903146 SNP was associated with T2D. Moreover, the MedDiet interacted significantly with rs7903146 on fasting glucose at baseline. Thus, when adherence to the MedDiet was low, TT subjects had higher fasting glucose concentrations than C-allele carriers (CC+CT). Conversely, when adherence to the MedDiet was high, this increase in fasting glucose was not observed in TT subjects. Similar statistically significant interactions were noted for total cholesterol, LDL cholesterol, and triglycerides (p interaction < 0.05 for all). Moreover, during the randomized trial, TT subjects had a higher stroke incidence in the control group compared with CC carriers ($p = 0.006$), whereas in the groups consuming the MedDiet no differences in stroke incidence were observed between TT and CC homozygotes ($p = 0.892$). These results support the concept that MedDiet reduces the otherwise increased fasting glucose and lipids in TT subjects, but most importantly also lowers the incidence of stroke to a level similar to that observed in CC subjects in both arms of the MedDiet intervention (extra-virgin olive oil and nuts).

Additional gene variants associated with increased T2D risk and insulin resistance found in the gene that encodes the Insulin Receptor Substrate 1 (IRS1)—a key player in insulin signaling pathways—were identified by GWAS. In particular, rs2943641 T-allele carriers and rs757826 G-allele carriers have been shown to be less susceptible to insulin resistance, T2D, and metabolic syndrome (MetS) than noncarriers. Over the last few years, several research groups have found interactions between these SNPs and different macronutrient intakes. Our results from GOLDN and BPRHS (Zheng et al., 2013) showed that carriers of both protective alleles (G-T haplotype) may only experience lower insulin resistance and MetS risk when their saturated fatty acid-to-carbohydrate ratio is low (SFA:CHO ≤ 0.24). Similarly, we also found that the rs757826 G-allele was only associated with a reduced risk of developing MetS when MUFA intake was lower than the median of each population.

Additional evidence comes from the POUNDS LOST trial (Qi et al., 2011) ($n = 738$, predominantly White Americans, 2-year follow-up) regarding the fairly well-studied rs2943641 SNP: carriers of two risk alleles (CC) randomized into the highest-carbohydrate (lower fat) diet group were found to experience a greater decrease in plasma insulin concentrations, BMI, and insulin resistance (HOMA-IR). Gender effects have also been shown to affect variables associated with this genotype, particularly adiposity for which the interaction only held significance in men. The aforementioned MDCS (Ericson et al., 2013) results provided further insight into gender-specific gene–environment interactions for this locus by suggesting that the minor T-allele interacted with diet in a sex-dependent manner affecting T2D risk (significantly decreased T2D incidence only in women in the lower tertiles of carbohydrate intake, and men in the lowest tertile of fat intake). The latter results, despite coming from an observational study and thus not providing the highest level of evidence to support this effect, may help us recognize the potential complexity of gene–environment interactions, in which parameters like gender could completely shift the optimal dietary approach needed to neutralize a genetic susceptibility.

Gene–Diet Interactions and Lipid Metabolism

Some pioneering studies in the field of gene–diet interactions and cardiometabolic health relate to candidate genes in the path of lipoprotein metabolism, specifically associated with the APOE and the APOA1/APOC3/APOA4/APOA5 gene cluster. However, whereas there are clear and consistent associations between some of these loci and plasma lipid concentrations, the results from gene–diet interactions suffer from the similar lack of replication found for other metabolic pathways.

In this section, we will focus on the lipoprotein lipase (LPL) gene, a key player in plasma lipoprotein metabolism and more specifically in the catabolism of triglyceride-rich lipoproteins. Similar to other candidate genes (i.e., APOE, APOA5), there are clear and consistent associations between common LPL variants and plasma lipid levels. However, the functionality and mechanisms involved in these associations are, for the most part, unknown. We will use this locus to illustrate the cross talk between genetics (LPL), epigenetics (microRNAs), and diet (PUFA) and to demonstrate how this new knowledge is helping to assign functionality to SNPs identified through candidate gene or GWAS approaches.

MicroRNAs (miRNAs) are small, 20–24 nucleotide, noncoding RNAs that function as posttranscriptional inhibitors of gene expression by binding to miRNA recognition elements (MRE) within the 3′UTR of their target mRNAs (Bartel, 2009). The most critical region for binding and repression of mRNA by a miRNAs are positions 2–7 of the MRE, called the "seed site." SNPs in MRE seed sites (MRESS) have been shown to decrease or eliminate miRNA-mediated repression (Brennecke et al., 2005). Moreover, some epidemiological evidence is mounting supporting that SNPs within an MRE or MRESS are associated with phenotypic variation (Saunders et al., 2007; Sethupathy and Collins, 2008; Richardson et al., 2011).

MicroRNAs have emerged as important epigenetic regulators in CVD. Therefore, based on previous findings related to gene–diet interactions for obesity and the results of a genome-wide search for SNPs in MREs and MRESS, we decided to explore the rs13702T>C SNP (rs13702) in the 3′ untranslated region of the LPL gene for functionality based on miRNA-related mechanisms. This SNP has an extensive literature over the past decade and a solid track record of associations with plasma triglyceride and HDL-C concentrations. Furthermore, the rs13702 is in linkage disequilibrium with several SNPs identified by GWAS associated with HDL-C and TG. In our *in silico* prediction, the rs13702 minor allele had been found to disrupt an MRESS for the human miRNA-410.

We used the CHARGE consortium to perform a meta-analysis and, consistent with the literature, we found a highly statistically significant association of the rs13702 SNP with low triglyceride ($p = 3.18 \times 10(-42)$) and high-HDL-C ($p = 1.35 \times 10(-32)$) with each copy of the minor allele associated with 0.060 mmol/L lower triglyceride and 0.041 mmol/L higher HDL-C (Richardson et al., 2013). Then, we carried out *in vitro* functionality tests and demonstrated that the expression of an LPL 3′ UTR luciferase reporter carrying the rs13702 major T-allele was reduced by 40% in response to a miR-410 mimic. Finally, we examined the interaction between intake of dietary fatty acids and the LPL-rs13702 SNP. Our meta-analysis involving 10 of the CHARGE cohorts demonstrated a highly significant interaction between the rs13702 SNP and dietary PUFA with respect to plasma triglyceride concentrations (p = 0.00153). Thus, the protective effect of this SNP on plasma triglyceride levels was further enhanced by an additional reduction of −0.007 mmol/L in the presence of high PUFA intake. The same applied to the HDL-C raising effect that was further increased by dietary PUFA. Our results demonstrate that the rs13702 SNP induces the allele-specific regulation of LPL by miR-410 in humans and these effects (lowering TGs and increasing HDL-C) were enhanced as the habitual intake of PUFA increased in the participants.

In a follow-up study, we intended to extend and solidify these findings by assessing the interaction between the rs13702 SNP and fat intake on triglycerides at baseline and longitudinally by using the PREDIMED dietary intervention design (Corella et al., 2014). We also examined as a primary outcome the association of this variant with CVD incidence and its modulation by the MedDiet. Gene–diet interactions for triglyceride were analyzed at baseline (n = 6880) and after a 3-year intervention (n = 4131). As in previous populations, the rs13702 SNP was significantly associated with lower plasma triglycerides in C-allele carriers. Moreover, we found a significant dietary interaction at baseline with unsaturated fat similar to the one reported in the CHARGE cohorts. After 3 years of intervention with MedDiet, high in unsaturated fat, the C-allele was associated with an even greater reduction in triglyceride concentrations. Consistent with the protective lipoprotein profile associated with the C-allele, we found an association with lower stroke risk that reached statistical significance only in the combined MedDiet intervention groups but not in the control group (p interaction = 0.044).

Therefore, in addition to validating our previous study in terms of lipid associations and gene–diet interactions, our findings in PREDIMED revealed a new association between rs13702 and stroke incidence, which is modulated by diet in terms of decreasing stroke risk in rs13702 C-allele carriers following a high-unsaturated fat MedDiet intervention.

CVD Risk Has Rhythm

The interest in chronobiology is experiencing a dramatic increase. This is in part due to the realization that chronodisruption is associated with most chronic diseases including CVD. Moreover, we should not forget that our metabolism and vital signs such as body temperature, respiratory rate, and blood pressure present circadian variations that may affect the risk of suffering cardiovascular events. For instance, myocardial infarctions do not occur evenly throughout the day, but rather they concentrate during specific time frames (i.e., early morning). Therefore, when it comes to gene–diet interactions—and particularly, personalized nutrition—time needs to be included in the equation. Our own research shows that CLOCK SNPs (i.e., rs4580704 and rs1801260) are associated with BMI and glucose-metabolism-related traits. Moreover, we found a modulation of the associations of these SNPs with plasma glucose, insulin resistance, and anthropometric traits by MUFA and SFA intakes (Garaulet et al., 2009). Furthermore, variation at the CLOCK locus was also associated with energy intake (Garaulet et al., 2010).

TRANSLATION OF KNOWLEDGE

Further research into gene–diet interactions is crucial to generate solid knowledge that will allow us to launch clinical applications aimed at early prediction of CV risk. The conceptual process is straightforward. Once genetic variants associated with CVD or an intermediate phenotype (i.e., dyslipidemia, dysglycemia, obesity) are found and we know that a certain diet can counteract that genetic risk, then one can forecast that CVD risk could be effectively reduced through recommendation of a personalized diet. To date, studies like PREDIMED have focused on primary prevention, but there is also great interest in discovering gene–diet interactions in secondary CVD prevention in order to provide appropriate dietary recommendations for individuals who have already had a non-fatal CVD event, as will be possible with studies like CORDIOPREV (Garcia-Rios et al., 2014). The results of this research can provide us with the much needed knowledge to achieve more successful prevention and therapy of CVD.

REFERENCES

Ahmad S., Rukh G., Varga T.V., Ali A., Kurbasic A., Shungin D. et al. Gene × physical activity interactions in obesity: Combined analysis of 111,421 individuals of European ancestry. *PLoS Genet.* 2013;9(7):e1003607.

Bartel D.P. MicroRNAs: Target recognition and regulatory functions *Cell.* 2009;136:215–233.

Bauer F., Elbers C.C., Adan R.A., Loos R.J., Onland-Moret N.C., Grobbee D.E., van Vliet-Ostaptchouk J.V., Wijmenga C., van der Schouw Y.T. Obesity genes identified in genome-wide association studies are associated with adiposity measures and potentially with nutrient-specific food preference. *Am J Clin Nutr.* 2009 Oct;90(4):951–959.

Bis J.C., Glazer N.L., Psaty B.M. Genome-wide association studies of cardiovascular risk factors: Design, conduct and interpretation. *J Thromb Haemost.* 2009;7(Suppl. 1):308–311.

Bouhaha R., Choquet H., Meyre D., AbidKamoun H., Ennafaa H., Baroudi T. et al. TCF7L2 is associated with type 2 diabetes in nonobese individuals from Tunisia. *Pathol Biol (Paris).* 2010;58:426–429.

Brennecke J., Stark A., Russell R.B., Cohen S.M. Principles of microRNA-target recognition. *PLoS Biol.* 2005;3:e85.

Casas-Agustench P., Arnett D.K., Smith C.E., Lai C.Q., Parnell L.D., Borecki I.B. et al. Saturated fat intake modulates the association between an obesity genetic risk score and body mass index in two US populations. *J Acad Nutr Diet.* 2014;114(12):1954–1966.

Cecil J.E., Tavendale R., Watt P., Hetherington M.M., Palmer C.N. An obesity-associated FTO gene variant and increased energy intake in children. *N Engl J Med.* 2008;359(24):2558–2566.

Chu A.Y., Workalemahu T., Paynter N.P., Rose L.M., Giulianini F., Tanaka T. et al. Novel locus including FGF21 is associated with dietary macronutrient intake. *Hum Mol Genet.* 2013;22(9):1895–1902.

Corella D., Arnett D.K., Tucker K.L., Kabagambe E.K., Tsai M., Parnell L.D. et al. A high intake of saturated fatty acids strengthens the association between the fat mass and obesity-associated gene and BMI. *J Nutr.* 2011a;141(12):2219–2225.

Corella D., Carrasco P., Sorlí J.V., Estruch R., Rico-Sanz J., Martínez-González M.Á. et al. Mediterranean diet reduces the adverse effect of the TCF7L2-rs7903146 polymorphism on cardiovascular risk factors and stroke incidence: A randomized controlled trial in a high-cardiovascular-risk population. *Diabetes Care.* 2013;36(11):3803–3811.

Corella D., Ordovas J.M. Nutrigenomics in cardiovascular medicine. *Circ Cardiovasc Genet.* 2009a;2:637–651.

Corella D., Peloso G., Arnett D.K., Demissie S., Cupples L.A., Tucker K. et al. APOA2, dietary fat, and body mass index: Replication of a gene-diet interaction in 3 independent populations. *Arch Intern Med.* 2009b;169(20):1897–1906.

Corella D., Qi L., Sorlí J.V., Godoy D., Portolés O., Coltell O., Greenberg A.S., Ordovas J.M. Obese subjects carrying the 11482G>A polymorphism at the perilipin locus are resistant to weight loss after dietary energy restriction. *J Clin Endocrinol Metab.* 2005;90(9):1521–1526.

Corella D., Qi L., Tai E.S., Deurenberg-Yap M., Tan C.E., Chew S.K., Ordovas J.M. Perilipin gene variation determines higher susceptibility to insulin resistance in Asian women when consuming a high-saturated fat, low-carbohydrate diet. *Diabetes Care.* 2006;29(6):1313–1319.

Corella D., Sorlí J.V., Estruch R., Coltell O., Ortega-Azorín C., Portolés O. et al. MicroRNA-410 regulated lipoprotein lipase variant rs13702 is associated with stroke incidence and modulated by diet in the randomized controlled PREDIMED trial. *Am J Clin Nutr.* 2014;100(2):719–731.

Corella D., Tai E.S., Sorlí J.V., Chew S.K., Coltell O., Sotos-Prieto M., García-Rios A., Estruch R., Ordovas J.M. Association between the APOA2 promoter polymorphism and body weight in Mediterranean and Asian populations: Replication of a gene-saturated fat interaction. *Int J Obes (Lond).* 2011b;35(5):666–675

Cornelis M.C., Qi L., Kraft P., Hu F.B. TCF7L2, dietary carbohydrate, and risk of type 2 diabetes in US women. *Am J Clin Nutr.* 2009;89:1256–1262.

Cornelis M.C., Rimm E.B., Curhan G.C., Kraft P., Hunter D.J., Hu F.B., van Dam R.M. Obesity susceptibility loci and uncontrolled eating, emotional eating and cognitive restraint behaviors in men and women. *Obesity.* 2014;22(5):E135–E141.

Dove F.W. A study of individuality in the nutritive instincts and of the causes and effects of variations in the selection of food. *Am Nat.* 1935 Sept.–Oct.;69(Suppl. 724):469–544.

Ericson U., Rukh G., Stojkovic I., Sonestedt E., Gullberg B., Wirfält E., Wallström P., Orho-Melander M. Sex-specific interactions between the IRS1 polymorphism and intakes of carbohydrates and fat on incident type 2 diabetes. *Am J Clin Nutr*. 2013;97(1):208–216.

Fildes A., Charlton J., Rudisill C., Littlejohns P., Prevost A.T., Gulliford M.C. Probability of an obese person attaining normal body weight: Cohort study using electronic health records. *Am J Public Health*. 2015;105(9):e54–e59.

Fisher E., Boeing H., Fritsche A., Doering F., Joost H.-J., Schulze M.B. Whole-grain consumption and transcription factor-7-like 2 (TCF7L2) rs7903146: Gene–diet interaction in modulating type 2 diabetes risk. *Br J Nutr*. 2009;101:478–481.

Fisher E., Meidtner K., Angquist L., Holst C., Hansen R.D., Halkjær J. et al. Influence of dietary protein intake and glycemic index on the association between TCF7L2 HapA and weight gain. *Am J Clin Nutr*. 2012;95(6):1468–1476.

Fredriksson R., Hägglund M., Olszewski P.K., Stephansson O., Jacobsson J.A., Olszewska A.M., Levine A.S., Lindblom J., Schiöth H.B. The obesity gene, FTO, is of ancient origin, up-regulated during food deprivation and expressed in neurons of feeding-related nuclei of the brain. *Endocrinology*. 2008;149(5):2062–2071.

Garaulet M., Lee Y.C., Shen J., Parnell L.D., Arnett D.K., Tsai M.Y., Lai C.Q., Ordovas J.M. CLOCK genetic variation and metabolic syndrome risk: Modulation by monounsaturated fatty acids. *Am J Clin Nutr*. 2009;90:1466–1475.

Garaulet M., Lee Y.C., Shen J., Parnell L.D., Arnett D.K., Tsai M.Y., Lai C.Q., Ordovas J.M. Genetic variants in human CLOCK associate with total energy intake and cytokine sleep factors in overweight subjects (GOLDN population). *Eur J Hum Genet*. 2010;18:364–369.

Garcia-Rios A., Gomez-Delgado F.J., Garaulet M., Alcala-Diaz J.F., Delgado-Lista F.J., Marin C. et al. Beneficial effect of CLOCK gene polymorphism rs1801260 in combination with low-fat diet on insulin metabolism in the patients with metabolic syndrome. *Chronobiol Int*. 2014 Apr;31(3):401–408.

Grant S.F., Thorleifsson G., Reynisdottir I., Benediktsson R., Manolescu A., Sainz J. et al. Variant of transcription factor 7-like 2 (TCF7L2) gene confers risk of type 2 diabetes. *Nat Genet*. 2006;38:320–323.

Harbron J., van der Merwe L., Zaahl M.G., Kotze M.J., Senekal M. Fat mass and obesity-associated (FTO) gene polymorphisms are associated with physical activity, food intake, eating behaviors, psychological health, and modeled change in body mass index in overweight/obese Caucasian adults. *Nutrients*. 2014;6(8):3130–3152.

Hardy D.S., Racette S.B., Hoelscher D.M. Macronutrient intake as a mediator with FTO to increase body mass index. *J Am Coll Nutr*. 2014;33(4):256–266.

Haupt A., Thamer C., Staiger H., Tschritter O., Kirchhoff K., Machicao F., Häring H.U., Stefan N., Fritsche A. Variation in the FTO gene influences food intake but not energy expenditure. *Exp Clin Endocrinol Diabetes*. 2009;117(4):194–197.

Hindy G., Sonestedt E., Ericson U., Jing X.J., Zhou Y., Hansson O., Renström E., Wirfält E., Orho-Melander M. Role of TCF7L2 risk variant and dietary fibre intake on incident type 2 diabetes. *Diabetologia*. 2012;55(10):2646–2654.

Huang T., Huang J., Qi Q., Li Y., Bray G.A., Rood J., Sacks F.M., Qi L. PCSK7 genotype modifies effect of a weight-loss diet on 2-year changes of insulin resistance: The POUNDS LOST trial. *Diabetes Care*. 2015;38(3):439–444.

Hurley L.S. Nutrients and genes: Interactions in development. *Nutr Rev*. 1969;27:3–6.

Jang Y., Kim O.Y., Lee J.H., Koh S.J., Chae J.S., Kim J.Y., Park S., Cho H., Lee J.E., Ordovas J.M. Genetic variation at the perilipin locus is associated with changes in serum free fatty acids and abdominal fat following mild weight loss. *Int J Obes (Lond)*. 2006;30(11):1601–1608.

Kalnina I., Geldnere K., Tarasova L., Nikitina-Zake L., Peculis R., Fridmanis D. et al. Stronger association of common variants in TCF7L2 gene with nonobese type 2 diabetes in the Latvian population. *Exp Clin Endocrinol Diabetes*. 2012;120:466–468.

Locke A.E., Kahali B., Berndt S.I., Justice A.E., Pers T.H., Day F.R. et al. Genetic studies of body mass index yield new insights for obesity biology. *Nature*. 2015 Feb 12;518(7538):197–206.

Mattei J., Qi Q., Hu F.B., Sacks F.M., Qi L. TCF7L2 genetic variants modulate the effect of dietary fat intake on changes in body composition during a weight-loss intervention. *Am J Clin Nutr*. 2012;96(5):1129–1136.

McCaffery J.M., Papandonatos G.D., Peter I., Huggins G.S., Raynor H.A., Delahanty L.M. et al. Obesity susceptibility loci and dietary intake in the Look AHEAD Trial. *Am J Clin Nutr*. 2012;95(6):1477–1486.

Mottagui-Tabar S., Rydén M., Löfgren P., Faulds G., Hoffstedt J., Brookes A.J., Andersson I., Arner P. Evidence for an important role of perilipin in the regulation of human adipocyte lipolysis. *Diabetologia*. 2003;46(6):789–797.

Ordovas J.M., Corella D. Nutritional genomics. *Annu Rev Genom Hum Genet*. 2004;5:71–118.

Ouhaibi-Djellouli H., Mediene-Benchekor S., Lardjam-Hetraf S.A., Hamani-Medjaoui I., Meroufel D.N., Boulenouar H. et al. The TCF7L2 rs7903146 polymorphism, dietary intakes and type 2 diabetes risk in an Algerian population. *BMC Genet.* 2014;15:134.

Parnell L.D., Blokker B.A., Dashti H.S., Nesbeth P.D., Cooper B.E., Ma Y. et al. CardioGxE, a catalog of gene-environment interactions for cardiometabolic traits. *BioData Mining*. 2014;7:21.

Qi L., Gene-diet interaction and weight loss. *Curr Opin Lipidol.* 2014;25(1):27–34.

Qi Q., Bray G.A., Smith S.R., Hu F.B., Sacks F.M., Qi L. Insulin receptor substrate 1 gene variation modifies insulin resistance response to weight-loss diets in a 2-year randomized trial: The Preventing Overweight Using Novel Dietary Strategies (POUNDS LOST) trial. *Circulation.* 2011;124(5):563–571.

Qi Q., Chu A.Y., Kang J.H., Huang J., Rose L.M., Jensen M.K. et al. Fried food consumption, genetic risk, and body mass index: Gene-diet interaction analysis in three US cohort studies. *BMJ.* 2014a;348:g1610.

Qi L., Corella D., Sorlí J.V., Portolés O., Shen H., Coltell O., Godoy D., Greenberg A.S., Ordovas J.M. Genetic variation at the perilipin (PLIN) locus is associated with obesity-related phenotypes in White women. *Clin Genet.* 2004a Oct;66(4):299–310.

Qi Q., Durst R., Schwarzfuchs D., Leitersdorf E., Shpitzen S., Li Y. et al. CETP genotype and changes in lipid levels in response to weight-loss diet intervention in the POUNDS LOST and DIRECT randomized trials. *J Lipid Res.* 2015;56(3):713–721.

Qi Q., Kilpeläinen T.O., Downer M.K., Tanaka T., Smith C.E. et al. FTO genetic variants, dietary intake and body mass index: Insights from 177,330 individuals. *Hum Mol Genet.* 2014b;23(25):6961–6972.

Qi L., Shen H., Larson I., Schaefer E.J., Greenberg A.S., Tregouet D.A., Corella D., Ordovas J.M. Gender-specific association of a perilipin gene haplotype with obesity risk in a white population. *Obes Res.* 2004b;12(11):1758–1765.

Qi L., Tai E.S., Tan C.E., Shen H., Chew S.K., Greenberg A.S., Corella D., Ordovas J.M. Intragenic linkage disequilibrium structure of the human perilipin gene (PLIN) and haplotype association with increased obesity risk in a multiethnic Asian population. *J Mol Med (Berl).* 2005;83(6):448–456.

Richardson K., Louie-Gao Q., Arnett D.K., Parnell L.D., Lai C.Q., Davalos A. et al. The PLIN4 variant rs8887 modulates obesity related phenotypes in humans through creation of a novel miR-522 seed site. *PLoS ONE.* 2011;6:e17944.

Richardson K., Nettleton J.A., Rotllan N., Tanaka T., Smith C.E., Lai C.Q. et al. Gain-of-function lipoprotein lipase variant rs13702 modulates lipid traits through disruption of a microRNA-410 seed site. *Am J Hum Genet.* 2013;92(1):5–14.

Roswall N., Ängquist L., Ahluwalia T.S., Romaguera D., Larsen S.C., Østergaard J.N. et al. Association between Mediterranean and Nordic diet scores and changes in weight and waist circumference: influence of FTO and TCF7L2 loci. *Am J Clin Nutr.* 2014;100(4):1188–1197.

Saunders M.A., Liang H., Li W.H. Human polymorphism at microRNAs and microRNA target sites. *Proc Natl Acad Sci USA.* 2007;104:3300–3305.

Sethupathy P., Collins F.S. MicroRNA target site polymorphisms and human disease. *Trends Genet.* 2008;24:489–497.

Shungin D., Winkler T.W., Croteau-Chonka D.C., Ferreira T., Locke A.E., Mägi R. et al. New genetic loci link adipose and insulin biology to body fat distribution. *Nature.* 2015 Feb 12;518(7538):187–196.

Smith C.E., Ordovás J.M. Update on perilipin polymorphisms and obesity. *Nutr Rev.* 2012 Oct;70(10):611–621.

Smith C.E., Tucker K.L., Arnett D.K., Noel S.E., Corella D., Borecki I.B. et al. Apolipoprotein A2 polymorphism interacts with intakes of dairy foods to influence body weight in 2 U.S. populations. *J Nutr.* 2013;143(12):1865–1871.

Smith C.E., Tucker K.L., Yiannakouris N., Garcia-Bailo B., Mattei J., Lai C.Q., Parnell L.D., Ordovás J.M. Perilipin polymorphism interacts with dietary carbohydrates to modulate anthropometric traits in hispanics of Caribbean origin. *J Nutr.* 2008;138(10):1852–1858.

Stunkard A.J., Messick S. The Three-Factor Eating Questionnaire to measure dietary restraint, desinhibition and hunger. *J Psychosom Res.* 1985;29:71–83.

Tanaka T., Ngwa J.S., van Rooij F.J., Zillikens M.C., Wojczynski M.K., Frazier-Wood A.C. et al. Genome-wide meta-analysis of observational studies shows common genetic variants associated with macronutrient intake. *Am J Clin Nutr.* 2013;97(6):1395–1402.

Tanofsky-Kraff M., Han J.C., Anandalingam K., Shomaker L.B., Columbo K.M., Wolkoff L.E. et al. The FTO gene rs9939609 obesity-risk allele and loss of control over eating. *Am J Clin Nutr.* 2009;90(6):1483–1488.

Tucker K.L., Smith C.E., Lai C.Q., Ordovas J.M. Quantifying diet for nutrigenomic studies. *Annu Rev Nutr.* 2013;33:349–371.

van Ooijen A.M., van Marken Lichtenbelt W.D., van Steenhoven A.A., Westerterp K.R. Seasonal changes in metabolic and temperature responses to cold air in humans. *Physiol Behav.* 2004;82(2–3):545–553.

Voight B.F., Scott L.J., Steinthorsdottir V., Morris A.P., Dina C., Welch R.P. et al. Twelve type 2 diabetes susceptibility loci identified through large-scale association analysis. *Nat Genet*. 2010;42:579–589.

Warodomwichit D., Arnett D.K., Kabagambe E.K., Tsai M.Y., Hixson J.E., Straka R.J. et al. Polyunsaturated fatty acids modulate the effect of TCF7L2 gene variants on postprandial lipemia. *J Nutr*. 2009; 139(3):439–446.

Wirström T., Hilding A., Gu H.F., Östenson C.G., Björklund A. Consumption of whole grain reduces risk of deteriorating glucose tolerance, including progression to prediabetes. *Am J Clin Nutr*. 2013;97(1):179–187.

Xu M., Ng S.S., Bray G.A., Ryan D.H., Sacks F.M., Ning G., Qi L. Dietary fat intake modifies the effect of a common variant in the LIPC gene on changes in serum lipid concentrations during a long-term weight-loss intervention trial. *J Nutr*. 2015;145(6):1289–1294.

Yanovski J.A., Yanovski S.Z., Sovik K.N., Nguyen T.T., O'Neil P.M., Sebring N.G. A prospective study of holiday weight gain. *N Engl J Med*. 2000;342(12):861–867.

Zheng J.S., Arnett D.K., Parnell L.D., Smith C.E., Li D., Borecki I.B., Tucker K.L., Ordovás J.M., Lai C.Q. Modulation by dietary fat and carbohydrate of IRS1 association with type 2 diabetes traits in two populations of different ancestries. *Diabetes Care*. 2013;36(9):2621-2627.

Zheng Y., Huang T., Zhang X., Rood J., Bray G.A., Sacks F.M., Qi L. Dietary fat modifies the effects of FTO genotype on changes in insulin sensitivity. *J Nutr*. 2015;145(5):977–982.

30 Gut Microbiome

Its Relationship to Health and Its Modulation by Diet

Brian J. Bennett and Katie A. Meyer

CONTENTS

ABSTRACT

Recent advances in sequencing technologies and analytics have dramatically improved our understanding of the gut microbiota. We now have a solid foundation for studying the microbiota and thus recent efforts have focused on identifying how perturbations to the microbiota composition and function affect disease risk. This chapter focuses on the relationship between the microbiota and cardiometabolic risk with an emphasis on how diet modulates these effects.

INTRODUCTION

Alterations in the composition of the gut microbiome have been identified to increase susceptibility to several chronic metabolic diseases including diabetes (Larsen et al. 2010), obesity (Turnbaugh et al. 2008), and cardiovascular disease (Karlsson et al. 2012, Robles Alonso and Guarner 2013). These findings have generated enthusiasm since they point to a largely unstudied contributor to biologic variability that may have large effects on human health. Furthermore, the microbiome appears to be modifiable through diet, pre-/probiotics, and transplantation, opening avenues for strategic intervention. At the same time, genetics appears important, as does early-life establishment of the gut community. We are still in the infancy of the science, and much remains to be understood/discovered, including the causal importance of the microbiome. Clearly, a better understanding of the microbiome's role in disease, and modifiability by dietary nutrients, could be useful as we begin to design nutritional interventions that target an individual's personal risk.

A developing body of literature indicates that microbial dysbiosis, an altered or unhealthy microbiome, including low microbial diversity, low abundance of bacteria considered beneficial, and increased presence of pathobionts, resident microbes with pathogenic potential (Chow et al. 2011), in the digestive tract (Vijay-Kumar et al. 2010, Ridaura et al. 2013) may influence systemic inflammation by altering gut permeability and thus increasing circulating lipopolysaccharide (Ostos et al. 2002, Cani et al. 2008, 2009)—a powerful trigger for immune response. Another line of literature reveals the microbiome to be a metabolically active, complex organ, producing many metabolites that can directly influence disease susceptibility, including those metabolites derived from nutrients. The hypothesized mechanisms of action relating the microbiome to disease are not exclusive, nor necessarily independent of each other, and there is evidence that diet and perhaps specific food components can affect disease risk directly or indirectly.

GUT MICROBIOME

The potential role for gut microbiota in our biology has long been recognized and studied via culture-based methods (Falk et al. 1998), but recent developments in next-generation sequencing (NGS) technology and bioinformatics methods have accelerated discoveries and expanded understanding of the health relevance of our microbial symbionts. These "culture-free" methods do not rely on the ability to grow bacteria in a laboratory and the microbial species identified through NGS have not been successfully cultured. These technological advances have promoted an explosion of research into the microbiome over the past decade, including the creation of major cooperative projects such as the NIH Common Fund's Human Microbiome Project (HMP) (Human Microbiome Project, Consortium 2012) and the European Metagenomics of the Human Intestinal Tract (MetaHIT) (Arumugam et al. 2011), designed to delineate the composition and function of human microbial communities across multiple sites in representative samples of healthy human adults. These studies have revealed 10–100 trillions of symbiotic microbial cells residing across and within the human body. Microbial ecosystems have coevolved to provide specific local functions, with distinct microbial communities populating body compartments such as the gut, oral cavity, and vagina, and contributing unique functions that enhance our biology. The digestive system is one of the largest reservoirs of these microbes, and the microbial community of the lower intestine is particularly relevant with respect to diet, nutrition, and cardiometabolic disease.

As with many new fields, there is some confusion regarding the terminology used to describe the gut community. *Microbiota* and *microbiome* are often used interchangeably; for the purposes of this chapter, we use *microbiota* to specifically refer to the taxonomic membership of the gut community, and *microbiome* to refer to the genomic information embodied in that community. We reserve the use of the term *metagenomics* for shotgun sequencing of total DNA to distinguish it from analysis of microbial community composition by sequencing marker genes (e.g., 16S ribosomal RNA). We focus specifically on the gut microbiome due to its close relation to nutrition and its association with cardiometabolic risk, but note that there are multiple microbial communities throughout the body, each with distinct ecologic characteristics. Most studies in humans that we will discuss use stool samples as a proxy for the lower-gut microbiome, while studies in model organisms may profile cecal contents or specific regions of the intestinal tract. Furthermore, we will largely restrict our discussion to bacterial members of the gut community, but increasing research includes viral and archaeal components (Hoffmann et al. 2013).

Much study of the gut microbiome to date has focused on the composition of the gut microbial community, while there has been less work employing measures of genetic potential or functional activity. The emphasis on community composition has been driven by both technical and analytical practicalities, as many of the individual bacteria comprising the microbiota have not yet been successfully cultured in the laboratory. The inability to culture these bacteria limits the functional characterization of specific microbiota because they cannot be specifically tested *in vitro* or *in vivo*.

Gut community composition is typically estimated by sequencing regions of the 16S ribosomal RNA (rRNA) marker gene, which is sufficiently conserved to identify bacteria, yet includes hypervariable regions to distinguish taxonomic groups (Doi and Igarashi 1966, Colli and Oishi 1969). In these analyses, 16S rRNA sequences are assigned to taxonomic groups (called operational taxonomic units, OTUs) (Schloss and Westcott 2011), from which statistical metrics of the ecologic community are derived, including clusters of taxonomic groups, and measures of diversity and richness (Legendre and Legendre 2012). Several analytical tools have been developed for 16S analysis and have been reviewed elsewhere (Kuczynski et al. 2012, Goodrich et al. 2014a).

One goal of the HMP and MetaHIT was to serve as reference samples for describing a core or optimal microbiome among healthy individuals. Based on results from these and other studies, we now know that members of phyla Firmicutes and Bacteroidetes dominate the gut microbiota with lesser representation from Actinobacteria, Proteobacteria, Verrucomicrobia, Fusobacteria, and other phyla (Mahowald et al. 2009). In both HMP and MetaHIT, *Bacteroides* was the dominant genus (Arumugam et al. 2011). These characterizations of the core composition of the microbiota are robust. In one comparative analysis, taxa with an OTU prevalence of 0.50 or greater in the HMP sample were confirmed in at least 90% of non-HMP samples (Fodor et al. 2012). Still, in spite of these relatively consistent taxa in humans, studies have revealed large variability within and across populations in the composition of the gut microbiome (Human Microbiome Project, Consortium 2012), and very few OTUs occurred in 95% of the HMP sample (Huse et al. 2012). Thus, there is a core of microbes found in the microbiota of humans alongside considerable variation in the overall makeup of the microbial community. This individual variability in the microbiome is particularly apparent with respect to the relative abundance of taxonomic groups. For example, the most abundant OTU in HMP gut microbiome samples accounted for an average of 23% of total sequences across cohort members, but ranged from 0.02% to 84% across individuals (Huse et al. 2012). Some studies have proposed that individuals may be distinguished through enterotypes, loosely defined as similar clusters of taxonomic groups (Turnbaugh et al. 2009, Arumugam et al. 2011). However, these clusters have not been consistently observed across studies (Wu et al. 2011, Yatsunenko et al. 2012, Human Microbiome Project, Consortium 2012), and it now appears more likely that a multitude of possible distinct clusters exist and that microbial composition may be better conceptualized as a gradient or through continuous measures of compositional pattern (Huse et al. 2012, Knights et al. 2014). Studies of age- (Biagi et al. 2010, 2012, Yatsunenko et al. 2012) and geographically diverse (Yatsunenko et al. 2012) populations have revealed large between-person differences in microbial composition, further illustrating the enormous natural variability of microbial communities. Together, these findings do not provide strong support for a single core group of microbiota across healthy populations. These studies also point to current limitations, despite detailed studies in hundreds of humans, in creating a definitive classification scheme of the microbial community among healthy humans.

The classification schemes described earlier focus on 16S rRNA characterizations of the microbiota. An alternative approach is to focus on the overall functional characteristics of the microbiota. Although relatively fewer in number, studies that have conducted whole-genome metagenomics have shown that the large variation observed in compositional measures of the microbiota does not imply large variability in the functional potential or activity of the microbiota. In fact, these studies point to clear redundancy in gene presence and expression, suggesting a core set of activities that can be fulfilled by different microbiota (Turnbaugh et al. 2009, Qin et al. 2010, Human Microbiome Project, Consortium 2012). We know from shotgun metagenomics studies that the total microbial community DNA encompasses a rich set of genes involved with carbohydrate and amino acid metabolism, illustrating a core functional role of the gut microbiome in digestion and metabolism. The presence of specific microbial genes only reflects functional potential, and to truly characterize functional activity of the microbiome, it will be necessary to employ microbial measures of messenger RNA (metatranscriptomics), proteins (metaproteomics), and metabolites (metametabolomics) (Integrative 2014). These approaches may reveal variability related to health and disease not captured through 16S rRNA characterization of the microbiota and contribute to understanding a healthy core microbiome from a functional perspective. For example, a study utilizing metagenomics and metatranscriptomics analysis revealed that there is greater variability in gene expression than in gene presence (Franzosa et al. 2014). Similarly, proteins related to carbohydrate metabolism have been shown to be expressed at a level greater than expected from metagenomics profiles (Verberkmoes et al. 2009). Furthermore, there is an indication that copy-number variation may also impact the functional capacity of the microbiota (Greenblum, Carr, and Borenstein 2015). Understanding the factors that regulate differences in microbiota gene expression and their relationship to disease is still a critical gap in our knowledge.

Despite the lack of a clear compositional definition of a healthy microbiome, with respect to specific patterns of community membership, certain objective features are often cited as consistent with dysbiosis. Diversity is generally considered a component of healthy ecology, contributing to an ecosystem that is more stable and less susceptible to experiencing long-term altered responses to external perturbations (such as—in the case of the gut community—treatment with antibiotics), and it is possible to consider diversity in terms of microbial composition or functional activity. Thus, in the absence of specific patterns of community membership fitting into a notion of a core healthy microbiome, diversity—of either microbial composition or functional activity—may be an important feature. It is important to note that there are different approaches to defining dysbiosis. For example, dysbiosis is often defined relative to health, using features that distinguish unhealthy individuals from healthy individuals as the measure of dysbiosis. Applying such a definition, characteristics of dysbiosis will likely vary depending on the outcome considered.

The gut microbiome of healthy adults is remarkably stable in the absence of large perturbations—such as dramatic weight loss or gain, dietary changes, or antibiotic use (Costello et al. 2009, Jakobsson et al. 2010, Caporaso et al. 2011, Dethlefsen and Relman 2011, Faith et al. 2013). In a U.S. study of 27 healthy adults, sampled between 2 and 13 times over 5 years, 60% of microbial strains were consistently observed over the study period (Faith et al. 2013). Samples collected over time reveal greater between-person than within-person variability, and support a relatively stable individual profile. While it is true that the resilience of diverse ecosystems reflects a healthy stability, it is also true that microbial communities can degrade into unhealthy, but stable, patterns. Furthermore, an unstable microbiota does not always reflect poor health, as in infancy or if rebounding from a perturbation, such as antibiotic use or dietary changes. In addition to returning to a previous steady state following a perturbation, the microbiome can rebound to a new steady state, which may differ from the original state. The time course of acute changes and the return to a steady state is still currently under investigation. For example, in a dietary crossover study, gut microbial changes were observed within 24 h after administration of a vegetable- or meat-based diet, and reverted to the prestudy microbiome after 2 days of returning to the original diet (David et al. 2014). Gut microbial changes have also been observed within 1 week of antibiotic use; in some instances, antibiotic-related changes remain after 4 years of observation (Jakobsson et al. 2010). Much work is needed to delineate gut microbial changes in response to exposure changes. In addition, these patterns of change vary by individual and we do not as yet understand the predictors of response patterns (Jakobsson et al. 2010, Dethlefsen and Relman 2011).

INFLAMMATION AND THE MICROBIOME

Inflammation plays a unifying role in cardiometabolic disease (Gorjao et al. 2012), affecting atherosclerosis (Libby 2002), insulin resistance (Glass and Olefsky 2012, Romeo, Lee, and Shoelson 2012), and obesity (Cancello and Clement 2006). In addition, there is growing recognition for the importance of the gut in immune system regulation, with subsequent metabolic effects. Details of this system remain to be delineated, but evidence supports a complex interplay between immune and gut microbial systems. For example, it has been shown that mutations in single genes related to host immunity can have dramatic effects on the microbial community structure (Wen et al. 2008, Thompson et al. 2010). Thus, specific deletion of gut mucosal expression of TLR-5 (toll-like receptor 5), an innate immune system modulator, results in insulin resistance (Vijay-Kumar et al. 2010). In addition to genetic manipulation of immune-related genes in mice, specific tests are used to identify inflammation in the gut. There is evidence that high fecal levels of calprotectin, an S100-related protein found in neutrophils and granulocytes, is indicative of an inflammatory colonic environment (Hildebrand et al. 2013). In addition to the identification of secreted proteins (such as calprotectin), several taxa, such as members of the *Clostridiales* order, are known to be decreased in intestinal inflammatory environments (Schwab et al. 2014). These findings suggest that differences in immune response and chronic inflammatory disease susceptibility may result from differences in microbiota composition.

Barrier function is crucial to guard against bacterial translocation from the gut into the circulation. Impaired barrier function with subsequent endotoxemia has been linked to risk factors for cardiometabolic disease, notably increased fasting glycemia, decreased glucose tolerance, increased body and liver weight, increased liver triglyceride content, and increased energy intake (Cani et al. 2007). Studies utilizing knockout mice for specific antigen recognition receptors on immune cells residing in the intestine, such as *Cd14* and *Nod1,* demonstrate a critical link between phagocytosis of bacteria in the microbiota and increased bacteria in the plasma and tissues of high-fat-fed mice (Amar et al. 2011).

Specific bacteria may impact barrier function of the intestine and physiological traits. *Bifidobacterium longum*, known to promote tight junction integrity, was associated with decreased plasma triglycerides suggesting a protective role (Ulluwishewa et al. 2011). On the other hand, *Rumminococcus gnavus*, a mucin-degrading species associated with reduced barrier integrity and bile acid metabolism, was positively related to plasma triglycerides and plasma glucose. Reduced bacterial translocation results in improved glycemic control and reduced adiposity, indicating perhaps a causal role for the microbiota in cardiometabolic disease through effects on the intestinal barrier integrity. Specific comparisons of the microbiota of the oral cavity, fecal samples, and carotid endarterectomy samples indicate that there are notable differences in the composition of each of these sites, but also highlight the possibility that some of the specific bacteria present in the atherosclerotic plaque could also be derived from the distal gut or the oral cavity (Koren et al. 2011). Interestingly, altered Proteobacteria:Firmicutes ratios have been observed in circulating bacteria among patients with CVD as compared to "healthy"

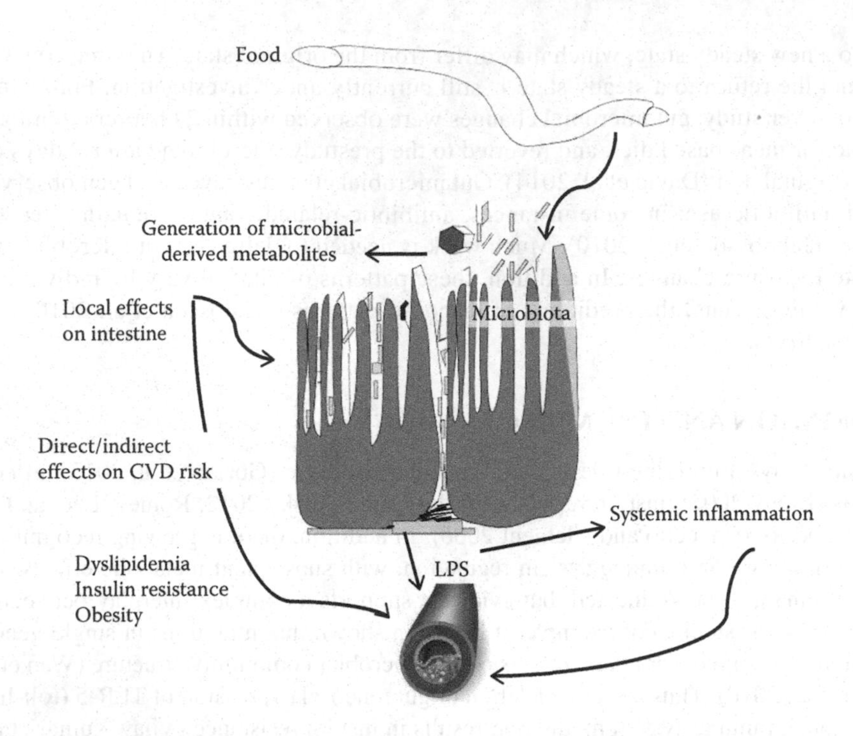

FIGURE 30.1 (See color insert.) Potential mechanisms by which the gut microbiota affects cardiovascular risk. Changes in microbial community structure can change gut permeability and allow microbes to enter the bloodstream (leaky gut syndrome). *Lps* or other bacterial products can induce low-grade systemic inflammation. Alternatively, the microbiota can metabolize nutrients in food to specific metabolites that either increase or decrease susceptibility to cardiometabolic disease.

controls with detectable bacteria in their blood (Rajendhran et al. 2013). We have outlined the inflammatory and gut permeability pathways in Figure 30.1.

THE GUT AS A METABOLICALLY ACTIVE TISSUE

The gut is a primary site of digestion and we now recognize the complex role the microbiome has in the metabolism of many individual foods and nutrients that compose our diet. Part of this renewed appreciation is driven by technological advances in metabolomics, which now allow the detection of many small compounds that were previously undetectable.

For example, the colonic metabolome of patients with nonalcoholic fatty liver disease (NAFLD), as compared to healthy controls, contains increased fecal ester volatile organic compounds, such as butanoic acid, and altered levels of certain Lactobacillus and Firmicutes bacteria (Raman et al. 2013). This presents the possibility that altered microbiota may affect the levels of endogenously produced toxins that increase susceptibility to metabolic disease. These results are supported by studies comparing germ-free (GF) mice with conventionalized mice. Dozens of circulating molecules were detected only in conventionalized mice, and ~10% of commonly observed molecules differed significantly in concentration between GF and conventionalized mice (Wikoff et al. 2009). A high-fat diet has also been shown to affect both the global metabolome and microbiota community as well as perturb specific taxa and metabolic pathways such as bile acid and hormone metabolism (Daniel et al. 2014). Consistent with these findings are those from a 2-week dietary intervention among African-Americans and Africans in which African-Americans were allocated a high-fiber, low-fat diet, more typical of a standard native African diet, and Africans were allocated a high-fat, low-fiber diet, more typical of an African-American diet. Changes in microbiota were apparent, with increased pathogenic proteobacteria among Africans after consuming the high-fat/low-fiber diet, but compositional changes in microbiota were less pronounced than changes in microbial metabolites following the dietary intervention, with increased butyrate production associated with the high-fiber, low-fat diet and proinflammatory metabolites associated with the low-fiber, high-fat diet (O'Keefe et al. 2015). The approach of linking health-related metabolites to the gut microbial community in diseased and healthy states allows us to delineate mechanisms through which the microbiome influences disease and identify potential clinical targets for intervention.

This meta-organismal approach was recently applied to cardiovascular disease and led to the discovery of an association between a specific bacterial metabolite, trimethylamine N-oxide, and cardiovascular risk in humans and mice (Brown and Hazen 2014). We describe this pathway and its relationship to cardiometabolic disease in detail later in this chapter.

MICROBIOTA AND THEIR METABOLITES CAN AFFECT CVD RISK

It is important to note that in order to design novel therapies for CVD based on microbiota, it is important to identify specific microbes and their biologic products that can affect disease. In 2011, *Trimethylamine N-oxide* (TMAO) was identified as a novel risk factor for CVD in humans and a series of animal and human studies have subsequently characterized several genetic polymorphisms, dietary components, and microbial factors affecting TMAO levels (Wang et al. 2011, Bennett et al. 2013, Koeth et al. 2013, Tang et al. 2013, Hartiala et al. 2014). Plasma TMAO levels show a dose-dependent association with the severity of coronary atherosclerosis in cardiac patients. Subjects in the upper quartile for TMAO levels (compared with the lowest quartile) had a significant, approximately threefold increased risk of experiencing a major adverse cardiac event (MACE), such as death, myocardial infarction (MI), and stroke, as well as overall poorer event-free survival, over a 3-year period (Tang et al. 2013). Notably, this relationship was independent of traditional CVD risk factors, renal function, and medication use. Atherosclerosis-susceptible $ApoE^{-/-}$ mice fed a diet supplemented with choline, L-carnitine, or TMAO had increased lesion size (Wang et al. 2011, Koeth et al. 2013). Additionally, studies with multiple inbred strains of mice suggest that TMAO explains about 11% of the total variation of atherosclerosis (Bennett et al. 2013). Since the initial reports, several studies have replicated the association of TMAO with CVD, including studies of patients with chronic heart failure (Troseid et al. 2014), diabetes mellitus (Lever et al. 2014), and renal disease (Tang et al. 2015).

Thus, this meta-organismal pathway may be an important new paradigm to consider for an improved understanding of atherosclerotic heart disease and perhaps other cardiometabolic disease processes (Tang and Hazen 2014). We give a brief overview of this pathway with a focus on the metabolism of dietary nutrients. One route for the initial catabolism of dietary choline and L-carnitine (a nutrient important for fat metabolism) is mediated by intestinal microbes and leads to the formation of trimethylamine (TMA). Foods rich in choline and L-carnitine, such as eggs, milk, and red meat, can thus lead to increased TMA production (Zeisel et al. 2003). TMA is efficiently absorbed from the gastrointestinal tract and oxidized in the liver by the flavin-containing monooxygenase (FMO) enzymes to form trimethylamine N-oxide (TMAO) (Bennett et al. 2013). Studies have shown that *Fmo3* is indeed the primary FMO responsible for hepatic metabolism of TMA to TMAO through a series of experiments that modulated *Fmo3* mRNA levels using adenoviral overexpression, transgenic overexpression, and *in vivo* antisense oligonucleotides and examined the effect on circulating levels of TMAO (Bennett et al. 2013).

Recent efforts have focused on the link between the microbiome and the atherogenic metabolite TMAO. The microbiome plays an obligate role in the formation of TMA (from trimethylamine-containing nutrients choline and carnitine), and antibiotic knockdown studies show clearly that TMAO is not formed in the absence of the microbiome (Tang et al. 2013). Bacterial species harboring putative choline utilization gene clusters (*cut-c*) have been suggested to play a central role in enteric TMA formation(Craciun and Balskus 2012) (and therefore down-stream TMAO production); however, the specific microbiota have not been fully ascertained.

Mice receiving cecal microbes from atherosclerosis-prone donors demonstrated dietary choline-dependent enhancement in atherosclerotic plaque burden compared to atherosclerosis-resistant donors. Using adoptive transfer approaches, cecal contents from distinct inbred donor strains with differing atherosclerosis potential and TMAO production capacity were identified and then introduced via gastric gavage into recipient mice in which endogenous gut microbes were initially suppressed through use of an oral antibiotic cocktail. A global 16S analysis revealed successful transplantation of donor microbiota, which tended to show coincident proportions with plasma TMAO levels (Gregory et al. 2015).

MICROBIOTA AND CARDIOMETABOLIC RISK FACTORS

In addition to TMA and cardiovascular risk, it is important to note that the microbiota's influence on other cardiometabolic risk factors such as dyslipidemia, insulin resistance, diabetes, and obesity has been extensively investigated.

Several elegant studies have clearly established a role for the microbiome in regulation of body weight and adiposity (Backhed et al. 2004, Ridaura et al. 2013). A shared genetic regulation has also been reported, with loci regulating complex traits of body composition coinciding with loci regulating microbial abundances (McKnite et al. 2012, Parks et al. 2013). The negative relationship of *Roseburia*, *Blautia*, and other unclassified genera of the Lachnospiraceae family with body weight and fat mass, and their positive relationship with lean mass suggest a relationship between butyrate production in the intestine and adiposity. In addition to providing a nutrient source for the enteric epithelium (De Vadder et al. 2014), increased butyrate levels may also increase host energy expenditure (Gao et al. 2009). Additionally, butyrate can influence gut peptide secretion, such as glucagon-like peptide 1 (GLP-1) and peptide YY (PYY), with the potential secondary effect of increased satiety (Hosseini et al. 2011). These effects may be mediated via short-chain fatty acid (SCFA) receptors such as GPR43 (Kimura et al. 2013).

Studies of humans identified a bimodal distribution of the microbiota composition with individuals having either low gene counts or high gene counts. Interestingly, there was increased adiposity in the low gene count group, and this was associated with increased serum leptin, decreased serum adiponectin, insulin resistance, increased levels of plasma triglycerides, and increased inflammation as determined by highly sensitive C-reactive protein (hsCRP) levels and higher white blood cell counts (Le Chatelier et al. 2013).

Blood profiling of patients identified that an increase in the proportion of Proteobacteria phylum was associated with long-term cardiovascular risk; from initial analysis, CVD risk appears to be independent of plasma lipoprotein levels (Amar et al. 2013).

FUNCTIONAL STUDIES OF THE MICROBIOME AND CARDIO-METABOLIC HEALTH: STUDY DESIGNS TO UNDERSTAND AND TEST MECHANISMS

One challenge in understanding the role of the microbiome in health is the difficulty establishing causality between actual microbes within the microbiota and disease. The basic framework for establishing causality of a microbe and disease was laid forth by Robert Koch in the late 1880s and they are called "Koch's postulates" (Fredricks and Relman 1996):

1. The parasite occurs in every case of the disease in question and under circumstances that can account for the pathological changes and clinical course of the disease.
2. The parasite occurs in no other disease as a fortuitous and nonpathogenic parasite.
3. After being fully isolated from the body and repeatedly grown in pure culture, the parasite can induce the disease anew.

This framework states that if the disease-causing entity is a microbe, differences in disease susceptibility should follow transplantation of the microbe into a new host. Using adoptive transfer approaches, it has been possible to identify pathogenic microbes that cause disease. Obviously, as medicine and technology have evolved, these principles have been refined (Falkow 2004). In the case of the microbiota, establishing causality is more difficult as these bacteria may not be uniformly associated with the disease. In spite of this limitation, the basic concept of experimental validation of the relationship between a specific entity in the microbiota and cardiometabolic disease is important.

There are several additional challenges in order to apply these principles to the microbiota. The first difficulty is that microbiota are a complex community and the effects observed on human health may be the result of the interactions among multiple taxa. Secondly, the association between the gut and cardiovascular health is spatially separated, and thus changes in the microbiota most likely affect disease risk through complex pathways with potentially many susceptibility factors that vary among people. Lastly, many of the bacteria in the microbiota have not yet been cultured successfully, and thus functional tests to establish causality remain technologically challenging. Obviously, establishment of causality is a high threshold of scientific work and thus many of the studies described throughout this chapter are associative in nature. What is clear from the vast number of associative studies is that there are strong impacts of the gut microbiome on disease susceptibility, but the underlying bacterial species, or gene sets from multiple species, causing disease remain elusive.

Gnotobiotics to Test Microbiota

One tool that has been particularly useful in demonstrating specific effects of the microbiome are gnotobiotic animals, defined as an animal stock or strain derived by aseptic cesarean section (or sterile hatching of eggs) that is reared and continuously maintained with germ-free techniques under isolator conditions (Gordon and Pesti 1971). Gnotobiotic techniques have been used for well over 50 years in microbial research, but recent advances have facilitated creation of several large facilities for using gnotobiotic mice. By using adoptive transfer approaches, various microbes can be transferred from humans, mice, or specific cultured microbes into gnotobiotic mice. Most often the adoptive transfer is performed using gastric gavage. These tools have been extremely useful to demonstrate that a phenomenon observed in an associative study is due to specific differences in the microbiome.

There are significant resource barriers to the development and use of gnotobiotic mice as this approach requires specialized techniques, facilities, and equipment. These challenges have spurred researchers to develop other methods to address causality in model organisms. A primary approach is to use broad-spectrum antibiotic treatment to dramatically and effectively reduce the microbial population of the gastrointestinal tract in rodents and then to perform an adoptive transfer experiment using gastric gavage. These experiments are partially confounded by the nonspecific effects of antibiotic treatment, but when utilized with appropriate controls, they have been used to demonstrate the effects of microbiota on a number of clinically relevant phenotypes.

As development of high-throughput and cost-effective sequencing technologies expands, it is possible to consider other experimental designs to demonstrate causality of the microbiota. For example, mice are coprophagic or feces-consuming rodents, and thus cohoused animals may adopt a similar microbiome. Therefore, one study design is to combine mice of differing genotypes, either different inbred strains or gene targeted knockout mice, to test if one "microbiota" is dominant amongst them. These studies can identify the invasive nature of microorganisms and the stability of changes over time among mice with variable genetic makeup.

Human Fecal Transplants

In addition to the use of model organisms, there is evidence that perturbing, and even transplanting, the microbiome between humans may have therapeutic benefit. For example, individuals with persistent and recurrent *Clostridium difficile* infection have been treated with fecal transplants. Several clinical studies have been performed and a recent meta-analysis of these data identified that 245 of the 273 patients receiving fecal transplants resolved their *Clostridium difficile* infection (Kassam et al. 2013). This initial success has prompted the design of studies investigating treatment of a variety of diseases, including cardiometabolic disease (Smits et al. 2013). One report demonstrated that transplant of microbiota from lean individuals improved insulin sensitivity of patients with metabolic syndrome (Vrieze et al. 2012). It is important to note that the clinical efficacy and potentially unintended adverse effects of such approaches needs to be fully evaluated before these therapies are moved into mainstream clinical practice.

EFFECTS OF DIET ON MICROBIOTA

The human microbiome utilizes both dietary and host-derived nutrients for survival. Thus, changes in host diet can have a profound impact on the microbiome (Cotillard et al. 2013, Spor, Koren, and Ley 2011), including altering the overall bacterial composition, influencing gene expression, or promoting a bloom or inhibition of certain taxa. These dynamic changes have been shown in both mouse and human microbial populations in response to dietary intervention (Spor, Koren, and Ley 2011). As noted earlier, changes in the diet generally yielded changes in the adult microbiome within 24 h, and a return to the baseline microbiome can be observed within 2 days following an individual's resumption of their usual diet (David et al. 2014). Interestingly, alterations beginning early in life may have long-lasting effects on multiple phenotypes (Cox et al. 2014).

National comparisons have revealed significant differences in gut microbial composition with distinct microbial patterns by country (Yatsunenko et al. 2012). These differences are apparent across all age groups (0–70 years) (Yatsunenko et al. 2012) and appear as early as 6 months of age (Grzeskowiak et al. 2012). Broadly, data indicate that Western adult populations may have on average lower microbial diversity as compared to African or South American populations. In addition, taxonomic differences are apparent, with higher *Prevotella* abundance among Africans (De Filippo et al. 2010, Yatsunenko et al. 2012, Ou et al. 2013, Schnorr et al. 2014) and South American (Yatsunenko et al. 2012) samples, as compared to Americans (Yatsunenko et al. 2012, Ou et al. 2013) or Europeans (De Filippo et al. 2010, Schnorr et al. 2014). These studies support diet-related differences, such as the enrichment of fiber-degrading microbiota in non-Western populations, but likely reflect a multitude of nondiet differences as well.

Observational and intervention studies support differences in the gut microbiome related to macronutrient consumption. Among 178 elderly adults, a healthy food diversity index was significantly associated with measures of microbial diversity, with higher microbial diversity among individuals consuming a diet high in fruits, vegetables, and whole grains, and low in red meat and snacks/sweets (Claesson et al. 2012). In another study, gut microbiota clustered into 3 taxonomic groups among 98 adults based on their habitual dietary consumption patterns of predominantly carbohydrate or predominantly high protein and fat (Wu et al. 2011). Cyclical changes in diet may affect microbiota composition fairly quickly; a randomized control trial of high-fat/low-fiber or low-fat/high-fiber diets found there were changes in the microbial composition within 24 h. However, these changes within individuals are insufficient to overcome the taxonomic differences between subjects observed at baseline (Wu et al. 2011). Similarly, in an intervention study of three diets high in resistant starch, high in nonstarch polysaccharides (wheat bran), or high in protein/low in carbohydrate, gut microbial changes were observed within days, but failed to overcome initial between-person differences (Walker et al. 2011). These findings illustrate the strength of an individual microbial pattern, but do not necessarily support a lack of large dietary effects on the gut microbiome, particularly given data indicating clear functional redundancies among microbiota. For example, a crossover study in 10 adults allocated to exclusively plant- or animal-based diets revealed significant differences in functional measures, even in the absence of large compositional changes in microbial pattern. After 24 h, bacterial gene expression changes distinguished subjects based on their assigned diet, rather than their individual baseline microbiome, with enrichment of microbial enzymes reflecting the needs of the specific diet (e.g., bile-acid enzymes increased with animal-based diet) (David et al. 2014). Studies in gnotobiotic mice reconstituted with known human microbiota and fed a variety of diets demonstrate significant plasticity in gene expression that is rapid, reproducible, and reversible in response to changes in diet (McNulty et al. 2013). These studies further illustrate the need for functional measures in studies of diet, the gut microbiome, and health.

SPECIFIC EFFECTS OF DIET AND POTENTIAL INTERACTION WITH CARDIOMETABOLIC HEALTH

Much of the efforts to understand the interactions of diet and the microbiome have focused on the effects of a high-fat, calorie-rich diet. In model organisms, there has been a focus on identifying the changes to the microbiota when a high-fat diet is consumed, and how altered composition of the microbiota relates to susceptibility or resistance to disease. Clinical studies in humans have focused on microbiota changes during weight loss interventions (Cotillard et al. 2013). In addition to increased energy density or alterations in macronutrient composition, specific nutrients or dietary components may have effects on the microbiota that are associated with cardiometabolic health.

FIBER

A large literature supports a protective role for fiber in various aspects of cardiometabolic diseases, including insulin sensitivity, glucose homeostasis, circulating lipids, and body weight. Fiber includes nondigestible carbohydrates or lignin that may be fermented by microbiota in the large intestine. Fiber encompasses many compounds—including resistant starch and oligosaccharides—that differ in their potential for microbial fermentation, as well as their ability to alter the composition and function of the gut microbial community. Extensive epidemiological evidence has led to the broad recommendation to consume a diet high in fiber to reduce risk of cardiovascular disease (American Heart Association Nutrition et al. 2006). The impact of fiber on cardiometabolic disease may be partially mediated by products of gut microbial fermentation of fiber and through fiber-induced ("prebiotic") microbial changes to a more health-promoting microbial profile.

Interestingly, the use of germ-free mice with a humanized microbiota determined that gastrointestinal transit time was faster when mice were fed a high-fiber (cellulose) diet, compared to mice fed a polysaccharide-deficient diet. Additional tests with a diet containing a fermentable fructo-oligosaccharide resulted in increased gastrointestinal transit time. These data suggest that a fiber-enriched diet improves gastrointestinal motility due to the presence of insoluble, nonfermentable fiber that reduces microbe-mediated carbohydrate fermentation (Kashyap et al. 2013a).

Microbe-mediated carbohydrate fermentation may be of particular interest. SCFAs (butyrate, propionate, and acetate) are products of microbial fermentation of fiber that may influence cardiometabolic health through local colonic as well as systemic pathways. Locally, SCFAs, in particular butyrate, enhance colonic membrane integrity, limiting inflammatory responses due to lipopolysaccharide movement from the gut to the circulation. In the periphery, SCFAs act as signaling molecules for glucose homeostasis and insulin sensitivity in the liver, skeletal muscle, and adipose tissues; influence concentrations of appetite-related hormones (peptide YY, glucagon-like peptide 1, and leptin); and suppress the release of proinflammatory mediators. A clinical study investigating diet alterations in obese subjects showed that reduced carbohydrate intake increases butyrate-producing bacteria in the feces (Duncan et al. 2007).

The production of SCFAs varies according to the type, amount, and compositional form of available fiber substrate, and the composition and function of the gut microbial community (Walker et al. 2011). There is evidence for some patterns of enzymatic specificity within taxonomic groups, such as greater acetate-producing bacteria within the Firmicutes phylum and greater butyrate-producing bacteria within the Bacteroidetes phylum, but there is also much overlap in function across phyla.

Furthermore, SCFAs that are produced by some microbiota are further degraded by other microbiota, highlighting the enormous complexity of the gut microbiome as an ecologic system.

Polyphenols

Polyphenols have been widely investigated due to their antioxidant and anti-inflammatory properties. Several risk factors associated with cardiometabolic disease are influenced by inflammation or oxidative stress and therefore polyphenols have been hypothesized to potentially reduce cardiovascular disease (CVD) risk. One area that is often overlooked is that an estimated 90%–95% of dietary polyphenols can be metabolized by microbiota in the lower gut prior to entering the bloodstream (Clifford 2004). Thus, the microbial community can directly influence the extent to which bioactive polyphenol metabolites are available to the host, potentially explaining observed individual variability in metabolite production (Atkinson et al. 2008).

In addition, the health benefits of polyphenols may partly be mediated through polyphenol-induced changes on the gut community. In fact, several studies have demonstrated microbial changes following feeding interventions with polyphenol-rich foods. For example, cranberry extracts enriched for polyphenols affected the levels of *Akkermansia* spp., a taxa associated with insulin sensitivity and intestinal inflammation (Anhe et al. 2015). Increases in butyrate-producing bacteria *Bifidobacterium* or *Lactobacillus* have been observed in interventions of isoflavones (Clavel et al. 2005), cocoa flavanol (Tzounis et al. 2011), almonds (Liu et al. 2014), wild blueberries (Vendrame et al. 2011), coffee (Jaquet et al. 2009), red wine (Queipo-Ortuno et al. 2012), green tea (Jin et al. 2012), apples (Shinohara et al. 2010), and bananas (Mitsou et al. 2011).

Pre-/Probiotics

There has been tremendous interest in the role that pre- and probiotics have in modulating the effects of the microbiome. For example, prebiotic feeding with oligofructose in ob/ob mice, a genetically obese strain, had broad effects on the microbiota affecting >100 distinct taxa and resulting in improved glucose tolerance and reduced fat-mass (Everard et al. 2011). Prebiotic feeding normalized abundance of *A. muciniphila*, a taxa increased in obese and diabetic mice, and the change correlated with an improved metabolic profile (Everard et al. 2013). Further analysis of metagenomic sequencing data revealed that high-fat diets and prebiotics affected the microbiota at different taxonomic levels and that prebiotics counteracted high-fat-diet-induced metabolic disorders (Everard et al. 2014). Similar effects of improved adiposity and plasma lipid levels have been seen with administration of wheat arabinoxylans (Neyrinck et al. 2011).

Food Additives

A less frequently studied area of research is the effects of processed foods and specific food products on the microbiome. A recent study identified that noncaloric artificial sweeteners had negative effects on insulin sensitivity that were nullified by antibiotic treatment (Suez et al. 2014), indicating that specific alterations in the microbiota induced by sweeteners may cause this effect. The robust nature of this specific interaction remains to be corroborated, but it does point to a limitation in our current understanding of the health effects of food additives.

INTERACTIONS BETWEEN HOST GENETICS AND MICROBIOTA

Genetic factors are clearly important to determine the risk of cardiometabolic disease. What is not clear is how the microbiota can buffer the risk of cardiometabolic disease or increase risk independently of the underlying genetic composition of the individual and if these deleterious or positive effects of the microbiota work in conjunction with the consumption of a specific diet. An interesting possibility is that specific genetic loci in the host may affect microbial composition and thereby modulate risk of cardiometabolic disease. We outline some of these concepts here.

Host Genetics and Microbial Composition

Considering the interindividual variability at the level of the microbiome (Eckburg et al. 2005, Qin et al. 2010), detailed studies integrating the intestinal microbiome with disease risk complement genome-wide association studies (GWAS), and other efforts seeking to assess the basis for heterogeneity in health and disease status. Importantly, understanding how microbial diversity and specific microbial species affect clinical phenotypes and risk of CVD will be beneficial as we begin to focus on personalized approaches to nutrition and medicine. As our interest in the microbiome's role in chronic disease has expanded, so has interest in how host genetics influences microbial diversity. Several groups have reported that enteric microbial composition is a heritable trait (Turnbaugh et al. 2010, Tims et al. 2013), although results from twin studies have shown evidence for discordance of heritability (Turnbaugh et al. 2009). One limitation of the initial characterization of the heritability of the composition of the microbiota is the limited population sample sizes available. Recently, 1000 fecal samples from the TwinsUK population were characterized. This cohort of ~416 twin pairs demonstrated that specific members of the microbiota are influenced, at least in part, by underlying host genetic factors. Interestingly, one highly heritable taxon, Christensenllaceae, is enriched in individuals with low BMI and potential effects of this taxa on adiposity were confirmed in germ-free gnotobiotic mice (Goodrich et al. 2014b).

Studies using naturally occurring genetic variation among panels of inbred mouse strains, in addition to single gene mutations in genetically modified mice, have consistently shown an effect of host genetics on intestinal microbial community structure (Toivanen, Vaahtovuo, and Eerola 2001, Benson et al. 2010, Kovacs et al. 2011, Spor, Koren, and Ley 2011, McKnite et al. 2012, Parks et al. 2013) and provide increased power to detect genotype-driven microbial differences. This is especially relevant since murine studies allow for tight control over environmental factors including diet (Benson et al. 2010) For example, numerous genetic studies in mice, including those using genetic reference panels (Benson et al. 2010, Campbell et al. 2012, McKnite et al. 2012, Hildebrand et al. 2013) have demonstrated an effect of genetic background on microbial diversity. Inbred strain surveys in mice also demonstrate a significant effect of host genetic makeup on microbial diversity (Campbell et al. 2012), and some of these differences have been linked to cardiometabolic phenotypes (O'Connor et al. 2014). Interestingly, using an advanced intercross population of mice, Benson and coworkers demonstrated that a single genetic locus may regulate the abundance of several taxa (Benson et al. 2010).

However, the relative strength of environmental versus genetic signals on microbial regulation remains unclear. Much of our knowledge about the environmental effects on the microbiome has been derived from studies in mice (Spor, Koren, and Ley 2011). Several studies have shown how the maternal environment, litter effects, cage mates, the location that the mice are housed, and the commercial vendor can influence microbial populations (Benson et al. 2010, Friswell et al. 2010, Campbell et al. 2012, Hildebrand et al. 2013, McCafferty et al. 2013). Uterine implantation studies have also shown that mice of different genetic backgrounds have similar microbial composition when reared by the same foster mother, indicating that in certain circumstances, environmental drivers can overpower genetic influences at least for nonadherent bacterial populations (Friswell et al. 2010). These findings are further supported by studies that have demonstrated that bacteria from diverse sources can colonize the gut of gnotobiotic mice and compete with "normal" microbiota (Seedorf et al. 2014). Clearly, more work is needed to understand the interactions between host genetics and microbial diversity.

Although gene by diet interactions influencing the microbiome is a relatively new field of investigation (Joseph and Loscalzo 2015), studies using mouse genetic reference populations (Parks et al.

2013) or single gene knockout models (Kashyap et al. 2013b) have demonstrated an interaction between microbiota and diet that is influenced by host genotype. These investigations have extended beyond studies utilizing mice to use of novel model organisms such as stickleback fish, in which there was a modest association between major histocompatibility complex polymorphisms and gut microbial composition and diversity (Bolnick et al. 2014a). The acceptance of interactions is not universal as a study of inbred mice showed that diet intervention has reproducible changes on microbiome, and overwhelms genetic differences between strains (Carmody et al. 2015). Moreover, gene–diet interactions on the microbiome have not been clearly documented in humans. A clinical study reported that despite retained variation in taxonomy following dietary intervention, microbial gene expression, as assessed by RNA-seq, clustered by diet group and exhibited less between-subject variation than at baseline (David et al. 2014).

In addition to specific genetic effects, there is also emerging evidence of gender differences in the composition of the microbiome. In a study of fish, mice, and humans, there were significant interactions between diet and sex on gut microbiome (Bolnick et al. 2014b). These studies indicate that attention to gender may be critical to delineating dietary effects on the microbiome. How gender differences in the microbiome relate to the established gender differences known to occur in cardiovascular disease remains to be determined.

ALTERED MICROBIOTA ACROSS LIFE SPAN

Age is an independent risk factor for cardiovascular disease and many of its risk factors. We are beginning to appreciate the changes to the microbiota that occur as we age, and how perturbations at specific time points may affect microbial composition of the microbiota.

Newborns and Early Childhood

Among other factors, infants experience tremendous alterations in their microbiome across the first few years of life. It has been noted that the microbiota are influenced by the type of birth (vaginal or Cesarean). For example, shortly after birth, the microbiota of vaginally delivered infants resembles the microbiota of their mother's vagina, while infants delivered via Cesarean section harbor microbial communities typically found on human skin (Penders et al. 2006). As an infant progresses through various milestones over the first year of life, such as the initial introduction of solid foods and transition to table foods, there are significant changes in the microbiota composition (Yatsunenko et al. 2012). One perturbation that clearly affects the microbiota is antibiotics, and there is evidence that treatment of newborn mice with antibiotics alters the microbiome and increases adiposity (Cho et al. 2012). However, whether alterations of the microbiome in childhood affect cardiometabolic health later in life is unclear.

In addition to changes in microbiota diversity, there is also an effect of age on microbiota gene ontology. For example, bacterial genes involved in B vitamin metabolism develop over the time course of early childhood, perhaps in response to the broad changes in diet (Yatsunenko et al. 2012). This notion of early diet changes driving microbiota diversity is supported by ecological studies comparing African and European children (De Filippo et al. 2010). In these studies, unique abundance of bacteria from the genus Prevotella and Xylanibacter, known to contain a set of bacterial genes for cellulose and xylan hydrolysis, were overrepresented in the African population. One can hypothesize that this particular bacteria coevolved with the microbiota of the African subjects in response to their diet that is enriched in polysaccharides. Similar effects of coevolution or perhaps horizontal gene transfer, where bacteria from food invade the microbiota of individuals consuming that food, are novel and need rigorous testing. It should be noted that at least one group has identified specific bacteria-associated genes that may be transferred to humans when they consume diets enriched in seafood (Hehemann et al. 2010).

Maternal Diet

Perhaps one of the most interesting concepts regarding horizontal gene transfer and other influences on the microbiome of children are the effects of the maternal microbiome and perhaps the effects of maternal diet and exposure to environmental factors. For example, treatment of pregnant mice with low-dose antibiotics results in a disruption of the microbiota. These altered microbiota in the offspring affect clinical traits such as body composition and adiposity (Cox et al. 2014). However, to date these maternal effects have not been thoroughly segregated from potential epigenetic effects such as DNA methylation.

Microbiota and Elderly Populations

As compared to other age groups, there are relatively few studies of gut microbiomes among the elderly. Alterations in gut microbial community homeostasis are anticipated based on age-related physiologic and behavioral changes, including diet, comorbidities, medication use, and gastrointestinal functioning. Studies have documented significant microbial compositional differences between young and older adults, though reported patterns of difference are not consistent. For example, diversity appears to decrease with age (Biagi et al. 2010), and several studies have shown an increased abundance of Proteobacteria with aging (Biagi et al. 2010, Claesson et al. 2011). In contrast, there are discordant results with respect to age-related shifts in the Firmicutes:Bacteriodetes ratio (Biagi et al. 2010, Claesson et al. 2011). The gut microbiome among healthy, community-dwelling older adults is similar to that of younger adults, with large population-level variability and high within-person temporal stability (Claesson et al. 2011). The gut microbiome among samples from older individuals is significantly associated with diet and health status, including measures of adiposity and inflammation, as well as frailty and cognitive function (Claesson et al. 2012), and is responsive to probiotic intervention (Eloe-Fadrosh et al. 2015). In contrast to healthy community-dwelling older adults, significant changes in the microbiome are apparent among older adults who reside in rehabilitative or residential care facilities (Claesson et al. 2012, Jeffery, Lynch, and O'Toole 2016), with facility-dwelling individuals having significantly lower microbial diversity and significant differences in functional measures, such as decreased SCFA production (Claesson et al. 2012).

SUMMARY

The microbiota represents a critical mediator of the effects of diet on human health and disease susceptibility. Advances in –omics scale technologies and analysis have provided the fundamental understanding of the composition of the microbiome and how specific bacteria and overall community composition change when cardiometabolic disease risk is high, such as in obese individuals or diabetic patients. Integrating culture-free microbial diversity analysis with metabolomics has identified interesting pathways and hypotheses to link dietary changes with specific disease risk factors. Over time, the goal is that these analyses can be used to refine our dietary recommendations to improve health. These are particularly important as we move toward a personalized medicine model.

GLOSSARY

HMP Human microbiome project
MetaHIT Metagenomics of the human intestinal tract
OTU Operational taxonomic unit

REFERENCES

Amar, J., C. Chabo, A. Waget, P. Klopp, C. Vachoux, L. G. Bermudez-Humaran, N. Smirnova et al. 2011. Intestinal mucosal adherence and translocation of commensal bacteria at the early onset of type 2 diabetes: Molecular mechanisms and probiotic treatment. *EMBO Mol Med* 3 (9):559–572. doi: 10.1002/emmm.201100159.

Amar, J., C. Lange, G. Payros, C. Garret, C. Chabo, O. Lantieri, M. Courtney et al. 2013. Blood microbiota dysbiosis is associated with the onset of cardiovascular events in a large general population: The D.E.S.I.R. study. *PLoS One* 8 (1):e54461. doi: 10.1371/journal.pone.0054461.

American Heart Association Nutrition Committee, A. H. Lichtenstein, L. J. Appel, M. Brands, M. Carnethon, S. Daniels, H. A. Franch et al. 2006. Diet and lifestyle recommendations revision 2006: A scientific statement from the American Heart Association Nutrition Committee. *Circulation* 114 (1):82–96. doi: 10.1161/CIRCULATIONAHA.106.176158.

Anhe, F. F., D. Roy, G. Pilon, S. Dudonne, S. Matamoros, T. V. Varin, C. Garofalo et al. 2015. A polyphenol-rich cranberry extract protects from diet-induced obesity, insulin resistance and intestinal inflammation in association with increased *Akkermansia* spp. population in the gut microbiota of mice. *Gut* 64 (6):872–883. doi: 10.1136/gutjnl-2014-307142.

Arumugam, M., J. Raes, E. Pelletier, D. Le Paslier, T. Yamada, D. R. Mende, G. R. Fernandes et al. 2011. Enterotypes of the human gut microbiome. *Nature* 473 (7346):174–180. doi: 10.1038/nature09944.

Atkinson, C., K. M. Newton, E. J. Bowles, M. Yong, and J. W. Lampe. 2008. Demographic, anthropometric, and lifestyle factors and dietary intakes in relation to daidzein-metabolizing phenotypes among premenopausal women in the United States. *Am J Clin Nutr* 87 (3):679–687.

Backhed, F., H. Ding, T. Wang, L. V. Hooper, G. Y. Koh, A. Nagy, C. F. Semenkovich, and J. I. Gordon. 2004. The gut microbiota as an environmental factor that regulates fat storage. *Proc Natl Acad Sci USA* 101 (44):15718–15723. doi: 10.1073/pnas.0407076101.

Bennett, B. J., T. Q. de Aguiar Vallim, Z. Wang, D. M. Shih, Y. Meng, J. Gregory, H. Allayee et al. 2013. Trimethylamine-N-oxide, a metabolite associated with atherosclerosis, exhibits complex genetic and dietary regulation. *Cell Metab* 17 (1):49–60. doi: 10.1016/j.cmet.2012.12.011.

Benson, A. K., S. A. Kelly, R. Legge, F. Ma, S. J. Low, J. Kim, M. Zhang et al. 2010. Individuality in gut microbiota composition is a complex polygenic trait shaped by multiple environmental and host genetic factors. *Proc Natl Acad Sci USA* 107 (44):18933–18938.

Biagi, E., M. Candela, S. Fairweather-Tait, C. Franceschi, and P. Brigidi. 2012. Aging of the human metaorganism: The microbial counterpart. *Age* 34 (1):247–267. doi: 10.1007/s11357-011-9217-5.

Biagi, E., L. Nylund, M. Candela, R. Ostan, L. Bucci, E. Pini, J. Nikkila et al. 2010. Through ageing, and beyond: Gut microbiota and inflammatory status in seniors and centenarians. *PLoS One* 5 (5):e10667. doi: 10.1371/journal.pone.0010667.

Bolnick, D. I., L. K. Snowberg, J. G. Caporaso, C. Lauber, R. Knight, and W. E. Stutz. 2014a. Major histocompatibility complex class IIb polymorphism influences gut microbiota composition and diversity. *Mol Ecol* 23 (19):4831–4845. doi: 10.1111/mec.12846.

Bolnick, D. I., L. K. Snowberg, P. E. Hirsch, C. L. Lauber, E. Org, B. Parks, A. J. Lusis, R. Knight, J. G. Caporaso, and R. Svanback. 2014b. Individual diet has sex-dependent effects on vertebrate gut microbiota. *Nat Commun* 5:4500. doi: 10.1038/ncomms5500.

Brown, J. M. and S. L. Hazen. 2014. Metaorganismal nutrient metabolism as a basis of cardiovascular disease. *Curr Opin Lipidol* 25 (1):48–53. doi: 10.1097/MOL.0000000000000036.

Campbell, J. H., C. M. Foster, T. Vishnivetskaya, A. G. Campbell, Z. K. Yang, A. Wymore, A. V. Palumbo, E. J. Chesler, and M. Podar. 2012. Host genetic and environmental effects on mouse intestinal microbiota. *ISME J* 6 (11):2033–2044. doi: 10.1038/ismej.2012.54.

Cancello, R. and K. Clement. 2006. Is obesity an inflammatory illness? Role of low-grade inflammation and macrophage infiltration in human white adipose tissue. *BJOG* 113 (10):1141–1147. doi: 10.1111/j.1471-0528.2006.01004.x.

Cani, P. D., J. Amar, M. A. Iglesias, M. Poggi, C. Knauf, D. Bastelica, A. M. Neyrinck et al. 2007. Metabolic endotoxemia initiates obesity and insulin resistance. *Diabetes* 56 (7):1761–1772. doi: 10.2337/db06-1491.

Cani, P. D., R. Bibiloni, C. Knauf, A. Waget, A. M. Neyrinck, N. M. Delzenne, and R. Burcelin. 2008. Changes in gut microbiota control metabolic endotoxemia-induced inflammation in high-fat diet-induced obesity and diabetes in mice. *Diabetes* 57 (6):1470–1481. doi: 10.2337/db07-1403.

Cani, P. D., S. Possemiers, T. Van de Wiele, Y. Guiot, A. Everard, O. Rottier, L. Geurts et al. 2009. Changes in gut microbiota control inflammation in obese mice through a mechanism involving GLP-2-driven improvement of gut permeability. *Gut* 58 (8):1091–1103. doi: 10.1136/gut.2008.165886.

Caporaso, J. G., C. L. Lauber, E. K. Costello, D. Berg-Lyons, A. Gonzalez, J. Stombaugh, D. Knights et al. 2011. Moving pictures of the human microbiome. *Genome Biol* 12 (5):R50. doi: 10.1186/gb-2011-12-5-r50.

Carmody, R. N., G. K. Gerber, J. M. Luevano, Jr., D. M. Gatti, L. Somes, K. L. Svenson, and P. J. Turnbaugh. 2015. Diet dominates host genotype in shaping the murine gut microbiota. *Cell Host Microbe* 17 (1):72–84. doi: 10.1016/j.chom.2014.11.010.

Cho, I., S. Yamanishi, L. Cox, B. A. Methe, J. Zavadil, K. Li, Z. Gao et al. 2012. Antibiotics in early life alter the murine colonic microbiome and adiposity. *Nature* 488 (7413):621–626. doi: 10.1038/nature11400.

Chow, J., H. Tang, and S. K. Mazmanian. 2011. Pathobionts of the gastrointestinal microbiota and inflammatory disease. *Curr Opin Immunol* 23 (4):473–480. doi: 10.1016/j.coi.2011.07.010.

Claesson, M. J., S. Cusack, O. O'Sullivan, R. Greene-Diniz, H. de Weerd, E. Flannery, J. R. Marchesi et al. 2011. Composition, variability, and temporal stability of the intestinal microbiota of the elderly. *Proc Natl Acad Sci USA* 108 (Suppl 1):4586–4591. doi: 10.1073/pnas.1000097107.

Claesson, M. J., I. B. Jeffery, S. Conde, S. E. Power, E. M. O'Connor, S. Cusack, H. M. Harris et al. 2012. Gut microbiota composition correlates with diet and health in the elderly. *Nature* 488 (7410):178–184. doi: 10.1038/nature11319.

Clavel, T., M. Fallani, P. Lepage, F. Levenez, J. Mathey, V. Rochet, M. Serezat et al. 2005. Isoflavones and functional foods alter the dominant intestinal microbiota in postmenopausal women. *J Nutr* 135 (12):2786–2792.

Clifford, M. N. 2004. Diet-derived phenols in plasma and tissues and their implications for health. *Planta Med* 70 (12):1103–1114. doi: 10.1055/s-2004-835835.

Colli, W. and M. Oishi. 1969. Ribosomal RNA genes in bacteria: Evidence for the nature of the physical linkage between 16S and 23S RNA genes in *Bacillus subtilis*. *Proc Natl Acad Sci USA* 64 (2):642–649.

Costello, E. K., C. L. Lauber, M. Hamady, N. Fierer, J. I. Gordon, and R. Knight. 2009. Bacterial community variation in human body habitats across space and time. *Science* 326 (5960):1694–1697. doi: 10.1126/science.1177486.

Cotillard, A., S. P. Kennedy, L. C. Kong, E. Prifti, N. Pons, E. Le Chatelier, M. Almeida et al. 2013. Dietary intervention impact on gut microbial gene richness. *Nature* 500 (7464):585–588. doi: 10.1038/nature12480.

Cox, L. M., S. Yamanishi, J. Sohn, A. V. Alekseyenko, J. M. Leung, I. Cho, S. G. Kim et al. 2014. Altering the intestinal microbiota during a critical developmental window has lasting metabolic consequences. *Cell* 158 (4):705–721. doi: 10.1016/j.cell.2014.05.052.

Craciun, S. and E. P. Balskus. 2012. Microbial conversion of choline to trimethylamine requires a glycyl radical enzyme. *Proc Natl Acad Sci USA* 109 (52):21307–21312. doi: 10.1073/pnas.1215689109.

Daniel, H., A. Moghaddas Gholami, D. Berry, C. Desmarchelier, H. Hahne, G. Loh, S. Mondot et al. 2014. High-fat diet alters gut microbiota physiology in mice. *ISME J* 8 (2):295–308. doi: 10.1038/ismej.2013.155.

David, L. A., C. F. Maurice, R. N. Carmody, D. B. Gootenberg, J. E. Button, B. E. Wolfe, A. V. Ling et al. 2014. Diet rapidly and reproducibly alters the human gut microbiome. *Nature* 505 (7484):559–563. doi: 10.1038/nature12820.

De Filippo, C., D. Cavalieri, M. Di Paola, M. Ramazzotti, J. B. Poullet, S. Massart, S. Collini, G. Pieraccini, and P. Lionetti. 2010. Impact of diet in shaping gut microbiota revealed by a comparative study in children from Europe and rural Africa. *Proc Natl Acad Sci USA* 107 (33):14691–14696. doi: 10.1073/pnas.1005963107.

De Vadder, F., P. Kovatcheva-Datchary, D. Goncalves, J. Vinera, C. Zitoun, A. Duchampt, F. Backhed, and G. Mithieux. 2014. Microbiota-generated metabolites promote metabolic benefits via gut-brain neural circuits. *Cell* 156 (1–2):84–96. doi: 10.1016/j.cell.2013.12.016.

Dethlefsen, L. and D. A. Relman. 2011. Incomplete recovery and individualized responses of the human distal gut microbiota to repeated antibiotic perturbation. *Proc Natl Acad Sci USA* 108 (Suppl 1):4554–4561. doi: 10.1073/pnas.1000087107.

Doi, R. H. and R. T. Igarashi. 1966. Heterogeneity of the conserved ribosomal ribonucleic acid sequences of Bacillus subtilis. *J Bacteriol* 92 (1):88–96.

Duncan, S. H., A. Belenguer, G. Holtrop, A. M. Johnstone, H. J. Flint, and G. E. Lobley. 2007. Reduced dietary intake of carbohydrates by obese subjects results in decreased concentrations of butyrate and butyrate-producing bacteria in feces. *Appl Environ Microbiol* 73 (4):1073–1078. doi: 10.1128/AEM.02340-06.

Eckburg, P. B., E. M. Bik, C. N. Bernstein, E. Purdom, L. Dethlefsen, M. Sargent, S. R. Gill, K. E. Nelson, and D. A. Relman. 2005. Diversity of the human intestinal microbial flora. *Science* 308 (5728):1635–1638. doi: 10.1126/science.1110591.

Eloe-Fadrosh, E. A., A. Brady, J. Crabtree, E. F. Drabek, B. Ma, A. Mahurkar, J. Ravel et al. 2015. Functional dynamics of the gut microbiome in elderly people during probiotic consumption. *mBio* 6 (2): e00231–e002315. doi: 10.1128/mBio.00231-15.

Everard, A., C. Belzer, L. Geurts, J. P. Ouwerkerk, C. Druart, L. B. Bindels, Y. Guiot et al. 2013. Cross-talk between *Akkermansia muciniphila* and intestinal epithelium controls diet-induced obesity. *Proc Natl Acad Sci USA* 110 (22):9066–9071. doi: 10.1073/pnas.1219451110.

Everard, A., V. Lazarevic, M. Derrien, M. Girard, G. G. Muccioli, A. M. Neyrinck, S. Possemiers et al. 2011. Responses of gut microbiota and glucose and lipid metabolism to prebiotics in genetic obese and diet-induced leptin-resistant mice. *Diabetes* 60 (11):2775–2786. doi: 10.2337/db11-0227.

Everard, A., V. Lazarevic, N. Gaia, M. Johansson, M. Stahlman, F. Backhed, N. M. Delzenne, J. Schrenzel, P. Francois, and P. D. Cani. 2014. Microbiome of prebiotic-treated mice reveals novel targets involved in host response during obesity. *ISME J* 8(10):2116–2130. doi: 10.1038/ismej.2014.45.

Faith, J. J., J. L. Guruge, M. Charbonneau, S. Subramanian, H. Seedorf, A. L. Goodman, J. C. Clemente et al. 2013. The long-term stability of the human gut microbiota. *Science* 341 (6141):1237439. doi: 10.1126/science.1237439.

Falk, P. G., L. V. Hooper, T. Midtvedt, and J. I. Gordon. 1998. Creating and maintaining the gastrointestinal ecosystem: What we know and need to know from gnotobiology. *Microbiol Mol Biol Rev* 62 (4):1157–1170.

Falkow, S. 2004. Molecular Koch's postulates applied to bacterial pathogenicity—A personal recollection 15 years later. *Nat Rev Microbiol* 2 (1):67–72. doi: 10.1038/nrmicro799.

Fodor, A. A., T. Z. DeSantis, K. M. Wylie, J. H. Badger, Y. Ye, T. Hepburn, P. Hu et al. 2012. The "most wanted" taxa from the human microbiome for whole genome sequencing. *PLoS One* 7 (7):e41294. doi: 10.1371/journal.pone.0041294.

Franzosa, E. A., X. C. Morgan, N. Segata, L. Waldron, J. Reyes, A. M. Earl, G. Giannoukos et al. 2014. Relating the metatranscriptome and metagenome of the human gut. *Proc Natl Acad Sci USA* 111 (22):E2329–E2338. doi: 10.1073/pnas.1319284111.

Fredricks, D. N. and D. A. Relman. 1996. Sequence-based identification of microbial pathogens: A reconsideration of Koch's postulates. *Clin Microbiol Rev* 9 (1):18–33.

Friswell, M. K., H. Gika, I. J. Stratford, G. Theodoridis, B. Telfer, I. D. Wilson, and A. J. McBain. 2010. Site and strain-specific variation in gut microbiota profiles and metabolism in experimental mice. *PLoS One* 5 (1):e8584. doi: 10.1371/journal.pone.0008584.

Gao, Z., J. Yin, J. Zhang, R. E. Ward, R. J. Martin, M. Lefevre, W. T. Cefalu, and J. Ye. 2009. Butyrate improves insulin sensitivity and increases energy expenditure in mice. *Diabetes* 58 (7):1509–1517. doi: 10.2337/db08-1637.

Glass, C. K. and J. M. Olefsky. 2012. Inflammation and lipid signaling in the etiology of insulin resistance. *Cell Metab* 15 (5):635–645. doi: 10.1016/j.cmet.2012.04.001.

Goodrich, J. K., S. C. Di Rienzi, A. C. Poole, O. Koren, W. A. Walters, J. G. Caporaso, R. Knight, and R. E. Ley. 2014a. Conducting a microbiome study. *Cell* 158 (2):250–262. doi: 10.1016/j.cell.2014.06.037.

Goodrich, J. K., J. L. Waters, A. C. Poole, J. L. Sutter, O. Koren, R. Blekhman, M. Beaumont et al. 2014b. Human genetics shape the gut microbiome. *Cell* 159 (4):789–799. doi: 10.1016/j.cell.2014.09.053.

Gordon, H. A. and L. Pesti. 1971. The gnotobiotic animal as a tool in the study of host microbial relationships. *Bacteriol Rev* 35 (4):390–429.

Gorjao, R., H. K. Takahashi, J. A. Pan, and S. Massao Hirabara. 2012. Molecular mechanisms involved in inflammation and insulin resistance in chronic diseases and possible interventions. *J Biomed Biotechnol* 2012:841983. doi: 10.1155/2012/841983.

Greenblum, S., R. Carr, and E. Borenstein. 2015. Extensive strain-level copy-number variation across human gut microbiome species. *Cell* 160 (4):583–594. doi: 10.1016/j.cell.2014.12.038.

Gregory, J. C., J. A. Buffa, E. Org, Z. Wang, B. S. Levison, W. Zhu, M. A. Wagner et al. 2015. Transmission of atherosclerosis susceptibility with gut microbial transplantation. *J Biol Chem* 290 (9):5647–5660. doi: 10.1074/jbc.M114.618249.

Grzeskowiak, L., M. C. Collado, C. Mangani, K. Maleta, K. Laitinen, P. Ashorn, E. Isolauri, and S. Salminen. 2012. Distinct gut microbiota in southeastern African and northern European infants. *J Pediatr Gastroenterol Nutr* 54 (6):812–816. doi: 10.1097/MPG.0b013e318249039c.

Hartiala, J., B. J. Bennett, W. H. Tang, Z. Wang, A. F. Stewart, R. Roberts, R. McPherson et al. 2014. Comparative genome-wide association studies in mice and humans for trimethylamine N-oxide, a proatherogenic metabolite of choline and L-carnitine. *Arterioscler Thromb Vasc Biol* 34(6):1307–1313. doi: 10.1161/ATVBAHA.114.303252.

Hehemann, J. H., G. Correc, T. Barbeyron, W. Helbert, M. Czjzek, and G. Michel. 2010. Transfer of carbohydrate-active enzymes from marine bacteria to Japanese gut microbiota. *Nature* 464 (7290):908–912. doi: 10.1038/nature08937.

Hildebrand, F., T. L. Nguyen, B. Brinkman, R. G. Yunta, B. Cauwe, P. Vandenabeele, A. Liston, and J. Raes. 2013. Inflammation-associated enterotypes, host genotype, cage and inter-individual effects drive gut microbiota variation in common laboratory mice. *Genome Biol* 14 (1):R4. doi: 10.1186/gb-2013-14-1-r4.

Hoffmann, C., S. Dollive, S. Grunberg, J. Chen, H. Li, G. D. Wu, J. D. Lewis, and F. D. Bushman. 2013. Archaea and fungi of the human gut microbiome: Correlations with diet and bacterial residents. *PLoS One* 8 (6):e66019. doi: 10.1371/journal.pone.0066019.

Hosseini, E., C. Grootaert, W. Verstraete, and T. Van de Wiele. 2011. Propionate as a health-promoting microbial metabolite in the human gut. *Nutr Rev* 69 (5):245–258. doi: 10.1111/j.1753-4887.2011.00388.x.

Human Microbiome Project, Consortium. 2012. Structure, function and diversity of the healthy human microbiome. *Nature* 486 (7402):207–214. doi: 10.1038/nature11234.

Huse, S. M., Y. Ye, Y. Zhou, and A. A. Fodor. 2012. A core human microbiome as viewed through 16S rRNA sequence clusters. *PLoS One* 7 (6):e34242. doi: 10.1371/journal.pone.0034242.

Integrative, H. M. P. Research Network Consortium. 2014. The Integrative Human Microbiome Project: Dynamic analysis of microbiome-host omics profiles during periods of human health and disease. *Cell Host Microbe* 16 (3):276–289. doi: 10.1016/j.chom.2014.08.014.

Jakobsson, H. E., C. Jernberg, A. F. Andersson, M. Sjolund-Karlsson, J. K. Jansson, and L. Engstrand. 2010. Short-term antibiotic treatment has differing long-term impacts on the human throat and gut microbiome. *PLoS One* 5 (3):e9836. doi: 10.1371/journal.pone.0009836.

Jaquet, M., I. Rochat, J. Moulin, C. Cavin, and R. Bibiloni. 2009. Impact of coffee consumption on the gut microbiota: A human volunteer study. *Int J Food Microbiol* 130 (2):117–121. doi: 10.1016/j.ijfoodmicro.2009.01.011.

Jeffery, I. B., D. B. Lynch, and P. W. O'Toole. 2016. Composition and temporal stability of the gut microbiota in older persons. *ISME J* 10 (1):170–182. doi: 10.1038/ismej.2015.88.

Jin, J. S., M. Touyama, T. Hisada, and Y. Benno. 2012. Effects of green tea consumption on human fecal microbiota with special reference to Bifidobacterium species. *Microbiol Immunol* 56 (11):729–739. doi: 10.1111/j.1348-0421.2012.00502.x.

Joseph, J. and J. Loscalzo. 2015. Nutri(meta)genetics and cardiovascular disease: Novel concepts in the interaction of diet and genomic variation. *Curr Atheroscler Rep* 17 (5):505. doi: 10.1007/s11883-015-0505-x.

Karlsson, F. H., F. Fak, I. Nookaew, V. Tremaroli, B. Fagerberg, D. Petranovic, F. Backhed, and J. Nielsen. 2012. Symptomatic atherosclerosis is associated with an altered gut metagenome. *Nat Commun* 3:1245. doi: 10.1038/ncomms2266.

Kashyap, P. C., A. Marcobal, L. K. Ursell, M. Larauche, H. Duboc, K. A. Earle, E. D. Sonnenburg et al. 2013a. Complex interactions among diet, gastrointestinal transit, and gut microbiota in humanized mice. *Gastroenterology* 144 (5):967–977. doi: 10.1053/j.gastro.2013.01.047.

Kashyap, P. C., A. Marcobal, L. K. Ursell, S. A. Smits, E. D. Sonnenburg, E. K. Costello, S. K. Higginbottom et al. 2013b. Genetically dictated change in host mucus carbohydrate landscape exerts a diet-dependent effect on the gut microbiota. *Proc Natl Acad Sci USA* 110 (42):17059–17064. doi: 10.1073/pnas.1306070110.

Kassam, Z., C. H. Lee, Y. Yuan, and R. H. Hunt. 2013. Fecal microbiota transplantation for *Clostridium difficile* infection: Systematic review and meta-analysis. *Am J Gastroenterol* 108 (4):500–508. doi: 10.1038/ajg.2013.59.

Kimura, I., K. Ozawa, D. Inoue, T. Imamura, K. Kimura, T. Maeda, K. Terasawa et al. 2013. The gut microbiota suppresses insulin-mediated fat accumulation via the short-chain fatty acid receptor GPR43. *Nat Commun* 4:1829. doi: 10.1038/ncomms2852.

Knights, D., T. L. Ward, C. E. McKinlay, H. Miller, A. Gonzalez, D. McDonald, and R. Knight. 2014. Rethinking "enterotypes". *Cell Host Microbe* 16 (4):433–437. doi: 10.1016/j.chom.2014.09.013.

Koeth, R. A., Z. Wang, B. S. Levison, J. A. Buffa, E. Org, B. T. Sheehy, E. B. Britt et al. 2013. Intestinal microbiota metabolism of L-carnitine, a nutrient in red meat, promotes atherosclerosis. *Nat Med* 19 (5):576–585. doi: 10.1038/nm.3145.

Koren, O., A. Spor, J. Felin, F. Fak, J. Stombaugh, V. Tremaroli, C. J. Behre et al. 2011. Human oral, gut, and plaque microbiota in patients with atherosclerosis. *Proc Natl Acad Sci USA* 108 (Suppl 1):4592–4598. doi: 10.1073/pnas.1011383107.

Kovacs, A., N. Ben-Jacob, H. Tayem, E. Halperin, F. A. Iraqi, and U. Gophna. 2011. Genotype is a stronger determinant than sex of the mouse gut microbiota. *Microb Ecol* 61 (2):423–428. doi: 10.1007/s00248-010-9787-2.

Kuczynski, J., C. L. Lauber, W. A. Walters, L. W. Parfrey, J. C. Clemente, D. Gevers, and R. Knight. 2012. Experimental and analytical tools for studying the human microbiome. *Nat Rev Genet* 13 (1):47–58. doi: 10.1038/nrg3129.

Larsen, N., F. K. Vogensen, F. W. van den Berg, D. S. Nielsen, A. S. Andreasen, B. K. Pedersen, W. A. Al-Soud, S. J. Sorensen, L. H. Hansen, and M. Jakobsen. 2010. Gut microbiota in human adults with type 2 diabetes differs from non-diabetic adults. *PLoS One* 5 (2):e9085. doi: 10.1371/journal.pone.0009085.

Le Chatelier, E., T. Nielsen, J. Qin, E. Prifti, F. Hildebrand, G. Falony, M. Almeida et al. 2013. Richness of human gut microbiome correlates with metabolic markers. *Nature* 500 (7464):541–546. doi: 10.1038/nature12506.

Legendre, P. and L. Legendre. 2012. *Numerical Ecology*, 3rd edn., Vol. 24, Developments in Environmental Modelling. Oxford, U.K.: Elsevier.

Lever, M., P. M. George, S. Slow, D. Bellamy, J. M. Young, M. Ho, C. J. McEntyre et al. 2014. Betaine and trimethylamine-N-oxide as predictors of cardiovascular outcomes show different patterns in diabetes mellitus: An observational study. *PLoS One* 9 (12):e114969. doi: 10.1371/journal.pone.0114969.

Libby, P. 2002. Inflammation in atherosclerosis. *Nature* 420 (6917):868–874.

Liu, Z., X. Lin, G. Huang, W. Zhang, P. Rao, and L. Ni. 2014. Prebiotic effects of almonds and almond skins on intestinal microbiota in healthy adult humans. *Anaerobe* 26:1–6. doi: 10.1016/j.anaerobe.2013.11.007.

Mahowald, M. A., F. E. Rey, H. Seedorf, P. J. Turnbaugh, R. S. Fulton, A. Wollam, N. Shah et al. 2009. Characterizing a model human gut microbiota composed of members of its two dominant bacterial phyla. *Proc Natl Acad Sci USA* 106 (14):5859–5864. doi: 10.1073/pnas.0901529106.

McCafferty, J., M. Muhlbauer, R. Z. Gharaibeh, J. C. Arthur, E. Perez-Chanona, W. Sha, C. Jobin, and A. A. Fodor. 2013. Stochastic changes over time and not founder effects drive cage effects in microbial community assembly in a mouse model. *ISME J* 7 (11):2116–2125. doi: 10.1038/ismej.2013.106.

McKnite, A. M., M. E. Perez-Munoz, L. Lu, E. G. Williams, S. Brewer, P. A. Andreux, J. W. Bastiaansen et al. 2012. Murine gut microbiota is defined by host genetics and modulates variation of metabolic traits. *PLoS One* 7 (6):e39191. doi: 10.1371/journal.pone.0039191.

McNulty, N. P., M. Wu, A. R. Erickson, C. Pan, B. K. Erickson, E. C. Martens, N. A. Pudlo et al. 2013. Effects of diet on resource utilization by a model human gut microbiota containing *Bacteroides cellulosilyticus* WH2, a symbiont with an extensive glycobiome. *PLoS Biol* 11 (8):e1001637. doi: 10.1371/journal.pbio.1001637.

Mitsou, E. K., E. Kougia, T. Nomikos, M. Yannakoulia, K. C. Mountzouris, and A. Kyriacou. 2011. Effect of banana consumption on faecal microbiota: A randomised, controlled trial. *Anaerobe* 17 (6):384–387. doi: 10.1016/j.anaerobe.2011.03.018.

Neyrinck, A. M., S. Possemiers, C. Druart, T. Van de Wiele, F. De Backer, P. D. Cani, Y. Larondelle, and N. M. Delzenne. 2011. Prebiotic effects of wheat arabinoxylan related to the increase in bifidobacteria, Roseburia and Bacteroides/Prevotella in diet-induced obese mice. *PLoS One* 6 (6):e20944. doi: 10.1371/journal.pone.0020944.

O'Connor, A., P. M. Quizon, J. E. Albright, F. T. Lin, and B. J. Bennett. 2014. Responsiveness of cardiometabolic-related microbiota to diet is influenced by host genetics. *Mamm Genome* 25 (11–12):583–599. doi: 10.1007/s00335-014-9540-0.

O'Keefe, S. J., J. V. Li, L. Lahti, J. Ou, F. Carbonero, K. Mohammed, J. M. Posma et al. 2015. Fat, fibre and cancer risk in African Americans and rural Africans. *Nat Commun* 6:6342. doi: 10.1038/ncomms7342.

Ostos, M. A., D. Recalde, M. M. Zakin, and D. Scott-Algara. 2002. Implication of natural killer T cells in atherosclerosis development during a LPS-induced chronic inflammation. *FEBS Lett* 519 (1–3):23–29.

Ou, J., F. Carbonero, E. G. Zoetendal, J. P. DeLany, M. Wang, K. Newton, H. R. Gaskins, and S. J. O'Keefe. 2013. Diet, microbiota, and microbial metabolites in colon cancer risk in rural Africans and African Americans. *Am J Clin Nutr* 98 (1):111–120. doi: 10.3945/ajcn.112.056689.

Parks, B. W., E. Nam, E. Org, E. Kostem, F. Norheim, S. T. Hui, C. Pan et al. 2013. Genetic control of obesity and gut microbiota composition in response to high-fat, high-sucrose diet in mice. *Cell Metab* 17 (1):141–152. doi: 10.1016/j.cmet.2012.12.007.

Penders, J., C. Thijs, C. Vink, F. F. Stelma, B. Snijders, I. Kummeling, P. A. van den Brandt, and E. E. Stobberingh. 2006. Factors influencing the composition of the intestinal microbiota in early infancy. *Pediatrics* 118 (2):511–521. doi: 10.1542/peds.2005-2824.

Qin, J., R. Li, J. Raes, M. Arumugam, K. S. Burgdorf, C. Manichanh, T. Nielsen et al. 2010. A human gut microbial gene catalogue established by metagenomic sequencing. *Nature* 464 (7285):59–65. doi: 10.1038/nature08821.

Queipo-Ortuno, M. I., M. Boto-Ordonez, M. Murri, J. M. Gomez-Zumaquero, M. Clemente-Postigo, R. Estruch, F. Cardona Diaz, C. Andres-Lacueva, and F. J. Tinahones. 2012. Influence of red wine polyphenols and ethanol on the gut microbiota ecology and biochemical biomarkers. *Am J Clin Nutr* 95 (6):1323–1334. doi: 10.3945/ajcn.111.027847.

Rajendhran, J., M. Shankar, V. Dinakaran, A. Rathinavel, and P. Gunasekaran. 2013. Contrasting circulating microbiome in cardiovascular disease patients and healthy individuals. *Int J Cardiol* 168 (5):5118–5120. doi: 10.1016/j.ijcard.2013.07.232.

Raman, M., I. Ahmed, P. M. Gillevet, C. S. Probert, N. M. Ratcliffe, S. Smith, R. Greenwood et al. 2013. Fecal microbiome and volatile organic compound metabolome in obese humans with nonalcoholic fatty liver disease. *Clin Gastroenterol Hepatol* 11 (7):868–875.e1-3. doi: 10.1016/j.cgh.2013.02.015.

Ridaura, V. K., J. J. Faith, F. E. Rey, J. Cheng, A. E. Duncan, A. L. Kau, N. W. Griffin et al. 2013. Gut microbiota from twins discordant for obesity modulate metabolism in mice. *Science* 341 (6150):1241214. doi: 10.1126/science.1241214.

Robles Alonso, V. and F. Guarner. 2013. Linking the gut microbiota to human health. *Br J Nutr* 109 (Suppl 2):S21–S26. doi: 10.1017/S0007114512005235.

Romeo, G. R., J. Lee, and S. E. Shoelson. 2012. Metabolic syndrome, insulin resistance, and roles of inflammation—Mechanisms and therapeutic targets. *Arterioscler Thromb Vasc Biol* 32 (8):1771–1776. doi: 10.1161/ATVBAHA.111.241869.

Schloss, P. D. and S. L. Westcott. 2011. Assessing and improving methods used in operational taxonomic unit-based approaches for 16S rRNA gene sequence analysis. *Appl Environ Microbiol* 77 (10):3219–3226. doi: 10.1128/AEM.02810-10.

Schnorr, S. L., M. Candela, S. Rampelli, M. Centanni, C. Consolandi, G. Basaglia, S. Turroni et al. 2014. Gut microbiome of the Hadza hunter-gatherers. *Nat Commun* 5:3654. doi: 10.1038/ncomms4654.

Schwab, C., D. Berry, I. Rauch, I. Rennisch, J. Ramesmayer, E. Hainzl, S. Heider et al. 2014. Longitudinal study of murine microbiota activity and interactions with the host during acute inflammation and recovery. *ISME J* 8(5): 1101–1114. doi: 10.1038/ismej.2013.223.

Seedorf, H., N. W. Griffin, V. K. Ridaura, A. Reyes, J. Cheng, F. E. Rey, M. I. Smith et al. 2014. Bacteria from diverse habitats colonize and compete in the mouse gut. *Cell* 159 (2):253–266. doi: 10.1016/j.cell.2014.09.008.

Shinohara, K., Y. Ohashi, K. Kawasumi, A. Terada, and T. Fujisawa. 2010. Effect of apple intake on fecal microbiota and metabolites in humans. *Anaerobe* 16 (5):510–515. doi: 10.1016/j.anaerobe.2010.03.005.

Smits, L. P., K. E. Bouter, W. M. de Vos, T. J. Borody, and M. Nieuwdorp. 2013. Therapeutic potential of fecal microbiota transplantation. *Gastroenterology* 145 (5):946–953. doi: 10.1053/j.gastro.2013.08.058.

Spor, A., O. Koren, and R. Ley. 2011. Unravelling the effects of the environment and host genotype on the gut microbiome. *Nat Rev Microbiol* 9 (4):279–290. doi: 10.1038/nrmicro2540.

Suez, J., T. Korem, D. Zeevi, G. Zilberman-Schapira, C. A. Thaiss, O. Maza, D. Israeli et al. 2014. Artificial sweeteners induce glucose intolerance by altering the gut microbiota. *Nature* 514 (7521):181–186. doi: 10.1038/nature13793.

Tang, W. H. and S. L. Hazen. 2014. The contributory role of gut microbiota in cardiovascular disease. *J Clin Invest* 124 (10):4204–4211. doi: 10.1172/JCI72331.

Tang, W. H., Z. Wang, D. J. Kennedy, Y. Wu, J. A. Buffa, B. Agatisa-Boyle, X. S. Li, B. S. Levison, and S. L. Hazen. 2015. Gut microbiota-dependent trimethylamine N-oxide (TMAO) pathway contributes to both development of renal insufficiency and mortality risk in chronic kidney disease. *Circ Res* 116 (3):448–455. doi: 10.1161/CIRCRESAHA.116.305360.

Tang, W. H., Z. Wang, B. S. Levison, R. A. Koeth, E. B. Britt, X. Fu, Y. Wu, and S. L. Hazen. 2013. Intestinal microbial metabolism of phosphatidylcholine and cardiovascular risk. *N Engl J Med* 368 (17):1575–1584. doi: 10.1056/NEJMoa1109400.

Thompson, C. L., M. J. Hofer, I. L. Campbell, and A. J. Holmes. 2010. Community dynamics in the mouse gut microbiota: A possible role for IRF9-regulated genes in community homeostasis. *PLoS One* 5 (4):e10335. doi: 10.1371/journal.pone.0010335.

Tims, S., C. Derom, D. M. Jonkers, R. Vlietinck, W. H. Saris, M. Kleerebezem, W. M. de Vos, and E. G. Zoetendal. 2013. Microbiota conservation and BMI signatures in adult monozygotic twins. *ISME J* 7 (4):707–717. doi: 10.1038/ismej.2012.146.

Toivanen, P., J. Vaahtovuo, and E. Eerola. 2001. Influence of major histocompatibility complex on bacterial composition of fecal flora. *Infect Immun* 69 (4):2372–2377. doi: 10.1128/IAI.69.4.2372-2377.2001.

Troseid, M., T. Ueland, J. R. Hov, A. Svardal, I. Gregersen, C. P. Dahl, S. Aakhus et al. 2015. Microbiota-dependent metabolite trimethylamine-N-oxide is associated with disease severity and survival of patients with chronic heart failure. *J Intern Med* 277(6):717–726. doi: 10.1111/joim.12328.

Turnbaugh, P. J., F. Backhed, L. Fulton, and J. I. Gordon. 2008. Diet-induced obesity is linked to marked but reversible alterations in the mouse distal gut microbiome. *Cell Host Microbe* 3 (4):213–223. doi: 10.1016/j.chom.2008.02.015.

Turnbaugh, P. J., M. Hamady, T. Yatsunenko, B. L. Cantarel, A. Duncan, R. E. Ley, M. L. Sogin et al. 2009. A core gut microbiome in obese and lean twins. *Nature* 457 (7228):480–484.

Turnbaugh, P. J., C. Quince, J. J. Faith, A. C. McHardy, T. Yatsunenko, F. Niazi, J. Affourtit et al. 2010. Organismal, genetic, and transcriptional variation in the deeply sequenced gut microbiomes of identical twins. *Proc Natl Acad Sci USA* 107 (16):7503–7508.

Tzounis, X., A. Rodriguez-Mateos, J. Vulevic, G. R. Gibson, C. Kwik-Uribe, and J. P. Spencer. 2011. Prebiotic evaluation of cocoa-derived flavanols in healthy humans by using a randomized, controlled, double-blind, crossover intervention study. *Am J Clin Nutr* 93 (1):62–72. doi: 10.3945/ajcn.110.000075.

Ulluwishewa, D., R. C. Anderson, W. C. McNabb, P. J. Moughan, J. M. Wells, and N. C. Roy. 2011. Regulation of tight junction permeability by intestinal bacteria and dietary components. *J Nutr* 141 (5):769–776. doi: 10.3945/jn.110.135657.

Vendrame, S., S. Guglielmetti, P. Riso, S. Arioli, D. Klimis-Zacas, and M. Porrini. 2011. Six-week consumption of a wild blueberry powder drink increases bifidobacteria in the human gut. *J Agric Food Chem* 59 (24):12815–12820. doi: 10.1021/jf2028686.

Verberkmoes, N. C., A. L. Russell, M. Shah, A. Godzik, M. Rosenquist, J. Halfvarson, M. G. Lefsrud et al. 2009. Shotgun metaproteomics of the human distal gut microbiota. *ISME J* 3 (2):179–189. doi: 10.1038/ismej.2008.108.

Vijay-Kumar, M., J. D. Aitken, F. A. Carvalho, T. C. Cullender, S. Mwangi, S. Srinivasan, S. V. Sitaraman, R. Knight, R. E. Ley, and A. T. Gewirtz. 2010. Metabolic syndrome and altered gut microbiota in mice lacking Toll-like receptor 5. *Science* 328 (5975):228–231. doi: 10.1126/science.1179721.

Vrieze, A., E. Van Nood, F. Holleman, J. Salojarvi, R. S. Kootte, J. F. Bartelsman, G. M. Dallinga-Thie et al. 2012. Transfer of intestinal microbiota from lean donors increases insulin sensitivity in individuals with metabolic syndrome. *Gastroenterology* 143 (4):913–916.e7. doi: 10.1053/j.gastro.2012.06.031.

Walker, A. W., J. Ince, S. H. Duncan, L. M. Webster, G. Holtrop, X. Ze, D. Brown et al. 2011. Dominant and diet-responsive groups of bacteria within the human colonic microbiota. *ISME J* 5 (2):220–230. doi: 10.1038/ismej.2010.118.

Wang, Z., E. Klipfell, B. J. Bennett, R. Koeth, B. S. Levison, B. Dugar, A. E. Feldstein et al. 2011. Gut flora metabolism of phosphatidylcholine promotes cardiovascular disease. *Nature* 472 (7341):57–63. doi: 10.1038/nature09922.

Wen, L., R. E. Ley, P. Y. Volchkov, P. B. Stranges, L. Avanesyan, A. C. Stonebraker, C. Hu et al. 2008. Innate immunity and intestinal microbiota in the development of Type 1 diabetes. *Nature* 455 (7216):1109–1113. doi: 10.1038/nature07336.

Wikoff, W. R., A. T. Anfora, J. Liu, P. G. Schultz, S. A. Lesley, E. C. Peters, and G. Siuzdak. 2009. Metabolomics analysis reveals large effects of gut microflora on mammalian blood metabolites. *Proc Natl Acad Sci USA* 106 (10):3698–3703. doi: 10.1073/pnas.0812874106.

Wu, G. D., J. Chen, C. Hoffmann, K. Bittinger, Y. Y. Chen, S. A. Keilbaugh, M. Bewtra et al. 2011. Linking long-term dietary patterns with gut microbial enterotypes. *Science* 334 (6052):105–108. doi: 10.1126/science.1208344.

Yatsunenko, T., F. E. Rey, M. J. Manary, I. Trehan, M. G. Dominguez-Bello, M. Contreras, M. Magris et al. 2012. Human gut microbiome viewed across age and geography. *Nature* 486 (7402):222–227. doi: 10.1038/nature11053.

Zeisel, S. H., M. H. Mar, J. C. Howe, and J. M. Holden. 2003. Concentrations of choline-containing compounds and betaine in common foods. *J Nutr* 133 (5):1302–1307.

31 Alcohol
Associations with Blood Lipids, Insulin Sensitivity, Diabetes, Clotting, CVD, and Total Mortality

Charlotte Holst and Janne Schurmann Tolstrup

CONTENTS

ABSTRACT

Alcohol is linked to more than 200 diseases, conditions, and injuries. However, extensive scientific literature indicates that alcohol has beneficial effects on health as well. For example, the association between alcohol intake and mortality is found to be J-shaped, indicating that moderate consumption of alcohol is associated with a lower risk, when compared to heavy consumption or abstention. Also, alcohol has been linked to a lower risk of type 2 diabetes mellitus and cardiovascular disease. Several epidemiological studies suggest that alcohol's protective effects are due to favorable changes in anti-inflammatory effects, blood lipids, such as high-density lipoprotein (HDL) cholesterol and apolipoprotein A1, as well as in insulin sensitivity. Alcohol has also been associated with the level of fibrinogen, a plasma protein important for the coagulation of blood, which contributes to part of the protective effects of alcohol on cardiovascular disease by decreasing the risk of thrombosis.

INTRODUCTION

Alcohol (ethanol) drinking has been a part of the human civilization for millennia. It is used worldwide, and in most Western societies, abstainers constitute the minority. Globally, individuals above 15 years of age drink on average 6.2 L of pure alcohol per year, corresponding to 13.5 g of pure alcohol per day. However, there is wide variation in the total alcohol consumption across the world with the highest consumption levels to be found in the developed world (World Health Organization 2014).

The use of alcohol is often linked with pleasure and sociability, but it also has potentially harmful consequences. Hence, alcohol contributes substantially to the global burden of disease

(Rehm et al. 2010) and in 2012, 5.9% of all deaths were attributable to alcohol (7.6% for men and 4.0% for women) (World Health Organization 2014). Also, alcohol is identified as a causal factor for more than 200 diseases, conditions, and injuries (Rehm et al. 2010). However, in the context of public health, the effects of alcohol are not only negative. The association between alcohol intake and all-cause mortality is J-shaped, indicating that light to moderate drinkers, corresponding to consumers of approximately 1 drink a day in women and 2 drinks a day in men, have a lower mortality risk, when compared to heavy drinkers (corresponding to consumers of more than 1 drink a day for women and more than 2 drinks a day for men) and abstainers (Di Castelnuovo et al. 2006, Shekelle 2007, Wang et al. 2014). This reduced mortality risk reflects a relatively lower risk of diabetes and cardiovascular disease, in particular coronary heart disease, among light to moderate drinkers compared to abstainers (Roerecke and Rehm 2012, Ronksley et al. 2011) (the definition of a drink varies from 8 to 14 g, but often a standard drink is defined as containing 12 g of pure alcohol). However, the authors of a recent study based on more than 150,000 American men and women from a large nationally representative survey reported that among White men and women, consumption of moderate levels of alcohol on most days of the week was associated with lowest mortality risk, but the same risk reduction was not observed among Black men and women with similar drinking patterns (Jackson et al. 2015).

Alcohol is generally consumed as beer (about 2.5%–6% alc. vol.), wine (about 12% alc. vol.), or spirits (about 40% alc. vol.). It is quickly absorbed through passive diffusion, primarily in the small intestine from where it is distributed throughout the total water compartment in the body. The main part of the absorbed alcohol is oxidized in the body, and the energy liberated from this oxidation corresponds to 29 kJ/g. Additionally, small amounts (5%–10%) are lost through expired air and in the urine.

BLOOD LIPIDS

The protective effects of a low to moderate alcohol intake on cardiovascular disease are partly thought to be attributable to an increase in high-density lipoprotein (HDL) cholesterol levels. HDL acquires cholesterol from peripheral tissue and facilitates its transport to the liver for removal in the bile. HDL cholesterol is secreted as small particles by the liver and the gut and changes composition in the circulation by exchanging lipids with other lipoproteins or by absorption of cholesterol from peripheral cells. HDL particles include multiple apolipoproteins, primarily apolipoprotein A1 (Hannuksela et al. 2002).

Substantial evidence from epidemiological studies suggests that HDL cholesterol levels increase monotonically with the level of consumed alcohol (Foerster et al. 2009, Marques-Vidal et al. 2010, Tolstrup et al. 2009a). In a comprehensive high-quality meta-analysis of 44 intervention studies by Brien et al. (2011), the effect of alcohol intake on several biological markers associated with the risk of coronary heart disease was investigated. In accordance with the findings reported earlier, the pooled analysis of the effect of alcohol intake on mean HDL cholesterol levels showed a significant dose–response relationship (33 studies), and the authors reported that 30 g alcohol consumed a day was associated with an increase in HDL cholesterol levels of 3.66 mg/dL (95% confidence interval: 2.22–5.13). Similar to the effect on HDL cholesterol levels, apolipoprotein A1 also significantly increased (16 studies). These favorable changes in cardiovascular biomarkers, presumed to be induced by a low to moderate alcohol intake, provide indirect pathophysiological support for a protective effect on certain aspects of cardiovascular disease, and in particular coronary heart disease.

However, a high intake of alcohol has been associated with increased levels of nonfasting triglycerides, which, on the contrary, is associated with increased risk of cardiovascular disease. Among 9584 men and women from the Danish general population, Tolstrup et al. (2009a) found a significantly U-shaped association between alcohol intake and nonfasting triglycerides, with consumption of more than 14 drinks a week for women being associated with the highest risk. In their meta-analysis, Brien et al. (2011) also reported a significant increase in the levels of triglycerides among consumers of more than 60 g alcohol a day, but not at amounts of alcohol intake below 60 g alcohol a day.

INSULIN SENSITIVITY

A light to moderate intake of alcohol is associated with a lower risk of type 2 diabetes (Baliunas et al. 2009, Koppes et al. 2005), an effect possibly mediated by an increase in insulin sensitivity, which might work through several possible mechanisms, including modulation of the inflammatory status of several organs, modulation in intermediary metabolism, or modulation of changes in the endocrine functioning of fat tissue (Hendriks 2007). On the other hand, individuals with reduced insulin sensitivity (insulin resistance) require larger amounts of insulin, either from the pancreas or from injections of exogenous insulin, in order to maintain euglycemia.

Epidemiological studies suggest that the relationship between alcohol intake and insulin sensitivity is either an inverted U-shape, indicating that a moderate alcohol intake is associated with an increased insulin sensitivity compared to abstention or heavy drinking, or a positive linear relationship, indicating increased insulin sensitivity by increased alcohol consumption (Ting and Lautt 2006). However, results of intervention studies examining the relation between alcohol intake and insulin sensitivity are inconsistent. The inconsistency might be due to methodological issues such as differences in amount of alcohol intake, duration of alcohol consumption, and duration of the abstention period (Ting and Lautt 2006). The authors of a systematic review and meta-analysis including 14 intervention studies, which were all based on nondiabetic study populations, found that alcohol intake tends to improve insulin sensitivity among women, but not among men (Schrieks et al. 2015). Furthermore, the authors reported that alcohol intake reduces glycated hemoglobin (HbA1C, a measure of long-term glycemic control), and fasting insulin concentrations compared with abstention, but that alcohol intake does not influence fasting glucose. Increasing HbA1c levels has also been associated with a greater risk of diabetes-related complications and cardiovascular disease among individuals with type 1 diabetes in the Diabetes Control and Complications trial (DCCT) (Diabetes Control and Complications Trial (DCCT)/Epidemiology of Diabetes Interventions and Complications (EDIC) Study Research Group 2016, Stratton et al. 2006) and with mortality among individuals with type 2 diabetes in the United Kingdom Prospective Diabetes Study (UKPDS) (Orchard et al. 2015).

RESEARCH ON ALCOHOL AND MORBIDITY AND MORTALITY

As mentioned initially, the scientific literature on alcohol and diseases is extensive. However, for ethical and logistic reasons, long-term randomized trials have not been performed. The best evidence thus comes from high-quality studies consisting of prospective cohort studies. In such studies, individuals, often from samples of the general population, have completed a questionnaire about alcohol intake as well as other lifestyle habits. By correlating this information with incidence of coronary heart disease in the years following collecting of the baseline data, risk for coronary heart disease according to alcohol intake can be estimated. Since alcohol is associated with other lifestyle habits, taking other information into account when calculating such risk estimates is extremely important. For example, heavy drinkers are more often smoking daily compared with light drinkers.

Concern has also been raised about the validity of self-reported alcohol intake. Are people really able to report their alcohol intake in a questionnaire? Findings suggest that this is really so. For instance, correlating self-reported alcohol intake to biomarkers that are known to associate with alcohol such as alanine aminotransferase, gamma glutamyl transpeptidase, erythrocyte volume, and alkaline phosphatase shows that stepwise increments of the self-reported alcohol consumption consistently corresponded to stepwise increments in factors expected to correlate with amount of alcohol consumption (Tolstrup et al. 2009b). This finding speaks in favor of the validity of self-reported alcohol consumption—using a questionnaire to assess alcohol intake seems to be effective in separating individuals with different levels of alcohol intake. Further, the use of self-reported methods (questionnaire and personal interviews) has been reviewed extensively and seems to offer a reliable and valid approach to measuring alcohol consumption (Del Boca and Darkes 2003).

DIABETES

The worldwide prevalence of type 2 diabetes mellitus is rapidly rising with an increase from 382 million individuals in 2013 to an estimated 592 million by 2035 (Guariguata et al. 2014). A light to moderate alcohol intake (approximately 1 drink a day for women and 2 drinks a day for men) has been suggested to be a lifestyle factor that might reduce the risk of developing type 2 diabetes mellitus (Baliunas et al. 2009, Koppes et al. 2005), an effect that has been proposed to be explained by factors such as increased insulin sensitivity (Pietraszek et al. 2010), anti-inflammatory effects or effects on adiponectin (Hendriks 2007). A meta-analysis of 44 intervention studies has shown that alcohol intake significantly increases adiponectin levels, but does not affect inflammatory factors (Brien et al. 2011), while Schrieks et al. (2015) reported that moderate alcohol consumption decreases fasting insulin concentrations and HbA_{1c}, but does not affect insulin sensitivity or fasting glucose levels.

Most studies report a J- or U-shaped association between alcohol consumption and the risk of developing type 2 diabetes, indicating that moderate drinkers have a lower risk of diabetes compared to abstainers and heavy drinkers (Pietraszek et al. 2010). Pooling data from 38 observational studies, Knott et al. (2015) identified a peak risk reduction at 10–14 g alcohol per day with an 18% decrease in hazards, relative to lifetime and current abstainers. However, the authors reported that reductions in risk of developing diabetes at moderate levels of alcohol consumption may be restricted to women and non-Asian populations. A U-shaped relationship for both men and women was found in a systematic review and meta-analysis undertaken by Baliunas et al. (2009) who examined alcohol intake as a risk factor for type 2 diabetes based on 20 prospective cohort studies. In comparison with lifetime abstainers, men consuming 22 g alcohol per day obtained the most protective effect of alcohol intake with 13% reduced risk of type 2 diabetes. Among women, 24 g alcohol per day was associated with the lowest risk, corresponding to a 40% reduced risk of type 2 diabetes. For men consuming above 60 g alcohol per day, the intake became harmful in regard to the risk of type 2 diabetes, whereas this limit was about 50 g alcohol per day for women (Baliunas et al. 2009). The results from this meta-analysis confirm previous research findings that moderate alcohol intake is associated with a lower risk of type 2 diabetes in men and women (Carlsson et al. 2005, Howard et al. 2004, Koppes et al. 2005). Recently, however, it has been suggested that reductions in risk of developing diabetes may be overestimated in epidemiologic studies by comparing drinkers to a less healthy current nondrinking reference population (Knott et al. 2015).

CLOTTING

In the blood clotting process (coagulation), the blood forms a clot by changing state from liquid to gel. This might result in hemostasis, where the blood loss from a damaged vessel stops, followed by a repair period. Current evidence suggests that alcohol intake is associated with a decrease in levels of fibrinogen (Brien et al. 2011), a plasma protein that plays an important role in coagulation by being transformed into an insoluble network of filamentous molecules called fibrin. Alcohol's effect on fibrinogen is not well understood; however, a decrease in fibrinogen levels is assumed to impair the coagulation process and thereby contribute to part of the protective effects of a low to moderate alcohol intake on cardiovascular disease by decreasing the risk of thrombosis.

Studies investigating the effects of increased alcohol intake on coagulation and fibrinolysis have mostly been performed on components of blood, rather than on whole blood, with inconsistent results across studies (Engstrom et al. 2006). Hence, some studies have found that alcohol impairs primary hemostasis (i.e., the part of hemostasis in which the platelets immediately form a plug at the site of injury), but that the humoral coagulation factors and the fibrinolytic system are not affected (this falls under the heading of secondary hemostasis in which additional coagulation factors respond in a complex cascade to form fibrin strands, which strengthen the platelet plug) (Elmer et al. 1984, El-Sayed et al. 1999, Serebruany et al. 2000, Zoucas et al. 1982). However, an acute impairment of the fibrinolytic system by increased ethanol intake has been suggested (Olsen and Osterud 1987, van de Wiel et al. 2001). A single study has also described an increase in fibrinolytic activity in chronic alcoholics after they have stopped drinking alcohol (Delahousse et al. 2001), and other authors report that binge drinking increases platelet aggregation (de Lange et al. 2004). Finally, in whole blood, ethanol intake has been proposed to increasingly impair both coagulation and fibrinolysis (Engstrom et al. 2006).

CARDIOVASCULAR DISEASE

Cardiovascular disease involves the heart, arteries, and veins. Coronary heart disease accounts for a major fraction of cardiovascular diseases.

CORONARY HEART DISEASE

The literature on the association between alcohol and coronary heart disease is massive and the subject has been and still is much debated both in the medical literature and the popular media. The reason for the controversy is that light to moderate alcohol drinkers have consistently been found to have a lower risk of coronary heart disease compared to individuals who abstain from alcohol. This has given rise to the hypothesis that alcohol has a cardioprotective effect.

Evidence linking alcohol with a lower risk of coronary heart disease comes from a high number of prospective cohort studies, many of which are of high quality. A meta-analysis conducted in 2011 comprised data from 84 prospective cohort studies, totaling 3,159,720 study participants (Ronksley et al. 2011). This study was conducted following the Meta-analysis of Observational Studies in Epidemiology (MOOSE) guidelines and is of high quality. The overall adjusted relative risk for alcohol drinkers relative to nondrinkers was 0.71 (95% CI: 0.66–0.77) for incident coronary heart disease, that is, the risk for coronary heart disease among drinkers was 29% lower among drinkers compared with nondrinkers. In analyses exploring dose–response, categories of 2.5–14.9, 15–29.9, and 30–60 g/day were associated with similar and statistically significant reduction in the relative risk of coronary heart disease relative to nondrinkers. The highest category (>60 g/day) was associated with a relative risk of 0.76 (0.52–1.09). Hence, there is evidence of a maximal upper range of intake for the cardioprotective effect, but no indication of a higher risk among individuals who drink the most heavily. In contrast, an earlier meta-analysis of 51 studies and a total of 49,640 cases found that the association between alcohol and coronary heart disease risk is J-shaped, implying a minimum relative risk of 0.80 at 20 g/day, a significant protective effect up to 72 g/day, and a significant increased risk at intakes above 89 g/day (Corrao et al. 2000). At this level, the statistical power was limited, which may explain why the larger meta-analysis by Ronksley and colleagues reported a different association at high levels of alcohol intake (Ronksley et al. 2011). In the Ronksley meta-analysis, the lower risk for coronary heart disease among drinkers was unchanged after exclusion of former drinkers from the reference category of nondrinkers, or in practical terms, when the reference category was changed from nondrinkers to lifelong abstainers (Ronksley et al. 2011). This is an important result because it is often speculated that individuals who go from drinking to abstaining do so in response to rising health problems. For instance, an individual who has drank heavily for years may start feeling malaise due to first symptoms of an underlying disease, caused by the high alcohol intake, which in turn may lead to reduced alcohol intake. Such a mechanism would lead to an apparent high risk among the nondrinkers, resulting in a relatively lower risk among the light to moderate drinkers that would not have anything to do with a cardioprotective effect but simply reflect a systematic bias. This so-called sick quitting hypothesis has been intensely discussed and tested in the scientific literature, but the overall results do not support the idea that the lower risk among drinkers is caused by a movement of former drinkers in poor health to the category of nondrinkers.

Gender generally impacts the way alcohol is metabolized and, hence, the risks associated with levels of intake. For a given alcohol intake, blood alcohol levels will be higher for women than for men because women have smaller body sizes and relatively more body fat. This means that any dose of alcohol will imply a higher effective dose for women than for men, and women are thus generally more sensitive to any alcohol-related effect. In line with this, a meta-analysis by Corrao and coworkers indicates differences in the cardioprotective effect of alcohol between men and women (Corrao et al. 2000). In women, the risk of coronary heart disease decreased for up to 6 drinks/week, showed evidence of protective effects (i.e., the risk was significantly lower compared with nondrinkers) for up to 18 drinks/week, and reached statistical significance of harmful effects (i.e., the risk was significantly higher compared with nondrinkers), at 30 drinks/week. In comparison, the risk in men decreased for up to 15 drinks/week, showed evidence of protective effects for up to 51 drinks/week, and reached statistical significance of harmful effects at 67 drinks/week. Hence, both the protective and the detrimental effects of alcohol on coronary heart disease are achieved at lower levels in women than in men.

Drinking pattern has been defined in various ways. These include drinking with meals, on weekends only, to intoxication, to a certain blood alcohol level, more than a certain amount per session (6 drinks, 13 drinks, half a bottle of spirits, etc.), and amount and frequency combined. Evidence has emerged over the last decade that drinking pattern plays a large role in the association between alcohol and coronary heart disease. In studies of drinking pattern, the focus is not to compare nondrinkers and drinkers, but rather to compare drinkers characterized by different drinking patterns. In a meta-analysis of six epidemiological studies (n = 63,848 participants), the dose–response relation between alcohol intake and coronary heart disease risk was significantly different in irregular and regular drinkers. In irregular drinkers who consumed alcohol for two or less days per week, a J-shaped curve was obtained, with an increasing risk at intakes over 11 drinks/week—a pattern consistent with a large amount of alcohol consumed per session. In contrast, in regular drinkers who consumed alcohol on three or more days of the week, a protective effect was observed, even at high amounts of alcohol intake (Bagnardi et al. 2008). Another meta-analysis concludes that episodic and chronic heavy drinking does not provide any beneficial effect against coronary heart disease at all (Roerecke and Rehm 2014).

It has been suggested that wine drinking—especially red wine—is especially beneficial for the cardiovascular system. This idea originated from the observation that the incidence of coronary heart disease in wine-loving France was low despite a high prevalence of smoking and high fat intake, the so-called French paradox (Criqui and Ringel 1994, Renaud and de Lorgeril 1992). Biological explanations for a more cardioprotective effect of wine compared with beer and spirits include the fact that substances in wine—besides the ethanol such as resveratrol (Bonnefont-Rousselot 2016)—have been shown to inhibit platelet aggregation and reduce oxidation of low-density lipoproteins (Bonnefont-Rousselot 2016, Frankel et al. 1993, Pace-Asciak et al. 1995, 1996, Ramprasath and Jones 2010, Renaud and Ruf 1996). In support of this appealing theory, it was found in the Copenhagen City Heart Study that wine drinkers had a much lower mortality than beer and spirit drinkers (Grønbæk et al. 1995). However, there is evidence that the apparent favorable effect of wine is an artifact resulting from characteristics of the drinker rather than of the drink itself. Differences in results from country to country according to wine, beer, and spirit intake may be attributable to socioeconomic or behavioral characteristics of those individuals who drink wine, beer, and spirits. In line with this, studies have shown that wine drinkers are more likely to report optimal health, score higher in intelligence tests, and to eat a more healthy diet than beer and spirits drinkers (Barefoot et al. 2002, Johansen et al. 2006, Mortensen et al. 2001, Tjønneland et al. 1999). Further speaking against that wine should have specific effects compared to other beverage types is that randomized studies found no difference in alcohol's effect on biomarkers according to type of alcohol (Brien et al. 2011). In contrast to more popular media where wine is often praised for its health-promoting effects, the theory that wine has special cardioprotective effects only has a few advocates in the scientific literature.

ALL-CAUSE MORTALITY

The association between alcohol and all-cause mortality is J-shaped (Di Castelnuovo et al. 2006); the nadir of the J reflects a relatively lower risk of coronary heart disease among light to moderate drinkers compared with abstainers, and the ascending leg of the J is reflecting an increased risk of alcohol-related diseases such as cardiomyopathy (Guzzo-Merello et al. 2014), pancreatitis (Irving et al. 2009), liver cirrhosis, upper gastrointestinal cancers, and deaths from accidents and violence among excessive alcohol users (Rehm and Shield 2013). Since the association between alcohol and all-cause mortality thus represents the sum of numerous diseases and outcomes that are related to alcohol, the shape and nadir of the risk curve depends upon the distribution of other variables such as age, relative incidences of diseases, the prevalence of drunk-driving, and so on. Hence, the association between alcohol and all-cause mortality does not have the same causal interpretation as associations between alcohol and singular endpoints.

A J-shaped relationship between alcohol and total mortality was found in adjusted studies, in both men and women. The finding that the relative risk of mortality is ≤1 for light to moderate alcohol intake is consistently observed in population-based cohort studies (Di Castelnuovo et al. 2006). Consumption of alcohol, up to 4 drinks/day in men and 2 drinks/day in women, was inversely associated with total mortality, maximum protection being 18% in women (99% confidence interval, 13%–22%) and 17% in men (99% confidence interval, 15%–19%). Higher doses of alcohol were associated with increased mortality. The inverse association of alcohol and total mortality disappeared at doses lower in women than in men. The same was observed in subanalyses where ex-drinkers and light drinkers were excluded from the reference category.

Age plays an important role for the association between alcohol and mortality. Since the relative incidence of alcohol-related diseases and outcomes differs by age, the J-shaped association between alcohol and all-cause mortality also differs by age. The nadir (representing the alcohol intake at the lowest risk of mortality) is achieved at a lower alcohol intake in younger individuals; in a British study, the lowest mortality risk among women 16–34 years old and men 16–24 years old was observed among the nondrinkers (White et al. 2002). Hence, a beneficial effect of alcohol is not observed among the young, where alcohol is directly associated with mortality, mainly due to injuries.

Alcohol drinking pattern is also an important consideration and some studies have investigated its relationship to the risk of all-cause mortality. Results consistently imply an increased mortality risk associated with drinking large amounts of alcohol per session. Further, there is good evidence that the protective effect of alcohol on cardiovascular disease only occurs if the pattern of drinking is not binging (Rehm et al. 2010). Hence, the J-shaped association between alcohol intake and all-cause mortality depends upon the drinking pattern.

To conclude, light to moderate drinking is not associated with increased mortality risk, or at best is associated with a lower risk, except among the young. A binge-like drinking pattern may not be associated with a decrease in risk of mortality among moderate drinkers.

CONCLUSION

Alcohol is linked to a wide range of diseases, conditions, and injuries. In 2012, 5.9% of all deaths globally were attributable to alcohol. However, the association between alcohol intake and all-cause mortality is J-shaped, indicating that alcohol consumption at moderate levels is associated with a lower risk of diseases such as diabetes and cardiovascular disease among light to moderate drinkers when compared to heavy consumers or abstainers. Beneficial effects on biological markers such as HDL cholesterol, nonfasting triglycerides, and apolipoprotein A1 are proposed to provide indirect pathophysiological support for protective effects on certain aspects of cardiovascular disease, and in particular coronary heart disease among moderate alcohol drinkers. Further, a moderate intake of alcohol is associated with a decrease in levels of fibrinogen, which is assumed to impair the coagulation process, and thereby decrease the risk of thrombosis. Red wine has previously been suggested to have especially beneficial effects for the cardiovascular system; however, the scientific literature is inconclusive. Drinking patterns, on the other hand, have been found to be of importance, in that there is good evidence that no protective effects of alcohol consumption in relation to cardiovascular disease are observed among binge drinkers.

REFERENCES

Bagnardi, V., W. Zatonski, L. Scotti, C. La Vecchia, and G. Corrao. 2008. Does drinking pattern modify the effect of alcohol on the risk of coronary heart disease? Evidence from a meta-analysis. *J Epidemiol Community Health* 62 (7):615–619.

Baliunas, D. O., B. J. Taylor, H. Irving, M. Roerecke, J. Patra, S. Mohapatra, and J. Rehm. 2009. Alcohol as a risk factor for type 2 diabetes: A systematic review and meta-analysis. *Diabetes Care* 32 (11):2123–2132. doi: 10.2337/dc09-0227.

Barefoot, J. C., M. Gronbaek, J. R. Feaganes, R. S. McPherson, R. B. Williams, and I. C. Siegler. 2002. Alcoholic beverage preference, diet, and health habits in the UNC Alumni Heart Study. *Am J Clin Nutr* 76 (2):466–472.

Bonnefont-Rousselot, D. 2016. Resveratrol and cardiovascular diseases. *Nutrients* 8 (5): 250. doi: 10.3390/nu8050250.

Brien, S. E., P. E. Ronksley, B. J. Turner, K. J. Mukamal, and W. A. Ghali. 2011. Effect of alcohol consumption on biological markers associated with risk of coronary heart disease: Systematic review and meta-analysis of interventional studies. *BMJ* 342:d636. doi: 10.1136/bmj.d636.

Carlsson, S., N. Hammar, and V. Grill. 2005. Alcohol consumption and type 2 diabetes meta-analysis of epidemiological studies indicates a U-shaped relationship. *Diabetologia* 48 (6):1051–1054. doi: 10.1007/s00125-005-1768-5.

Corrao, G., L. Rubbiati, V. Bagnardi, A. Zambon, and K. Poikolainen. 2000. Alcohol and coronary heart disease: A meta-analysis. *Addiction* 95 (10):1505–1523.

Criqui, M. H. and B. L. Ringel. 1994. Does diet or alcohol explain the French paradox? *Lancet* 344 (8939–8940):1719–1723.

Delahousse, B., F. Maillot, I. Gabriel, F. Schellenberg, F. Lamisse, and Y. Gruel. 2001. Increased plasma fibrinolysis and tissue-type plasminogen activator/tissue-type plasminogen activator inhibitor ratios after ethanol withdrawal in chronic alcoholics. *Blood Coagul Fibrinolysis* 12 (1):59–66.

de Lange, D. W., M. L. Hijmering, A. Lorsheyd, W. L. Scholman, R. J. Kraaijenhagen, J. W. Akkerman, and A. van de Wiel. 2004. Rapid intake of alcohol (binge drinking) inhibits platelet adhesion to fibrinogen under flow. *Alcohol Clin Exp Res* 28 (10):1562–1568.

Del Boca, F. K. and J. Darkes. 2003. The validity of self-reports of alcohol consumption: State of the science and challenges for research. *Addiction* 98 (Suppl 2):1–12.

Diabetes Control and Complications Trial (DCCT)/Epidemiology of Diabetes Interventions and Complications (EDIC) Study Research Group. 2016. Intensive diabetes treatment and cardiovascular outcomes in type 1 diabetes: The DCCT/EDIC study 30-year follow-up. *Diabetes Care* 39 (5): 686–693. doi: 10.2337/dc15-1990.

Di Castelnuovo, A., S. Costanzo, V. Bagnardi, M. B. Donati, L. Iacoviello, and G. de Gaetano. 2006. Alcohol dosing and total mortality in men and women: An updated meta-analysis of 34 prospective studies. *Arch Inter Med* 166 (22):2437–2445. 166/22/2437 [pii].

Elmer, O., G. Goransson, and E. Zoucas. 1984. Impairment of primary hemostasis and platelet function after alcohol ingestion in man. *Haemostasis* 14 (2):223–228.

El-Sayed, M. S., P. Eastland, X. Lin, and A. M. Rattu. 1999. The effect of moderate alcohol ingestion on blood coagulation and fibrinolysis at rest and in response to exercise. *J Sports Sci* 17 (6):513–520. doi: 10.1080/026404199365821.

Engstrom, M., U. Schott, and P. Reinstrup. 2006. Ethanol impairs coagulation and fibrinolysis in whole blood: A study performed with rotational thromboelastometry. *Blood Coagul Fibrinolysis* 17 (8):661–665. doi: 10.1097/MBC.0b013e32801010b7.

Foerster, M., P. Marques-Vidal, G. Gmel, J. B. Daeppen, J. Cornuz, D. Hayoz, A. Pecoud et al. 2009. Alcohol drinking and cardiovascular risk in a population with high mean alcohol consumption. *Am J Cardiol* 103 (3):361–368. doi: 10.1016/j.amjcard.2008.09.089.

Frankel, E. N., J. Kanner, J. B. German, E. Parks, and J. E. Kinsella. 1993. Inhibition of oxidation of human low-density lipoprotein by phenolic substances in red wine. *Lancet* 341 (8843):454–457.

Grønbæk, M, A. Deis, T. I. Sorensen, U. Becker, P. Schnohr, and G. Jensen. 1995. Mortality associated with moderate intakes of wine, beer, or spirits. *BMJ* 310 (6988):1165–1169.

Guariguata, L., D. R. Whiting, I. Hambleton, J. Beagley, U. Linnenkamp, and J. E. Shaw. 2014. Global estimates of diabetes prevalence for 2013 and projections for 2035. *Diabetes Res Clin Pract* 103 (2):137–149. doi: 10.1016/j.diabres.2013.11.002.

Guzzo-Merello, G., M. Cobo-Marcos, M. Gallego-Delgado, and P. Garcia-Pavia. 2014. Alcoholic cardiomyopathy. *World J Cardiol* 6 (8):771–781. doi: 10.4330/wjc.v6.i8.771.

Hannuksela, M. L., M. K. Liisanantti, and M. J. Savolainen. 2002. Effect of alcohol on lipids and lipoproteins in relation to atherosclerosis. *Crit Rev Clin Lab Sci* 39 (3):225–283. doi: 10.1080/10408360290795529.

Hendriks, H. F. J. 2007. Moderate alcohol consumption and insulin sensitivity: Observations and possible mechanisms. *Ann Epidemiol* 17:S40–S42.

Howard, A. A., J. H. Arnsten, and M. N. Gourevitch. 2004. Effect of alcohol consumption on diabetes mellitus: A systematic review. *Ann Intern Med* 140 (3):211–219.

Irving, H. M., A. V. Samokhvalov, and J. Rehm. 2009. Alcohol as a risk factor for pancreatitis. A systematic review and meta-analysis. *JOP* 10 (4):387–392.

Jackson, C. L., F. B. Hu, I. Kawachi, D. R. Williams, K. J. Mukamal, and E. B. Rimm. 2015. Black-White differences in the relationship between alcohol drinking patterns and mortality among US men and women. *Am J Public Health* 105 (Suppl 3):S534–S543. doi: 10.2105/AJPH.2015.302615.

Johansen, D., K. Friis, E. Skovenborg, and M. Gronbaek. 2006. Food buying habits of people who buy wine or beer: Cross sectional study. *BMJ* 332 (7540):519–522.

Knott, C., S. Bell, and A. Britton. 2015. Alcohol consumption and the risk of type 2 diabetes: A systematic review and dose-response meta-analysis of more than 1.9 million individuals from 38 observational studies. *Diabetes Care* 38 (9):1804–1812. doi: 10.2337/dc15-0710.

Koppes, L. L., J. M. Dekker, H. F. Hendriks, L. M. Bouter, and R. J. Heine. 2005. Moderate alcohol consumption lowers the risk of type 2 diabetes: A meta-analysis of prospective observational studies. *Diabetes Care* 28 (3):719–725.

Marques-Vidal, P., M. Bochud, F. Paccaud, D. Waterworth, S. Bergmann, M. Preisig, G. Waeber, and P. Vollenweider. 2010. No interaction between alcohol consumption and HDL-related genes on HDL cholesterol levels. *Atherosclerosis* 211 (2):551–557. doi: 10.1016/j.atherosclerosis.2010.04.001.

Mortensen, E. L., H. H. Jensen, S. A. Sanders, and J. M. Reinisch. 2001 Better psychological functioning and higher social status may largely explain the apparent health benefits of wine: A study of wine and beer drinking in young Danish adults. *Arch Intern Med* 161 (15).1844–1848.

Olsen, H. and B. Osterud. 1987. Effects of ethanol on human blood fibrinolysis and coagulation. *Alcohol Alcohol Suppl* 1:591–594.

Orchard, T. J., D. M. Nathan, B. Zinman, P. Cleary, D. Brillon, J. Y. Backlund, and J. M. Lachin. 2015. Association between 7 years of intensive treatment of type 1 diabetes and long-term mortality. *JAMA* 313 (1):45–53. doi: 10.1001/jama.2014.16107.

Pace-Asciak, C. R., S. Hahn, E. P. Diamandis, G. Soleas, and D. M. Goldberg. 1995. The red wine phenolics trans-resveratrol and quercetin block human platelet aggregation and eicosanoid synthesis: Implications for protection against coronary heart disease. *Clin Chim Acta* 235 (2):207–219.

Pace-Asciak, C. R., O. Rounova, S. E. Hahn, E. P. Diamandis, and D. M. Goldberg. 1996. Wines and grape juices as modulators of platelet aggregation in healthy human subjects. *Clin Chim Acta* 246 (1–2):163–182.

Pietraszek, A., S. Gregersen, and K. Hermansen. 2010. Alcohol and type 2 diabetes. A review. *Nutr Metab Cardiovasc Dis* 20 (5): 366–375. doi: 10.1016/j.numecd.2010.05.001. S0939-4753(10)00106-7 [pii].

Ramprasath, V. R. and P. J. Jones. 2010. Anti-atherogenic effects of resveratrol. *Eur J Clin Nutr*.

Rehm, J., D. Baliunas, G. L. Borges, K. Graham, H. Irving, T. Kehoe, C. D. Parry et al. 2010. The relation between different dimensions of alcohol consumption and burden of disease: An overview. *Addiction* 105 (5):817–843. doi: 10.1111/j.1360-0443.2010.02899.x.

Rehm, J. and K. D. Shield. 2013. Global alcohol-attributable deaths from cancer, liver cirrhosis, and injury in 2010. *Alcohol Res* 35 (2):174–183.

Renaud, S. and M. de Lorgeril. 1992. Wine, alcohol, platelets, and the French paradox for coronary heart disease. *Lancet* 339 (8808):1523–1526.

Renaud, S. C. and J. C. Ruf. 1996. Effects of alcohol on platelet functions. *Clin Chim Acta* 246 (1–2):77–89.

Roerecke, M. and J. Rehm. 2012. The cardioprotective association of average alcohol consumption and ischaemic heart disease: A systematic review and meta-analysis. *Addiction* 107 (7):1246–1260. doi: 10.1111/j.1360-0443.2012.03780.x.

Roerecke, M. and J. Rehm. 2014. Alcohol consumption, drinking patterns, and ischemic heart disease: A narrative review of meta-analyses and a systematic review and meta-analysis of the impact of heavy drinking occasions on risk for moderate drinkers. *BMC Med* 12:182. doi: 10.1186/s12916-014-0182-6.

Ronksley, P. E., S. E. Brien, B. J. Turner, K. J. Mukamal, and W. A. Ghali. 2011. Association of alcohol consumption with selected cardiovascular disease outcomes: A systematic review and meta-analysis. *BMJ* 342:d671. doi: 10.1136/bmj.d671.

Schrieks, I. C., A. L. Heil, H. F. Hendriks, K. J. Mukamal, and J. W. Beulens. 2015. The effect of alcohol consumption on insulin sensitivity and glycemic status: A systematic review and meta-analysis of intervention studies. *Diabetes Care* 38 (4):723–732. doi: 10.2337/dc14-1556.

Serebruany, V. L., D. R. Lowry, S. Y. Fuzailov, D. J. Levine, C. M. O'Connor, and P. A. Gurbel. 2000. Moderate alcohol consumption is associated with decreased platelet activity in patients presenting with acute myocardial infarction. *J Thromb Thrombolysis* 9 (3):229–234.

Shekelle, P. 2007. Review: High alcohol intake increases mortality in both men and women. *ACP J Club* 146 (2):48. ACPJC-2007-146-2-048 [pii].

Stratton, I. M., C. A. Cull, A. I. Adler, D. R. Matthews, H. A. Neil, and R. R. Holman. 2006. Additive effects of glycaemia and blood pressure exposure on risk of complications in type 2 diabetes: A prospective observational study (UKPDS 75). *Diabetologia* 49 (8):1761–1769. doi: 10.1007/s00125-006-0297-1.

Ting, J. W. and W. W. Lautt. 2006. The effect of acute, chronic, and prenatal ethanol exposure on insulin sensitivity. *Pharmacol Ther* 111 (2):346–373. doi: 10.1016/j.pharmthera.2005.10.004.

Tjønneland, A., M. Gronbaek, C. Stripp, and K. Overvad. 1999. Wine intake and diet in a random sample of 48763 Danish men and women. *Am J Clin Nutr* 69 (1):49–54.

Tolstrup, J. S., M. Gronbaek, and B. G. Nordestgaard. 2009a. Alcohol intake, myocardial infarction, biochemical risk factors, and alcohol dehydrogenase genotypes. *Circ Cardiovasc Genet* 2 (5):507–514. doi: 10.1161/CIRCGENETICS.109.873604.

Tolstrup, J. S., M. Gronbaek, A. Tybjaerg-Hansen, and B. G. Nordestgaard. 2009b. Alcohol intake, alcohol dehydrogenase genotypes, and liver damage and disease in the Danish general population. *Am J Gastroenterol* 104 (9):2182–2188.

van de Wiel, A., P. M. van Golde, R. J. Kraaijenhagen, P. A. von dem Borne, B. N. Bouma, and H. C. Hart. 2001. Acute inhibitory effect of alcohol on fibrinolysis. *Eur J Clin Invest* 31 (2):164–170.

Wang, C., H. Xue, Q. Wang, Y. Hao, D. Li, D. Gu, and J. Huang. 2014. Effect of drinking on all-cause mortality in women compared with men: A meta-analysis. *J Womens Health* 23 (5):373–381. doi: 10.1089/jwh.2013.4414.

White, I. R., D. R. Altmann, and K. Nanchahal. 2002. Alcohol consumption and mortality: Modelling risks for men and women at different ages. *BMJ* 325 (7357):191.

World Health Organization. 2014. Global status report on alcohol and health 2014. World Health Organization, Geneva, Switzerland.

Zoucas, E., D. Bergqvist, G. Goransson, and S. Bengmark. 1982. Effect of acute ethanol intoxication on primary haemostasis, coagulation factors and fibrinolytic activity. *Eur Surg Res* 14 (1):33–44.

32 Endocrine Disrupting Chemicals, Obesogens, and the Obesity Epidemic

Raquel Chamorro-Garcia and Bruce Blumberg

CONTENTS

ABSTRACT

Obesity and related disorders have become a significant burden worldwide. In 2014, the World Health Organization estimated that ~2 billion people around the world were overweight and of those, 600 million people were obese. Obesity is also associated with metabolic conditions such as hypertension, cardiovascular disease, and type 2 diabetes. The additional health care costs for the treatment of these conditions are estimated to be $2 trillion annually worldwide. Thus, understanding the factors that are contributing to this epidemic becomes timely and important. The causal factors associated with obesity were traditionally ascribed to positive energy balance. More recently, evidence linking obesity with certain genetic mutations and the balance of bacterial flora in the gut microbiome is mounting. However, the prevalence of obesity and overweight in infants and in other animal species that live in urban areas indicates that there may be other environmental factors that should not be overlooked. In this chapter, we review the possible contributions of chemical obesogens to the obesity epidemic and other obesity comorbidities such as cardiovascular diseases. We discuss *in vitro* approaches currently used to determine the molecular mechanisms through which chemicals might act as obesogens as well as *in vivo* approaches using animal models to test the capability of obesogens to promote obesity. Since obesity is a condition with a developmental origin, we particularly focus on the effect of obesogens during *in utero* development and the potential transgenerational consequences of this exposure. We review the current knowledge about two different obesogens: the organotin tributyltin (TBT), whose mode of action is at least partly understood, and the estrogenic chemical bisphenol A (BPA), whose widespread use makes exposure ubiquitous. We provide an overview of the direction this field is following to better understand the relationship between obesogen exposure and the obesity epidemic.

ABBREVIATIONS

BADGE	Bisphenol-A diglycidyl ether
BPA	Bisphenol A
DDT	Dichloro-diphenyl-trichloroethane
DES	Diethylstilbestrol
EDCs	Endocrine disrupting chemicals
F1–F3	First–third filial generation
FABP4	Fatty acid binding protein-4
LPL	Lipoprotein lipase
MSCs	Mesenchymal stem cells
NAFLD	Nonalcoholic fatty liver disease
NHANES	National Health and Nutrition Examination Survey
NOAEL	No observable adverse effect levels
PCBs	Polychlorinated biphenyls
PPARγ	Peroxisome proliferator activated receptor gamma
RXR	Retinoid X receptor
TBT	Tributyltin
TPT	Triphenyltin
ZFP423	Zinc finger protein 423

ENDOCRINE DISRUPTING CHEMICALS (EDCs) AND HUMAN HEALTH

In the last 60 years, the number of artificial chemicals introduced in our environment has dramatically increased. There is a growing body of research in laboratory animals and in wildlife showing that some of these chemicals used in industry and agriculture may negatively modulate the endocrine system and, therefore, may be involved in the increasing rates of various health conditions worldwide (Diamanti-Kandarakis et al. 2009). As defined by the Endocrine Society, the term endocrine disrupting chemicals (EDCs) refers to "an exogenous chemical, or mixture of chemicals, that interferes with any aspect of hormone action" (Zoeller et al. 2012). This differs from the definitions promulgated by the United States Environmental Protection Agency and the World Health Organization that add the qualifier, "and causes adverse health effects in an intact organism, its progeny or subpopulations" (WHO/UNEP 2013). The difference is one of perspective and training. To an endocrinologist, disrupting the normal function of the endocrine system is *de facto*, adverse, even if the results might be subtle and take years to be manifested. To a regulatory toxicologist, adverse consequences must be demonstrated in a short time frame and subtle changes are typically ignored or deemphasized. These different perspectives have led to much debate in the scientific literature between regulators and industrial toxicologists on one side, and the endocrine/environmental health community on the other side. We adopt the view of the Endocrine Society in the review that follows.

In mammals, the endocrine system consists of a complex network of glands and organs that regulate physiological functions such as appetite, circadian rhythms, or reproduction. The classical glands include but are not limited to the pituitary gland, thyroid gland, pancreas, gonads, and adrenal glands (Melmed et al. 2011). However, other organs such as fat tissue, liver, and intestines also have endocrine functions that are critical for the maintenance of body functions, including metabolic homeostasis (Kershaw and Flier 2004). The link between the classical endocrine glands and other organs with endocrine functions lies in the fact that all of them secrete hormones into the bloodstream in response to certain environmental stimuli and will generate a physiological response in a (usually distant) target tissue. Although the endocrine system has the ability to adapt in response to hormonal fluctuations, if the changes occur at critical windows in life (e.g., embryonic development) or last for long periods (e.g., insulin resistance), they may have permanent detrimental effects on the physiological response of the individual (reviewed by Gore et al. 2015).

The mechanisms through which EDCs act are diverse and include their interactions with nuclear and nonnuclear hormone receptors (e.g., nuclear and membrane estrogen receptors, respectively), nonsteroid receptors (e.g., neurotransmitter receptors), or enzymatic pathways involved in the synthesis and metabolism of hormones (e.g., cytochrome P450s). These interactions may activate or inhibit the pathway they regulate by mimicking or blocking the action of the endogenous molecules (Gore et al. 2015).

THE OBESITY EPIDEMIC

The endocrine system may participate in the regulation of energy homeostasis by modulating neuroendocrine circuits involved in the control of appetite and satiety (Mackay et al. 2013); therefore, agents altering hormone levels and activity may contribute to the development of obesity. The most commonly accepted factors involved in obesity are generally ascribed to positive energy balance (Hall et al. 2012). Other factors such as genetics or gut microbiome may not be directly associated with lifestyle but their effects can be exacerbated by it (McAllister et al. 2009, Turnbaugh et al. 2006). However, the continuous worldwide increase in global obesity rates is difficult to explain by only considering the traditional factors associated with this health condition (Ng et al. 2014, Ogden et al. 2014). These trends open the debate regarding what are all of the major causes contributing to the obesity epidemic. More alarming is the fact that this increased tendency toward obesity has also been shown for children below 5 years of age, who, in 2013, numbered at least 40 million worldwide (Ng et al. 2014). In parallel to the trends observed in humans, it has been shown that wild and domestic animal populations living in proximity to humans have also undergone significant average increases in body weight in recent years (Klimentidis et al. 2011). An easy explanation for this trend would be to assume that animals living around industrialized areas have easy access to unhealthy food wasted by humans. Interestingly, laboratory animals that are maintained on what are thought to be tightly controlled, optimal diets are also following the same trend (Klimentidis et al. 2011), suggesting the existence of additional, unidentified factors that are contributing to the increasing rates in overweight in different species.

In 2006, our laboratory introduced the "obesogen hypothesis" that proposes the existence of a subset of EDCs that alter lipid metabolism to inappropriately stimulate an increase in the number of adipocytes or the amount of fat stored within these cells, which may contribute to disturbances in metabolic homeostasis (Janesick and Blumberg 2011). This alteration in energy balance may ultimately lead to the development of obesity.

OBESOGENS, ADIPOGENESIS, AND OBESITY

Since the introduction of the obesogen hypothesis, the effects of a growing list of obesogens have been characterized using both *in vitro* and *in vivo* approaches.

Although not all obesogens act through the same pathways, a subset of obesogens act through the peroxisome proliferator activated receptor gamma (PPARγ), which is considered to be the "master regulator of adipogenesis" (Tontonoz and Spiegelman 2008). PPARγ is highly expressed in fat tissue and functions as an obligate heterodimer with the retinoid X receptor (RXR) (Kliewer et al. 1992). Upon ligand binding, this heterodimer transcriptionally activates downstream genes involved in lipid synthesis and metabolism such as fatty acid binding protein-4 (FABP4), lipoprotein lipase (LPL), and leptin.

IN VITRO EXPOSURE TO OBESOGENS AND ADIPOGENESIS

The organotins tributyltin (TBT) and triphenyltin (TPT) were the first obesogens described and they both activate PPARγ (Grun et al. 2006, Janesick et al. 2016, Kanayama et al. 2005). More recently, the pesticides triflumizole, quinoxyfen, spirodiclofen, and zoxamide have been shown to activate PPARγ and to increase lipid accumulation using *in vitro* models such as the murine pre-adipocyte 3T3-L1 cell line and mouse and human mesenchymal stem cells (MSCs) (Janesick et al. 2016, Li et al. 2012). In the same study, we found that the fungicide fludioxonil is not a PPARγ activator, but it activates RXR and increases lipid accumulation in 3T3-L1 cells and MSCs (Janesick et al. 2016). MSCs are able to differentiate into a variety of cell types, including adipocytes, osteoblasts, chondrocytes, and myocytes, depending upon the stimuli they receive (Cristancho and Lazar 2011). By exposing 3T3-L1 cells or MSCs to obesogen candidates in the presence of an adipogenic cocktail, it is possible to assess the adipogenic capabilities of individual chemicals by analyzing lipid accumulation and mRNA expression levels of adipogenic marker genes such as those described earlier (Chamorro-Garcia et al. 2012, Grun et al. 2006, Janesick et al. 2016, Kirchner et al. 2010). There is a subset of candidate obesogens whose mechanisms of action remain unknown. One example is bisphenol-A diglycidyl ether (BADGE), which is used in the manufacture of epoxy resins, paints, and as a coating in food cans. BADGE induces lipid accumulation in 3T3-L1 pre-adipocytes and MSCs, but the inhibition of PPARγ with the specific antagonists T0070907 or GW9663 does not interfere with BADGE-induced accumulation of lipids (Chamorro-Garcia et al. 2012). Other potential obesogens whose mechanisms of action remain unknown are imazalil, tebupirimfos, florchlorfenuron, flusilazole, acetamiprid, and pymetrozine, which are not PPARγ or RXR activators but induce adipogenesis in 3T3-L1 cells (Janesick et al. 2016). These studies indicate that further analyses are needed to more fully understand the mechanisms through which obesogens act.

In Vivo Exposure to Obesogens during Adulthood and Obesity

Epidemiological studies showed a positive association between the presence of some EDCs in blood and an increase in fat storage. Multiple independent epidemiological studies have linked high plasma levels of polychlorinated biphenyls (PCBs) with obesity (Dhooge et al. 2010, Donat-Vargas et al. 2014, Lee et al. 2011). Cross-sectional analyses showed that increased urine levels of phenols (e.g., bisphenol A; BPA), whose use is widespread in industry, and phthalates, used as plasticizers and in personal care products, are associated with an increase in fat content in the adult human (Carwile and Michels 2011, Song et al. 2014). In many cases, the increase in fat storage is accompanied by other metabolic conditions such as insulin resistance, type 2 diabetes, and cardiovascular disease (James-Todd et al. 2012, Lind, Zethelius, and Lind 2012, Shankar and Teppala 2011).

Likewise, studies performed using laboratory animals have also demonstrated a positive association between obesogen exposure during adolescence and adulthood, and obesity and related diseases. Adult exposure to PCB-153 in mice led to increased fat storage, liver steatosis, and abnormal levels of adipokines in plasma when animals were fed with a high-fat diet (Wahlang et al. 2013). Mice chronically exposed to a mixture of different PCB congeners and dichloro-diphenyl-trichloroethane (DDT) developed insulin resistance, glucose intolerance, and visceral adiposity (Ibrahim et al. 2011). Adult mice exposed to BPA had a significant increase in body weight, hyperglycemia, and insulin resistance (Alonso-Magdalena et al. 2006, Marmugi et al. 2014). Female mice exposed to phthalates showed increased body weight, visceral adiposity, and food intake (Schmidt et al. 2012). Juvenile exposure to organotins such as TBT induces fat storage, fatty liver, and insulin resistance in rodents (Penza et al. 2011, Zuo et al. 2011). Taken together, both human epidemiological studies and studies performed in animal models show the positive association between the presence of obesogens in the body in adult individuals and an increase in fat storage and obesity.

DEVELOPMENTAL ORIGINS OF OBESITY

Energy Balance during Development

There is a growing body of evidence showing that obesity during adulthood may have a developmental origin (Janesick and Blumberg 2011).The developing organism possesses plasticity to adapt to environmental stimuli and this plasticity may be detrimental for the organism later in life, since it may promote the development of a variety of health conditions. Thus, environmental insults such as under- or overnutrition or the presence of artificial chemicals during embryogenesis may lead to detrimental effects later in life.

Epidemiological studies found a correlation between maternal overweight during pregnancy and increased body weight at birth (Surkan et al. 2004). Experiments performed in rodents showed that high-fat diets during pregnancy and lactation lead to obesity, hypertension, and insulin resistance in the offspring even if they were maintained on a normal diet after weaning (Armitage et al. 2005, Khan et al. 2003, Taylor et al. 2005). Experiments performed with cross-fostering approaches between control dams and dams exposed to a high-fat diet showed that both *in utero* and lactational exposure to a high-fat diet are critical factors in the development of metabolic syndrome later in life and that these effects can be transmitted to subsequent generations (Hoile et al. 2015, Khan et al. 2005). More strikingly, rats exposed to cafeteria-style "junk-food" during *in utero* development showed a biased preference toward palatable high-fat diets compared to animals exposed to control rat diet, which indicates that high-fat and high-sugar exposure during critical windows of development cause an alteration on the central reward pathways that will condition diet choices and food intake later in life (Ong and Muhlhausler 2011).

Paradoxically, as reviewed in Chapter 28 of this book, undernutrition during critical windows of development also leads to obesity later in life. Epidemiological observations performed in men and women born during the "Dutch famine winter" at the end of World War II in the Netherlands showed that malnutrition during early stages of development led to increased body mass index and waist circumference in women but not men later in life (Ravelli et al. 1999). Analyses of the same cohort showed that, when the famine period occurred at later stages of development, both men and women had lower glucose tolerance, suggesting that undernutrition during development led to permanent changes in metabolic homeostasis (Ravelli et al. 1998). In line with these findings, studies of a British cohort in Hertfordshire showed that poor nutrition during perinatal development was positively associated with cardiovascular disease and type 2 diabetes during adulthood (Hales and Barker 1992). These observations led David Barker to propose the "Barker hypothesis," also known as the "thrifty phenotype hypothesis." The fundamental tenet of this hypothesis is that nutritional deprivation during a very energy-demanding period of life, such as *in utero* development, will lead to metabolic adaptations in the fetus that favor energy storage; thus, the metabolism "learns" to be thrifty with calories. This enables some degree of adaptation to poor nutrition throughout life. However, if instead this "thrifty phenotype" individual encounters adequate or excess nutrition, the metabolic adaptations made during fetal life will lead to inappropriate storage of ingested calories, altering glucose homeostasis and ultimately leading to obesity and related disorders (Hales and Barker 2001). Thus, the "thrifty adaptations" become detrimental only when the postnatal environment differs from the prenatal setting.

Obesogens and the Developmental Origins of Obesity

The "obesogen hypothesis" introduces another level of complexity to the developmental origins of obesity. There is a growing body of research showing that exposure to obesogens during critical windows of development such as *in utero* development and during lactation lead to obesity later in life (Heindel, Newbold, and Schug 2015).

The organotin TBT belongs to the group of obesogens whose *in utero* effect has been more deeply characterized (Janesick, Shioda, and Blumberg 2014). In rodents, TBT causes masculinization of females and infertility in mollusks and fish (Bryan et al. 1986, McAllister and Kime 2003) as well as toxicity in liver, nervous system, and immune system (Boyer 1989). More recently, it was shown that exposure to low doses of TBT during tadpole stages in *Xenopus laevis* and larvae stages in *Danio rerio* (zebrafish) increases fat storage (Grun et al. 2006, Tingaud-Sequeira, Ouadah, and Babin 2011). Human studies have shown that the presence of TBT in placenta is positively associated with weight gain in the first months of life (Rantakokko et al. 2014). Experiments performed in mice demonstrated that prenatal exposure to TBT increases adiposity, nonalcoholic fatty liver disease (NAFLD), and the reprogramming of the MSCs compartment favoring their differentiation into adipocytes at the expense of the bone in the offspring (Chamorro-Garcia et al. 2013, Grun and Blumberg 2006, Kirchner et al. 2010).

There are other EDCs with shorter half-lives that are in widespread industrial use, such as BPA. BPA is used in the manufacture of polycarbonate plastics, epoxy resins, and thermal papers; therefore, it can be found in a variety of products the public encounters on a daily basis, including plastic containers, food packaging, thermal papers, medical devices, dental sealants, and so on (Vandenberg et al. 2010). Despite its ephemeral existence, the widespread use of BPA makes it ubiquitously present. BPA has been detected in human samples including urine, serum, breast milk, and fat and is associated with increased body weight, breast and prostate cancer, and alterations in the reproductive system (reviewed by Rubin 2011). Data from the National Health and Nutrition Examination Survey (NHANES), a cross-sectional study with over 2500 participants ≥ 6 years of age, revealed that BPA was present in 92.6% of the samples at an average level in urine of 2.6 ng/mL (Calafat et al. 2008). Interestingly, participants between 6 and 11 years of age showed an average BPA level of 4.5 ng/mL. These data raise concern about the impact of obesogens during childhood, when metabolic setpoints are being programmed and are, therefore, more susceptible to environmental insults. Although BPA is an estrogen, its mechanism of action in promoting obesity is not known but it is notable that perinatal estrogen exposure can predispose animals to obesity later in life (Newbold et al. 2007). Experiments performed using animal models showed that *in utero* exposure to low doses of BPA leads to increased body weight and abdominal fat and the disruption of lipid homeostasis later in life (Alonso-Magdalena et al. 2010, Howdeshell et al. 1999, Somm et al. 2009). Similar results regarding increased body weight during adulthood were found in rodents exposed to the estrogen diethylstilbestrol (DES) during *in utero* development (Newbold et al. 2004).

Obesogens and the Transgenerational Transmission of Obesity

Recent studies performed in animal models have revealed that ancestral perinatal exposure to obesogens leads to obesity in subsequent generations (Chamorro-Garcia et al. 2013, Manikkam et al. 2013). The transgenerational transmission of diseases implies that the germ line genome has been modified in nucleotide sequence (mutations) in epigenomic marks (epimutations) or both. As discussed more extensively in Chapter 28, the mechanisms involved in the modification of the epigenomic profile include covalent modifications of the DNA (e.g., methylation and hydroxymethylation of cytosines) and histones (e.g., methylation of lysines), and the presence of noncoding RNAs (Xin, Susiarjo, and Bartolomei 2015). By modifying the epigenomic profile of the cell, it is possible to modulate the functional output of the information stored in the genome sequence. During early stages of the development, the primordial germ cells go through a genome-wide demethylation/remethylation cycle before implantation. At this stage, the genome is extremely sensitive to the exposure of agents that may permanently change the original methylation pattern (Heard and Martienssen 2014). Thus, any changes in the epigenomic profile in the germ line at these developmental stages and the biological traits associated with them may be transmitted to subsequent generations, although, the precise mechanisms remain to be elucidated.

Experiments performed in our laboratory showed that *in utero* exposure to environmentally relevant doses of TBT (5.42, 54.2, and 542 nM) of the first generation (F1) led to the development of obesity in subsequent generations with a sexually dimorphic penetrance (Chamorro-Garcia et al. 2013). F1 female mice exposed to TBT exhibited increased adiposity in a dose-dependent manner, whereas in F1 male mice this effect was not as strong as in subsequent generations. Both males and females developed nonalcoholic fatty liver with the phenotype stronger in females. F2 females and F2 and F3 males derived from TBT-exposed animals showed a dramatic increase in adiposity, whereas F3 females did not show significant changes. Gene expression analyses in the MSCs showed a significant increase in the gene expression levels of adipogenic markers such as ZFP423, FABP4, LPL, and PPARγ in both genders. These effects were stronger in the F3 males than in previous generations, suggesting the existence of an epigenetic mechanism involved in the regulation of this phenotype (Chamorro-Garcia and Blumberg 2014, Chamorro-Garcia et al. 2013). It is worth noting that two of the TBT concentrations used in this experiment (5.42 and 54.2 nM) were lower than the established no observable adverse effect levels (NOAEL) (Vos et al. 1990). Other obesogens involved in the transgenerational inheritance of obesity include BPA, phthalates, hydrocarbons, and DDT. In all cases, the exposure to obesogens led to sperm epimutations in regions associated to obesity (Manikkam et al. 2013, Skinner et al. 2013, Tracey et al. 2013).

A recent study showed that surgery-induced weight loss in obese men led to a significant change in the DNA methylation profile of genes involved in central control of appetite in the sperm (Donkin et al. 2016). Studies performed in a different cohort of obese men showed that noncoding RNA expression levels and DNA methylation profiles in sperm were significantly different when compared to the profiles in lean men (Donkin et al. 2016). These data indicate that the epigenome of the male germ line is susceptible to environmental changes.

OBESOGENS AND CARDIOVASCULAR DISEASE

Obesity, NAFLD, and type 2 diabetes are just a few examples of risk factors for future cardiovascular diseases such as heart failure, coronary heart disease, or atrial fibrillation (Mozaffarian et al. 2016). Therefore, it should come as no surprise that factors that are contributing to obesity, NAFLD, and type 2 diabetes also contribute to cardiovascular comorbidities.

In the last two decades, there is increasing evidence showing an association between obesogen exposure and cardiovascular disease. Independent cross-sectional and longitudinal epidemiological studies revealed that urine BPA levels in adults is associated with an increasing risk for future coronary artery disease and high blood pressure (Bae et al. 2012, Lang et al. 2008, Melzer et al. 2010, 2012). *Ex vivo* analyses of rat cardiomyocytes showed that exposure to low doses of BPA alters electrical conduction causing arrhythmias in females; moreover, this effect was exacerbated when other conditions such as stress and previous heart damage were also present (Posnack et al. 2014, Yan et al. 2011, 2013). Two independent experiments showed that chronic BPA exposure in adult mice caused increased blood pressure and atherosclerosis (Saura et al. 2014, Sui et al. 2014), whereas perinatal chronic exposure to low doses of BPA modified the epigenetic profile of cardiac cells, leading to remodeling of cardiac structure and function (Patel et al. 2013). Although the mechanism underlying this phenotype remains unclear, alterations in the activity of the estrogen receptor and the pregnane X receptor are two hypotheses under investigation (Sui et al. 2014, Yan et al. 2013).

As mentioned earlier, our lab showed that *in utero* exposure to TBT causes increased fat storage and NAFLD in mice and that this phenotype is transmitted to future generations (Chamorro-Garcia et al. 2013). It has been reported that TBT alters cardiac function by increasing coronary perfusion pressure and cardiac hypertrophy in adult Wistar rats exposed to TBT for 15 days via gavage feeding (dos Santos et al. 2012). There is a notable lack of epidemiological studies associating TBT with cardiovascular disease, but these experiments performed in rodents suggest the potential contribution of TBT to the development of these health conditions.

Other EDCs that have been shown to alter cardiac function are dioxins, whose presence in blood in humans has been associated with artery disease when combined with other risk factors such as obesity (Min et al. 2011).

CONCLUSION AND FUTURE DIRECTIONS

Evidence is mounting regarding the existence of factors relevant to the obesity epidemic other than nutrition and exercise, which have been typically considered to be the most important factors in obesity. However, understanding the potential interactions between nutrition and other factors such as stress, exercise, genetics, and so on has become an important challenge.

The obesogen hypothesis introduces another level of complexity to the current understanding of obesity and related disorders and offers a different perspective. One key point is that there is now abundant evidence showing that obesogens are ubiquitously present in industrialized societies, occurring in water pipes, personal care products, food packaging, and agriculture. As a result, it makes sense to devote resources to understanding how obesogens act in biological systems in order that their effects on human, animal, and wildlife health be better assessed.

Experiments performed using *in vitro* models such as cell lines and primary cultures are contributing to the detection of new EDCs with obesogenic properties. Although such experiments have obvious limitations, they can contribute to a deeper, mechanistic understanding of how obesogens act. *In vivo* experiments performed in animal models will be required to definitively prove that chemicals are *bona fide* obesogens. Moreover, transgenerational studies in animal models are changing the genetic determinism dogma that the inheritance of certain phenotypes results solely from genomic mutations by providing evidence that epigenomic changes in DNA and histone methylation also play an important role in phenotypic inheritance. These new approaches demonstrate that, despite efforts to reduce or ban the use of certain artificial chemicals, the effects of such chemicals could last for generations not only as residues in nature but even more alarming, in our epigenome.

Further studies are needed to determine what interactions exist between obesogens and traditional factors involved in obesity such as diet. We currently know very little about the effects of exercise in fat mobilization and thermogenesis after obesogen exposure, the interactions of obesogens with diet composition, or the potential effects of obesogens on the balance of bacterial strains present in the gut microbiome.

Obesity is a multifactorial disease that is difficult to treat once it has developed. Obesity affects a significant fraction of the world population irrespective of the country, average income, age, gender, or lifestyle (Ng et al. 2014). The prevalence of other conditions associated with obesity (e.g., type 2 diabetes, hypertension, and cardiovascular disease) continues to increase in parallel with the obesity epidemic. Since obesity is largely refractory to treatment, new approaches are needed to prevent obesity from developing. The obesogen hypothesis offers a new perspective for understanding this global problem and proposes that the reduction of chemical exposure during critical windows of development may offer an additional approach for prevention.

REFERENCES

Alonso-Magdalena, P., S. Morimoto, C. Ripoll, E. Fuentes, and A. Nadal. 2006. The estrogenic effect of bisphenol A disrupts pancreatic beta-cell function in vivo and induces insulin resistance. *Environ Health Perspect* 114(1):106–112.

Alonso-Magdalena, P., E. Vieira, S. Soriano, L. Menes, D. Burks, I. Quesada, and A. Nadal. 2010. Bisphenol A exposure during pregnancy disrupts glucose homeostasis in mothers and adult male offspring. *Environ Health Perspect* 118(9):1243–1250. doi: 10.1289/ehp.1001993.

Armitage, J. A., L. Lakasing, P. D. Taylor, A. A. Balachandran, R. I. Jensen, V. Dekou, N. Ashton, J. R. Nyengaard, and L. Poston. 2005. Developmental programming of aortic and renal structure in offspring of rats fed fat-rich diets in pregnancy. *J Physiol* 565(Pt 1):171–184. doi: 10.1113/jphysiol.2005.084947.

Bae, S., J. H. Kim, Y. H. Lim, H. Y. Park, and Y. C. Hong. 2012. Associations of bisphenol A exposure with heart rate variability and blood pressure. *Hypertension* 60(3):786–793. doi: 10.1161/HYPERTENSIONAHA.112.197715.

Boyer, I. J. 1989. Toxicity of dibutyltin, tributyltin and other organotin compounds to humans and to experimental animals. *Toxicology* 55(3):253–298.

Bryan, G. W., P. E. Gibbs, L. G. Hummerstone, and G. R. Burt. 1986. The decline of gastropod *Nucella lapillus* around south-west England: Evidence for the effect of tributyltin from antifouling paints. *J Mar Biol Assoc UK* 66(03):611–640.

Calafat, A. M., X. Ye, L. Y. Wong, J. A. Reidy, and L. L. Needham. 2008. Exposure of the U.S. population to bisphenol A and 4-tertiary-octylphenol: 2003–2004. *Environ Health Perspect* 116(1):39–44. doi: 10.1289/ehp.10753.

Carwile, J. L., and K. B. Michels. 2011. Urinary bisphenol A and obesity: NHANES 2003–2006. *Environ Res* 111(6):825–830. doi: 10.1016/j.envres.2011.05.014.

Chamorro-Garcia, R., and B. Blumberg. 2014. Transgenerational effects of obesogens and the obesity epidemic. *Curr Opin Pharmacol* 19:153–158. doi: 10.1016/j.coph.2014.10.010.

Chamorro-Garcia, R., S. Kirchner, X. Li, A. Janesick, S. C. Casey, C. Chow, and B. Blumberg. 2012. Bisphenol A diglycidyl ether induces adipogenic differentiation of multipotent stromal stem cells through a peroxisome proliferator-activated receptor gamma-independent mechanism. *Environ Health Perspect* 120(7):984–989. doi: 10.1289/ehp.1205063.

Chamorro-Garcia, R., M. Sahu, R. J. Abbey, J. Laude, N. Pham, and B. Blumberg. 2013. Transgenerational inheritance of increased fat depot size, stem cell reprogramming, and hepatic steatosis elicited by prenatal exposure to the obesogen tributyltin in mice. *Environ Health Perspect* 121(3):359–366. doi: 10.1289/ehp.1205701.

Cristancho, A. G., and M. A. Lazar. 2011. Forming functional fat: A growing understanding of adipocyte differentiation. *Nat Rev Mol Cell Biol* 12(11):722–734. doi: 10.1038/nrm3198, nrm3198 [pii].

Dhooge, W., E. Den Hond, G. Koppen, L. Bruckers, V. Nelen, E. Van De Mieroop, M. Bilau et al. 2010. Internal exposure to pollutants and body size in Flemish adolescents and adults: Associations and dose-response relationships. *Environ Int* 36(4):330–337. doi: 10.1016/j.envint.2010.01.005.

Diamanti-Kandarakis, E., J. P. Bourguignon, L. C. Giudice, R. Hauser, G. S. Prins, A. M. Soto, R. T. Zoeller, and A. C. Gore. 2009. Endocrine-disrupting chemicals: An Endocrine Society scientific statement. *Endocr Rev* 30(4):293–342. doi: 10.1210/er.2009-0002, 30/4/293 [pii].

Donat-Vargas, C., A. Gea, C. Sayon-Orea, S. Carlos, M. A. Martinez-Gonzalez, and M. Bes-Rastrollo. 2014. Association between dietary intakes of PCBs and the risk of obesity: The SUN project. *J Epidemiol Community Health* 68(9):834–841. doi: 10.1136/jech-2013-203752.

Donkin, I., S. Versteyhe, L. R. Ingerslev, K. Qian, M. Mechta, L. Nordkap, B. Mortensen et al. 2016. Obesity and bariatric surgery drive epigenetic variation of spermatozoa in humans. *Cell Metab* 23(2):369–378. doi: 10.1016/j.cmet.2015.11.004.

dos Santos, R. L., P. L. Podratz, G. C. Sena, V. S. Filho, P. F. Lopes, W. L. Goncalves, L. M. Alves et al. 2012. Tributyltin impairs the coronary vasodilation induced by 17beta-estradiol in isolated rat heart. *J Toxicol Environ Health A* 75(16–17):948–959. doi: 10.1080/15287394.2012.695231.

Gore, A. C., V. A. Chappell, S. E. Fenton, J. A. Flaws, A. Nadal, G. S. Prins, J. Toppari, and R. T. Zoeller. 2015. EDC-2: The Endocrine Society's second scientific statement on endocrine-disrupting chemicals. *Endocr Rev* 36(6):E1–E150. doi: 10.1210/er.2015-1010.

Grun, F., and B. Blumberg. 2006. Environmental obesogens: Organotins and endocrine disruption via nuclear receptor signaling. *Endocrinology* 147(6 Suppl):S50–S55. doi: 10.1210/en.2005-1129, en.2005-1129 [pii].

Grun, F., H. Watanabe, Z. Zamanian, L. Maeda, K. Arima, R. Cubacha, D. M. Gardiner, J. Kanno, T. Iguchi, and B. Blumberg. 2006. Endocrine-disrupting organotin compounds are potent inducers of adipogenesis in vertebrates. *Mol Endocrinol* 20(9):2141–2155. doi: 10.1210/me.2005-0367, me.2005-0367 [pii].

Hales, C. N., and D. J. Barker. 1992. Type 2 (non-insulin-dependent) diabetes mellitus: The thrifty phenotype hypothesis. *Diabetologia* 35(7):595–601.

Hales, C. N., and D. J. Barker. 2001. The thrifty phenotype hypothesis. *Br Med Bull* 60:5–20.

Hall, K. D., S. B. Heymsfield, J. W. Kemnitz, S. Klein, D. A. Schoeller, and J. R. Speakman. 2012. Energy balance and its components: Implications for body weight regulation. *Am J Clin Nutr* 95(4):989–994. doi: 10.3945/ajcn.112.036350, 95/4/989 [pii].

Heard, E., and R. A. Martienssen. 2014. Transgenerational epigenetic inheritance: Myths and mechanisms. *Cell* 157(1):95–109. doi: 10.1016/j.cell.2014.02.045.

Heindel, J. J., R. Newbold, and T. T. Schug. 2015. Endocrine disruptors and obesity. *Nat Rev Endocrinol.* 11:653–661. doi: 10.1038/nrendo.2015.163.

Hoile, S. P., L. M. Grenfell, M. A. Hanson, K. A. Lillycrop, and G. C. Burdge. 2015. Fat and carbohydrate intake over three generations modify growth, metabolism and cardiovascular phenotype in female mice in an age-related manner. *PLoS One* 10(8):e0134664. doi: 10.1371/journal.pone.0134664.

Howdeshell, K. L., A. K. Hotchkiss, K. A. Thayer, J. G. Vandenbergh, and F. S. Vom Saal. 1999. Exposure to bisphenol A advances puberty. *Nature* 401(6755):763–764. doi: 10.1038/44517.

Ibrahim, M. M., E. Fjaere, E. J. Lock, D. Naville, H. Amlund, E. Meugnier, B. Le Magueresse Battistoni et al. 2011. Chronic consumption of farmed salmon containing persistent organic pollutants causes insulin resistance and obesity in mice. *PLoS One* 6(9):e25170. doi: 10.1371/journal.pone.0025170.

James-Todd, T., R. Stahlhut, J. D. Meeker, S. G. Powell, R. Hauser, T. Huang, and J. Rich-Edwards. 2012. Urinary phthalate metabolite concentrations and diabetes among women in the National Health and Nutrition Examination Survey (NHANES) 2001–2008. *Environ Health Perspect* 120(9):1307–1313. doi: 10.1289/ehp.1104717.

Janesick, A., and B. Blumberg. 2011. Endocrine disrupting chemicals and the developmental programming of adipogenesis and obesity. *Birth Defects Res C Embryo Today* 93(1):34–50. doi: 10.1002/bdrc.20197.

Janesick, A. S., G. Dimastrogiovanni, L. Vanek, C. Boulos, R. Chamorro-Garcia, and B. Blumberg. 2016. On the utility of ToxCast and ToxPi as methods for identifying new obesogens. *Environ Health Perspect* 124(8):1214–1226. doi: 10.1289/ehp.1510352 ehp.1510352 [pii].

Janesick, A. S., T. Shioda, and B. Blumberg. 2014. Transgenerational inheritance of prenatal obesogen exposure. *Mol Cell Endocrinol* 398(1–2):31–35. doi: 10.1016/j.mce.2014.09.002.

Kanayama, T., N. Kobayashi, S. Mamiya, T. Nakanishi, and J. Nishikawa. 2005. Organotin compounds promote adipocyte differentiation as agonists of the peroxisome proliferator-activated receptor gamma/retinoid X receptor pathway. *Mol Pharmacol* 67(3):766–774. doi: 10.1124/mol.104.008409, mol.104.008409 [pii].

Kershaw, E. E., and J. S. Flier. 2004. Adipose tissue as an endocrine organ. *J Clin Endocrinol Metab* 89(6):2548–2556. doi: 10.1210/jc.2004-0395.

Khan, I. Y., V. Dekou, G. Douglas, R. Jensen, M. A. Hanson, L. Poston, and P. D. Taylor. 2005. A high-fat diet during rat pregnancy or suckling induces cardiovascular dysfunction in adult offspring. *Am J Physiol Regul Integr Comp Physiol* 288(1):R127–R133. doi: 10.1152/ajpregu.00354.2004.

Khan, I. Y., P. D. Taylor, V. Dekou, P. T. Seed, L. Lakasing, D. Graham, A. F. Dominiczak, M. A. Hanson, and L. Poston. 2003. Gender-linked hypertension in offspring of lard-fed pregnant rats. *Hypertension* 41(1):168–175.

Kirchner, S., T. Kieu, C. Chow, S. Casey, and B. Blumberg. 2010. Prenatal exposure to the environmental obesogen tributyltin predisposes multipotent stem cells to become adipocytes. *Mol Endocrinol* 24(3):526–539. doi: 10.1210/me.2009-0261, me.2009-0261 [pii].

Kliewer, S. A., K. Umesono, D. J. Mangelsdorf, and R. M. Evans. 1992. Retinoid X receptor interacts with nuclear receptors in retinoic acid, thyroid hormone and vitamin D3 signalling. *Nature* 355(6359):446–449. doi: 10.1038/355446a0.

Klimentidis, Y. C., T. M. Beasley, H. Y. Lin, G. Murati, G. E. Glass, M. Guyton, W. Newton et al. 2011. Canaries in the coal mine: A cross-species analysis of the plurality of obesity epidemics. *Proc Biol Sci* 278(1712):1626–1632. doi: 10.1098/rspb.2010.1890, rspb.2010.1890 [pii].

Lang, I. A., T. S. Galloway, A. Scarlett, W. E. Henley, M. Depledge, R. B. Wallace, and D. Melzer. 2008. Association of urinary bisphenol A concentration with medical disorders and laboratory abnormalities in adults. *JAMA* 300(11):1303–1310. doi: 10.1001/jama.300.11.1303.

Lee, D. H., P. M. Lind, D. R. Jacobs, Jr., S. Salihovic, B. van Bavel, and L. Lind. 2011. Polychlorinated biphenyls and organochlorine pesticides in plasma predict development of type 2 diabetes in the elderly: The prospective investigation of the vasculature in Uppsala Seniors (PIVUS) study. *Diabetes Care* 34(8):1778–1784. doi: 10.2337/dc10-2116.

Li, X., H. T. Pham, A. S. Janesick, and B. Blumberg. 2012. Triflumizole is an obesogen in mice that acts through peroxisome proliferator activated receptor gamma (PPARgamma). *Environ Health Perspect* 120(12):1720–1726. doi: 10.1289/ehp.1205383.

Lind, P. M., B. Zethelius, and L. Lind. 2012. Circulating levels of phthalate metabolites are associated with prevalent diabetes in the elderly. *Diabetes Care* 35(7):1519–1524. doi: 10.2337/dc11-2396.

Mackay, H., Z. R. Patterson, R. Khazall, S. Patel, D. Tsirlin, and A. Abizaid. 2013. Organizational effects of perinatal exposure to bisphenol-A and diethylstilbestrol on arcuate nucleus circuitry controlling food intake and energy expenditure in male and female CD-1 mice. *Endocrinology* 154(4):1465–1475. doi: 10.1210/en.2012-2044.

Manikkam, M., R. Tracey, C. Guerrero-Bosagna, and M. K. Skinner. 2013. Plastics derived endocrine disruptors (BPA, DEHP and DBP) induce epigenetic transgenerational inheritance of obesity, reproductive disease and sperm epimutations. *PLoS One* 8(1):e55387. doi: 10.1371/journal.pone.0055387, PONE-D-12-15587 [pii].

Marmugi, A., F. Lasserre, D. Beuzelin, S. Ducheix, L. Huc, A. Polizzi, M. Chetivaux et al. 2014. Adverse effects of long-term exposure to bisphenol A during adulthood leading to hyperglycaemia and hypercholesterolemia in mice. *Toxicology* 325:133–143. doi: 10.1016/j.tox.2014.08.006.

McAllister, B. G., and D. E. Kime. 2003. Early life exposure to environmental levels of the aromatase inhibitor tributyltin causes masculinisation and irreversible sperm damage in zebrafish (Danio rerio). *Aquat Toxicol* 65(3):309–316. doi: S0166445X03001541 [pii].

McAllister, E. J., N. V. Dhurandhar, S. W. Keith, L. J. Aronne, J. Barger, M. Baskin, R. M. Benca et al. 2009. Ten putative contributors to the obesity epidemic. *Crit Rev Food Sci Nutr* 49(10):868–913. doi: 10.1080/10408390903372599.

Melmed, S., K.S. Polonsky, P. R. Larsen, and H. M. Kronenberg. 2011. *Williams Textbook of Endocrinology*. Philadelphia, PA: Elsevier/Saunders.

Melzer, D., N. J. Osborne, W. E. Henley, R. Cipelli, A. Young, C. Money, P. McCormack et al. 2012. Urinary bisphenol A concentration and risk of future coronary artery disease in apparently healthy men and women. *Circulation* 125(12):1482–1490. doi: 10.1161/CIRCULATIONAHA.111.069153.

Melzer, D., N. E. Rice, C. Lewis, W. E. Henley, and T. S. Galloway. 2010. Association of urinary bisphenol a concentration with heart disease: Evidence from NHANES 2003/06. *PLoS One* 5(1):e8673. doi: 10.1371/journal.pone.0008673.

Min, J. Y., J. S. Cho, K. J. Lee, J. B. Park, S. G. Park, J. Y. Kim, and K. B. Min. 2011. Potential role for organochlorine pesticides in the prevalence of peripheral arterial diseases in obese persons: Results from the National Health and Nutrition Examination Survey 1999–2004. *Atherosclerosis* 218(1):200–206. doi: 10.1016/j.atherosclerosis.2011.04.044.

Mozaffarian, D., E. J. Benjamin, A. S. Go, D. K. Arnett, M. J. Blaha, M. Cushman, S. R. Das et al.; Committee American Heart Association Statistics, and Subcommittee Stroke Statistics. 2016. Heart disease and stroke statistics-2016 update: A report from the American Heart Association. *Circulation* 133(4):e38–e360. doi: 10.1161/CIR.0000000000000350.

Newbold, R. R., W. N. Jefferson, E. Padilla-Banks, and J. Haseman. 2004. Developmental exposure to diethylstilbestrol (DES) alters uterine response to estrogens in prepubescent mice: Low versus high dose effects. *Reprod Toxicol* 18(3):399–406. doi: 10.1016/j.reprotox.2004.01.007.

Newbold, R. R., E. Padilla-Banks, R. J. Snyder, and W. N. Jefferson. 2007. Perinatal exposure to environmental estrogens and the development of obesity. *Mol Nutr Food Res* 51(7):912–917. doi: 10.1002/mnfr.200600259.

Ng, M., T. Fleming, M. Robinson, B. Thomson, N. Graetz, C. Margono, E. C. Mullany et al. 2014. Global, regional, and national prevalence of overweight and obesity in children and adults during 1980–2013: A systematic analysis for the Global Burden of Disease Study 2013. *Lancet* 384(9945):766–781. doi: 10.1016/S0140-6736(14)60460-8.

Ogden, C. L., M. D. Carroll, B. K. Kit, and K. M. Flegal. 2014. Prevalence of childhood and adult obesity in the United States, 2011–2012. *JAMA* 311(8):806–814. doi: 10.1001/jama.2014.732.

Ong, Z. Y., and B. S. Muhlhausler. 2011. Maternal "junk-food" feeding of rat dams alters food choices and development of the mesolimbic reward pathway in the offspring. *FASEB J* 25(7):2167–2179. doi: 10.1096/fj.10-178392.

Patel, B. B., M. Raad, I. A. Sebag, and L. E. Chalifour. 2013. Lifelong exposure to bisphenol a alters cardiac structure/function, protein expression, and DNA methylation in adult mice. *Toxicol Sci* 133(1):174–185. doi: 10.1093/toxsci/kft026.

Penza, M., M. Jeremic, E. Marrazzo, A. Maggi, P. Ciana, G. Rando, P. G. Grigolato, and D. Di Lorenzo. 2011. The environmental chemical tributyltin chloride (TBT) shows both estrogenic and adipogenic activities in mice which might depend on the exposure dose. *Toxicol Appl Pharmacol* 255(1):65–75. doi: 10.1016/j.taap.2011.05.017.

Posnack, N. G., R. Jaimes, III, H. Asfour, L. M. Swift, A. M. Wengrowski, N. Sarvazyan, and M. W. Kay. 2014. Bisphenol A exposure and cardiac electrical conduction in excised rat hearts. *Environ Health Perspect* 122(4):384–390. doi: 10.1289/ehp.1206157.

Rantakokko, P., K. M. Main, C. Wohlfart-Veje, H. Kiviranta, R. Airaksinen, T. Vartiainen, N. E. Skakkebaek, J. Toppari, and H. E. Virtanen. 2014. Association of placenta organotin concentrations with growth and ponderal index in 110 newborn boys from Finland during the first 18 months of life: A cohort study. *Environ Health* 13(1):45. doi: 10.1186/1476-069X-13-45.

Ravelli, A. C., J. H. van der Meulen, R. P. Michels, C. Osmond, D. J. Barker, C. N. Hales, and O. P. Bleker. 1998. Glucose tolerance in adults after prenatal exposure to famine. *Lancet* 351(9097):173–177.

Ravelli, A. C., J. H. van Der Meulen, C. Osmond, D. J. Barker, and O. P. Bleker. 1999. Obesity at the age of 50 y in men and women exposed to famine prenatally. *Am J Clin Nutr* 70(5):811–816.

Rubin, B. S. 2011. Bisphenol A: An endocrine disruptor with widespread exposure and multiple effects. *J Steroid Biochem Mol Biol* 127(1–2):27–34. doi: 10.1016/j.jsbmb.2011.05.002, S0960-0760(11)00106-3 [pii].

Saura, M., S. Marquez, P. Reventun, N. Olea-Herrero, M. I. Arenas, R. Moreno-Gomez-Toledano, M. Gomez-Parrizas et al. 2014. Oral administration of bisphenol A induces high blood pressure through angiotensin II/CaMKII-dependent uncoupling of eNOS. *FASEB J* 28(11):4719–4728. doi: 10.1096/fj.14-252460.

Schmidt, J. S., K. Schaedlich, N. Fiandanese, P. Pocar, and B. Fischer. 2012. Effects of di(2-ethylhexyl) phthalate (DEHP) on female fertility and adipogenesis in C_3H/N mice. *Environ Health Perspect* 120(8):1123–1129. doi: 10.1289/ehp.1104016.

Shankar, A., and S. Teppala. 2011. Relationship between urinary bisphenol A levels and diabetes mellitus. *J Clin Endocrinol Metab* 96(12):3822–3826. doi: 10.1210/jc.2011-1682.

Skinner, M. K., M. Manikkam, R. Tracey, C. Guerrero-Bosagna, M. Haque, and E. E. Nilsson. 2013. Ancestral dichlorodiphenyltrichloroethane (DDT) exposure promotes epigenetic transgenerational inheritance of obesity. *BMC Med* 11:228. doi: 10.1186/1741-7015-11-228.

Somm, E., V. M. Schwitzgebel, A. Toulotte, C. R. Cederroth, C. Combescure, S. Nef, M. L. Aubert, and P. S. Huppi. 2009. Perinatal exposure to bisphenol a alters early adipogenesis in the rat. *Environ Health Perspect* 117(10):1549–1555. doi: 10.1289/ehp.11342.

Song, Y., R. Hauser, F. B. Hu, A. A. Franke, S. Liu, and Q. Sun. 2014. Urinary concentrations of bisphenol A and phthalate metabolites and weight change: A prospective investigation in US women. *Int J Obes (Lond)* 38(12):1532–1537. doi: 10.1038/ijo.2014.63.

Sui, Y., S. H. Park, R. N. Helsley, M. Sunkara, F. J. Gonzalez, A. J. Morris, and C. Zhou. 2014. Bisphenol A increases atherosclerosis in pregnane X receptor-humanized ApoE deficient mice. *J Am Heart Assoc* 3(2):e000492. doi: 10.1161/JAHA.113.000492.

Surkan, P. J., C. C. Hsieh, A. L. Johansson, P. W. Dickman, and S. Cnattingius. 2004. Reasons for increasing trends in large for gestational age births. *Obstet Gynecol* 104(4):720–726. doi: 10.1097/01.AOG.0000141442.59573.cd.

Taylor, P. D., J. McConnell, I. Y. Khan, K. Holemans, K. M. Lawrence, H. Asare-Anane, S. J. Persaud et al. 2005. Impaired glucose homeostasis and mitochondrial abnormalities in offspring of rats fed a fat-rich diet in pregnancy. *Am J Physiol Regul Integr Comp Physiol* 288(1):R134–R139. doi: 10.1152/ajpregu.00355.2004.

Tingaud-Sequeira, A., N. Ouadah, and P. J. Babin. 2011. Zebrafish obesogenic test: A tool for screening molecules that target adiposity. *J Lipid Res* 52(9):1765–1772. doi: 10.1194/jlr.D017012.

Tontonoz, P., and B. M. Spiegelman. 2008. Fat and beyond: The diverse biology of PPARgamma. *Annu Rev Biochem* 77:289–312. doi: 10.1146/annurev.biochem.77.061307.091829.

Tracey, R., M. Manikkam, C. Guerrero-Bosagna, and M. K. Skinner. 2013. Hydrocarbons (jet fuel JP-8) induce epigenetic transgenerational inheritance of obesity, reproductive disease and sperm epimutations. *Reprod Toxicol* 36:104–116. doi: 10.1016/j.reprotox.2012.11.011, S0890-6238(12)00348-6 [pii].

Turnbaugh, P. J., R. E. Ley, M. A. Mahowald, V. Magrini, E. R. Mardis, and J. I. Gordon. 2006. An obesity-associated gut microbiome with increased capacity for energy harvest. *Nature* 444(7122):1027–1031. doi: 10.1038/nature05414.

Vandenberg, L. N., I. Chahoud, J. J. Heindel, V. Padmanabhan, F. J. Paumgartten, and G. Schoenfelder. 2010. Urinary, circulating, and tissue biomonitoring studies indicate widespread exposure to bisphenol A. *Environ Health Perspect* 118(8):1055–1070. doi: 10.1289/ehp.0901716.

Vos, J. G., A. De Klerk, E. I. Krajnc, H. Van Loveren, and J. Rozing. 1990. Immunotoxicity of bis(tri-n-butyltin) oxide in the rat: Effects on thymus-dependent immunity and on nonspecific resistance following long-term exposure in young versus aged rats. *Toxicol Appl Pharmacol* 105(1):144–155.

Wahlang, B., K. C. Falkner, B. Gregory, D. Ansert, D. Young, D. J. Conklin, A. Bhatnagar, C. J. McClain, and M. Cave. 2013. Polychlorinated biphenyl 153 is a diet-dependent obesogen that worsens nonalcoholic fatty liver disease in male C57BL6/J mice. *J Nutr Biochem* 24(9):1587–1595. doi: 10.1016/j.jnutbio.2013.01.009.

WHO/UNEP. 2013. *State of the Science of Endocrine Disrupting Chemicals (2012)*. A. Bergman, J. J. Heindel, S. Jobling, K. A. Kidd and R. T. Zoeller, eds. Geneva, Switzerland: United Nations Environmental Program, World Health Organization. ISBN: 978-92-807-3274-0, 978-92-4-150503-1.

Xin, F., M. Susiarjo, and M. S. Bartolomei. 2015. Multigenerational and transgenerational effects of endocrine disrupting chemicals: A role for altered epigenetic regulation? *Semin Cell Dev Biol* 43:66–75. doi: 10.1016/j.semcdb.2015.05.008.

Yan, S., Y. Chen, M. Dong, W. Song, S. M. Belcher, and H. S. Wang. 2011. Bisphenol A and 17beta-estradiol promote arrhythmia in the female heart via alteration of calcium handling. *PLoS One* 6(9):e25455. doi: 10.1371/journal.pone.0025455.

Yan, S., W. Song, Y. Chen, K. Hong, J. Rubinstein, and H. S. Wang. 2013. Low-dose bisphenol A and estrogen increase ventricular arrhythmias following ischemia-reperfusion in female rat hearts. *Food Chem Toxicol* 56:75–80. doi: 10.1016/j.fct.2013.02.011.

Zoeller, R. T., T. R. Brown, L. L. Doan, A. C. Gore, N. E. Skakkebaek, A. M. Soto, T. J. Woodruff, and F. S. Vom Saal. 2012. Endocrine-disrupting chemicals and public health protection: A statement of principles from The Endocrine Society. *Endocrinology* 153(9):4097–4110. doi: 10.1210/en.2012-1422.

Zuo, Z., S. Chen, T. Wu, J. Zhang, Y. Su, Y. Chen, and C. Wang. 2011. Tributyltin causes obesity and hepatic steatosis in male mice. *Environ Toxicol* 26(1):79–85. doi: 10.1002/tox.20531.

Index

A

B

C

E

F

G

H

I

L

P

R

S

Printed in the United States
by Baker & Taylor Publisher Services